KU-615-229

THIRD EDITION

HUMAN SEXUALITY
and its
PROBLEMS

This volume is dedicated to Alfred Kinsey

Commissioning Editor: **Alison Taylor**
Development Editor: **Janice Urquhart**
Project Manager: **Emma Riley**
Designer/Design Direction: **Sarah Russell / Stewart Larking**
Illustration Manager: **Bruce Hogarth**

THIRD EDITION

HUMAN SEXUALITY and its PROBLEMS

John Bancroft MD FRCP FRCPE FRCPsych

Formerly Director and currently Senior Research Fellow,
The Kinsey Institute for Research in Sex, Gender and Reproduction,
Bloomington, Indiana, USA

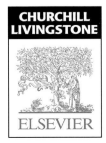

EDINBURGH   LONDON   NEW YORK   OXFORD   PHILADELPHIA   ST LOUIS   SYDNEY   TORONTO 2009

CHURCHILL LIVINGSTONE
ELSEVIER

© Longman Group Limited 1983
© Longman Group UK Limited 1989
© Elsevier Science Limited 2002. All rights reserved.
© 2009, Elsevier Limited. All rights reserved.

No part of this publication may be reproduced or transmitted in any form or by any means, electronic or mechanical, including photocopying, recording, or any information storage and retrieval system, without permission in writing from the publisher. Permissions may be sought directly from Elsevier's Rights Department: phone: (+1) 215 239 3804 (US) or (+44) 1865 843830 (UK); fax: (+44) 1865 853333; e-mail: healthpermissions@elsevier.com. You may also complete your request on-line via the Elsevier website at http://www.elsevier.com/permissions.

First published 1983
Second edition 1989
Third edition 2009

ISBN: 9780443051616

British Library Cataloguing in Publication Data
A catalogue record for this book is available from the British Library

Library of Congress Cataloging in Publication Data
A catalog record for this book is available from the Library of Congress

Notice
Knowledge and best practice in this field are constantly changing. As new research and experience broaden our knowledge, changes in practice, treatment and drug therapy may become necessary or appropriate. Readers are advised to check the most current information provided (i) on procedures featured or (ii) by the manufacturer of each product to be administered, to verify the recommended dose or formula, the method and duration of administration, and contraindications. It is the responsibility of the practitioner, relying on their own experience and knowledge of the patient, to make diagnoses, to determine dosages and the best treatment for each individual patient, and to take all appropriate safety precautions. To the fullest extent of the law, neither the Publisher nor the Author assumes any liability for any injury and/or damage to persons or property arising out of or related to any use of the material contained in this book.

The Publisher

ELSEVIER your source for books, journals and multimedia in the health sciences

www.elsevierhealth.com

Working together to grow
libraries in developing countries

www.elsevier.com | www.bookaid.org | www.sabre.org

ELSEVIER   BOOK AID International   Sabre Foundation

The Publisher's policy is to use **paper manufactured from sustainable forests**

Printed in Europe

Preface

This long-awaited third edition provides a comprehensive and authoritative cross-disciplinary approach to understanding human sexuality that is unusual in the literature. Close attention is paid to the following: the physiological mechanisms central to sexual experience and the psychological processes that precede and react to them; how these psychophysiological interactions fit into sexual relationships; the influence of socio-cultural factors, the sexual development of young people and how sexuality changes with ageing. In addition to heterosexuality, variations in sexual expression, including homosexuality and transgender, are considered. A recurring theme is the comparison of male and female sexuality, their similarities and differences.

In the second half of the book, the principal problems related to sexuality are closely examined, and detailed guidelines provided for their clinical assessment and treatment. Further chapters cover sexual aspects of medical practice, HIV, AIDS and other sexually transmitted infections, sexual aspects of contraception and infertility, and sexual offences.

It is 20 years since the last edition of this book, and there has been a huge increase in the research and evidence that needs to be considered. As a consequence, major revision has been required. A new feature is the emphasis on theory and its role in sex research, and a theoretical framework is used to organize much of the book.

This book is written principally for academics and clinicians who deal with human sexuality in their professional work, but it is written in a clear and straightforward manner that will be of value to graduate students and anyone else with a scholarly interest in the subject.

J.B.   2008

Contents

Acknowledgements   ix

CHAPTER 1 Introduction   1

CHAPTER 2 Models of human sexuality: the role of theory

Introduction   5
Models of human sexuality: some examples   8
What is human sexuality?   18

CHAPTER 3 Sexual differentiation and the development of gender identity

Introduction   20
The fundamental roles of reproductive hormones   20
Anatomical sexual differentiation   24
Hormone levels during childhood and adolescence and their effects on development   25
The development of gender identity   30
Genital anatomy in adult women and men   32
Biological rhythms and normal patterns of change in reproductive hormones   39
Anomalies of sexual differentiation – sex chromosome aneuploidies and intersex conditions   44

CHAPTER 4 Sexual arousal and response – the psychosomatic circle

Our sources of information   56
The brain and sexuality   56
Central control of sexual excitation and inhibition   65
Genital response (anatomy and physiology) in men and women   74
Orgasm, seminal emission and ejaculation   84
Information processing: response to sexual stimuli, cognitive mechanisms and the relevance of mood   96
The role of hormones in sexual arousal and response   111
Making sense of gender differences   130

CHAPTER 5 Sexual development

The developmental process   144
The development of sexual behaviour and sexual relationships   146

Sexual preferences and the development of sexual identity   159
Conclusions   169

CHAPTER 6 Heterosexuality

The history of sex surveys   174
Masturbation   183
Sex and the unmarried   186
Marriage and co-habitation   200
The impact of social class   213
The impact of culture   214
Sexual desire and sexual fantasy   220
Response to erotica   225
Sex and the Internet   226
Personality and individual differences in sexuality   228
Comparison of men and women   231

CHAPTER 7 Sexuality and ageing

Changes in sexual behaviour with age   238
Ageing and sexual function in men   240
Ageing and sexual function in women   243
Conclusions   250

CHAPTER 8 Homosexuality and bisexuality

The historical background   253
The concept of sexual identity   259
Cross-cultural comparisons   265
The prevalence of homosexual and bisexual behaviours and identities   268
The characteristics of homosexual men and women: gender identities, personalities and mental health   270
The status of relationships in the gay male and lesbian world   275

CHAPTER 9 Sexual variations

Terminology: sexual minorities, variations, deviance, perversions or paraphilias?   280
Asexuality   281
Fetishism   283
Sadomasochism   286
'Multivariant sexuality' and conclusions   287

CHAPTER 10 Transgender, gender non-conformity and transvestism

Introduction   289
Socio-cultural factors   289
The incidence of transgender identity   291
An interactive explanatory approach   292
The medical management of gender reassignment   296
Standards of care   300

CHAPTER 11 The nature of problematic sexuality

Sexuality in the context of a relationship   303
The medicalization of sexual problems   304
Conceptualizing sexual problems – the fundamental role of inhibition   305
Problems of reduced sexual interest or responsiveness   307
Prevalence of problems in the community   310
People who attend sexual problem clinics and their problems   313
Understanding problems of reduced interest or responsiveness   316
Problematic sexual behaviour   329
Problems with sexual or gender identity   335
The classification of sexual problems   336
The benefits of being sexual   338

CHAPTER 12 Helping people with sexual problems: assessment and treatment options

Treatment of sexual problems – the historical background   344

PART 1 Problems of reduced sexual interest or response

Sex therapy for the couple   346
Sex therapy for the individual   353
The outcome of sex therapy for couples   355
Pharmacological and hormonal treatments   360
Other non-pharmacological methods of treatment   366
Outcome of integrated psychological and medical treatment   366
The current status of treatment for problems of impaired sexual response or interest   367
Assessment for treatment – when to treat and which treatments to use   367
Clinical illustrations   374
Treatment of same-sex couples   375

PART 2 Problematic sexual behaviour

'Out of control' sexual behaviour   376

PART 3 Sexual or gender identity problems

Sexual identity problems   377
Gender identity problems   377

CHAPTER 13 Sexual aspects of medical practice

Some general principles   381
Andrology   382
Gynaecology   385
Psychiatry   387
General medicine   390
Neurology   397
Sexual side effects of medication   401
Sexual aspects of alcohol and drug addiction   405

CHAPTER 14 HIV/AIDS and other sexually transmitted infections

Venereal disease: a historical background   413
The story of HIV and AIDS   414
The nature of sexually transmitted infections and associated diseases   414
The prevalence of sexually transmitted infections in community surveys   419
The HIV/AIDS pandemic   420
HIV/AIDS prevention programmes   423
Understanding sexual risk taking – the 'individual differences' component   429
The impact of HIV/AIDS on sexual behaviour   435

CHAPTER 15 Sexual aspects of fertility, fertility control and infertility

Pregnancy and the post-partum period   439
Fertility control and contraception   442
Sterilization   454
Induced abortion   457
Infertility   458

CHAPTER 16 Sexual offences

Introduction   464
Sexual offences as defined in the UK   465
What is the true incidence of sexual offences?   468
The socio-cultural context of sexual offending   471
The sexual offender   478
The victims of sexual offences   489
The management of sex offenders   501
Conclusions   505

Glossary of abbreviations   511

Index of referenced authors   515

Index   525

Acknowledgements

I am very grateful to a large number of friends and colleagues who have promptly responded to my e-mail questions and requests. They include, in alphabetical order, Henry Burger, Jacques Buvat, Susan Davis, Lorain Dennerstein, Alan Dixson, Anke Ehrhardt, Paul Federoff, Richard Green, Don Grubin, Dean Hamer, Elaine Hatfield, Keith Hawton, Joe Herbert, Melissa Hines, Roger Ingham, Anne Johnson, Barry Keverne, Barry Komisaruk, Prakash Kothari, Ellen Laan, Ed Laumann, Sandy Leiblum, Roy Levin, Bill Marshall, Arnold Melman, Heino Meyer-Bahlburg, Brian Mustanski, Ebo Neischlag, Richard Parker, Jim Pfaus, Ray Rosen, David Rubinow, Ben Sachs, Peter Schmidt, Koos Slob, Serge Stoleru, Aleksander Stulhofer, Leonore Tiefer, Martin Tovee, Randolph Trumbach, Eric Vilain, Gorm Wagner, Kim Wallen, Kay Wellings, Fred Wu, Claire Yang and Ken Zucker.

I am also indebted to my colleagues at the Kinsey Institute, who have helped me in many ways; in particular Shawn Wilson, Tom Albright, Liana Zhou, Erick Janssen and Julia Heiman.

Cynthia Graham has given me valuable feedback on much of this book, and, in particular, I want to thank her and our two children, Rosie and Jack, for coping with my almost total preoccupation with this book over the past 3 years.

I am also grateful to Vaughn Call, Cynthia Graham, Roger Gorski, Erick Janssen, Tillmann Krüger, Helen O'Connell and Claire Yang for their permission to reproduce or adapt figures from their publications.

Introduction

The thread of sexuality is woven densely into the fabric of human existence. There are few people for whom sex has not been important at some time and many for whom it has played a dominant part in their lives. Sex is a motive force leading two people to intimate contact. They may have nothing in common except mutual sexual interest. Their encounter may be brief or it may lead on to the principal relationship in their lives, and often the formation of a family.

The preceding paragraph opened the introduction to the last edition of this book in 1989. Twenty years later it is no less relevant. Sexuality continues to play a fundamental part in the lives of many of us. However, there are ongoing changes in the sexual world. Interestingly, a turning point relating to these changes happened around the date of the second edition of this book. In the two to three decades before 1989 there had been noticeable changes, most marked in the sexuality of women. It seemed that the longstanding societal repression of women's sexuality was lessening, enabling them to express their sexualities more openly, and revealing a much greater variability among women than had previously been apparent. This pattern and the challenge of comparing and contrasting the sexuality of men and women is an important theme in this third edition, and I have ventured into potential political incorrectness in my attempts to theorize about this gender comparison. Since 1989 we have not seen any reversal of this change in relation to women's sexuality, but in general the previous phase of increasing sexual permissiveness, described as the era of sexual liberation or revolution, depending on one's perspective, has not been so evident. This is most noticeably apparent in the cessation and to some extent reversal of the trend towards younger age at sexual initiation (see Chapter 5, p. 155). The trend towards more premarital sexual experience, on the other hand, has continued, at least in the Western world, largely because people are getting married later and less often (see Chapter 6, p. 205), and sexuality has become accepted as a manifestation of a 'sexual relationship' rather than of marriage per se.

By 1989, HIV and AIDS were having a major impact and have continued to do so ever since. In the early days of this epidemic, attention was focused on AIDS as a 'gay disease', with an associated intensification of anti-homosexual attitudes. The subsequent worldwide pandemic, however, has shown this to be a predominantly heterosexual problem, with more recent attention focused on the particular vulnerabilities of heterosexual women, an important demonstration of the consequences of gender inequality in human societies (see Chapter 14). We have also seen how HIV infection is characterized by relatively low infectivity, a long latency, but a major health consequence, AIDS. This is in striking contrast to the event-related and usually treatable nature of other sexually transmitted infections (STIs), and has added further complexity to the issues of responsible sexual behaviour.

The new phase of sex survey research, reviewed in this volume, has been largely driven by this pandemic. Whereas it remains very difficult to obtain funding for sex research in general, the need to carry out large-scale surveys that would be informative about behaviours and attitudes relevant to HIV transmission has been acknowledged. This, however, has not gone unchallenged; the continuing political opposition to sex research is considered in Chapter 6 and is reviewed more comprehensively in Bancroft (2004). The view that it is better to ignore sex than to attempt to understand it, for fear that in the process you somehow encourage it, has persisted in various forms, particularly in the USA.

The final phase of my career brought me into close contact with this 'sex negativism'. In 1995 I moved to the USA to become Director of the Kinsey Institute for Research in Sex, Gender and Reproduction at Indiana University. From the first day, I was contending with the ongoing anti-Kinsey campaign. Kinsey had become a scapegoat for what these campaigners regarded as a decline in sexual morality (Bancroft 2004).

Fortunately, beyond that, my time at the Kinsey Institute had many positive consequences for me. I became much more aware of Kinsey's work on individual variability, a central theme in much of my research in the subsequent 10 years. Through the amazing collections at the Kinsey Institute, I experienced the many ways that sexuality has been expressed in the arts and literature. Above all, I had 10 years of working with a wonderful team of colleagues at the Institute. Only since retiring from that wholehearted investment, and returning to the UK, have I been able to work on this third edition.

The past 20 years have influenced my thinking in many ways that will be evident in this new edition. There has been a huge increase in the literature relating to human sexuality and its problems. Given that the objective of this book is to provide a broad cross-disciplinary perspective, the literature has been close to overwhelming. There are, I have no doubt, many important gaps in the next

15 chapters, and to those scholars and researchers whose work I have inadequately addressed, I can only apologize. I have, however, experienced a major transformation that I will try to explain. In the last edition I wrote that human sexuality was an enigma or a riddle. Since then this enigma has become endowed with even more significance for me. Scientific progress, while it may bring clear practical benefits, more often than not makes the human condition more rather than less difficult to understand. No doubt there are exceptions, but in my experience they have been few. One particularly telling example, which I will revisit at several points in this book, is brain imaging. We may use brain imaging to study what happens in the brain when we become sexually aroused, or to compare and contrast individuals with normal and low levels of sexual desire. What we find is a multiplicity of interactive brain functions that do not slot easily into our preconceived concepts of 'sexual arousal' or 'sexual desire'. And why should they? The common assumption that we can work out, with our brains, how those brains work, is one aspect of the arrogance of human beings. There are many, beyond the field of brain science, who believe that it is only a matter of time before science gets everything worked out. This has not made me nihilistic about scientific research, far from it; the practical benefits of research continue to be considerable. But it has made me more humble, and in the process has intensified my sense of spirituality.

As part of this process, it has become clearer to me that, rather than pursuing the 'truth' or the 'reality' of brain function, or hormone function, or neurotransmitter function, or by contrast, the impact of culture, we should endeavour to devise simplified models of reality. Their purpose is not only to help us grapple with the seemingly endless increase in complexity, of human sexuality and a lot more besides, but also to have heuristic value in various ways, such as making it easier to write a book like this, and hopefully for the reader to make sense of it. When we look back over the history of science we can find many examples of such models, which served to help the process of making sense, but after a while gave way to new models which could better deal with the next stage. In the field of medicine, where scientific understanding is of particular importance, and its heuristic value readily demonstrated, this process has been very evident.

I have therefore become more theoretical, which has not only influenced my research over the past 10 years, but also the structuring and writing of this third edition. This is explored closely in Chapter 2, one of the new components of this book. Through the other chapters the reader will encounter a variety of theories, ranging from testable hypotheses, to models intended to aid in the organization of our thinking. I feel somewhat frustrated, as this late emergence of a more theoretical approach has generated numerous researchable questions when it is too late for me to attempt to answer them. I have included many of them in this book, in the hope that others might want to pursue them.

As with the previous two editions, I have struggled over the best way of structuring this book. This reflects the core theme; that human sexuality results from an interaction between the psychobiological mechanisms inherent in the individual and the culture in which he or she lives. To some extent, it is possible to focus on the fundamentally biological process of sexual differentiation, as in Chapter 3, and on the psychobiological mechanisms involved in sexual response, as in Chapter 4. But the development of gender identity, sexual identity and our emerging patterns of sexual behaviour require more attention to socio-cultural factors. I have considered these more closely in Chapters 5 and 6, and in relation to homosexual identity in Chapter 8.

There are two other chapters that are new. HIV and AIDS, together with other STIs, now have a chapter to themselves (Chapter 14), as do transgender and gender non-conformity (Chapter 10). The assessment of sexual problems, previously a separate chapter, is now incorporated into the chapter on their treatment (Chapter 12). This reflects changes in this clinical field. With the introduction of the 'Viagra era' there has been a major shift away from surgical interventions for erectile dysfunction. This has resulted in much less use of the physiological methods of assessment (e.g. arteriography) that had previously been considered appropriate to demonstrate the organic nature of an erectile problem before embarking on irreversible surgical procedures to correct it. In parallel, there has been a shift towards integration of psychological and pharmacological approaches to treatment (see Chapter 12), which has reinforced my view that the early stages of psychological 'sex therapy' are particularly effective at assessing the likely causes of the sexual problem, and hence the best approach to treatment.

There have been some direct and striking impacts of information technology on the writing process. When I wrote the first edition of this book, published in 1983, I had a typewriter and a box full of index cards to help me organize the references. When I wrote the second edition, published in 1989, I had a word processor; a big difference. For this third edition, as well as the many advantages of a modern laptop and a wealth of helpful software programmes, I have had access to the Internet. As I am no longer at the Kinsey Institute, with its unique library and wonderful librarians just up the stairs, I have been amazed how many of the papers I need can be obtained online. Increasingly, I find myself searching less through books on my shelves to find the answer to a question, and turning to Google instead. And then I have had e-mail. It has been wonderful how responsive my friends and colleagues around the world have been, answering my questions and sending papers and references almost as soon as I dispatched my message to them. A long list of their names is given in the acknowledgments.

The Internet, however, is of much more significance than helping authors write their books. It is a major new factor in the modern sexual world, crossing age, cultural and geographic boundaries, and with effects on human sexuality, both bad and good, which we have hardly begun to understand (see Chapter 6).

Personal statement

This new introduction has been something of a personal statement from start to finish, reflecting increased introspection as I age. But the importance of being explicit about my values, so that those reading this book are better able to judge how they might have influenced or biased my analysis and presentation of the evidence, is as important as ever.

In most respects, little has changed in my value system. The importance of responsibility in our sexual lives I see as paramount. In the human species, sexuality has come to serve more than the reproductive function. I feel positively about some of these non-reproductive functions, but not all. The ways that sex can bind a couple and foster intimacy are, for me, the most positive non-reproductive aspects of sexuality. I have no problem with sex as a source of pleasure, providing that the pleasure is mutual and is responsibly obtained. I am not comfortable with the use of sex as a way of asserting one's masculinity or femininity. That is not to suggest that what we need is an elimination of gender differences, even if that were possible. It may be that for both men and women to enjoy the full non-reproductive benefits of being sexual, some distinction between 'maleness' and 'femaleness' will continue to be an advantage, at least as far as heterosexual sex is concerned. This is one example of gender differences, which, if used appropriately, complement each other. But any way in which sex is used to reinforce stereotypes of masculine dominance and exploitation causes me concern.

Using sex to bolster self-esteem is potentially problematic. The quality of sexual attractiveness has a wide influence. In the materialistic societies of the modern world, sex is used to impart appeal to non-sexual objects; the commercial exploitation of sex is all around us. This stems from the powerful link between sexual attractiveness and self-esteem. For many, sexual appeal will be or will be seen to be the most powerful asset they possess. That is all the more reason for them to use it responsibly. Given that we are all, including our children, bombarded with sexual messages, mainly from the media and from advertising, it is crucial that there are counterbalancing messages emphasizing the importance of responsibility in our sexual lives, combined with good information. There continues to be much ignorance and misinformation about sex. Sex education is not only important for the young adolescent.

Sex as an expression of hostility is clearly unacceptable. The complex relationships between anger, sexual arousal and sexual violence are explored in Chapters 4 and 16. The use of sex as a mood regulator is now receiving research attention, and is increasingly being seen as potentially problematic. This is considered more closely in Chapters 4 and 11.

Sex for material gain raises complex issues. Traditional 'arranged' marriages, in most cultures, entail a complex set of motives, in which the 'bartering' of sex for non-sexual benefits, while not explicit, cannot be excluded. Only with the emergence of the 'companionate marriage' in the 20th century were we able to assume that sexuality was primarily for mutual pleasure and intimacy, and such relationships have often shown themselves to be difficult to maintain (see Chapter 6). I can also understand that poverty drives some individuals to use sex for material gain, and I can only wish that there were better solutions for their poverty. I have once again failed to address the important issue of prostitution in this edition, which probably reflects my difficulty in getting it into perspective.

I continue to hold my somewhat idiosyncratic view of the binding effect of sexuality. Whereas the shared experience of sexual pleasure strengthens a sexual relationship, I see the vulnerability inherent in the sexual interaction as equally, if not more, important. To enjoy sex requires us to let go, to become abandoned to a degree, undefended. In such a state we are vulnerable. For many species this vulnerability is probably an important reason why sexual behaviour is biologically controlled and limited to the minimum time required for the purposes of reproduction; otherwise animals would be exposing themselves to undue danger. For humans, it is not physical but psychological or emotional hazards that are most likely — the risks of being exploited, rejected or humiliated. These are some of the bad consequences of sex. But to be able to expose oneself to such a risk and yet remain safe reinforces the feelings of security in a relationship, and has a binding effect. To a considerable extent, the emotional security of a sexual relationship is undermined when sex is used for other purposes such as asserting masculinity or dominance, or bolstering self-esteem, or even as a mood regulator.

The need for sexuality to be expressed and dealt with responsibly is profoundly important. This book documents many of the negative consequences of irresponsible sexual behaviour, including unwanted pregnancies, sexually transmitted infections, and emotional and physical trauma. I was privileged to be part of a multidisciplinary group of advisors organized by the Surgeon General of the US Government in 2000, Dr David Satcher. The group process was informative because it involved individuals with a wide range of values relating to sexual behaviour, yet it proved possible, with sufficient discussion, to reach consensus about the basic requirements for responsible sexual behaviour. This resulted in the Surgeon General's *Call to Action to Promote Sexual Health and Responsible Sexual Behavior* issued in July 2001 (Satcher 2001). The following is an extract from the introduction:

Sexual responsibility should be understood in the broadest sense. While personal responsibility is crucial to any individual's health status, communities also have important responsibilities. Individual responsibility includes understanding and awareness of one's sexuality and sexual development: respect for oneself and one's partner; avoidance of physical or emotional harm to either oneself or one's partner; ensuring that pregnancy occurs only when welcomed; and recognition and tolerance of the diversity of sexual values within any community. Community responsibility includes assurance that its members have access to developmentally and culturally appropriate sexuality education, as well as sexual and reproductive health care and counseling; the latitude to make appropriate sexual and reproductive choices; respect for diversity; and freedom from stigmatization and violence on the basis of gender, race, ethnicity, religion or sexual orientation (p. 1)

This Call to Action (CTA) highlights that sexual responsibility has to be considered at two levels: the individual and the community. It is appropriate to expect the individual to take responsibility as long as the community does as well. The crucial issue of diversity is also raised. It becomes easier to accept diversity of sexual expression providing that it is expressed responsibly. The intention of the Surgeon General was to use this CTA to 'stimulate respectful, thoughtful, and mature discussion in our communities and in our homes. While sexuality may be difficult to discuss for some, and there are certainly many different views and beliefs regarding it, we cannot afford the consequences of continued or selective silence' (p. 2).

It is uncertain to what extent it has succeeded in this respect. Not long after this CTA was issued there was a change of government, from Democrat to Republican. Perhaps not surprisingly, there has been no further evidence of government involvement. However, David Satcher, since leaving his government post, has continued his efforts to build on this initiative. After becoming Director of the National Center for Primary Care at Morehouse School of Medicine, in Atlanta, Georgia, he established the Center of Excellence for Sexual Health, with funding from the Ford Foundation. This has brought together leaders of various diverse groups in the USA to continue this discussion, resulting in the ongoing National Consensus Process on Sexual Health and Responsible Sexual Behavior (Satcher 2006). Hopefully, they will make progress.

There are two specific issues that are, according to my value system, in particular need of change. One is the tendency, reinforced by patriarchal societies in various ways, for men to see the need for sexual containment and the prevention of unwanted pregnancies as the responsibilities of women. Men and women should be equally responsible in their sexual lives. There are no grounds for maintaining that the status quo is justified for biological or evolutionary reasons. Given the history of patriarchal societies, it is surprising that they have not yet eliminated themselves. If the human species has any potential for adaptation, then a shift towards more gender equal societies, with shared responsibilities between men and women, is an obvious way forward.

The other issue is the importance of instilling the need for sexual responsibility into young males and females as they enter adolescence. This is dealt with to a variable extent across communities and families. All too often there is an avoidance of explicit consideration of sex beyond the simple message that it is something that should be postponed until marriage, and the more specific guidance is directed at the young females more than the males. With the clear increase in the age at marriage and lowering of the age at puberty and hence the onset of fertility as well as increased sexual arousability, this issue has increased in importance. The relevance to sex education is considered further in Chapter 5.

In a social species such as ours, socially imposed limits for sexual behaviour are necessary. The cultural assertion of sexual morality is an important way to set such limits. But sexual morality may be 'good' or 'bad' and the history of human societies shows us many bad examples, often reflecting the difficulties that the societal or religious system had in acknowledging the existence of sexuality. Thus sex is grudgingly accepted on the grounds that it is necessary for reproduction, an inescapable part of God's plan, and with the condition that it is restricted to marriage. This is usually combined with the rejection of homosexual relationships on the grounds that they cannot reproduce. There are many heterosexual women, and perhaps some men, who are only comfortable with sex if there is some possibility that reproduction might result. In any case, God's plan, in this respect, has apparently changed as, with the growing world population, the need for our species now is less reproduction not more.

According to my values, we need a new form of sexual morality based on responsibility and gender equality, and the acceptance of responsible diversity. This would, it is hoped, involve a more honest form of sexual constraint that would not only steer our teenagers away from sexual danger without spoiling their unfolding joy of sexual intimacy, but also help us to avoid much of the distress and bitterness that accompanies the breakdown of sexual relationships. For sexual relationships between men and women, I would hope for a responsible attitude to parenthood by both partners, so that children will not be born because 'that is the normal thing to do' or because no suitable alternative to parenthood is available, or because taking contraceptive precautions would indicate an unacceptable degree of sexual intention, but because two people have a genuine and shared desire to experience parenthood.

REFERENCES

Bancroft J 2004 Kinsey and the politics of sex research. Annual Review of Sex Research 15: 1–39.

Satcher D 2001 The Surgeon General's Call to Action to Promote Sexual Health and Responsible Sexual Behavior. http://www.surgeongeneral.gov/library/sexualhealth/default.htm

Satcher D 2006 The National Consensus Process on Sexual Health and Responsible Sexual Behavior. Interim Report. Morehouse School of Medicine, Atlanta.

Models of human sexuality: the role of theory

2

Introduction.. 5
Essentialism and the tolerance of uncertainty 5
Reality... 6
Political correctness 7
The individual versus society 7
Reductionism... 8
Models of human sexuality: some examples...................... 8

Sexual strategy theory.. 8
Sexual scripting theory... 10
The big picture 13
The Dual Control model 15
What is human sexuality?... 18

Introduction

In 1998, *The Journal of Sex Research* published a special issue on the use of theory in sex research and scholarship. In his introductory paper, Weis (1998a), having reviewed the evidence, concluded that the majority of the sex research literature had no explicit theoretical base. In his concluding paper, Weis (1998b) gave his personal evaluation of a wide range of theoretical models which were of potential relevance to sex research. Although he found many of them relevant, very little use had been made of them by sex researchers. This widespread lack of a theoretical base can be regarded as a major limitation to the field. This chapter is not intended to review the relevant theoretical models, but rather to explore the role that theory can play in sex research, and provide a rationale for the theoretical approaches used in this book.

In 1993 Paul Abramson, Gilbert Herdt and Steven Pinkerton organized a conference entitled 'Theorizing sexuality: evolution, culture and development'. Papers were circulated in advance, and the conference was spent discussing them. Most of the papers from this meeting were published as a book, *Sexual Nature, Sexual Culture* (Abramson & Pinkerton 1995), which included an overview of the discussions by Okami & Pendleton (1995). It had been the organizers' hope to 'move past the influence of constricting dichotomies of sex/gender (biology/culture) and essentialism/constructionism' (p. 388), and facilitate a paradigm shift towards a broader interdisciplinary study of human sexuality, which attaches appropriate importance to non-reproductive sex. In considering non-reproductive sex they pointed out the neglect of scholarly attention to sexual pleasure. Clearly, there was vigorous debate and little agreement. Tuzin (1995), one of the anthropologist participants, stood out as someone advocating an interactionist perspective, seeing human sexuality as an interaction between biological mechanisms and cultural processes.

In 1998, a workshop was held at The Kinsey Institute on 'The Role of Theory in Sex Research'. In this case, the objective was to select a series of themes and to invite participants with contrasting theoretical perspectives to address each theme. The four themes covered were sexuality across the life cycle, sexual orientation, individual differences in sexual risk taking and adolescent sexuality. The proceedings of this meeting, including edited versions of the extensive discussion, were published as a book (Bancroft 2000a). The contrasts were very evident both in the papers and the discussion, and the book includes an overview and my personal conclusions as organizer and editor.

A number of themes emerged from this meeting that will be examined closely.

Essentialism and the tolerance of uncertainty

Much of the epistemological divide in the field of sex research stems from a postmodern reaction to the alleged 'certainty' of conventional science. This divide has typically been characterized as a conflict between essentialism and social constructionism. However, as DeLamater & Hyde (1998) pointed out, the concept of essentialism, in much of the relevant literature, has come to be used in an ill-defined and variable fashion, often by those critical of mainstream sex research, including the postmodernists. Essentialism in science, which can be regarded as the search for the 'truth', forms only part of mainstream sexual science. Popper (1957, 1977) distinguished between methodological nominalists and methodological essentialists. The nominalist seeks conjectural explanation, and tests the conjecture by exploring its consequences, aware of the fact that any such conjecture or assumption can never be proved correct, or 'established' as Popper put it (1977). The method of the essentialist, in sharp contrast, is 'the intuitive grasp of the essence ... here intuition implies infallible insight' (Popper 1977, p. 172). I would argue, however, that both types of researcher are to be found amongst conventional *and* social constructionist sex researchers. The factors that lead to an individual becoming a conventional researcher or social constructionist are of interest, and Weis (1998b) listed them on his research agenda for the future. But I am also intrigued by what determines whether an individual is a nominalist or an essentialist.

Is it a matter of disciplinary background and influence, personality, cognitive style or, more specifically, tolerance of uncertainty?

Reality

Stemming from essentialism is the issue of reality. What is 'real' and how it is recognized as such has been one of the most fundamental issues in philosophy. In recent years we have seen a growing divide between conventional sex researchers and social constructionists. Conventional sexual scientists are alleged to attribute reality to the biological basis of human sexuality. The social constructionists, in countering this, point to the social construction of sexuality and how it has changed through history. Popper's (1957) views are again relevant. 'Methodological essentialists are inclined to formulate scientific questions in such terms as "what is matter?" ... Methodological nominalists, as opposed to this, would put their problems in such terms as "how does this piece of matter behave?" ... that the task of science is only to describe how things behave.' (p. 29). Some social constructionists point out that sexuality, at least for humans, is a social construct, (the 'what is' approach). It is noteworthy that in the last few years there has been an increased attention to the 'what is' type of question among conventional sex researchers, possibly a consequence of the social constructionist critiques, e.g. 'what is sexual desire', with the somewhat embarrassed acknowledgment that we can't really say, although there are many related 'how' and 'why' questions that have been and are being addressed. We will confront this issue explicitly later in this chapter, when we ask the question, 'What is human sexuality?'. Hopefully, in the process, this will demonstrate that there can be benefits from both the essentialist and nominalist approaches provided their limitations are kept in mind.

There is good anthropological evidence that sexuality and gender have been constructed differently across societies and through history (e.g. Ortner & Whitehead 1981). But let us look at this concept of construction more closely. We can see that how we have conceptualized most aspects of nature and our environment has been 'constructed' dependent on the level of relevant knowledge available. Thus the idea that the world was flat persisted until convincing evidence that it was not influenced common knowledge. More recently, and at least in more educated social groups, we can see constructs of gender difference become shaped by the accumulation of scientific evidence, e.g. the work of Jost (1965) demonstrating the bi-potentiality of gender development with, at least in the mammal, female development being the default mode. However, as long ago as 1939, Frank Lillie wrote in the introduction to the second edition of *Sex and Internal Secretions*, 'There is no such biological entity as sex. What exists is a dimorphism ... into male and female individuals ... in any given species we recognize a male form and a female form, whether these characters be classed as of biological, or psychological or social orders. Sex is not a force that produces these contrasts. It is merely a name for our total impression of the differences.' (Lillie 1939, p. 3). This statement is still pertinent today and, interestingly, is as pertinent to a biological as it is to a social constructionist perspective.

This confronts us with different kinds of knowledge. Harris (1979), in his anthropological conceptualization of culture (cultural materialism), proposed the distinction between 'emic' knowledge, that 'the native accepts as real, meaningful and appropriate', and 'etic', referring to concepts and categories used by the expert or scientist. This distinction has given way in anthropology to the insider versus outsider distinction of Geertz (1983). Escoffier (1999) proposed that vernacular knowledge, common sense, everyday knowledge and local knowledge were all equivalent to insider knowledge, and pointed out that the difference between insider and outsider knowledge is much more blurred in a modern industrial society. He quotes Gramsci: 'Every philosophical current leaves behind a sedimentation of "common sense": this is the documentation of its historical effectiveness ... Common sense is not something rigid or immobile, but is continually transforming itself, enriching itself with scientific ideas and philosophical opinions that have entered everyday life' (Gramsci 1971, p. 316).

We can look back over history and see how science has informed common sense only to be shown to be wrong by later scientific progress. We should therefore keep in mind that whether we are a 'native' or a social constructionist, or a conventional scientist, we construct our view of reality, and as a conjectural scientist, we should remain humble and uncertain about that 'reality', judging its worth not by its truth but by the benefits that it brings.

As a behavioural endocrinologist, I am interested in the interface between psychological and physiological mechanisms in human sexuality. We are increasingly aware of extensive discoveries in many aspects of brain function with, for example, increasing knowledge of neurotransmitters, new methods for tracking neural pathways, new techniques for identifying hormone receptors, and the introduction of brain imaging to explore localization of brain activity during response to sexual stimuli. However, from our perspective, this new information increases the complexity rather than our comprehension of what we are trying to grasp. Each phase of scientific progress, it would seem, uncovers a new layer of complexity, challenging us with the question, 'Will we ever really understand how our brains work?' We are aware that this reaction to scientific progress is far from new, and is in no way an argument against further scientific research. But there is a need to counter the fragmentation that inevitably results, with researchers becoming more and more specialized in their focus and increasingly distanced from any holistic view of brain function and its relationship to human behaviour. There are places for at least two types of sexual scientist (and indeed of any scientist studying human behaviour), one focusing in depth on specific aspects, the other striving for some broad conceptualization of human sexuality. For the latter, there is a need to seek explanatory models or 'conceptual systems', which are, at best, simplifications of reality, and whose validity depends on their enabling us to deal more effectively with the growing complexity. Any such model, therefore, should be shown to have heuristic value. If it does not, then it should be modified, adapted or abandoned for a better model. There is nothing new about such models. In relation to the brain, Hebb (1949) introduced the conceptual nervous system, as a way of conceptualizing brain activity to account for behaviour without knowing all the precise brain mechanisms involved. Gray (1971) built on this with his conceptual nervous system of behavioural approach and inhibition, the basis of a highly fruitful programme of research, and which very much influenced the Dual Control model of sexual response elaborated later in this chapter. Such models not only allow the formulation of testable hypotheses, they also provide a structure for organizing our thinking on related topics.

Political correctness

By the end of the Kinsey theory workshop, we were left with the distinct impression that a substantial source of the conflict between the conventional sexual scientist and the postmodernist was political. Many postmodernists follow Foucault in believing that conventional science is used to gain social control, particularly control of sexual aspects of life, and is hence politically suspect. At the Kinsey workshop, this was most comprehensively evident in the paper by John Gagnon on sexual risk taking. He pointed out that problems such as sexual risk were typically defined by ideological and political interests, and warned that, as a result, the scientist could unwittingly (or deliberately) be reinforcing undesirable social control. 'Treating the problem of risky sex as a property of the individual often blames the individual for structural conditions about which they can do nothing. In this way the situation is justified by placing the blame for risk taking on the individuals in the situation' (Gagnon 2000, p. 169). In his conclusions, Gagnon calls for extreme caution. 'Sexual theorizing *is* consequential. It is part of the day-to-day struggle to direct, manage, control and invent human sexuality.' (p. 172). From this perspective, the solution appeared to be scholarly inaction, perhaps an example of what Tuzin (1995) described as a form of nihilism: 'a special exemption . . . granted to those sophisticated few who grasped the significance of cultural differences and could use this knowledge to soar above the confines of their own cultural traditions' (p. 263). There are, however, other 'calls to inaction' that have emerged in recent years. Within clinical psychology there is a strong movement to avoid any kind of clinical intervention which has not been empirically validated, on the grounds that such intervention is unethical (e.g. McFall 1991). As few clinical interventions have such validation, and as many types of intervention, because of the complexity of what is involved, are difficult to validate unequivocally, this is a recipe for withholding clinical help in many situations of need. For those of us who are committed to action either in a clinical, a socio-cultural or political context, such inaction is not an option.

We must strive to get our action 'right' and learn from our mistakes. In that sense we must be prepared to take risks, knowing full well that if we do not, someone else, less cautious, certainly will.

Social control of sexual behaviour is a justifiable cause for concern, and indeed many of the problems people experience in their sexual lives can be attributed to the negative effects of social control, as Alfred Kinsey concluded from his major study. But on the other hand, sexual behaviour in a social species such as the human requires social control of some kind. The issue, therefore, is determining what is 'good' social control, and what is 'bad'. We doubt that many postmodernists would fundamentally disagree on this point, but it would seem that for the time being they are more concerned about deconstructing existing forms of social control, than proposing preferable alternatives. As part of this process, they are preoccupied with discrediting conventional scientific method, perhaps demonstrating Foucault's idea that power leads to systems of resistance as well as systems of oppression.

Much of the social control of sexuality is imposed on women, and of course is also used to suppress homosexuality. It is therefore no surprise that many academics in the sexual postmodern field are feminist, gay or lesbian. In addition to benefits from the resulting dialectic discourse, this has brought into the field of sex research and scholarship a considerable amount of intellectual ability, which previously had been in short supply. However, it leaves us with the challenge of sorting out the scientific from the political.

The individual versus society

As exemplified by Gagnon's comments above, one aspect of political correctness that was much in evidence at the Kinsey workshop was criticism of focus on the individual, which is the core of much conventional sex research. Such focus was rejected at two levels. First, attempting to understand sexual risk-taking by theorizing about individual differences in the propensity for taking sexual risks (Bancroft 2000b) was seen to be flawed because sexual interactions involve more than one person. Secondly, theorizing about why some teenage girls are more at risk of unplanned pregnancy was focusing on the individual as the responsible agent, whereas often it was poverty and hence society that were to blame. At both levels, it was argued, holding the individual responsible could lead to further social control. This postmodern position was expressed more recently by Flowers & Duncan (2002). In criticizing the tendency to distinguish between risk takers and risk avoiders, they commented 'it is easy to appreciate how such dichotomous understandings can be extended to construct "good" and "bad" individuals; . . . In contrast, a more social understanding of sexual health embraces a more diffuse notion of responsibility.' (p. 234). There is a paradox here in that pluralism in terms of human experience is central to much of postmodern thinking. According to (Simon 1996, p. 12) 'part, but not all, of the pluralism of the postmodern world is the increased significance or empowering of individual differences, both genetic and contextual'.

The reluctance to focus on the individual is crucial. We have no problem with the ideas that situational factors can increase the likelihood of risky sexual behaviour, that such situations may be socio-culturally determined (e.g. as a result of poverty) and that we should be looking for ways to promote less problematic socio-cultural contexts. But deliberate avoidance of the promotion of individual responsibility is unacceptable and contrary to many of our basic principles of education. I strongly endorse the *Call to Action to Promote Sexual Health and Responsible Sexual Behavior*, issued in June 2001 by the then Surgeon General of the US Government, Dr David Satcher (2001), as a fine example of government seeking 'good' social control by encouraging community as well as individual responsibility (see Chapter 1). The fact that focus on the individual may, if done badly, lead to culpability or inappropriate social control, is not a reason for avoiding any such individual focus, although it may justify careful monitoring of such interventions.

Reductionism

This takes us to another core issue. The unacceptability of focusing on an individual's propensities or traits relates to the accompanying assumption that such traits allow one to predict how an individual will behave in the future. This conflicts with the view that future behaviour will depend on the full range of circumstances, which cannot be foreseen. This has led, in the postmodern world, to a preference for theorizing the situation and not the individual, and not the situation in general but the specific situation. At the Kinsey workshop, Ken Plummer elaborated this point: 'Previously we could take particular sets of Eurocentric and North American theories and use them to generalize around the world; but we must now learn from the failures of all that over the past couple of centuries or so. The time has arrived for a multiplicity of much more localized specific theories.' (Bancroft 2000a, p. 54). This comment appropriately points out the error of taking an explanatory model developed in one culture and applying it in another without consideration of the cultural differences. This was particularly evident in the early stages of the AIDS epidemic (Abramson & Herdt 1990). But it also points to a postmodern reaction against identifying generalities, and avoiding what has become a pejorative term: 'reductionism'. However, as we shall see in the next section, reductionism can occur in both conventional science and postmodern social constructionism.

Models of human sexuality: some examples

The assault of postmodern academia on conventional sexual science, whilst paying more attention to 'de-construction' than 're-construction', has served a dialectic purpose. It has caused at least some of us who are conventional scientists to reflect on our scientific methods; to remind ourselves, as Thomas Kuhn (1970) pointed out, that relatively little conventional science meets the desired criteria of falsifiability, and to become more open to the idea that our biases could be distorting our results. In the spirit of Popperian conjecture, we should be open to the use of varying theoretical approaches, on the understanding that they will be judged on their heuristic value, both to the understanding of the human condition and to attempts to improve it, both individually and societally.

With this in mind, we will look more closely at two theoretical models: sexual strategy theory from evolutionary psychology and sexual scripts theory from social constructionist sociology. I have chosen these for two reasons: they are unusual in being developed specifically to look at human sexuality, and they come from opposite ends of the epistemological spectrum. I will then move on to elaborate and justify the theoretical approaches used in this book.

Sexual strategy theory

Sexual strategy theory (SST) was first expounded by Buss & Schmitt (1993) and was reviewed by Buss (1998) in the previously mentioned theory issue of *The Journal of Sex Research*. What distinguishes evolutionary psychology from the mainstream of evolutionary biology is its focus on psychological mechanisms, rather than the wider spectrum of biological mechanisms, as examples of adaptations. A key premise of such theory is that adaptive psychological mechanisms relevant to sexuality are not part of a more 'domain general' psychological responsiveness, but are particular and numerous. In describing SST, which is an application of such evolutionary psychology principles, Buss (1998) postulates that desire lies at the foundation of sexuality and human mating, although he does not, in this review, define what he means by 'desire'. SST focuses on desire 'and all of its interpersonal ramifications'. These include attraction tactics, conflict between the sexes, mate-expulsion tactics, causes of conjugal dissolution, mate retention tactics, and harmony between the sexes. The implication is that there are a myriad of psychological mechanisms that deal with these interpersonal ramifications, each of which can be regarded as an adaptation. However, these mechanisms are 'activated selectively and sequentially, depending on context. They are functional, which means that they exist in the form that they do because they solved in ancestral environments specific problems of survival or reproduction . . . ' (p. 24).

Buss goes on to explain that such specific adaptive mechanisms can be divided into short-term and long-term strategies, involving different adaptive challenges. Because of gender differences in 'minimum obligatory parental investment', men are more involved in short-term strategies than women. For men, there are four relatively distinct short-term adaptive strategies: (i) desire for a variety of partners, (ii) assessment of sexual accessibility, (iii) assessment of physical cues linked with fertility and (iv) strategies for keeping time and investments to a minimum. Men who lack the ability to pursue these strategies would have been out-reproduced by men with such adaptive skills. Women, although less likely to engage in such short-term strategies, can nevertheless reap a host of adaptive benefits from them, including (i) immediate resources for her and her children, (ii) 'mate insurance' should she lose her regular mate and (iii) genetic benefits from mating with superior men. 'Because it is clear that women engage in short-term mating and likely have done so throughout human evolutionary history, it is unlikely that they would have done so in the absence of benefits' (p. 24).

Long-term strategies deal with a different set of problems. Men need to identify reproductively valuable women, ensure paternity (avoid the evolutionary pitfall of being cuckolded), and identify women with good parenting skills. Women, on the other hand, need to identify men with ability to acquire resources, who display a willingness to invest those resources in them and their children, are willing to commit to a long-term relationship, have good parenting skills, and are able to protect the women and children from aggressors. Each of these short- and long-term objectives is met by an evolutionary adaptive mechanism originating during the longest period of human evolution, known as the 'environment of evolutionary adaptiveness' (EEA; Allgeier & Wiederman 1994).

Buss is able to report on an extensive range of studies that are consistent with his theory, although all of his examples involve gender differences. Men, on average, desire more sexual partners than women, and see themselves as more likely to engage in sex early in a relationship than women. Cross-culturally, men attach more importance to physical attractiveness and youth in potential partners than women do. Women attach more importance to financial prospects of their partners, and are more likely to show a preference for partners older rather than younger than themselves. Men and women typically differ in the determinants of sexual jealousy; men are more disturbed by the thought of their partner being sexually active with another man; women are more disturbed by the thought of their partner being emotionally involved with another woman.

Buss (1998) comments that SST has been far more successful at predicting and explaining gender differences in human sexuality than gender similarities, the features of sexuality that men and women have in common. It has been even less successful in explaining individual differences in human sexuality. How does one account for such huge variability, which (Kinsey et al 1948, 1953) first reported, when it is assumed that psychological mechanisms related to sex which are not adaptive will have been selected out of existence. This fundamental issue, which is of general relevance to evolutionary psychology, was addressed by Allgeier & Wiederman (1994). Based on previous writings by Buss (1991), they propose four explanatory models to account for individual differences:

1. Heritable alternative strategies: some individuals would possess psychological mechanisms for a particular strategy, whereas others would not. This is regarded as difficult to apply to humans, the one exception being biological sex; mechanisms that are possessed by males but not females, and vice versa. However, they do not give examples of such mechanisms. Of the many aspects of behaviour relevant to sexuality where gender differences are found, most nevertheless show considerable overlap of males and females (Oliver & Hyde 1993).
2. Heritable calibration of psychological mechanisms: the hypothesis that the optimally adaptive strategy may have fluctuated across time and/or place, resulting in current heritable variability with regard to the threshold for eliciting a particular strategy.
3. Developmental calibration of the psychological mechanism: earlier experience results in differential calibration of thresholds for elicitation of a particular mating strategy at a later time.
4. Situationally contingent alternative strategies: each individual must possess mechanisms for gathering and processing the relevant information that subsequently produces a decision as to which mating strategy to employ.

Allgeier & Wiederman (1994) regard (3) and (4) as having the best potential for accounting for individual differences in human sexuality.

Evolutionary psychology, in general, has been highly controversial, mainly on the grounds of political incorrectness, in particular the alleged gender differences being taken to justify the status quo of gender relationships (Allgeier & Wiederman 1994). As discussed earlier, political correctness has to be taken into account and cannot be ignored. However, putting such political issues on one side, to what extent can SST be shown to have heuristic value?

The importance of evolutionary principles, I would agree, is beyond question. But it can be argued that the theoretical models based on such principles have varied considerably in their heuristic value. Specific criticisms of SST can be made. One implication of the theory is that psychological adaptations, which evolved to deal with some ancestral problem, remain adaptive today, even though the social as well as natural contexts of human existence have changed enormously. Noteworthy is the absence of any mention of the role of culture, and in particular patriarchal social systems, when considering the explanation for gender differences. Virtually nothing is known about patterns of human sexual behaviour during the EEA. Whereas it is conceivable (though by no means certain) that certain aspects of human sexuality, having evolved as adaptations during the EEA, remained largely unaffected by the subsequent evolution of human societies (and characteristics of sexual attractiveness offer feasible if unsubstantiated examples), it is likely that most of the numerous methods of adapting sexually, listed by Buss, will have altered or even disappeared. The possibility that various behaviours related to sex could have occurred throughout evolutionary history whose immediate benefits may have been out-weighed by longer-term costs, certainly a feature of much human sexual behaviour today, is not considered.

But there are more fundamental criticisms. SST as described, particularly with its postulated methods for accounting for individual differences, seems able to explain just about any phenomenon in human sexual behaviour. Most, if not all, of the gender differences cited as supporting SST were well known before this theoretical model was proposed. So in terms of its heuristic value, what can it *predict* that is not already predictable from other theoretical approaches? And in what ways can it be shown to be refutable? We therefore present this as an example of a theory which portrays 'infallible insight' in an essentialist fashion, set up according to Hrdy's description so that the alternative to accepting it is rejecting evolutionary theory in general, i.e. 'if you don't accept my evolutionary interpretation that means you reject Darwinian logic regarding natural selection' (Hrdy 2000, p. 36).

Comparable bias in evolutionary science is not restricted to evolutionary psychology. An interesting example is the evolutionary explanation for female orgasm. Lloyd (2005), a scholar of the history and philosophy of science, has published a book dedicated to examining in great detail the various evolutionary explanations for female orgasm as an adaptation, by promoting pair-bonding or sperm retention or influencing sperm competition. All of these explanations, in her view, reveal bias and misuse of evidence. She favours the 'by-product' explanation, proposed by Symons (1979); the capacity for orgasm is a potential which is crucial for the male to reproduce, but which is not suppressed in the course of female differentiation. Hence the female develops with this capacity retained, and orgasm is elicited if the female is appropriately stimulated (not necessarily during vaginal intercourse). Thus the female orgasm, however rewarding it might be, is not an adaptation that promotes successful reproduction. The parallel example is the presence of nipples in men and the fact that if men are exposed to high levels of oestrogens they get some degree of breast development. The function of orgasm in women will be considered more closely later in the book.

Sexual scripting theory

This model was first proposed by Gagnon & Simon in 1973 and they have written extensively about it since (e.g. Gagnon 1990; Simon 1996). It derives from three major intellectual traditions: symbolic interactionism, and the works of Kenneth Burke and Sigmund Freud (Simon & Gagnon 1987). It is one of the, if not *the* most frequently cited theoretical models in post-psychoanalytic sexual science. It uses the dramaturgical metaphor of 'script' to describe the sequence followed by an 'actor' engaged in sexual behaviour. It also requires that the script precedes the behaviour: 'The term script might properly be invoked to describe virtually all human behavior in the sense that there is very little that can in

a full measure be called spontaneous' (Gagnon & Simon 1973, p. 19). Gagnon describes the concept of script as 'a unit large enough to comprehend symbolic and non-verbal elements in an organized and time-bound sequence of conduct through which persons both envisage future behavior and check on the quality of ongoing conduct'. He goes on: 'the flexibility of scripts in terms of their internal order and their capacity to be assembled or disassembled in creative or adaptive responses to new circumstances is a critical element in our capacity to manage a changing internal and external environment' (Gagnon 1974, p. 61–62).

Sexual scripting theory clearly locates the origins of sexual meanings and desire in the social context. Thus 'virtually all the cues that initiate sexual behavior are embedded in the social routines of the external environment — just as the absence of external cues serve to mute desire' (Simon 1996, p. 47). And because sexual scripts have this social origin, individuals must call on shared meanings and expectations to produce them. Gender, however, is regarded as being fundamental to the organization of sexual scripts (Mahay et al 2001).

Sexual scripts are defined at 'three analytically distinct levels: *cultural scenarios* (paradigmatic assemblies of the social norms that impinge on sexual behavior), *interpersonal scripts* (where social convention and personal desire must meet), and *intrapsychic scripts* (the realm of the self-process)' (Simon & Gagnon 1987, p. 364).

Interpersonal scripting 'serves as the primary text if only because it is the script that is readable by others' (Simon & Gagnon 1987, p. 374). It involves translating 'abstract cultural scenarios into scripts appropriate for particular situations' (Mahay et al 2001, p. 198).

'Intrapsychic scripts represent the content of mental life. Such scripts can range from the most orderly cognitive narratives to fragments of desire, memories and plans' (Gagnon 1990, p. 10).

At the interface between the interpersonal and the intrapsychic, 'the individual is actor, critic and play-wright' (Gagnon 1990, p. 10), while the intrapsychic script allows a 'meaningful internal rehearsal' (Simon 1996, p. 41).

While sexual script theory provides an all-embracing model to account for human sexual behaviour, the complexity of what it is trying to account for is acknowledged. Thus 'even in the seemingly most traditional social settings, cultural scenarios are rarely predictive of actual behavior' (Gagnon 1990, p. 11) and cultural scenarios are 'too abstractly generic to be mechanically applied in all circumstances. Improvisation . . . conditions all social interactions' (Simon 1996, p. 40). Sexual scripts are 'often relatively incomplete — they do not specify each act and the order in which it is to occur' (Gagnon 1974, p. 61).

In a recent reflection on their sexual scripts approach, Simon & Gagnon (2003) commented that the evolution in their thinking had moved from a social learning towards a social constructionist position. In the *Sexual Conduct* book (Gagnon & Simon 1973) they referred occasionally to sexual learning. More recently we find 'It should be clear that the term scripted is not merely a synonym or codeword for "learned"' (Simon 1996, p. 45). McCormick (1987) commented that psychologists and sociologists lacked awareness of overlap in their literatures, a problem that, in her view, had to some extent been remedied by script theorists. Simon & Gagnon, on the other hand seem to have gradually distanced themselves from psychology, striving to provide an explanatory model of human sexuality, which does not require understanding of psychological mechanisms. This distancing is even more evident in relation to biological factors in human sexuality. From the start 'our preference was to yield as little as possible to the explanatory powers of biology in any of its guises' (Simon & Gagnon 2003). In their earlier papers, some attention was paid to the biological component of sexual experience. They commented on Schachter's widely accepted view that the meaning attributed to physiological arousal (not necessarily sexual) depends on the situation in which it is experienced (Gagnon & Simon 1973), but they qualified the connection where sex is concerned as follows: 'Undeniably, what we conventionally describe as sexual behavior is rooted in biological capacities and processes, but no more than other forms of behavior — the sexual area may be precisely that realm wherein the super-ordinate position of the socio-cultural over the biological level is most complete.' (Gagnon & Simon 1973, p. 15) They go on: 'The sources of sexual arousal are to be found in socio-cultural definitions. It is not the physical but the social aspects that generate the arousal and organize the action, or, in other words, provide the script.' (p. 262). By 1987 they were writing: 'Scripting implies rejection of the idea of a permanent mandate for the sexual rooted in the biological substratum . . . ' (Simon & Gagnon 1987, p. 363). Biological approaches to understanding sexuality are reduced to two sets of theories: instinct theories (which are basically theories of genetic determination) and drive theories (Laumann & Gagnon 1995). Both sets are described as 'folk theories', which presumably means that they principally exist as part of vernacular knowledge. And if biology has any relevance at all, it is qualified by their assertion that 'no biological factor finds its way into the behavior of an individual except through socio-cultural mediation' (Laumann & Gagnon 1995, p. 212).

In 1990 Gagnon was asked to review the impact of sexual scripting theory on sex research for the *Annual Review of Sex Research*. Early in the article he expressed his reservations about the value of research:

' . . . *In a post-positivist world the same sets of acceptable findings can be given quite different explanations and . . . the choice between these explanations cannot be ultimately submitted to an empirical or philosophical test . . . it is always possible to offer a defense for a strongly held theory in the face of any set of evidence and . . . any "program" of scientific work is ultimately non-refutable.*'

(Gagnon 1990, p. 131)

When Gagnon moved on to consider how his theory had influenced sex research, he pointed out that in the majority of cases the presence of scripting is implicit rather than explicit. Gagnon & Simon (1987) published a paper entitled 'The sexual scripting of oral genital contacts.' This examined data showing changing patterns of oral sex outside marriage, with earlier studies showing this activity only likely to occur in relationships in which coitus was already established, and later studies showing oral sex increasing as a pre-coital form of sexual activity. However, it was assumed that this change in behaviour indicated a change in sexual scripts — no evidence directly relevant to any of the three levels of script was reported, only evidence on behaviours as typically reported in surveys.

In the National Health and Social Life Survey (NHSLS; Laumann et al 1994) three models were given as the theoretical background to the study: scripting theory, choice theory and network theory, of which only scripting had direct sexual connotations. However, it was pointed out that 'studying scripts directly is difficult since it requires detailed data not only on what activities occur during a sexual encounter, but also on the order in which those activities occur . . . impossible to implement in a national cross cultural survey . . . our approach is to use detailed questions about specific activities during the last encounter and make inferences about the nature of the scripts being used' (Laumann et al 1994, p. 7). However, almost no attention was paid to such inferences in reporting the results. In a subsequent secondary analysis Mahay et al (2001) examined the extent to which sexual scripts varied by race, gender and class. For this purpose, cultural scripts or scenarios were represented by sexual attitudes (e.g. at what age is it appropriate to have sex?); intrapersonal scripts were represented by actual sexual practices and intrapsychic scripts by sexual preferences, i.e. how appealing did the respondent find each of three activities: vaginal intercourse, fellatio and cunnilingus. For cultural scenarios and interpersonal scripts, responses were assigned to one of three categories: traditional, relational and recreational. No consideration is given to the extent to which such aspects of human sexuality are meaningful illustrations of sexual scripts, and one is left with the distinct impression that this was a post-hoc attempt to use the NHSLS data to support a scripting approach rather than evidence that scripting theory had influenced the design of the survey in the first place. It is certainly questionable whether the basically interesting and informative data that emerged from this survey would have been any different or less informative without the influence of sexual script theory.

There has been research where the script concept was more explicitly incorporated. Two of the better examples involved qualitative studies of women's and men's narratives about real or imaginary sexual encounters. Ortiz-Torres et al (2003) examined women's gender scripts via descriptive narratives of their ideal romantic encounters. Thus, the subjects were told: 'I'd like you to imagine that you are out with a guy — you may have dated him once, or several times. You know you're both attracted to each other. You can feel each other's sexual interest. I'd like you to tell me your most attractive, most romantic way you'd end up together, starting with your first feelings about why you would want to be with this person, and taking it step by step up to where you'd end up together sexually.' (Ortiz-Torres et al 2003, p. 5). Most of the women were subsequently asked how this ideal scenario compared to what actually occurred with their current partner. Around half of the women reported more differences than similarities, leading the authors to conclude that relying on narratives of the ideal scenario was a limitation of their study. Seal & Ehrhardt (2003), in a comparable narrative study of men, did not use the ideal scenario but combined questions about how they typically behave with narratives about the current relationship thus:

'*Courtship*. Tell me how you meet and get to know women ... Tell me how you met and got to know your current (last steady) partner.

Romance. If you wanted to do something romantic for a woman, what would you do ... Tell me about the most romantic thing you've done for a woman (your partner)?

First sex. How does sex occur for the first time? Tell me about the first time you had sex with your current (last steady) partner — what was going on, who was doing what, etc.

Ongoing sex. Tell me how sexual relationships with steady partners change over time ... Tell me about changes in your current (last steady) sexual relationship.' (Seal & Ehrhardt 2003, p. 300).

Seal & Ehrhardt (2003) concluded that the men's narratives revealed gender role and gender script uncertainty as they attempted to understand and internalize changing societal norms. With these two studies we see a clear use of the sexual script approach. It is noteworthy that they employ qualitative methodology, and it is probably the case that script theory needs a considerable amount of such qualitative application before it can hope to lead to useful developments in quantitative research.

Another interesting application of the scripting approach is in sex therapy. McCormick (1987) pointed out that scripts are highly relevant to therapy because the therapist can explicitly negotiate them, e.g. what words to use, what sequences to follow. It can be said that much of sex therapy involves giving the couple or individual scripted assignments to follow. Gagnon et al (1982) explained how a scripting approach can be used in the treatment of sexual dysfunctions such as premature ejaculation and orgasmic difficulty. Rosen & Leiblum (1988) took this further by pointing out that a detailed comparison of the 'sexual scripts' of the two people in a problematic sexual relationship is a powerful way of identifying reasons for low sexual desire in one or other partner.

Weis, who has carried out a number of studies relevant to sexual scripts, uses sexual script theory, as defined by Gagnon & Simon, as an example of 'the failure to build an explanatory model to identify correlates of the primary construct' (Weis 1998b, p. 107). He points out that there is still little understanding of how scripts become institutionalized, the process of social change, the relationship between scripts and behaviour, the associations among scripts at the three levels of analysis and how scripts are internalized. He goes on to make proposals for how such questions should be addressed which to a large extent employ mechanisms from psychology.

What are my conclusions about Gagnon & Simon's sexual script approach? I consider their dramaturgical metaphor to be useful as a way to grasp what are otherwise highly complex psychological processes; in other words, a good example of a simplified model of reality. On several occasions, Gagnon & Simon have described their approach as metaphor rather than theory. Thus: '... not a theory of sexual behavior, but rather a conceptual apparatus ...' (Simon & Gagnon 1987, p. 381); '... essentially a metaphor for conceptualizing the production of behavior within social life' (Simon 1996, p. 40). But most of their writing on this subject presents sexual scripting as a theoretical model, albeit 'a way of constructing or inventing a world rather than discovering it' (Gagnon 1990, p. 131). Instinct and drive models in their dismissal are contrasted with a 'strong sociocultural theory of sexual action which is based on the theory of sexual scripts' (Laumann & Gagnon 1995, p. 212). In addition to rejecting biological explanations, they effectively distance themselves from the use of psychological mechanisms which, as Weis (1998b) pointed out, are needed to explain their scripting concepts. Their sole use of a dramaturgical model, which has the advantage of being comprehensible in a vernacular sense, effectively puts their work into the folk-theory category. Furthermore, their writing is permeated with strong assertions which are not justified by evidence. The following are examples: '... all human sexual behavior is socially scripted behavior' (Gagnon & Simon in 1973, p. 262); 'The probability of something sexual happening will under normal circumstances remain exceedingly small until either one or both actors organize the behavior into an appropriate script' (p. 19); 'All the cues that initiate sexual behavior are embedded in the external environment' (Simon & Gagnon 1987, p. 367). There is no uncertainty in their writing; it is a clear example of Popper's 'intuitive grasp of the essence' discussed earlier. Gagnon & Simon are essentialists as much as Buss with his sexual strategies theory, and it is notable that through the three decades of its existence, they have shown little inclination to put their theoretical model to the test.

This critical evaluation of these two theoretical models of human sexuality, from the two ends of the epistemological spectrum but similar in several respects, is intended to set the scene for presenting my own theoretical approaches, in particular setting criteria of worth which must be considered in relation to my own ideas. Overall, I am proposing that models of sexuality can have a number of roles. More conventionally, they can have explanatory value in terms of testable hypotheses, and adhere to the Popperian standard of refutability, while acknowledging that this is not always feasible. I have yet to be persuaded that this form of scientific method should be abandoned — although there are good and bad ways of using it. The crucial point is that it is not sufficient for our task. More often than not, rigorous implementation of scientific method requires control of the circumstances, experimentation in other words, which removes the factor under study from the ordinary world. Interpreting the results in terms relevant to the ordinary world can then be difficult. Nevertheless, in my opinion, the rigour of striving to formulate hypotheses that are in some sense refutable is an important and valuable part of scientific discipline.

More broadly we can provide simplified models of otherwise overwhelmingly complex situations, which, at a minimum, provide a useful way for organizing our thinking. All such models need to be judged in terms of their heuristic value. Evidence derived from good scientific method while of likely explanatory value, still needs to be justified in terms of its practical value. In this way we evade many of the epistemological conflicts about reality. For example, a research finding which results in clinical benefits can be demonstrably useful without necessarily helping us to understand how the beneficial changes were achieved. We can extend this pragmatism to the less individual-oriented, more group-oriented area of social policy. A theoretical model could conceivably be validated by the extent to which it leads to effective policies. This is in some respects a radical suggestion. It might cause anxiety in those who fear science becoming modified to sustain a political ideology. But informing the policy maker should be an important part of our objective. The theoretical model that we choose to use may make that task harder or easier. But on the other hand, the eclectic approach that still currently prevails may make it easier for policy makers to pick and choose the pieces of evidence that suit their agendas. That possibility is something we should keep in mind.

The big picture

There can be little doubt that the determinants of human sexuality and its behavioural manifestations are many and varied. The prevailing culture shapes in a powerful way the sexual mores and taboos, and the social expectations of appropriate sexual behaviour, which in turn shape the sexual behaviour itself. Sexual relationships between men and women are determined to a considerable extent by the gender roles and gender power differences that are themselves culturally determined; gender power and sexual roles become entangled with political and economic factors.

However, the socio-cultural, political and economic factors do not shape human sexuality in a biological vacuum. This does not mean a biological 'given', but rather the potential for considerable individual variation, and possibly also ethnic variation in biological factors. We need to take the individual biological variability into account when striving to explain the fact that in a given cultural setting, individuals vary considerably in the extent to which they conform to the cultural pattern.

We therefore need a basic model that acknowledges the full range and complexity of human sexual expression and its determinants, whilst allowing us to focus on specific parts of it without losing sight of the whole.

My starting point is Marvin Harris's account of cultural materialism (Harris 1979). Harris is a controversial and provocative figure in anthropology; at the Kinsey Theory workshop, Herdt described Harris's work as *passé* in anthropology because he wasn't really interested in culture, but rather the material resources around which culture and social structure are created (Bancroft 2000a, p. 234). But from my perspective, his ideas are attractive because they provide scope for a broad interactive explanatory model, which also allows us to identify and focus on its specific components. Harris's cultural materialism model has three parts: infrastructure, structure and superstructure. Each part has various components:

Infrastructure
  (a) mode of production (especially of food and
      energy)
  (b) mode of reproduction (methods for expanding,
      limiting or maintaining population size)

This can be seen as the principal interface between culture and nature. Harris (1997) considers the pursuit of sexual pleasure to be an aspect of reproductive infrastructure.

Structure
  (a) domestic economy (e.g. family structure, age
      and sex roles, domestic division of labour,
      education)
  (b) political economy (e.g. division of labour, class
      system, police, war)

Superstructure
  e.g. shared beliefs, symbolism, taboos, religion,
  epistemologies and expressions of culture
  (e.g. music, dance, etc)

The guiding principle in Harris's model is that of infrastructural determinism, an adaptation of the fundamental Marxist principle, i.e. the modes of production and reproduction probabilistically determine the domestic and political economy, which in turn probabilistically determine the superstructure. It is conceded that aspects of the structure and superstructure can achieve a degree of autonomy from the infrastructure, but this should only be considered if the possibility of infrastructural determinism has been thoroughly explored first. Although Harris does not say this, it seems reasonable to assume that some components of the superstructure are going to be more determined by the infrastructure than others.

Not surprisingly, this model is most convincing when dealing with relatively primitive and small cultures. It gets increasingly difficult to apply as we move to complex modern industrial states. However, our principal aim is to use the model to structure and order our thinking about human sexuality and how it varies cross-culturally, and how biological factors may interact with socio-cultural factors. But let us first illustrate how cultural materialism can help us understand comparatively simple early cultures, taking examples from Harris' writing.

The hunter-gatherer society illustrates a cultural pattern, which while now almost disappeared, had the longest history of any type of human society during the very prolonged period before domestication of plants and animals. The 'mode of production' of the hunter-gatherer involved hunting, fishing and collection of wild seeds, nuts, fruit and other sources of food available in the environment. This aspect of the infrastructure accounted for their mobile, nomadic existence. Bands of 20–50 people were typical. There was inter-marriage between neighbouring bands which fostered various levels of inter-band cooperation. Food production was shared, ownership of property and social stratification were minimal. These were egalitarian groups, with relatively slight sexual dimorphism and relatively equal relationships between men and women. Children were a liability for the first few years of their life, contributing little to food foraging and restricting the mother's activity within the group. Long periods of adolescent infertility and later lactational anoestrus are assumed to be secondary to the high protein low carbohydrate diet that prevailed. The birth rate was relatively low so that methods of controlling population (e.g. infanticide) were not needed.

Harris (1979) emphasized population density and population growth as key determining factors in the infrastructure, pointing out that prior to 3000 BC there was a very long period of relative population stability. When social groups turned to agriculture and stock raising, fundamental changes occurred. Harris postulated that the change in diet (less protein and more carbohydrate) may have reduced lactational infertility, with the associated increase in birth rate resulting in children who, in contrast to the hunter-gatherer life style, could now provide useful child labour. However, in these circumstances population pressure was more likely; women's roles were necessarily altered by more child rearing, warfare between villages increased, emphasizing the importance of male children, leading to selective female infanticide and the establishment of sexual stratification. Polygynous patterns were encouraged by awarding females to dominant senior males; the property status of women became established and the gender power differential was reinforced. The acquisition of wealth, in the form of land or domestic animals, raised issues of inheritance, leading to a variety of devices to ensure appropriate transfer of property and raising the need for the dominant male to protect himself from cuckoldry, with resulting emphasis on virginity, a characteristic of the female property transfer from father to husband.

There is certainly a need to explain the substantial increase in population after a long period of stability. Harris' explanations, while speculative, are interesting, and it is the emphasis on population control and reproductive behaviour that makes cultural materialism of potential relevance to the understanding of human sexuality.

So how can we use cultural materialism as a foundation for building our theoretical model of human sexuality? There is an important difference between establishing a science of culture, which aims to explain differences and similarities between different cultures, and a science of human sexuality, which aims to explain differences and similarities between cultures but also between individuals within those cultures. For this purpose the original model is modified by incorporating the individuals that make up a cultural group, in terms of their innate characteristics and capacities, as an element of the infrastructure of that culture. Obviously, those individuals will be shaped in many respects by the culture in which they live. But each individual has innate or early determined characteristics which may or may not be useful to the process of conforming to or fitting in to the culture, or occasionally shaping it. We can regard such characteristics as the human resources within the infrastructure, or the 'individual infrastructure'. Let us, therefore, elaborate the concept of reproductive infrastructure with the following subheadings:

(a) demographics of population
　　e.g. population density, sex ratios and age distribution
(b) neurobiological basis of sexual responsiveness (individual differences genetically determined or acquired)
　● sexual activation (propensity for sexual arousal)
　● sexual inhibition (propensity for sexual inhibition)
　● other relevant physiological mechanisms (e.g. sexual signalling systems)
(c) age-related developmental processes
　● aspects of cognitive development which delay certain types of learning until the relevant developmental stage has been reached
　● aspects of emotional development which may be influenced by the developmental stage (both cognitive and neurobiological)
(d) development of patterns of sexual attraction
　● factors, which may involve genetic as well as early learning processes, which influence subsequent development of sexual preferences and how these preferences are experienced is further elaborated by socio-cultural processes in the superstructure (i.e. shared constructs of sexual identity)
(e) methods of fertility regulation
　● inherent (interaction between environment and biology)
　　e.g. age at puberty, age when fertile, factors affecting fertility such as STDs, nutrition and lactation
　● technology available for use
　　e.g. contraception, sterilisation, abortion, infanticide.

This then leads us to identify and elaborate reproductive components of the structure:

(a) mating patterns (e.g. polygyny, monogamy, incest taboos)
(b) levels of sexual stratification
(c) levels of sexual segregation
(d) age at marriage
(e) family structure (matri- or patrilinearity, fatherless families)
(f) social management of adolescence and transition to sexual adult
　　e.g. induction rituals, separation from parents, teen culture
(g) reactions to cultural norms
　　i.e. counter cultures, sexuality as a form of dissent
(h) communication systems (see below).

and reproductive components of the superstructure:

(a) shared concepts of masculinity, femininity and male-female relationships
(b) shared constructs of sexual identity
(c) shared beliefs about appropriate patterns of sexual behaviour
(d) shared beliefs or attitudes about:
  - fertility versus virginity before marriage
  - importance of marriage versus family ties
  - sex as commodity/exchange
(e) sexual conformity
  - individual differences in need to conform/ rebel
(f) identification with sexual counter cultures.

Together, these interactive components of the model lead us to a variety of 'reproductive individuals'.

This modified model of cultural materialism continues to assume the principle of infrastructural determinism, and therefore challenges the evidence to show that superstructural changes can be primary and dominant. It does, however, acknowledge that cultural conflict can, through the development of counter-cultures — 'the rules for breaking rules' — add diversity to the culture at both structural and superstructural levels. Sexuality has been a highly relevant vehicle for expressing social conformity and non-conformity. It may well be this non-conformity that is the aspect of the superstructure least determined by the infrastructure. This model also assumes that reproduction and sexuality are closely interdependent, counter to the fashion which has prevailed in the social sciences for some time now, which sees them as essentially separate. It does, however, allow for the development and establishment of sexual patterns that are not determined by reproduction. An important factor, which needs to be incorporated, is communication, in particular the methods by which ideas and values are disseminated within a culture. Although this has always been of fundamental importance, it represents a component of the model which has changed dramatically in the past 100 years, and which has and is still having a major impact on patterns of sexuality. Given that it is, at least more recently, dependent on evolving technologies, we are proposing that it should be incorporated as part of the structure.

As we proceed through the book we will return to this model at each stage, primarily as a way of organizing our thinking and presentation of evidence, but also, to a limited extent, as a challenge to see to what extent the evidence supports the model.

One of our aims with this 'big picture' is to have a model incorporating components that we can focus on. In particular, the individual, and various sources of individual variability, has been added to the reproductive infrastructure. (Note: The individual could also be added in this way to the productive infrastructure, but this is of less relevance to human sexuality.) One component of the reproductive infrastructure I have proposed is the neurobiological basis of sexual responsiveness, including the propensities for sexual arousal or excitation and sexual inhibition. This component is the theme of a more specific theoretical model that will feature substantially in this book. We will now focus our attention on this model.

The Dual Control model

For the past 10 years, much of the research at the Kinsey Institute has been guided and shaped by a new theoretical model, the Dual Control model (Bancroft & Janssen 2000). This postulates that whether sexual response and associated arousal occurs in a particular individual, in a particular situation, is ultimately determined by the balance between two systems in that individual's brain, the sexual activation or excitation system and the sexual inhibition system, each of which has a neurobiological substrate (see review of the relevant evidence in Bancroft 1999). This model, which we have called the Dual Control model, makes three basic assumptions:

1. Although sexual arousal typically occurs in interactions between two or more individuals, and the context and cultural scenario associated with the interaction are important sources of stimulation, both excitatory and inhibitory, the effects of such stimulation depend ultimately on neurobiological characteristics of the individuals involved.
2. Neurobiological inhibition of sexual response is an adaptive pattern, of relevance across species, which reduces the likelihood of sexual response, and the distracting effects of sexual arousal and appetite, from occurring in situations when sexual activity would be disadvantageous or dangerous, or would distract the individual from dealing appropriately with other demands of the situation.
3. Individuals vary in their propensity for both sexual excitation and sexual inhibition. Although for the majority these propensities would be adaptive or non-problematic, individuals with an unusually high propensity for excitation and/or low propensity for inhibition would be more likely to engage in high risk or otherwise problematic sexual behaviour, and individuals with a low propensity for sexual excitation and/or high propensity for sexual inhibition would be more likely to experience problems with sexual response (i.e. sexual dysfunctions).

Our initial research using this model focused on the male. In order to measure the postulated variance in the two components of the Dual Control model, a questionnaire was developed and psychometrically established (the SIS/SES; Janssen et al 2002). Questions were focused on the extent to which the respondent would become sexually aroused, lose sexual arousal or fail to become sexually aroused in a variety of situations. This resulted in three factors or scales, rather than the two we had anticipated: a Sexual Excitation Scale (SES) and two Sexual Inhibition Scales. On the basis of the questions contributing to these latter two scales, they were called 'sexual inhibition due to the threat of performance failure' (SIS1) and 'sexual inhibition due to the threat of performance consequences' (SIS2). Two examples of questions from each scale are:

'When I think of a very attractive person, I easily become sexually aroused.'
'When I start fantasizing about sex, I quickly become sexually aroused.' (SES)
'If I feel that I'm expected to respond sexually, I have difficulty getting aroused.'
'When I have a distracting thought, I easily lose my erection.' (SIS1)
'If I realize there is a risk of catching a sexually transmitted disease, I am unlikely to stay sexually aroused.'
'If I can be heard by others while having sex, I am unlikely to stay sexually aroused.' (SIS2)

There are 20 items and four subscales in SES, 14 items and three subscales in SIS1, and 11 items and three subscales in SIS2.

We have now collected data using this questionnaire from several large samples of men and the results, and the extent to which we have found support for our predictions, will be discussed at various stages of this book. We did, however, find close to normal distributions of scores on each of the three scales, consistent with our aim to measure normal individual variability (see Chapter 6, Fig. 6.11).

More recently, a questionnaire — the Sexual Excitation/Sexual Inhibition Inventory for Women (SESII-W) — has been developed for measuring these individual propensities in women (Graham et al 2006). The expectation was that women, on average, would show higher propensities for inhibition than men and that there would also be gender differences in the situations which evoked inhibition of sexual response. A series of focus groups involving women of different ages, ethnic and racial backgrounds, and sexual orientation were used to elicit women's ideas about factors that enhanced and inhibited sexual arousal (Graham et al 2004). The qualitative data obtained from these groups was used to inform questionnaire development.

Initial validation of the original 115-item SESII-W was carried out on a sample of 655 women. Factor analysis identified eight factors (five related to excitation and three to inhibition) and two higher-order factors, one related to sexual excitation and one to sexual inhibition. The excitation factors were sexual arousability (the tendency to become sexually aroused in a variety of situations), partner characteristics (the tendency for a partner's personality or behaviours to enhance arousal), sexual power dynamics (the tendency to become sexually aroused by force or domination in a sexual situation), smell (the tendency for olfactory cues to enhance arousal) and setting (the tendency for arousal to be increased by the possibility of being seen or heard while having sex). The three inhibition factors were relationship importance (reflecting the need for sex to occur within a specific type of relationship), concerns about sexual function (the tendency for worries about sexual functioning to impair arousal) and arousal contingency (the potential for arousal to be easily inhibited or disrupted by situational factors). The resultant 36-item measure

demonstrated good test–retest reliability and discriminant and convergent validity. As found with the male SIS/SES measures, the SESII-W also showed close to normal distributions of scores (see Chapter 6, Fig. 6.12).

A fundamental question is whether this putative sexual inhibitory system is a sexual manifestation of a more general behavioural inhibitory system, such as that postulated by Jeffrey Gray (1971), or whether we are dealing with a form of central inhibition, which is specific to sexual response, or possibly a combination of the two. Gray's model and the considerable amount of animal research and more recently the human research that it has stimulated do provide us with a rich source of ideas and putative mechanisms in our explorations. Carver & White (1994) developed a questionnaire, the Behavioural Inhibition/Activation Behavioural Scales (BIS/BAS), to quantify Gray's two components in human subjects. We have compared our SIS/SES scales with the BIS/BAS (Janssen et al 2002) and found significant but modest correlations between SES and the three BAS subscales ($r = +0.31$, $+0.22$ and $+0.25$, all significant at $p < 0.001$), and between SIS2 and BIS ($r = +0.22$; $p < 0.001$). Similarly, for the female SESII-W measure, low to moderate correlations were found between the BAS subscales and all of the SESII-W excitation scales. As expected, the higher-order and all lower-order inhibition factors showed small to modest positive correlation with BIS. Thus, whereas there may be some overlap of these questionnaires and conceptual models, these correlations are consistent with the two components of our Dual Control model being, at least in part, specifically related to sexual response.

How does the Dual Control model fit into our larger model? First, how might this dual control system interact with other aspects of the infrastructure?

Let us first consider the developmental process. In our male studies we have found correlations with age. SES tends to be lower in older men ($r = -0.24$; $p < 0.001$), consistent with a negative effect of the aging process on sexual responsiveness. SIS1 tends to be higher in older men ($r = +0.34$), which raises some key questions about the aging process (see Chapter 7, p. 243 for further discussion). SIS2 has shown no relationship to age. In the studies involving women, there was a significant negative correlation between age and the higher-order factor of SE ($r = -0.29$), but, interestingly, no relationship between age and SI.

Do the activation and inhibition systems develop at the same time? If we are dealing with a specifically sexual form of inhibition, is this present before puberty and the hormonal amplification of the sexual activation system? There is a hint of evidence that, at least in the male, the inhibitory mechanisms are lacking prior to puberty, with the pubertal increase in androgens playing a role in organizing and activating both the sexual excitation and inhibition systems (see Chapter 4, p. 91 for further discussion). As yet we can say little about this in relation to females. The crucial stage of adolescent brain development is likely to be relevant here, and this is considered in Chapter 4 (see p. 60).

To what extent are these propensities for excitation and inhibition genetically determined or the result of early learning? So far we have one study addressing this question (Varjonen et al 2007). In this Finnish study of 1289 male twins, a modest heritability was found for both SIS1 and SIS2, whereas SES appeared to be more determined by the shared environment. It will be interesting to look at female twins in this way.

To what extent have we demonstrated gender differences in the Dual Control model? Our instruments for measuring individual variability in excitation and inhibition propensities have been developed for men and women separately but in each case we have adapted the wording to make the questionnaire usable by the opposite sex. Comparison of male and female student samples using the SIS/SES shows significantly higher group means for excitation in men and inhibition in women, as predicted (Carpenter et al 2008). In a similar comparison using the SESII-W, significant gender differences were found on all of the factor scales (Milhausen 2006). Women were significantly more likely to report that their arousal was enhanced by positive partner characteristics and by hormonal changes. Men, on the other hand, were more likely to indicate that a variety of sexual stimuli and negative mood states could increase sexual arousal. Turning to the inhibition factors, women were much more likely than men to report that sexual arousal was reduced in situations not characterized by trust and intimacy (the relationship importance factor). Women also had higher scores than men on the inhibition factors, 'Concerns about sexual functioning' and 'Setting'; higher scores on these scales indicate that worries about sexual functioning or performance, or about being seen or heard while having sex are likely to dampen sexual arousal.

Is there a link with fertility regulation? There is an extensive biological literature on mechanisms for controlling population density in other species. One important aspect of this is the capacity for inhibition of sexual behaviour in situations of overcrowding. In social animals this is usually mediated via the dominance hierarchy — it is the low dominance animals whose sexual behaviour is inhibited. Is there a relationship between low dominance and *high* propensity for sexual inhibition? Most sexually transmitted diseases have their main impact on fertility rather than mortality (see Chapter 14). Maybe *low* propensity for sexual inhibition increases the likelihood of sexual transmission of disease. It is worth keeping in mind that if any genetically determined mechanisms are involved in the control of population density, then there would need to be more than one — otherwise the single mechanism would eventually be bred out. The relevance of the Dual Control model to high risk sexual behaviour, leading to both unplanned pregnancies and sexual transmission of infections and to 'out of control' sexual behaviour, are considered in Chapters 11 and 14.

When we consider our Dual Control model in relation to reproductive structure and superstructure, a number of relevant links suggest themselves. The impact of high propensity for sexual inhibition may vary according to the prevailing patterns of male–female relationships (i.e. whether there is a gender power difference) and the shared beliefs about masculinity and male–female relationships. Accordingly, in any phallocentric culture which promotes the idea that an erect penis is a symbol of manhood and potency (and the USA is a good modern example), the man with high propensity for sexual inhibition will be more likely to experience sexual dysfunction as a result.

On the other hand, for the man with a low propensity for sexual inhibition, who finds himself sexually aroused even in situations that are manifestly risky, the impact of this tendency will vary according to whether he is in a culture or, more likely, subculture which tends to view sexual risk taking as an admirable masculine trait. Indeed, the balance of our putative dual control system may help to determine which set of beliefs about appropriate sexual behaviour are shared and adopted, and which type of sexual subculture the individual identifies with. Depending on how age-related developmental processes impinge upon our theoretical mechanisms, propensities for sexual inhibition and excitation may help determine the pattern or style of sexual unfolding during adolescence, and whether sexual expression is used as a form of adolescent rebellion. As yet these interactions between the Dual Control model, the socio-cultural context and the subculture that an individual identifies with are researchable questions awaiting study.

The Dual Control model is therefore presented as an explanatory model of certain basic neurophysiological aspects of individual variability, which is open to testing and is relatively refutable. While focusing on putative neurophysiological mechanisms, potential interactions with socio-cultural factors are recognized and are open to investigation. As I discuss our results in more detail, at various points in this book, we will be confronted by the potential limitations of the questionnaire methods we are using to measure this variability. It is clearly important to keep in mind that such instruments are relatively imperfect, ad hoc methods for exploring the model, and should not be equated with the postulated underlying mechanisms that they are intended to measure. In addition to demonstrating the need to modify and improve the basic model, we may also encounter the need to develop or change the methods of measurement that we use. However, the model also offers a template for organizing our ideas and our review of available evidence that is used in several parts of this book.

Other simple organizing models of this kind are also used. The Psychosomatic Circle of Sex, which featured in the second edition of this book, remains as a model of how cognitive, central and peripheral neurophysiological mechanisms interact (see Chapter 4), which has now been augmented by incorporation of the Dual Control model. The three-strand model of sexual development is a further example. This considers three aspects of development — sexual responsiveness, gender identity and the capacity for dyadic relationships — as being relatively independent strands of development during childhood, which become integrated to a varying extent as individuals enter adolescence and adulthood (see Chapter 5).

What is human sexuality?

The title of this book is *Human Sexuality and Its Problems*. This appropriately confronts us with the question 'What is human sexuality?'. At the same time that also confronts us with the distinction Popper made between methodological essentialists, who ask 'what is ...?' questions, and methodological nominalists, who ask 'how' and 'why' questions. The social constructionists will say, with little doubt, that human sexuality is a social construct, which has evolved and changed across history, and to some extent is a relatively recent construct. Rather than evade the 'what is' question and stick to the 'how' and 'why' responses, let me attempt an answer. Consistent with what has been said through the course of this chapter, I am aware of our need, as sexual scientists, to impose a construction on to the complexity of what we encounter. It has been acknowledged that this is a construction of reality, rather than true reality, and the need to demonstrate its heuristic value has been emphasized, if we are to continue to use it. Within those limitations, I see human sexuality as that aspect of the human condition, which is manifested as sexual desire or appetite, associated physiological response patterns, and behaviour which leads to orgasm, or at least pleasurable arousal, often between two people, but not infrequently by an individual alone. I am aware of a fundamental link between such sexuality and reproduction, even though the large majority of human sexual behaviour is not reproductive in its consequences. Across cultures and through most of human history, we see the association between 'sexual' and 'reproductive' as a key organizing principle in marriage, although the institution of marriage takes many forms and is undergoing major changes in the Western world. We see evidence of social mechanisms, in the form of mores and associated attitudes, and rules of conduct and laws, which are intended to control human sexual expression, most typically aiming to contain it within marriage. We see the sexual expression of two people in a relationship as having the potential for either bonding or weakening the relationship. Overall, from this multi-faceted construct, we see a range of issues of major importance to both individuals and society and a common source of problems which are, more often than not, ill-understood; hence our justification for attempting to pursue and grapple with this construct. If we take one facet of this picture — sexual desire — we are immediately confronted with difficulty in defining what it is that we are dealing with. This 'I know it when I feel it' experience has been conceptualized as desire or appetite because of an associated motivation to 'do something about it'. But when we get to grips with such experience, we have to acknowledge that what forms its basis is unclear and evasive. This is being brought home to sexual scientists by the advent of brain imaging. This new technology will probably be the most important and illuminating component of sexual science for the next several decades. Yet already it is confronting us with the fact that our constructs, such as sexual desire, do not fit with patterns of brain activity — any more than the ideas of phrenology did in the 19th century. This should serve as a reminder of our need for humility and the pursuit of useful simplifications of the real world.

REFERENCES

Abramson PR, Herdt G 1990 The assessment of sexual practices relevant to the transmission of AIDS: a global perspective. Journal of Sex Research 27: 215–232.

Abramson PR, Pinkerton SD 1995 Sexual Nature/Sexual Culture. University of Chicago Press, Chicago.

Allgeier ER, Wiederman MW 1994 How useful is evolutionary psychology for understanding contemporary human sexual behaviour. Annual Review of Sex Research 5: 218–256.

Bancroft J 1999 Central inhibition of sexual response in the male: a theoretical perspective. Neuroscience and Biobehavioral Reviews 23: 763–784.

Bancroft J (ed) 2000a The Role of Theory in Sex Research. Indiana University Press, Bloomington, Indiana.

Bancroft J 2000b Individual differences in sexual risk taking. In Bancroft J (ed) The Role of Theory in Sex Research. Indiana University Press, Bloomington, Indiana.

Bancroft J, Janssen E 2000 The dual control model of male sexual response: a theoretical approach to centrally mediated erectile dysfunction. Neuroscience and Biobehavioral Reviews 24: 571–579.

Buss DM 1991 Evolutionary personality psychology. Annual Review of Psychology 42: 459–491.

Buss DM 1998 Sexual strategies theory: historical origins and current status. Journal of Sex Research 35: 19–31.

Buss DM, Schmitt DP 1993 Sexual strategies theory: a contextual evolutionary analysis of human mating. Psychological Review 100: 204–232.

Carpenter DL, Janssen E, Graham CA 2008 Women's scores on the Sexual Excitation/Sexual Inhibition Scales (SIS/SES): gender similarities and differences. Journal of Sex Research 45: 36–48.

Carver CS, White TL 1994 Behavioral inhibition, behavioral activation, and affective responses to impending reward and punishment: the BIS/BAS Scales. Journal of Personality and Social Psychology 67: 319–333.

DeLamater JD, Hyde JS 1998 Essentialism versus social constructionism in the study of human sexuality. Journal of Sex Research 35: 10–18.

Escoffier J 1999 The invention of safer sex: vernacular knowledge, gay politics and HIV prevention. Berkeley Journal of Sociology 43: 1–30.

Flowers P, Duncan B 2002 Gay men and sexual decision making. Journal of Community & Applied Social Psychology 12: 230–236.

Gagnon J 1974 Scripts and the coordination of sexual conduct. Reprinted in Gagnon J (2004) An Interpretation of Desire. University of Chicago Press, Chicago, pp. 59–87.

Gagnon J 1990 The explicit and implicit use of the scripting perspective. Annual Review of Sex Research 1: 1–44.

Gagnon J 2000 Theorizing risky sex. In Bancroft J (ed) The Role of Theory in Sex Research. Indiana University Press, Bloomington, Indiana, pp. 149–176.

Gagnon J, Simon W 1973 Sexual Conduct: the Social Sources of Human Sexuality. Aldine, Chicago.

Gagnon JH, Simon W 1987 The sexual scripting of oral genital contacts. Archives of Sexual Behavior 16: 1–26.

Gagnon JH, Rosen RC, Leiblum SR 1982 Cognitive and social aspects of sexual dysfunction: sexual scripts in sex therapy. Journal of Sex and Marital Therapy 8: 44–56.

Geertz C 1983 Local Knowledge. Basic Books, New York.

Graham CA, Sanders SA, Milhausen R, McBride K 2004 Turning on and turning off: a focus group study of the factors that affect women's sexual arousal. Archives of Sexual Behavior 33: 527–538.

Graham CA, Sanders SA, Milhausen R 2006 The sexual excitation and sexual inhibition inventory for women: psychometric properties. Archives of Sexual Behavior 35: 397–410.

Gramsci A 1971 Selections from the Prison Notes. International Publishers, New York.

Gray JA 1971 The Psychology of Fear and Stress. Weidenfeld & Nicholson, New York.

Harris M 1979 Cultural Materialism: The Struggle for a Science of Culture. Random House, New York.

Harris M 1997 Culture, People, Nature: an Introduction to General Anthropology. 7th edn. Longman, New York.

Hebb DO 1949 The Organization of Behavior. Wiley, New York.

Hrdy SB 2000 Discussion paper. In Bancroft J (ed) The Role of Theory in Sex Research. Indiana University Press, Bloomington, Indiana, p. 36.

Janssen E, Vorst H, Finn P, Bancroft J 2002 The sexual inhibition (SIS) and sexual excitation (SES) scales: I. Measuring sexual inhibition and excitation proneness in men. Journal of Sex Research 39: 114–126.

Jost A 1965 Gonadal hormones in the sex differentiation of the mammalian fetus. In DeHaan RL, Ursprung H (eds) Organogenesis. Holt, Rinehart & Winston, New York.

Kinsey AC, Pomeroy WB, Martin CE 1948 Sexual Behavior in the Human Male. WB Saunders, Philadelphia.

Kinsey AC, Pomeroy WB, Martin CE, Gebhard PH 1953 Sexual Behavior in the Human Female. WB Saunders, Philadelphia.

Kuhn TS 1970 The Structure of Scientific Revolutions. 2nd edn. University of Chicago Press, Chicago.

Laumann EO, Gagnon J 1995 A sociological perspective on sexual action. In Parker RG, Gagnon JH (eds) Conceiving Sexuality. Routledge, New York, pp. 183–214.

Laumann EO, Gagnon JH, Michael RT, Michaels S 1994 The Social Organization of Sexuality. University of Chicago Press, Chicago.

Lillie FR 1939 General biological introduction. In Allen E (ed) Sex and Internal Secretions. Williams & Wilkins, Baltimore, pp. 3–14.

Lloyd EA 2005 The Case of the Female Orgasm: Bias in the Science of Evolution. Harvard University Press, Cambridge.

Mahay J, Laumann EO, Michaels S 2001 Race, gender and class in sexual scripts. In Laumann EO, Michael RT (eds) Sex, Love and Health in America. University of Chicago Press, Chicago, pp. 197–238.

McCormick NB 1987 Sexual scripts: social and therapeutic implications. Sexual and Marital Therapy 2: 3–27.

McFall R 1991 Manifesto for a science of clinical psychology. The Clinical Psychologist 44: 75–88.

Milhausen R 2006 Factors that inhibit and enhance sexual arousal in college men and women. PhD Thesis, Indiana University, Indiana.

Okami P, Pendleton L 1995 Appendix: theorizing sexuality. In Abrahamson PR, Pinkerton SD (eds) Sexual Nature/Sexual Culture. University of Chicago Press, Chicago, pp. 387–397.

Oliver MB, Hyde JS 1993 Gender differences in human sexuality: a meta-analysis. Psychological Bulletin 114: 29–51.

Ortiz-Torres B, Williams SP, Ehrhardt AA 2003 Urban women's gender scripts: implications for HIV prevention. Culture, Health & Sexuality 5: 1–17.

Ortner SB, Whitehead H 1981 Sexual Meanings: The Cultural Construction of Gender and Sexuality. Cambridge University Press, Cambridge.

Popper KR 1957 The Poverty of Historicism. Routledge & Kegan Paul, London.

Popper KR 1977 The Self and Its Brain: An Argument for Interactionism. Part I. In Popper KR, Eccles JC (eds). Springer International, New York.

Rosen RC, Leiblum SR 1988 A sexual scripting approach to problems of desire. In Rosen RC, Leiblum SR (eds) Sexual Desire Disorders. Guilford, New York, pp. 168–191.

Satcher D 2001 Call to action to promote sexual health and responsible sexual behavior. www.surgeongeneral.gov/library/sexualhealth

Seal DW, Ehrhardt AA 2003 Masculinity and urban men: perceived scripts for courtship, romantic, and sexual interactions with women. Culture, Health & Sexuality 5: 295–319.

Simon W 1996 Postmodern Sexualities. Routledge, New York.

Simon W, Gagnon J 1987 A sexual scripts approach. In Geer JH, O'Donohue WT (eds) Theories of Human Sexuality. Plenum, New York.

Simon W, Gagnon J 2003 Sexual scripts: origins, influences and changes. Qualitative Sociology 26: 491–497.

Symons D 1979 The Evolution of Human Sexuality. Oxford University Press, New York.

Tuzin D 1995 Discourse, intercourse, and the excluded middle: anthropology and the problem of sexual experience. In Abrahamson PR, Pinkerton SD (eds) Sexual Nature/Sexual Culture. University of Chicago Press, Chicago, pp. 257–275.

Varjonen M, Santtila P, Hoglund M, Jern P, Johansson A, Wager I, Witting K, Algars M, Sandnabba NK 2007 Genetic end environmental effects on sexual excitation and sexual inhibition in men. Journal of Sex Research 44: 359–369.

Weis DL 1998a The use of theory in sexuality research. Journal of Sex Research 35: 1–9.

Weis DL 1998b Conclusions: The state of sexual theory. Journal of Sex Research 35: 100–114.

Introduction.. 20

The fundamental roles of reproductive hormones........... 20
Peptides 21
The anterior pituitary–gonadal system 22
Steroid hormones... 22

Anatomical sexual differentiation 24
Chromosomal gender.. 24
Gonads 25
Hormones 25
Internal sexual organs 25
External genitalia 25

Hormone levels during childhood and adolescence
and their effects on development.................................. 25
The post-natal period 25
Adrenarche and pre-puberty 28
Puberty 28
Effects of steroid hormones on the reproductive tract and
secondary sexual characteristics 29

The development of gender identity................................ 30

Genital anatomy in adult women and men 32
The woman.. 32
The man 36
Nerve supply to the genitalia in men and women.......... 38

Biological rhythms and normal patterns of change
in reproductive hormones 39
The menstrual cycle 40
Pregnancy... 40
Parturition and lactation 41
The menopause... 42

Anomalies of sexual differentiation — sex chromosome
aneuploidies and intersex conditions............................ 44
Sex chromosome aneuploidies 44
Inborn errors of metabolism 47
The effects of exogenous hormones during pregnancy 50
Other congenital abnormalities of the genitalia............ 51
Conclusions from evidence of abnormalities of sexual
development... 52
Clinical management of intersex conditions 52

Introduction

Gender difference has become a sensitive issue, which is discussed later in this chapter. However, we develop as either female or male because of a fundamental process, reproduction. While it may be politically incorrect at the present time to view human sexuality as an aspect of reproduction, the reproductive purpose of our sexual differentiation into male or female is beyond dispute. In this chapter, the process of sexual differentiation is considered, together with the typical male and female genital anatomy that results. The process of gender identity development is also reviewed. Abnormalities of sexual differentiation or intersex conditions are also reviewed, not only because they are of interest in their own right, but also because they have taught us a lot about normal mechanisms of sexual differentiation. The mechanisms involved in sexual arousal, including brain mechanisms, and how they compare in men and women, are considered in Chapter 4. Sexual differentiation of the brain, which is difficult to summarize without first looking at the role of brain function, is also considered in Chapter 4. Reproductive hormones play a crucial role in many aspects of our sexual differentiation, development and function. First, therefore, we will consider some basic endocrinology.

The fundamental roles of reproductive hormones

A hormone is a form of chemical messenger, which typically travels from its cell of origin to its target cell via the bloodstream. Some hormones are broken down so quickly by local or circulating enzymes that their effects are confined close to their site of origin. Prostaglandins, for example, are rendered inactive as they pass through the lungs. These are called *local hormones*. Other substances circulating in the blood are inactive until altered chemically in the vicinity of the target cell. These *pre-hormones* also allow the site of hormone action to be selective.

There are two main chemical types of hormone to be considered: steroids (e.g. oestradiol, testosterone (T)) and peptides (e.g. gonadotrophins, prolactin). Steroid hormones, although produced in various tissues, are, to some extent, stored in the blood since they are bound to plasma proteins. Testosterone, for example, is present in three forms in the plasma: bound firmly to a specific globulin, called sex hormone binding globulin (SHBG; in the male around 45% of total T is in this form), bound more loosely to albumin (around 50% in this form), and unbound or free (less than 4%). The function of SHBG remains controversial, but the most widely held view is that it is the free and to some extent relatively available albumin-bound fractions which are biologically active, whereas the firmly bound SHBG fraction, which is in dynamic equilibrium with the other fractions, is protected from metabolic clearance and provides a store of steroid (Winters & Clark 2003).

Peptide hormones, on the other hand, are stored in the cell or gland that makes them and are released when required, often in a pulsatile fashion. Consequently, in contrast to steroids, their level in the blood may fluctuate considerably or may only be detectable for a brief period after release. Many peptides function as neurotransmitters in some contexts, and as classical hormones in others. Some of them function principally as *releasing hormones*, i.e. releasing other peptides from their cells of origins (e.g. luteinizing hormone-releasing hormone (LHRH)). Most have been found to be widely distributed in the body, suggesting that they arose at a primitive stage of development and have been adapted in some cases to serve specialized functions, and in others to be involved in more varied processes. A number of these peptides will need further consideration in relation to the hormonal control of sexuality and reproduction.

Most cells will only be affected by a hormone if they contain its specific receptor. Receptors for steroids lie within the cytoplasm and when activated lead to the unique steroid pattern of protein synthesis. There is evidence that some steroids also act at the cell membrane to alter excitability of the cell. Thus oestradiol has an excitatory and progesterone an inhibitory effect (Dufy & Vincent 1980). Receptors for peptides are mainly found in the cell membrane, and involve a variety of second messenger pathways, such as cyclic AMP.

The principal hormone system concerned with reproduction and sexual behaviour is the anterior pituitary–gonadal axis, which will be considered more closely. The anterior pituitary–adrenal cortex system is also relevant, though it is concerned with a much wider range of functions than the reproductive or sexual ones. The adrenal cortex produces a proportion of the steroids related to sex, and it is partly through this pathway that acute stress may influence sex steroid levels.

Peptides

The posterior pituitary releases two peptide hormones: vasopressin (or antidiuretic hormone) and oxytocin (OT). OT causes milk ejection in the suckling woman and contraction of uterine muscle. OT has also been proposed as a key factor in affiliative behaviour (Insel 1992). We will consider the potential sexual functions of OT in the chapter on sexual arousal (Chapter 4). Both these hormones are of interest as they are synthesized in the brain (the paraventricular and supraoptic nuclei of the hypothalamus) and then transported along the axons of the supraoptico-hypophyseal nerve tract to the posterior pituitary where they are stored, bound to a specific protein, until they are released in pulsatile fashion into the blood. The posterior pituitary is thus merely a storage extension of the hypothalamus. However, in addition to these more classical 'hormonal' functions, when a neuropeptide like OT is released into the bloodstream to act in specific ways on target organs around the body (e.g. breast, uterus), peptides are engaged in a variety of brain mechanisms as neurotransmitters or modulators. It also seems that many of these functions can be carried out by a variety of peptides. Thus in gene ablation studies of mice, OT knockout mice have a clear impairment of milk let down but no apparent impairment of mating or parturition (Nishimori et al 1996; Young et al 1996). The specific peripheral impact on the breast obviously requires OT. But with other OT-related functions the animal can manage without OT, presumably making use of alternative neuropeptides. This distinction between classical hormone and local neurotransmitter effects of neuropeptides in mammals has probably been facilitated by the evolution of the blood–brain barrier. To what extent these intra-cerebral neurotransmitter effects involve synaptic transmission, 'parasynaptic' transmission through local diffusion, or dissemination via the cerebro-spinal fluid is not clear, but all may be involved, together with considerable potential for interaction with other neurotransmitters, as well as steroid hormones. The emotional brain, as we shall see, is characterized by peptidergic neurotransmission, contrasting with the synaptic neuronal structure of the neo-cortex (Herbert 1993) and consistent with the more primitive phylogenetic origins of the brainstem. The specific effect of a peptide may depend on its site of action, or even the context in which it is acting.

The *endogenous opioids* are a relatively recent addition to the list of peptides. They are called opioids because they share affinity for receptors with morphine-like substances. Their discovery caused great excitement as it was thought possible that they were the 'natural analgesic'. However, their effects are very widespread and they are probably best understood as peptide neurotransmitters. They undoubtedly play an important part in the hypothalamic–pituitary–gonadal system, probably modulating the feedback effects of steroids on the hypothalamus and pituitary.

Prolactin remains a mystery peptide. As its name implies, it has a definite function in stimulating growth and activity of the milk-secreting system of the breast. But it probably has other effects that are less well understood. A certain amount of prolactin seems to be necessary for normal steroid synthesis in the ovary, whereas too much is associated with inhibition of both ovarian and testicular function. Part of the difficulty in understanding prolactin function is that, as a hormone, it is controlled by an inhibitory substance, dopamine, which is itself a central neurotransmitter of widespread significance. Anything that leads to a generalized reduction of dopaminergic activity in the hypothalamus will result in increased prolactin secretion. It then becomes difficult to distinguish between the effects of the raised prolactin itself and other possible effects of reduced dopaminergic activity. In other words, in such situations prolactin may simply be a marker hormone. Prolactin release is also stimulated by serotonin and thyrotrophin-releasing hormone (TRH). The function of prolactin is especially obscure in the male, though, as we shall see, high levels of prolactin are usually associated with impaired sexual function in men.

Inhibin is a relatively new peptide hormone, though its existence has been assumed for some time. It is produced in very small quantities by both the ovary and the testis and is believed to exert negative feedback on the hypothalamic pituitary system, specifically reducing the release of follicle stimulating hormone (FSH). Two types of inhibin have been recognized, inhibin A and B, though their respective functions are still not clearly understood (Hall 2004).

The local hormones of most reproductive significance are the various prostaglandins, which, though widespread in the body, do have a special and as yet incompletely understood role in the reproductive system.

The anterior pituitary–gonadal system

The main components of this system are shown schematically in Figure 3.1. Let us look more closely at the various levels involved.

Hypothalamus

This mediates control of the system by other parts of the brain such as the cortex and pineal gland. The hypothalamus itself directly influences the system by means of controlling hormones, which it secretes and transports through the blood–brain barrier to the anterior pituitary gland by means of special blood vessels called the hypophyseal portal system. In addition to the regulation of prolactin, discussed above, a key control mechanism from the hypothalamus is the regulation of gonadotrophin production by the anterior pituitary, i.e. luteinizing hormone (LH) and FSH. This is carried out by gonadotrophin releasing hormone (GnRH).

GnRH is a decapeptide released in a pulsatile fashion from the ventromedial and anteromedial areas of the hypothalamus resulting in sharp pulses of LH and rather more gradual release of FSH from the basophilic cells of the anterior pituitary into the blood. The frequency of GnRH pulses differentially regulates LH and FSH, with higher frequency pulses favouring LH and lower frequency pulses, FSH release (Boime et al 2004). GnRH is an example of a local hormone, which is broken down rapidly in the blood and probably does not reach the general circulation in detectable amounts. Receptors for GnRH, or a very similar peptide, are found in other parts of the body, and, in particular, in the ovary and testis. GnRH may serve other functions in those areas either as a result of its local production or by small amounts from the hypothalamus circulating in the blood.

Gonadotrophins

Once the glycoproteins LH and FSH are released from the anterior pituitary, they affect the gonads after reaching them via the bloodstream. Both play key roles in reproductive function in both men and women. In women, FSH stimulates follicular growth in the ovary and the proliferation of granulosa cells. It also induces aromatase activity. LH stimulates synthesis of androgens in thecal cells, which are converted to oestradiol in the granulosa cells by the aromatase. The resulting increase in oestradiol in the late follicular phase is responsible for the pre-ovulatory LH surge, known as the 'positive feedback' mechanism, considered below (Boime et al 2004). In the male, LH and FSH interact to promote spermatogenesis, and LH is responsible for activating T synthesis in the Leydig cells of the testis (Winters & Clark 2003).

Steroid hormones

Sex steroids (oestrogens, progestagens and androgens) are produced principally by the gonads and the adrenal cortex. They can be synthesized in the central nervous system, adipose tissue and skin, but to a more limited extent (Strauss 2004). They have a wide variety of metabolic effects, but have a particular role in reproduction. Androgens play a key role in sexual differentiation, and both androgens and oestrogens are responsible for most of the development of secondary sexual characteristics at puberty. These mechanisms are considered below. Oestrogens and progestagens are necessary for the establishment and maintenance of pregnancy and lactation in the female, and androgens for spermatogenesis in the male. It is the possible effects of androgens and oestrogens on sexual desire and response or sexual arousability that are of particular relevance to this book, and these are considered in Chapter 4.

A crucial step in the control of the hypothalamo–pituitary–gonadal system is the feedback effects of steroids on the hypothalamus. Most of the principal sex steroids exert a negative feedback effect, probably both on the release of GnRH and the response of the anterior pituitary to GnRH. This provides a homeostatic mechanism in both the male and the female in which any rise in circulating steroid is followed by a decreased LH release (FSH is affected in a comparable way).

However, we must allow for the additional and somewhat mysterious feedback mechanism that is responsible for ovulation in the female. In certain circumstances, as the level of oestrogen and possibly progesterone rises, the negative feedback switches into a positive feedback

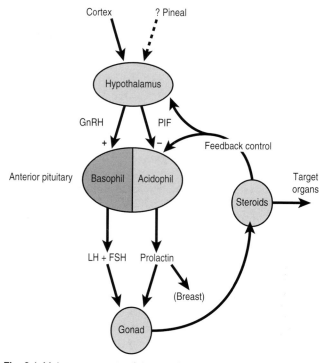

Fig. 3.1 Main components of the anterior pituitary–gonadal system. GnRH, gonadotrophin releasing hormone; PIF, prolactin-inhibiting factor; FSH, follicle-stimulating hormone; LH, luteinising hormone.

on either the hypothalamus, anterior pituitary or both. This explains the characteristic LH surge which precedes ovulation and which will be considered in more detail when we discuss the normal menstrual cycle.

The three principal types of sex steroid, oestrogens, progestagens and androgens, all have a common basic structure that is similar to cholesterol. There is considerable inter-conversion between different steroids, with a number of intermediate stages that may be present in the blood but are relatively inactive until further conversion (i.e. pre-hormones). The principal steroids and their intermediates are shown in Figure 3.2. Recent evidence has suggested that much earlier in our phylogenetic history the function of T was a precursor of oestradiol (Thornton 2001). Sex steroids are also closely related chemically to adrenocortical steroids. 17α-OH progesterone, for example, is a precursor of hydrocortisone and aldosterone.

The principal oestrogens are oestradiol-17β and oestrone; oestrone probably depends on conversion to oestradiol for most of its oestrogenic activity. In the female, the ovary is the principal source of oestradiol. Some oestrogens are produced by the adrenal cortex, and in both men and women, particularly post-menopausal women, peripheral aromatization, mainly in adipose tissue, of either androstenedione or T, is an important source of oestradiol.

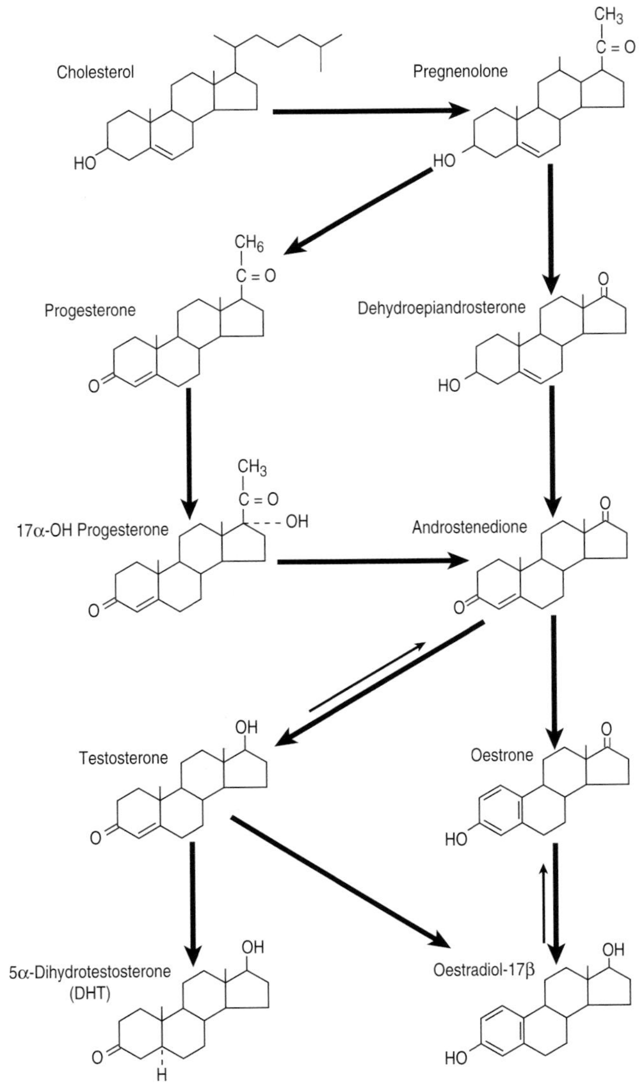

Progesterone, the principal progestagen, is produced mainly by the corpus luteum of the ovary, though it occurs as an intermediate stage in the production of other steroids by both the gonads and the adrenal cortex. It is present in the circulation of the male in negligible amounts.

The principal androgens are T, dihydrotestosterone (DHT), androstenedione, dehydroepiandrosterone (DHEA) and DHEA sulphate (DHEAS). In women, androstenedione can be converted in the tissues into oestradiol, but is also an important source of T and DHT. Approximately 50% of a woman's androstenedione comes from the ovary; the other half comes from the adrenal cortex.

In the male, the most important circulating androgen is T, which is mainly produced by the testes, although small amounts come from the adrenal cortex. Circulating DHT comes from both sources but is mainly produced peripherally in the tissues, and the amount in the circulation is comparatively low.

In the female, the adrenal source of androgens is much more important than in the male. In a consensus document (Bachmann et al 2002) it was concluded that approximately 25% of androgen production in women takes place in the ovaries, 25% in the adrenal glands and the remainder is produced at tissue sites in the periphery.

DHEA and DHEAS present a particular challenge, as there is little certainty and some confusion about their function and purpose. In both men and women, DHEA and DHEAS are produced by the adrenal cortex, but they are also regarded as neurosteroids, i.e. synthesizable within the brain (Yen 2004). DHEA is also made by the placenta. Concentrations decline from the first few months post-natally, until 5 years of age, then rise rapidly from age 7 years in girls and around 9 years in boys as the earliest manifestations of adrenarche. In pre-menopausal women the normal range for DHEA is 7.0–52.0 nmol/L; in men it is 2.8–34.6 nmol/L. The levels of DHEAS are substantially higher; 2.2–9.2 mmol/L in pre-menopausal women and 5.4–9.1 mmols/L in men. They reach a peak between 20 and 30 years of age in both women and men and then decline. By age 70–80, the level of DHEA is approximately 20% of that in a 20-year-old. DHEA can be converted into androstenedione and therefore subsequently into either T or oestradiol and is regarded by some as a major precursor of these principal sex steroids (Arlt & Hewison 2004), based on an intracrine process, i.e. conversion within the same cell as the main steroid effect. Labrie et al (2003) go further, stating that as a result of this conversion of DHEA, women produce around two-thirds of the total androgens synthesized by men, but only about 10% of the T produced intracellularly leaks into the general circulation. If there is any validity in these revolutionary claims, we will need to fundamentally revise our approach to the endocrinology of human sexuality. But as yet, apart from agreement that DHEA is a more important source of T in women than in men, there appears to be little consensus on how much of these

Fig. 3.2 Sex steroids and their intermediate stages.

principal steroids is derived from DHEA and DHEAS (e.g. Buvat 2003), or whether DHEA has any primary function other than as a precursor for other steroids. DHEAS, present in much higher concentrations than DHEA, is assumed to be the more stable storage form of DHEA. There is support for the idea that DHEAS acts as a $GABA_A$ antagonist at the membrane level (Yen 2004). There is growing evidence of a role for DHEA and DHEAS in maintaining the immune system, with an association between declining levels and impaired immunity in the elderly (Arlt & Hewison 2004). This may be related to a dissociation between DHEA and corticosteroids in the adreno-cortical response to depression and stress. Whereas cortisol tends to go up in these negative states, DHEA goes down, particularly in older age groups (Goodyer et al 2000). Recently, evidence of specific DHEA receptors has been reported, on the plasma membrane of bovine aortic endothelial cells (Liu & Dillon 2002) where the receptor is coupled to the G protein family and in human vascular smooth muscle cells (Williams et al 2002). As Buvat (2003) points out, given the history of other steroid receptors, these findings may lead on to discovery of intracellular receptors. With their unusually high concentrations in the circulation, DHEA and DHEAS remain an intriguing mystery, which is in serious need of solution.

Steroids are metabolized mainly by the liver and kidney to water-soluble conjugates of sulphuric and glucuronic acid. These are then excreted in the urine. Conjugates of both oestrone and oestradiol appear in the urine and can be measured as such, thus providing an index of the daily production of oestrogens. The main urinary products of T are androsterone and aetiocholanolone, and of progesterone, pregnanediol.

The functions of sex steroids

The functions of sex steroids are complex and varied; few systems are immune to their metabolic effects. There are, however, three main sites of action of relevance to this book:

1. sexual differentiation and subsequent function of the reproductive tract and genital organs
2. secondary sexual characteristics
3. the central nervous system, particularly those parts of the emotional brain which subserve sexual behaviour.

These will be looked at more closely later in this chapter and in Chapter 4.

Anatomical sexual differentiation

Along with other mammals, human beings develop as either female or male, with rare exceptions when the differentiation is in some respects ambiguous (i.e. intersex). However, each human embryo has the initial capacity to develop either as male or female. The mechanisms involved are gradually becoming better understood. Current thinking on this issue started with the pioneering work of Alfred Jost in the 1940s, who concluded that

the key process was the development of the primitive gonad into a testis (Jost 1947). Hormones produced by the testis were, in Jost's view, responsible for the development of the fetus as male. Without normal testes, the fetus would develop as female. This conceptualization, that femaleness is the default position whereas maleness requires an active intervention, has prevailed ever since, though not without controversy. Reactions of feminists have been mixed. Fausto-Sterling (2000) saw this as a further example of sexism in science: 'Jost failed to notice that his theory adopted wholesale the metaphor of female lack and male presence' (p. 202). Angier (1999), on the other hand, concluded that 'from a biological perspective women are not the runners up; women are the original article' (p. 38). Further research, however, is revealing a much greater complexity, which will be briefly summarized.

Sexual differentiation and the development of gender identity can be summarized in seven stages:

1. chromosomes
2. gonads
3. hormones
4. internal sexual organs
5. external genitalia and secondary sexual characteristics
6. the gender assigned at birth (e.g. 'It's a boy')
7. gender identity (e.g. 'I am a girl').

Each of these levels leads on to the next during this fascinating developmental process. An eighth stage, sexual differentiation of the brain, develops in parallel with the other later stages (see Chapter 4).

Problems are fortunately rare, but can occur at any of these stages. We will look at the normal process as far as we understand it and then consider some of the anomalies.

Chromosomal gender

The most basic manifestation of gender lies in our sex chromosomes, which are present in every cell of the body. The normal female has two X chromosomes (46XX); the normal male has one X and one Y (46XY). The Y chromosome determines maleness (in some animals, e.g. birds, it is the other way round; the female is XY). There are 23 pairs of chromosomes (i.e. 46 chromosomes) of which the XY pair in the male is unique in being of very different size; the Y chromosome is much smaller than the X. After many years of research, mainly based on studies of intersex conditions, the key gene in the Y chromosome was identified in 1990. This is known as SRY, which is the testis determining factor. A key question, as yet unanswered, is how SRY works; in particular, does it work by activating a genetic sequence leading to male development or does it repress an 'anti-testis' gene? The activating pathway is consistent with Jost's model of female development as the default mode. In the repressive pathway, the anti-testis gene could be a 'pro-ovary' gene, which puts a different spin on Fausto-Sterling's 'female lack' (see above). So far the evidence is not consistent, but overall it is in favour of the repressive model (Vilain 2000). Also, there are a number of other non-Y genes which are being recognized (Vilain 2000), providing us with a classic example of how, when you look closely enough, biology just gets more complex.

Gonads

The next stage is the differentiation of the primitive gonad into testis or ovary. In either case the developed gonad will have two functions: production of hormones and germ cells (oocytes or spermatozoa). The presence of a normal testis will lead, in the large majority of occasions, to sexual differentiation as a male. The absence of a testis will, in the large majority of cases, be associated with sexual differentiation along female lines.

The primitive gonad evolves from the genital ridge, which is derived from the mesonephros. In the presence of the SRY gene, there is a migration and proliferation of cells from the mesonephros in the genital ridge that will form testes. This process starts in about the eighth week of fetal life. If SRY is absent, the genital ridge will differentiate into an ovary, with migration of germ cells. This happens a little later, starting in the 12th week. The full development of the gonad and its functioning depends on the presence of both somatic and germ cells within the gonad. Germ cell development depends on a different set of genes. Thus individuals who are 46XX males, who are male because they carry SRY on one of their X chromosomes, are not fertile because they lack the spermatogenic genes located on the long arm of the Y chromosome. In Turner's syndrome, where one X chromosome is missing (i.e. 45X) or deficient, the remaining X chromosome is sufficient for female somatic development and a primitive ovary forms. However, the absence of the second X chromosome results in no oocyte formation and without these the ovary does not develop as a hormonally secreting organ and eventually atrophies.

Hormones

In the male fetus, the Leydig cells of the testis start to produce steroids, in particular T, from about the 8th week, reaching a maximum between the 10th and 18th weeks. Following this, steroidogenesis is much reduced, though the testis continues to grow in size. This phase of maximal fetal steroid production is a crucial time for differentiation of the male internal and external genitalia. The fetal testis is stimulated by the placental human chorionic gonadotrophin (HCG), but also by fetal gonadotrophins, which predominate during the second half of pregnancy.

In the female fetus, differentiation of the reproductive tract does not depend on steroids and in fact ovarian steroidogenesis is minimal. Oestrogens circulating in the fetus are largely derived from the placenta.

Internal sexual organs

The early fetus has the potential for developing both male and female internal sexual organs (Fig. 3.3). The Wolffian duct can develop into the vas deferens, seminal vesicles and ejaculatory ducts of the male. The Müllerian duct can develop into a uterus, fallopian tube and upper vagina. The fetal testis secretes two types of hormone: T, which stimulates male development of the Wolffian duct, and a large molecular weight protein, produced by the Sertoli cells of the testis, which causes regression of the Müllerian duct, and hence is called Müllerian-inhibiting factor (MIF). The Müllerian duct will develop normally along female lines unless MIF is present, and it does not require oestrogenic or any other hormonal stimulation, in the way that the Wolffian duct requires T.

External genitalia

The continuation of an androgen milieu leads to the development of male *external* genitalia. Prior to this differentiation, the external genitalia are the same regardless of genetic sex. There is a genital tubercle, a genital groove and a urethro-labial fold and labio-scrotal swelling on each side (Fig. 3.4). In the presence of androgens, these will develop respectively into penis and scrotum. For this purpose, T needs to be converted by 5α reduction into DHT. In cases of 5α reductase deficiency where T is present but DHT is not formed, normal development of the external genitalia does not occur (Fig. 3.5). In normal development, the testis descends from its original position in the abdomen, close to the kidneys, to its final position in the scrotum. This descent depends not only on normal development of the scrotum to receive it, but probably also other specific hormonal mechanisms.

In normal female development the upper part of the vagina derives from the fused Müllerian ducts and the lower part from the urogenital sinus (O'Rahilly 1977).

Hormone levels during childhood and adolescence and their effects on development

The post-natal period

At birth the male infant has circulating levels of T that are approximately half that of the normal adult (i.e. approximately 240 ng/100 mL), whereas the levels in the female infant are similar to those in the adult, and much lower than in the male (i.e. approximately 30 ng/100 mL). In both sexes there is a dramatic drop within the first few days, presumably due to the withdrawal of HCG. Oestrogen levels also drop to pre-pubertal levels in both sexes (see Fig. 3.6).

The sensitivity of the hypothalamus to negative feedback has still not reached its maximum at birth, so that with the withdrawal of HCG there is a further rise in LH and FSH.

In the male, there is a secondary rise in circulating T starting in the second or third post-natal week, reaching a maximum similar to the levels at birth (approximately 260 ng/100 mL) between the 30th and 60th day, and

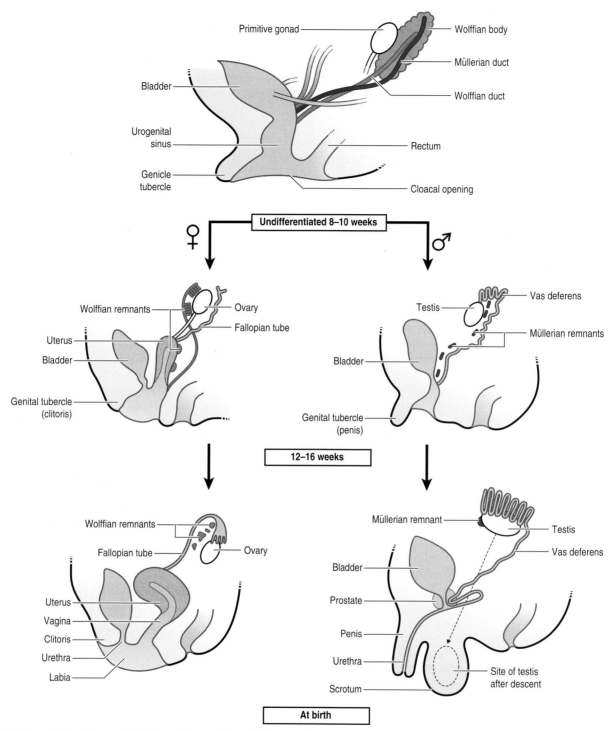

Fig. 3.3 Differentiation of the genitalia. The existence of a primitive gonad capable of developing into either a testis or ovary and both Wolffian (male) and Müllerian (female) systems gives the potential for either male or female differentiation. The presence of androgens and Müllerian-inhibiting factor leads to male development. The absence of both leads to female development.

then gradually declining to low pre-pubertal levels. There is no such post-natal androgen surge in the female; levels similar to those of the pre-pubertal male are established and maintained from the end of the first post-natal period. At birth they are relatively low in both sexes with approximately 3% of the total T being unbound. There is then a rise in SHBG over the next few days in both boys and girls, resulting in the unbound fraction dropping to about 0.7%, which is lower than in the adult (i.e. 2% in males, 1% in females). The

effective post-natal androgen surge is not therefore quite as dramatic as it appears from the total T levels, but it nevertheless represents a striking difference between the sexes at this stage, the significance of which is not yet understood. This secondary surge of androgens may play a role in the masculinization of the central nervous system, and as it occurs post-natally is potentially open to investigation.

Sensitivity of the hypothalamus to negative feedback continues to increase markedly so that by 6 months both

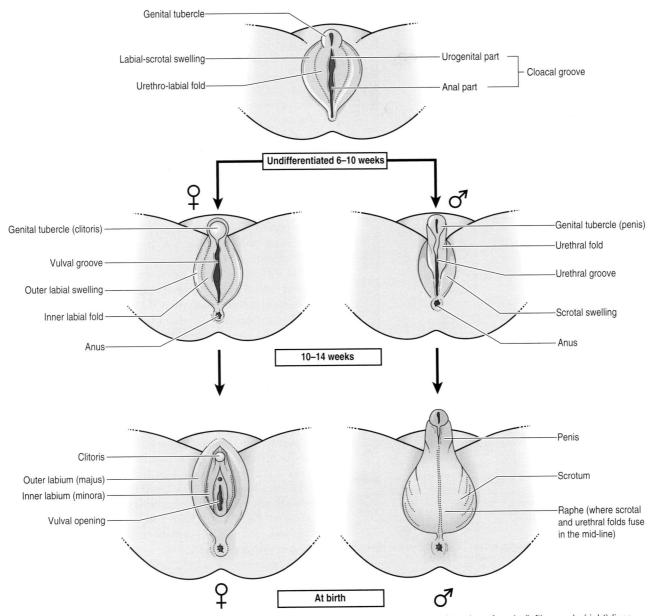

Fig. 3.4 Differentiation of the external genitalia. The undifferentiated structures at 6–10 weeks develop along female (left) or male (right) lines, depending on whether androgens are present or absent.

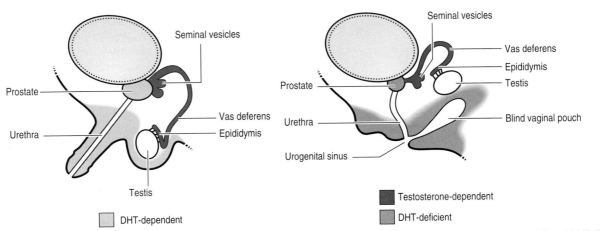

Fig. 3.5 The possible role for T and DHT in the development of the male genitalia. Left: normal development in the presence of T and DHT. Right: incomplete development when DHT is missing or insufficient, as in 5α-reductase deficiency. (From Imperato-McGinley et al 1974.)

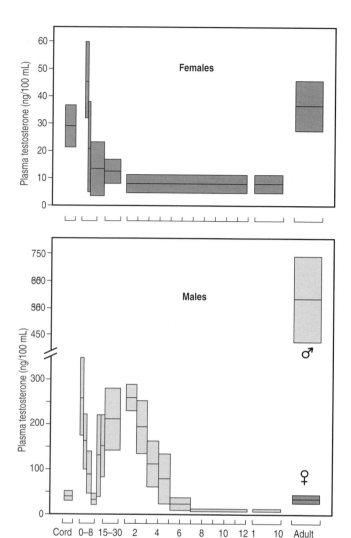

Fig. 3.6 Plasma T levels at different stages of the life cycle in males and females — means and SD. (From Forest et al 1976.)

gonadotrophins and steroid levels are low in both males and females. No sign of a positive feedback effect, characteristic of the ovulating female (see p. 40), appears in the female until well after the onset of puberty.

This pattern of low endocrine activity, with little difference between males and females, persists for several years during early childhood.

Adrenarche and pre-puberty

The next endocrine change involves the adrenal cortex. From about the age of 6 years in girls and 8 years in boys, there is an increased production of DHEAS followed by DHEA and, somewhat later, androstenedione. These steroids are of adrenal origin, but what triggers this change in adrenal function is not known, although it may be a matter of genetically determined tissue maturation. Increased thickness of the zona reticularis, the part of the adrenal cortex involved in androgen production, occurs in association with these hormonal changes, and there is also increased enzyme activity of the kind necessary for DHEA/DHEAS production. Insulin, insulin-like growth

factor (IGF-I) and growth hormone may be involved (Witchell & Plant 2004). There is no associated change in ACTH levels, and no apparent relationship to changes in the hypothalamo–pituitary–gonadal axis. The purpose of this so-called adrenarche, which is only found in humans and the Great Apes, is also not clear. This increase in adrenal androgens is probably responsible for early axillary and pubic hair growth in both sexes.

Between the ages of 6 and 10 years there is a very gradual rise in LH and FSH, but as yet this is not reflected in rising gonadal steroid levels.

Puberty

The precise mechanism controlling the onset of puberty is still uncertain. It involves a change in the production and release of GnRH, but whether this results from a decrease of an inhibitory signal or increase in stimulatory drive is not yet clear. This change is associated with a progressive reduction in the sensitivity of the hypothalamus to negative feedback, resulting in a more substantial rise in gonadotrophins and steroids until a new gonadostat level is set (Cameron 1990; Hopwood et al 1990). A number of factors, relatively species-specific, have been identified which permit puberty to occur or progress. These include metabolic indicators that the body can cope nutritionally with the next stage of growth and development. The current view is that these are not causes of the onset of puberty, but have a 'permissive' effect. Sensors in the hypothalamus and hindbrain monitor these signals. Behind this permissive process is a GnRH 'clock' which develops to the state when it initiates high-frequency GnRH release once the permissive signals reach appropriate levels. Genetic factors are involved; GPR54 has been proposed as a 'puberty gene'. This gene encodes a G-protein-coupled receptor, and mutations in this gene lead to absence of increased GnRH secretion when puberty should be occurring. However, it is not clear that such genes are a sufficient explanation for regulation of puberty, and may simply represent specific components of a complex system (Sisk & Foster 2004).

The response of the testis to HCG administration has been shown to increase closer to puberty, indicating that some maturation of the testis is also involved. The pituitary response to GnRH administration also increases. However, the rise in gonadotrophins also occurs in individuals without gonads. Obviously more is involved than a reduction of negative feedback. Presumably some maturational process in the hypothalamus is taking place.

The earliest signs of pubertal endocrine changes are nocturnal surges of gonadotrophins before there is any noticeable change in daytime levels.

Puberty in the female

The timing of pubertal changes in girls is well documented. Breast development and growth of pubic hair usually starts between the ages of 9 and 13 years, whilst menarche occurs normally between 11.5 and 15.5 years (Marshall & Tanner 1969). The mean age at menarche has declined by about 1 year between the beginning of the 20th century and the late 1970s to about 12.5 years (MacMahon 1973). The trend towards earlier puberty onset has levelled out as far as menarche is concerned, but there is some evidence of earlier onset in breast development and pubic hair growth. Ethnic differences have been well documented. In the USA, each stage of pubertal development occurs earlier, on average, in African American girls than white girls, with Mexican American girls coming midway (Witchel & Plant 2004) (see Chapter 6 for further discussion of this issue).

The growth spurt starts about 2 years earlier in girls than in boys. The girls' growth therefore ends earlier, contributing to the sex difference in size. The relationship between these events and hormonal changes is less well documented. Brown et al (1978) found that breast development coincides with a rise of oestrogen from earlier childhood levels and that oestrogen levels then start to fluctuate, often irregularly at first, causing bleeding when levels are high enough. Probably the commonest sequence of events is a series of anovulatory cycles before a full ovulatory cycle occurs, though the time between onset of menstruation and ovulation must be very variable (see Chapter 6, section on adolescent infertility; p. 191).

Once normal regular cycles are established — and this may take several months — they usually continue in a predictable way, normally interrupted only by pregnancy and lactation. A minority of women continue to have irregular cycles and unpredictable ovulation.

Puberty in the male

In the male it is not until a bone age of approximately 12 years is reached that there is any increase in T production. Thereafter it rises steeply until the age of 15–17 years, after which there is a further slight rise to adult levels by the early or mid-20s. The LH and FSH levels, having risen at puberty, decline in late adolescence until they reach lower adult levels, presumably reflecting the increased steroidogenic and spermatogenic potential of the fully grown testis. There is also a fall in SHBG during adolescence to adult levels.

Oestrogens in the male are predominantly in the form of oestrone. Though the testis secretes oestradiol and small amounts of oestrone, the majority of oestrogen comes from the peripheral conversion of androgens to oestrone.

The development of the secondary sexual characteristics accompanying the hormonal change of puberty is varied in its timing. The earliest change is accelerated growth of the testes and scrotum (9.5–13.5 years). Shortly after this pubic hairs begin to appear. About a year later the penis starts to grow (10.5–14.5 years) accompanied by development of the internal structures, the seminal vesicles and prostate. About a year after the start of penile growth the first ejaculation occurs. The growth spurt in boys starts between 10.5 and 16 years with deceleration of growth starting about 18 months later. The voice starts to break and deepen towards the end of the growth spurt (Marshall & Tanner 1970). About one-third of boys show noticeable enlargement of the breasts around the middle of puberty that normally recedes after about a year.

The considerable difference in timing and speed of these pubertal changes contributes to the uncertainty about body image that adds to the adolescent's problems. The age of onset of puberty has also declined over the past 200 years. Daw (1970) in a study of J.S. Bach's choir in Leipzig, found that the average age at which boys' voices changed from treble to alto was 17–17.5 years. In London today it is 13.3 years. However, the secular changes and ethnic differences in age at puberty onset during the 20th century have been less striking in boys than in girls.

Effects of steroid hormones on the reproductive tract and secondary sexual characteristics

Androgens

The fundamental part androgens play in sexual differentiation and early anatomical development has already been considered. In the male, the increases in these hormones at puberty are responsible for the enlargement of the penis, scrotum and possibly testes as well as for the greater responsiveness of these tissues to tactile stimulation (Fig. 3.17). Androgens also determine the characteristic pattern of masculine body hair growth, which is not usually fully expressed until well into adult life. They affect the larynx, resulting in deepening of the voice, which is characteristic of male puberty. The sweat and sebaceous glands are activated, sometimes leading to acne, common at this age. Androgens promote increased muscle bulk and influence bone growth in a way not completely understood. The adolescent growth spurt in boys probably depends on intermediate levels of T characteristic of pre- and early puberty. As higher levels develop they lead to epiphyseal closure and cessation of the growth spurt. In the post-pubertal male, T is necessary for normal spermatogenesis and secretory activity of the prostate gland and seminal vesicles.

In the female, the somatic function of androgens is less well understood. Androgens obviously contribute to body hair growth and sebaceous gland activity. They may be necessary in small amounts for the normal pubertal development of the external genitalia, especially the labia majora and clitoris, which are the embryological homologues of the scrotum and penis. We know that high doses of exogenous androgens may produce enlargement and increased sensitivity of the clitoris in adult women. Androgens may also contribute to epiphyseal closure in the female, though the levels involved are much smaller, and oestradiol probably has a more important role.

Oestrogens

In the pubertal girl, oestrogens cause enlargement of the breasts. They also influence pubertal growth of the uterus and fallopian tubes, vagina and vulva, and are largely responsible for the adolescent growth spurt in girls (Short 1980). Of particular importance to normal sexual response is the effect oestrogens have on the vaginal epithelium. They are necessary for the normal vaginal transudate which follows erotic stimulation, though the mechanism involved is only partially understood (see p. 79).

Oestrogens may influence pubic and axillary hair growth, though this is not certain. They stimulate the endometrium to proliferate and they indirectly provoke ovulation; these effects will be considered in more detail when we deal with the menstrual cycle.

The functions of oestrogens in the male are not understood. They may be responsible for the slight and transient breast enlargement that occasionally occurs at puberty (gynaecomastia of puberty). They may also play an important part in the control of normal bone growth and epiphyseal closure in the male. As we will see in the next chapter, many of the actions of T in the brain may depend on aromatization to oestradiol.

Progesterone

As its name implies, progesterone has a special function in maintaining pregnancy, which will be considered further below. In the non-pregnant woman it is mainly produced by the corpus luteum. In most of its effects it acts synergistically with other hormones, in particular oestrogens. It acts on breast tissue that has been primed with oestrogen to promote the growth of alveoli and subsequent milk production. In the endometrium, the proliferative state produced by oestrogens in the first half of the menstrual cycle is changed into the secretory endometrium by the addition of progesterone.

The development of gender identity

How a child, once born, is treated by its parents and other people depends to a considerable extent on whether they see the child as a boy or a girl. That in turn depends on the initial observation of anatomical gender at birth — 'It's a boy' or 'It's a girl'. This seemingly obvious remark in the delivery room is therefore noteworthy, although the extent to which parental and societal influences determine an individual's gender identity following birth is a matter of debate (Ruble et al 2006). In the vast majority of births, anatomical development has proceeded normally, and the gender of assignment will be consistent with other, earlier and subsequent gender differentiating influences. But, in rare cases there are varying degrees of ambiguity of the external genitalia. The gender of assignment is then based on a somewhat arbitrary decision with far-reaching consequences. Some of the causes of such ambiguity will be considered later in this chapter. We have learnt a lot from these clinical conditions about factors, both pre- and post-natal, that influence gender identity development, and they indicate that at least some forms of typically male behaviour are influenced by pre-natal androgen effects, being more likely in females with high pre-natal androgen levels. They are less helpful, however, in our understanding the determinants of gender identity.

There are two components to gender identity development: the recognition that 'I am a girl' or 'I am a boy', which Stoller (1968) called 'core gender identity', and a sense of masculinity or femininity, which is expressed in typically masculine or feminine behaviour. Gender is one of the earliest and most salient social categories, and of fundamental importance to a child's sense of self. Core

gender identity is relatively straightforward, although there are some who question whether there are two distinct sexes. Fausto-Sterling (2000), for example, proposes that '...complete maleness and complete femaleness represent the extreme ends of a spectrum of body types. That these extreme ends are the most frequent, has lent credence to the idea that they are not only natural (that is produced by nature) but normal (that is, they represent both a statistical and a social ideal)' (p. 76). But it is the issue of 'masculinity' versus 'femininity' that generates the fiercest arguments. In our society, there are differences between the behaviour of boys and girls, but also considerable overlap between the sexes. The controversy surrounds the extent to which these gender roles are socially or innately determined. Do boys become typical boys because they are taught to be so? Hyde (2005), in putting forward her 'gender similarities' hypothesis, was able to show, on the basis of meta-analyses of 46 studies comparing males and females, that for the large majority of functions assessed, there were, on average, more similarities than differences between men and women. With several functions, a gender difference was apparent if the respondents believed that they were being assessed as a male or a female, but when the same questions were asked with respondents believing themselves to be anonymous, gender differences in, for example, aggressive behaviour, disappeared. There were two consistent areas of gender difference, motor performance (e.g. throwing) and certain aspects of sex (e.g. masturbation).

The issue of the presence or absence of gender difference is at the heart of the political campaign to liberate women. Much of the control of women by men in our society has been a societal exploitation of stereotyped roles. Women have been expected to stay at home, look after the children and the house, and do the cooking. This has effectively tied women, making it more difficult for them to develop their own careers or even separate identities. There have been some improvements in this respect, at least within the Western world, with a substantial increase in the number of mothers having careers beyond mothering. NORC's General Social Surveys have shown a shift towards more egalitarian gender role attitudes in the USA from 1974 to 1994 (Harris & Firestone 1998). There are many parts of the world, however, where patriarchal gender inequality is as strong as ever.

Those who defend the imbalance of gender power often justify it on the basis of innate determinants of basic gender roles. Those who reject it tend to rely on the argument that gender role stereotypes are simply the products of a culture that has a vested (male) interest in fostering such roles. The result is that what appears to be a scientific argument is often a political one with a consequent loss of scientific objectivity. I have no doubt that alteration of the balance of power and opportunities between men and women is one of the most fundamental needs for human societies at the present time. But this need for change exists whether sex roles are constitutionally or socially determined, and arguing about the relative importance of nature or nurture seems politically irrelevant. The constitutional origins of a disadvantage do not justify its exploitation. But, on the other hand, it may be foolish to ignore or even inhibit constitutionally determined advantages on the grounds that everybody ought to have the same opportunities. We should therefore be acknowledging and respecting those abilities and aptitudes which are female or male characteristics. Recently, twin studies have been used to assess the relative contributions of genetic and shared environmental factors in gender identity development. Assessment of gender typical and atypical behaviour of 3–4-year-old twin pairs from the British Twin Early Development Study showed that both shared environment and heritability contributed, though the heritability factor was more marked in gender atypical girls (Iervolino et al 2005; Knafo et al 2005). In a longitudinal study using The Netherlands Twin Registry, twin pairs were assessed at 7 and again at 10 years of age. Though gender atypical behaviour lessened over the 3 years, 70% of the variance in gender atypical behaviour could be explained by genetic factors, at both ages and for both boys and girls (van Beijsterveldt et al 2006). The differences between these two studies may reflect the different ages studied and different methods of assessing gender-atypicality.

It is therefore inescapable that genetic factors as well as intrauterine experiences all determine how we interact later with our environment (see p. 44 for further discussion). We have much to learn, however, about the relative importance of different determinants at specific stages of development.

The last edition of this book relied heavily on a comprehensive review by Maccoby & Jacklin (1974). But there has been an enormous amount of research into gender differences since that publication, and a recent comprehensive review of this literature has been provided by Ruble et al (2006), and used to a considerable extent in the summary that follows.

Many children have gained some understanding of gender labels, and the stereotypical behaviours that go with them, by their second birthday and continue to do so between ages 3 and 5 years. Most children can correctly label their own gender, and that of others, between 2 and 3 years of age. Thus 'core gender identity' is established early. Once this happens, children seek information and 'scripts' about same-sex activities and become sensitive to gender differences. The first signs of gender non-conformity may be evident at this age. By 5 years, children spontaneously categorize people by gender. Not surprisingly they are able to distinguish gender in adults before they can do so in other children. When asked to describe the characteristics of the two sexes, girls are more likely to focus on what they look like, and both boys and girls focus more on appearance when describing girls. After the age of around 7 years, children start to become more flexible in how they apply gender stereotypes, and to recognize that men and women can vary in their manifestations of masculinity and femininity. Negative reactions to gender non-conformity include ridicule, rejection and teasing, and they tend to get stronger as children get older, more so when it is boys who are not conforming, and stronger, apparently, with non-conforming children, compared to non-conforming adults. There is limited cross-cultural evidence suggesting that in comparison with children of European origin,

Hispanic and Asian children show greater and African American children less gender stereotyping.

At what stage a child learns that being male or female is a constant characteristic, which does not change, remains uncertain, but is likely to be important for the development of the child's own gender identity. Kohlberg (1966) stressed the importance of this sense of permanence about gender: 'a child's gender identity can provide a stable organizer of the child's psychosexual attitudes only when he is categorically certain of its unchangeability' (p. 95). There is also the possibility that once permanence of core gender identity is recognized, children feel freer to defy gender norms.

There is some evidence to suggest that after pre-school years, girls are more flexible in their acceptance of gender stereotypes, whereas boys hold stereotypic views more rigidly. Girls show the least stereotypical behaviours around age 13 years, but increasingly withdraw from male-typical activities after that age. Variability is a result of increasing cognitive flexibility interacting with increasing pressures to conform to gender stereotypes in preparation for sex roles and adult status.

Preschool children typically prefer same-sex friends and playmates, a pattern which becomes apparent by around 2 years for girls and 3 years for boys, and increases as the child gets older until adolescence, when changes in peer group structure occur. This pattern of childhood sex segregation appears to be cross-cultural, and is also observed in non-human primates (Wallen 1996).

Typical boy activities, like rough-and-tumble play, increase when boys are in groups, accentuating the gender separation, as girls avoid such behaviour. Interestingly, boys are more likely to engage in group activities, such as sports; girls are more likely to do things in pairs. Group activities, particularly large groups, promote competition and conflict. The dyadic activities more typical of girls, in contrast, promote consideration of others.

By middle to late childhood girls give more importance to intimacy and closeness in their friendships and spend more time talking to their friends than boys do. When conflicts arise within friendships, girls attach more importance to maintaining the relationship whereas boys are more likely to strive for control.

In early adolescence, children initially form small same-sex groups, but by middle adolescence, although same-sex preferences are still apparent, various types of cross-sex interactions and networks emerge, paving the way for dating and romantic relationships. Greater comfort with same-sex friends typically continues, however. Gender-related issues may take on a new importance in adolescence as sexual issues emerge.

Parents clearly vary in their reaction to gender conformity and non-conformity. However, the extent to which a child's gender stereotypical behaviour is influenced by parental behaviour or attitudes remains uncertain. It is noteworthy that no marked or consistent differences in the gender identity development of children in non-traditional families (single parent, gay or lesbian) have been reported, although the relative lack of traditional gender role attitudes among African American children may be related to the increased likelihood of being reared by a single mother, an effect complicated by the fact that most such mothers will also be working outside the home, reflecting another difference between African American and white American cultures. Siblings may contribute to gender stereotyping. Children with no siblings are more likely to have gender egalitarian beliefs.

Gender differences in emotional reactions and vulnerability to mental health problems are well documented, although the reasons for such differences are not clear and are likely to be complex. Boys engage in more aggressive behaviours than girls, a difference that is evident in early childhood and cross-culturally. Females are considered to be more emotionally expressive than males. During elementary school years boys start to conceal negative emotions, and girls become more concerned about hurting other's feelings. Boys and girls show clearly different themes in the stories they tell, with girls focusing on affectionate themes, and boys on aggressive themes. In adolescence, girls report more negative emotions, whereas boys are more likely to deny them.

Body image is an important predictor of low self-esteem, depression and eating disorders. Between the ages of 6 and 8 years girls start to show more dissatisfaction with their bodies and more desire to be thin than boys do. Boys focus more on how muscular they are, girls on their weight. By adolescence a substantial proportion of girls, particularly those with earlier puberty, are unhappy with their body image, an effect linked to media and cultural emphasis on physical attractiveness and thinness for females.

Early onset of puberty in girls is associated with more emotional distress, and 'maladaptive' behaviour patterns, including sexual behaviour, problems which persist into adulthood. Early puberty in boys is also associated with maladaptive behaviours, but at least until their peer group catch up with them, early puberty boys are more popular and have a better self-image. Late onset boys tend to have low self-esteem.

The media are of increasing importance to children's gender development, with the range of media options expanding rapidly, and the Internet adding a new interactive dimension. Not only do most media designed for children strongly reinforce gender stereotypes in various ways, including a marked under-representation of women, there are clear differences in the types of media watched or listened to by girls and boys. Boys spend more time playing video games (often violent), watching sports, cartoons, action-adventure and fantasy programming like *Dr Who*, whereas girls spend more time watching comedy and programmes about relationships, differences which increase as children get older. Children who watch the most television also have the more gender stereotyped attitudes, although the direction of causality has not yet been clearly demonstrated.

The peer group world of the pre-pubertal schoolchild is undoubtedly a powerful source of learning, though not an easy one to study. The fascinating work of Opie & Opie (1959; 1969) showed how ritualized and adult-free this world was at the time of their research, with rules, games and songs handed down through generations of children. The rules or scripts for successful boyhood and girlhood were clear, and although they clearly reflected adult sex role stereotypes, it was difficult to know how much they were determined by adult influences. It would be interesting to employ the unusual methodologies of the Opies with today's children, given the pervasive and cross-cultural impact of the media and Internet.

Girls have greater verbal ability than boys, though this is not obvious until about the age of 11. Boys, on the other hand, are superior in visual-spatial tasks, though again this is not apparent until adolescence. At a similar age, boys' mathematical skills grow faster than those of girls.

Genital anatomy in adult women and men

The woman

The appearance of the vulva or external genitalia of a nulliparous woman is shown in Figure 3.7. Only the labia majora are visible. These are well endowed with fat and covered, together with the mons, by pubic hair with a characteristically female distribution; an appearance of an inverted triangle with its base as a straight line across the mons. (The male distribution is rhomboidal with hair typically spreading up the midline towards the navel.) To observe the other structures it is necessary to separate the labia (Fig. 3.8), when the glans of the clitoris, labia minora and urethral and vaginal openings come into view. It is now possible to obtain images of the underlying genital anatomy from MRI scanning. The precise image obtained depends on the level at which the scan was taken, but a helpful view of the anatomical arrangement is shown in Suh et al (2003) (See Fig. 7.2, Chapter 7). They compared pre- and post-menopausal women (not on hormone treatment), and found that post-menopausal women had smaller width of the labia minora, bulb of the clitoris, and

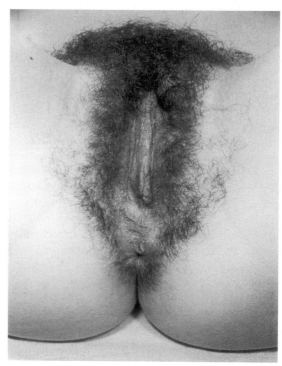

Fig. 3.7 The external genitalia of the female.

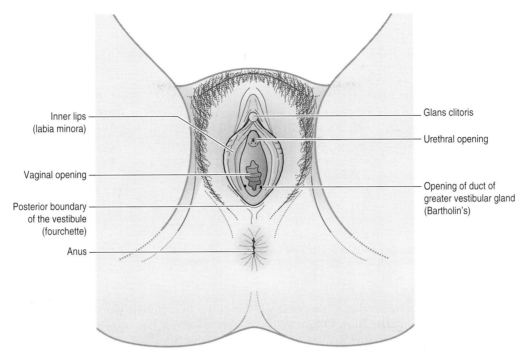

Fig. 3.8 The external genitalia of the female with the labia drawn apart.

vagina, thinner vaginal walls, without the infoldings or rugae of the vaginal lining, and smaller cervical diameter.

Clitoris

The clitoris is a much more extensive structure than its visible part, the glans, would suggest. Our understanding of its anatomy and neurovascular supply has been clarified by the recent histological studies of O'Connell and her colleagues (O'Connell et al 1998; 2005) and by MRI scanning (Suh et al 2003; O'Connell & DeLancey 2005), and its origins, homologous to those of the penis, are very apparent. Description of the clitoris presents a challenge because of the difficulty in capturing its three-dimensional form (see Figs 3.9 and 3.10). The clitoris consists of the glans and the erectile bodies. The glans is the small visible component, not particularly erectile but packed with sensory nerve endings. The main body of the clitoris, which lies just behind the glans, is formed by the fusion together in the midline of the two corpora cavernosa, which, as in the male, are firmly anchored to the underlying bone on either side by the attachment of their diverging crura, and the paired bulbs (with the same origin as the male corpus spongiosum, and previously called 'bulbs of the vestibule'). The distal parts of the urethra and vagina form a midline core in a pyramidal-shaped structure, which is packed into the perineum behind the labia minora and majora, projecting several centimetres in front of the pelvic bone. The apex of this pyramid is formed by the most superior part of the clitoral body, which is attached to the undersurface of the symphysis pubis by the deep suspensory ligament. The bulbs of the clitoris form the lateral margins of the base

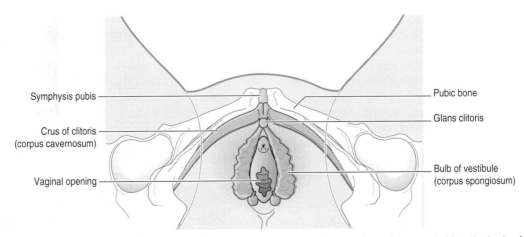

Fig. 3.9 Deep erectile structures of the clitoris. Homologous erectile structures, which in the male are incorporated into the body of the penis, are in the female displaced around the vaginal opening and urethra. The corpora cavernosa provide a cushion in their attachment to the pubic bone whereas the corpora spongiosa (divided in the female) form the deep erectile tissues behind the labia on each side.

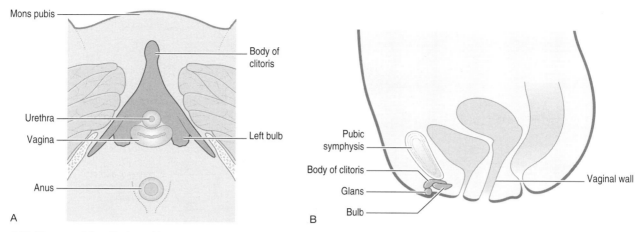

Fig. 3.10 Diagram of the clitoris and its component in axial plane **(A)** and mid-sagittal plane **(B)**, based on MRI scanning of a pre-menopausal nulliparous woman. (From O'Connell & Delancey 2005, with permission from Helen O'Connell.)

of the pyramid, which extends between the ischio-pubic rami on either side, and is ventral to the anus (O'Connell et al 2005). The body of the clitoris is surrounded by a thick tunica albuginea, and contains erectile tissue similar to that of the penis. The crura are similar to the body except they do not have the same surrounding neurovascular structures or internal vasculature. They are covered by ischiocavernosus muscles. The bulbs are covered by a thin layer of muscle, the bulbospongiosus, but no tunica, and contain spongy tissue with larger spaces and fewer nerves than found in the corpora.

Vulva

Flanking the vaginal opening are the labia minora, which are folds of skin much thinner than the labia majora, devoid of fat but also highly vascular. Anteriorly, as the labia minora converge towards the clitoris, they each bifurcate into two smaller folds, the inner of which merge together in the midline to form the frenulum of the glans of the clitoris. The outer folds form a fold of skin or prepuce enveloping the clitoris near its tip. Posteriorly, the labia minora are joined behind the vaginal opening by a sharp fold of skin, the fourchette. The area bounded by the clitoris, labia minora and fourchette is termed the vestibule and is normally moist. During sexual arousal not only do the erectile tissues of the deeper clitoral structures become engorged, but so do the labia minora, which consequently become a little everted, exposing their inner moist surfaces and further preparing the vestibule for entry of the penis. If penile entry is attempted in the sexually unaroused female, the flaccid labia minora may be carried into the vaginal opening, causing discomfort. In the aroused woman, reciprocal movement of the engorged labia minora during penile thrusting serves to stimulate the body and glans of the clitoris.

In multiparous women, the vascular engorgement of the labia minora, which occurs during pregnancy and childbirth, leads to a permanent enlargement due to a degree of varicosity of the contained vasculature. As a result, the labia minora are often visible between the labia majora, even in the unaroused state. This accounts for the considerable variability in external appearance of the vulva in different women, many of whom are self-conscious about this appearance and may be reassured to learn that such variation is usual after childbearing.

Between the clitoris and the vaginal opening — a distance of about 2 cm — lies the urethral opening.

In the virginal state, the vaginal opening is partially occluded by a thin fold of skin, the hymen. The size of the hymeneal orifice and the thickness and elasticity of the hymen are variable. Usually after puberty the orifice will admit a finger. In a woman who has had intercourse (or other forms of vaginal penetration) the hymen is generally torn in several places and its retracted remnants are represented by a fringe of skin tags (carunculae myrtiformes) which surround the vaginal opening. Very occasionally, the hymen is sufficiently elastic to allow penetration without rupturing. The hymen of some women is divided by a strand (i.e. with two or more orifices). This may become stretched rather than broken so that although intercourse or tampon insertion is possible, the strand remains and may become caught or stretched further, causing pain and sometimes vaginismus (Sarrel 1976).

Just external to the attachment of the hymen, on either side, are the openings of the ducts from the two greater vestibular (Bartholin's) glands. These discharge mucoid secretion late during sexual arousal.

Vagina and the pelvic floor

The vagina is a tube, which, in the non-aroused state, is collapsed, with a cross-section shaped like the letter H. It is usually 10–11 cm in length to the depth of the posterior fornix. The lumen of the vagina, when distended, is like an inverted flask. This is because the upper two-thirds are lax and capacious, whereas the lower third is closely invested by the surrounding pelvic floor muscles. Recent MRI studies of the pelvis have shown the pelvic floor muscles to be more complex than is suggested by many anatomical texts (Van Houten 2005). The pelvic floor is neither flat nor horizontal. What has typically been called the levator ani muscle, is in fact composed of several distinct muscle groups, the most important of which are the iliococcygeus and pubococcygeus, which in their resting state both support the vagina

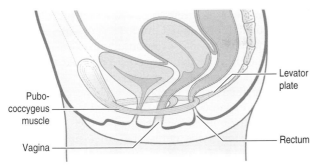

Fig. 3.11 The muscular supports of the vagina. This diagram shows the sling of muscle fibres surrounding the urethra, vagina and rectum, running from the pubic bone to the coccyx. The levator plate formed by these fibres supports the rectum and the vagina in its non-aroused horizontal position.

and rectum, combining with presacral fascia to form a levator plate. Contraction of the pubococcygeus elevates the vagina. Part of the pubococcygeus complex forms a sling around the vagina, known as the pubovaginalis muscle, contraction of which draws the vagina in an anterior and superior direction (Figure 3.11).

The need to understand the pelvic floor musculature has increased recently because of a re-appraisal of the concept of 'vaginismus', previously assumed to be a spasm of pelvic floor muscles surrounding the vagina, making vaginal penetration difficult or impossible. In contrast, poor tone in these muscles, or the inability to contract them voluntarily, has been blamed for loss of sexual pleasure and even orgasmic difficulties (Graber & Kline-Graber 1979) (see p. 85). These issues will be discussed in more detail in Chapter 11 (see discussion of vaginismus; p. 309).

In the non-aroused woman, the vagina is normally curved backwards over the pelvic floor (see Fig. 3.11) and is not straight, as is often portrayed in anatomical texts. The vaginal wall includes a thick rugose lining of squamous epithelium, layers of longitudinal and circular plain

muscle, and a very extensive plexus of veins, especially on the lower part. There is a rich arterial blood supply.

Blood supply

The clitoris receives its blood supply from the terminal part of the internal iliac artery, the common clitoral artery, which branches into the clitoral cavernosal and dorsal clitoral arteries. The inner part of the vagina is supplied from the uterine and hypogastric arteries; the outer part from the middle haemorrhoidal and clitoral arteries. The labia are supplied from the internal pudendal artery, as well as superficial branches of the femoral artery (Giraldi & Levin 2005).

Uterus

The uterus, a pear-shaped organ with a thick muscular wall, has a narrow lower part, the cervix or neck, which protrudes into the anterior wall of the vagina near its upper limit. The cervix is anchored securely in position by a dense fascial structure called the paracervical connective tissue, which is connected by a series of ligaments to various parts of the bony pelvis (Van Houten 2005). The narrow cervical canal linking the vagina with the uterine cavity is lined by mucus-secreting glands. The recesses at the upper end of the vagina surrounding the cervix are called the fornices. The body of the uterus is more mobile, necessary for pregnancy when it enlarges. Typically it lies anteriorly (see Fig. 3.11), in anteflexion, but in a minority of women the uterus points more posteriorly, known as retroversion or, if extreme, retroflexion. While usually non-problematic, retroversion can be associated with dyspareunia.

Ovaries

The fallopian tubes (oviducts) enter the upper part of the uterus on each side. The ovaries lie lateral to the uterus below the fallopian tubes (see Fig. 3.12). Each contains ova (egg cells) surrounded by a cluster of cells forming a

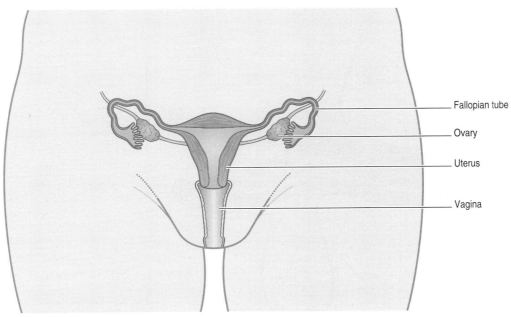

Fig. 3.12 Female internal genitalia.

follicle. Every month a single follicle ripens and the ovum is discharged, collected by the fimbria of the fallopian tube and transported down its length to the uterine cavity.

The man

Penis

The shaft or body of the penis is formed principally by a fused pair of corpora cavernosa, cylinders of tough fibrous tissue, the tunica albuginea, filled with a sponge-like lattice of vascular spaces or erectile tissue, which inflates with blood during erection. The detailed structure of this erectile tissue is of fundamental importance to the mechanism of erection, and will be considered in more detail in Chapter 4. The bulk of this tissue consists of vascular spaces or sinusoids containing smooth muscle in their walls. Beneath the two fused corpora cavernosa lies another erectile column, the corpus spongiosum, which envelops the urethra in its course along the lower surface of the penis (Figs 3.13 and 3.14). Because of the specialized surrounding fibrous architecture, and lower pressure than occurs in the corpora cavernosa, engorgement of the corpus spongiosum occurs without compression of the

urethral lumen, which remains sufficiently patent for the rapid ejaculation of seminal fluid. The corpora cavernosa are consequently the most important structures in establishing the rigidity of the fully erect penis. At the root of the penis the corpora cavernosa diverge to be firmly attached by their crura to the pelvic bones. The corpus spongiosum expands around the dilated part of the urethra to form the bulb of the urethra (see Fig. 3.18).

Near the root of the penis, the outer surfaces of the erectile columns are invested by layers of muscle, the bulbospongiosus and ischiocavernosus muscles, which contract rhythmically during orgasm and also semi-voluntarily during the development of erections (Figs 3.15 and 3.16). Contraction of these muscles may contribute to the development of the high pressures within the corpora cavernosa; however, their role in this respect has not been established (see caption for Fig. 3.16).

Near the tip of the penis, the corpus spongiosum expands to form the glans, a cushion-like expansion of the penile shaft, separated from it by a shallow groove. In the uncircumcised male, the glans is covered by a hood of lax skin, the prepuce or foreskin, that is wholly or partially removed in those males who have been circumcised

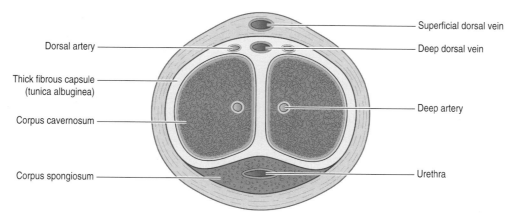

Fig. 3.13 Cross-section of the body of the penis, showing erectile spaces and principal blood vessels.

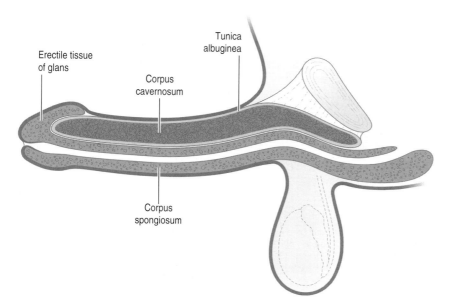

Fig. 3.14 Erectile tissues of the penis. Each crus of the corpora cavernosa is inserted into the pubic bone.

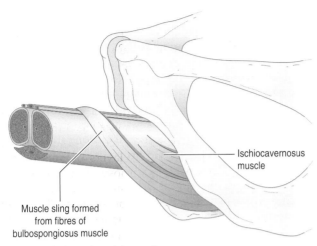

Ischiocavernosus muscle

Muscle sling formed from fibres of bulbospongiosus muscle

Fig. 3.15 The muscles of the penis.

(Fig. 3.17). On the lower surface, the prepuce is attached to the glans by a longitudinal fold of skin, the frenum. The separation of the foreskin from the underlying glans is sometimes incomplete in the neonate and normally requires androgens for its completion. During erection of the penis, the foreskin is partially retracted by tension of the skin along the elongated penile shaft, exposing the tip of the glans and the urethral orifice. During coital thrusting, the foreskin is intermittently retracted further by friction with the vaginal walls, exposing the glans completely. If, however, the mobility of the preputial skin is restricted, difficulty and discomfort may result during intercourse (see p. 384).

Beyond the dilated urethral bulb, and before its junction with the urinary bladder, the male urethra traverses the prostate gland, a firm fibromuscular structure containing branching glands, which contribute accessory fluid to the seminal ejaculate. This is therefore called the prostatic part of the urethra (Fig. 3.18). In ageing males the prostate gland tends to enlarge and may have to be removed (prostatectomy) if it restricts the flow of urine. This operation should have no physical effect on erection or orgasm, providing that there is no damage to the nerve supply to the penis, but the prostatic removal may impair the capacity to ejaculate or lead to retrograde ejaculation into the bladder (see Chapter 13).

Testes

The male gonads or testes lie in a superficial pouch of skin and muscle, the scrotum. The testes develop during fetal life in the abdominal cavity and migrate down into the scrotum during the latter part of fetal development. This 'externalisation' of the testes provides them with a cooler environmental temperature, which is essential for normal spermatogenesis. In boys in whom there is a failure of testicular descent, i.e. undescended testes or cryptorchidism, damage to the testes both in their germinal and endocrine functions will result unless the condition is treated. Within the scrotum, the level of the testes is controlled by two muscles, the dartos, that can corrugate and shrink the scrotal wall, and the cremaster muscle, which forms a sling encircling the testis and spermatic cord within the scrotum.

The testes contain two principal types of cells, the interstitial (Leydig) cells which produce steroid hormones, principally T, and the tubular cells from which spermatozoa are derived. The sperm pass from the seminal tubules into a long convoluted tubule, which forms the epididymis of the testis. The structure is linked on each side to the urethra by a long fibromuscular tube, the vas deferens, which at its upper end expands to form the ampulla of the vas. This is a storage chamber for sperm, lying behind the bladder.

The seminal vesicles are two elongated sacs, which also lie behind the bladder and prostate gland. They secrete a significant volume of accessory fluid, which is discharged along the ejaculatory duct, together with the contents of the ampullae of the vas, into the prostatic part of the urethra. Further secretion during sexual arousal comes from the bulbo-urethral (Cowper's) glands, which lie on each side of the urethra near its bulbous portion, and the urethral glands, along the penile part of the urethra. This can lead to discharge of fluid before ejaculation occurs, and may occur at a relatively early stage of sexual arousal. Such fluid is clear and viscous and varies considerably in amount in different men. Some 22% of Kinsey's subjects reported no such secretion whereas about 18% normally experienced fairly excessive secretion, sufficient to drip from the penis (Gebhard & Johnson 1979). In some men this is a source of embarrassment. The function of this fluid is not known, but it has sometimes been found to contain a few sperm.

Blood supply

The blood supply of the penis is important since disease in these vessels may be an important cause of erectile failure (see Chapter 13). Although there is considerable variation, the commonest arrangement is as follows. The internal pudendal artery, which is one of the two terminal branches

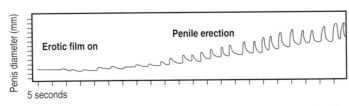

Penis diameter (mm)

Erotic film on

Penile erection

5 seconds

Fig. 3.16 Rhythmic contractions of the penile muscles (bulbospongiosus and ischiocavernosus) during the development of an erection. About one in four men tested in the laboratory shows this pattern. Most are aware of these contractions and can prevent them if asked. In the case illustrated here, the subject was unable to stop them and the contractions were also observed during his nocturnal erections. Their functional significance is not known, but some men try to 'pump up' their erection in this way. It is not yet clear whether this helps or hinders the erection. With a full erection such contractions produce transient dramatic increases in intracavernosal pressure that increase the rigidity of the erect penis (see p. 76).

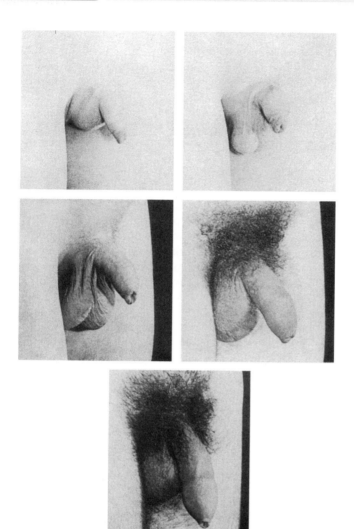

Fig. 3.17 Normal male genitalia showing the five stages of development of genitals and pubic hair as defined by Marshall & Tanner (1970). (From van Wieringen et al 1971.)

of the anterior trunk of the internal iliac artery, passes round the side of the pelvis until it reaches the inner side of the lower part of the pubic bone. Close to the midline, just before it pierces the perineal membrane, the internal pudendal artery gives off a large calibre but short branch to supply the bulb of the corpus spongiosum. The main artery then divides into the deep artery and the dorsal artery of the penis. The deep artery runs through the corpus cavernosum; and the dorsal artery runs along the dorsum of the penis, within the loose fibrous tissue surrounding the tunica to the glans, where it divides into two branches. Along its length the dorsal artery may give off small branches which penetrate the fibrous sheath of the corpus cavernosum and anastomose with the deep artery of the penis. When the penis is flaccid, the penile arteries are tortuous, straightening as an erection develops (Fig. 3.19).

Venous drainage of the foreskin and skin of the penile shaft is via the superficial dorsal vein which, noticeable on the surface of the penis, turns either to the right or left before joining the external pudendal vein, a tributary of the long saphenous vein. Drainage of the glans penis and the corpora cavernosa is mainly via the deep dorsal vein. The small emissary veins from within the corpora cavernosa empty into 5–10 sets of circumflex veins which run round the outside of the tunica albuginea before joining the deep dorsal vein, which itself eventually drains into the prostatic plexus.

Nerve supply to the genitalia in men and women

Four components of the nerve supply need to be considered: the sensory and motor somatic, and the parasympathetic and sympathetic autonomic components. (The autonomic nervous system will be considered in more detail in Chapter 4.)

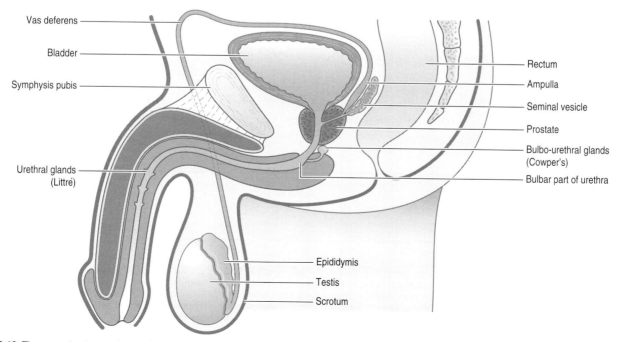

Fig. 3.18 The reproductive anatomy of the male.

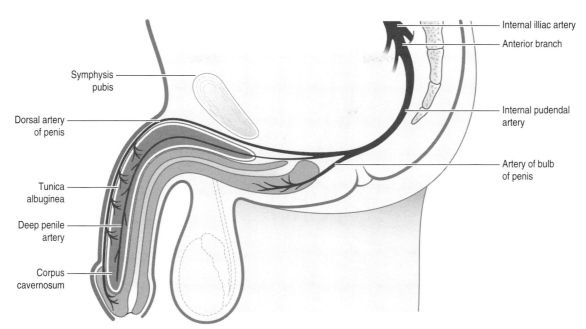

Fig. 3.19 Arterial supply of erectile tissues of penis. The dorsal artery, which supplies the erectile tissue of the glans and distal part of the corpus spongiosum, also sends fine branches through the tunica albuginea into the corpus cavernosum.

Somatic

Sensory innervation. The genitalia of both men and women are richly supplied with sensory nerve endings. Many of them are specialized in type, though their precise function is not always understood. Some are concentrated around blood vessels and may be important in monitoring vasocongestion (Levin 1980). Others may be peculiar to erotic perception. The clitoris is particularly rich in nerve endings, containing a similar number to those found in the penis, though obviously concentrated into a much smaller space. There is nevertheless considerable variation between individuals in the number and distribution of these specialized nerve endings, which could account for some of the variation in the degree and localisation of erotic sensitivity (Krantz 1958).

These sensory fibres leave the second and third sacral roots of the spinal cord to run in the pudendal nerve in both the male and female. In the male, a branch of the pudendal nerve, the dorsal nerve of the penis, provides sensory supply to the penis. In the female, the equivalent is the remarkably large dorsal clitoral nerve, which mainly supplies the clitoral glans. In both male and female, other branches of the pudendal nerve provide cutaneous nerves to the perineum.

Somatic motor innervation of the striped musculature of the penis derived from the second, third and fourth sacral segments of the cord, runs in the internal pudendal nerve, alongside the sensory fibres, and finally reaches the bulbocavernous, ischiocavernous and other perineal muscles via the perineal nerve.

Somatic innervation of the pelvic floor muscles, in men and women, is mainly via the pudendal nerves, with the iliococcygeus also receiving innervation directly from the S2, 3 and 4 segments.

Autonomic

Parasympathetic innervation of the blood vessels and erectile tissues of the genitalia also derive from the second,

third and fourth sacral segments (in the male the third segment is most important for control of erection). Parasympathetic fibres run in the pelvic splanchnic nerves to the pelvic plexus, which is usually situated immediately in front of the bifurcation of the abdominal aorta, from which the cavernous nerves emerge to supply the corpora cavernosa and spongiosum in the male. In the female, the cavernous nerves originate from the vaginal component of the pelvic plexus, and supply the clitoris by joining the dorsal clitoral nerve, adding neurons which stain positive for nitric oxide synthase, providing a nitrergic component to the innervation of the clitoral bodies (Yucel et al 2004).

Sympathetic fibres from the thoracic and the upper lumbar rami pass to the pelvic plexus. From there, fibres run to the genitalia as well as other pelvic viscera, including the bladder. They may be organized in discrete nerves throughout their course or be scattered as a complex network of fibres for part of their course, finally passing to the genitalia within the cavernous nerve, alongside the parasympathetic supply. This anatomical distribution in both men and women, more variable in the sympathetic than the parasympathetic pathways, poses a problem for the surgeon operating in this area who strives to avoid damaging this important nerve supply (Fig. 3.20).

The functional significance of the sympathetic and parasympathetic fibres to sexual arousal and response will be considered further in the next chapter.

Biological rhythms and normal patterns of change in reproductive hormones

An important source of information about hormonal effects on behaviour in humans stems from the patterns of hormone change which normally occur. We have already considered adrenarche and puberty, and the

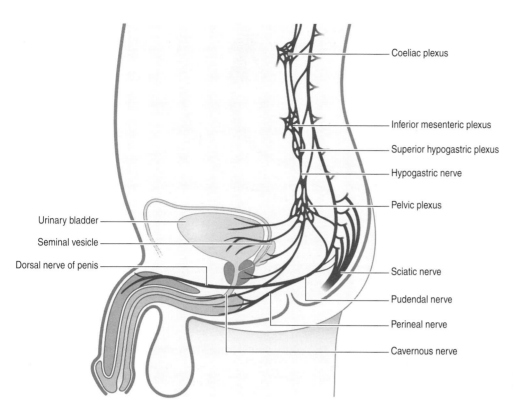

Coeliac plexus

Inferior mesenteric plexus

Superior hypogastric plexus

Hypogastric nerve

Pelvic plexus

Urinary bladder

Seminal vesicle

Dorsal nerve of penis

Sciatic nerve

Pudendal nerve

Perineal nerve

Cavernous nerve

Fig. 3.20 Autonomic innervation of the urinary bladder and male genitalia. (Modified from de Groat & Booth 1984.)

changes associated with ageing are reviewed in Chapter 7. Of the various endocrine rhythms or cycles in the human the most important is the menstrual cycle. Others are the diurnal rhythm and a possible seasonal rhythm. We will also consider the patterns of hormonal change associated with reproduction, i.e. pregnancy and lactation. The impact of these basic patterns on sexuality will be considered in Chapters 4 and 15.

The menstrual cycle

This fascinating aspect of endocrine function is fundamental not only to our reproduction, but also to the state of womanhood, being, apart from anatomy, the most distinct female characteristic. At a time when methods are available for controlling or stopping the menstrual cycle, its biological and psychological significance become of great topical interest. As yet there are still many mysteries surrounding this phenomenon, though the gaps in our knowledge are gradually being filled.

By convention the first day of menstruation is regarded as the first day of a new cycle. This is the beginning of the follicular or proliferative phase — the first term referring to the growth of a new follicle in the ovary, the second to the proliferation of the endometrium (the lining of the uterus) that accompanies it. From the beginning there is a gradual rise in levels of FSH and LH due to an increase in the frequency of pulsatile release of these hormones from the pituitary. This leads to the development of a new follicle and secretion of steroids (oestradiol-17β, androstenedione and 17α-OH progesterone, a precursor) by the theca interna cells. As the oestradiol rises, so the FSH level starts to fall because of negative feedback. The LH does not fall as one might expect; instead, when the

oestradiol reaches a certain level it triggers the characteristically female 'positive feedback response', which produces the pre-ovulatory surge of LH. This then provokes ovulation from the by now ripe follicle, a mature ovum being released into the fallopian tube. Once this takes place the follicle becomes a corpus luteum, which secretes large amounts of progesterone as well as oestradiol. There is thus a peak of oestrogen in the late follicular phase, followed by the LH peak, followed by ovulation, a rise in progesterone and a second rise in oestrogen. These are shown in Figure 3.21. After ovulation we enter the second phase of the cycle, called luteal (i.e. dependent on the corpus luteum) or secretory, referring to the further change in the endometrium induced by the combination of progesterone and oestrogen. This prepares the endometrium for implantation of the ovum if it is fertilized. The corpus luteum has a limited life and when it starts to regress the progesterone and oestrogen levels fall, followed by spasm of the endometrial arteries and the consequent shedding of the endometrial lining, called menstruation. This brings us to the beginning of the next cycle.

How this system switches from negative to positive feedback in the case of LH and what produces the luteal regression are the two principal mysteries of the menstrual cycle. The impact of the menstrual cycle on women's sexuality is considered in Chapter 4.

Pregnancy

The pregnant condition has special endocrine characteristics, largely due to the presence of an additional endocrine gland, the placenta. The endocrine function of this organ does depend, however, on its collaboration with both the mother and the fetus. It relies on a maternal supply of

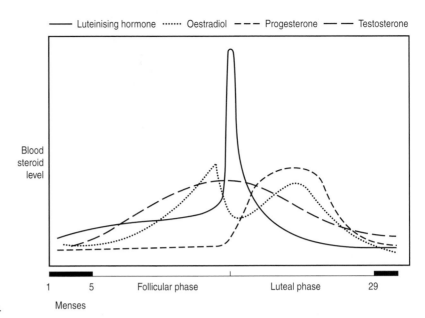

Fig. 3.21 Hormone changes during the menstrual cycle.

cholesterol for steroid synthesis and on fetal liver enzymes for some of the later stages of steroid production, in particular that of oestriol, the oestrogen of pregnancy. The placenta is capable of producing huge quantities of progesterone, and is also unusual in being apparently autonomous, i.e. not controlled by either negative or positive feedback.

The earliest and still mysterious phenomenon of pregnancy is the recognition by the mother's reproductive system that fertilization or implantation has occurred. This in some way prevents the usual monthly regression of the corpus luteum and hence allows continued production of progesterone, which is essential for the continuation of pregnancy. In the human female the self-protective effect of the conceptus is probably due to the action of human chorionic gonadotrophin (HCG), a peptide hormone produced by it. HCG is very similar in structure to LH and is produced in large quantities by the trophoblastic layer of the placenta early in pregnancy, providing the basis for the usual forms of pregnancy test. When injected into non-pregnant women or men it acts like LH. In the pregnant woman, in addition to maintaining the corpus luteum of pregnancy, it probably stimulates steroid synthesis by the placenta itself. The endocrinology of the placenta is extraordinarily complex, with many peptides, steroids and monoamines being produced (Mesiano & Jaffe 2004).

In the human, the essential role of the corpus luteum of pregnancy is short-lived because by the 20th week the placenta takes over and its production of progesterone and oestrogens continues to rise substantially until the end of pregnancy, reflecting the lack of any regulation by the hypothalamic pituitary system.

As previously mentioned, progesterone usually acts synergistically with other hormones, especially oestrogen. Understanding its effects is complicated by the fact that this synergism varies with the progesterone:oestrogen ratio, probably being maximal when the ratio is approximately threefold. As the ratio declines the effects of the two steroids tend to become mutually antagonistic.

Progesterone reduces the excitability of the myometrium and its responses to oxytocin and this may play an important part in maintaining pregnancy. Unlike other species, e.g. sheep, the onset of labour in the human is not preceded by a fall in progesterone level.

Oestrogen and progesterone together stimulate growth of the pregnant uterus and breast. Oestrogens probably increase blood flow through the uterus. Both hormones have other far-reaching metabolic effects during pregnancy that are only partially understood. Although there is a modest rise of T levels in pregnant women, there is a marked rise in the binding protein SHBG, with the result that free unbound T falls slightly. The impact of pregnancy on women's sexuality is considered in Chapter 15.

Parturition and lactation

The process of parturition begins before the onset of labour. For most of pregnancy, the myometrium of the uterus is relaxed and relatively insensitive to hormones that promote uterine contraction, such as prostaglandins and oxytocin. This state is maintained by a range of inhibitory compounds including progesterone and prostacyclin. The 'awakening' of the uterus leading to the contractions of labour, which in many species is determined by a relative withdrawal of progesterone and increase in oestradiol, is less well understood in humans. The hormonal changes following parturition are more relevant to our subject. These provide a dramatic example of gross changes in endogenous steroid levels. The principal and most immediate change obviously follows the expulsion of the placenta, the principal source of steroids in late pregnancy. The progesterone level drops precipitously within 24 h of delivery and continues to decline until it reaches a low level from 7 to 14 days onwards. The oestrogens also drop precipitously but after the initial fall further change depends on whether or not the woman breastfeeds. If lactation is established, the oestrogen levels continue to decline and are then maintained at a low level. If lactation is not established, oestrogens rise to more normal levels from the third post-partum week until normal menstruation resumes. Prolactin, which is at a high level in late pregnancy, dips only slightly during the early stages of breastfeeding, whereas in the non-lactating woman it declines to within the normal range by the end of the third week (Fig. 3.22).

Thus the hormonal pattern continuing during the puerperium depends on whether lactation is established. We see the ingenious way in which parturition allows lactation to start in the well-prepared, but previously non-lactating, breast. During pregnancy, the placenta, as already mentioned, acts autonomously and produces large quantities of oestrogen. This acts synergistically with progesterone and prolactin to produce full development of the milk-secreting mechanism, but the oestrogens also inhibit actual milk production. In addition they have a positive feedback effect on the acidophilic cells of the anterior pituitary, stimulating prolactin production. Once the placenta is expelled, oestrogen production is largely dependent on the ovary, which, in contrast to the placenta, is always susceptible to external control. Part of this control is by prolactin or at least the changes in the dopaminergic system related to prolactin, which inhibit oestrogen production, whilst being maintained by the reflex effects of suckling. Consequently prolactin levels are maintained whilst oestrogen levels fall, allowing milk production and release to ensue. It may be the maintenance of prolactin levels during lactation and the consequent ovarian suppression that underlies the amenorrhoea and infertility of the lactating woman (see Chapter 15). This effect weakens, however, as lactation continues. After the 10th week or so, prolactin levels gradually fall and ovulation may occur in spite of continued breastfeeding (Bonnar et al 1975). The frequency of suckling may be an important factor. The return to ovulatory cycles is most likely to occur after there has been a substantial drop in suckling frequency and the introduction of supplementary feeds (Howie et al 1982). During exclusive breastfeeding, approximately 40% of women will remain amenorrheic at 6 months post-partum (Barbieri 2004).

The impact of lactation and the post-partum period on women's sexuality is considered in Chapter 15.

The menopause

The reproductive span of women is quite different to that of men. Whereas both sexes attain fertility at roughly similar ages, men continue to be fertile into late life. Women, by comparison, have a relatively abrupt cessation of fertility around the menopause. The life cycle of reproductive hormones also differs in the two sexes. In men the gamete-producing and hormonal functions of the testis are relatively independent. A man can lose the capacity to produce sperm and continue with normal T production from the Leydig cells. In women the ovarian hormone production is intimately associated with the growth of the follicle and maturation of the ovum during each menstrual cycle, as described above. Furthermore, the ovary has a limited number of primitive ova present at birth,

and these undergo some form of ageing so that follicles become increasingly resistant to gonadotrophic stimulation, to the point when ovarian activity and menstruation cease. This change is associated with a dramatic change in the ovarian output of steroids.

This is, however, a gradual process. The most discrete marker is the last menstrual bleed (literally the 'menopause') — an event that can only be identified in retrospect (by convention, a woman should have ceased to menstruate for at least a year before being considered post-menopausal; the average age for the last menstrual bleed is 51 in the Western world). This last menstruation is preceded by a gradual slowing down of ovarian responsiveness over a variable number of years. However, this process continues for a time *after* the last menses, before the woman reaches a stable post-menopausal state. In 2001 a consensus was achieved at a workshop aimed at defining stages of the menopausal transition (Soules et al 2001). The reproductive period was divided into early, peak and late stages, each with variable duration, and with varying degrees of reduced fertility in the late stage. Then follows the menopausal transition with an early stage characterized by variable cycle length (more than 7 days different from normal), and a late stage (with 2 or more skipped cycles and an interval of amenorrhoea of 60 or more days). Each of these two stages varies in duration across women. Then the last menstrual bleed occurs, confirmed a year later. The post-menstrual stage is divided into early, i.e. the first 5 years after the final menses, and late thereafter.

The age at last menses is quite variable, and genetic factors probably account for more than 80% of the variance. There are also clear ethnic differences. In the USA, in African American and Hispanic women, the post-menstrual stage starts approximately 2 years earlier than in white women. Age at menopause also tends to be earlier in some Eastern countries (Lobo 2004).

During the menopausal transition, oestradiol levels decline, although the major reduction does not occur until approximately the last 6 months of the menopausal transition (Lobo 2004). FSH levels start to rise even during the late reproductive phase (as early as age 38), and fluctuate considerably during the menopausal transition, typically not stabilizing till the end of the early post-menopausal stage, when levels are consistently greater than the peri-ovulatory peak of the young woman. LH levels rise less substantially. Ovarian androgens, in particular androstenedione and T, which tend to rise during mid-cycle in the early and peak reproductive stages, thereafter show a gradual decline although they are not predictably affected by the subsequent menopausal transition. This is considered more closely in Chapter 7 (see pp 244–245).

The post-menopausal ovary virtually ceases to secrete oestradiol, although appreciable quantities of androstenedione and T continue to be produced by the ovarian stroma, under the stimulation of the increased LH levels, and together with adrenal androgens provide an important source of oestrogen by peripheral aromatization.

The symptoms most characteristic of the menopausal transition are vasomotor phenomena of hot flushes and

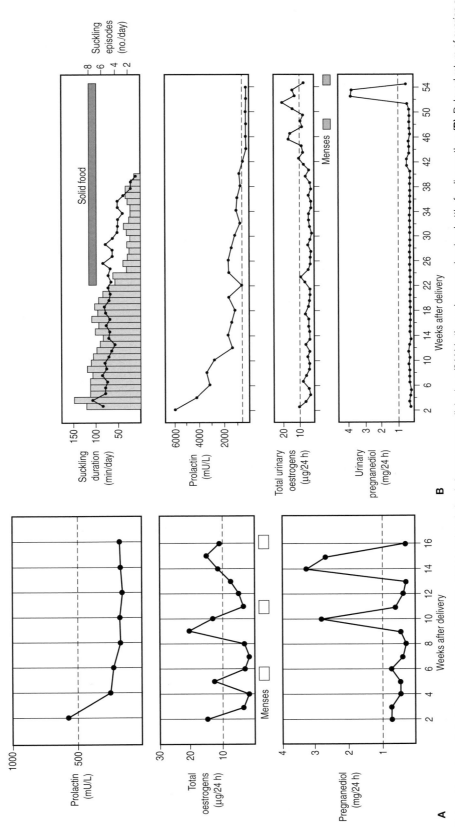

Fig. 3.22 (A), Return of ovarian activity (urinary total oestrogens >10 μg/24 h) and ovulation (urinary pregnanediol >10 μg/24 h) in the early puerperium in a bottle-feeding mother. **(B)**, Delayed return of ovarian activity and ovulation in a breast-feeding mother. (Courtesy of AS McNeilly; Howie & McNeilly 1982.)

night sweats. Their endocrine basis remains elusive, and although typically they are suppressed by exogenous oestrogen administration, their severity is not correlated with circulating oestrogen levels. These are transitional phenomena, which disappear after a variable period of time, and presumably reflect some adaptation process in the brain. A more persistent negative effect of the reduction in oestrogens, which is of obvious relevance to women's sexual health, is vaginal dryness, an important cause of dyspareunia. This will be considered more closely in Chapters 7 and 11.

The overall impact of the menopause on the sexuality of women in mid-life and later will be discussed in Chapter 7.

Anomalies of sexual differentiation — sex chromosome aneuploidies and intersex conditions

While the various anomalies of sexual differentiation are rare, they have proved to be very relevant to understanding normal sexual differentiation and for that reason alone warrant close examination. They also present the clinician, and indeed the parent, with difficult decisions about how the intersex child should be raised, and to what extent and when surgical interventions are appropriate. This has become a controversial issue in the last few years and is undergoing vigorous debate. From a scientific perspective it confronts us with the need to understand normal gender identity development, which tends to be taken for granted in the vast majority growing up as boys or girls. When dealing with an infant whose gender is in some respect ambiguous, we are faced with the question of what determines our gender identity and at what stage in development. In the 1950s, John Money interpreted the available evidence as indicating that, in terms of gender identity, we are born with the potential for developing either a male or a female gender identity, which is subsequently organized during the first 3 to 4 years of the child's development. It was therefore feasible to reassign gender, if there was a good reason, providing that this was done early (Money et al 1957). In 1972 Money & Ehrhardt reported on a pair of monozygotic twin boys, one of whom, at the age of 7 months, lost his penis in a circumcision procedure that went disastrously wrong. Money's recommendation to the family was to bring the child up as a girl, and gender reassignment was done at the age of 17 months, followed by surgical feminization. Money continued to report on the apparently successful progress of this child until 9 years of age. Much was made of this case, in both the scientific literature as well as the media, and it was used by a number of feminists to support the view that gender is socially constructed. Then in 1982, Diamond, who for some years had been a strong critic of Money's position on the bi-potentiality of gender identity, revealed that this child's development was in trouble (Diamond 1982). In the mid-1990s it became known that this individual, brought up as girl, had, in early adulthood, changed his gender back to male (Colapinto 2000). This outcome was taken to show that the bi-potentiality of gender identity depended on the conditions of pre-natal development. If these are normal, then reassignment of gender contrary to the genetic sex is unlikely to be successful, whereas in infants who have undergone abnormal pre-natal development, reassignment is an option providing it is started early enough (which according to Money was before the age when gender identity is clearly established in a child, i.e. from age 2 to 4 years. More recently this stage occurs between 2 and 3 years in the majority; see above). However, this case is not the end of the story. In another similar case, where the penis was lost as a result of faulty circumcision, reassignment to female has apparently been successful, even though behaviour during childhood was masculine, and the final sexual orientation was bi-sexual (Bradley et al 1998). Zucker (1999) has suggested that one possible explanation for these two different outcomes was that the latter case was reassigned at an earlier age (between 2 and 7 months versus 17 months), plus an apparently greater uncertainty about the gender reassignment in the parents of the first case.

Over recent years, there has been mounting criticism from the intersex community of early surgical interventions (ISNA 2005) for infants with ambiguous genitalia, and we are now in a phase of thoughtful circumspection. A new feminist perspective has been proposed by Fausto-Sterling (2000), who takes the existence of intersex conditions as evidence that there is no simple gender dichotomy, but a spectrum with typical male and typical female at each end. For these various reasons, we will be paying some attention to these anomalies and what we can learn from them. The issue of clinical management will also be briefly discussed.

There are five categories of anomalous development to consider:

1. sex chromosome aneuploidies
2. other sex chromosome abnormalities
3. inborn errors of metabolism affecting the reproductive hormones
4. exposure to exogenous steroids during fetal development
5. abnormal genital development of other kinds.

Sex chromosome aneuploidies

Variations from the normal sex chromosome karyotype (i.e. 46-XY or 46-XX) are complex, with mosaicism, where a variation is only present in a proportion of cells, adding to the complexity. We will confine our attention to the simplest and most common: 45-XO, 47-XXY, 47-XYY and 47-XXX. Although chromosomal status may influence development in a variety of ways, some of the most obvious effects are mediated through the gonads and sex endocrine system.

45-XO: Gonadal dysgenesis or Turner's syndrome

Although this is the commonest sex chromosome anomaly to arise, the large majority of fetuses so affected are aborted and consequently this karyotype occurs in less than 1 in 5000 live births. The specific genetic anomaly varies, with 50–60% lacking the second X chromosome completely, and others having mosaicisms or abnormalities of the second X chromosome (Collaer & Hines 1995).

Ovarian development starts normally, but presumably because of the absence of normal oocytes (which require two X-chromosomes, see p. 25) the ovaries soon regress and by birth are no more than streaks of connective tissue. There is thus a marked deficiency of sex steroids, including an absence of the normal increase in oestrogens during the first post-natal year. This results in absence of breast development and secondary sexual characteristics, and amenorrhoea. The genitalia are otherwise normally female. The most consistent feature is short stature, usually less than 58 inches (1.45 m) in height. This has now been attributed to a genetic deficiency; with absence or rearrangement of part of the X chromosome that is relevant to linear growth (Jaffe 2004). A variety of other somatic anomalies may occur, the best known being webbing of the neck (see Fig. 3.23). There are also a number of other health problems that may occur, including coarctation of the aorta and diabetes.

Intelligence is usually normal, though spatial aptitude may be impaired. Gender identity is unequivocally female (Money & Ehrhardt 1972), with some indications of enhanced femininity in some cases (Collaer & Hines 1995). Menstruation can be initiated and maintained with long-term oestrogen substitution therapy. The available evidence does not provide information about the development of sexual preferences, sexual appetite or response in these girls, though Money & Ehrhardt (1972) stress that without hormone substitution therapy it is difficult for them to establish psychosocial maturity. (For a more substantial review see Collaer & Hines 1995.)

This syndrome tells us little about the role of hormones in sexual development except that female prepubertal genitalia and gender identity develop in the absence of any ovarian steroid production.

47-XXX: Triple X

This has a frequency of about 1 in 1250 live female births. Sexual development appears to be normal in most cases although puberty may be delayed and a proportion do not menstruate normally. At least some of these women are fertile (producing normal children). They tend to be tall, and there may be learning disabilities.

47-XXY: Klinefelter's syndrome

About 1 in 700 newborn males has this karyotype. In some cases there may be three or even four X chromosomes. This is not an inherited condition, but results from non-disjunction during a meiotic or mitotic phase, which occurs more frequently with increased maternal age (Abruzzo & Hassold 1995). Development is invariably along male lines. The full picture of Klinefelter's syndrome includes small testes (about 2–6 mL) with tubular dysgenesis, hypogonadism, infertility, tall stature and gynaecomastia. There may be intellectual impairment, more likely with each additional X chromosome, personality problems and abnormal sexual preferences. Considering the frequency of this condition at birth, the full syndrome is rare. This presumably means that the majority of such men must be relatively free from such stigmata. This is borne out by their relative frequency amongst otherwise normal men attending infertility clinics (approximately 5% of male clinic attenders).

The endocrine pattern in this condition shows a somewhat low plasma T concentration (though overlapping the normal range) and raised gonadotrophins (both LH and FSH). Although the raised FSH is to be expected in view of the tubular dysgenesis, the high LH is probably not simply due to impaired Leydig cell function, as it is difficult to suppress the LH level to the normal range with exogenous androgens. These men usually have a relatively high oestrogen:T ratio which may account for their tendency to gynaecomastia.

The variability of phenotypes associated with 47-XXY may well be explained by recent research on the X-linked androgen receptor gene carrying the CAGn

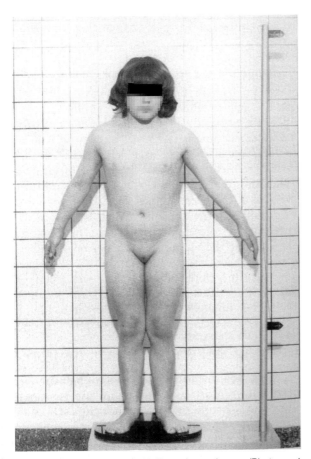

Fig. 3.23 Twelve-year-old girl with Turner's syndrome. (Photograph courtesy of Dr Shirley Ratcliffe.)

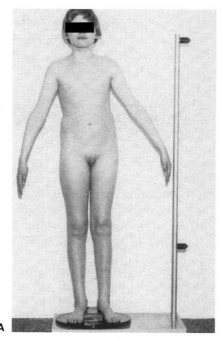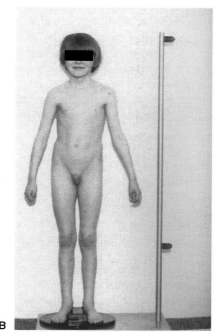

A   B

Fig. 3.24 Ten-year-old twins. The taller one **(A)** has an XXY chromosome constitution; his penis is proportionally smaller and he has increased fat deposition on the hips and more marked increase in leg length. (Photograph courtesy of Dr Shirley Ratcliffe.)

repeat polymorphism, the length of which is inversely related to androgen action (Zitzman et al 2004).

The tall stature, which is by no means invariable, is not fully understood. It is detectable throughout childhood before epiphyseal closure normally occurs, and is therefore not simply a result of delayed closure (see Fig. 3.24).

Tubular degeneration in the testes proceeds throughout childhood and it is only in late childhood that the testis size and consistency is noticeably different from normal.

Raboch et al (1979) found evidence of delayed development of heterosexual interest and socio-sexual behaviour in XXY males attending clinics. A study of adolescent boys with 47-XXY karyotypes identified at birth found them to have slightly lower intelligence than a group of normal matched controls (Ratcliffe et al 1982). Most developed normally except for being behind their peer group in the onset of adolescent sexual interest, relatively impaired in peer group relationships and with more tender-minded personalities than the controls (Bancroft et al 1982).

One study found evidence of a positive feedback response in five adult males with Klinefelter's syndrome (Barbarino et al 1979). This may reflect a relative lack of adult T rather than impaired early defeminization as, in contrast to the rat, suppression of positive feedback in the human male appears to depend on the prevailing hormonal milieu rather than on early defeminizing organization of the hypothalamus (Gooren 1986).

There is no evidence that XXY males are more likely to develop homosexual preferences. Gender identity problems and trans-sexuality have been reported in a number of XXY individuals (Diamond & Watson 2004), though it has not yet been conclusively shown that the likelihood of this is increased by an XXY constitution.

A rarer and possibly related condition is that of the 46-XX male. This is thought to be due to transfer of SRY from the Y chromosome to an X chromosome or autosome (Vilain 2000). These men are similar in many ways to the 47-XXY male, though not showing a tall stature to the same extent. The converse, when SRY is missing from the Y chromosome, leads to XY female development.

47-XYY

This condition has approximately the same incidence as 47-XXY, i.e. 1 in 700–1000 live male births. There are no obvious sexual consequences except that testicular abnormalities with impaired spermatogenesis and tubular atrophy may occur (Polani 1972). They are often fertile, fathering chromosomally normal children, though their fertility is apparently reduced by a low incidence of marriage. Hormonally, they have slightly raised gonadotrophins (both LH and FSH). The FSH may well reflect the tubular atrophy. The raised LH is more difficult to explain. Most studies have reported normal T levels, though one study found raised T compared with matched controls (Schiavi et al 1978).

These men show tall stature, similar to the XXY male, though their body shape is somewhat different. They first attracted attention because of their apparently high incidence amongst patients of special hospitals (i.e. for mentally disturbed offenders). It was suggested at one time that they had a tendency to high aggression, presumably a naive extrapolation from their extra Y chromosome. In fact the XYY men found in the special hospital populations were characterized by offences against property rather than people. They showed inadequacy rather than aggression. It may be that they have an increased incidence of behavioural problems of various kinds, though the risk of an XYY male becoming convicted, although increased, is very small. As with

XXY males, the majority live their lives without obvious problems or stigmata. There is no evidence of an increased likelihood of homosexual development.

Inborn errors of metabolism

Of the various types of innate metabolic anomalies, there are some which directly affect the production of, or receptor responsiveness to, sex hormones. They are all rare and we will consider only the most important. Those affecting individuals with 46XY karyotype will be considered first.

Androgen insensitivity syndrome (AIS)

The basic defect in this condition is a reduced affinity of cellular receptors for androgens. This results in a more or less complete failure of androgenic effects at cellular level and probably in all cells of the body. The clearest example of this condition is known as complete androgen insensitivity syndrome (CAIS). Partial AIS (PAIS) presents a more variable and, in several respects, more complex and less well understood picture. Because CAIS and PAIS never occur in the same family they are considered to be distinct entities, rather than PAIS being a less complete version of CAIS (Zucker 1999).

Complete androgen insensitivity syndrome

A variety of types of mutation in the androgen receptor gene have been linked to CAIS. The syndrome is transmitted either as an X-linked recessive trait or a male-limited dominant trait, so only genetic males are affected. Its prevalence has been estimated at 1 in between 13 158 and 40 800 live births (Minto et al 2003). According to Jaffe (2004), over 50% of individuals with CAIS have other affected relatives.

During embryonic development, the Müllerian-inhibiting factor is produced normally so that no fallopian tubes, uterus or upper vagina develop. In other respects the body develops along female lines. Their vaginas are short but their external genitalia are indistinguishable by their outward appearances from those of a normal female. Such children are therefore reared as girls.

Testes are found in the abdominal cavity or more commonly in the groin or labia. These testes have a tendency to neoplastic change and are usually removed during adulthood. They secrete normal male amounts of T and also relatively large quantities of E, which is responsible for the feminization (hence the original term 'testicular feminization', used before the actual mechanism was understood). LH levels are raised, presumably reflecting a failure of negative feedback by T. E is both secreted by the testes and converted from the plentiful supply of T. At puberty, good breast development and feminine contours arise, though there is a deficiency of body and pubic hair even by female standards (Fig. 3.25).

Gender identity and sexual orientation

The first sign of something wrong may be failure to menstruate. In spite of this, psychological development is along female lines. Money & Ehrhardt (1972) reported 10 such women. Nine 'conformed to the

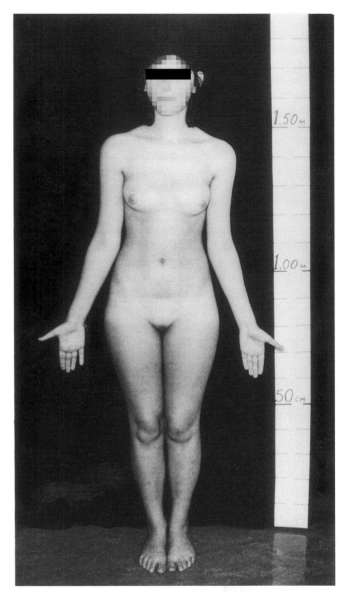

Fig. 3.25 Woman with complete androgen insensitivity syndrome. Notice the normal breast development and absence of sexual hair. (Photograph courtesy of Professor David Baird.)

idealized stereotype of what constitutes femininity in our culture' (p. 112). One woman reported some bisexual fantasies, but none reported homosexual experience as adults. Hines et al (2003) reported on 22 CAIS women and an age-matched control group. They found no difference between the two groups in measures of quality of life and self-esteem, personality traits that usually show gender differences, or patterns of gender role behaviour during childhood, gender identity or sexual orientation. In a review of articles covering 156 women with CAIS (Mazur 2005), there were no cases of self-initiated gender reassignment. So far, therefore, the evidence shows that such individuals have fairly normal female gender identities and are sexually attracted to men.

An unpublished study of CAIS

In view of the relative paucity of data about CAIS and its considerable theoretical relevance to sexual development,

I have revisited a series of 14 women with CAIS who I interviewed in their homes in 1981. They were all patients of Professor Polani, at Guy's Hospital, London. This study was never completed because the plan to recruit a comparison group of women with primary infertility ran into problems. There are limitations to this data. At that time, modern methods of genetic diagnosis were not available and one cannot therefore be absolutely certain about the diagnosis, in particular whether it was complete or partial AIS, although in no case was there any suggestion of ambiguity of the external genitalia, and hence partial AIS was unlikely. An advantage, however, was that each subject was interviewed by a sex researcher not involved in her clinical management. Various questionnaires were used in addition to the interview, but will not be reported here.

Ages ranged from 19 to 61 (mean 33.1). Ten were married, three of them twice, two were divorced and three were single. All but two had undergone gonadectomy. Age at surgery ranged from 15 to 30 years (mean 19.25 years). In four women it was unclear whether they had ever had hormone replacement (HR). The other 10 had HR but for very variable periods of time; mostly since gonadectomy, usually starting some time after surgery, although one started HR before gonadectomy. There is no clear explanation for this variability. Two women had been given vaginal dilators to use; only one woman had undergone surgical vaginoplasty.

None of the women reported any wish to be male at any time in their lives. Eight women described themselves as 'tomboys' during childhood; of these one also regarded herself as a tomboy when a teenager. Most, however, changed as a teenager. As one woman (subject A) put it: 'I was a tremendous tomboy; loved joining in with boys, climbing trees, "scrumping" apples and getting into trouble, until I was 12. Then I suddenly grew up and became a lady.' Two women, tomboys as children, described themselves in 'gender neutral' terms as teenagers. One (subject G) 'didn't feel like a tomboy or a girl. I just felt I didn't belong.' At age 15 'I regarded myself as coming from planet Venus.' She continued to feel uncomfortable about her lack of femininity and 'ugliness' until she started a relationship with a 'big tough guy' who made her feel attractive. 'He was so powerful and strong, I felt feminine alongside him.' Another woman (subject N) who was very much a tomboy as a child, felt less of a tomboy as a teenager, but not a particularly typical teenage girl. Boys were not interested in her. Her body shape was 'straight', with large waist and less noticeable hips, she wore short hair and dull clothes, and was often mistaken for a boy. But she was happy to be a woman. These self-descriptions of tomboyishness were consistent with answers to systematic questioning about play and activity preferences.

There were a number of factors which had psychological impact on many of these women, and which have to be taken into account when considering their gender, sexual and general personality development. All of them found themselves 'behind' their peer group in not having menstruated, and feeling 'different' as a consequence. Most of them had to deal with prolonged periods of medical investigation, including surgery, typically ending by being told that they would be infertile throughout their life. The issue of infertility, not important for some women, had a very traumatic effect on others, and indeed proved in two cases to be a barrier to the continuation of a relationship, because of the partner's wish to have children. The understanding of the nature of their abnormality seemed very variable, and indicated a very inconsistent and usually inadequate process of explanation by the doctors involved. One woman (subject J) had regarded herself as a 'freak', being half female and half male, because of what she had heard doctors saying to each other about her. Another woman (subject N) had the experience of her gynaecologist teaching about her to medical students as XY, but never discussing this with her. She had remained wanting to know why she did not develop as a male. These cases demonstrate the crucial importance of appropriate information as a part of clinical management.

Two women had family histories of AIS, with two other relatives affected in each case. For one of these women, this made her to some extent prepared for what was happening to her, although her mother apparently never discussed it with her. The other woman had a mother with a sister and cousin affected. Her mother knew that her daughter was affected when she was only 9 months old, because of an inguinal hernia. She would never discuss the diagnosis with anyone, and withdrew from any sexual activity with her husband for fear of having another affected child, resulting in long-term marital problems. This did not help her daughter deal with the problem.

Eight women had significant problems with being overweight, which in most cases were most marked in their mid-teens, and which usually influenced their self-esteem and sense of attractiveness. Several women, having been told that they had short vaginas, were apprehensive about having sexual intercourse, and some of them were pleasantly surprised to find that it was not a problem.

How do these findings compare with the other reports in the literature? They are consistent in terms of adult gender identity; all of these women were unequivocally female. In terms of childhood gender role behaviour, more than half of these women described themselves as tomboys, and gave detailed evidence about preferred activities consistent with this. This is somewhat at variance with the published literature. As Green (1974) has pointed out, tomboyishness in girls is considerably more common than the equivalent in boys, and in the majority of such cases can be regarded as a normal passing phase, which gives way to a more clearly feminine pattern once adolescence is reached. Nevertheless, not all girls are tomboys as children, and one is left wondering to what extent CAIS individuals do 'conform to the idealized stereotype of what constitutes femininity in our culture' as claimed by Money & Ehrhardt (1972). Such relatively masculine behaviour in childhood is taken to be a marker of androgenization in conditions such as congenital adrenal hyperplasia (Meyer-Bahlburg et al 2006).

Sexuality

Less attention has been paid to the sexual histories of women with CAIS. However, this is of considerable theoretical relevance to the role of androgens in women's sexuality. For that reason, the available evidence on sexuality of CAIS women is considered in Chapter 4 (see p.122).

Partial androgen insensitivity syndrome

This category involves 46XY individuals, who, as with CAIS, are born with intra-abdominal or inguinal testes, and who have breast development at puberty, but differ in having varying degrees of phallic enlargement at birth. Probably the best studied form of PAIS is a familial condition, Riefenstein's syndrome, which shows considerable variability in the degree of masculinization of the external genitalia, ranging from a minimal defect with micropenis and bifid scrotum, a more marked defect with perineo-scrotal hypospadias, to the most severe form with absent vas deferens, perineo-scrotal hypospadias and a vaginal orifice (Jaffe 2004). Because of this variability, gender of assignment may be either male or female, and there is a relatively high likelihood of gender problems. In reviewing 99 cases of PAIS reported in the literature, Mazur (2005) found nine who had undergone gender reassignment at some stage, and one had gender dysphoria. When last assessed, 47 identified as female, the remainder male. There is very little information about the sexuality of PAIS individuals.

5α-reductase 2 deficiency (5-ARD)

5α-reductase 2 is necessary for the conversion of T to DHT in early development. DHT is necessary for the male development of the urogenital sinus into normal external genitalia (see Fig. 3.5). The role of DHT in the human brain is less certain. There do not appear to be separate receptors for T and DHT in the brain and, although DHT has higher affinity for the androgen receptor (Grino et al 1990), T appears to be effective. Gooren (1985), in a small study of hypogonadal men, found that switching from T replacement to DHT replacement produced no change in their level of sexual interest or behaviour.

Imperato-McGinley et al (1974) studied a small community in the Dominican Republic in which there were 24 genetic males all related to one another and with 5-ARD. They were all born with ambiguous genitalia. The vas deferens, epididymis and seminal vesicles developed normally, being dependent on T. The urogenital sinus, however, remained as a blind vaginal pouch, with a clitoral-like phallus, labia-like scrotum and inguinal or labial testes. Most of these individuals were reared as girls, but at puberty not only did growth of the penile stump and scrotum occur, associated with deepening of the voice and masculine muscle development, there was also a change to a masculine gender identity with sexual feelings directed at females. Why T should show this effect at puberty and not cause normal development earlier is still somewhat uncertain. It has been suggested that it results from an increase in 5α-reductase 1, which is less effective early in development, but becomes more effective with age (Wilson 2001).

The change of gender identity in these individuals was striking and generated considerable debate. The initial reaction was to see this as evidence of androgenic masculinization over-riding the gender of rearing. It was then realized that, in this Dominican community, most if not all of these individuals were recognized as having this abnormality when they were small children (because it had been seen in previous relatives) and hence the gender of rearing was somewhat ambiguous. It is said that these children were socially labelled as *guavedoce*, which means 'penis at 12'. Herdt & Davidson (1988) reported a comparable situation among communities in Papua New Guinea where a number of individuals with 5-ARD were identified. They emphasized the male dominance of this culture, and whereas individuals with this syndrome may remain stigmatized even when adopting the male role, those identifying as female would be even more disadvantaged. They thus concluded that the gender socialization in this relatively primitive culture played a key role in the identification as male. Although rare, cases of 5-ARD have been reported from various parts of the world, including industrialized societies. The long-running debate on the interpretation of the associated inconsistencies in gender identity formation has been well summarized by Zucker (1999). Cohen-Kettenis (2005) reviewed the literature covering 129 cases of 5-ARD aged over 12. Of the 127 cases with relevant information, the gender assignment at birth was female in 99 and male in 17. Of the 99 female assigned individuals, 66 (67%) were reassigned to male, mostly during adolescence or early adulthood, whereas 32 (32%) remained female. There was little evidence to suggest that it was the degree of masculinization of the genitalia which determined the final gender identity, and Cohen-Kettenis (2005) concluded that a more general bodily masculine appearance, in association with masculine behaviour, both of which could have been, at least in part, determined by pre-natal exposure to T, make a gender role change more likely once further masculinization occurs at puberty, reinforcing an already existing gender discomfort. There is virtually no systematically collected evidence in the literature on the sexuality of individuals with 5-ARD.

17β-Hydroxysteroid dehydrogenase deficiency

17β-Hydroxysteroid dehydrogenase (17βHSD) is required for the conversion of androstenedione to T and for conversion of oestrone to oestrogen. Males with this deficiency are therefore susceptible to impaired masculinization in early development. This is an autosomal recessive trait (Jaffe 2004). Genital ambiguity at birth is similar to that found with 5-ARD, and some degree of pubertal virilization also occurs. Exposure of the brain to androgens during early development is, however, likely to be different in these two conditions, as the 5-ARD individual has no shortage of T. Increased virilization at puberty probably depends on augmentation of alternative enzyme pathways (Wilson 2001). Cohen-Kettenis (2005) found evidence in the literature from 35 cases of this condition. Five were assigned as female at birth, but reassigned to male within the first 3 years of life. Of the remainder, 28 were assigned as female and 2 as male. When last assessed, 18 of those assigned as female had been re-assigned as male. As with 5-ARD, most of these re-assignments occurred during adolescence or early adulthood. There is virtually no systematic evidence available on their sexuality. Cohen-Kettenis (2005) reached the same conclusions as with 5-ARD, about the relative importance of genital ambiguity and other aspects of masculinization in determining the final gender identity.

Metabolic anomalies affecting sexual differentiation of 46-XX females are of two types: congenital adrenal hyperplasia (CAH) and exposure to exogenous hormones during fetal development.

Congenital adrenal hyperplasia (or adrenogenital syndrome)

This is the result of an autosomal recessive gene defect in cortisol synthesis, usually due to a deficiency of the 21-hydroxylase enzyme. If severe, serious electrolytic disturbance and Addisonian crises occur. Usually the defect is less severe, and adequate cortisol production is maintained by means of excessive adreno-corticotrophic hormone stimulation, but at the expense of considerable hyperplasia of the adrenal cortex and a resulting excess of androgenic steroids. The classic 21-hydroxylase deficiency is detected in approximately 1 in 16 000 births (Speiser & White 2003). Classical CAH is present in utero, whereas non-classical CAH has an onset in childhood or later, and hence is less relevant to early sexual differentiation. CAH varies in severity, probably due to variation in the degree of enzyme deficiency (Jaffe 2004). In the more severe forms of CAH, there is a deficiency of the mineralocorticoid, aldosterone, as well as deoxycorticosterone, resulting in the 'salt-wasting' (SW) form, which can be fatal if untreated. The less severe forms are mainly manifested by the effects of increased androgens, and are known as the 'simple virilizing' (SV) variety.

Classical CAH in the male causes precocious puberty. In girls it leads to pre-natal virilization with varying degrees of masculinization of the external genitalia (i.e. clitoral enlargement and labioscrotal fusion) evident at birth. Some such children have been reared as males, and have apparently adapted successfully, though needing surgery both during childhood and later to remove the uterus.

Usually, however, the anomaly is correctly diagnosed and the child is reared as a female. In recent years, effective treatment, in the form of corticosteroids, has been available. Previously, lack of appropriate treatment led to androgen excess not only during fetal development but throughout childhood as well.

Money & Ehrhardt (1972) studied two groups of such women: those who were effectively treated from birth and thus only suffered excess androgens in utero, and those who were already adult or adolescent when treatment became available and who therefore continued to be androgenized throughout childhood. In both groups there was definite evidence of tomboy behaviour during childhood, significantly more than in a matched control group. The women also showed other features more consistent with a male than a female stereotype, e.g. preference for male clothes and avoidance of self-adornment, and putting career before marriage. In these respects, the early- and late-treatment groups did not differ, presumably indicating that these effects reflected pre-natal androgenization. The two groups did show some sexual differences, however. The late-treated group were more likely to report homosexual or bisexual fantasies than those treated early, though definite homosexual orientation did not occur. Also the late-treated group reported possibly greater sexual arousability (Money & Ehrhardt 1972; Lev Ran 1977). Thus we have some evidence from this source that androgens may influence sexual appetite and sexual preference, although in the latter case this could once again be via effects on gender identity.

Meyer-Bahlburg et al (2003) reported on the long-term outcome in 28 women with SW CAH, 10 with SV CAH, 35 with non-classical CAH and 30 normal control women. Measures of masculinized gender role behaviour in childhood were significantly higher in the SW group, and did not differ between the other three groups. This indicates that the severity of the CAH, and hence the degree of excess androgen production is related to the degree of masculinization of behaviour, presumably resulting from pre-natal effects, as the SW cases of CAH would have started treatment early in the post-natal period. Dessens et al (2005) reviewed the literature on gender identity in 46-XX individuals with CAH, finding evidence from 250 individuals raised female and 33 raised male. Of those raised female, the large majority had no problems with their female gender identity. Nevertheless, 5% (13 cases) did have serious gender identity problems; this is higher than the prevalence of female-to-male transgendered individuals in the general population. Among those raised male, 12% (4 cases) had serious gender identity problems. This underlines the point that whereas pre-natal androgenization is commonly associated with some degree of masculinization of behaviour during childhood, it affects gender identity development only in a small minority, and we do not understand why those individuals in particular are affected in this way.

The limited evidence of the effects of CAH on sexuality in women is of considerable theoretical interest, and is considered further in Chapter 4 (p. 123).

Much less is known about CAH in males, though precocious puberty is its main manifestation. Money & Alexander (1969), describing a series of such cases, found a relatively early onset of sexual interest, although the content of sexual imagery tended to be consistent with the boys' social and emotional age. Sexual behaviour problems did not arise in these boys. This is consistent with androgens 'energizing' the sexual experience, with the form it takes being more determined by social learning.

The effects of exogenous hormones during pregnancy

The administration of steroid hormones to the mother during pregnancy, and hence to the fetus, provides us with further evidence of the effects of steroids on physical and behavioural development. Of particular interest, therefore, are those children born to mothers given synthetic steroids during pregnancy in order to prevent spontaneous abortion. The early progestagens used for this purpose had androgenic properties. Pre-natal exposure of girls to these compounds was associated with increases in some male-typical characteristics: higher levels of tomboyism, preferences for male-typical toys and male playmates, and more physical aggression. These effects are comparable to those of CAH. The effects of androgenic progestagens in boys and of progestagens without androgenic properties in boys and girls are less clear cut (Collaer & Hines 1995).

The effects of oestrogenic steroids present us with a more challenging puzzle. Diethylstilboestrol (DES), a synthetic oestrogen, was given to many pregnant women as a protection against threatened miscarriage, until it was shown to be ineffective as well as increasing the risk of subsequent vaginal and cervical cancer. Female children, exposed to DES pre-natally in this way, were found to show no increase in male-type behaviours or gender identity, but they did have an increased likelihood of developing homosexual preferences (Ehrhardt et al 1985; Collaer & Hines 1995). No such effects on sexual orientation and no clear effects on male-type behaviour patterns have been reported in males exposed to DES pre-natally. The animal evidence suggests that the organizational effects of androgens depend on aromatization of T to oestradiol within the brain cells. This could be the case in the human, although the evidence of lack of masculinization in CAIS, discussed above, questions this. The fetus, however, is normally exposed to high levels of oestrogen and progesterone from the placenta (see p. 40). So the question remains why do not these high levels of oestrogen masculinize the brain, whether male or female? The favoured answer has been that there is some barrier which prevents the fetal and maternal oestrogens from entering the brain cells to masculinize them; either a placental barrier, or a mechanism by which oestradiol is prevented from entering the cell, a restriction which does not apply to T, e.g. by being bound to α-feto-protein (McEwan 1976). DES, because it is a synthetic oestrogen, was assumed not to be blocked in this way. Gorski (2000) has countered this 'protection hypothesis' with a very different explanation — 'the delivery hypothesis'. Based on the work of Toran-Allerand (1976) showing how oestradiol promotes neural growth in cultures of cells from the hypothalamus, and evidence that anti-oestrogen treatment of neonatal female rats defeminizes the brain but does not masculinize it, he proposes that the rat brain is basically neuter and is not, as is the reproductive tract, female by default. He suggests that α-fetoprotein-bound oestradiol not only can enter certain brain cells, it delivers the oestradiol in the process. The reader is entitled to feel confused, and Gorski is talking about the rat brain. Where the human brain fits into this scheme is another matter. Why the oestrogenic effects of DES should be confined to sexual orientation, and only in females, is puzzling.

Other congenital abnormalities of the genitalia

A number of developmental abnormalities of the genitalia, although rare, are receiving increased attention because of improved surgical techniques for correcting

them and the current controversies about assignment of gender and whether and when to intervene surgically in such cases. Cloacal exstrophy, which occurs in both genetic males and females, is a complex disorder of anatomic development involving both the genitourinary and intestinal tracts, which until recently had been regarded untreatable, resulting in early death of the affected infant. Micropenis and failure of penile development (penile agenesis) are two additional conditions. Reviews of the gender identity and psychosexual implications of these rare conditions are given by Zucker (1999) and Meyer-Bahlburg (2005). The most common disorder in this category is hypospadias.

Hypospadias

This results from an incomplete development of the anterior urethra. Normally, the urethra becomes surrounded by the corpus spongiosum during development, emerging as the urethral meatus at the tip of the penile glans. Varying degrees of hypospadias occur, ranging from a minor form where the meatus is at the level of the coronal sulcus, to the most severe form where the urethra opens in the perineum. The incidence of this anomaly has ranged from 0.8 to 8.2 per 1000 live births.

The cause for this anomaly is not known, except that in some cases it forms part of a more extensive endocrine abnormality, such as testicular dysgenesis, or partial androgen insensitivity, or is associated with pre-natal exposure to exogenous progestagens. It is generally assumed, however, that it results from at least transient abnormality of androgenization during fetal development.

Berg et al (1982) studied 34 men aged 21–34 years who had been born with hypospadias. Compared to a control group, they were more likely to recall depression and anxiety as well as poorer adjustment with peers during childhood. They tended to have an 'insecure gender identity' and were also delayed in their sexual development (e.g. age at first kiss and first sexual intercourse). From a retrospective study of this kind, it is difficult to distinguish between understandable reactions to the hypospadias and indications of other related pre-natally determined abnormalities (such as 'insecure gender identity'). Sandberg et al (1995) studied a sample of 175 boys with hypospadias, aged between 6 and 10 years, relying on parental reports. They found no increase in feminized behaviours and, unexpectedly, a slight but significantly higher level of masculine-type behaviour in the boys with hypospadias. They also found no relation between the severity of the hypospadias and degree of feminine or masculine-type behaviours, although they did find that a higher number of hospitalizations were associated with increased 'gender-atypical' behaviour. They had predicted that the assumed deficiency of androgenic stimulation during fetal development would lead to a lack of behavioural masculinization, and they found no support for this. They postulated that the androgen deficiency leading to the hypospadias may have been restricted to a limited and early phase of fetal development, whereas hormonal influences on behavioural development occur later. However, they cited studies indicating a persistent defect in androgen production continuing into the post-natal period, which does not support that particular explanation. Clearly, psychological and stress-related effects on development associated with a condition of this nature have to be taken into account. As yet the determinants of hypospadias and its relevance to sexual differentiation in a more general sense remain uncertain.

Conclusions from evidence of abnormalities of sexual development

Perhaps the least equivocal conclusion is that in the absence of pre-natal androgen effects, and particularly if there are unambiguous female external genitalia, a stable female gender identity develops. This is most clearly seen in Turner's syndrome and CAIS. There is also strong evidence that pre-natal exposure to androgens results in some masculinization of behaviour, though this depends on the extent of exposure (e.g. more likely with the salt-wasting than simple virilizing forms of CAH). Problems with gender identity are slightly more likely in such cases, but we have no indication of why such cases are affected in this way. It is conceivable that the effects of androgenization interact with some other factor (perhaps genetic) to determine gender identity. These developmental abnormalities throw little light on the determinants of sexual orientation or identity, with the exception of the increased likelihood of bisexual or homosexual identity in women exposed to DES in utero (see Chapter 5, p. 162).

Clinical management of intersex conditions

As indicated at the start of this section, there is now considerable uncertainty and disagreement about how to manage children with intersex conditions. There are two key issues; the gender of assignment and the use of surgery to increase consistency with gender of assignment. The evidence is sufficiently inconsistent that clear black and white criteria remain elusive. However, there is enough uncertainty to justify avoidance of genital surgery in the infant stage before any evidence of innately determined gender role or identity preferences have become apparent. The Intersex Society of North America strongly advocates avoidance of such surgery, and promotes the use of 'intersex' as an alternative identity, at least until the individual is mature enough to indicate preferences. CAIS is an interesting exception, as individuals with this condition have apparently unambiguous external genitalia at birth, and develop female gender identities in spite of their Y chromosome. Their constitution is usually not discovered until well into childhood, although with a strong family history this might happen earlier. The clinical challenge in these cases is one of information. At what point during development should individuals with CAIS know about the nature of their condition, and how should they be informed (e.g. should it be in stages?). Keeping them uninformed is clearly unacceptable.

For those with genital ambiguities at birth or early in infancy (e.g. ablatio penis), an important distinction is whether there is any reason to suspect abnormal pre-natal hormone exposure. Cloacal exstrophy is a further example. This is believed to be a developmental abnormality restricted to one section of the body, not involving the brain. In this case, however, there are sufficiently marked anatomical abnormalities that a normal childhood, free from uncertainties or related health problems, is out of the question. In such cases one can argue that assigning gender according to the chromosomal constitution is to be preferred, in the knowledge that this could be changed at a later stage.

Warne et al (2005) published a long-term outcome study of men and women with intersex conditions. This was a heterogeneous group; of 17 males, 11 had severe hypospadias; of 31 females, 14 had CAH and 5 vaginal agenesis. This combined group was compared with two other groups with chronic health problems from childhood or adolescence, 27 with Hirschsprung disease, a congenital condition affecting the digestive system and requiring early surgery, and 19 with early onset insulin-dependent diabetes. A limitation of this study is the combined control groups, which included 63% males whereas the intersex group had 65% females. All subjects were between 18 and 30 years of age, with an average age of 25–26 years in both groups. A range of standardized questionnaires was used. The intersex group did not differ from controls in physical or mental health. Intersex participants were satisfied with their overall body appearance, although the intersex males were less satisfied than controls with the size and appearance of their genitalia. The intersex group did not differ from controls in level of sexual desire or enjoyment of sexual activities, but were more likely to have difficulty or pain with vaginal intercourse and less likely to experience orgasm.

Overall, we are at a stage of vigorous debate on these issues, and it is to be hoped that with further unbiased, objective evaluations of the various options over the next few years, and further outcome research with well-matched groups, the criteria for clinical management (and parental choice) will become clearer.

REFERENCES

Abruzzo M, Hassold TJ 1995 Etiology of non-disjunction in humans. Environmental and Molecular Mutagenesis 25 (suppl 26): 38–47.

Angier N 1999 Woman: an Intimate Geography. Houghton Mifflin, New York.

Arlt W, Hewison M 2004 Hormones and immune function: implication of aging. Aging Cell 3: 209–216.

Bachman G, Bancroft J, Braunstein G, et al 2002 Female androgen insufficiency: the Princeton consensus statement on definition, classification, and assessment. Fertility and Sterility 77: 660–665.

Bancroft J, Axworthy D, Ratcliffe SG 1982 The personality and psychosexual development of boys with 47 XXY chromosome constitution. Journal of Child Psychology and Psychiatry 23: 169–180.

Barbarino A, DeMarinis L, Lafuente G, Muscatello P, Matterici BR 1979 Presence of positive feedback between estrogen and LH in patients with Klinefelter's syndrome and Sertoli-cell-only syndrome. Clinical Endocrinology 10: 235–242.

Barbieri RL 2004 The breast. In Strauss JF, Barbieri RL (eds) Yen & Jaffe's Reproductive Endocrinology, 5th edn. Elsevier, Philadelphia, pp. 307–326.

Berg R, Berg G, Svensson J 1982 Penile malformation and mental health. A controlled psychiatric study of men operated for hypospadias in childhood. Acta Psychiatrica Scandinavica 66: 398–416.

Boime I, Garcia-Campayo V, Hsueh AJW 2004 The glycoprotein hormones and their receptors. In Strauss JF, Barbieri RL(eds) Yen & Jaffe's Reproductive Endocrinology, 5th edn. Elsevier, Philadelphia, pp. 75–92.

Bonnar J, Franklin M, Nott PN, McNeilly A S 1975 Effect of breast feeding on pituitary-ovarian function after childbirth. British Medical Journal 4: 82–84.

Bradley SJ, Oliver GD, Chernick, AB, et al 1998 Experiment of nurture: ablatio penis at 2 months, sex reassignment at 7 months, and a psychosexual follow-up in young adulthood. Pediatrics 102: E91–E95.

Brown JB, Harrisson P, Smith MA 1978 Oestrogen and pregnanediol excretion through childhood, menarche and first ovulation. Journal of Biosocial Science 10 (suppl 5): 43–62.

Buvat J 2003 Androgen therapy with dehydroepiandrosterone. World Journal of Urology 21: 346–355.

Cameron J 1990 Factors controlling the onset of puberty in primates. In Bancroft J, Reinisch J (eds) Adolescence and Puberty. The Third Kinsey Symposium. Oxford University Press, New York.

Cohen-Kettenis PT 2005 Gender change in 46,XY persons with 5-alpha-reductase deficiency and 17-beta-hydroxysteroid dehydrogenase-3 deficiency. Archives of Sexual Behavior 34: 399–410.

Colapinto J 2000 As nature made him: The boy who was raised as a girl. Harper Collins, New York.

Collaer ML, Hines M 1995 Human behavioral sex differences: a role for gonadal hormones during early development? Psychological Bulletin 118: 55–107.

Daw SF 1970 Age of boys' puberty in Liepzig, 1729-49 as indicated by voice breaking in J.S. Bach's choir members. Human Biology 42: 87–89.

De Groot WC, Booth AM 1984 Peripheral Neuropathy, Vol I. Saunders, Philadelphia.

Dessens AB, Slijper FME, Drop SLS 2005 Gender dysphoria and gender change in chromosomal females with congenital adrenal hyperplasia. Archives of Sexual Behavior 34: 389–398.

Diamond M 1982 Sexual identity, monozygotic twins reared in discordant sex roles and a BBC follow up. Archives of Sexual Behavior 11: 181–186.

Diamond M, Watson LA 2004 Androgen insensitivity syndrome and Klinefelter's syndrome: sex and gender considerations. Child and Adolescent Psychiatric Clinics of North America, 13: 623–640.

Dufy B, Vincent JD 1980 Effects of sex steroids on cell membrane excitability: a new concept for the action of steroids on the brain. In de Wied D, van Keep PA (eds) Hormones and the Brain. MTP, Lancaster.

Ehrhardt AA, Meyer-Bahlburg HFL, Rosen LR, et al 1985 Sexual orientation after prenatal exposure to exogenous estrogen. Archives of Sexual Behavior 14: 57–78.

Fausto-Sterling A 2000 Sexing the Body. Basic Books, New York.

Forest HG, Deperetti E, Bertrand J 1976 Hypothalamic-pituitary-gonadal relationships from birth to puberty. Clinical Endocrinology 5: 551–569.

Gebhard PH, Johnson AB 1979 The Kinsey data: Marginal tabulations of the 1935-1965 interviews conducted by the Institute for Sex Research. Saunders, Philadelphia.

Giraldi A, Levin RJ 2005 Vascular physiology of female sexual function. In Goldstein I, Meston CM, Davis SR, et al (eds) Women's Sexual Function and Dysfunction: Study, Diagnosis and Treatment. Taylor & Francis, London, pp. 174–180.

Goodyer IM, Tamplin A, Herbert J, Altham PME 2000 Recent life events, cortisol, dehydroepiandrosterone and the onset of major depression in high risk adolescents. British Journal of Psychiatry 177: 499–504.

Gooren LJG 1985 Human male sexual functions do not require aromatization of testosterone: a study using tamoxifen, testolactone and dihydrotestosterone. Archives of Sexual Behavior 14: 539–549.

Gooren LJG 1986 The neuroendocrine response of luteinizing hormone to estrogen administration in the human is not sex specific but dependent on the hormonal environment. Journal of Clinical Endocrinology and Metabolism 63: 589–593.

Gorski RA 2000 Sexual differentiation of the nervous system. In Kandel ER, Schwartz JH, Jesell TM (eds) Principles of Neural Science, 4th edn. McGraw-Hill, New York, pp. 1131–1148.

Graber B, Kline-Graber G 1979 Female orgasm — role of pubococcygeus. Journal of Clinical Psychiatry 40: 34–39.

Green R 1974 Sexual Identity Conflict in Children and Adults. Basic Books, New York.

Grino PB, Griffin JE, Wilson JD 1990 Testosterone at high concentrations interacts with the human androgen receptor similarly to dihydrotestosterone. Endocrinology 126: 1165–1172.

Hall JE 2004 Neuroendocrine control of the menstrual cycle. In Strauss JF, Barbieri RL (eds) Yen & Jaffe's Reproductive Endocrinology, 5th edn. Elsevier, Philadelphia, pp. 195–212.

Harris RJ, Firestone JM 1998 Changes in predictors of gender role ideologies among women: a multivariate analysis. Sex Roles 38: 239–252.

Herbert J 1993 Peptides in the limbic system: neurochemical codes for co-ordinated adaptive responses to behavioural and physiological demand. Progress in Neurobiology 41: 723–791.

Herdt GH, Davidson J 1988 The Sambia 'Turnim-Man' sociocultural and clinical aspects of gender formation in male pseudohermaphroditism with 5-alpha-reductase deficiency in Papua New Guinea. Archives of Sexual Behavior 187: 33–56.

Hines M, Ahmed SF, Hughes I 2003 Psychological outcomes and gender-related development in complete androgen insensitivity syndrome. Archives of Sexual Behavior 32: 93–101.

Hopwood NJ, Kelch RP, Hale PM, et al 1990 The onset of human puberty— biological and environmental factors. In Bancroft J, Reinisch JM (eds) Adolescence and Puberty, the Third Kinsey Symposium. Oxford University Press, New York, pp. 29–49.

Howie PW, McNeilly AS 1982 Effects of breast feeding patterns on human birth intervals. Journal of Reproduction and Fertility 65: 545–557.

Howie PW, McNeilly AS, Houston MJ, et al 1982 Fertility after childbirth: post partum ovulation and menstruation in bottle and breast feeding mothers. Clinical Endocrinology 17: 323–332.

Hyde JS 2005 The gender similarities hypothesis. American Psychologist 60: 581–592.

Iervolino AC, Hines M, Golombok SE, et al 2005 Genetic and environmental influences on sex-typed behavior during the preschool years. Child Development 76: 826–840.

Imperato-McGinley J, Guerrero L, Gautier T, Peterson RE 1974 Steroid 5a-reductase deficiency in man; an inherited form of male pseudo-hermaphroditism. Science 186: 1213–1215.

Insel TR 1992 Oxytocin — a neuropeptide for affiliation: evidence from behavioral, receptor autoradiographic, and comparative studies. Psychoneuroendocrinology 17: 3–35.

ISNA 2005 Intersex Society of North America. www.isna.org

Jaffe RB 2004 Disorders of sexual development. In Strauss JF, Barbieri RL (eds) Yen & Jaffe's Reproductive Endocrinology, 5th edn. Elsevier, Philadelphia, pp. 463–492.

Jost A 1947 Recherches sur la differentiation sexualle de l'embryon de lapin. 3. Role des gonads foetales dans la differentiation sexuelle somatique. Archives D'Anatomie Microscopique et de Morphologie Experimentale 36: 271–315.

Knafo A, Iervolino AC, Plomin R 2005 Masculine girls and feminine boys; genetic and environmental contributions to atypical gender development in early childhood. Journal of Personality and Social Psychology 88: 400–412.

Kohlberg L 1966 A cognitive-developmental analysis of children's sex role concepts and attitudes. In Maccoby EE (ed) The Development of Sex Differences. Stanford University Press, Stanford.

Krantz KE 1958 Innervation of the human vulva and vagina. Obstetrics and Gynecology 12: 382–396.

Labrie F, Luu-The V, Labrie C, et al 2003 Endocrine and intracrine sources of androgens in women; inhibition of breast cancer and other roles of androgens and their precursor dehydroepiandrosterone. Endocrine Reviews 24: 152–182.

Levin RJ 1980 Physiology of sexual function in women. Clinics in Obstetrics and Gynaecology 7: 213–252.

Lev-Ran A 1977 Sex reversal as related to clinical syndromes in human beings. In Money J, Musaph H (eds) Handbook of Sexology. Excerpta Medica, Amsterdam, pp. 157–171.

Liu D, Dillon JS 2002 Dehydroepiandrosterone activates endothelial cell nitric-oxide synthase by a specific plasma membrane receptor coupled to $G\alpha_{i\ 2,3}$. Biological Chemistry 277: 21379–21388.

Lobo RA 2004 Menopause and aging. In Strauss III JF, Barbieri RL (eds) Yen & Jaffe's Reproductive Endocrinology, 5th edn. Elsevier, Philadelphia, pp. 421–462.

Maccoby EE, Jacklin CN 1974 The Psychology of Sex Differences. Stanford University Press, Stanford.

MacMahon B 1973 Age at menarche. Vital and Health Statistics (Series 11, No 133). National Center for Health Statistics, Rockville, MD.

Marshall EA, Tanner JM 1969 Variations in patterns of pubertal changes in girls. Archives of Diseases of Childhood 44: 291–303.

Marshall EA, Tanner JM 1970 Variations in patterns of pubertal changes in boys. Archives of Diseases of Childhood 45: 13–23.

Mazur T 2005 Gender dysphoria and gender change in androgen insensitivity or micropenis. Archives of Sexual Behavior 34: 411–422.

McEwan BS 1976 Interactions between hormones and nerve tissue. Reprinted in Silver R & Feder HH (eds) Hormones and Reproductive Behavior. Readings from Scientific American. W H Freeman, San Francisco, pp. 106–116.

Mesiano S, Jaffe RB 2004 The endocrinology of human pregnancy and fetal-placental neuroendocrine development. In Strauss JF, Barbieri RL (eds) Yen & Jaffe's Reproductive Endocrinology, 5th edn. Elsevier, Philadelphia, pp. 327–366.

Meyer-Bahlburg HFL 2005 Gender identity outcome in female-raised 46,XY persons with penile agenesis, cloacal exstrophy of the bladder, or penile ablation. Archives of Sexual Behavior 34: 423–438.

Meyer-Bahlburg HFL, Baker SW, Dolezal C, et al 2003 Long-term outcome in congenital adrenal hyperplasia: gender and sexuality. The Endocrinologist 13: 227–232.

Meyer-Bahlburg HFL, Dolezal C, Zucker KJ, et al 2006 The recalled childhood gender questionnaire-revised: a psychometric analysis in a sample of women with congenital adrenal hyperplasia. Journal of Sex Research 43: 364–367.

Minto CL, Liao KL-M, Conway GS, Creighton SM 2003 Sexual function in women with complete androgen insensitivity syndrome. Fertility and Sterility 80:157–164.

Money J, Alexander D 1969 Psychosexual development and absence of homosexuality in males with precocious puberty: a review of 18 cases. Journal of Nervous and Mental Diseases 148: 111–123.

Money J, Ehrhardt A 1972 Man and woman: boy and girl. Johns Hopkins Press, Baltimore.

Money J, Hampson JG, Hampson JL 1957 Imprinting and the establishment of gender role. Archives of Neurology and Psychiatry 77: 333–336.

Nishimori K, Young LJ, Guo Q, et al 1996 Oxytocin is required for nursing but not essential for parturition or reproductive behavior. Proceedings of the National Academy of Science, USA 93: 1699–1704.

O'Connell HE, DeLancey JOL 2005 Clitoral anatomy in nulliparous healthy premenopausal volunteers using unenhanced magnetic resonance imaging. Journal of Urology 173: 2060–2063.

O'Connell HE, Hutson CR, Anderson CR, Plenter RJ 1998 Anatomical relationship between urethra and clitoris. Journal of Urology 159: 1892–1897.

O'Connell HE, Sanjeevan KV, Hutson JM 2005 Anatomy of the clitoris. Journal of Urology 174: 1189–1195.

Opie I, Opie P 1959 The Lore and Language of Schoolchildren. Clarendon Press, Oxford.

Opie I, Opie P 1969 Children's Games in Street and Playground. Clarendon Press, Oxford.

O'Rahilly R 1977 The development of the vagina in the human. In Blandau RJ, Bergsma D (eds) Morphogenesis and Malformation of the Genital System. The National Foundation — March of Dimes. Birth defects: original article series, vol 13, no 2. Alan Liss, New York.

Polani PE 1972 Sex chromosome anomalies. In Ounsted C, Taylor DC (eds) Gender Differences: Their Ontogeny and Significance. Churchill Livingstone, Edinburgh, pp. 13–40.

Raboch J, Mellan I, Starka L 1979 Klinefelter's syndrome: sexual development and activity. Archives of Sexual Behavior 8: 333–339.

Ratcliffe SG, Bancroft J, Axworthy D, McLaren W 1982 Klinefelter's syndrome in adolescence. Archives of Diseases of Childhood 57: 6–12.

Ruble DN, Martin CL, Berenbaum SA 2006 Gender development. In Eisenberg N (ed) Handbook of Child Psychology, vol 3, 6th edn. Wiley, New York, pp. 858–932.

Sandberg DE, Meyer-Bahlburg HFL, Yager TJ, et al 1995 Gender development in boys born with hypospadias. Psychoneuroendocrinology 20: 693–709.

Sarrel PM 1976 Biological aspects of sexual function. In Gemme R, Wheeler CC (eds) Progress in Sexology. Plenum, New York, pp. 227–244.

Schiavi RC, Owen D, Fogel M, et al 1978 Pituitary-gonadal function in XXY and XYY men identified in a population survey. Clinical Endocrinology 9: 233–239.

Short RV 1980 Hormonal control of growth at puberty. In Lawrence TLJ (ed) Growth in Animals. Butterworth, London, pp. 25–45.

Sisk CL, Foster DL 2004 The neural basis of puberty and adolescence. Nature Neuroscience 7: 1040–1047.

Soules MR, Sherman S, Parrott E, et al 2001 Executive summary: stages of reproductive aging workshop (STRAW). Fertility and Sterility 76: 874–878.

Speiser PW, White PC 2003 Congenital adrenal hyperplasia. New England Journal of Medicine 349: 776–788.

Strauss JF 2004 The synthesis and metabolism of steroid hormones. In Strauss JF, Barbieri RL (eds) Yen & Jaffe's Reproductive Endocrinology, 5th edn. Elsevier, Philadelphia, pp. 125–154.

Stoller R 1968 Sex and Gender. On the Development of Masculinity and Femininity. Hogarth, London.

Suh DD, Yang CC, Cao Y, et al 2003 Magnetic resonance imaging anatomy of the female genitalia in premenopausal and postmenopausal women. Journal of Urology 170: 138–144.

Thornton JW 2001 Evolution of vertebrate steroid receptors from an ancestral estrogen receptor by ligand exploitation and serial genome expansions. PNAS 98: 5671–5676.

Toran-Allerand CD 1976 Sex steroids and the development of the newborn mouse hypothalamus and preoptic area in vitro: implications for sexual differentiation. Brain Research 106: 407–412.

Van Beijsterveldt CEM, Hudziak JJ, Boomsma DI 2006 Genetic and environmental influences on cross-gender behavior and relation to behavior problems: a study of Dutch twins at ages 7 and 10 years. Archives of Sexual Behavior 35: 647–658.

Van Houten T 2005 Anatomy of the pelvic floor and pelvic organ support system. In Goldstein I, Meston CM, Dacis SR, Traish AM (eds) Women's Sexual Function and Dysfunction: Study, Diagnosis and Treatment. Taylor & Francis, London, pp. 134–150.

Van Wieringen JC, Wafelbakker F, Verbrugge HP, De Haas JH 1971 Growth Diagrams 1965, The Netherlands. Wolters-Noordhoff, Groningen.

Vilain E 2000 Genetics of sexual development. Annual Review of Sex Research 11: 1–25.

Wallen K 1996 Nature needs nurture: the interaction of hormonal and social influences on the development of behavioral sex differences in rhesus monkeys. Hormones and Behavior 30: 364–378.

Warne G, Grover S, Hutson J, et al 2005 A long-term outcome study of Intersex conditions. Journal of Pediatric Endocrinology and Metabolism 18: 555–567.

Williams MRI, Ling S, Dawood T, et al 2002 Dehydroepiandroterone inhibits human vascular smooth muscle cell proliferation independent of ARs and ERs. Journal of Clinical Endocrinology and Metabolism 87: 176–181.

Wilson JD 2001 Androgens, androgen receptors and male gender role behavior. Hormones and Behavior 40: 358–366.

Winters SJ, Clark BJ 2003 Testosterone synthesis, transport and metabolism. In Bagatell CJ, Bremner WJ (eds) Androgens in Health and Disease. Humana Press, Totowa, NJ, pp. 3–22.

Witchel SF, Plant TM 2004 Puberty: gonadarche and adrenarche. In Strauss JF, Barbieri RL (eds) Yen & Jaffe's Reproductive Endocrinology, 5th edn. Elsevier, Philadelphia, pp. 463–492.

Yen SSC 2004 Neuroendocrinology of reproduction. In Strauss JF, Barbieri RL (eds) Yen & Jaffe's Reproductive Endocrinology, 5th edn. Elsevier, Philadelphia, pp. 3–74.

Young WS, Shepard E, Amico J, et al 1996 Deficiency in mouse oxytocin prevents milk ejection, but not fertility or parturition. Journal of Neuroendocrinology 8: 847–854

Yucel S, DeSouza A Jr, Baskin LS 2004 Neuroanatomy of the human female lower urogenital tract. Journal of Urology 172: 191–195.

Zitzman M, Depenbusch M, Gromoll J, Nieschlag E 2004 X-Chromosome inactivation patterns and androgen receptor functionality influence phenotype and social characteristics as well as pharmacogenetics of testosterone therapy in Klinefelter patients. Journal of Clinical Endocrinology and Metabolism 89: 6208–6217.

Zucker KJ 1999 Intersexuality and gender identity differentiation. Annual Review of Sex Research 10: 1–69.

Sexual arousal and response — the psychosomatic circle

4

Our sources of information 56

The brain and sexuality.. 56
A brief introduction to the brain 57
Development and sexual differentiation of the brain 59
Brain development during childhood and adolescence............. 60
The emotional brain.. 61
Where does sex fit in? 64
And what about love? 65

Central control of sexual excitation and inhibition 65
The need for inhibitory mechanisms 65
Animal evidence 67
Human evidence... 69
Brain imaging during sexual stimulation 71
Brain imaging and romantic love 73
Neurological lesions 74

**Genital response (anatomy and physiology) in men
and women**.. 74
Genital response in men 74
Genital response in women.. 78

Orgasm, seminal emission and ejaculation...................... 84
Genital and pelvic responses during orgasm.......................... 84
General muscular responses during orgasm 85
Cardiovascular and respiratory responses associated
with orgasm.. 85
The somatic sensations of orgasm 86
Altered consciousness 86
The psychological components of the orgasmic experience 86
Types of female orgasm.. 86

Mechanisms underlying orgasm, seminal emission
and ejaculation 87
After the orgasm: the refractory period....................... 90
Female ejaculation.. 93
The functions of orgasm 94

**Information processing: response to sexual stimuli,
cognitive mechanisms and the relevance of mood** 96
Response to sexual stimuli 96
Models of information processing....................................... 98
EEG and brain-imaging studies... 101
Conditioning, learning and habituation.............................. 104
Sexual fantasy 105
The role of inhibition.. 105
Individual differences and the relevance of personality............ 106
Mood and sexuality 106

**The role of hormones in sexual arousal and
response**... 111
Gonadal steroids — androgens in the male 111
Androgens in the female 114
Oestrogens 124
Mode of action of androgens and oestrogens in the brain 124
Comparison of gonadal steroid effects in men and women...... 127
Peptides 128
Hormones and passionate love... 130

Making sense of gender differences 130
Towards an explanatory model of gender differences
in sexuality... 131
Conclusion... 133

The biological characteristics of an essentially sexual experience include changes in our genitalia, in particular erection of the penis in a male and tumescence of the clitoris and lubrication of the vagina in a female, heightened awareness of pleasurable erotic sensations and changes in our subjective state that we call sexual excitement or arousal. An important element is 'information processing'; cognitive processes that attend to the sexual meaning of what is happening by focusing on external events and relating them to memory, internal processes such as imagery, or perceptions of bodily changes that have sexual meaning. Such processes can be conscious or unconscious. It is through this cognitive component that the whole gamut of social and interpersonal influences impinges on our sexuality. In a proportion of occasions, orgasm will occur.

The whole body is involved in this interplay of psychological and somatic processes; the sexual experience is par excellence psychosomatic. The genital responses, as we shall see, depend on specific local vascular mechanisms. But sexual excitement is accompanied by a more generalized form of arousal that, in addition to central manifestations of increased alertness, includes peripheral changes in blood pressure and heart rate, and increased blood flow to the skin. Orgasm, still largely a neurophysiological mystery, involves both central processes in the brain and widespread peripheral effects, experienced as acute increases in the intensity of erotic sensation, and muscle contractions that are largely involuntary. In the male, orgasm is associated with seminal emission, and these two things together result in ejaculation. Following orgasm, at least in the male, there is a period of reduced arousability, the refractory period.

The extent to which our awareness of what is happening in our bodies impacts on the experience allows us to conceptualize a 'psychosomatic circle', as shown in Figure 4.1. We can recognize links between (i) cognitive processes, conscious and unconscious, (ii) the emotional brain, (iii) the spinal cord and reflex centres within it, which, via peripheral somatic and autonomic nerves, control (iv) genital responses as well as (v) other peripheral manifestations of sexual excitement. Perception, awareness and cognitive processing of these peripheral and genital changes complete the circle. Fitting somewhat uncertainly in this schema is (vi) the orgasm, which has been given a central position in the diagram as much for symbolic as physiological reasons, though the orgasm probably involves mechanisms within both the brain and the spinal cord. The post-orgasm refractory period, the physiology of which is not well understood, involves

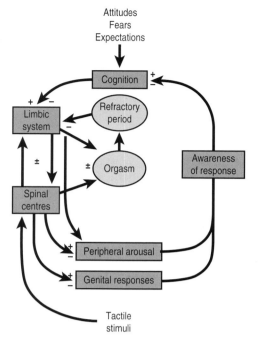

Fig. 4.1 The psychosomatic circle of sex. The post-orgasmic refractory period is of greater significance in the male.

an inhibitory phase, possibly affecting several components of the circle.

Although the process leading to a sexual experience may start in the periphery (e.g. some unanticipated tactile stimulation), the processes that impart 'sexuality' to the experience are in the brain, both conscious and unconscious. A fundamental aspect of the whole system is represented in Figure 4.1 by a + and − sign at each interface in the circle, representing the balance of excitatory and inhibitory influences at each point. This has been elaborated in the Dual Control model of sexual response, presented in Chapter 2, and provides the organizing template for much of this chapter.

Our sources of information

Much of the conventional wisdom about brain mechanisms and sexual response is based on animal studies, where invasive techniques can be used to relate specific actions or responses to specific parts of the brain. Although the precise behaviours involved in sexual activity vary across species, it is possible to identify appropriate animal homologues for many aspects of human sexuality. It is evident that basic neurophysiological mechanisms involved in reproductive behaviour are similar across mammalian species (Pfaus et al 2003), and most of the evidence relating to neurotransmitter mechanisms and pathways reported here has come from animal studies.

In the human, we can study the role of hormones in various ways. There is limited evidence of the distribution of steroid receptors in the brains of men and women taken from post-mortem studies, which can be compared with somewhat more extensive evidence from non-human primates. We can examine the relations between circulating levels of sex steroids, such as

testosterone (T), and aspects of sexual response and behaviour. We can also examine the effects of lowering gonadal steroids (e.g. the lowering of free T by oral contraceptives) and administering exogenous steroids. The effects of sexual stimulation and orgasm on hormonal levels in the peripheral blood are being researched, and there is a growing literature on the effects of various pharmacological agents, either from experimental studies or from reports of side effects of drug administration.

There is also an extensive literature on psychophysiological studies in both men and women, mainly using measurement of genital response and relating it to other measures, either physiological (e.g. blood pressure) or subjective.

The most important methodological advance in studying the neurophysiology of human sexuality in recent years is functional brain imaging, which allows identification of sites in the brain where activation or deactivation occurs in response to sexual stimulation. In its application to sexual response, this is still at an early stage of development. In a useful review, Mouras & Stoleru (2007) reported on 16 studies of brain imaging during response to sexual stimulation. There are two techniques that have been mainly used, both based on measurement of regional cerebral blood flow (rCBF); activation of a brain area is reflected in increased and deactivation in reduced local blood flow. Positron emission tomography (PET) scanning involves the intravenous injection of water containing a proportion of molecules with an isotope of oxygen (^{15}O). As blood flow increases in a specific area, there is increased disintegration of the ^{15}O-containing molecules, resulting in the release of positrons, which can be identified by detectors applied to the head. Functional magnetic resonance imaging (fMRI) is based on the blood-oxygen level-dependent (BOLD) contrast. Haemoglobin, which carries the oxygen in the blood, exists under two forms: deoxyhaemoglobin and oxyhaemoglobin. These two molecules present different magnetic properties: when placed in a magnetic field, the deoxyhaemoglobin acts as an endogenous tracer for the fMRI technique, making fMRI non-invasive as compared to PET. When a brain area gets activated, the increased concentration of oxyhaemoglobin leads to a relative decrease in the local blood deoxyhaemoglobin concentration. This constitutes the basis of the BOLD response. Localization of brain activity or deactivation during response to sexual stimuli has been assessed in two ways. One method compares the increase or decrease in rCBF during a sexual stimulus with the changes during a neutral (or non-sexual stimulus). Here the derived variable results from subtraction of rCBF during the non-sexual stimulus from rCBF during the sexual stimulus. A second method is to correlate changes in rCBF with some other measure of sexual response, e.g. penile erection. Results from such studies will be reported at various points in this chapter.

The brain and sexuality

The history of brain neurophysiology has gone through interesting phases (Kandel 2000). The phrenologists of the late 18th and early 19th centuries, most notably

Gall, a German neuroanatomist, assumed that complex traits such as spirituality and hope were controlled by specific brain areas, which expanded as the trait developed. As a result, they believed that an individual's character could be determined by examining the bumps in that person's skull, which reflected the enlarged functional brain areas underneath. This gave way to a 19th-century version of the aggregate-field view, which basically reduced brain mechanisms to one over-riding function, more compatible with the idea of a soul. By the late 19th century, neuroscientists such as Hughlings Jackson, Wernicke and Sherrington were promoting cellular connectionism whereby individual neurons are signalling units, organized in functional interconnecting groups. Evidence to support this view was accumulating, yet during the first half of the 20th century a more modern version of the aggregate-field view was dominant. Lashley's experiments with rats learning to run a maze seemed to indicate that the severity of defective learning following brain lesions depended more on the size than on the site of the lesions. This led to the mass action view; it is brain mass not its neuronal components that is crucial to brain function. Since then there has been a return to a distributed processing view based on Wernicke's cellular connectionism. Thus, according to Kandel (2000), 'specific brain regions are not concerned with faculties of the mind, but with elementary processing operations. Perception, movement, language, thought and memory are all made possible by the serial and parallel interlinking of several brain regions, each with specific functions' (p. 15). When we turn our attention to brain mechanisms and sexual behaviour, we indeed find a range of processing operations that are not specific to sex but that combine, in ways that are still not well understood, to create what we call a 'sexual experience', hence the need, discussed in Chapter 2, to develop simplified conceptual systems underlying the faculty of sexual responsiveness.

A brief introduction to the brain

At several places in this book, including the previous chapter, we consider aspects of brain function and evidence of the localization of such function in the brain. For those not familiar with the details of brain structure (which includes the author!) such evidence can be confusing. This section is therefore intended to provide a simple guide to brain structure, which can be revisited to clarify the location of specific brain areas when they arise in the text. Also, because of the complexity of brain function we are following this introduction with the section on development and sexual differentiation of the brain, which otherwise might have been included in Chapter 3 or Chapter 5.

The central nervous system has seven main structural divisions (Amaral 2000): the cerebral hemispheres, diencephalon, cerebellum, midbrain, pons, medulla and spinal cord. The midbrain, pons and medulla are together referred to as the brain stem (Fig. 4.2).

The *cerebral hemispheres* consist of the cerebral cortex, divided on each side into four lobes (frontal, parietal, temporal and occipital), the underlying white matter, the basal ganglia, the amygdala and the hippocampus. There are three principal structures in the subcortical basal ganglia: striatum, globus pallidus and subthalamic nucleus. The substantia nigra is also regarded as a basal ganglion but is situated in the midbrain. The striatum is made up of the caudate nucleus, putamen and ventral striatum (which includes the nucleus accumbens). The two hemispheres are connected by the corpus callosum.

The hemispheres are concerned with perceptual, motor and cognitive functions, including memory and emotion. The basal ganglia are mainly involved in the control of fine movements, the hippocampus with memory and the amygdala with the expression of emotion and social behaviour.

The *diencephalon* has two components, the thalamus and hypothalamus. The *thalamus* is a crucial intermediary between sensory receptors in the periphery and motor information from the cerebellum and basal ganglia, and relevant processing areas in the cerebral cortex. The *hypothalamus* plays a central role in regulation of behaviours crucial to homeostasis and reproduction. It is involved in the motivational system, initiating and maintaining behaviours that are rewarding, as well as control of many aspects of the endocrine system (see Fig. 4.3).

The cerebral hemispheres and diencephalon are together known as the *forebrain*.

The *cerebellum*, long known to be involved in posture and fine motor coordination, has recently been recognized to be involved also in language and other cognitive functions.

The *midbrain*, the smallest part of the brain stem, has, in addition to the substantia nigra, components of the auditory and visual systems.

The *pons*, which protrudes from the ventral surface of the brain stem, is involved as an intermediary between the cerebellum and cortex in the processing of movement and sensation, and contains neuronal clusters involved in respiration, taste and sleep.

The *medulla*, which resembles the spinal cord in organization and function, is involved in the regulation of blood pressure and respiration, and also includes some early relay nuclei involved in taste, hearing, balance and control of neck and facial muscles.

The medulla, pons and cerebellum are together known as the *hindbrain*. The hindbrain (excluding the cerebellum) and midbrain are together known as the *brain stem*. Some neuroscientists include the diencephalon in the brain stem.

The *spinal cord* extends from the base of the skull to the first lumbar vertebra. The grey matter of the cord is divided into dorsal and ventral horns; the dorsal horn includes the sensory neurons entering the cord and the ventral horn includes the motor neurons that leave the cord. The white matter is made up of ascending and descending pathways between the cord and brain.

Also to be considered is the *autonomic nervous system*, a visceral sensory and motor system with widespread

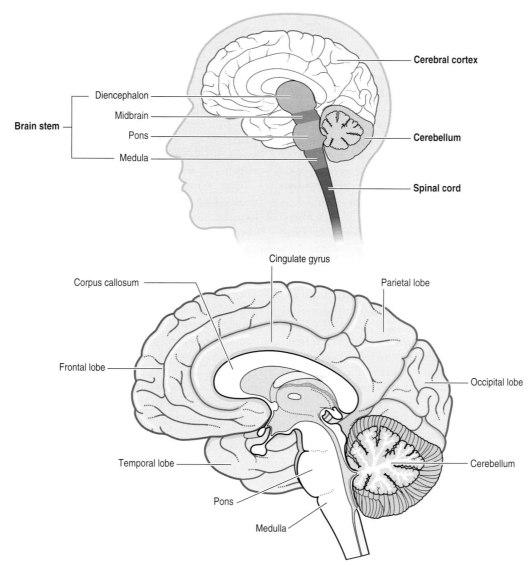

Fig. 4.2 The structural divisions of the central nervous system. (Adapted from Amaral 2000.)

effects, which include control of the heart, smooth muscle and glandular structures. It is regulated by a network of nuclei in the brain stem, hypothalamus and other parts of the forebrain. It has three divisions: *sympathetic, parasympathetic* and *enteric*.

The enteric division, which contributes to regulation of the gastrointestinal tract, is self-contained, with minimal connections to the rest of the nervous system. However, the gastrointestinal tract also has sympathetic and parasympathetic innervation, which presumably can over-ride the control of the enteric system. The motor neurons of the sympathetic and parasympathetic systems originate in the autonomic ganglia (and are called post-ganglionic), where they connect with the pre-ganglionic fibres that emerge from the brain stem and spinal cord.

The pre-ganglionic neurons of the sympathetic system form a column within the spinal cord from the first thoracic spinal segment to the lower lumbar segments. They exit the spinal cord at each vertebral level, initially with the spinal nerves, and then separate, either to form the ganglia of the sympathetic chains, which run along

each side of the spinal cord, or to pass through the splanchnic nerves to the prevertebral ganglia, which include the celiac and the superior and inferior mesenteric ganglia. Post-ganglionic fibres from the inferior mesenteric ganglia supply the reproductive organs, in addition to the bladder, large intestine and rectum. Some pre-ganglionic fibres in the splanchnic nerves supply the adrenal medulla, the central part of the adrenal gland, which, instead of issuing post-ganglionic fibres, secretes adrenaline (A) and, to a lesser extent, noradrenaline (NA) directly into the circulation (see below).

The pre-ganglionic neurons of the parasympathetic nervous system (PNS) originate mainly in the brainstem, exiting through cranial nerves, and also from the second to fourth sacral segments of the cord. The 10th cranial nerve, or *vagus* nerve, contains the main parasympathetic supply to the lungs, heart and upper parts of the gastrointestinal tract. The sacral outflow supplies the large intestine, bladder and reproductive organs.

The sympathetic system innervates throughout the body, whereas the PNS is more restricted. The parasympathetic ganglia are distributed close to the organs

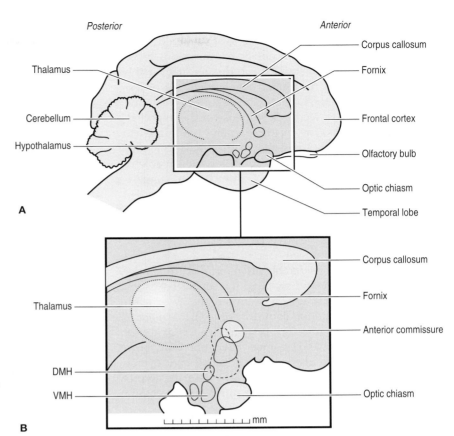

Fig. 4.3 **(A)**, Sagittal section of the brain of the rhesus monkey showing hypothalamic area. **(B)**, Enlarged view of the hypothalamic area: the dotted line indicates the medial preoptic area (MPOA). DMH, dorsomedial nucleus of the hypothalamus; VMH, ventro medial nucleus of the hypothalamus.

supplied. This means that the pre-ganglionic parasympathetic neurons are long (e.g. vagus nerve), with the post-ganglionic neurons much shorter. In the sympathetic system, it is the other way round, with the ganglia close to the spinal cord and the post-ganglionic fibres long as they extend to most parts of the body. Both sympathetic and PNSs include sensory fibres, the functions of which are not fully understood, but which probably contribute to visceral reflexes together with other sensory inputs. These are believed to be integrated, and dispersed, via the *nucleus of the solitary tract*, which runs through most of the medulla.

Development and sexual differentiation of the brain

In lower animals, particularly rodents, which have been the most intensively studied, there are fairly clear differences between the brains of males and females. In some species, structural differences can even be observed with the naked eye and there is now good evidence that the neural architecture of certain parts of the brains of rodents, especially in the hypothalamus, is determined by exposure to steroid hormones, both androgens and oestrogens (E) (Gorski 2000). For some time, this organizing effect of steroids has been assumed to occur early in development, in most rodents in the first few days following birth. T injected into female rats within the first postnatal week alters the function of the medial pre-optic area (MPOA) of the hypothalamus. Such masculinized female rats, as well as normal male rats, are unable to respond to the pre-ovulatory surge of oestradiol with the positive

feedback response that is fundamental to ovulation. This effect is an example of organizational defeminization of the brain. Castrating a male rat post-natally suppresses later adult masculine sexual behaviour and enhances feminine behaviour (e.g. lordosis). However, there is now evidence that there may be a second sensitive period for organizational effects of androgens, around puberty and during adolescence. Whether E has this pubertal organizing impact on the brain is not yet known (Sisk 2006).

Structural sex differences in the rat brain, which are most likely to be relevant to sexual and reproductive behaviour, include the bed nucleus of the stria terminalis (BNST), medial nucleus of the amygdala, MPOA of the hypothalamus, and sexually dimorphic nucleus (SDN) of the pre-optic area (POA), which are all larger in the male rat, and the anteroventral periventricular nucleus and locus coeruleus (l.c.) (see p. 68), which are larger in the female rat. There are other sex differences in brain structure that are less clearly relevant to sexual or reproductive behaviour (Gorski 2000). There are also clear examples of such neuronal sex differentiation in the spinal cord, most notably the spinal nucleus of the bulbocavernosus (penile muscle), which disappears in the female rat during the first few weeks of life (Gorski 2000). The most important mechanism by which steroids produce these sex differences in brain and nervous system structure is probably their effect in preventing apoptosis or programmed cell death, although androgens and E may have different effects on apoptosis depending on the particular brain structure involved (Gorski 2000).

So much for the rat; when we consider the human, and indeed non-human primates, we have much less evidence and greater uncertainty about sexual differentiation of the brain and its relevance to sexual and reproductive behaviour. The concept of organization, based on early exposure to steroids producing irreversible structural as well as functional development, is of less certain relevance to the human. The organized defeminization of the positive feedback response of the hypothalamus in the male, for example, may not apply to humans. Gooren (1986) has shown that male-to-female transsexuals after surgical castration become capable of a positive feedback response to E provocation, suggesting that the absence of positive feedback in the human male is an activational effect of the prevailing hormonal milieu. On the other hand, 46XY women, with CAIS, show no evidence of positive feedback and have been in some sense 'defeminized' (see p. 47).

There has been considerable attention paid to gender differences in the size and shape of the corpus callosum, the main connecting pathway between the two hemispheres, and the anterior commissure, which connects the two sides of the olfactory system. Reports of differences between men and women have not only been inconsistent but have also generated much controversy (Fausto-Sterling 2000; Hines 2004). In any case, the corpus callosum may be relevant to gender differences in certain aspects of cognitive function, but these are not of obvious relevance to sexual behaviour. The anterior commissure, because of its involvement in olfaction, may have some reproductive or sexual relevance, but probably of an indirect kind. Of more direct relevance is the anterior hypothalamic/preoptic area (AH/POA), which contains many androgen and E receptors, which are considered later in this chapter. In the human, four subregions of the AH/POA, named the interstitial nuclei of the anterior hypothalamus 1 to 4 (INAH 1–4), have been studied in the search for gender differences. INAH 1, which is closest to the SDN of the rat in its position, has not been consistently shown to differ in size between men and women. INAH 3, however, has been consistently shown to be larger in men and to contain more neurons in men than in women. The relevance of this difference to sexuality is unclear (Hines 2004) (see Fig. 4.4).

The BNST, which also contains steroid-concentrating neurons, has attracted attention. The postero-medial region of the BNST has been found to be larger in men (Allen & Gorski 1990) and has been shown to be activated during ejaculation in male rats, but so far such activation has not been demonstrated in brain-imaging studies of men (Stoleru & Mouras 2007). The central region of the BNST has been shown to be smaller in six male to female transsexuals than in heterosexual or homosexual men, and more similar to the size in women, raising the possibility that it is related in some way to core gender identity (Zhou et al 1995). In animals, the BNST is involved in some way with sexual behaviour, but its precise function is not understood (Allen & Gorski 1990). The gender difference in the size of the BNST may not become established until adolescence (Chung et al 2002).

A possible human equivalent of the spinal nucleus of the bulbo-cavernosus, which is bigger in the male rat than in the female, is Onuf's nucleus, which controls

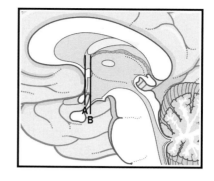

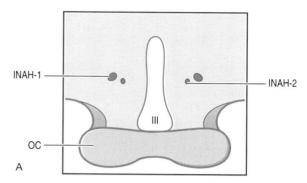

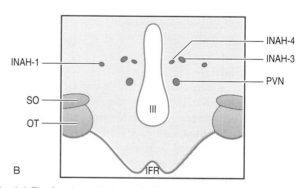

Fig. 4.4 The four interstitial nuclei of the anterior hypothalamus (INAH-1 to INAH-4) in the human brain. The section shown in **(A)** is about 800 μm anterior to the one in **(B)**. IFR, infundibular recess; OT, optic tract; OC, optic chiasm; PVN, paraventricular nucleus; SO, supraoptic nucleus; III, third ventricle. (Adapted from Gorski 2000 with permission.)

striated muscles of the penis (Steers 2000) and has been found to be bigger in the male (Hines 2004).

Brain-imaging studies of activation in response to sexual stimuli in men and women are considered later in this chapter.

Brain development during childhood and adolescence

In the past decade there have been substantial advances in human and primate neuroscience, helped by new techniques of structural and functional brain imaging (see p. 56). It is now clear that there are major changes in the brain during the second decade of life. These have been summarized in an excellent review by Weinberger et al (2005), comprehensible to non-experts, and a basis for the following account.

The brain doubles in size from birth to young adulthood, and the surface folds become more complex, reflecting a substantial change in the number of synapses, with both development of new synapses and regression of earlier ones. The first 5 years post-natally is a time of major plasticity in this respect. Most synapses are either excitatory, mediated by glutamate, or inhibitory, mediated by gamma-aminobutyric acid (GABA) (see p. 24). The balance between excitatory and inhibitory synapses changes during childhood and adolescence, with the predominance shifting from excitatory, during early childhood, to inhibitory by early adulthood. There are also increased connections between different brain regions, with greater myelination of neurons increasing the speed of neuronal transmission. These maturational processes occur earliest in the brain areas dealing with more fundamental mechanisms, such as limb and eye movements. The prefrontal cortex, in contrast, is not fully myelinated until well into the third decade of life. Neuronal mechanisms involved in response to alerting and orienting signals become more efficient. This is shown in dopaminergic (DA) pathways to the prefrontal cortex, which are crucial for focusing attention on relevant stimuli when choosing between alternative options for responding, especially when memory is required for making the choice. According to Weinberger et al (2005), dopamine inputs to the prefrontal cortex increase dramatically during adolescence, probably contributing to increased capacity for more mature judgments and impulse control. The hippocampus is involved in the establishment of new memory, and changes in synaptic organization, myelination and DA neurotransmission also occur in the hippocampus during adolescence. The way that the prefrontal cortex, hippocampus and amygdala interact in the processing of environmental stimuli changes during adolescence, leading to greater control of previously automatic response patterns. The connection between the hippocampus and the cingulate cortex, involved in emotions, increases, with a doubling of myelin content during adolescence, facilitating connections between gut feelings and intellectual processes. Brain-imaging studies with fMRI have assessed how adolescents and adults process emotional stimuli (Baird et al 1999). When asked to identify the emotion expressed in the picture of a face, adolescents show activation of the amygdala, involved in the primal assessment of fear. Adults, in contrast, activate the frontal lobes and identify the expressed emotions more correctly. This is seen to indicate that adults ask questions first, whereas adolescents reach more intuitive conclusions.

These functional changes are relevant to a series of fundamental developments. Adults whose frontal lobes are damaged often lack inhibitory control. In comparison with normal adults, children show less inhibitory control, and adolescents perform relatively inefficiently in coping with inhibitory tasks, pointing to the emergence of these functions through adolescence. The ability to work out complex plans, using working memory, is also impaired by frontal lobe damage and has not reached adult levels during adolescence. Decision making, which requires the assessment of both long-term and short-term probabilities and is particularly important in the appraisal of risk, is again impaired as a result of frontal lobe damage in adults and is not fully developed during adolescence.

It is easy to see how such brain development is of fundamental importance to adolescent development. Adolescence is not just a matter of learning new skills, but also of developing brain mechanisms to facilitate such learning. In addition, this developmental phase may involve increased difficulty in carrying out some tasks (e.g. avoiding distraction) before a more adult function is achieved, contributing to the increased risk-taking characteristic of adolescence (Powell 2006). The factors that influence such brain development are as yet not well understood. Genetic factors may play a part, but experience is also likely to be relevant, following the principle that new synaptic networks evolve in response to their need. On that basis it is important that the adolescent strives to grapple with these challenges. The relevance of pubertal hormonal changes to these developments are not yet clear in humans, but there is some indication that age at puberty may have important consequences, presumably because hormonal changes may occur at different stages of brain development (Sisk 2006).

As yet no direct relationships between such brain development and sexual development have been demonstrated. However, we should not expect to find specifically sexual brain mechanisms, but rather complex interactions of more general mechanisms, such as impulse control and risk assessment, influencing our sexual behaviour. The progress from a gut feelings response to a more intellectually-based appraisal may be important for understanding how we attribute meaning to otherwise gut-feeling sexual experiences, which may themselves be hormone dependent. When do we recognize, for example, that the physiological changes in our genitalia and their association with general arousal constitute sexual arousal? The ability to do this probably increases as we enter and progress through adolescence. Even a young adult may occasionally have experiences of bodily change that are wrongly assigned to anxiety rather than sexual arousal. We therefore need to keep these cognitive developmental stages, based on brain development, in our mind as we strive to understand sexual arousal in adult life in this chapter, and as we tackle the process of sexual development through childhood and adolescence in Chapter 5.

The emotional brain

We will be arguing later that the sexual experience is, at least in part, an emotional experience, and, for that reason, we need to consider the brain mechanisms underlying the various kinds of emotion before focusing on the sexual experience. There has been a long-running debate in neuropsychology about the nature of emotions. This has mainly centred around whether conscious feelings follow bodily changes (the James–Lange approach) or vice versa. Current thinking allows for both sequences to be involved, and there is support for Arnold's (1960) conceptualization, i.e. emotions are generated by an unconscious, implicit evaluation of a stimulus, which is followed by a tendency to act in a particular way (i.e. action tendency), which is followed by peripheral responses, and finally conscious experience. The unconscious evaluation, the action tendency and the conscious experience or 'feeling' are considered to be mediated by the cerebral cortex, whereas the peripheral (autonomic) responses, which prepare the body for action, are mediated by the hypothalamus, with the amygdala probably playing a crucial organizing role in the interaction between these central and peripheral components. It is the phylogenetically more primitive areas of the cerebral cortex that are mainly involved in the central processing, i.e. the prefrontal limbic cortex and the limbic lobe, which surrounds the brain stem, composed of the cingulate gyrus and the hippocampal formation (i.e. hippocampus, dentate gyrus and subiculum). It is these parts of the brain that were originally identified by Papez in the 1930s as the limbic system. This concept was extended by MacLean in the 1950s to incorporate parts of the hypothalamus, the septal area, the nucleus accumbens in the ventral striatum, the orbitofrontal cortex and the amygdala. The current view differs principally by seeing the amygdala and not the hippocampus as playing the integrating role between the central (cortical) and peripheral (autonomic) components. The hippocampus is involved, however, in the memorizing of emotional experience (Iversen et al 2000). This revised version of the limbic system has been labelled the 'emotional brain' by LeDoux (1996).

Crucial to the emotional brain is the neurochemistry mediating its various functions. Peptides and monoamines are crucial to the emotional brain and will be considered further. Steroid hormones, such as T and oestradiol, are also important, with substantial evidence of their receptors in the emotional brain, as well as in other parts of the cerebral cortex. As these are of obvious relevance to sexuality, they will be considered in detail later in this chapter.

Peptides

The basic neurochemistry of peptides was summarized in Chapter 3. Although peptides are released in many different parts of the body, neuropeptides are produced in substantial amounts within the CNS. With the evolution of the blood–brain barrier, the mammalian brain has been able to develop peptidergic communication independent of classically hormonal effects that may occur from the same peptides in the peripheral circulation. The emotional brain is characterized by peptidergic neurotransmission, contrasting with the synaptic neuronal structure of the cortex (Herbert 1993) and consistent with the more primitive phylogenetic origins of the structures involved in the emotional brain. The specific effect of a peptide may depend on its site of action or even the context in which it is acting. We will consider the relevance of oxytocin (OT), β-endorphin and prolactin (PRL) on sexual response and orgasm in this chapter.

Monoamines

Most of the monoaminergic innervation of the emotional brain comes from five fibre systems ascending from the brain stem. These are the (i) noradrenergic (or norepinephric[1]) (NA), (ii) dopaminergic (DA), (iii) serotonergic (5HT), (iv) cholinergic (ACh) and (v) histaminergic systems (Role & Kelly 1991).

1. *The NA system*, which in terms of numbers of neurons is the smallest, originates principally in dorsal and ventral columns in the brain stem. The dorsal column includes the l.c., also known as the A6 group, sitting dorsally and laterally in the periaqueductal and periventricular grey matter of the pons. The ascending projections from the l.c. terminate quite widely in the dorsal thalamus, hypothalamus, basal forebrain, including hippocampus, and the frontal cortex. The descending projections from the l.c. go to the spinal cord (mainly ventral horn) and to sensory nuclei in the brain stem. The l.c. receives two major inputs, from the nucleus paragigantocellularis, in the rostral medulla, and the nucleus prepositus hypoglossi, also in the brain stem. The ventral column in the brain stem includes the A5 and A7 groups, located in the ventrolateral reticular formation of the pons and projecting mainly to the spinal cord.

   The l.c. is activated by novel sensory input, with a role in orienting and attending to sudden contrasting or aversive sensory input. The NA neurons from the l.c. have both excitatory (e.g. in the hippocampus) and inhibitory effects (in other cortical areas). The A5 and A7 components of the NA system are involved in integration of autonomic function in brain stem and spinal cord nuclei. Direct activation of these neurons reduces blood pressure and heart rate (Saper 2000).

   There are five different NA receptors: α1 and 2, and β1, 2 and 3. α1 receptors mediate the contractile effect of NA on smooth muscle, including that in the erectile tissues of the penis and clitoris; α2 receptors are mainly presynaptic, i.e. their stimulation increases reuptake of NA at the synapse and hence reduces NA post-synaptic transmission. However, α2 receptors are also found post-synaptically, where their function is not well understood. β1 receptors are involved in the stimulatory effect of NA on the heart; β2 receptors mediate smooth muscle relaxation in the lungs, gastrointestinal tract and urogenital system, relevant to the sexual side effects of β2 blockers; β3 receptors are involved in fat metabolism.

2. *The dopaminergic system* contains three to four times as many neurons as the NA systems but is less diffuse, being highly organized topographically into five subsystems. The first three are the meso-striatal system (projecting from the substantia nigra and ventral tegmentum to the striatum), the meso-limbic system (from the ventral tegmentum to limbic and cortical areas) and the meso-cortical system. In addition, there are two smaller and more localized DA systems, the incerto-hypothalamic (or A14) periventricular (which projects from DA neurons along the wall of the third ventricle to the MPOA) and the tubero-infundibular

---

[1]The term noradrenaline (NA) rather than norepinephrine (NE) is used in this book.

(from the arcuate nucleus of the hypothalamus to the pituitary stalk), which are important for reproductive behaviour and neuroendocrine control, respectively (Role & Kelly 1991).

3. *The serotonergic system.* In terms of numbers of neurons, the 5HT system is the most extensive of the three. The majority of neurons are located within the raphe nuclei (named because of their midline position near the raphe or seam of the brainstem). The more caudal of these nuclei provide the descending serotonergic projections to the spinal cord, whereas the upper raphe nuclei project rostrally through the median forebrain bundle to a variety of target sites, the dorsal raphe nucleus mainly to the frontal cortex and striatum, and the median raphe nucleus mainly to the septum and hippocampus. These neurons are mainly inhibitory in their effects.

4. *The cholinergic system.* The two largest ACh cell groups in the midbrain, the pedunculopontine and laterodorsal tegmental nuclei, innervate the brain stem and thalamus, and are involved in regulating sleep–wake cycles. In the basal forebrain, neurons from the nucleus basalis of Meynert project to the cerebral cortex where they enhance responses to sensory input.

5. *The histaminergic system* has neurons from the tuberomammilary nucleus of the posterior lateral hypothalamus projecting to most parts of the brain, similar to the NA neurons from the l.c. They are also involved in maintaining arousal (Saper 2000).

The autonomic nervous system

The principal neurotransmitters in the autonomic nervous system are acetylcholine (ACh) and NA, although at each level a variety of other neurotransmitters and neuromodulators are involved, including adenosine triphosphate (ATP), vasoactive polypeptide (VIP) and neuropeptide Y. As we shall see later, nitric oxide (NO) is a key neurotransmitter involved in vasodilatation and smooth muscle relaxation in various parts of the body, including the genitalia. At the level of the autonomic ganglion, whether sympathetic or parasympathetic, ACh is the principal neurotransmitter, by means of nicotinic receptors. At the distal end of the post-ganglionic neuron, ACh is the principal neurotransmitter for the parasympathetic (via muscarinic receptors) and NA for the sympathetic system.

Emotional excitation and inhibition

The concept of a balance between excitation and inhibition is fundamental to neurophysiology, although in most respects at the neuronal level, i.e. each neuron, at least within the CNS, has both excitatory and inhibitory neurons acting on it. But at that level, the interplay between positive and negative inputs can have a wide variety of outcomes, e.g. an inhibitory signal can have a disinhibiting effect by acting on an inhibitory neuron. The issue becomes more relevant to our purpose when we consider excitatory and inhibitory systems within the CNS.

Emotion, as considered so far, can have negative or positive valence. Gray (1994) has proposed three fundamental emotion systems: a behavioural approach system (BAS), a fight/flight system (F/FLS) and a behavioural inhibition system (BIS). The first two involve action, i.e. approach for reward or fight/flight to avoid punishment. The third involves inhibition or inaction, accompanied by increased arousal and attention, as a way of coping with threat. We will be considering these three types of emotion in relation to the Dual Control model. Arousal mechanisms are relevant to all three of Gray's emotional systems. We need to consider *general arousal*, which activates the individual in a non-specific way. This appears to be influenced by the NA, ACh and histaminergic systems. We also need to consider *specific arousal*, which prepares the body for specific types of action. Here the neurochemical basis is less well understood. This is clearly of relevance to sexual arousal, and we will return to this concept later.

Gamma-aminobutyric acid (GABA) and 5HT are major inhibitory neurotransmitters in the brain and spinal cord. GABA is widely, though unevenly, distributed in the mammalian central nervous system. Because of its ubiquitous nature, it can be expected to play a role in inhibiting inhibitory as well as excitatory processes. This is well demonstrated by Gray's (1987) Behavioral Inhibition System, the effects of which can be reversed by drugs such as benzodiazepines, which amplify effects of GABA by their action on the GABA$_A$–benzodiazepine receptor complex. As discussed above, the extensive 5HT system projecting from the brainstem has predominantly inhibitory effects in many parts of the brain.

The first of Gray's systems, BAS, raises a key question. What determines approach behaviour and to what extent are such determinants separate and different from the experience of reward that may follow? This, in other words, asks about the neurophysiology of pleasure and the anticipation of pleasure, of central relevance to the experience of sexual arousal. Much consideration has been given to the effects of drugs of addiction as providing insight into the basic mechanisms of incentive and reward. This has resulted in a vigorous debate about whether the addiction process results from an effect of the drug on incentive or from the hedonic, pleasurable effects of the drug (Robinson & Berridge 2000). In the animal literature, attention has focused on the distinction between appetitive and consummatory behaviour. The assumption is that appetitive behaviour indicates incentive or motivation whereas consummatory behaviour involves reward. Unfortunately, one cannot ask animals about the very subjective experience of 'pleasure', which can be regarded as the conscious manifestation of the reward process, whether the reward involves food, water or sex. Nevertheless, Robbins & Everitt (1996), in reviewing the relevant animal literature, concluded that there is a basic distinction between appetitive and consummatory behaviours in terms of the brain mechanisms involved, with activation of the mesolimbic DA system projecting from the ventral tegmentum to the ventral striatum, in particular the nucleus accumbens, being more relevant to appetitive behaviour. Salamone & Correa (2002) presented evidence that, with eating behaviour, low doses of DA antagonists and depletion of DA in the nucleus accumbens reduce the likelihood of an animal working to obtain food (i.e. reduction of 'instrumental responses that have a high degree of work related response costs') without impairing appetite to consume food. How the reward, or 'liking', as distinct from 'wanting', is mediated remains an open question. We will return to this issue when considering the role of the DA systems in sexual arousal and response and subsequently orgasm.

Where does sex fit in?

In the view of many sex researchers (e.g. Rosen & Beck 1988), and in this book, sexual arousal is seen as a specific example of an emotional response. In a positive sexual context, this is a sexual example of Gray's BAS. We can assume that this involves an unconscious, implicit evaluation of a stimulus, associated with a tendency to act in a particular way (i.e. action tendency), which can be regarded as a form of incentive motivation, accompanied by a state of general arousal, centrally and peripherally, and the occurrence of specific genital responses. This, sooner or later, will be experienced consciously as a sexual event. In a negative sexual context, or a context when it is adaptive to avoid sexual response and behaviour, we may see an example of Gray's third system, with inhibition of the more specifically sexual components, but with varying degrees of general arousal or 'alertness'. These two response patterns have been embodied in our Dual Control model, presented in Chapter 2, which postulates that the occurrence of sexual arousal will depend on a balance between the activating or excitatory system of sexual response and the inhibition of sexual response. Our model assumes that positive and negative aspects of a sexual, or potentially sexual, context can coexist. And we will examine these two arms of the model more closely.

But first we need to acknowledge two possible differences between the human experience and how we, as observers, conceptualize the sexual experience in other species. First, is the distinction between appetitive and consummatory sexual behaviour, central to much of animal sex research, as considered above. Such distinctions, in the experimental context, are based on the difference between a behaviour aimed at gaining access to the sexual partner (appetitive) and, once access is gained, the process of mounting or accepting being mounted (consummatory). When we consider the distinction between appetitive and consummatory behaviour in relation to human sexual experience, we can perhaps distinguish between states that only involve desire for sexual contact, where the anticipation of reward is the incentive motivation, or behaviours that, explicitly or implicitly, are in pursuit of some kind of sexual reward and involve engagement in some form of sexual activity that is pleasurable and hence rewarding. However, this is not necessarily a clear-cut distinction, as the imagination of

impending sexual reward (the fantasy) may in itself be rewarding. Once consummatory behaviour starts, either with a partner or on one's own during masturbation, the process of sexual stimulation may be pleasurable and hence rewarding, as well as arousing. In addition, however, there is the anticipation of possible further rewarding interaction as well as the ultimate reward, at least for some individuals, associated with the experience of orgasm. We will consider the neurobiology of orgasm later in this chapter.

Secondly, we should consider the range of possible rewards of sexual behaviour, which are likely to influence the incentive motivation. Certainly there is a wide range of rewards or motives for human sexual behaviour apart from sexual pleasure and orgasm (Bancroft 1994). The range of what might be called functions of sexual behaviour and their relevance to sexual development are discussed more fully in Chapter 5 (p. 146).

In the human, we also have to consider more closely the distinction between conscious and unconscious processing. This has been well summarized by Janssen et al (2000), who contrasted automatic processes, which are fast and unconscious, with controlled or attentional processes, which are conscious. The automatic processes are nevertheless cognitive and are fundamental to the appraisal of emotional events. In sex research much more attention has been paid to the conscious, attentional processes, than the automatic appraisal. We will return to this crucial issue in the section on information processing. In the meantime, we should keep in mind that a sexual experience, which is characterized by general arousal and incentive motivation, requires involvement of the emotional brain and cannot result simply from conscious, attentional processing.

The distinction between sexual arousal and sexual desire

This has become a vexed issue in the sexological literature. I would argue that, rather than attempting to distinguish between sexual arousal and sexual desire, we should consider varying degrees of involvement of the emotional processes at any one time. Thus with full-blown sexual arousal we have unconscious appraisal, controlled or attentional processing, incentive motivation (a desire to 'do something about it', i.e. seek the potential reward), central and peripheral arousal of a general kind, and genital response, which is part of the sexual essence of the experience. (I prefer not to regard genital response per se as arousal, as it can occur without other aspects of arousal.) 'Sexual desire', as incentive motivation, could be experienced with only part of this pattern of response, or at least with some parts being much more evident than others. Thus, an individual might be aware of the incentive motivational state with little in the way of general arousal or genital response. Experiences of desire may also vary in the extent to which attentional processes are involved, although the assumption is that some automatic appraisal, of external, internal or peripheral cues, has taken place. Thus, I am proposing that the conventional distinction between sexual arousal and sexual desire involves constructs that we have attempted to impose rather than a useful way of conceptualizing reality. Instead, I prefer to see these two constructs as two 'windows' into the complexity of sexual arousal as described above, one focusing on the incentive motivation component (desire) and the other on the arousal component (excitement).

And what about love?

One of the prevailing criticisms of Alfred Kinsey's work was his focus on sex and his apparent neglect of love. He found sex, as a subject of scientific inquiry, difficult enough. He was probably overwhelmed by the idea of researching love. Later in the chapter we will look at the limited amount of evidence from brain-imaging studies of people looking at pictures of their loved ones. In this case, even more so than sexual desire, we are dealing with a human construct, which has uncertain connections to basic psychobiological processes. In other words, is 'love', as we see it, a discrete emotional state, or is it a composite of various interacting components, which when combined together, set it apart as 'something special'? A common distinction, at least among scholars, is between 'passionate' (or 'romantic') love and 'companionate' love. Clearly, it is passionate love which is most likely to overlap with sexual arousal or sexual desire, although the extent to which sex fosters intimacy may well make it relevant to companionate love as well. Hatfield & Rapson (1993) defined passionate love as follows:

'A state of intense longing for union with another. Passionate love is a complex functional whole including appraisals or appreciations, subjective feelings, expressions, patterned physiological processes, action tendencies, and instrumental behaviors. Reciprocated love (union with the other) is associated with fulfillment and ecstasy. Unrequited love (separation) is associated with feelings of emptiness, anxiety and despair'

(p. 5).

The interesting cultural differences and similarities in the role that passionate love plays in people's lives will be considered further in Chapter 6. There are various terminologies used in attempts to conceptualize love, and these will be briefly considered in Chapter 6. However, romantic love seems to carry the same meaning as passionate love, with perhaps a different nuance; possibly the need for reciprocation to make the experience 'romantic'. These concepts will be considered further later in this chapter (p. 130).

As we shall see from the brain-imaging evidence, various types of brain activity are involved in relation to passionate or romantic love. As with sexual arousal and desire, we are dealing with a complex emotional state resulting from the interplay between a range of functions. It is our need to have a unitary concept such as 'passionate love' or 'sexual desire' that gets us into difficulties. At best, they are our attempts to simplify the complexity of emotional experience.

Central control of sexual excitation and inhibition

The need for inhibitory mechanisms

It has been assumed for some time that an interaction between excitatory and inhibitory mechanisms determines the species-specific pattern of sexual behaviour (Beach 1967; Kurtz & Adler 1973; Sachs & Barfield 1976). However, evidence for such inhibitory mechanisms has been largely indirect and has received much less research attention than the excitatory mechanisms. Such paired systems are very familiar in neurophysiology, although they vary in complexity and in the type of purpose they serve. There are purely homeostatic systems, such as those that control body temperature or blood pressure, where the interplay between positive and negative feedback signals is designed to maintain a steady state, within relatively narrow limits. Control of food intake is a further interesting example, more complex than temperature regulation, and having some features in common with control of sexual behaviour. This can also be seen as a feedback system maintaining a steady state, in this case body weight, although in contrast to temperature, the system can be set to achieve widely differing body weights across individuals, and even within the same individual over time. When we consider the control of sexual behaviour, there is no direct individual-based homeostatic parallel. The occurrence of sexual activity carries a cost, at least in terms of risk, whereas the absence of sexual activity has no cost to the individual (apart from the lack of reward from sexual interaction, and the problem of frustration from unfulfilled sexual desire). However, the fact that sexual activity may result in reproduction, and inhibition of sexual activity avoids reproduction, raises the issue of homeostatic control of population density (i.e. a homeostat for the group rather than the individual). For most mammals studied in this respect, there is maintenance of a fairly stable population density, which is only destabilized by major environmental changes. In Chapter 2, we considered Marvin Harris's explanations for the major change in human population size that followed the change from hunter-gatherer-type human social groups to agricultural social systems, and, in one way or another, this probably reflected some form of homeostat for human groups. But for some reason not as yet understood, it is difficult to find evidence of such regulation of human population density in more recent times.

Bjorklund & Kipp (1996) made the persuasive case that inhibitory mechanisms became necessary in small groups of hominids for the purposes of cooperation, group cohesion and individual political success. The two response patterns most in need of inhibition for these purposes, they suggest, are sexual and aggressive behaviour. The comparison of these two is of interest. While, with aggression, inhibition is beneficial in many social situations, in other situations lack of aggression is dangerous. Inhibition of sex is not quite like that, although it can be likened to the inhibition of aggressive behaviour. Certainly, in many social primates there is evidence of inhibition of sexual behaviour organized around the dominance hierarchy (Dixson 1998). It is potentially dangerous for a low-dominance animal to be sexually active in the presence of a high-dominance member of the group. There are no obvious risks from avoiding sexual activity, apart from the aggressive response it might induce in a potential partner whose sexual needs are thwarted. Furthermore, beyond the social context, engagement in sexual activity reduces vigilance and therefore may increase vulnerability to a variety of threats and, if pursued excessively, may reduce attention to other important adaptive functions.

Fertility is also dependent on inhibition of sexual response in a variety of ways. The simplest example is the inhibition of sexual arousal following ejaculation in the male, the refractory period, to avoid excessive sexual activity and repeated ejaculations, which, over a short time period, result in lowering of the available sperm store. More complex is the organization of sexual behaviour, by hormonal mechanisms, to occur around the time of ovulation, the oestrous pattern, which maximizes the chance of fertile mating. It has been proposed that the main effect of reproductive hormones on sexual behaviour is to reduce inhibition of sexual responses in a permissive fashion (Beach 1967). This is of particular relevance to the female who, in most species, has to expose herself to mounting and penetration by another animal, a situation that in other circumstances would be threatening and potentially dangerous. In addition, such penetration has the potential to cause pain, and recent research has shown specific pain-reducing mechanisms in females associated with coitus, possibly mediated by OT (Komisaruk & Sansone 2003). These mechanisms will be considered further in the section on genital response (p. 83).

A threat to fertility, and in some cases survival, is sexual transmission of disease. This is an issue of paramount importance to humans. Sexually transmitted diseases are also common in animals and are of particular importance in agricultural breeding as a cause of infertility and abortion (Oriel & Hayward 1974). The possibility that such infections in other species may have evolutionary significance, influencing, for example, mating patterns, is receiving increasing attention (e.g. Lockhart et al 1996). The role of inhibition of sexual response as an adaptive mechanism to avoid such risks has, as far as I am aware, not been considered or studied in other species, but obviously forms a large part of the relevance of this theoretical model to humans.

The biological benefits of incest avoidance may also rely on inhibition of sexual response. Keverne & Vellucci (1988) described the family groups of the marmoset that appear to involve some form of incest taboo. The father will not mate with his daughter until she has been living outside the family group for several months. Goodall (1986) also provides relevant evidence for chimpanzees, in whom sexual activity between mother and son is strikingly absent and between siblings or between father and daughter is seldom seen. The mechanisms underlying incest avoidance are not well understood and will be considered more fully in Chapter 16. Increased inhibition of sexual responsiveness, however, may well be involved.

The threat of population overcrowding, as already mentioned, is important. How do different species deal with problems of population density? Mechanisms studied include migration outward, increased mortality in some individuals, reduction of fertility and actual suppression of sexual behaviour (Wynne-Edwards 1964; Christian 1970; Wilson 1975; Gray 1987). Most, if not all, of these mechanisms are often manifested via the dominance hierarchy, with the low dominance animal being more susceptible to the stress-related increase in mortality, reduction of fertility and suppression of sexual behaviour. The likelihood that such mechanisms are, at least in part, genetically determined poses a problem for evolutionary biologists, which, as yet, remains unresolved. If a genetically determined susceptibility to overcrowding is involved then such genes would soon disappear. The best attempt to get round this dilemma is the concept of coupled genetic oscillators discussed by Wilson (1975), which proposes that there is more than one genetically determined mechanism, so that as one begins to be 'non-bred' out of existence, another mechanism takes over, allowing the first to reappear.

This fundamentally important notion of inhibition of sexual behaviour or suppression of fertility as a method of controlling population density does not translate easily into human terms (Freedman 1998). Furthermore, it confronts us with an apparent paradox, i.e. the existence of two contradictory adaptive goals: maintaining fertility and, in situations of overcrowding, reducing fertility or at least reproduction. Yet this paradox, ironically, is captured by two of the principal threats facing the human race at the present time — overpopulation and the threat of sexually transmitted diseases to both fertility and survival.

It is therefore relatively easy to make the case for the adaptive function of inhibition of sexual response and behaviour and, furthermore, to regard it as having a fundamental cross-species role. Thus, we might expect to find physiological mechanisms involved, of relevance across species.

Functions of sexual inhibition

At this stage we can recognize four situations in which inhibition of sexual activity may be adaptive for both males and females: (i) when sexual activity carries some threat or danger (e.g. attack from other more dominant males, or risk of sexually transmitted disease, or unwanted pregnancy); (ii) where a non-sexual threat exists, and inhibition of otherwise distracting response patterns, including sexual, is necessary for focusing on the appropriate avoidance response; (iii) when excessive involvement in the pursuit of sexual pleasure distracts from other important adaptive functions; and (iv) when social or environmental pressures result in suppression of reproductive behaviour and reduction of population density. For the male, an additional situation is when the consequences of continued 'excessive' sexual behaviour includes reduction of fertility due to excessive ejaculation and, for the female, when a potential sexual partner is unsuitable for reproductive purposes, reflected in the relationship factor from the SESII-W described in Chapter 2 (p. 16). We should keep in mind that these six different needs for inhibition of sexual behaviour may involve different inhibitory mechanisms or systems.

Now let us return to the animal evidence and consider to what extent the neurochemistry of the emotional brain relates to sexual excitation and sexual inhibition.

Animal evidence

Peptides

There is some evidence that OT plays a role in the sexual excitation system. Most notable is a direct hypothalamic–spinal pathway originating in the parvocellular region of the paraventricular nucleus (PVN) of the hypothalamus, stimulation of which induces erection, with OT as the neurotransmitter (McKenna 2000). Injection of OT into the PVN elicits penile erection. Hypothalamic–hippocampal oxytocinergic pathways may also be involved in control of penile erection (Heaton 2000).

β-Endorphin is the endogenous opiate that has received the most research attention, and this is considered more closely in the section on hormones and sexual response. While β-endorphin clearly has inhibitory effects, these do seem to be dose dependent, with certain levels producing enhancing effects of sexual response, probably because of actions in a different part of the brain (see p. 129).

The monoaminergic systems and sexual response

Dopamine

Dopaminergic mechanisms are involved in aspects of the sexual excitation system. There is a substantial body of evidence showing that DA agonists enhance and DA antagonists impair male sexual behaviour (Bitran & Hull 1987). Experiments in which specific D1 or D2 DA receptors were selectively involved, or where local infusion of drugs or dialysis allowed investigation of DA action in discrete areas of the brain, have contributed to a more complex picture of DA activity as it relates to male sexual behaviour (Everitt & Bancroft 1991; Melis & Argiolas 1995). Hull et al (1998) concluded that three of the five DA systems impact on sexual behaviour, two of them in a relatively non-specific way and one more specifically sexual. First, the nigro-striatal tract (from the substantia nigra to the dorsal striatum), degeneration of which causes Parkinson's disease — this is involved in the organization of motor behaviour, particularly initiation of motor responses and 'readiness to respond', which includes copulatory, but also many other integrated motor patterns. Second, the meso-limbic tract (from the ventral tegmentum to the ventral striatum, and other parts of the emotional brain) — this promotes appetite for a variety of appetitive behaviours, including sexual. It is therefore involved in the incentive motivational process. Third, the DA input to the MPOA from the A14 periventricular system — the MPOA

receives sensory input from many parts of the brain and is involved in a number of response patterns, apart from sexual, including maternal behaviour, temperature regulation, thirst and water balance, and some aspects of cardiovascular function (McKenna 2000). When serving a more specifically sexual function, it helps to orchestrate genital responses and stereotyped sexual motor patterns such as mounting or thrusting. While there is a remarkable consistency across species in the role that the MPOA plays in the orchestration of consummatory responses, there is less agreement about its possible role in appetitive responses (e.g. Everitt 1995; Baum 1995 and following discussion). If the MPOA does have a role in sexual motivation, then its DA activity may be relevant to this (Hull et al 1995). DA therefore plays a role in our sexual excitation system, though its effects on the MPOA may depend on disinhibition of inhibitory tone (Hull et al 1998).

Apomorphine is a dopamine agonist with mainly D2 receptor effects, and its administration can lead to penile erection, probably via interaction with the oxytocinergic mechanisms of the PVN and possibly via effects on the MPOA (Heaton 2000).

Noradrenaline

The NA systems present us with a complex and seemingly paradoxical picture. Evidence of effects of β receptors in the reproductive organs is inconclusive, though their role in bladder control presents an interesting comparison with genital response. In the bladder, contraction of the bladder wall necessary for emptying of the bladder results from parasympathetic activation, whereas activation of β receptors relaxes the bladder wall (Iversen et al 2000). In the periphery, α receptor activation blocks genital response, at least in the male, by contracting erectile smooth muscle (Riley 1994). This is relatively straightforward in the case of α1 receptors that are post-synaptic and that induce smooth muscle contraction. It is less straightforward with α2 receptors; as discussed above, these are predominantly pre-synaptic, their activation resulting in reabsorption of NA, effectively reducing NA activation of the post-synaptic receptors. However, α2 receptors are also found post-synaptically. The fact that intracavernosal injection of idazoxan, an α2 antagonist, has little or no effect on the erectile tissues (see Table 4.1) has been taken to suggest that the pre- and post-synaptic effects of α2 receptor activation in these tissues cancel each other out.

By contrast with these peripheral effects, drugs that increase central NA transmission or availability at α receptors increase various aspects of male rat sexual behaviour consistent with an enhancing effect on central arousal relevant to sexual activity (Bitran & Hull 1987; Wilson 1993). Central α effects appear to be complex, however. Sala et al (1990) demonstrated an inverted U dose–response curve, with middle range doses producing maximal enhancing effects and high doses inhibitory effects. Dose–response relationships of this kind are not well understood. They may reflect a shift from predominantly pre- to post-synaptic effect as the dosage increases, either involving, in this case, α2 receptors both

TABLE 4.1	Effects of intracavernosal injections of drugs (from Brindley 1984)	
Effect		**Duration**
PRODUCING FULL ERECTION		
Phenoxybenzamine		1–6 h
Papaverine		2–2.5 h
Phentolamine		5–10 min
Verapamil		2–2.5 min
Thymoxamine		1–2.5 min
CAUSING SWELLING OF PENIS BUT NEVER FULL ERECTION		
Guanethidine		
Naftidrofuryl oxalate		
CAUSING SHRINKAGE OF ERECTILE TISSUE		
Metaraminol		
Imipramine		
Clonidine		
CAUSING LITTLE OR NO EFFECT		
Atropine		
Neostigmine		
Morphine		
Dextromoramide		
Lignocaine		
Hydralazine		
Idazoxan		

pre- and post-synaptically or, alternatively, shifting from pre-synaptic α2 to post-synaptic α1 receptor action with the higher dose (Andersson 1995). Sala et al (1990) also suggest that the NA system may have very complex inter-relationships with the DA and 5HT systems, accounting for these apparently inconsistent effects. Perhaps, as a result of this complexity, much less attention has been paid to the central role of NA transmission in relation to sexual behaviour, compared with other neurotransmitters. We will consider later how NA α2 receptor activity may be involved in mediating the central effects of T on sexual response.

As discussed above, the NA system is involved in inhibition of male genital response in the periphery. The descending neurons from the l.c. may contribute to this. In the rat, transneuronal labelling with the pseudorabies virus demonstrated a clear link between neurons in the penis and the l.c. However, these studies also showed a link between other somatic and autonomic, non-sexual neurons and the l.c., indicating that the l.c. has more downstream functions than sexual (McKenna 1999). While supraspinal inhibition of genital reflexive response is likely to result from direct inhibition of the spinal reflex centres (mediated in part by 5HT), inhibitory influences on erectile response are also implemented by an antierectile sympathetic outflow, originating in the caudal sympathetic chain (see p. 58). The evidence also suggests that there may be two sets of such fibres, one acting on the arterial blood supply to the penis and the other on the sinusoidal smooth muscle in the corpora cavernosa. It is likely that both sets involve NA neurotransmission.

Hence the paradox; central effects of NA on sexual response are excitatory and peripheral effects are inhibitory, mediated via the α1 receptor, causing smooth muscle contraction. The first fundamental point in tackling this paradox is to remember that the excitatory central effects of the NA system are not confined to sexual arousal (see above). In many circumstances, it is entirely appropriate that elicitation of general central arousal should require localized peripheral inhibition of genital response. Thus, if the NA system generates arousal in response to the threat of punishment, an emotional state that in those circumstances Gray (1987) would call 'anxiety', then inhibition of other response patterns, such as sexual response, which might interfere with an appropriate avoidance response, would be adaptive. Conversely, when central arousal is in response to sexual stimuli, we might expect peripheral inhibition of genital response to be reduced. The integrating component of the system is presumably the l.c., with both its upward and downward projections. However, one of the principal mysteries of the central NA system is how it is mobilized to serve sexual function in some situations and avoidance behaviour in others. Testosterone may be relevant to this selective process (see below).

The situation is further complicated by the uncertain role of β2 receptors, through which NA causes smooth muscle relaxation in the urogenital system. How relevant this is to genital response is not clear, but β blockers, particularly those that are not specifically β1 blockers, are likely to cause erectile problems and possibly lowered sexual interest (Bochinski & Brock 2001). The relevance of β2 receptors in the brain to sexual arousal is also not clear.

In conclusion, whereas it is clear that the central NA system is of fundamental importance to sexual arousal and response, we have many uncertainties about how it functions in that respect.

Histamine and acetylcholine

As yet there is no clear evidence that the histaminergic system is relevant to sexual response and only limited evidence that the ACh system in the emotional brain is involved; ACh neurons in the hippocampus facilitate erections (Steers 2000).

Serotonin

For our inhibitory system, we find evidence for a role of serotonin. Studies of the male rat show that drugs that increase serotonergic transmission inhibit and those that disrupt serotonergic transmission enhance male sexual behaviour (see reviews by Bitran & Hull 1987; Wilson 1993). However, there are a number of complexities that have to be borne in mind. First, most such drugs also affect a variety of other behaviours such as eating, aggression and general motor activity (Everitt & Bancroft 1991). Hence, we are considering serotonergic inhibition of a non-specific kind. Second, there are a variety of 5HT receptors; central inhibition of behaviour, including sexual, is most clearly related to the 5HT2 receptor, whereas, by contrast, the 5HT1A variety is predominantly an auto-receptor on the cell body and dendrites, activation of which reduces 5HT transmission through that neuron. Third, drug effects are often complex and apparently contradictory depending on their site of action or dose. Thus, 8-OH-DPAT, in addition to decreasing 5HT release by its 5HT1A agonist effect, also increases 5HT in the MPOA (Lorrain et al 1998). Also, experiments with lysergic acid diethylamide (LSD), a 5HT1A agonist, indicate a U-shaped dose–response curve, with low doses facilitating and high doses inhibiting behaviour. As with central NA effects, this complex picture can be explained by low doses preferentially affecting the auto-receptors and high doses predominantly affecting post-synaptic receptors (Bitran & Hull 1987).

Localization of the specifically sexual inhibitory effects of 5HT is evident in the lateral hypothalamic area where, following ejaculation, an increase in 5HT has been reported (Lorrain et al 1997), and in the nucleus paragigantocellularis, situated in the medulla (Marson & McKenna 1992). This nucleus, via its descending serotonergic neurons to the lumbosacral cord, is probably involved in the maintenance of inhibitory tone in the erectile tissues, which requires to be reduced if erection is to occur.

There is a consistent body of evidence showing that GABA and drugs with GABAergic effects have an inhibitory effect on male sexual behaviour in the rat (Bitran & Hull 1987). GABA$_B$ agonists injected intrathecally around the lumbo-sacral cord inhibit ex copula reflexive erections without apparently interfering with mounting and intromission (Bitran et al 1989). GABAergic effects may also be particularly significant during the post-ejaculatory refractory period and will be considered further in the section on orgasm.

Human evidence

In the human, we have evidence of a different and more fragmented kind. This includes the effects of pharmacological agents used to enhance sexual response, as well as the sexual side effects of drugs. The phenomenon of nocturnal penile tumescence (NPT) is of potential relevance. We also have a limited amount of evidence from brain-imaging studies and some long-established clinical evidence of the effects of spinal cord damage.

Dopamine

Evidence from clinical trials of apomorphine, a DA agonist, show effects in enhancing erectile response, which are comparable to those found in animal studies. The main difference appears to be the side-effect profile. Nausea is a common side effect in humans, and apparently in dogs, but not in rats (Heaton 2000). Evidence from clinical studies of other DA drugs, e.g. bromocriptine, or precursors, e.g. l-dopa, is somewhat inconsistent, partly because of DA side effects, such as nausea (Crenshaw & Goldberg 1996). Sexual side effects are also common in men and women using dopamine antagonists for the treatment of psychotic conditions such as schizophrenia, although the complexity of such conditions, together with the mixed pharmacological actions of most psychotropic drugs, makes interpretation

difficult (Mustanski & Bancroft 2006; see Chapter 13). However, the evidence from both agonists and antagonists is consistent with DA being involved in the human sexual excitation system, without allowing any more specific conclusions about DA's role.

Noradrenaline

In men

When considering the NA system, the phenomenon of NPT gives us some interesting insights, at least as far as the male is concerned. Spontaneous erections occurring during sleep (i.e. NPT) are largely confined to REM or 'paradoxical' sleep. Until recently, however, little attention has been paid to why there should be this particular temporal association between erection and REM. It appears that for REM to occur, certain inhibitory signals need to be switched off. Probably most important for REM are the 5HT REM-off cells from the raphe nuclei, but also histaminergic neurons from the posterior hypothalamus and, of particular relevance here, NA neurons from the l.c. (Rechtschaffen & Siegel 2000). There is also animal evidence that during REM, peripheral sympathetic activity decreases in the renal and splanchnic (which would include genital) circulation, while increasing in the vasculature of skeletal muscles. Less is known about REM sleep in the human, although so-called 'autonomic storms' occur during human REM sleep, with bursts of increased heart rate, blood pressure and respiratory rate (Mancia 1993; Somers et al 1993). As yet we have no evidence of what happens to NPT during such bursts of peripheral sympathetic activity, although, typically, erection during NPT is well sustained. However, it is distinctly possible that switching off of the l.c. during REM is part of a wider reorganization of peripheral autonomic activity, which includes decreased sympathetic activity in the splanchnic (and renal) vessels, and which therefore results in reduction or cessation of the inhibitory tone in the smooth muscle of the erectile tissue. If so, that would have a permissive effect on erection during REM but would not be a sufficient explanation for why erections occur at that time.

The central effects of NA are probably best shown pharmacologically by α2 adrenoceptor antagonists, which increase NA at the synapse by blocking reuptake. The NA cell bodies in the l.c., as well as their presynaptic terminals throughout the brain, are populated with α2 receptors (Stahl 1996, p. 159). The effects on NPT of intravenous infusion through the night of a specific α2 antagonist, delaquamine, which would be expected to have an excitatory effect on the NA arousal system, were studied in both sexually functional and sexually dysfunctional men (Bancroft et al 1995). As mentioned above, α2 antagonists (e.g. idazoxan) injected into the corpora cavernosa have little or no effect on erection, either positive or negative. It is therefore reasonable to assume that any effects of such drugs when given intravenously are centrally rather than peripherally mediated. The results in this study were complex, as might be expected from the complex picture of NA effects in the animal literature, presented above. In the sexually functional men, there was a curvilinear dose–response curve; in comparison with placebo, the lower dose produced an increase in erection *outside REM sleep*, whereas the higher dose produced a reduction of erection *during REM*. In the dysfunctional men who received the same dosages the positive effect of the drug on non-REM erection was apparent, but only with the higher dose; the lower dose had no effect and the disruptive effect on REM-related erection was not apparent. This complex picture was interpreted as follows: the curvilinear dose–response curve in the functional men, which is reminiscent of that reported by Sala et al (1990) on rat sexual behaviour (see above), was seen as an example of a dose-related shift of maximum receptor impact, with the higher dose having a disruptive effect on the REM related 'switch off' of l.c. NA neurons and the lower dose producing an arousal effect that was apparent only during non-REM. It is also of interest that the higher dose produced an increase in spontaneous erections in the 'lights out' period preceding sleep onset. The pattern observed in the dysfunctional men was seen as a shift in the dose–response curve to the right, consistent with a higher degree of $\alpha2$ inhibitory tone in the dysfunctional subjects (Bancroft 1995). If that interpretation is correct then we would predict a similar curvilinear dose–response curve in the dysfunctional men when higher doses are used. If there is any validity in such an interpretation it raises the possibility of increased central $\alpha2$ tone as being a causal factor in certain cases of psychogenic erectile dysfunction (ED).

An interesting comparison is to be made with the effects of trazadone on NPT reported by Saenz de Tejada et al (1989). Trazadone increased NPT in a dose-related fashion, but this effect was largely confined to the period following REM-related erections. In other words, when the centrally derived peripheral inhibition was 'switched on' again following an REM-related erection, the drug blocked the resulting detumescence, prolonging the erection. This was not the pattern with delequamine, which increased erection during non-REM sleep predominantly in the period between sleep onset and first REM. Nor was there any evidence of trazadone disrupting NPT during REM sleep, though there might conceivably have been with a higher dose. It is also relevant that delequamine had a marked effect in delaying sleep onset, which trazadone did not. These contrasting effects are consistent with trazadone having a peripheral $\alpha1$ antagonist effect and delequamine a central $\alpha2$ antagonist effect. Trazadone, however, has a complex pharmacological action, which also includes serotonergic effects, and it remains a possibility that these effects may have been responsible or contributed to the pattern observed. Other studies of the effects of drugs on NPT have been reviewed by Rosen (1995).

Effects of $\alpha2$ antagonists in men have also been studied in the waking state. Yohimbine is the drug in this category that has received the most attention. A series of studies of its effects in treating ED, while limited by methodological shortcomings, consistently showed, on average, a modest positive effect on erectile function (Riley 1994). Other $\alpha2$ antagonists, idazoxan and fluporaxan, have received limited attention with borderline positive effects in men with erectile problems. In experimental studies, yohimbine induces anxiety (Charney et al 1983) and, combined with naloxone, it produces both anxiety and penile erection (Charney & Heninger 1986). Anxiety has not been a problem as a side effect in the treatment studies cited above, and it remains a question of some interest why anxiety has been evoked in such experimental studies, but not in treatment studies. It may be a matter of acute dosage contrasted with chronic dosage or it may be dependent on the context in which the drug is taken.

More experimental evidence was obtained from a placebo-controlled acute dosage study in which the specific $\alpha2$ antagonist, delequamine, was infused intravenously in both functional and dysfunctional men while responding to erotic stimuli (Munoz et al 1994a,b). The dysfunctional men had significantly smaller erectile responses than the functional men during the placebo condition, with partial normalization during the drug administration. Of particular interest was the finding that in younger dysfunctional men, blood pressure and heart rate responses to erotic stimuli were also blunted during placebo administration and normalized by the $\alpha2$ antagonist. This evidence, together with that from the sleep study mentioned earlier (Bancroft et al 1995), suggests that, in psychogenic ED, there is central inhibition of autonomic response to erotic stimuli, involving both erection and cardiovascular responses, which is based, at least in part, on increased central $\alpha2$ tone. The lack of effects of the drug in the older dysfunctional subjects raises the interesting possibility that these central inhibitory mechanisms (and presumably their excitatory counterparts) decline with advancing age.

In women

There is more limited evidence for women, which has largely relied on vaginal pulse amplitude (VPA) as the measure of genital response. The relevance of this measure will be considered more closely in the section on women's genital response later in this chapter. Meston & Heiman (1998) used a placebo-controlled study in young sexually functional women to assess the effects of ephedrine, a sympathomimetic agent. Increase in VPA while watching erotic stimuli was significantly greater with ephedrine than with placebo. Heart rate was higher with ephedrine. There were no significant differences in subjective reports of sexual arousal or affect, although there was a significant correlation between VPA change and subjective ratings of 'mental sexual arousal' following ephedrine administration, which was not evident with placebo. The principal effect of ephedrine is to release NA from presynaptic neurons. The authors interpreted these findings as evidence that NA enhances VPA, which would be contrary to how NA is understood to work in the periphery, at least in the male. It is conceivable that the observed effects resulted from central action, increasing general arousal and hence facilitating genital response. This would have been more likely if there had been significant increases in subjective ratings of arousal, but the observed correlation between subjective arousal and VPA is noteworthy. Meston et al (1997) used a comparable design to assess the effects of clonidine, an α2 agonist, although they also incorporated exercise to precede exposure to the erotic and neutral stimuli. The use of exercise by Meston and her colleagues, in a number of studies of this kind, will be considered later in the chapter. In this particular study, clonidine was associated with reduced VPA and subjective sexual arousal responses to erotic stimuli, findings consistent with clonidine-lowering central NA-induced arousal. Meston & Worcel (2002) compared yohimbine, which is predominantly an α2 antagonist, used on its own, with a combination of yohimbine and L-arginine, and placebo in post-menopausal women with 'sexual arousal disorder'. L-arginine is a precursor of NO, and the rationale for this combination was evidence that stimulation of prejunctional α2 receptors in horse penile vasculature inhibits NO release (Simonsen et al 1997). Thus, by blocking such α2 receptors, yohimbine might facilitate the action of NO. However, as yet there is no conclusive evidence of such an effect in human males. In this study of women, the combination was associated with significantly greater VPA increase in response to erotic stimuli than with placebo, with the yohimbine on its own coming midway, but not significantly different to either the combination or the placebo. As there was no assessment of the effects of L-arginine on its own, these findings are of interest but not conclusive.

An early study by Levi (1969), which has not been replicated but remains of considerable interest, has relevance to possible gender differences in the role of the NA system in sexual arousal. Erotic films were shown to a group of 50 males and 50 females, together in a cinema. Urine was collected from each participant before and after the film, and the urinary catecholamine excretion measured. In addition, self-ratings of sexual arousal in response to the films were obtained. Both male and female groups reported significant increases in sexual arousal, though the increase for the males was significantly greater than that for the females. Both groups showed increases in urinary A and NA excretion, but whereas for NA this was similar for the two groups, for A it was substantially higher in the men. In addition, self-ratings of sexual arousal correlated with catecholamine excretion in the females but did not do so for the males. One possible explanation is that the males judged their level of arousal by their perceived degree of erection, whereas, for females, less aware of genital changes, they were influenced by their state of general arousal that would be determined, in part, by adrenal medullary activity.

Serotonin
Serotonin reuptake inhibitors (SSRIs) are now extensively used for depressive and anxiety symptoms, often for long periods. Their use provides us with the best evidence of manipulation of the 5HT system in humans. Sexual side effects with SSRIs, as with most other types of antidepressants, are common. However, Montgomery et al (2002), in reviewing the relevant literature, concluded that the majority of the reported evidence was inconclusive because of methodological shortcomings and in many cases an inadequate distinction between different types of adverse sexual effects (of particular importance when questions about ejaculatory or orgasmic difficulties were not asked). In the more recent studies of SSRIs, however, one side effect stands out: delayed ejaculation or orgasm is the most commonly reported sexual side effect in men and in women. Across studies, 30–60% of patients on SSRIs report orgasmic or ejaculatory difficulty, substantially more than those reporting other types of dysfunctional sexual response. Although this relatively predictable effect of SSRIs on orgasm and ejaculation is consistent with a serotonergic inhibitory effect, it is not clear why inhibition of orgasm/ejaculation is so much more predictable than inhibition of erection or other components of genital response, considering that the most clearly established sexually relevant action of 5HT is via the nucleus paragigantocellularis in inhibiting erectile response. Given the rise in 5HT in the lateral hypothalamus following ejaculation in rats (Lorrain et al 1997), SSRIs may be having a more predictable 5HT effect in this part of the hypothalamus. This uncertainty reflects our relative lack of understanding of inhibitory systems as they affect sexuality, as well as specific receptor effects of different drugs.

Brain imaging during sexual stimulation
In Mouras and Stoleru's (2007) review of brain-imaging studies of cerebral responses to visual sexual stimuli (VSS), the most consistent, reproducible patterns of response tend to involve areas of the neo-cortex concerned with information processing, and these will be looked at later in this chapter. However, there are a number of other response patterns more relevant to the 'emotional brain' component of sexual arousal.

Anterior cingulate cortex
Here a distinction needs to be made between the rostral and caudal parts of the anterior cingulate cortex (ACC). In brain-imaging studies of non-sexual emotions, the rostral division has strong connections to the amygdala and hypothalamus. The caudal division is regarded as having a more cognitive function, including processing of contradictory signals or intentions, which could include the conflict between 'go' and 'no-go' signals in response to sexual stimuli. Both divisions of the ACC have shown activation in response to VSS, which could involve both excitatory and inhibitory sexual response patterns.

Putamen
This basal ganglion was activated in two studies based on correlations between rCBF and penile erection. This is consistent with early evidence from Macaque monkeys that electrical stimulation of the putamen evoked erection and/or genital manipulation (Robinson & Mishkin 1968).

Amygdala

Four studies have reported activation of the amygdala in response to VSS. Given the crucial role of the amygdala in emotional responses in general, it is not clear that these observed patterns were specifically related to sexual stimulation. Activation of the claustrum in response to VSS has been more consistent. This structure, a thin plate of grey matter lying between the basal ganglia and the insular cortex, is believed to be involved in visual attention but has not featured in the literature on the emotional or the sexual brain. However, Mouras & Stoleru (2007) speculate that as the claustrum and amygdala have the same embryological origin, in humans the role of the amygdala in more positive emotional states could have been taken over by the claustrum.

Overall, there has been less evidence of activation in subcortical than in cortical areas, and there may well be methodological reasons for this. Evidence of activation in the hypothalamus has been inconsistent, though three studies have found a correlation between penile tumescence and rCBF in the posterior hypothalamus. Only one study has reported activation of the midbrain (Bocher et al 2001). This was based on correlation between rCBF and subjective rating of penile erection. Also, this study involved longer exposure to the sexual stimuli than other studies, which may be important for eliciting identifiable activation in brain stem structures.

Evidence of inhibition may be apparent when specific brain areas are deactivated during a response to VSS. This is consistent with there being some inhibitory tone present, which needs to be reduced to allow a sexual response to occur. Brain-imaging studies have not been consistent in this respect, but a number have found deactivation of the temporal lobes and medial orbito-frontal cortex (MOFC). Some patterns of deactivation may not indicate reduction of inhibition but rather a change in focus. Thus, in non-sexual brain-imaging studies there has been a consistent finding that the posterior cingulate cortex becomes deactivated during active visual tasks when compared to passive visual tasks, reminding us that in most respects measurement of activation or deactivation depends on 'subtraction' of the rCBF in one stimulus condition compared to another.

A negative correlation between rCBF and penile erection has been found in some brain areas. This was shown in the temporal lobes in one study using PET but was not apparent in another study using fMRI. Two studies of apomorphine administration in men with ED showed a negative correlation between rCBF in the temporal cortex (medial inferior in one study) and penile erection 50 min after drug administration. This could indicate a reduction in inhibition initiated by the apomorphine.

Gender differences

Most of this limited data on brain imaging come from male subjects, but the small amount of evidence from women indicates some similarities and also some potentially important differences. Karama et al (2002), using fMRI, found similar bilateral activation, in men and women, of the medial prefrontal, orbitofrontal, insular and occipitotemporal cortices, as well as in the anterior cingulate gyrus, ventral striatum and the amygdala. Activation of the thalamus and hypothalamus, on the other hand, was only evident in the men, who also showed a significant correlation between the hypothalamic rCBF and subjective ratings of sexual arousal. Hamann et al (2004), using fMRI, found similar patterns of activation in men and women in multiple brain regions, including the ventral striatum, which is involved in the DA incentive motivation system. The amygdala and hypothalamus, however, were more strongly activated in men than in women. They concluded that the amygdala accounts for gender differences in responses to appetitive and biologically salient stimuli. Other studies have found the amygdala to be larger in men than in women (Hines 2004). Park et al (2001), also using fMRI, studied women only. They found significant activation in the inferior frontal and inferior temporal lobes, the cingulate cortex and insula, the caudate nucleus, globus pallidus and thalamus. Other evidence of gender differences in brain-imaging studies has been reviewed by Hines (2004).

Thus, we are gradually accumulating evidence about brain action from these brain-imaging studies, which shows a reasonable degree of common ground, but also a fair amount of variance (Stoleru & Mouras 2007). Brain imaging is probably going to be the most important source of information about the neural basis of human sexuality in the next few decades, but as yet it is at an early stage of development. There is still substantial variation in key aspects of methodology, in particular the types of stimulus presentations. In addition, such studies inevitably involve small numbers of participants and so far only two studies have compared and contrasted different types of individual: in one, hypogonadal vs eugonadal men (Redouté et al 2005; see p. 126) and in the other men with hypoactive sexual desire disorder (HSDD) vs controls (Stoleru et al 2003; see p. 103), and so far there has been no attempt to assess the potentially relevant types of non-clinical individual variability, which could impact on how a person reacts to sexual stimuli in a brain scanner. Hence, it is impossible to know how comparable these various small samples are. There is also the issue of participation bias, which again warrants some form of assessment, such as the sexual inhibition/sexual excitation scales, to allow comparison with non-participants. We have much to look forward to in this field.

A model of excitation and inhibition

On the basis of the evidence so far, Redoute et al (2000) proposed a four-component model of brain processing involved in sexual excitation and a three-component model of sexual inhibition.

Sexual excitation

1. A cognitive component that involves (i) appraisal that leads to stimuli being categorized as sexually relevant and their intensity evaluated; this initial step, they

postulate, is related to activation of the right lateral orbitofrontal cortex; (ii) attentional processes that focus on the stimuli categorized as sexual and are related to activation of the superior parietal cortex; and (iii) the activation of areas involved in motor imagery networks (e.g. the inferior parietal lobes, the left ACC, the supplementary motor areas, the ventral premotor areas and the caudate nuclei).

2. A motivational component that directs behaviour to a sexual goal. This, they postulate, involves activation of the caudal part of the left ACC and the claustrum bilaterally; this component is also closely related to motor imagery processing and its supporting neural network.

3. An autonomic and neuroendocrine component, including cardiovascular, respiratory and genital responses, related to activation of the rostral portion of the left ACC, the hypothalamus and possibly the insular control of testicular hormone production.

4. An emotional component involving the pleasure associated with rising arousal and penile tumescence, and related to activation of the right insula and secondary somatosensory cortex.

Sexual inhibition

1. Inhibitory processes operating in the resting state and imposed by the temporal lobes, which inhibit the initiation of sexual excitation.

2. Processes that limit the development of sexual excitation once it has been initiated, particularly in terms of its active expression. This form of inhibition is conceived as mediated by the caudate nucleus and the putamen.

3. Cognitive processes, relevant to problems of low sexual desire, which involve devaluation of potential sexual partners, resulting from a lack of deactivation of the MOFC.

It will be interesting to see how this model fares with future research.

Brain imaging and romantic love

Bartels & Zeki (2000) used fMRI to assess brain activity in young people who were 'in love' and looking at pictures of their loved ones. They went on to use a similar method to assess mothers' reactions to pictures of their children and compared the effects of 'romantic' and 'maternal' love (Bartels & Zeki 2004). They found similarities and differences in the areas of activation and similar areas of deactivation. Similar cortical areas of activation included the medial insula, previously shown to be activated by pleasant touch, and anterior cingulate cortex, involved in emotive processing. Similar subcortical areas of activation included various parts of the striatum (putamen, globus pallidus and head of the caudate nucleus, and, to some extent, the substantia nigra), also overlapping structures too small to be reliably identified, including subthalamic nuclei, the BNST and the ventral tegmental area (VTA). These subcortical areas are activated by a variety of incentive/reward stimuli (e.g. monetary, drug and sex). However, Bartels & Zeki (2004) concluded that the components of this 'incentive/reward' system involved in these two forms of attachment were those with high density of receptors for OT and vasopressin, both of which are regarded as crucial neuropeptides for affiliation and attachment (Insel 1992).

Areas activated by romantic but not maternal love stimuli included the dentate gyrus/hippocampus and the hypothalamus, possibly representing an overlap with sexual arousal. Areas activated by maternal but not romantic stimuli included the lateral orbitofrontal and prefrontal cortices, especially on the right, the posterior ventral thalamus and the periaqueductal grey in the midbrain, an area known to be involved in maternal attachment in other species.

Deactivation was similar in the romantic and maternal studies, involving areas of the prefrontal, parietal and middle temporal cortices, and the amygdala. This pattern was interpreted as 'switching off' processes involved in critical social assessment, such as moral judgment, social observation, and judgment of trustworthiness of faces, and negative emotions, such as depression and anger.

Aron et al (2005) reported a comparable fMRI study of men and women in love, one difference from the previous study being, on average, a shorter duration of the love relationship (7 vs 29 months in Bartels & Zeki 2000). They concluded that the dorsal caudate nuclei and VTA, both part of the incentive/reward system, and involving DA transmission, were activated in both studies, although there was more extensive activation of the caudate in the more recent study. The mid-insular, anterior and posterior cingulated cortices were activated in both studies, though they attributed difference in degree of activation in these areas to the effect of length of relationship. Within their own study, there was a positive correlation between length of relationship and degree of activation in a number of areas, including mid-insular and anterior cingulate cortices and some areas of the striatum, and a negative correlation with activity in the posterior cingulate. In comparison with Bartels & Zeki (2000), they found more extensive activation in the septum and retrosplenial cortex and no activation in the dorsal hippocampus or putamen. They found deactivation of the amygdala, but not the other cortical areas reported as deactivated by Bartels & Zeki (2000).

Aron et al (2005) concluded that 'rather than being a specific emotion, romantic love is better characterized as a motivation or goal-oriented state that leads to various specific emotions such as euphoria or anxiety'. This motivation state results from the convergence of neural systems in the region of the caudate, representing motivating stimuli and relevant memories. The differences they found between their study and that of Bartels & Zeki (2000) may be the result of differences in the duration of the love relationships but could also reflect other sources of variance, such as individual and methodological differences.

How do these findings compare with those presented earlier for response to sexual stimuli? Such comparisons are not easy, but there appears to be some overlap, most notably involving the components of incentive/motivation system, such as the caudate nucleus and anterior cingulate cortex, but also the insula, involved in emotive processing. There also appear to be differences in the types of information processing activity involved, which requires closer scrutiny.

Overall, these findings, as well as the somewhat more extensive evidence of responses to sexual stimuli, should be seen as preliminary, and considerably more research, including direct comparison of sexual and romantic stimuli, will be needed before we can make more than tentative suggestions about relevant brain mechanisms involved (Cacioppo et al 2003).

Neurological lesions

Early and extensive clinical studies of men with spinal cord injuries (SCI), many of them during the period following World War II, have demonstrated that provided the lumbosacral part of the cord, which contains the reflexive centres for penile erection, is not damaged, reflexive erections occur in many cases, often requiring minimal tactile stimulation to be elicited (see Higgins 1979, for review). This evidence suggests the reduction or absence of inhibitory signals from the brain, which are unable to get past the cord lesion to reach the reflexive centres in the cord and is entirely consistent with the animal evidence from spinal transection.

Lesions in the brain, whether traumatic or due to cerebrovascular accidents, tumours or other pathologies, are commonly associated with a decline in sexual interest and response, more so when certain brain areas, such as the temporal lobes or limbic system, are involved. Increased sexual responsiveness or interest following brain lesions, however, is rare (Lundberg 1992).

Genital response (anatomy and physiology) in men and women

The most fundamental function of genital response in the male and the female is to enable entry of the penis into the vagina, with the consequent deposition of semen in the vagina. In addition to the obvious reproductive consequences of such a sequence, which explain the existence of these responses, are the rewarding consequences of genital pleasure and orgasm. In the human, unlike most other species, the separation of sexual activity for the purpose of sexual pleasure from the reproductive consequences has become an important aspect of the human condition, with a range of benefits but also costs; hence the need for a book such as this. Even though currently this is politically incorrect in some circles, it remains important not to lose sight of the fundamental reproductive purpose of sex, as this has determined how our patterns of genital response have evolved.

The changes in the genitalia of both the male and the female during a sexual response mainly result from localized vasocongestion, but, as we will see, the purposes of this vasocongestion, and its determinants, may differ to some extent in men and women. However, these local vascular changes can start within 10–30 s of the onset of sexual stimulation, whether psychic (i.e. mediated via the brain) or reflexive (i.e. via reflex pathways in the spinal cord), and before any other discernible physiological changes have occurred.

Genital response in men

In the male, the principal response is erection of the penis. This is the most crucial of the male genital responses, often the subject of much concern and self-observation, and its failure is the most important form of sexual dysfunction reported by men. We will therefore consider this response in considerable detail.

In addition to penile erection, the testes become somewhat enlarged, presumably due to vascular engorgement, and elevated due to retraction of the spermatic cords and contraction of the associated cremaster muscle. The wall of the scrotum becomes thicker and tighter, due in part to local vasocongestion but also to contraction of the dartos muscle in its wall. If stimulation is prolonged or intensified, the testes are pulled up to the perineal floor and increase further in size. The purpose of these changes is not clear, in terms of either reproduction or sexual pleasure. Masters & Johnson (1966) suggested that elevation of the testes is necessary if the full force of ejaculation is to occur, though it is not clear why this should be so. Contraction of the scrotum may serve to support the elevated testes. The purpose of the testicular enlargement, if any, is not understood.

Penile erection

The function of penile erection in the male is obvious. Adequate entry of the penis into the vagina, and consequent deposition of semen, is difficult without full erection. The erect penis also acts to stimulate the genitalia of the female, whilst providing the main tactile erotic input for the male.

The stiffness of an erect penis depends on the filling with blood of the erectile tissues within the corpora cavernosa and the increase in intracavernosal pressure to around systolic levels. The tough fibrous tunica albuginea surrounding the corpora cavernosa contains the increased pressure, and the integrity of the resulting hydraulic system produces the rigidity. Vascular engorgement of the glans and corpus spongiosum also occurs during erection but does not contribute to the crucial rigidity of the organ.

Traditional physiological textbooks have, perhaps out of a sense of propriety, shown scant attention to the phenomenon of erection, usually describing the process as simply one of increased arterial inflow to the penis resulting from parasympathetically induced arterial dilatation. The sympathetic nervous system (SNS), it has been assumed, causes reversal of erection or detumescence. For some time this has been considered an inadequate explanation by many physiologists and anatomists. To produce the pressure necessary for rigidity, reduced emptying, as well as increased filling, of the erectile tissues is obviously required. The history of attempts to understand penile erection is an interesting one and will be briefly reviewed.

Dickinson, in his *Human Sex Anatomy* (1933, p. 79–80) translates the description of Fritz Kahn (1931), which includes the following:

Blood flows from the supply arteries through the caverns from the front part of the organ, the glans, and thence streams through the great dorsal vein back to the body ... the urethra is protected from constriction by a peculiar suspensory apparatus. From the cavernous bodies run numerous bundles of fibres like the spokes of a wheel, from periphery to wall of urethra. In proportion to the swelling of the cavernous body and the increasing distance of its outer wall from the urethra, this canal is drawn open by the fibres and so closure by mounting pressure of blood is prevented. To permit length wise extension of the urethra it lies when flaccid in pleats like an accordion, and so can unfold without discomfort.

*The tissues of the relaxed corpora cavernosa are pressed closely together. The arteries lie in the chamber walls in sharp curves. These meanderings or elbows slow the current, and like bent rubber tubing they lie, empty during normal blood pressure. Access of blood is still further hampered because in the bends the arterial wall is greatly thickened by a bolster of cells (Zellpolster) so that recurrent corking obstructions shut off the lumen ... in these arteries ... the bolsters close the lumen-like valves so only the least blood needed for nutrition passes. When the cramp of the vessel wall relaxes to allow the cavernous bodies to fill, the tube expands, the bolster moves away from the wall, and blood streams through the opened vessels. The sharp curves are flattened out, and the caverns fill. **It was a surprising paradox to discover that erection, or hardening was started by a process of relaxation of spasm!***

(Kahn 1931, p. 182) (bold added).

The concept of 'bolsters' was subsequently abandoned, but Kahn's final 'surprising paradox' still reverberates with current thinking. Entrapment of the blood by compression of the veins beneath the tunica albuginea as intracavernosal pressure increases became the favoured explanation. Whilst this may contribute to hydraulic efficiency of the system, it was unlikely to be a sufficient explanation. Reduction in venous outflow can be observed early in the development of an erection, before any appreciable increase in intracavernosal pressure has occurred. The importance of substantially reducing venous outflow has been further emphasized in recent years by the discovery that erectile failure is sometimes caused by venous 'leaks' in the system.

Deysach (1939), commenting on the histological difference between erectile tissue of animals with an os penis (i.e. most mammals and primates) and those without (e.g. humans), described 'sluice channels' in the human-type penis, which, he suggested, diverted blood into the erectile spaces during erection. Other specialized vascular structures have been described by Wagner et al (1982), who, studying plastic injection casts of post-mortem specimens, found vessels passing from the corpora cavernosa through the tunica into the spongiosum. It was postulated that these act as shunts allowing large quantities of blood to pass quickly through the erectile spaces in the flaccid condition. Closure of the muscular walls of these vessels, they suggested, then diverts blood into the corpora cavernosa in response to erotic stimulation.

The simple concept of a balance between the parasympathetic and SNSs has been challenged in various ways. It has been known for some time that sympathetic pathways carry fibres involved in the development of erection as well as in detumescence (Bancroft 1970). In the cat, the lower part of the sympathetic chain is responsible for 'psychic' erections, with the sacral, parasympathetic outflow controlling reflexive responses (Root & Bard 1947). There is some suggestion of a similar division of function in men from studies of paraplegic patients (Bors & Comarr 1960; Kuhn 1950).

Further problems arose in establishing which neurotransmitters are involved. Electrical stimulation of the cavernous nerves leads to arterial dilatation and increased blood flow, but in most species studied this effect is not blocked by atropine, making a simple cholinergic mechanism unlikely (Brindley 1983). Human erections in response to erotic stimuli are also unaffected by atropine (Wagner & Brindley 1980). Active searching for other possible neurotransmitters focused attention on vasoactive intestinal polypeptide (VIP), a neuropeptide, which is undoubtedly present in the erectile tissues, its concentration increasing as an erection develops (Virag et al 1982). However, in several species it also increases with simple handling of the penis without erection (Dixson et al 1984) and injection of VIP into the cavernosal spaces does not produce erection (Ottesen et al 1984).

A crucial development was the recognition of the large amount of smooth muscle within the corpora cavernosa, mainly within the walls of the sinusoids (trabeculae). A number of reports of the effects of drugs and neurotransmitters on strips of such smooth muscle tissue appeared in the literature, providing a useful in vitro method for studying pharmacological effects (Benson 1983). It was also shown that both cholinergic and adrenergic receptors are present in cavernosal tissue, but the latter are mainly in the smooth muscle walls of the sinusoids and are about 10 times more frequent than the former (Benson et al 1980) with a greater proportion of α than β receptors (Levin & Wein 1980).

The next important source of evidence of the physiology of erection was the studies of drugs injected into the corpora cavernosa in human subjects. Brindley (1983) and Virag (1982) pioneered this technique, initially as a method of investigating erectile failure but subsequently as a possible method of treatment. A variety of drugs were shown by this method to produce erection in men (Table 4.1), though with varying duration of erections resulting. Pharmacologically, this is a heterogeneous group of compounds but they all share in common the capacity for relaxing smooth muscle, some by adrenergic blockade (e.g. phenoxybenzamine), some by calcium channel blocking (e.g. verapamil) and others by as yet unknown mechanisms (e.g. papaverine). We thus have to incorporate these findings into any explanatory model of erectile function.

In the last edition of this book the following model of erection was presented based on the available evidence at that time. Relaxation of the smooth muscle in the sinusoidal walls occurs. This is normally constricted by an active process of adrenergic tone. Reduction of this tone and consequent relaxation then result in filling and enlargement of the spaces with blood (Fig. 4.5). Passive compression of the venules running between the sinusoidal spaces impedes venous outflow and further increases sinusoidal filling (Fig. 4.6). Dilatation of arteries results in increased inflow. It was not clear whether this dilatation preceded, accompanied or followed the sinusoidal relaxation. The possibility of some additional active reduction of venous outflow had not been excluded. The combination of these processes, it was assumed, leads to an effective sealing off of the corpora cavernosa and a build-up of intracavernosal pressure to levels around systolic, which is probably sufficient to produce rigidity. Additional stiffening may result from transient contraction of the ischiocavernosus and bulbospongiosus muscles, which has been shown to produce grossly elevated intracavernosal pressure. This mechanism can be elicited by the bulbocavernosus reflex. During neurological examination this reflex is elicited by squeezing the glans penis. It is possible that contact of the erect penis with the vaginal introitus also elicits this reflex, resulting in a further stiffening and easier entry. When erectile responses are measured in the laboratory, it is common to find these contractions occurring as a semivoluntary attempt to 'pump up' an erection (see Fig. 3.16).

There remained, however, a number of uncertainties. While there was general agreement that reduction of NA tone allowed the relaxation of the smooth muscle in the sinusoidal wall, the neurotransmitters involved in the increase in blood flow were less well understood. The earlier assumption that this was a parasympathetic effect mediated by ACh had been challenged by the finding that atropine, an ACh muscarinic receptor blocker, did not prevent erection. It was becoming increasingly recognized that a variety of neurotransmitters or neuromodulators were probably involved. The end of this section in the previous edition read as follows:

'This remains a fascinating area of vascular physiology and it is to be hoped that in the next few years many of the remaining uncertainties will be resolved. The possibility of a major breakthrough in the pharmacological treatment of erectile failure remains a tantalizing possibility.'

(Bancroft 1989, p. 61)

This breakthrough was soon to follow.

The Viagra story

Ignarro et al (1990), at UCLA, reported that NO and cyclic guanesine monophosphate (cGMP) caused relaxation of the smooth muscle in the corpus cavernosum.

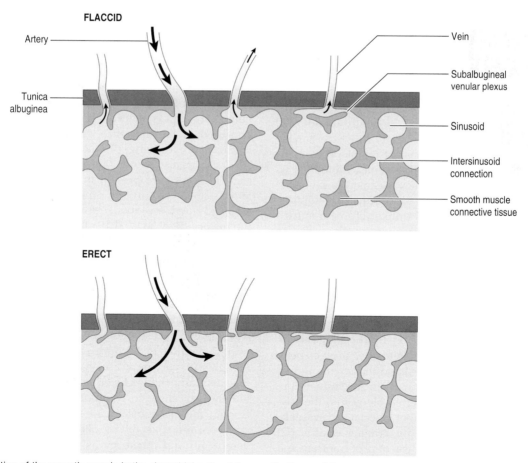

Fig. 4.5 Relaxation of the smooth muscle in the sinusoidal walls of the erectile tissue of the corpora cavernosa. These are normally constricted by an active process of adrenergic tone. Reduction of this tone and consequent relaxation then result in filling and enlargement of the spaces with blood and reduced venous drainage. (Modified from Fournier et al 1987.)

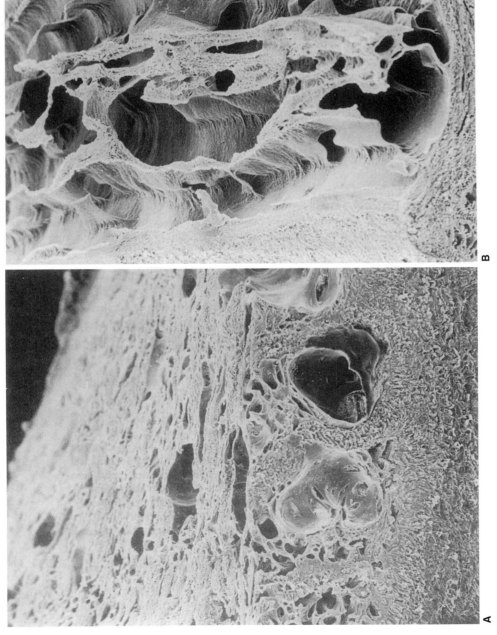

Fig. 4.6 Comparison of architecture of corpora cavernosum and spongiosum in the dog. Electron micrographs of flaccid state. **(A)**, corpus cavernosum. **(B)**, corpus spongiosum from same specimen. (Courtesy of C. Carati.)

Cyclic GMP is normally broken down by phosphodiesterase, of which there are several varieties in the human. Around the same time, Pfizer Inc., in their laboratories in the UK, developed a phosphodiesterase 5 (PDE5) inhibitor called sildenafil and were testing it as a possible treatment for angina. It proved to be only modestly effective, with not inconsiderable side effects. However, one unexpected side effect was an increased likelihood of penile erection. The exploration of the use of sildenafil for treating ED started in 1993, and the first, positive results were published in 1996 (Boolell et al 1996). The era of Viagra was born (Katzenstein 2001), and there has been intense interest, both from basic research and from clinical perspectives, in the related mechanisms ever since. (For further review of clinical implications see Chapter 12.)

In light of these new developments and understandings, we can consider the current views on the mechanisms of erection. The basic steps, presented above, are still considered relevant. But now we can say much more about the mechanisms involved. The following account is largely based on the review by Rehman & Melman (2001).

Whether a penis is flaccid or erect depends to a considerable extent on the state of the smooth muscle in the corpus cavernosum (CC). The flaccid penis requires maintenance of inhibitory tone in the smooth muscle of the CC. The crucial intracellular factor is the level of calcium in the muscle cell. The inhibitory tone depends on maintenance of high levels of calcium, which are induced by NA from the sympathetic nerve supply acting principally on $\alpha 1$ receptors (β receptors are of little significance in the erectile process). Injection of $\alpha 1$ blockers, phenoxybenzamine and phentolamine, into the CC causes erection, indicating that reduction of adrenergic inhibitory tone is one component of erectile response, and such reduction presumably results normally from reduced inhibitory signals from the brain. There is also the possibility that endothelin, a peptide, is involved. Endothelin-1 is synthesized by the endothelium in the corpus cavernosum, and in vitro elicits strong sustained contraction of CC smooth muscle (Rehman & Melman 2001).

Development of an erection, however, normally depends on active relaxation by decreasing intracellular calcium as well as reduction of the inhibitory effect. Because erection can occur in the presence of both parasympathetic (i.e. atropine) and sympathetic blockers, attention was focused on what became known as the nonadrenergic–noncholinergic neuroeffector system (NANC). This reduces intracellular calcium by increasing cGMP and cAMP. NO plays a key role in increasing the availability of cGMP when, in response to sexual stimulation, it is released from autonomic neurons, as well as from vascular endothelium in the erectile tissues. cGMP is broken down by PDE5, the predominant isoform of phosphodiesterase in the penile tissues. PDE5 inhibitors, such as sildenafil (Viagra), act by slowing the breakdown of cGMP so that its muscle-relaxing effect is prolonged. Other neurotransmitters presumably work via the cAMP pathway; prostaglandin E1 (PGE1), which is released from the endothelium, elicits

erection in two ways: it promotes relaxation via the cAMP pathway and it also blocks α-adrenergic inhibition.

ACh, which for a long time was believed to be the sole neurotransmitter causing erection, is now to seen to have a more limited and subtle role. ACh acts as a neuromodulator in at least two ways: it inhibits adrenergic nerves in the CC and it probably stimulates release of NO from the endothelium. VIP is probably a co-transmitter with ACh but does not produce erection when injected on its own into the CC. A number of other potential neurotransmitters have received attention in the literature. (For a more detailed account of this complex process see Rehman & Melman 2001.)

The other key component of the erectile process is the virtual cessation of venous drainage from the CC. It is now recognized that the early reduction of venous drainage that precedes the full development of intracavernosal pressure and rigidity of erection results from the compression of sinusoidal venules that follow increased sinusoidal filling. In addition, the emissary veins that leave the CC through the tunica albuginea travel obliquely between the two layers of the tunica before entering the deep dorsal vein and other venous drainage. The pressure of the CC enlarging inside the tunica, as its spaces dilate and fill with blood, leads to pressure on the tunica, which effectively blocks the emissary veins running through it. Other mechanisms, as yet not identified, may also be involved.

Genital response in women

The consequences of erotically induced local vasocongestion in the female are more extensive and complex than in the male. The conventional view of this process is as follows. The venous plexus, which surrounds the lower part of the vagina, the bulbs of the clitoris and the body and crura of the clitoris, become engorged (see Fig. 3.10). A turgid cuff thus forms, which narrows and elongates the outer third of the coital canal. If stimulation continues or is intensified, reaching the phase preceding orgasm, which Masters & Johnson (1966) called the plateau phase, congestive swelling of the vulva causes reddening and 'pouting' of the labia minora. Masters & Johnson (1966) also observed that the clitoris, which erects to a variable degree in the earlier stages of sexual response, now retracts into a less prominent attitude against the symphisis pubis. Less attention has been paid to this 'retraction process' in recent years.

In the deeper parts of the female genital tract (see Figs. 3.12 and 3.13), the uterus also becomes engorged and increases in size, at the same time rising in the pelvis. This displacement probably results from contraction of the smooth muscle fibres within the parametrial tissues supporting the uterus and upper vagina. Elongation of the vaginal canal is associated with a 'ballooning' of the upper two-thirds of the vagina. Slow irregular contractions of the vaginal vault may occur as sexual stimulation continues.

Recently, MRI scanning has started to be used to investigate the process of female genital response (Deliganis et al 2002; Maravilla et al 2005). This provides a more comprehensive method of assessing genital response than has been possible with other methods, including direct visual examination as used by Masters & Johnson (1966). The findings have been summarized by Maravilla (2006) and Heiman & Maravilla (2007). To assess changes during response to sexual stimulation, both contrast (Deliganis et al 2002) and non-contrast (T^2-weighted; Maravilla et al 2005) MRI techniques have been used. While the use of contrast methods allows measurement of genital blood volume, the results have so far been less robust than the direct measurement of tissue volume used with the non-contrast T^2-weighted method. This has the advantage of suppressing signals from subcutaneous and interstitial fat, allowing a clearer structural picture. Sequential three-dimensional images of the genital region are obtained at approximately 3 min intervals, while the participant views a sequence of neutral and erotic videos (15 min of each). In the small number of women assessed so far, enlargement of the body and crura of the clitoris is clearly evident; the bulbs of the clitoris enlarge to a lesser extent. The volume of the clitoris in the non-aroused state ranged from 1.5 to 5.5 mL in different women. In response to sexual stimuli, this volume increased on average by 90% to a maximum of 10 mL. No apparent changes were observed in the labia, the vaginal wall or the vaginal lining, possibly because any such changes would be below the limit of resolution of the MRI technique.

As erection of the penis in the male facilitates entry into the vagina, so do the genital changes in the female. The congested and 'pouting' labia and more patent introitus invite entry of the penis, whilst the vaginal transudate lubricates the vaginal barrel in readiness. The narrowing of the outer third of the vagina, the so-called 'orgasmic platform', adds to the stimulation of the penis and possibly to the erotic stimulation of the woman. The function of the ballooning of the inner third of the vagina is not clear, though, together with the orgasmic platform, it may aid conception by encouraging the formation of a seminal pool near the cervix and reducing drainage of semen out of the vagina. The elevation of the uterus effectively pulls the cervix out of the way of the deeply thrusting penis; buffeting of the cervix can cause discomfort. It follows that if vaginal entry is attempted without these genital responses having occurred, discomfort or pain may be experienced.

The purposes of these genital and pelvic responses in women present us with an interesting challenge. Clearly, they facilitate vaginal intercourse and hence have direct relevance to reproduction. But to what extent do they occur in order to enhance women's sexual pleasure? In the male, sexual pleasure, or the anticipation of it, is associated with penile erection, orgasm and ejaculation, all of obvious reproductive importance. But is sexual pleasure as fundamental to reproduction in women as it is in men? Does a woman require sexual pleasure for her to experience the vasocongestive changes in the vagina and labia necessary for comfortable penile entry? To what extent have pain suppression responses from vaginal and cervical stimulation (VCS) (see below) evolved to allow women, and indeed the females of other species, to participate in vaginal intercourse without discomfort, but

also without the need for sexual pleasure? We will consider these questions at various points in the remainder of this chapter (and see Chapter 6, p. 232). But we should keep in mind, as we grapple with the more complex picture of female sexual response which the current scientific evidence provides us, that certain parts of this picture may be unrelated to sexual pleasure.

However, even if sexual pleasure is not necessary for effective reproduction in women, there is no doubt that most women experience such pleasure to a greater or a lesser extent. It is generally assumed that the sole function of the clitoris, or at least the visible part of it, the glans, is to provide the principal source of erotic stimulation for the female. It is exquisitely sensitive and may contain as many nerve endings as are found in the glans penis, though the number does vary considerably from woman to woman (Krantz 1958). Later, we will ask why the woman has a clitoris that is so erotically sensitive. In a similar vein, we will consider whether the female orgasm, clearly a source of sexual pleasure, has reproductive significance and, if not, what has determined its existence, particularly as female orgasm is relatively unusual in other primates. In addition, we will consider the relationship between penile–vaginal intercourse and orgasm. In both cases it has been argued that these female features, a hypersensitive clitoris and the capacity for orgasm, exist because there is no biological purpose in suppressing them. If correct, this is a 'decision' by nature that will certainly be appreciated by many women.

Vaginal response

The lining of the vagina is normally moist. This results in part from fluid from the uterus and mucous secretion from the cervix, as well as fluid from the vaginal wall. The cervical fluid varies in amount and consistency through the ovarian cycle; close to ovulation there is a marked increase in volume and in watery consistency. This facilitates entry of sperm from the vagina into the uterus. During the luteal phase of the cycle, the cervical fluid reduces in volume, thickens and 'plugs' the cervical canal, reducing the likelihood of sperm entry (Levin 2003a). Without sexual stimulation, however, the vagina is not sufficiently lubricated for comfortable entry of an erect penis. In response to sexual stimulation, a fluid appears on the vaginal epithelium (usually at an early stage), quickly forming a lubricating coat, which was likened by Masters & Johnson (1966) to a sweating response. The characteristics of this fluid indicate that it is a modified plasma transudate. This transudation results from a substantial increase in vaginal blood flow (VBF). It is also likely that comparable lubrication of the labia occurs, though this has not as yet been clearly demonstrated (Levin 2003a). The vaginal transudate, by its effects on electrolyte content and pH of the vagina, may make the vaginal milieu more favourable to sperm, though the relative importance of this is still disputed.

In comparison to the male, genital response in the female, and in particular its neurophysiological control, presents an additional challenge. The clitoris, which is homologous to the penis, probably depends on similar mechanisms of control to the penis when responding to sexual stimulation, and is considered later. However, the vagina has no homologous counterpart in the male, and the control of VBF, necessary for vaginal lubrication as well as other manifestations of vasocongestion, is less well understood. As Levin (2003a) has pointed out, vaginal lubrication has an uncertain relationship to sexual arousal, and, whereas it typically increases in early stages of sexual response, it is often not sustained, particularly if stimulation is prolonged. Understanding the control of vaginal response, however, is of some importance to psychophysiological research because, until recently, the principal indicator of genital response in women has been increased pulse amplitude in the vaginal wall (VPA). This has the advantage of being relatively easily monitored by photometers incorporated in tampon-shaped cylinders inserted into the vagina.

Increase in VBF is mediated in part by release of VIP (Levin 2003a). Ottesen et al (1987) showed that intravenous infusion of VIP in normal women increased VBF and transudation of vaginal fluid. As discussed earlier, this neuropeptide has been implicated in penile erection but is now considered not to be of fundamental importance in that respect. There is evidence that nitrergic transmission is involved in vaginal response, but there is uncertainty about whether it is as important as it is in penile erection (Giuliano et al 2002). NA and neuropeptide Y are probably the main inhibitors of vaginal response (Giraldi & Levin 2005).

Let us consider vaginal pulse amplitude (VPA) more closely. There is now a substantial literature based on the measurement of VPA. What is striking about this literature is the basic assumption throughout that VPA is a measure of sexual *arousal* in women. There are two problems with such an assumption. First, it is not clear precisely what is measured by VPA. The vaginal photometer involves a methodology widely used in studies of peripheral circulation — mainly in the finger. The photometer shines red light into the vaginal wall and measures the amount of light reflected back. The amplitude of the vaginal pulse wave (the contrast between the peak and trough of light reflectance) is assumed to reflect the amount of flow of the blood with each pulse. How it does so has not been clearly established. It could be affected by increases in flow, but also by changes in the vascular bed. VPA is very much affected by changes in the general circulation. As Levin (2007) has pointed out, if you place a photometer on your finger, raising your finger above your head produces a large change in pulse amplitude as a result of changing venous tone. In addition, there is no absolute measure involved in VPA. As a result, one can only compare VPA within the same session in the same subject, which poses substantial problems when using this measure to generate group data or compare individuals. A more physiologically quantifiable measure of VBF is by means of a heated oxygen electrode, which is held by suction against the vaginal wall, enabling calculation of absolute flow (mLs/100 g vaginal tissue/min) (Levin & Wagner 1997). For some reason, possibly expense, this has been little used by researchers other than Levin & Wagner. Duplex Doppler ultrasound probes have also been used to a limited extent (e.g. Berman et al 1999) but have the disadvantage of being more intrusive, requiring continued positioning by the investigator.

A second major problem with VPA, and indeed any measure of VBF, stems from our lack of understanding of its relationship with sexual arousal. That VPA changes when women are exposed to sexual stimuli is beyond dispute; furthermore, increase in VPA typically starts within seconds of the onset of a sexual stimulus. But the relationships between VPA and other indices of sexual arousal are unpredictable. As Laan & Everaerd (1995) put it: 'Even when these explicit sexual stimuli are negatively evaluated, or induce little or no feelings of sexual arousal, genital (i.e. vaginal) responses are elicited' (p. 67). They also found that repeated exposure to the same erotic stimulus was associated with consistent VPA response, despite a decrease in positive affective response to the stimuli. What they never observed was a subjective experience of sexual arousal with no evidence of vaginal response. In a meta-analysis of their series of studies measuring VPA in women (combined n of 243), using multiple regression and a variety of potential predictor variables (including sexual history, situational variables and emotional responses), Laan & Everaerd (1995) were able to account for 26% of the variance in women's reports of subjective sexual arousal. Seven predictors entered the model; masturbation frequency was the strongest predictor and appraisal of the erotic stimulus was next; genital 'arousal' (i.e. VPA) and awareness of vaginal lubrication just entered the model as sixth and seventh (unique contribution to the variance, 1% each). In predicting 'genital physiological arousal' (i.e. VPA response), only 9% of the variance was accounted for; appraisal of the erotic stimulus was the strongest predictor (6%), subjective rating of sexual arousal did not enter the model. Overall, experimental manipulations (e.g. the type of erotic stimulus used) had most impact on subjective sexual arousal. These findings led Laan & Everaerd (1995) to wonder whether increased VBF was an 'automatized response mechanism'. We will return to this concept in the section on gender differences later in this chapter.

The inconsistency between vaginal response and subjective arousal is evident in other ways. Morokoff & Heiman (1980) found no difference in VPA response between women presenting for treatment with sexual problems and a control group. Meston & Gorzalka (1996a) found no difference in VPA response between functional women, women with low sexual desire and women with anorgasmia. Wouda et al (1998) compared women with dyspareunia with non-dyspareunic women and found no differences in their VPA response to erotic videos. However, when the videos depicted coitus rather than non-penetrative sex, the dyspareunic women showed less VPA response than the controls, although they did not differ in their subjective ratings of sexual arousal. This therefore appears to be an exception to the general rule arrived at by Laan & Everaerd (1995) that subjective sexual arousal does not occur in the absence of vaginal response. In this case, however, it was a matter of relative decrease in VPA rather than absence of vaginal response. What is interesting about this finding is the apparently specific effect of women with dyspareunia observing coitus. However, in a more recent study (Brauer et al 2006), women with superficial dyspareunia did not show less VPA response to images of coitus than to images of oral sex. In fact, they showed significantly more VPA response to coital images, and significantly less to images of oral sex, than the non-dyspareunic controls. It is nevertheless noteworthy how, overall, these studies show little difference between dysfunctional and functional women in their VPA response to erotic stimuli. It is difficult to reconcile this with the idea that increase in VBF in response to erotic stimuli is a genital manifestation of sexual arousal.

There is a striking contrast between this body of psychophysiological evidence from women, and evidence from men based on measurement of penile erection. In men, although circumstances such as distraction can have an impact, there is a relatively predictable correlation between the degree of penile response and subjective ratings of arousal, usually around $r = 0.6$, and tending to be higher with higher levels of erectile response (Rosen & Beck 1988). In women, the association varies across studies from negative to zero to positive. However, this may depend on what women are asked to focus on, when assessing their subjective sexual arousal. Brotto & Gorzalka (2002) asked women to make this assessment in two different ways: (i) by focusing on genital sensations and (ii) by assessing how 'sexually aroused' they felt. Correlations with VPA were higher with genital sensation appraisal. This underlines the importance of specifying this aspect of future research.

The possible significance of this gender difference, in relation to the subjective experience of sexual arousal, will be discussed further later in this chapter (p. 131).

As indicated earlier, the neurophysiological control of VBF is not well understood, though VIP and NO are probably involved in the increase and NA and neuropeptide Y in the reduction of VBF. Challenging this conclusion, however, is a series of studies by Meston and her colleagues. The theme running through these studies is that activation of the SNS produces sexual arousal in women, as evidenced by VPA increase. Let us look at this series more closely (for review see Meston & Bradford 2007). The studies are of two types: one involves physical exercise proceeding the measurement of VPA response to erotic stimuli and the other involves drug administration and its effect on VPA response to erotic stimuli (in some cases combined with the exercise procedure). What has been found consistently is that VPA response is increased if its measurement is preceded by 20 min of intense stationary cycling, with the workload involved set to maintain a heart rate at approximately 70% of maximum. Exercise, on the other hand, does not influence the lack of VPA response to a non-sexual stimulus. This is an interesting phenomenon, which would be good to explain. However, the explanation that it is a consequence of exercise-induced activation of the SNS is questionable on a number of grounds. There is no doubt that intense physical exercise involves activation of the SNS, and one manifestation of this is an increase in plasma levels of A and NA. But this is part of a complex process of control of cardiovascular function to facilitate the exercise. The idea that activation of the SNS is a unitary phenomenon, which will affect all mechanisms influenced by the SNS, stems from the early

concept of a sympathetic system counterbalanced by a PNS. This is an example of a 'simple model' that may have served a useful purpose when neurophysiologists were first grappling with autonomic function but that no longer has heuristic value (Paton et al 2005). Sympathetic and parasympathetic processes interact in an exceedingly complex fashion, which varies according to the response being controlled and the part of the body affected (Nakamura et al 1993). As proposed earlier (see p. 63), central arousal together with its autonomically mediated peripheral manifestations, such as increased heart rate or blood pressure, and increased plasma levels of A and NA, is fundamental to many emotional states, including sexual arousal. And as shown for the male, 'sexual arousal' is a combination of non-specific peripheral arousal together with the specific sexual component, genital response. And this involves a reduction of 'sympathetic' tone in the penile erectile tissues — confronting us with the apparent paradox that NA can be involved in both excitatory and inhibitory mechanisms at the same time (see p. 67). There is as yet no reason to assume that women are different in this respect.

In addition, it is far from clear how the vascular consequences of a bout of intense exercise would affect the ill-understood phenomenon of VPA. It is well established that a single bout of exercise reduces arterial pressure for some hours. Kenney & Seals (1993) suggest that possible mechanisms involved 'include decreased stroke volume and cardiac output; reductions in limb vascular resistance, total peripheral resistance and muscle sympathetic nerve discharge; group III somatic afferent activation; altered baroreceptor reflex circulatory control; reduced vascular responsiveness to α-adrenergic receptor-mediated stimulation; and activation of endogenous opioid and serotonergic systems' (p. 653). Interestingly, a study of rats (Rao et al 2002) found a sex difference in the mechanisms involved. In male rats, $\alpha 1$-adrenergic receptor responsiveness was reduced following exercise due to a counteractive effect of NO. This mechanism was not apparent in female rats, even though they showed the post-exercise hypotension.

So what is happening to the cardiovascular system and the vascular bed in Meston and colleagues' female participants after exercise? And to what extent might this change over time following the bout of exercise? Meston & Gorzalka (1996b) addressed this last question. They compared the effects of exercise on VPA response at 5, 15 and 30 min following the exercise. They were interested to see if the effects of SNS activation would be maximal soon after exercise, decreasing as the SNS activation subsided. They found the reverse. The VPA response 5 min after exercise was diminished ($p = 0.026$); after 15 min it was increased ($p = 0.004$). At 30 min the mean VPA increase was substantially higher than at 15 min, but the variance was greater, so it was less significant ($p = 0.04$). The authors were not deterred by these findings. They concluded that there was an optimal level of SNS activation 'beyond and below which physiological sexual arousal is suppressed or unaffected'. They did not entertain the idea that their basic hypothesis might be wrong.

A consistent finding in these studies has been absence of any effect of the exercise on subjective ratings of sexual arousal, in contrast with the enhancing effect on VPA. What these researchers have not adequately considered is the issue of 'excitation transfer' (Zillmann 1972), whereby central arousal induced by one situation (e.g. exercise or anxiety) can, at least in some individuals, enhance the arousal experience to other situations (e.g. sexual). Such an effect, as far as subjective arousal is concerned, depends on the subject's attribution of the source of the arousal. Cantor et al (1975) used physical exercise as the primary arouser and assessed subjective sexual arousal in response to erotic slides at three time intervals following exercise. The subjects were told that the experiment was to study the effects of distraction and were asked at one of the three intervals following exercise (short by comparison with the Meston & Gorzalka 1996b study) to indicate whether they still felt affected by the exercise. Subjects tested after the first interval, when the effects of exercise were present, recognized that they were still present. Subjects tested after the second interval believed that the effects of exercise had gone whereas, in physiological terms, they were still present. Subjects tested after the third longest interval correctly recognized that the exercise effects were no longer present. Subjects tested after the second interval reported higher levels of subjective sexual arousal than those in the other two groups. This raises the question of what the participants in Meston and colleagues' research believed the purpose of the study to be and the extent to which they recognized that they were still affected by the exercise when responding to the erotic film.

The other series of studies involving pharmacological manipulations included assessment of the effects of ephedrine, an α and β adrenergic agonist (Meston & Heiman 1998), and clonidine, an $\alpha2$ adrenergic agonist (which reduces NA release at the synapse; Meston et al 1997). Interpretation of the results was limited by the uncertainty of whether observed effects were due to peripheral or central action of the drug.

This research has revealed an interesting aspect of vaginal response but unfortunately, in spite of considerable diligence and perseverance, it has not helped us to clarify the control mechanisms of vaginal response. Meston & Bradford (2007), in their recent review, are starting to acknowledge some of the limitations of their basic theoretical model. This returns us to the issue of how we use the concept of 'arousal'. I am firmly of the opinion that this concept should only be used to describe the total pattern of sexual arousal, or the central processes of non-specific arousal and its peripheral non-specific manifestations. As proposed earlier in this chapter (p. 64), genital response, whether vaginal, clitoral or penile, should be regarded as one component of the total pattern, and, while it is the most obviously sexual component, it is not sexual arousal per se. In the meantime, the weight of experimental evidence, while much of it is from animal research, points to an adrenergic inhibitory control of VBF.

Erotic sensitivity of the vagina

Our understanding of how stimulation of the vagina contributes to sexual arousal makes an interesting history. Psychoanalytic conventional wisdom in the 1930s and 1940s was that the clitoris and the vagina were both erotically sensitive, and normal maturation from girlhood to womanhood involved a transference of importance from clitoris to vagina. 'The clitoris in the girl ... is in every way equivalent during childhood to the penis ... the transition to womanhood very much depends upon the early and complete relegation of this sensitivity from the clitoris over to the vaginal orifice' (Freud 1935, p. 278). Failure to make this transition and reliance on 'clitoral orgasm' rather than 'vaginal orgasm' were seen as evidence of immaturity as well as an explanation for 'frigidity'.

Kinsey et al (1953) challenged this view. They had five experienced gynaecologists, two of them women, carry out systematic tests of both touch and pressure sensitivity in the genital regions of 879 women (p. 577). With the labia majora and minora, the clitoris and the vestibule, 92–98% of women indicated tactile sensitivity. In the vagina (578 women tested), 11–14% indicated tactile sensitivity in the anterior, posterior, right or left walls. 'Most of those who did make some response had the sensitivity confined to certain points, in most cases on the upper (anterior) walls of the vagina just inside the vaginal entrance' (p. 580). Kinsey et al (1953), on the basis of this evidence, questioned the concept of 'vaginal orgasm'. pointing out that the occurrence of vaginal contractions during orgasm was not evidence that the orgasm was dependent on vaginal stimulation (VS).

Masters & Johnson (1966) stated unequivocally that 'from an anatomic point of view, there is absolutely no difference in the responses of the pelvic viscera to effective sexual stimulation' (p. 66) whatever type of erotic stimulation is involved. They did not, however, report evidence of vaginal tactile sensitivity, as Kinsey did. They have, nevertheless, been credited with dispelling the 'myth of the vaginal orgasm', although such credit should really go to Kinsey.

Perry & Whipple (1981) revisited an earlier paper by Grafenberg (1950) reporting an area of erotic sensitivity in the anterior wall of the vagina in some women, naming this area 'the G spot', after Grafenberg. There has been considerable controversy about the relevance of this area to women's sexual response ever since. It is noteworthy that this is comparable to the area cited by Kinsey et al (1953) as being sensitive in a minority (11%) of women, raising the question if such an area of erotic sensitivity exists, in how many women is it present? Current thinking presents no consensus on this issue. The urethra runs for part of its course close to the anterior vaginal wall (see Chapter 3). O'Connell & Sanjeevan (2006) comment that 'it is likely that the increased area of sensitivity reported in some women in relation to the urethra is due to the fact that the urethra is surrounded by erectile tissue' (p. 109). Jannini et al (2006) comment that there are more than 250 papers on the G spot, but only a few in peer-reviewed journals — a reason for scepticism. A particularly sceptical review, 'The G-spot: a modern gynecological myth'. was written by Hines (2001). Maravilla (2006) found no evidence of tumescence in this region during MRI scanning of sexual response. On the other hand, Hilliges et al (1995) examined specimens of vaginal wall from the anterior and posterior fornices, the anterior vaginal wall at the bladder neck level and the vaginal introitus. All these regions revealed a 'profound innervation', though the extent of this varied. The more distal areas had more nerve fibres than the more proximal areas, and the anterior wall more than the posterior wall. To what extent these findings could account for localized erotic sensitivity in the anterior wall, and what proportion of women would have such innervation, remain uncertain. However, the types of nerve fibres identified would suggest that pressure is a more important stimulus than touch. Levin (2003b) points out that there are three putative erogenous sites, Halban's fascia, the urethra and clitoral tissue, each or all of which would be stimulated by strong stimulation of this part of the anterior vaginal wall, which he refers to as the 'anterior wall erogenous complex'.

At the present time it is probably prudent to conclude that localized erotic sensitivity in the anterior vaginal wall, possibly dependent on pressure stimulation, occurs in some women, but in what proportion of women is not yet known.

Analgesic effect of vaginal stimulation

An intriguing phenomenon in the sensory system of women's genitalia is a mechanism by which pressure on the anterior vaginal wall or the cervix produces an increase in pain threshold; in other words, an analgesic effect. The relevant evidence, which started with female rats and has now been extended to women, largely comes from Komisaruk and his colleagues (the following is based on a review by Komisaruk & Whipple 1995). In the female rat, pressure on the vaginal wall and cervix (VS), from a vaginal probe, induces sexual receptivity in previously unreceptive rats and a range of other effects, including immobilization, extension of all limbs, lordosis and suppression of responses to painful stimuli. This pain suppression has also been demonstrated with VS due to penile intromission. The pain-blocking effect of intromission has been estimated to be at least five times greater than a standard analgesic dose of morphine. A combination of receptivity and lordosis induction combined with reduced pain sensitivity increases the likelihood that a female rat will accept the multiple intromissions necessary for impregnation.

The three pain responses particularly studied are the tail flick (mediated at the spinal cord level), vocalizations (mediated at the brain stem level) and a sympathetically mediated autonomic reflex, pupil dilatation. Section of the pelvic nerve abolished the suppression of the tail flick response to pain, while leaving vocalizations and pupillary dilatation still suppressed following VS. Section of the hypogastric nerve abolished suppression of vocalizations. This left intact the suppression of autonomic reflex responses such as pupil dilatation,

indicating that some neural pathway, other than the sensory input into the spinal cord, was involved in this component of the analgesic effect of VS. This was eventually shown to be sensory fibres in the vagus nerve, section of which abolished these autonomic manifestations of analgesia.

Studies in women showed an analgesic effect of self-induced continuous pressure on the anterior vaginal wall, as shown by increased pain thresholds in the finger, an effect not produced by comparable pressure on the posterior vaginal wall or clitoris. Further studies in women with complete spinal cord transection at various levels indicated that the analgesic effect of anterior vaginal pressure was still present, consistent with there being sensory pathways to the pain centres in the brain which circumvent the spinal cord. Based on the evidence from the rat, this is assumed to be via the vagus nerve. The possibility that such analgesic effects of VS may reduce pain during parturition was also discussed by Komisaruk & Whipple (1995).

This picture, as applied to women, is somewhat complicated by the finding that, in women with intact spinal cords, self-stimulation of the vaginal wall (anterior and posterior) or clitoris, which is not simply continuous pressure but which produces sexual pleasure, also increases pain thresholds. This has not been shown in rats with stimulation of their external genitalia. In addition, orgasm, in both men and women, can produce analgesia, and some women, including some with SCI, can elicit orgasm with imagery alone (Komisaruk & Whipple 1995). However, in their studies of women with SCI, the analgesic effect in most women was observed without the occurrence of orgasm. Furthermore, there was no significant correlation between the degree of analgesia and the level of subjective arousal. Komisaruk & Whipple (1995) suggest that the pain reduction resulting from pleasurable genital stimulation is mediated differently, via brain centres and associated cognitive processing, compared to the somewhat more robust effect of continuous pressure on the anterior vaginal wall. The spinal cord-mediated analgesic effect of VS may in part result from suppression of the release of substance P in the spinal cord (Steinman et al 1994).

As yet the relationship between these analgesic mechanisms and erotic sensitivity remains unknown. Also, little attention has been paid to the possible clinical relevance of these analgesic mechanisms in women, and in particular how they relate to the common occurrence of pain during sexual intercourse.

Clitoral response

There is no argument about the erotic sensitivity of the clitoris, and its rich supply of sensory nerve fibres (Hoyt 2006), although clitoral response has been less well studied, mainly because it is methodologically more difficult to do so. Now that techniques of ultrasound and MRI scanning are available, more evidence about clitoral response is being obtained (see above), although the greater intrusiveness of the methodologies involved imposes limitations on the experimental methods that can be used. Given the uncertain relationship between

VPA and other aspects of sexual arousal, discussed above, it is of obvious interest to know how clitoral tumescence relates to other aspects of sexual arousal. At the time of writing there is one relevant study. Maravilla et al (2005) compared change in clitoral volume, measured by non-contrast MRI, with ratings of subjective sexual arousal in eight women. There was no correlation ($r = 0.01$). However, there was one substantial outlier, with volume change two to three times greater than the remainder. When she was excluded the correlation was $r = 0.71$, which in comparison with VPA studies is high. There was also a strikingly high correlation between the clitoral volume change on two occasions in the same woman ($r = 0.99$), which is promising for the future of this method. The outlier raises an interesting methodological issue, however, which will need to be addressed in future studies. If the maximum increase in clitoral volume was assessed for each subject and the percentage of maximum change used as the outcome variable, then the outlier would not have had the same effect. This issue is relevant to measurement of penile response, and in some studies percentage of maximum erection has been used. This approach has limitations, however, as in studies of dysfunctional subjects, maximum response may be difficult to establish. We await further studies with interest to see if there is a predictably higher correlation between clitoral and subjective response than has been found with vaginal response.

Orgasm, seminal emission and ejaculation

Of all the various sexual responses, orgasm remains the most mysterious and the least well-understood. It is difficult to define because it is such a subjective experience in which one's powers of observation are impaired, if not suspended. For the post-pubertal male the event is clearly marked by the occurrence of ejaculation. For the female, no such unequivocal event occurs (see later for further discussion of this point), and it is therefore more common for a woman than for a man to be uncertain whether an orgasm has happened.

And yet the orgasm is endowed with considerable importance. Its occurrence is often regarded as the goal of sexual activity and the natural conclusion; the pleasure and reduction of tension associated with it are important reinforcers in the learning of sexual behaviour; lack of orgasm is a cause of concern for many people.

Kinsey et al (1953) regarded an orgasm as an 'explosive discharge of neuromuscular tension' and described it as follows: 'as the individual approaches the peak of sexual activity he or she may suddenly become tense, momentarily maintain a high level of tension, rise to a new peak of maximum tension — and then abruptly and instantaneously release all tensions and plunge into a series of muscular spasms or convulsions through which he or she returns to a normal or even subnormal physiologic state'. There are many other definitions in the literature but they have in common a peak of tension, which is then dramatically reduced. But such a definition begs several questions — what sort of tension? How could it be measured? What triggers the reduction? Clearly this is definition by analogy and is not descriptive in a scientifically adequate sense.

Much has been written about orgasms. Mah & Binik (2001), in their extensive review of this literature, cite around 300 publications. Their review reveals that orgasm is a phenomenon of considerable interest, which is, however, difficult to study, and we are left with some fundamental questions unanswered. Let us, nevertheless, attempt to identify the key components of orgasm and work towards a conceptual model that might aid further research. Building on the model of sexual arousal previously presented, we can conceptualize orgasm as follows:

1. An increase in both the central and the peripheral aspects of sexual arousal to a peak at which some neurophysiological process is triggered with the following manifestations:
   a. Intense feeling of pleasure, or what Mah & Binik (2001) call 'ecstasy'.
   b. Some degree of altered consciousness with reduced awareness and information processing.
   c. Specific sensations, typically felt in the genital regions but spreading through the body to a variable extent.
   d. Muscle contractions: in the female involving pelvic floor, perivaginal and possibly uterine muscles, and in the male bulbocavernosus and bulbospongiosus plus some degree of involvement of pelvic floor muscles.
   e. Other non-genital changes such as rhythmic body movements, vocalization and skin flushing.
2. A post-orgasmic state in which the above manifestations return to a non-aroused state, but with a speed that suggests an active rather than passive process, resulting in a 'refractory period' when further sexual arousal is inhibited.

These manifestations are similar in men and women except that in men the orgasm is usually accompanied by seminal emission. Also the refractory period is more predictable and substantial in men than in women. Seminal emission, ejaculation, female 'ejaculation' and the refractory period will be considered in more detail below.

Genital and pelvic responses during orgasm

The male

It is relatively rare for a man to be unable to ejaculate and experience orgasm, although men vary considerably in the ease with which orgasm is attained, and its intensity, and also in their ability to be able to control ejaculation. Also, whereas it is commonly assumed that ejaculation and orgasm is the goal for men engaging in sexual activity, Laumann et al (1994) found that only 75% of men reported always ejaculating during sexual activity with their primary partner.

Usually, before any of the other phenomena of orgasm occurs, the male becomes aware that ejaculation is imminent — the point of the so-called 'ejaculatory inevitability', when ejaculation follows inevitably within 1–3 s. Ejaculation means forceful expulsion of semen from the urethra, sometimes propelled for a distance of 50 cm or more. If semen drains from the urethra without this force it is called emission. The processes underlying this response are complex and not fully understood. Masters & Johnson (1966) divided it into two stages. In stage I, smooth muscle contraction occurs in the vas efferens of the testis, the epididymis, and vas deferens, together with the seminal vesicle, prostate and ampulla. A substantial part of the seminal fluid comes from the prostate. Accumulation of fluid builds up in the prostatic urethra, whilst the urethral bulb dilates in anticipation. Retrograde passage of the fluid into the bladder is prevented by closure of the internal sphincter, which also prevents urine from joining the semen. Stage II starts with a relaxation of the external bladder sphincter, allowing the pent-up fluid into the urethral bulb. The semen is then propelled along the penile urethra by rhythmic contractions of the bulbospongiosus and ischiocavernosus muscles, the sphincter urethrae and the urethral bulb.

The volume of semen ejaculated varies considerably, usually between 1 and 6 mL. With repeated ejaculations over a short period, the volume and sperm content progressively lessen. The largest volumes typically occur after relatively long periods of ejaculatory abstinence.

The female

In comparison with men, women are much more variable in their capacity for experiencing orgasm. While the large majority of men experience their first orgasm and ejaculation close to the onset of puberty, women report a much more varied age of onset of orgasmic experience, ranging from well before puberty to sometime in adulthood. Kinsey et al (1953) found that 23% had experienced orgasm by age 15, 53% by age 20, 77% by age 25 and about 90% by age 35. They concluded that around 9% of women remain unable to experience orgasm throughout their lives. It is likely that there has been some change in this respect, with women in more recent years tending to have their first orgasmic experience earlier (Bancroft et al 2003a), but there is as yet no evidence that the 9% figure has lessened. Women also vary in the ease with which they achieve orgasm, some women experiencing orgasm from fantasy alone, or from stimulation of their breasts or other non-genital areas, whereas other women require very specific forms of genital stimulation. Laumann et al (1994) found that 29% of women always experienced orgasm during sexual activity with their primary partner, which contrasts with the 75% reported for men.

The limited evidence on the duration of the orgasmic experience also suggests considerable variability among women. Levin & Wagner (1985), measuring duration in the laboratory, reported an average duration of 20 s. A few seconds after the subjective experience of orgasm, there is an initial spasm of the muscles surrounding the outer third of the vagina (the 'orgasmic platform'), followed by a series of rhythmic contractions, usually five to eight in number. Synchronous contractions of the anal sphincter occur in some women (Bohlen et al 1982). Evidence of contractions of the uterine muscles is less consistent, though some researchers have suggested that uterine contractions occur in the 'terminal' orgasm (after which the woman has a relatively refractory period) (Meston et al 2004).

Masters & Johnson (1966) considered the perivaginal contractions to be the essence of the female orgasm, comparable to the rhythmic contractions that subserve ejaculation in the male. It has been contested that women may experience orgasm without these perivaginal contractions (Bohlen et al 1982) and this issue is still disputed (Meston et al 2004). Inadequate tone in the perivaginal muscles has been suggested as a cause of orgasmic dysfunction in women (Graber & Kline-Graber 1979), but Chambless et al (1982) found no relationship between the strength of the levator ani (pubococcygeus) muscle contraction and orgasmic responsiveness.

General muscular responses during orgasm

The pattern of general skeletal muscle activity during non-orgasmic sexual arousal varies considerably, though there is no obvious gender difference in this respect. Much of the motor activity is voluntary and depends on the body position adopted. As arousal increases, certain motor responses become more predictable and less voluntary, especially pelvic thrusting and contraction of the rectus abdominus muscles, sternomastoid and facial musculature, and sometimes carpopedal spasm. During orgasm, spasm of these various muscle groups is maximal, with muscle tension declining rapidly once orgasm has occurred. Not only the extent but also the intensity of these spasms, which have both tonic and clonic phases, vary considerably among individuals, and in their most extreme forms resemble generalized convulsions, leading Kinsey and his colleagues to liken such an orgasm to an epileptic fit (Kinsey et al 1953).

Cardiovascular and respiratory responses associated with orgasm

As already described, changes in heart rate and blood pressure, together with other peripheral vascular responses, may occur during sexual arousal, though to a very variable degree. With orgasm, however, there is a predictable though short-lived rise in both heart rate and blood pressure that starts shortly before the orgasm occurs. According to Littler et al (1974), rises in blood pressure during the arousal phase are inconsistent because of compensatory baroreceptor-induced bradycardia. This compensatory mechanism appears to be over-ruled at the time of orgasm, when the increase in heart rate ranges from 20 to 80 beats/min, systolic blood pressure from 25 to 120 mmHg and diastolic pressure from 25 to 50 mmHg.

Respiration rate, which also shows variable changes during the arousal phase, predictably shows hyperventilation shortly before orgasm. Masters & Johnson (1966) cite rates of around 40 breaths/min. One wonders whether carpopedal spasm that occasionally occurs at this time may be due to hyperventilation tetany. Singer (1973) emphasized a characteristic respiratory pattern of apnoea accompanying certain types of female orgasm. Physiological evidence of this pattern is given by Fox & Fox (1969). A characteristic 'sex flush'. an erythematous rash affecting the skin of the trunk, occurs shortly before orgasm in a proportion of women and men. The incidence of this phenomenon is not known, though of Masters & Johnson's laboratory subjects, 75% of the women and 25% of the men showed it.

The somatic sensations of orgasm

The somatic feelings experienced during orgasm are to some extent determined by the specific genital responses. Thus, the sensation of ejaculation is a characteristic part of the male and the vaginal or uterine contractions of the female experience. But apart from these sensations, the experience is felt or at least described in very different ways, with no clear gender difference. The sensation may be confined to the perineum or spread over part or all of the body. Subjective descriptions are so varied that any attempt to describe a typical orgasmic experience would be misleading. Vance & Wagner (1976) obtained written descriptions from a group of men and women and, when the obviously sex-linked features were removed, it was not possible to distinguish between male and female accounts.

The following are examples from this study:

'An orgasm . . . located (originating) in the genital area, capable of spreading out further . . . legs, abdomen. A sort of pulsating feeling − very nice if it can extend itself beyond the immediate genital area'.

'Begins with tensing and tingling in anticipation, rectal contractions starting series of chills up spine. Tingling and buzzing sensations grow suddenly to explosion in genital area, some sensation of dizzying and weakening almost loss of conscious sensation, but not really. Explosion sort of flowers out to varying distance from genital area, depending on intensity'.

'A heightened feeling of excitement with severe muscular tension especially through the back and legs, rigid straightening of the entire body for about 5 seconds, and a strong and general relaxation and very tired relieved feeling'.

'I really think it defies description by words . . . combination of waves of very pleasurable sensations and mounting of tensions culminating in a fantastic sensation and release of tension'.

'Often loss of contact with reality . . . all senses acute . . . sight becomes patterns of colour, but often very difficult to explain because words were made to fit in the real world'.

'Stomach muscles get "nervous" causing a thrusting movement with hips or pelvis . . . muscular contractions all over the body'.

Altered consciousness

Some of the descriptions given above imply altered consciousness. At its quietest, an orgasm may leave the subject completely in control; at its most extreme, there may be virtual loss of consciousness and certainly loss of control, similar to certain types of epileptic fit in both its convulsive quality and its alteration of consciousness. Although many of the sensory and motor components of orgasm may reflect spinally mediated mechanisms, this altered consciousness strongly suggests some central neurophysiological event. We will return to this point when considering underlying mechanisms.

The psychological components of the orgasmic experience

Mah & Binik (2001) developed a questionnaire to assess the psychological and psychosocial as well as the somatic components of the orgasmic experience. From their results they concluded that 'orgasmic pleasure and satisfaction were related more to (a) the cognitive-affective than the sensory aspects of the orgasm experience; (b) the overall physical and psychological intensity of orgasm but not the anatomical localization or orgasm sensations; and (c) relationship satisfaction' (p. 187). It is questionable whether these conceptual distinctions help in understanding orgasm. Given the varying degree of altered consciousness, and the likelihood of some pivotal central nervous system event, it may be difficult for the individual to recall more than a general 'evaluative' appraisal of the experience. The issue of ecstasy and intense pleasure will be considered further in the next section.

Types of female orgasm

One of the most intriguing debates in the field of human sexuality has concerned the existence and significance of different types of female orgasm, a debate that has been curiously lacking in relation to the male orgasm. The starting point was Freud's doctrine that the continued reliance of a woman on clitoral stimulation in order to experience orgasm is a sign of immaturity, a failure of the 'clitoral–vaginal transfer' that signals sexual maturity. The battle has raged ever since, in one way or another, fuelled in part by those large numbers of women who understandably question whether they should be regarded as immature on such grounds. Kinsey et al (1953) challenged the Freudian position by pointing to the insensitivity to touch of the vaginal wall in contrast to the clitoris and labia minora, concluding that vaginal as distinct from clitoral orgasms were a 'biological impossibility'. They may have underestimated the importance of pressure rather than touch as a vaginal stimulus. Masters & Johnson (1966) developed this theme, claiming that either direct or indirect stimulation of the clitoris is always necessary for orgasm and that the physiological changes accompanying it are the same whatever the method of stimulation. This led to the conclusion that instead of two types of female orgasm (clitoral and vaginal) there was only one. Evidence to the contrary continues to accumulate. The women in Fisher's study (Fisher 1973) described fundamentally different types of orgasmic experience, often in the same individual. Fox & Fox (1969) have physiological correlates of different types occurring in one particular woman. Bentler & Peeler (1979) found that young female students distinguished quite clearly between orgasm experienced during vaginal intercourse, and those resulting from direct clitoral stimulation, whether with their partners or alone. Singer (1973) considered the evidence and reached the conclusion that there are at least two basic patterns which may combine — he called these 'vulval' and 'uterine'. The vulval orgasm depends on clitoral stimulation, occurring either directly or indirectly during coitus or petting, and manifested by vaginal contractions. The uterine experience, he suggests, is characterized by more marked emotional reactions, by apnoea and without vaginal contractions. He speculated that this may depend on uterine or visceral buffeting, which occurs with deep vaginal penetration during coitus. It is this type of orgasm, which is more emotionally fulfilling, that he associated with a female refractory period. He explained the apparent absence of this type of orgasm from the observations of Masters & Johnson in the laboratory as being due to the difficulty in obtaining the necessary psychological conditions in that setting. The vulval orgasm, he suggested, is more mechanical and hence easier to produce. More recent has been the attention paid to stimulation of the anterior vaginal wall and the so-called 'G-spot' considered earlier. As yet there is limited evidence of a physiological difference between orgasms produced by anterior vaginal wall and clitoral stimulation, with different patterns of uterine pelvic floor muscular contractions (Levin 2001). The recent report of differences in post-orgasmic PRL levels in both women and men, when comparing orgasms from masturbation and those from sexual interaction with one's partner (Brody & Krüger 2006), opens up some new intriguing possibilities.

Although controversy about typologies of female orgasms continues, there is now general agreement that Freud's attribution of immaturity to clitoral orgasm is untenable. Kinsey and Masters & Johnson have done women a service in that respect. Findings from Fisher's (1973) study even suggest the opposite. Women who had a definite preference for vaginal orgasms were more prone to anxiety. He suggested that reliance on vaginal intercourse rather than direct clitoral stimulation could serve to avoid more intense sexual excitement that these women find threatening, perhaps because they are generally less comfortable about somatic changes in their own bodies. He also pointed out that vaginal intercourse might be a more acceptable form of behaviour for these women than stimulation, which has masturbatory connotations. Hite (1976), in her survey, found a substantial majority of women who required clitoral stimulation in order to experience orgasm and this has been found in a number of surveys (see Chapter 6). The continuing debate on these various aspects of female orgasm is a fascinating one in several respects, as it is not just a matter of sexual physiology. Doris Lessing (whose description of several types of female orgasm in her novel *The Golden Notebook* is often quoted in sexological texts) wrote the following: 'There can be a thousand thrills, sensations, etc. but there is only one real female orgasm and that is when a man, from the whole of his need and desire, takes a woman and wants all her response. Everything else is a substitute and a fake and the most inexperienced woman feels this instinctively' — not exactly the most politically correct conclusion! Of more recent origin is a vigorous ongoing controversy about the functions of female orgasm, and these will be considered later.

Mechanisms underlying orgasm, seminal emission and ejaculation

The male

In the male we face the challenge of distinguishing between orgasm, seminal emission and ejaculation. Semans & Langworthy (1938), following their study of sexual responses in cats, proposed a neurophysiological basis of emission and ejaculation, which is usually accepted as relevant to the human male. They postulated an ejaculation centre in the lumbar cord that produces emission via the sympathetic outflow from the first two lumbar roots and ejaculation via the sacral parasympathetic outflow (S2–4), and is presumably dependent on contraction of the ischiocavernosus, bulbospongiosus and contractor urethra muscles. Direct evidence of this kind from men is lacking. Effects on sexual responses of sympathectomy involving different parts of the sympathetic chain were reported by Whitelaw & Smithwick (1951) and they proved to be variable and inconsistent. It was, however, relatively common for emission to be impaired when lumbar parts of the cord were removed and unusual if only thoracic rami were affected.

The effects of various drugs may be relevant. It is important to distinguish between drugs that in some way impair sexual arousal, as this may secondarily reduce or delay the likelihood of orgasm without specifically blocking orgasm. Antiadrenergic compounds such as guanethidine may lead to failure of ejaculation. Typically the man experiences orgasm without the sensation of emission or ejaculation — the so-called 'dry-run orgasm' (Money & Yankowitz 1967). This has been attributed to failure of control of the internal bladder sphincter, leading to retrograde ejaculation into the bladder. However, whereas this undoubtedly happens after certain kinds of prostatectomy and as an occasional consequence of diabetic neuropathy, there is no evidence that this is the explanation in the case of antiadrenergic drugs. It thus seems possible that emission can be pharmacologically blocked without interfering with orgasm. Use of selective SSRIs commonly results in inability to ejaculate, and, currently, short-acting SSRIs are being developed as treatment for premature ejaculation. However, SSRIs can also impair orgasm in women (see Chapter 13, p. 403). We cannot yet exclude the possibility that the primary effect of SSRIs in this respect is to impair the arousal process, which would normally lead to triggering of orgasm and seminal emission. However, it is also possible that there is a direct pharmacological effect on orgasm rather than seminal emission. However, in such cases, seminal emission does not occur without orgasm, suggesting a link between the two mechanisms.

In men with severe premature ejaculation, it is common for them to describe a minimal or absent orgasm and no ejaculatory component; the semen just oozes out of the urethra. These men would appear to be experiencing emission with no ejaculation and little or no orgasm. The relationship between these three components therefore remains uncertain, except that they usually occur together. Levin (2005a) prefers to see these three components in the male as separate, if usually coordinated. However, he was unable to find evidence of any predictable pattern whereby seminal emission triggered ejaculation, such as the 'prostatic pressure chamber' concept, which had been suggested in the literature. The phenomenon of 'ejaculatory inevitability'. which probably depends on the initiation of seminal emission, suggests that seminal emission comes first and somehow triggers the other two components. But Levin has not presented evidence that the contractions, which are the crucial component of ejaculation, are other than those that are a component of orgasm. At the present time, therefore, it is reasonable to conclude tentatively that the muscular contractions that produce ejaculation are part of the motor component of orgasm, whereas emission, a smooth muscle response, is distinct and separable; this would conform with the neural separation of the two processes described by Semans & Langworthy (1938) in the cat.

The female

The most directly relevant evidence of the peripheral mediation of orgasm in the female comes from studies of women with SCI. Approximately 50% of women with SCI are able to experience orgasm following their injury, and their subjective descriptions of the orgasmic experience do not differ from those of women without SCI, although they usually take longer to achieve orgasm (Meston et al 2004). Sipski et al (2001) found that women with complete lower motor neuron injuries affecting their S2–5 reflex arc were significantly less likely to experience orgasm than women with other SCIs. They concluded that an intact sacral reflex arc is important for the ability to experience orgasm.

The brain

So far, we have considered mechanisms operating at a spinal level. But these uncertainties bring us to a fundamental question about orgasm. To what extent is it a spinal phenomenon, to what extent does it depend on central events, or to what extent is it an interaction between spinal and central events? Kinsey, it will be remembered, likened the more intense orgasm to an epileptic fit. Orgasmic sensations may be experienced as part of an epileptic aura, and this is most likely to occur when the epileptic focus is the area of the right temporal lobe, which includes the amygdala and hippocampus (Komisaruk et al 2007). EEG changes resembling petit mal or the late stage of a grand mal seizure have been recorded during self-induced orgasm (Mosovich & Tallafero 1954). Heath (1972) recorded changes from implanted electrodes in a man and woman, both epileptic patients, and each showed localized discharges from the septal region associated with orgasm. These were similar to epileptiform changes but were localized and did not reach scalp electrodes. Cohen et al (1976) used a change in laterality of the EEG as an indicator of a significant cerebral neurophysiological event and found that this occurred in the majority of their normal subjects during orgasm. When it did not occur, the orgasms were of low intensity. In contrast, Graber et al (1985) failed to find any distinctive EEG changes in four men during masturbation and ejaculation; the authors concluded that changes reported by other workers were at least in part the result of movement artefact.

With the advent of brain imaging, we may expect some progress in understanding the central mechanisms, although at the time of writing we have only limited evidence of this kind to consider. An early brain imaging study by Tiihonen et al (1994) used PET scanning in eight men who masturbated to orgasm and ejaculation. They found decreased cerebral blood flow in all areas of the cerebral cortex during orgasm, except in the right prefrontal cortex, where there was a significant increase. This corresponds roughly to Brodmann's area 10, the function of which remains uncertain.

Holstege et al (2003) used PET to assess eight men who ejaculated following manual stimulation by their female partners. They reported brain areas where there was significantly more blood flow during ejaculation than before it. Such activation was found in the transitional zone between the midbrain and diencephalon (thalamus and hypothalamus). The resolution of their method did not allow precise identification of the activated structures within that zone. However, within that cluster are the VTA, the subparafascicular nucleus, the midbrain lateral central tegmental field, and medial and ventral thalamic nuclei. The VTA is part of the mesolimbic (A10) DA system, which is involved in a variety of appetitive behaviours (see p. 67). Also to be found in this cluster is the A11 DA cell group. In rats and monkeys this projects throughout the spinal cord grey matter, but most strongly to the pelvic floor motor neurons in the upper sacral cord, the L2–3 motor neurons to the cremasteric muscle, and the T1–L2/3 sympathetic preganglionic motor neurons, including those innervating the genitalia.

Additional areas activated included the claustrum and adjoining parts of the rostral insula, striatum and anterior nucleus of the right thalamus. Activation in the neocortex was mainly on the right, involving the inferior frontal gyrus, parts of the parietal and inferior temporal cortex, and the precuneus (part of the medial surface of the parietal lobe). There was also marked activation in the left cerebellar hemisphere and an area of distinct *deactivation* in the anterior part of the left medial temporal lobe, including parts of the amygdala and entorhinal cortex (involved in memory). It is not possible from this report to identify those areas where some activation first occurred during the development of sexual arousal.

Komisaruk and colleagues (reviewed in Komisaruk & Whipple, 2005) used fMRI to explore brain activity during orgasm in women, including a number of women who were able to induce orgasm by thought processes alone. With orgasms induced by VCS, activation was observed in the hypothalamus, amygdala, hippocampus, cingulate and insular cortex, the region incorporating the nucleus accumbens, BNST and MPOA, the basal ganglia, especially the putamen, the parietal and frontal lobes of the neocortex, cerebellum, and parts of the lower brainstem (central grey, mesencephalic reticular formation and nucleus of the tractus solitarius). When activation during orgasm was contrasted with activation immediately before and after orgasm, areas most directly related to orgasm included the paraventricular area of the hypothalamus, amygdala, anterior cingulate region and nucleus accumbens. Activation during 'thought-induced' orgasms was mainly similar, the most interesting difference being a lack of activation of the amygdala, leading the authors to speculate that amygdala has a genital sensory role in orgasm whereas the other areas activated have a more cognitive role. The fact that activation of the cerebellum occurred in both 'thought' and VCS-induced orgasms suggests that cerebellar involvement is not a reflection of motor activity involved in genital stimulation. However, it could be involved in the integration of muscle contractions that are likely to occur in both types of orgasm. Komisaruk & Whipple (2005) also speculated that the cerebellum has a 'significant perceptual/cognitive–hedonic role in orgasm' (p. 17).

A comparison of these three studies shows limited agreement. The earliest imaging study (Tiihonen et al 1994) showing only one area of activation, the right prefrontal cortex, and otherwise deactivation in several other cortical areas is so different that methodological factors seem the most likely explanation. The two more recent studies differ in the method of imaging used, with the fMRI (Komisaruk & Whipple 2005) allowing greater resolution. In addition, one study is of men and the other of women. The similarities are activation of frontal and parietal cortical areas and of the cerebellum. The results in men, however, point more to the thalamus and midbrain, whereas in women there was more focus on the hypothalamus, particularly the PVN which is involved in the secretion of OT (see p. 128). The mesolimbic DA system was implicated in both studies, via the ventral tegmentum in the men and the nucleus accumbens in the women. An interesting difference is the suggestion of *deactivation* of the amygdala in the men and *activation* in the women, which contrasts with the finding of Hamann et al (2004) that the amygdala showed more activation in response to sexual stimuli in men than in women (p. 72). Activation of the insula was found during orgasm in the women and has been found in other studies in response to pain, leading Komisaruk et al (2007) to

consider whether processing of pleasure and pain had some features in common. Komisaruk & Whipple (2005) concluded that apart from the methodological differences between PET and fMRI, there is no simple way to account for the differences and that 'it seems more prudent to postpone such speculation pending information generated by "differential diagnostic" types of studies' (p. 16). This does not deter them, however, from indulging in some interesting speculations in their subsequent book (Komisaruk et al 2007).

How do these results compare to experimental findings from animals? Although there is persuasive evidence of orgasm occurring in a variety of female primates (Dixson 1998), there is no related evidence of brain activity. There is also no relevant evidence of female orgasm from lower mammals. In the male the emphasis has been on ejaculation, which can be clearly identified, and male orgasm, as a separate entity, has received scant attention. However, there is evidence from male rats relevant to the process of ejaculation. The subparafascicular nucleus (SPFp) of the male rat, found in the midbrain lateral central tegmental field, shows evidence of increased c-Fos after ejaculation. Neurons in the third and fourth lumbar segments of the spinal cord are connected to the SPFp. If these cells are ablated by selective toxins, ejaculatory behaviour is completely disrupted, while other components of sexual behaviour remain intact (Truitt & Coolen 2002). Brain imaging evidence from men (Holstege et al 2003) was consistent with SPFp activation during ejaculation. If we return to the earlier consideration of the neuromediation of seminal emission and ejaculation, the role of the SPFp may be the control of seminal emission. In rodent research no distinction is made between seminal emission and ejaculation.

The source of orgasmic pleasure

The explanation for the intense pleasure, only one component of orgasm but perhaps the most important, remains elusive. Holstege et al (2003) and Komisaruk & Whipple (2005) allude to the activation of the mesolimbic DA system as the explanation and draw comparisons with the 'rush' of addictive drugs. Holstege et al (2003) refer to brain-imaging studies involving administration of heroin (Sell et al 1999) and cocaine (Breiter et al 1997). Komisaruk & Whipple refer to a third study involving nicotine (Stein et al 1998). Because activation of the mesolimbic DA system was evident in all three of these studies, this is taken as evidence that this system is involved in the intense pleasure of the experience, and hence is relevant to the pleasure of orgasm. The vigorous debate about whether, with drugs of addiction, this DA system is involved in the 'appetitive' or 'reward' component was considered earlier (p. 63). Let us revisit that debate while considering the evidence from these brain-imaging studies more closely. In the studies involving heroin and cocaine, mesolimbic activation occurred in response to drug-salient cues as well as administration of the drugs per se. In the study involving nicotine there was no test of 'drug salient cues'. It is, however, important to keep in mind that all three studies involved individuals already addicted, who have already gone through a complex learning process associated with the establishment of addiction to a particular drug (Robbins & Everitt 2002). It would be more directly relevant to our purpose, although not ethically feasible, to assess brain activation in response to intravenous injections of such drugs in individuals not already addicted. What direct pharmacological effects might be expected? Heroin is an opiate that stimulates μ opioid receptors in addition to others. Animal studies have shown that the μ opioid effect results in an increased release of DA in the striatum and nucleus accumbens, due to inhibition of other neurons that tonically inhibit DA neurons (Chahl 1995). Cocaine is a reuptake inhibitor of NA and 5HT but most powerfully of DA, an effect that has been demonstrated in the mesolimbic DA system (Stahl 1996). Nicotine releases a variety of neurotransmitters (e.g. ACh). There are nicotinic receptors in the l.c., the centre for the NA arousal system, relevant to sexual as well as other types of central arousal (see p. 67). But nicotine also releases DA in the striatum and mesolimbic system (Wonnacott 1995). There are therefore pharmacological grounds for DA activation in the mesolimbic system with all three drugs.

Endogenous opiates have been clearly implicated in the inhibition of sexual response, but this may involve different opioid receptors. Of particular interest are the effects of opiate antagonists, such as naloxone and naltrexone. In humans, the limited research has produced inconsistent but, in some cases, interesting results. A dual dose-related effect was observed in women masturbating to orgasm (Gillman & Lichtigfield 1983); low doses of naloxone enhanced pleasure during orgasm, while higher doses had the opposite effect, reducing sexual arousal as well as orgasmic pleasure. This is consistent with the idea that endogenous opiates have both inhibitory and facilitatory effects, but the precise explanation for the relation to dose remains elusive. So far, no changes in plasma levels of β-endorphin have been found during sexual arousal or orgasm in men (Krüger et al 1998) or women (Exton et al 1999).

In the study involving nicotine, Stein et al (1998) concluded that the direct activation of the frontal and cingulate regions was responsible for the drug's primary behavioural and mood-altering effects. The nature of the nicotine 'rush', however, may be somewhat different to that from heroin or cocaine. Stein et al (1998) found that their subjects, all addicted to nicotine, reported a dose-dependent but 'moderate' intensity of 'rush' and a moderate liking of the experience (mean rating 4.1, SD 2.1, on a 0–10 scale for rating peak response).

In conclusion, there is no doubt that mesolimbic activation is associated with *anticipation* of intense pleasure and the 'incentive motivation' to obtain such reward. It clearly becomes involved in the complex process leading to the establishment of an addiction. But its role in mediating the intense pleasure of orgasm remains somewhat uncertain, and we should keep in mind the possibility that other brain areas, and possibly other neurotransmitters apart from DA, are involved.

We therefore remain uncertain about the nature of the central phenomena associated with orgasm, and how they are triggered. The considerable variation in intensity of orgasm could well be accounted for by variation in the intensity of such central components, which when intense would not only lead to alteration of consciousness but could also influence the perceived intensity of spinal responses. Given that, in most respects orgasm per se appears to be similar in men and women, the hint of gender differences in the central mechanisms involved is particularly intriguing.

After the orgasm: the refractory period

A characteristic of orgasm is the state of calm that follows it. There is a fairly rapid return of the various physiological manifestations of arousal and vasocongestion to normal, together with a subjective feeling of calm. Without orgasm, these changes take much longer to resolve, especially in women where congestion of the pelvic organs may remain for several hours, sometimes with a sense of discomfort, if no orgasm occurs.

The male following orgasm usually remains unresponsive to further sexual stimulation for a period of time known as the 'refractory period'. In the young male this may be a matter of minutes, whereas in the older male it may be many hours. Women, on the other hand, may be able to experience repeated multiple orgasms in a short period, and many were observed to do so by Masters & Johnson in their laboratory investigations, leading them to regard the refractory period as a uniquely male phenomenon.

This conclusion should not be too readily accepted. There are females who describe a definite refractory period, and this may be associated with certain types of female orgasm, possibly not the type that is likely to occur in a laboratory setting. Kinsey et al (1953) reported only 14% of their female sample as being multiply orgasmic on a regular basis. There may be many women who fail to realize their potential in this respect, though the proportion who do may be larger than 14% if Kinsey's survey were repeated now. Nevertheless, it is highly likely that the women in Masters & Johnson's study were not representative of women in general.

The refractory period is not invariable in the male either. There have been a few case reports of men who appear to lack normal post-ejaculatory refractoriness and are similar to women in their capacity for multiple orgasms. In an earlier report (Robbins & Jensen 1978), the pattern described suggested an avoidance of ejaculation to allow several orgasms to occur. This raised the question of whether it was repeated orgasms or rather peaks of arousal and sensation that were occurring. In a later report (Dunn & Trost 1989), some subjects clearly described ejaculating more than once during single episodes. Interestingly, several of the subjects interviewed by Dunn & Trost (1989) were in middle age and had developed this pattern relatively late. Kinsey et al (1948) presented evidence that a number of preadolescent boys were capable of multiple orgasm. This evidence came largely from the observations of one man who had been involved in sexual activity with or observing sexual activity in a large number of boys (see Kinsey et al 1948, Tables 31–34). This evidence has become the focus for recent attacks on Kinsey, with allegations that he engaged in or at least promoted child sexual abuse (see Bancroft 1998, 2004 for discussion of this controversy). While such allegations are unfounded, one has to raise questions about the scientific validity of these observations. Yet if they are valid they raise theoretical issues of considerable interest. Careful enquiries of adolescents and young adults about their pre-pubertal orgasmic experiences are required to throw light on this issue. In a recent study of students, asked to recall their childhood sexual experiences, 13.5% of males recalled their first orgasm occurring before puberty, defined as age at first ejaculation (Bancroft et al 2003a). Further studies are needed to explore carefully whether such individuals experienced multiple orgasms. If it is the case that some such boys are capable of repeated orgasm, with minimal or no refractory period, when they are pre-pubertal, it strongly suggests that something happens, developmentally, with the onset of puberty, to bring the refractory process into play. One possibility is that it is the onset of seminal emission that triggers the inhibitory mechanism. In rats, the normal refractory period that occurs after coitus does not occur after electroejaculation (Beach et al 1966). Another possibility is that the peri-pubertal increase in T leads to development of this inhibitory mechanism (Sachs 1995), at the same time as it is having obvious positive effects on the excitatory mechanisms.

A further characteristic of the post-ejaculatory refractory period that is widely accepted is that it typically increases with age (e.g. Kolodny et al 1979). Interestingly, it is difficult to find any systematic evidence to that effect, which is unfortunate because the explanation for this age effect could be of considerable theoretical interest. Is it due, for example, to an age-related decline in excitability? The commonly reported reduction in refractory period together with a general increase in arousability that older men may experience with a new partner is consistent with that explanation. Is there an age-related increase in inhibitory response post ejaculation, and if so why? Are both types of change involved, and, if so, is the age-related decline in responsiveness to T playing a part? The Dual Control model (p. 64) is of relevance here. Whatever inhibitory mechanism is involved, the duration and intensity of the refractory period may depend on the balance between excitation and inhibition at that point. Although there is a lack of systematic evidence on this point, it is likely that the degree of unarousability post ejaculation depends in part on the degree of excitation that preceded ejaculation. This is vividly illustrated in men with severe premature ejaculation, better described as premature emission, which occurs without obvious ejaculation and with a minimum of orgasmic sensation. Such rapid emissions, while often associated with anticipatory anxiety, are typically accompanied by low or minimal sexual arousal. Typically, after the premature emission the refractory state is prolonged and intense. This contrasts with the individual, typically a young man, who ejaculates quickly in a sexual encounter because he becomes rapidly and strongly aroused. His refractory period may be minimal.

The refractory period is one example of inhibition of sexual response, which in the male has an obvious reproductive benefit. If males ejaculate too frequently their sperm count declines and they become less fertile. Not surprisingly, the refractory period, or its equivalent, is found in other species, although most experimental evidence pertains to the male rat, where the refractory period is referred to as the 'post-ejaculatory interval'. Evidence of the underlying mechanisms is unfortunately limited. Lorrain et al (1997) showed in male rats that, during the post-ejaculatory interval, serotonin increased in the lateral hypothalamic area. Injecting an SSRI into the lateral hypothalamus produced behavioural effects similar to the post-ejaculatory interval. Serotonin does, therefore, appear to be involved in the refractory period of the male. Administration of the NA-synthesis inhibitor DDC produces a dramatic lengthening of the post-ejaculatory refractory period and intromission latencies as negative effects, and facilitation of copulation, with reduction in the number of intromissions preceding ejaculation and ejaculation latency as positive effects (McIntosh & Barfield 1984). This is a further example of the complexity of NA mechanisms in the brain, with NA being involved, depending on the context, in either inhibitory or excitatory effects. But as we will see below, the NA system may be of fundamental importance to the refractory period.

An interesting extension of the 'post-ejaculatory inhibition' model is the 'sexual satiation' or 'sexual exhaustion' of male rats. The unrestricted exposure of male rats to receptive females results in repeated copulation until a state of sexual satiation is established. The average number of such copulations required to establish this state is seven, and complete recovery takes around 15 days. The assumption that this state involves a specific inhibition of sexual responsiveness is supported by the otherwise normal behaviour shown by the sexually sated animal.

Although first described more than 40 years ago, only recently has this state been subjected to experimental evaluation. Rodriguez-Manzo & Fernando-Guasti (1994, 1995a) showed that the 5HT1A agonist, 8-OH-DPAT, which typically facilitates ejaculation by its reduction of serotonergic transmission, the $\alpha2$ adrenoceptor antagonist, yohimbine, which also typically has sexually enhancing effects by increasing NE at the synapse, and the opioid antagonists (naloxone and naltrexone), when given individually, all partially restore sexual behaviour in the sated rat. Furthermore, the positive effects of 8-OH-DPAT and the opioid antagonists were largely eliminated by neurotoxic lesioning of the central NA system, although the positive effects of yohimbine were not affected (Rodriguez-Manzo & Fernandez-Guasti 1995b), suggesting that the anti-opioid and anti-serotonergic effects were dependent on an intact central NA system. Taking a different experimental approach, Mas et al (1995) reported evidence of a blockade of DA neurotransmission resulting in an increase in DA turnover and DA metabolite levels. They found further support for this explanation by demonstrating a positive effect of apomorphine on sexual responsivity of the sated rat and postulated that the mediator of the DA blockade could be PRL, which is known to increase in male rats following ejaculation, and in humans also (Krüger et al 2002). This response in men will be considered further below. Fiorino et al (1997) found further evidence of the role of DA in sexual satiation in the rat, reporting an increase in DA transmission in the nucleus accumbens, as exposure to a novel receptive female resulted in re-initiation of sexual behaviour.

With 'sexual satiation' we therefore have an experimental model of probable relevance to normal adaptive sexual behaviour in rats, which demonstrates the involvement of most of the principal excitatory and inhibitory mediators that are currently known about (with the apparent exception of GABA), and that also appears to depend on the integrity of the NA arousal system. But it is consistent with the idea that both inhibitory and excitatory mechanisms affecting sexual behaviour depend on complex interactions between different neurotransmitters and neuromodulators and that experimental manipulation of single parts of this complex system is likely to produce an incomplete or inconsistent picture.

In the human, the most directly relevant evidence available comes from studies of hormone levels in the blood preceding and following orgasm in men and women. In a recent series of studies in which masturbation or sexual activity with a partner led to orgasm or ejaculation, continuous blood sampling was carried out both before and after orgasm, with assaying at 2 min intervals of epinephrine, NA, cortisol, OT, vasopressin, β-endorphin and PRL. The one compound that showed a clear and predictable increase following orgasm was PRL, a pattern observed in both men (Krüger et al 1998, 2003a) and women (Exton et al 1999), with levels still raised after 60 min (see Fig. 4.7). Levels both at baseline and following orgasm, however, were much higher in women than men. This pattern was not found in a parallel study of men who masturbated without ejaculating (Krüger et al 2003b).

These apparently consistent recent results have led these researchers to postulate that the post-orgasmic rise in PRL acts as a feedback control of sexual drive, contributing to the post-orgasmic refractory period (Krüger et al 2002). In a comparable fashion, sexual side effects of DA antagonistic psychotropic drugs, used for the treatment of schizophrenia, and of SSRI, used for the treatment of depression, have been explained as resulting from the associated and chronic increase in PRL (e.g. Halbreich et al 2003). Let us consider these claims

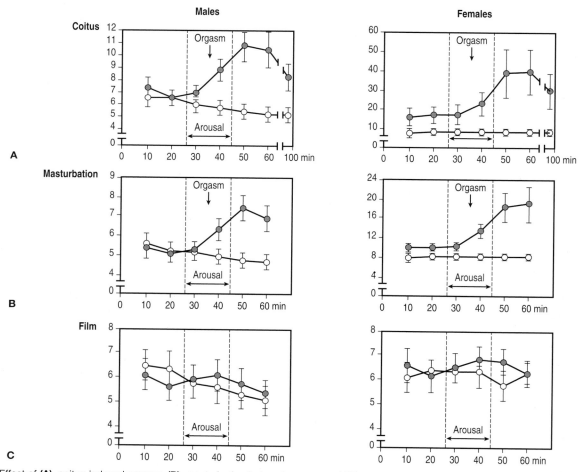

Fig. 4.7 Effect of **(A)**, coitus-induced orgasm, **(B)**, masturbation-induced orgasm and **(C)**, sexual arousal in response to an erotic film not leading to orgasm, on plasma PRL levels. These three 'experimental' conditions are depicted by filled circles. The control condition, depicted by hollow circles, involved no sexual stimuli. (From Krüger et al 2007.)

more closely. DA in the tuberoinfundibular DA system maintains inhibitory control of PRL release. Thus, any reduction of DA activity in this system will result in increased PRL release. Serotonin and thyrotrophin-releasing hormone increase PRL release. An important distinction in the experimental animal literature is between chronic and acute exposure to elevated PRL. The evidence from chronic exposure, typically implemented by means of transplants of pituitary glands, indicates that after a week or longer there is predictable impairment of sexual response with increased intromission and ejaculation latencies, and reduction in reflexive erections in male rats (Meisel & Sachs 1994). The more limited evidence of acute or short-term elevation of PRL indicates either no effect or a facilitatory effect (Melis & Argiolas 1995). A parallel can be drawn with chronic hyperprolactinaemia in humans. In cases of PRL-secreting tumours of the anterior pituitary, there is presumably a continuing release of PRL unaffected by the normal control mechanisms, such as DA. In other non-tumour cases, the mechanism underlying the hyperprolactinaemia is not well understood. But in both types of case, given the very high levels of PRL that usually prevail, and the interaction of PRL, DA, serotonin and β-endorphin, and most probably a number of other factors, it is reasonable to expect some more widespread dysregulation. With the transient and comparatively small increase in PRL observed following orgasm by Krüger and his colleagues, such dysregulation is less likely to be involved. Furthermore, given that the refractory period is more complete and sustained in men than in women, it is noteworthy that the PRL rise is more substantial in women. There are therefore alternative explanations to be considered. Thus, the increase in PRL following orgasm can be seen as an epiphenomenon of post-orgasmic inhibition of DA activity, and not a hormonal mechanism of functional significance. The evidence is also clear that PRL has a positive feedback on DA release from the arcuate nucleus; given the PRL inhibiting effect of DA this shows a negative feedback loop — the increased PRL results in an increase in DA inhibition of PRL release. Thus, the increased DA activity would be likely to have the opposite effect on the refractory period, which, at least in part, can be seen as manifestation of reduced DA activity. The assumption made by Halbreich et al (2003) that the negative sexual effects of PRL-elevating drugs result from the resulting hyperprolactinaemia is somewhat more valid, because of the sustained hyperprolactinaemia involved. But the case can also be made for the DA antagonistic or the serotonin agonistic drug effect as being the cause of the sexual side effects, with the raised PRL as an epiphenomenon.

If the above interpretation is correct, it points to a reduction of DA activity in the brain following orgasm. However, the fact that it occurs in both men and women to a similar extent suggests that it is not a fundamental component of the male-type refractory period. It may, however, contribute to a reduced sexual arousability in both men and women. In an interesting re-analysis of these studies (Brody & Kruger 2006), which had involved self-masturbation in some cases and sexual interaction with a partner in others, it was found that the post-orgasm increase in PRL was substantially greater (by around 400%) following sexual interaction with the partner than following masturbation, and in both men and women. This also points to the PRL increase resulting from some mechanism that is not simply post-ejaculatory. Brody & Kruger (2006) interpreted this difference as indicating greater 'satiety' following partner-induced orgasm, but the nature and function of this greater 'satiety' remains, as yet, unexplained. The possibility that it may be related to reproductive success is considered in the later section on PRL (p. 129).

As discussed earlier, OT has also been reported to increase after orgasm (Carmichael et al 1987), remaining raised for about 5 min in both men and women. However, more recent studies have shown less consistent results (Murphy et al 1987; Blaicher et al 1999; Krüger et al 2003a,b). There is no evidence of an increase of β-endorphin in the circulation following orgasm (e.g. Krüger et al 1998; Exton et al 1999).

As with 'sexual satiety' in rats, it so far appears that the refractory period in humans is a complex process involving a variety of mechanisms, as yet not well understood.

Female ejaculation

There is no doubt that a small number of women are worried by a tendency during orgasm to pass fluid, which they take to be urine. Probably in some cases urinary incontinence does occur. But are there other explanations? Such fluid has been reported to contain constituents, e.g. prostatic acid phosphatase, suggestive of prostatic secretion, raising the possibility that vestigial remnants of prostatic tissue may persist in some women and account for the fluid. Descriptions of some female 'ejaculators' include the development during sexual response of a swelling in the anterior vaginal wall close to the erotically sensitive area described earlier (p. 82), which disappears once 'ejaculation' has occurred. This is presumably the fluid collecting in the urethra at that point. It seems reasonable to conclude from the available evidence that a small proportion of women do produce fluid, which is not urine, from the urethra at the time of orgasm. Its ejection can in a literal sense be called ejaculation, but to what extent is the process homologous in physiological terms to male ejaculation, or in anatomical terms to the prostatic origin of male ejaculatory fluid?

As we saw in Chapter 3, the prostate gland is derived embryologically from the Wolffian duct system, which normally atrophies during female development. The female urethra is, however, surrounded by glandular tissue. In some women these glands are organized to feed into a paraurethral duct system, running along either side of the outer part of the urethra and opening just inside the urethral meatus. Such structures are normally called Skene's glands after the man who described them in 1880. Huffman (1948) in a more recent and detailed anatomical study found that these paraurethral duct systems were the exception rather than the rule. He found considerable variability between women in the extent and location of these glands, most of which open directly into the urethra along its course. That the embryological origin of these glands is similar or even homologous to that of prostatic tissue has been suggested for a long time. More recently these glands have been found to be immunologically similar to prostatic tissue and to secrete prostatic acid phosphatase (Pollen & Dreilinger 1984), though it should be pointed out that prostatic acid phosphatase is produced by tissues other than the prostate (e.g. the kidney). In addition, there are in the male comparable glands along most of the urethra. Although little attention has been paid to the anatomy and physiology of these male structures, it is probable that they (rather than Cowper's glands) are responsible for the pre-ejaculatory emission experienced by many men during sexual arousal. In the Kinsey survey (Gebhard & Johnson 1979), 78% of male subjects were aware of this pre-ejaculatory fluid, and, although in the majority this only involved a drop or two, in nearly 20% there was sufficient fluid to drip from the penis, causing embarrassment in some such men. It is possible that all the glandular structures along the urethra, including these periurethral glands and the prostate, have features in common. The comparable glands in the female may also share some features, including embryological origin, but there is little purpose in referring to them as the 'female prostate', any more than we call the periurethral glands in the male 'prostatic tissue'. If, however, the glands in the female do originate from the Wolffian system, then we should expect to find them to be much more developed in a few women than is usual in the majority, accounting for the occasional woman who produces an unusual amount of fluid. It is also interesting to speculate whether such tissue of Wolffian origin may respond to T and therefore be more developed in women with relatively high androgen levels. Such tissue has been shown to be T dependent in female rodents (Korenchevsky 1937), but there are no relevant data for women.

To what extent is ejection of such fluid homologous to male ejaculation? It is important to remind ourselves that ejaculation in the male has two components: the emission of fluid, which depends on smooth muscle contraction passing fluid along both the vas and the urethra, and the pumping effect of the rhythmic striped muscle contraction accompanying orgasm, adding to the emission a forceful ejaculatory spurt. In a woman who collects fluid, from whatever source, in her urethra, possibly contained during sexual stimulation by restriction of the perivaginal muscles, the onset of orgasm and the rhythmic muscle contractions that are basically similar to those in the male would lead to ejaculation of the fluid. Thus, the ejaculatory process may be found in both cases but the emission of fluid only in the male. In any case, rather more has been made of this issue than the subject warrants. What is of clinical importance is the recognition that some women do eject fluid during orgasm, which is not necessarily urine. This information could be very reassuring to those women who are deeply embarrassed by what they assume is urinary incontinence.

The functions of orgasm

The reproductive function of orgasm in the male is obvious because of the associated ejaculation of semen. The pleasure experience during orgasm will also act as a motivator for further reproductive acts. In the female, the function is not so obvious, although this has not discouraged attempts to suggest functions. Levin (1992) listed a number of such suggestions: (i) reward for allowing coitus to occur, (ii) bringing coitus to an end, (iii) resolving vaginal tenting and allowing the cervix to dip back into the seminal pool, (iv) resolving pelvic vasocongestion, (v) stimulating the male to ejaculate intravaginally by means of perivaginal muscular contractions, (vi) pair-bonding (resulting from the male who induces the orgasm having more appeal), (vii) uterine contractions leading to 'upsuck' of semen into the uterus and (viii) psychological resuscitation. Levin (1992) suggested that perhaps the first of these is sufficient, though he qualifies this by pointing out that no more than 50% of women experience orgasm as a result of coitus. More recently he has explained that any 'upsuck' effect of orgasm is likely to have a negative effect on the likelihood of fertilization by a specific ejaculate (Levin 2005b). Sperm transport into the uterus is most rapid in the sexually unaroused woman. It is sexual arousal, he argued, that is important for conception, by leading to vaginal tenting, pooling of semen, and providing the environment for capacitation of sperm, the maturing process that makes the sperm capable of conception. Orgasm, therefore, is likely to terminate this stage, perhaps too quickly for achieving optimum conditions for conception.

Several of these postulated functions have been presented in the literature as explanations for why the female orgasm should be regarded as an evolutionary 'adaptation'. Using West-Eberhard's (1992) definition, 'it is correct to consider a character an "adaptation" for a particular task only if there is some evidence that it has evolved (been modified during its evolutionary history) in specific ways to make it more effective in the performance of that task, and that the change occurred because of the increased fitness that results ... To be considered an adaptation a trait must be shown to be a consequence of selection for that trait' (p. 13). The extent to which some evolutionary psychologists apparently believe that they can meet this definition with one or other of these 'coping strategies', several of which contradict each other, prompted Lloyd (2005) to write a book as a critique of this literature. She, convincingly in my view, argues that, without exception, these cases for adaptation as the explanation for female orgasm are cases of 'bias in the science of evolution', other examples of which were considered in Chapter 2. Of the several 'upsuck' explanations, the most far-fetched is that of Baker & Bellis (1993). They claimed that orgasm allows the woman (presumably unwittingly) to influence which of the various men she copulates with, in a short period of time, gets his sperm into her reproductive tract. Ejaculates that occur from 45 min before until 1 min after the woman's orgasm are likely to have high sperm retention. Puts (2006), in his review of Lloyd's (2005) book, and his somewhat desperate attempt to counter her demolitions of the 'adaptation' literature on women's orgasms, emphasizes that the 'increased fitness' that resulted in 'adaptation' and the establishment of the female orgasm does not have to be currently evident but should have been evident at some stage in the earlier history of human development. He goes on ... 'Multiple lines of evidence suggest that female orgasm has been designed for the function of sire choice in species where the sperm of multiple males compete for fertilization in a single female ... '. Such patterns of sexual interaction do occur in some non-human primates (Dixson 1998). Interestingly, the occurrence of orgasm in female primates was disputed for many years, although there is now agreement that it does occur, at least in some individual females. While most obvious during female–female mounting or self-stimulation, there is limited evidence of its occurrence during coitus (e.g. stumptail macaques; Dixson 1998). One cannot yet exclude the possibility that in multi-male, multi-female mating systems, as found in macaques and chimpanzees, female orgasm may be relevant to sperm competition. But quite when, if ever, human mating came into this category remains obscure. In addition, for both human and non-human primates there is, as yet, no clear evidence that female orgasm in any way enhances fertility, although it should be said that the relationship between female orgasm and fertility has not yet been studied carefully enough to conclude that such an effect does not occur.

Lloyd (2005) offers an alternative explanation for the existence of female orgasm, the 'by-product' explanation first proposed by Symons (1979). This sees orgasm as a neurophysiological pattern that has evolved to allow orgasm and ejaculation in the male, for obvious reproductive reasons, but occurs as a 'potential' response pattern in the female because there has not been any evolutionary reason selectively to suppress its development. In Chapter 3 we considered sexual differentiation, mainly from an anatomical perspective. There we saw several types of differentiation. In one type where there are two potential systems, one male the other female (i.e. Wolffian and Müllerian systems), there is a specific mechanism (MIF), linked to the Y chromosome, for suppressing development of the female Müllerian system in the genetic male. The other type involved the same anatomic substrate, the genital tubercle, groove, etc., which develops into female external genitalia unless stimulated by androgens during development, in which case male external genitalia develop. The development of the gonads comes midway between these two types, with differentiation into ovary or testis dependent on whether the SRY gene is active. Another anatomical example is the breast; the capacity for female breast development depends on exposure to appropriate hormonal stimulation at puberty. In the male only the nipple is evident, although some degree of gynaecomastia sometimes occurs in boys around puberty as well as in adult men exposed to E (e.g. for the treatment of prostatic carcinoma). The male nipple is an example of a 'by-product' in Symon's terms. With the orgasm we are considering a neurophysiological response pattern (and one that is poorly understood). Other examples can be considered.

Lordosis is a complex neurophysiological motor response pattern in some lower mammals that occurs reflexively in response to mounting of the female by the male, providing the hormonal milieu of the female (i.e. oestrus) is right, a response that can also be elicited by stimulation of the oestrus female's cervix and her rectum. Though rarely mentioned in the literature, the lordosis response can also be elicited in a male rat primed with E (Komisaruk 1971). Komisaruk, in an unpublished early study, also found that rectal probing in male as well as female rats elevated pain thresholds measured by vocalization threshold and inhibition of tail flick to radiant heat (see p. 83), an effect enhanced by E treatment in both males and females. That observation raised the interesting question of the site of action of the E in this case (Komisaruk, personal communication). Here we are considering 'by-product' neurophysiological response patterns in the male, which are only observable if activated by female hormones. With orgasm we have another type of 'by-product' where the need for hormonal priming is less clear. If the limited evidence of prepubertal orgasms in human males and females is valid (see p. 152), then we have a neurophysiological response pattern that is not dependent on hormonal activation, at least in those individuals where the orgasmic 'potential' is sufficiently strong. This faces us with a challenge, similar to that faced earlier in the chapter when striving to explain the greater variability in women's responsiveness to T than in men's (see p. 127). After puberty, as reported earlier, males show a comparatively consistent capacity for orgasm, given appropriate stimulation and arousal, whereas women present a much more variable picture. As intimated earlier, the male pattern has the added component of seminal emission, and this clearly is dependent on hormonal activation at puberty. Although there is no conclusive evidence on this point, it is possible that the greater predictability of male orgasm post puberty depends on its link with seminal emission. In women, without that link, the greater variability in orgasmic 'potential' remains evident. In studies of androgen deficiency and replacement, the sexual arousability is clearly reduced with T deficiency, and if the deficiency is sustained, seminal emission becomes impossible (see p. 111). It is not clear, however, that there is no capacity for orgasm, keeping in mind that orgasm normally requires an adequate level of sexual arousal before it is triggered. As yet there is also no clear evidence that a woman's orgasmic potential, as distinct from her capacity for sexual arousal, is influenced by hormones. In a recent study, Dunn et al (2005) used a classical twin study format to compare orgasmic responsiveness in 4037 women. By comparison of identical and non-identical twin pairs, an estimated heritability of 34% (95% confidence interval 27–40%) for difficulty reaching orgasm during intercourse, and 45% (85% confidence interval 38–52%) for orgasm during masturbation was reported. This study was limited by the use of unclear questions about orgasm, obscuring the difference between orgasm induced by interaction with the partner and self-masturbation. However, the results indicate a genetic influence in some important aspect of orgasmic potential.

Without the 'controlling' link of seminal emission, a woman's experience of orgasm is likely to be affected by a range of factors, starting with a variable genetic disposition. The 'meaning' and acceptability of orgasm is likely to be influenced by socio-cultural factors, and there is limited evidence on this point (Meston et al 2004). Fisher (1973) suggested that some women felt more comfortable with orgasms that occurred during vaginal intercourse, either because of an association between clitoral orgasm and masturbation, a taboo activity, or because of concerns about more intense orgasmic experiences, which might threaten the intimacy of the sexual encounter (because with an intense orgasm the woman may feel she is 'abandoning' the sexual interaction for a highly individual 'orgasmic experience'). Personality factors as well as the influence of religion are likely to contribute to this complexity.

On the basis of the above discussion, I favour a 'by-product' rather than 'adaptation' explanation for women's orgasm. Regarding a woman's orgasm as a 'by-product' of male development is not 'politically correct', and Lloyd (2005) addressed a number of feminist criticisms of this perspective. Undoubtedly, if only as a source of pleasure, orgasm is an important and valued component of sexuality for many women. In a survey of women in heterosexual relationships, the main results of which were published by Bancroft et al (2003d), women were asked how important each of four factors was to their sexual happiness; the percentage of women answering very or extremely important for each factor were, in order of importance, (i) 'to feel emotionally close to your partner', 83.5%, (ii) 'that your partner be sexually satisfied', 78.9%, (iii) 'to feel comfortable talking to your partner about sex', 61.5% and (iv) 'to have an orgasm', 29.6% (previously unpublished results). This helps us to get the functions of orgasm in women in perspective.

Information processing: response to sexual stimuli, cognitive mechanisms and the relevance of mood

Response to sexual stimuli

The early experimental literature showed that many men and women can produce genital responses at will, usually by concentrating on sexual thoughts or fantasies (Laws & Rubin 1969; Henson & Rubin 1971; Heiman 1977; Stock & Geer 1982), and many also respond in the laboratory setting to non-tactile external erotic stimuli (e.g. visual or auditory; Bancroft & Mathews 1971; Heiman 1977; Bancroft & Bell 1985). There is now an extensive literature on the psychophysiological effects of such stimuli (Rosen & Beck 1988; Janssen 2007). Many men can also voluntarily inhibit erections in response to such stimuli (Laws & Rubin 1969; Henson & Rubin 1971; Rosen et al 1975).

Visual stimuli

Visual stimuli are among the most important in the elicitation of sexual interest, desire and arousal and have been the most frequently used in psychophysiological studies (Fig. 4.8). Generally, erotic films are more powerful in eliciting sexual responses in men than are fantasies or non-moving visual stimuli (e.g. slides; Bancroft 1978; Bancroft & Bell 1985) raising the question of how the information processing of moving visual erotic stimuli differs from that of non-moving visual stimuli (Bancroft & Mathews 1971; Bancroft 1978). The advent of brain imaging is starting to confront us with the complexity of this question, and this will be addressed further below.

What constitutes sexual attractiveness in terms of visual appearance is clearly complex and probably reflects different criteria in men and women. Such criteria are considered more closely in Chapter 6 (p. 200).

Non-visual stimuli

Smell

Olfactory stimuli are of considerable importance in the sexual behaviour of most non-human mammals (Keverne 1978). The word 'pheromone' is often used to describe such olfactory cues, though the term was originally used to describe a chemical attractant in insects and there is nothing of comparable specificity or potency in the mammalian world. Two types of olfactory effect must be considered: (i) olfactory priming, by which an olfactory stimulus has some gradual effect on the physiology of the recipient over a period of time — an example of such an effect is alteration of the timing of menstruation and (ii) olfactory signalling, by which olfactory stimuli have a more immediate effect on the behaviour of the recipient. Urinary and vaginal odours,

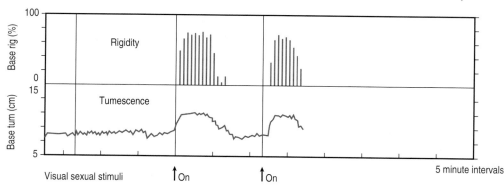

Fig. 4.8 Erectile response to two visual stimuli measured by Rigiscan, showing increased circumference and rigidity at the base of the penis. (Provided by Erick Janssen.)

indicating that the female is in oestrus and hence 'attractive', act in this way.

How important are such mechanisms in human sexuality? It is worth noting that most mammals have a dual olfactory system. One originates from the olfactory bulbs and communicates with the cortex. The other starts at the vomeronasal organ and communicates via the vomeronasal nerve with the limbic system. A vomeronasal system has been identified in humans (Garcia-Velasco & Mondragon 1991), but as yet its functional relevance is unknown.

There is some evidence that human females synchronize their menstrual cycles with one another, presumably via olfactory priming (McClintock 1971; Graham & McGrew 1980). Sleeping with a male partner also increases the incidence of ovulation (Veith et al 1983). This is not necessarily dependent on sexual activity, and it has been suggested that it is an effect of axillary odours from the male. Cutler and her colleagues (1986) claimed that the application of male axillary secretions to women tends to make their menstrual cycles more regular.

Signalling pheromones play an important role in primate sexual behaviour, in particular vaginal odours. These result from aliphatic acids produced by bacterial action in the vagina that varies according to the amount of E and the phase of the ovarian cycle. These odours inform the male that the female is in oestrus, receptive and hence 'attractive'. However, once a female is identified as attractive these olfactory signals are not necessary for sexual activity to be maintained (Keverne 1978). Such responses are not stereotypical; however, they vary in importance considerably from male to male. It is also possible that the signalling effect is acquired as the result of learning (i.e. experience of previous females in oestrus) rather than an innately programmed response.

Similar aliphatic acids are present in the vaginas of women and vary in a similar way with the menstrual cycle (Michael et al 1974). As yet no sexual signalling with these cues has been demonstrated in humans. There are other observations of possible relevance. Women vary through the menstrual cycle in their ability to perceive odours, with maximal sensitivity around ovulation. Women are more likely than men to smell androstenol, a steroid emitted by the boar that elicits a sexually receptive posture in the oestrous sow. But an attempt to render men more attractive to women using this odour was unsuccessful (Black & Biron 1982). Similarly, synthetic aliphatic acids, similar to those in the vagina, failed to influence sexual attractiveness or interaction between human pairs (Morris & Udry 1978).

It is nevertheless difficult to exclude the importance of olfaction in human sexuality. Our apocrine glands, which produce body odour, are well developed. Oral–genital contact is widespread. There is a substantial market for scents, perfumes and deodorants, though this may be as much concerned with masking unattractive odours as exploiting attractive ones. Anecdotal evidence suggests that for some people olfactory cues are extremely important, not only in initial attraction to a sexual partner but also in the maintenance of a stable relationship. But we do not know the proportion of people affected in this way or whether there is a sex difference in such sensitivity. A number of recent studies have started to explore these mechanisms in humans. Cutler et al (1998a) compared a 'synthesized human male pheromone' with placebo in a double-blind study of heterosexual men who kept a daily diary record of a number of 'sociosexual' behaviours. There was a significant increase in several of the sociosexual behaviours with the active compound compared to placebo. It should be noted that the nature of the active compound was not described, and this was explained in a response of the authors to a criticism by Wysocki & Preti (1998); the compound had been developed by Cutler's private company for commercial purposes and an application for a patent was in progress (Cutler et al 1998b). Graham et al (2000) assessed the effect of fragrances on sexual arousal and mood in women. Each fragrance was commercially available, one intended for use by men (male fragrance) the other by women (female fragrance). Participants were tested at two phases of the menstrual cycle: mid-follicular and periovulatory. No effect of either fragrance on mood was observed. Subjective and genital (VPA) responses to sexual fantasy and erotic films were assessed. An enhancing effect of the male fragrance on genital response to sexual fantasy (not sexual film) was observed, but only in the mid-follicular phase. This somewhat unexpected finding was explained as possibly indicating that olfactory stimuli might be used in the development of a sexual fantasy but be irrelevant or even distracting while watching an erotic film. Given the evidence of maximal sensitivity to olfactory stimuli around ovulation (Doty et al 1981), the authors speculated that the fragrance may have been too strong to be pleasant in the periovulatory phase of this study. More research in this area is required.

Touch

Touch is obviously an important source of erotic stimulation. The sensory pathways from the genitalia are described in Chapter 3 (p. 38). There are dramatic changes in the erotic tactile sensitivity of the genitalia during vasocongestive responses such as penile erection or labial engorgement. This may be secondary to structural changes induced by the tumescence, which alter the sensory mechanism so that ordinary cutaneous sensations become erotic in quality. As yet, particularly in the skin of the vulvar region, the relevant mechanisms are not well understood and may well be highly complex (Martin-Alguacil et al 2006).

In animal studies, sectioning of the dorsal nerve of the penis, which supplies much of the sensory area of the penis, appears to prevent erection and ejaculation in various species, indicating how important this sensory input is for normal genital response (Hart & Leedy 1985). In humans this becomes relevant in those cases of peripheral nerve damage affecting the genitalia (e.g. multiple sclerosis) where loss of sensation may contribute to erectile failure.

But clearly, erotic touch is not confined to the genitalia. In the right circumstances, tactile stimulation of many parts of the body can be intensely erotic. This reminds us that the input of sensory stimulation from the periphery has to be processed centrally and can be substantially influenced at this stage. An interesting and basically unexplained phenomenon occurs in many individuals with transection of the spinal cord. Having lost all sensation below the level of the injury, they may find that the skin region just above the level of sensory loss develops an erotic sensitivity that it did not previously possess. Some reorganization of the perception of tactile stimuli has presumably taken place. On a more dynamic level, central processes can influence whether genital stimulation is perceived as erotic. In some instances, erotic anaesthesia seems to develop in spite of non-erotic sensation being intact. The underlying mechanisms for such a pattern are not understood but presumably inhibition of erotic sensory input, or a failure to reduce inhibitory control, is taking place at some central level in the cord or above. Of possible relevance is the finding from a brain-imaging study of men with hypoactive desire disorder compared with normal controls. One feature of the low-desire men was a lack of *deactivation* of their MOFC in response to sexual stimuli (Stoleru et al 2003). This area is believed to be involved in the inhibitory control of motivated behaviours.

Effects of feedback and performance demand

Are our sexual responses enhanced by our paying attention to them? Masters & Johnson (1970) have blamed the spectator role as a crucial factor in causing or maintaining sexual dysfunction. What is the available evidence?

Price (1973) and Rosen et al (1975) found that in men the provision of feedback of their erectile response had, if anything, a slightly beneficial effect on their voluntary production of erection. A comparable effect was found in women (Hoon et al 1977). It is of course possible that people who develop sexual dysfunction are different in this respect or at least become so. In general terms, however, dysfunctional men have not differed from normal men in their response to laboratory-based feedback. Csillag (1976) compared six normal volunteers with six men with ED. In neither group did feedback apparently impair their erectile response, but whereas the normal men reached their peak response in the second testing session and thereafter declined somewhat, the dysfunctional men steadily improved with repeated testing. Perhaps something else was happening; perhaps they were becoming increasingly reassured by their responses, a form of deconditioning of performance anxiety. But clearly feedback was not having a negative effect on this process.

Sakheim et al (1984) considered the effect of visual feedback, i.e. what happens if you can see how your penis is responding? With normal volunteers, being able to see their penis had an enhancing effect if they were responding to a strong erotic stimulus but had the opposite effect in the case of a relatively weak stimulus. In other words, perceiving a good sexual response is in itself sexually arousing; perceiving a poor response is sexually inhibiting. Heiman & Rowland (1983) found that normal men were not adversely affected by demand for a response in the experimental situation, whereas dysfunctional men were.

Other studies have demonstrated that various aspects of feedback and self-awareness must be taken into consideration. Beck et al (1983) and Abrahamson et al (1985) investigated the possible effect of the partner's response. They compared two groups of sexually functional and dysfunctional men. If the partner was showing low sexual arousal, both groups of men responded better by concentrating on their own responses rather than the partner's. If, however, the partner was showing high arousal, the functional men responded better by focusing their attention on the partner, whereas with dysfunctional men the reverse applied. Here we see the meaning of the impact of a particular situation. High arousal in the partner of a dysfunctional man might be more threatening than low arousal.

Dekker et al (1984) conjectured whether information processing of sexual stimuli was effective simply by focusing on the external stimulus or whether it was necessary in some way to focus on or imagine the sexual response. Their male and female subjects listened to an erotic tape. In one condition they were asked not only to attend to the scene being described on the tape but also to concentrate on their own feelings and responses; in another condition they were asked simply to attend to what was being described in the tape. Their reported sexual arousal was greater in the first condition, and these workers concluded that cognitive mediation needs to focus on response if it is to lead to sexual arousal. However, no objective measure of sexual response was involved and the higher levels of sexual arousal reported during the first condition may have been simply because by focusing on their reactions they were more aware of them.

The most sensible conclusion we can draw from these various findings is that the effect of awareness, feedback, being a spectator and performance demand depend on the circumstances and how they are interpreted by the individual. Awareness of our genital responses and those of our partner can in some circumstances lead to a positive feedback loop, resulting in escalating sexual arousal, and in other circumstances may have a negative feedback effect with inhibition of sexual response.

Models of information processing

In this section we consider some simplified conceptual models that may have heuristic value in grappling with the complexity of information processing. The evidence relevant to the processing of emotional reactions has largely been restricted to negative emotions such as fear, and as yet relatively little relevant to the emotion of sexual arousal.

Explicit versus implicit memory

According to LeDoux (1996) 'explicit', conscious or declarative memory is mediated by the hippocampus and related cortical areas. 'Implicit' or unconscious forms of memory, on the other hand, are mediated by a number of different systems. The 'fear' memory system, he proposes, involves the amygdala and related systems. It is not yet clear which system is involved in 'implicit' or unconscious sexual memory.

Automatic versus attentional processing

The model that currently prevails in the cognitive literature on sexual arousal was described by Janssen et al (2000) and elaborated further by Spiering & Everaerd (2007). It has two components: (i) automatic or 'unconscious' processing and (ii) attentional or controlled 'conscious' processing.

Automatic cognitive processes are rapid, dynamic, but 'unconscious'; i.e. the individual is not aware of them, in part because they are so rapid. They should not, however, be confused with the psychoanalytic concept of 'the unconscious'. They are regarded by most contemporary emotion theorists as fundamental to the appraisal of events resulting in emotional reactions, even though attentional processes may also contribute to the appraisal. This is also seen to apply to the emotion of 'sexual arousal'. Conscious processing involves awareness and is linked to 'attention' (Spiering & Everaerd 2007). Attention can be divided into three systems: orienting to sensory stimuli, activation of ideas from memory and maintaining alertness (Posner 1994).

Thus, applying this distinction to our four-component model of sexual arousal, appraisal of a stimulus as sexual, initially automatic, leads to an emotional response that incorporates a degree of incentive motivation and a specifically sexual response (i.e. genital). The attentional component subsequently leads to the attribution of sexual meaning, while also influencing, in ways that will be considered later, the affective component and its valence. Attentional processing also appraises the responses to the original stimulus, specific and non-specific, completing our 'psychosomatic circle' in the process, whereby the emotional response, and in particular the genital component of it, becomes part of the sexual stimulus.

The automatic, 'preattentive' response to a sexual stimulus is assumed to depend on implicit sexual memory. Spiering & Everaerd (2007) define 'implicit sexual memory', however, as including innate sexual reflexes, learned (automatized) sexual scripts and classically conditioned sensations. The concept of 'memory' applies more obviously to 'learned scripts' than to innate sexual reflexes, or even classically conditioned responses.

We have four types of evidence relevant to information processing of sexual stimuli to consider: (i) cognitive (the effects of cognitive manipulations), (ii) electroencephalographic (EEG) evidence, (iii) brain-imaging evidence of brain activity in response to sexual stimuli and (iv) conditioning and habituation experiments.

Cognitive manipulations

As yet much less research attention has been paid to the 'automatic', preattentional, than to attentional, conscious processing of sexual stimuli. Spiering & Everaerd (2007) therefore drew on the much more extensive literature relating to automatic fear responses. Hansen & Hansen (1988), for example, introduced the 'face-in-the-crowd' effect. When presented with an array of faces and asked to detect the 'odd face out', an angry face is much more quickly identified in a group of happy faces than the reverse. The assumption is that identification of the angry face results from 'preattentional' automatic processing, whereas its recognition as an angry face requires attentional processing. Similar preattentive rapid identification of other potentially threatening stimuli have been demonstrated (e.g. snakes and spiders), and Spiering & Everaerd (2007) interpreted this as the selection of stimuli related to recurrent survival threats as automatic triggers of attention, a part of the process of evolutionary adaptation. It has also been shown that such triggering of attention may be more or less powerful depending on personality characteristics such as degree of fearfulness.

Sexual content-induced delay

As yet, the 'face-in-the-crowd' paradigm has not been used with 'sexual' faces, and it is not immediately obvious how one would do this. There is, however, an extensive parallel literature on other paradigms of 'attentional bias' (e.g. the emotional Stroop task), showing a bias, particularly but not exclusively in anxious individuals, to attend to threatening stimulus content. A number of comparable studies relating to sexual stimuli have been reported. Several of these have shown that, in both men and women, delay completing a task (usually categorizing a word or picture) occurs when an erotic element is present (known as sexual content-induced delay or SCID). Various manipulations of this paradigm, including the use of conscious and unconscious primes, have been reported (Geer & Bellard 1996; Geer & Melton 1997; Spiering et al 2002, 2003, 2004). It remains unclear, however, to what extent the observed effects on the assigned 'attentional' tasks are due to a distracting effect of automatic processing or to what Spiering & Everaerd (2007) call regulatory, or in other words, inhibitory mechanisms. Geer et al (1994) used a reading task, involving narratives incorporating sentences with 'sexual', 'romantic' and 'neutral' content. The Sexual Opinion Survey, which measures 'erotophilia and erotophobia' (Fisher et al 1988) was completed by participants. It was predicted that because 'erotophobics' avoid contact with sexual material, subjects high on erotophobia would spend less time reading erotic material. What they found was that they were significantly *slower* at reading all three types of sentence. Given that the 'high erotophobia' subjects had given informed consent to participate in this study, it is perhaps naïve to expect that they would then 'avoid' erotic content. In some way, they appeared to approach the whole exercise with increased caution. This potentially interesting and informative finding has not, unfortunately, led to any further studies incorporating measures of relevant individual difference.

Physiological responses to information processing

To what extent has there been experimental demonstration of the effect of 'automatic' unconscious information processing on physiological responses relevant to sexual arousal? Both et al (2003) used enhancement of a tendon reflex (T reflex from the Achilles tendon) as evidence of increased spinal excitability reflecting early motor preparation for motivated action. In both men and women, they found that, during observation of sexual, anxiety-provoking and sexually threatening films there was a significant enhancement of the T reflex compared to responses during a neutral film. This was taken as an illustration of similar 'preparedness for action' in both 'avoidant' and 'approach' emotional responses. What about genital response?

A series of experiments have measured genital response in association with a variety of cognitive manipulations, including 'subliminal priming', distraction, misattribution and misinformation and 'false feedback' of genital response.

Subliminal priming

Janssen et al (2000), in a study of men, measured erectile response to sexual stimuli, which had been subliminally primed either with sexual or neutral primes (i.e. preceding the main stimulus by the presentation of a priming stimulus, e.g. a sexual word, for a few milliseconds so that the subject is consciously unaware of it). They focused on the first 5 s of erectile response to the main stimulus. They unexpectedly found erectile response to be less following sexual than neutral primes. The explanation they gave for this was that in the first stages of erectile response there is lengthening of the penis, which may be accompanied by some transient reduction in circumference, and they had used a circumference measure. The possibility of an inhibitory effect was not discussed.

Effects of distraction

What effect does distraction by non-sexual stimuli have on response to sexual stimuli? Geer & Fuhr (1976), using a dichotic listening task, showed that the more difficult the task, which involved listening in one ear, the lower the erectile response to an auditory sexual stimulus in the other ear. Farkas et al (1979) found a comparable effect in response to erotic films, but also found that subjective arousal was not affected by the distraction. Przybyla & Byrne (1984) looked at the effect of distraction on both visual (erotic film) and auditory erotic stimuli. They found that distraction was relatively ineffective in reducing the response to visual stimuli in men, whereas, in women, responses to both auditory and visual stimuli were reduced by distraction, an interesting and potentially important sex difference.

Barlow and his colleagues (for reviews see Barlow 1986; Cranston-Cuebas & Barlow 1990) assessed the effects of distraction on erectile response in men with and without ED. They found that distraction impaired erectile response in the functional subjects but had no effect or a slightly enhancing effect on erectile response in the dysfunctional subjects. Barlow (1986) interpreted the negative effect of distraction in the functional men as evidence of the fundamental importance of 'attention to the sexual cues' for normal sexual response. The paradoxical effect of distraction in the dysfunctional men, he suggested, was because they were otherwise distracted by non-erotic cues even more negative in their effects on sexual response than the experimental distractors. Barlow viewed distraction as a 'process which is the mechanism of action through which many experiences act to inhibit sexual responsivity' (Cranston-Cuebas & Barlow 1990, p. 141). However, it remains unclear how these contrasting physiological patterns of response to distraction, in the functional and dysfunctional men, are mediated.

Van Lankveld & van den Houte (2004) also compared response to erotic stimuli in functional and dysfunctional men, using four markedly varying degrees of distraction: (i) being simply presented with a pair of digits, (ii) repeating them aloud, (iii) adding and verbalizing the sum of them and (iv) applying a complex formula to them. There was a clear effect of increasing degrees of distraction on erectile response, but no effect on ratings of subjective arousal. They found no difference between the functional and dysfunctional men, in striking contrast to the findings of Barlow's group (Barlow 1986). The restriction of effect to the erectile response is also noteworthy, though, overall, the subjective ratings of arousal were modest (from a scale of 0 to 100, around 30 for the stronger and 20 for the less strong erotic stimuli). The authors offer an alternative explanatory model to account for this: the distinction between 'referential' and 'expectancy' systems of emotional responding (Lang et al 1990). The referential system quickly assesses 'likes and dislikes', i.e. making the distinction between the need for approach or avoidance. This, it is postulated, requires little cognitive effort. In contrast, the expectancy system identifies reliable predictors of significant events and prepares for a cost-effective method of responding or coping. This requires substantial attentional capacity. According to this model, the genital response is part of the expectancy system, whereas subjective sexual arousal is a less demanding 'referent response'. This seems to evade the complexity of the process of rating subjective sexual arousal, which not only involves a subjective state but also cognitive as well as attitudinal factors involved in first the rating and then the communication of this rating to the experimenter (in this study by means of a continuous lever rating).

Salemink & van Lankveld (2006) went on to assess the effects of distraction in women with and without sexual dysfunction, using the same sequence of graded distraction as used in the above male study (Van Lankveld & van den Houte 2004). As with the men, increasing distraction reduced genital response (in this case VPA). The effects on subjective arousal depended on how it was assessed. 'Real-time' continuous assessment during presentation of the erotic stimulus was not affected by distraction; retrospective assessment, made after the stimulus presentation, showed subjective sexual arousal reduced by increasing distraction. The authors speculated that the 'real-time' assessment depended on contextual cues in the erotic stimuli, whereas the retrospective assessment may have depended on recall of perceived genital response, reflecting the contrast reported by Brotto & Gorzalka (2002).

Effects of misattribution and misinformation

The relevant studies exploring misattribution have involved giving the participant a pill, which in fact is inactive, but telling the participant that it will increase the sexual response whilst the participant looks at erotic stimuli. The participant is then likely to attribute any response that occurs to the pill and consequently to minimize their own arousal. Conversely, if the participant is given an inactive pill and told that it will *decrease* the response, the participant will be impressed by any response that does occur and hence will report greater subjective sexual arousal. Cranston-Cuebas & Barlow (1990), using this paradigm, found to their surprise that this effect was demonstrated strikingly in functional men, but in the actual erectile response and not in their report of subjective arousal. With dysfunctional men, however, the findings were different. When told that the pill would decrease their response, that is what in fact happened, again in the erectile and not in their subjective responses. The response-enhancing pill, on the other hand, was no different to placebo. Thus, there was a further difference between functional and dysfunctional men that again raises the question of whether it is a cause or an effect. Janssen & Everaerd (1993) went on to replicate these findings, although they looked only at functional and not dysfunctional men. They commented, however, on the remarkable difference between the clear effect of the misattribution procedure on the physiological response, the erection, and the lack of effect on the subjective response, the self-rating of arousal.

Whilst information processing was undoubtedly involved in these procedures, if it was conscious or controlled processing then it is difficult to account for the differential effects on the genital response and subjective experience. An alternative explanation is that the altered expectation produced by the misattribution effect was associated, in the functional men, with a reduction in the usual level of inhibitory tone, an effect resulting from automatic processing of which the subject was presumably unaware and which did not lead to any revision of his subjective state. In contrast, the dysfunctional men processed the information differently, resulting in either no reduction or an increase of inhibitory tone. As yet, it is difficult to say to what extent automatic and conscious processing was responsible for this difference.

False feedback

A comparable paradox was apparent in a series of studies from Barlow's group in which false feedback about the individual's response was given (reviewed in Wiegel et al 2007). Thus Bach et al (1999) told half of their male subjects, following viewing of an erotic film, that their erectile response had been less than average for subjects in their laboratory. They were then shown a further erotic film during which they showed less erectile response (and reported less expectation of response) but reported the same level of subjective arousal and no increase in negative affect. Weisberg et al (2001) went on to manipulate the explanation for the 'less than average response'; some subjects were told it was because of 'poor quality of the film' (external cause); others were told it was because they were not the type to become easily aroused in a laboratory setting (internal cause). Exposure to a further erotic film showed that the external cause group showed greater erectile response and subjective sexual arousal than the internal cause group, although the manipulation had no effect on the expected degree of response or on negative affect. This led Wiegel et al (2007) to emphasize the importance of 'attribution of cause' for a 'perceived sexual failure'. Although these false-feedback manipulations have not yet been reported in dysfunctional men, the same discrepancy between effects on genital and subjective responses was apparent in functional and dysfunctional men in the earlier studies. We should keep in mind, when attempting to interpret these interesting findings, that more conscious processing, which is clearly fundamental to the reporting of subjective sexual arousal, is likely to reflect the specific experimental context and hence may have limited or uncertain relevance to the real-life situation, a limitation that, unfortunately, pervades much of psychophysiological sex research.

EEG and brain-imaging studies

EEG studies

The use of event-related potential (ERP) from EEG electrodes to track brain reactions to external stimuli has an extensive literature. In a relevant study, Cuthbert et al (2000) compared ERPs, as well as peripheral indicators of autonomic arousal (e.g. skin conductance (SC)) and subjective ratings of arousal, in response to a series of images, neutral and affective, the affective stimuli having either negative (e.g. depictions of violence or mutilation) or positive valence (e.g. erotic). A late, slow and sustained positive voltage change was observed for all types of stimuli but was significantly greater to the affective stimuli (positive and negative) and was correlated to other indicators of arousal (e.g. SC and subjective arousal). The ERP was sustained throughout the 6 s of image exposure. The authors concluded that 'because of their motivational significance, emotional stimuli are selected by the brain for sustained attentive processing' (p. 106). This research group, in a separate study (Schupp et al 1997), had assessed the response to brief noise probes administered intermittently during a more sustained visual image. They found that ERPs to the noise probes were less while attending to an emotional than to a neutral stimulus. They interpreted this as showing that attentional resources are devoted to emotional images, resulting in less attention paid to other potentially distracting stimuli. This could be relevant to the SCID effect. Thus, the presence of a sexual stimulus could result in sustained emotional attention, limiting attentional resources for the additional conscious task, such as categorizing the word or image. Overall, they concluded that the sustained attention processing they had observed reflected activation of motivational systems in the brain that simultaneously prompt autonomic arousal and subjective affective experience.

Costa et al (2003) used magnetoencephalography (MEG) to measure CMV, the magnetic equivalent of contingent negative variation (CNV), and visual-evoked fields (VEF) in response to erotic pictures. MEG is regarded as having better temporal and spatial resolution than EEG. This study focused on how these MEG response patterns related to subjective arousal, and how they compared in men and women. Twenty neutral pictures were compared with 20 whole-body pictures of nude men and 20 of nude women all 'in frontal view, with visible genitalia and explicit provocative erotic pose'. The pictures were shown as pairs, the first for 1 s, and with a 3.5 s interval between (results are presented for the first stimulus only). The subject was asked to indicate whether the second image of the pair was the same or different. This was used as a method of controlling attention. Of the pairs shown, 50% were identical. With subjective rating of valence, male participants reported the pictures of women more positive than those of men, which were more positively rated than neutral pictures. The ratings of valence by female participants did not differ between the three types of image. For arousal, male participants showed the same pattern as for valence. The female participants rated the pictures of men more arousing than the neutral, but not significantly more so than the pictures of women. With both ratings, female participants showed greater variance than the males.

The CMV, analyzed as the mean level between 1.5 and 3.5 s, produced comparable results to those reported by Cuthbert et al (2000) for emotional (positive and negative) images. For both male and female participants, in comparison to the neutral stimuli, the CMV was significantly greater in response to opposite sex pictures (not same sex). The VEF, reflecting more immediate and anticipatory response patterns, revealed two components: M1, with a mean peak latency of 126 ms and M2, with a peak at 203 ms. The M2 peak was significantly higher in response to pictures of both men and women than to neutral images but did not differ between male and female participants. This was similar to patterns of response shown previously in the perception of human faces. The M1 peak, however, was significantly greater in male participants than female, across stimuli, and only in male participants was it significantly greater in response to nudes than to neutral stimuli (female nudes $p < 0.009$; male nudes $p < 0.04$). Because of the clear gender difference in the M1 peak, the authors concluded that this peak was not simply a reaction to human faces, but that in some way men were reacting more strongly than women to nude images, particularly opposite sex nude images. They saw this as evidence in support of the evolutionary theory of mate selection. These, and other gender differences, will be considered further later in this chapter. What we can conclude at this stage is that in addition to a more sustained emotional reaction to erotic stimuli, some immediate or anticipatory response is also involved, at least in men, the implications of which as yet remain obscure.

Brain imaging

Until now the majority of brain-imaging studies relevant to sexual arousal have focused on response to VSS (see p. 71). Not surprisingly, most of the evidence of brain activation in such studies has been in areas of the cerebral hemispheres involved in information processing, rather than the brain stem. Although this may, in part, reflect the greater methodological difficulties in identifying localized activation in the deeper brain areas, it also reflects an experimental paradigm that is focused on the early responses to exposure to visual stimuli. Obviously, many of the processes reflected in the activation are likely to be involved in the processing of various kinds of stimuli, not only sexual. Some, for example, seem to be specific to the process of evaluating human faces, an obviously basic human function (e.g. right orbitofrontal cortex; see below).

Interpretation of brain imaging is complicated by the fact that a series of brain processes becomes involved sequentially, and it is often difficult to know what happens first in this sequence. Recent studies of the early stages of penile erectile response to VSS, using volumetric measurement of erection that is more sensitive to early change than the usual circumferential measures, have been reported by Stoleru and his colleagues. Moulier et al (2006) using fMRI showed that early penile volumetric changes were correlated with the BOLD signal in the right medial prefrontal cortex, the right and left orbitofrontal cortices, the insula on both sides, the paracentral lobules, the right ventral lateral thalamic nucleus and the right anterior cingulate cortex and regions involved in motor imagery and motor preparation. They concluded that the penile response to static sexual stimuli is controlled by a network of frontal, parietal, insular and cingulate cortical areas and, as a feedback response, penile tumescence activates somatosensory regions of the brain. In the next study from this group, the role of the 'mirror neuron' system was explored. This relatively new concept in neuroscience is based on primate research showing that certain brain areas are activated when the animal makes a movement but are also activated when the animal sees the same movement made by another animal. This mirroring, initially of motor responses, has been extended to include emotional reactions associated with the motor response. Thus, observing fearful body expression results in activation of areas involved in both the motor and the emotional component, allowing the observer to 'empathize' with the observed. Mouras et al (in press) explored the mirror-neuron system in response to sexual stimuli, using the same volumetric measure of penile tumescence. Activation of two components of this system, the left frontal operculum and the inferior parietal lobules, were predictive of later erectile response. Previous studies have shown the frontal operculum to interact with the insula, and other studies have shown insular activation to be correlated with penile response. In a more general emotional sense, the insula is believed to play a fundamental role in relaying information about motor action to the limbic areas processing emotional content of a stimulus, thus enabling the empathic viewing of emotional facial expressions mentioned earlier. In this particular context, the insula could be playing a comparable role in relation to sexual 'emotion'.

So far, as with the cognitive manipulations considered earlier, there has been little attempt to compare and contrast different types of individual. There are two notable exceptions. Redouté et al (2005) compared brain-imaging response to VSS in hypogonadal men with and without T replacement and eugonadal controls. This study is considered in the section on T effects in the brain (p. 126). Stoleru et al (2003) compared brain-imaging responses, using PET, in seven men with HSDD and eight normal controls (Fig. 4.9). Here, the comparison has more potential relevance to our understanding

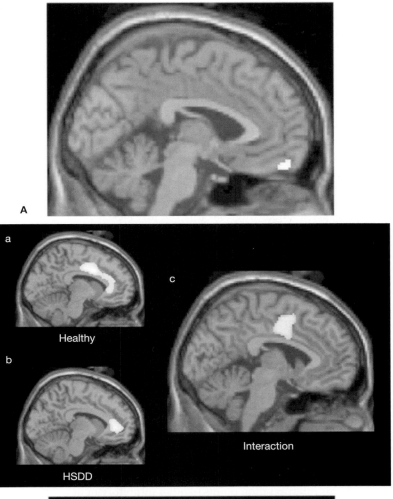

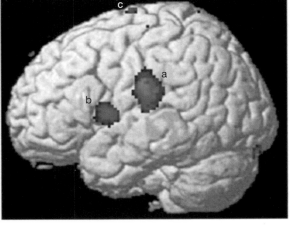

Fig. 4.9 Differences in brain activation and deactivation in response to visual sexual stimuli (VSS) in seven men with hypoactive sexual desire disorder (HSDD) and eight healthy controls. **(A)**, Significant group X condition interaction showing maintained activation in left gyrus rectus of the orbitofrontal cortex in HSDD men, implicated in the inhibitory control of motivated behaviour. **(B)**, Areas of activation in the left anterior cingulate gyrus, more extensive in the controls, with area of significant group X condition interaction also shown. This area is involved in premotor processes. **(C)** (left view of brain), Areas of higher activation in controls in (a), inferior parietal cortex and lower part of post central gyrus; (b), lower part of precentral gyrus; and (c), left supplementary motor area. These areas are involved in emotional and motor imagery processing. (From Stoleru et al 2003, with permission.)

of sexual information processing. The interesting discussion of their findings by Stoleru et al (2003) is closely considered here. There are some similarities and some differences between the two groups. The differences will be considered first.

1. Activity (as manifested by rCBF) was decreased in the left MOFC of the controls but did not change in the HSDD men. This part of the MOFC is involved in decision-making and emotional processing (Bechara et al 2000), holding links between a given situation or stimulus and previous emotional reactions to it. Individuals with lesions in this area tend to be tactless, lacking in social restraints, and to present with excessive pleasure seeking behaviour, especially, but not exclusively, in the sexual domain. Thus, deactivation of this area in the control group suggests a release from some form of inhibitory control by the MOFC. Interestingly, activation of this area is found during satiation of appetite for food. It has been suggested that the MOFC codes for anticipation of *lack* of reward and, in experimental animals, lesions in this area lead to continued response during extinction paradigms; in other words, the lesioned animal fails to recognize that reward, previously experienced, is no longer forthcoming. On the other hand, recent human studies have shown strong activation of the MOFC in response to emotionally aversive photographs, suggesting that it is not just lack of reward that is being indicated. Bechara et al (2000) described how the MOFC interacts with other structures, including the amygdala and somatosensory insular cortices, in contributing to decision-making processes, and we should not expect any simple function in relation to sexual stimuli. However, we are left with uncertainty about the relative importance of memory of lack of reward, a demotivating process, and some form of active regulation or inhibition of positive response.

2. Only in control subjects was there activation of the head of the right caudate nucleus. Redouté et al (2000) have suggested that once sexual arousal has been induced, this area is involved in the control of its overt behavioural expression. In the experimental context this reflects a conflict between feeling sexually aroused and not wanting to act on it (e.g. by masturbating). If valid, this interpretation points to other inhibitory or at least regulatory functions of this area in the management of sexual arousal. This is supported by evidence of hypersexuality in individuals with lesions in this area (Richfield et al 1987).

3. Other studies have shown, somewhat inconsistently, deactivation of some parts of the temporal lobes in response to VSS, raising the possibility that these temporal lobe structures exert an inhibitory tone, which needs to be reduced for sexual arousal to occur. However, in this particular study no difference was found between the HSDD and control men, suggesting that lack of reduction of inhibitory tone is not the key factor in HSDD. However, more evidence is needed on this issue.

4. When considering the excitatory or activating function of the information processing, the control men showed activation of the lower and rostral parts of the inferior parietal lobes. This area has been implicated in the activation of motor imagery (e.g. imagining performing movements with one's right hand). The lack of activation of this area in the HSDD men suggests less rehearsal of sexually motivated mental imagery. There were further differences in the groups in relation to motor imagery. The caudate nucleus and inferior parietal lobes, already considered, the left anterior cingulate gyrus, the supplementary motor areas and the ventral premotor area, all belong to a neural network activated in motor imagery and all showed less activation (or more deactivation) in the HSDD men. This raises the issue of cause or effect. The lack of motor imagery may have been a consequence of a lack of arousal response rather than its cause.

These very preliminary findings do not give us clear explanation of the mechanisms involved in sexual arousal or lack of arousal in HSDD, but they raise some interesting possibilities, and further research of this kind is eagerly awaited.

Conditioning, learning and habituation

Notwithstanding the ongoing contest between biological and cultural determinants of human sexuality (see Chapter 2), there is less disagreement about the importance of learning in sexual development, and this will be discussed more fully in Chapter 5. Where there is less certainty is with the nature of the learning process. In the 1960s the emergence of 'modern learning theory' focused attention on classical and operant conditioning. Rachman (1966) reported evidence of classical conditioning of erectile response to images of black boots, an example, he considered, of an experimentally induced fetish. Around that time, attention was also paid to the use of aversive conditioning to modify sexual preferences, to reduce the sexual impact of unwanted fetish objects (Marks et al 1970), or to change sexual orientation from homosexual to heterosexual (Bancroft 1974). Such techniques involved the association of unpleasant electric shocks simply with presentation of the 'unwanted' sexual stimulus, or sexual fantasy, or following development of an early erectile response to the deviant stimulus. Although some initial effects were observed, lasting changes were relatively unusual, more evident in cases of fetishism and transvestism and less with sexual orientation or gender identity (i.e. transgender). Such treatments raise ethical issues, are considered elsewhere in this book, and are no longer used. And whereas such aversive procedures produced some effects of theoretical interest, though rarely clear-cut conditioned anxiety (Bancroft 1974, p. 98), they throw little light on normal learning of sexual response patterns.

Other non-aversive, classical conditioning studies have been reported. O'Donohue & Plaud (1994) reviewed this earlier literature, almost all restricted to men, and pointed to a number of methodological deficiencies limiting their scientific value and concluded that evidence of the impact of either classical or operant conditioning on sexual learning was at best tenuous. Since then, attempts have been made to address the methodological issues, with varying success. In only the second study of classical conditioning in women, LeTourneau & O'Donohue (1997) found no evidence of conditioned VPA response, although the conditioned stimulus (CS) used, an amber light, was entirely 'neutral'. Lalumiere & Quinsey (1998), in a study of men, used a CS with some erotic significance, a picture of a moderately attractive, partially nude woman. This was then followed by an unconditional stimulus (US) showing a videotape of an arousing heterosexual interaction. The objective was to enhance the erectile response to the CS by association with the US. They found a small (10%) increase in subsequent response to the unreinforced CS. They suggested that the effect of such conditioning may vary with the developmental stage (e.g. puberty), although they presented no evidence in support of this. Hoffman et al (2004) reported the first study where the same conditioning paradigm was used in both men and women, though the comparison of men and women was limited by the different types of genital response measured (penile circumference increase in men and VPA increase in women). They compared and contrasted two types of response, one with erotic implications (image of an abdomen of the opposite sex), the other without (a gun), and two types of CS exposure, subliminal and more prolonged, and consciously perceived. With the subliminal CS, they found similar conditioning of genital response to the 'abdomen' in both men and women. With the consciously perceived CS, they found an interesting gender difference: the men showed the expected conditioned response, as found with the subliminal CS, whereas the women showed a conditioned VPA response to the gun, not the abdomen. They also measured SC as an indicator of autonomic arousal, and they found that women showed a greater SC response to the gun than the abdomen, whereas the men did not differ in this respect. On this basis, they speculated that the paradoxical VPA response to the gun in women was a result of 'excitation transfer' (see p. 111). The conditioning effects in this study were not robust, and it is not possible to say whether the paradoxical VPA response would be found in women in general, or whether there is a subset of women who are susceptible to such an effect, whether due to 'excitation transfer' or some other mechanism.

Habituation, by which response to a stimulus lessens with its repetition, could be relevant to learning of sexual response patterns. In particular, it confronts us with a key paradox in human sexuality: some individuals continue to show preference for and response to very specific sexual stimuli, whereas others require novelty to maintain sexual arousability. Both extremes are potentially problematic; long-term preference for very specific stimuli is often part of a fetishistic pattern. Conversely, a strong need for novelty may underlie difficulty in maintaining stable sexual relationships. An explanation of these contrasting patterns is therefore of some

importance. Variations in propensity for habituation may be relevant. As yet there is limited evidence of habituation of the effects of sexual stimuli, largely confined to experimental testing. This has been reviewed by Over & Koukanas (1995), who found substantial methodological difficulties measuring habituation of sexual arousal response to sexual stimuli, associated with inconsistencies in the evidence reported. As yet, there is more evidence for men than for women. However, Over & Koukanas (1995) make the interesting point that if one accepts the gender differences in reproductive strategies postulated by evolutionary psychologists (see Chapter 2), one might expect habituation, related to a need for novelty, to be more marked in men than in women. That remains to be demonstrated, though it is worth noting that the more extreme and deviant forms of 'specificity' of sexual preference, such as fetishism, implying minimal habituation, are rarely found in women.

Once again, for both conditioning and habituation of sexual response, we find a literature which, as yet, has paid no attention to individual differences, though Over & Koukanas (1995) review some such evidence related to habituation of non-sexual stimuli.

At the present time there is little support for classical conditioning as being of fundamental importance for normal sexual learning, but the possibility remains that some individuals may be susceptible to atypical learning, which might complicate their sexual development. Learning will be considered further in the chapter on sexual development.

Sexual fantasy

The issue of fantasy or internal imagery presents us with a challenging aspect of information processing: is a sexual fantasy a stimulus, a result of information processing of other stimuli or a combination of both? There is now an extensive literature on sexual fantasy, in terms of frequency, content and gender differences, which will be considered in Chapter 6 as an example of 'internalized' sexual behaviour. There is much less evidence relating to the above question. At this stage we can identify some key issues. What brain mechanisms are involved in fantasy and how do they differ from response to external sexual stimuli? This awaits relevant brain-imaging studies, which until now have been restricted to external stimuli or tactile stimulation. To what extent do individuals vary in the intensity and clarity of their sexual fantasies, and what possible explanations are there to account for such individual variability? For example, is the capacity for intense and vivid sexual images part of a more general capacity for intense internal imagery? What other cognitive or personality characteristics are related to this capacity?

The role of inhibition

The Dual Control model is based on the premise that, in some circumstances, appraisal of a sexual stimulus leads in an uncomplicated and relatively direct way to sexual arousal, but in other circumstances, due either to automatic or to attentional appraisal or a combination of both, the sexual arousal sequence is inhibited. Apart from awareness of a negative or at least 'mixed' valence, the inhibitory process per se is predominantly automatic, or at least not consciously or deliberately enacted. Whether or not such inhibition occurs will depend not only on the precise circumstances but also on individual differences in how they are appraised, reflecting the propensities for inhibition postulated in the Dual Control model.

This raises the issue of how such inhibition is enacted. As Spiering & Everaerd (2007) point out, central regulation of emotional responses is essential for adaptive functioning. The most directly relevant evidence comes from the limited brain-imaging literature reviewed earlier. This suggests that inhibition of sexual arousal involves a variety of brain mechanisms, some of which impact on information processing, and others more directly on genital response (Mouras & Stoleru 2007).

Individual differences and the relevance of personality

Considering the extensive work that has been carried out in the field of personality measurement, surprisingly little attention has been paid to the influence of personality variables on the patterns of information processing and sexual response considered in this chapter. The use of the Sexual Opinion Survey (SOS) by Geer et al (1994) was considered earlier (p. 99). The early distraction study by Farkas et al (1979) used the Eysenck Personality Inventory (Eysenck & Eysenck 1968), and an intriguing negative association between erectile response and scores on the Lie scale was found, plus a weak negative correlation between neuroticism score and latency to maximum tumescence. Becker & Byrne (1988) compared type A and type B males in a dichotic listening task, with a challenging numerical task played in one ear and an erotic audio tape in the other. The type A males performed better on the numerical task, while paying less attention and remembering less of the erotic material. It is difficult to escape the conclusion that individual differences could explain much of the variability and inconsistency across experimental studies, including an impact on participation biases. Yet, this aspect has been largely ignored up till now. Clearly there is a need for appropriate measures of individual variability to be used in such studies. The Dual Control model, introduced in Chapter 2, and discussed at various points in this book (e.g. Chapter 6, p. 229) is associated with methods of measuring individual variability that could be appropriately used in studies of information processing of sexual stimuli.

Mood and sexuality

It is conventional clinical wisdom that negative mood, whether experienced as anxiety, depression or anger, has a negative impact on sexual arousability. Given that sexual arousal can be appropriately regarded as an emotion, it is of some interest to consider how the processing of negative emotions differs from the processing of sexual arousal, and to what extent these two types of information processing interact.

Until recently it was widely assumed that anxiety had a disruptive effect on sexual response. A long-favoured explanation was that anxiety activated the peripheral SNS, which in turn had a vasoconstrictive effect on genital vasocongestion. This was an example of the dualistic model of the autonomic nervous system, which saw parasympathetic activity as associated with positive and sympathetic activity with negative states, a simplistic model of the autonomic nervous system, considered earlier in this chapter (see p. 81), which is no longer helpful. It has become clear that we need to confront a more complex and variable relationship between anxiety, genital response and subjective sexual arousal. Similarly, with depression we should not expect any simple predictable relationship with sexuality, and with anger we are also faced with a range of patterns. Once again, with each type of negative affect we are confronted with some key issues of individual difference.

The evidence will be considered under three headings: (i) the association between clinical mood disorders and sexual function, (ii) experimental manipulation of mood states and the impact on sexual response, and (iii) non-clinical variations in mood and their relation to sexual interest and response, with a particular emphasis on individual differences. Finally, in this section we will consider the possible mediating mechanisms that underlie the range of mood–sexuality relationships. The presence of negative mood in men and women with sexual dysfunctions or other sexual problems, and their possible aetiological role, will be considered more fully in Chapters 11 and 16.

Clinical mood disorders and sexual function

There is now a substantial literature showing sexual problems in men and women with depressive illness, most often loss of sexual interest, and a more limited literature showing an association in anxiety disorders. This literature is briefly reviewed in Chapter 13 (p. 387).

Frohlich & Meston (2002), in a study of women students, selected a depressed group on the basis of Beck Depression Inventory (BDI) scores of 20 or higher. In comparison with a non-depressed group, with BDI scores of 3 or less, they found the depressed women reported more inhibited sexual arousal and orgasm and less satisfaction and pleasure. In contrast, however, they also reported more interest than the control group in masturbating on their own. Further evidence of this kind was reported by Cyranowski et al (2004) in their study of women at midlife. Those with a history of recurrent MDD reported higher frequencies of masturbation than women with no history of MDD. This was not, however, related to the level of sexual pleasure in the relationship and therefore did not fit into a compensatory pattern. Frohlich & Meston (2002) speculated that masturbation may provide a form of self-soothing mood regulation.

To what extent are we seeing here the development of a paradoxical relationship between negative mood and sexuality?

There are indications in the clinical literature that relationships between mood and sexuality are not always in the same direction, although this mainly comes from studies of depression rather than anxiety. Thus Mathew & Weinman (1982) found in a mixed gender group of 57 depressives that, whereas 31% had loss of sexual interest, 22% reported increased sexual interest. Similarly, Angst (1998) found that, among depressed males, 25.7% reported decreased and 23.3% increased sexual interest, compared to 11.1% and 6.9%, respectively of their non-depressed group. In contrast, only 8.8% of the Angst females reported increased interest when depressed, compared to 35.3% with decreased sexual interest (with 1.7% and 31.6%, respectively, of their non-depressed group). In a study of depressed men receiving cognitive behaviour therapy, Nofzinger et al (1993) found that those who failed to respond to treatment had significantly higher levels of sexual interest than both those who remitted and their non-depressed control group. In addition, this high sexual interest, non-remitting group were more anxious as well as having more intermittent depression. So here we have an interesting link between anxiety and increased sexual interest, but in the context of a depressive disorder. It is apparent that asking about *increased* sexual interest in negative mood states in research has been very unusual, and if more studies had covered this possibility there may have been more consistency in the published evidence.

Relevant to this paradox is the recent evidence of comorbidity between compulsive sexual behaviour or 'sexual addictions' and mood disorders (Black et al 1997), an additional indication that the relationship between negative mood and sexuality is not always in the same direction.

Experimental manipulation of mood and its effect on sexual response

Here, there is substantially more evidence relating to anxiety than to depression, and this is considered in relation to men and women separately. Although some studies have shown a negative effect of anxiety on sexual arousal in men (e.g. Hale & Strassberg 1990), others have shown that by inducing anxiety, genital response to erotic stimuli can be enhanced. This has been done either by showing an anxiety provoking film prior to the erotic film (e.g. Wolchick et al 1980) or by using threat of electric shock (Barlow 1986). However, this paradoxical effect was observed in 'functional' men, whereas in dysfunctional men the induced anxiety was associated with a reduction of genital response (reviewed in Cranston-Cuebas & Barlow 1990). Barlow (1986) interpreted this phenomenon as an amplifying effect of arousal, whether it be negative, such as that associated with anxiety, or otherwise non-specific. Thus, arousal will enhance the focus of the information processing — if it is focused on sexual cues, then the sexual response will be enhanced, whereas if it is focused on

non-erotic or anti-erotic cues, such as worrying thoughts about failure, then the anti-erotic effect will be enhanced. In these ways he explained the discrepancy between the functional and dysfunctional men in his experiments, maintaining his focus on the central role of information processing.

In studies of women, Hoon et al (1977) found increased VBF response to an erotic film if it was preceded by an anxiety-provoking film. Beggs et al (1987) measured VPA while women listened to 100 s narratives of their own personal experiences, which were associated with either sexual anxiety or sexual pleasure. There was a significant increase in VPA from baseline with both types of narrative, but it was significantly greater with 'pleasure' than with 'anxiety' narratives. Palace & Gorzalka (1990) presented an anxiety provoking film (of threatened amputation) immediately before an erotic film and found that the VPA response to the erotic film was increased in both sexually functional and dysfunctional women. Beck & Bozman (1995) had women listen to personalized erotic scripts in which the content was varied to induce anxiety. The woman's level of sexual desire (not sexual arousal) was monitored continuously by her moving a lever. Less sexual desire was reported during the anxiety-inducing scripts.

It is difficult to draw any general conclusions about the role of anxiety in women's sexual arousal from these varied methodologies. They do, however, confront us with the complexity of the concept 'anxiety'. As Wiegel et al (2007) put it 'Anxiety is frequently (and mistakenly) used as a general term loosely referring to a number of affective states that include fear, panic and worry.... Anxiety defined more specifically refers to a state of 'anxious apprehension' that incorporates a sense of uncontrollability focused largely on future negative events, a strong physiological or somatic component (SNS), a vigilance (or hypervigilance) for threat-related cues, and a shift in attention to a self-focus (self-preoccupation) in which evaluation of one's (inadequate) capabilities to cope with threat is prominent' (p. 146). The various experiments reviewed above manipulate different aspects of this complex picture, not surprisingly with varied results.

There has been more limited evidence of the induction of depressed mood but it has been somewhat more consistent in producing a reduction in sexual response. Wolchick et al (1980), found that by first showing a film inducing a depressed mood, the sexual response to a later erotic film was reduced, in contrast to anxiety-provoking films, which, as already mentioned, had an enhancing effect. Meisler & Carey (1991) induced positive and negative mood immediately before showing an erotic film, during which erectile response and subjective arousal were monitored. Following depression induction there was a trend towards less and more delayed subjective arousal but no effect on erectile response. The method of mood induction (the Velten Mood Induction Procedure, in which a series of statements are made) may be less effective in inducing depressed mood than the film used by Wolchick et al (1980). Mitchell et al

(1998) used music to induce both positive and depressed mood before viewing erotic films. Positive mood induction resulted in enhanced erectile and subjective response in comparison to a neutral control condition, whereas negative mood induction reduced erectile response but did not alter subjective arousal. The above studies involved only men.

Kuffel & Heiman (2006) compared two groups of women, one with normal mood (BDI score less than 9, mean 3.6) and the other with mild to moderate depression (BDI score 10 or more, mean 17.0). Each woman watched two erotic films after being asked to adopt (i) a positive sexual schema script (starting with 'You like your sexuality a lot . . .') and (ii) a negative sexual schema script (starting with 'You do not like your sexuality . . .'), using one of these scripts with each film. The positive script was associated with significantly more subjective sexual arousal than the negative script. The effects on VPA were more complex. There was significantly more VPA response with the positive script if it had been preceded by the film with the negative script. If the film with the positive script came first, there was no difference in the VPA response, an effect not easily explained. In some way, the initial use of the positive script produced an effect on VPA responsiveness, which carried over to the sequence with the negative script. There was overall no correlation between subjective arousal and VPA response. Interestingly, there were no differences between the depressed and non-depressed groups in any of these effects.

The effect of anger on sexual response has also received little research attention, but there is some evidence to suggest that sexual response and anger may facilitate each other. Clark (1953) found that men who had looked at sexually stimulating pictures showed more evidence of aggressive fantasies in response to TAT cards. Jaffe et al (1974) instructed their subjects to punish with electric shocks confederates who had made incorrect responses to some task. After reading erotic literature they gave stronger shocks. Two studies (Barclay & Haber 1965; Barclay 1969) have shown that inducing anger leads to greater sexual imagery in response to TAT cards. Beck & Bozman (1995), in the study of men and women mentioned earlier, found that induced anger was associated with more negative effects on sexual desire than anxiety, more noticeably in the women than in the men studied. The relationship between anger and sexuality is profoundly important and will be discussed further in relation to both sexual violence (Chapter 16) and interpersonal sexual problems (Chapter 11).

What is notably absent from this literature is the idea that individuals may vary in how negative mood states affect their sexuality. This aspect will be considered in the next section.

Non-clinical variations in affect and their relationship to sexual interest and response

Clearly, many people experience episodes of depression or anxiety from time to time in their lives, and the question arises whether they also experience predictable changes in their sexuality during such mood change. The only predictable recurrent mood change that has been studied is that related to the menstrual cycle in women. The variation in sexual interest and arousability through the cycle in some women is considered in the last part of this chapter (p. 116). Sanders et al (1983) found that one-third of the variability in women's self-ratings of sexual interest through the cycle could be accounted for by changes in their well-being, with a positive association between well-being and sexual interest. In a retrospective study of more than 3000 women (Warner & Bancroft 1988), most of whom experienced perimenstrual mood change, the commonest time for their sexual interest to peak was the post-menstrual week, which was also the commonest time for their most positive mood. However, there was an interesting 13% who reported their peak of sexual interest in the premenstrual week, and for most of them this was also the time for their most negative mood. This is consistent with a paradoxical relationship between negative mood and sexuality in some women.

We have recently started to explore what typically happens to one's sexual interest and sexual responsiveness when experiencing more 'normal' depressed or anxious mood. A simple instrument, the Mood and Sexuality Questionnaire (MSQ) was devised (Bancroft et al 2003b). This first asks whether the individual has experienced enough (i) depression or (ii) anxiety to recognize a predictable pattern. Those who indicated this was not the case were separated as 'excluders', for depression, anxiety or both. For the non-excluders, two bipolar scales for depression (MS1 for sexual interest and MS2 for sexual response) and two for anxiety (MS3 for interest and MS4 for response) were presented; e.g. 'when you have felt depressed what typically happens to your sexual interest?', with answers on a 1–9 scale, 5 indicating 'no change', 1 'markedly decreased' and 9 'markedly increased'. There were thus four 1–9 scales (MS1–4) and a composite scale of 4–36. This questionnaire has now been completed by large samples of heterosexual men (Bancroft et al 2003b), self-identified gay men (Bancroft et al 2003c) and heterosexual women (Lykins et al 2006) (for MS1 and 3 scores for men and women see Fig. 4.10). The scores for each of the MS1–4 scales were reduced to three categories 'decreased' (1–3), 'no change' (4–6) and 'increased' (7–9). The percentage of excluders and distributions of responses of the includers from these three studies are shown together in Table 4.2.

This shows clearly that there is substantial variability in all three samples, with a paradoxical increase in sexual interest and/or response in negative mood states being reported by a minority in each case, more frequently in relation to sexual interest than response, and more frequently in relation to anxiety than depression. In each sample more than 20% reported increased sexual interest in states of anxiety. Direct comparison of these three samples has to be limited, because none is representative and there are some major relevant sampling differences. Age, for example, is very different for each sample and appears to be an important and interesting

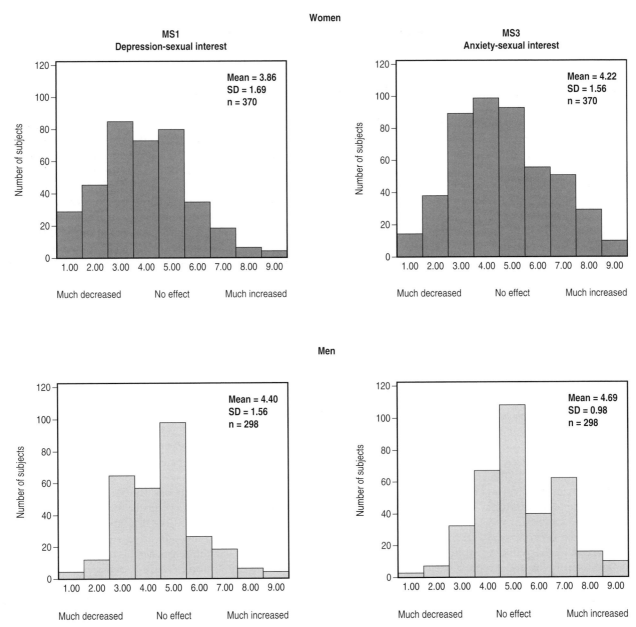

Fig. 4.10 Distribution of scores for mood and sexual interest in 370 female and 298 male students: MS1 depression and sexual interest; MS3 anxiety and sexual interest (Lykins et al 2006).

TABLE 4.2	The distribution of patterns of association between negative mood and sexuality in heterosexual and gay men and heterosexual women						
		Sexual interest (MS1 and MS3)			Sexual response (MS2 and MS4)		
	Excluded* (%)	Decreased (%)	No change (%)	Increased (%)	Decreased (%)	No change (%)	Increased (%)
DEPRESSION							
Heterosexual men	37.4	42	49	9	19	77.5	3
Gay men	19.8	47	37	16	37	56	7
Heterosexual women	36.5	50.5	40	9.5	34	57	8
ANXIETY							
Heterosexual men	20.2	28	51	21	21	73	11
Gay men	10.8	39	37	24	24	31	14
Heterosexual women	14.9	34	43	23	34	57	8

*Those reporting that they have not been depressed or anxious enough to recognize any predictable pattern
Total n and mean age for each group: heterosexual men, n = 919, 28.1 years (16–84); gay men, n = 662, 35.7 years (18–80); heterosexual women, n = 663, 18.9 years (17–32)

variable. In the heterosexual men, age was negatively correlated with each MS score and was the strongest predictor of the MS total score in multiple regression, indicating that paradoxical patterns of increased sexuality with negative mood were more likely in younger men. In the gay men, whereas negative correlations were present univariately, age was not predictive of MS total score in multiple regression. This interesting difference awaits replication and explanation but may reflect a different developmental history in the evolving relationship between negative mood and sexuality in straight and gay men. Not surprisingly, there were substantially fewer 'excluders' in the gay sample, consistent with the high rates of depression in homosexual men (e.g. Fergusson et al 1999; Sandfort et al 2001). In exploring the possible relationship between excitation and inhibition proneness and the paradoxical mood/sexuality pattern, we found SIS2, measuring the propensity for 'sexual inhibition due to the threat of performance consequences', negatively predictive of MS scores in both groups; SIS1, negatively predictive in the heterosexual but not the gay men; and SES, measuring sexual excitation proneness, positively predictive, although only weakly in the gay men. Overall, we accounted for more of the variance in the heterosexual men (19%) than in the gay men (4%).

The study of women was restricted to students and hence had a much lower and less variable age (Lykins et al 2006). This sample of women was therefore compared with a subsample of 399 male students from the heterosexual male study (Bancroft et al 2003b). Although there was substantial overlap in the distribution of MS scores from the female and male samples, women scored significantly lower on all the MS scores except MS4, i.e. sexual response with anxiety. In attempting to predict the MS scores in the women, multivariate analysis was only significant with the anxiety scales (MS3 and 4), and SES was most strongly predictive of the paradoxical mood sexuality pattern. Age was negatively predictive but only for MS4 (anxiety and sexual response). Only 3% of the variance in MS scores was accounted for.

In the two male studies described above (Bancroft et al 2003b,c), 43 heterosexual and 42 gay men were interviewed and asked to describe how they experienced the impact of mood on their sexuality. The complexity of their descriptions contrasted with the simplicity of the MSQ scales. Also some individuals were more clearly aware of the relationship between mood and sexuality than others. Overall, the impact of depression was more variable and complex than that of anxiety. Sexual activity when depressed was described as serving a variety of functions, e.g. establishing intimacy and self-validation or, more simply, as a mood regulator. Masturbation when depressed had contrasting effects across individuals. For some, the solitariness of the act reinforced a depressive sense of isolation and worthlessness; for others it allowed sexual expression without low self-esteem being amplified by a dyadic interaction. These differences are of possible relevance to the findings of increased interest in masturbation in depressed women, reported by Frohlich & Meston (2002) and considered

earlier. Such individual differences in the impact of depression probably reflect personality-related cognitive differences. Six gay men described what one of them called 'what the heck' — a pattern where feeling depressed increased the likelihood of taking sexual risks because of less concern about the consequences. This was not described by any of the heterosexual men and may reflect a greater sense of fatalism among gay men (e.g. Kalichman et al 1997). It may also reflect that it is simply easier for gay than straight men to find a casual partner when depressed.

With anxiety and stress, the patterns seemed, by comparison, straightforward. The term 'stress' was used to describe feeling under pressure, overwhelmed, anxious or worried about what needed to be done. The paradoxical increase in sexuality for some appeared to be principally a matter of benefiting from the arousal-reducing and calming effect of the post-orgasmic state.

Possible mediating mechanisms

It has become increasingly clear that the interaction between negative mood and sexuality is variable in both men and women. This probably reflects, in part, the context and cause of the negative mood, but also considerable individual variability. As we will see later in this book (Chapter 14) the impact of mood on sexuality is of obvious relevance to sexual risk taking, and also 'out of control' sexual behaviour, usually labelled 'sexual addiction' or 'sexual compulsion'. It is also likely to be relevant to sexual offences (Chapter 16). What mechanisms act to mediate these variable patterns?

Once again, we will use the Dual Control model to structure our thinking. What is the relative importance of excitation and inhibition in accounting for these patterns? With depression, we can consider two mechanisms: a reduction in excitation proneness or arousability, and an increase in inhibition. The reduced arousability can be seen as a manifestation of the metabolic changes that can accompany depression, particularly endogenous depressive illness. This is well illustrated in the reduction of NPT in depressive illness (Roose et al 1982; Thase et al 1987), an effect that is reversed by treatment, even psychological treatment of depression. NPT, which is considered more closely later in this chapter (p. 112) can be regarded as a manifestation of 'excitatory tone', which is allowed expression due to the reduction of inhibitory tone accompanying REM sleep. Depression, therefore, can reduce this 'excitatory tone' even during sleep. The nature of this effect and how it relates to other manifestations of depression remain unknown. Further research is needed to compare NPT in different types of depression.

The second mechanism involves elicitation of sexual inhibition as part of the depressive process. This may in part depend on the sexual salience of the depressive situation, which in turn involves information processing and the capacity for individual characteristics to influence this processing, in the manner described by Barlow and his colleagues (Wiegel et al 2007). It may also reflect the individual's propensity for inhibition, which may not be a direct function of cognitive processing. It is noteworthy that, at least in men, both SIS1 and SIS2 were negatively predictive of paradoxical mood relations. The failure to show this in women may be due to the use of the SIS/SES questionnaire, which, while modified for use by women, was designed originally for men. Further studies using the more recent SESII-W, designed specifically for women (see p. 16), may show that inhibition of a kind that is more relevant to women may be relevant to the effects of mood. So far, however, the indication is that in men, a low propensity for inhibition increases the likelihood of a paradoxical mood sexuality pattern. Conversely, a high propensity for inhibition increases the likelihood of negative effects of depression on sexuality.

With anxiety there is an additional factor: the impact of the increased arousal associated with anxiety. Here there is the possibility of 'excitation transfer' (Zillman 1983) whereby the central and peripheral activations associated with the anxiety augment the arousal response to the sexual stimulus. Once again we should consider: (i) the meaning of the anxiety-provoking stimulus; the more sexually salient, in a negative sense, the less likely is there to be excitation transfer; and (ii) the inhibition proneness of the individual. The presence of low inhibition proneness may allow excitation transfer without the counteracting effect of inhibition.

The tendency for paradoxical patterns of mood and sexuality being more likely in younger people is of interest. What happens, as we get older, to lessen this? And is there an increased likelihood that negative mood can become associated with sexual response at an early stage of sexual development? In an interesting study of prepubertal boys, which has never been replicated, Ramsey (1943) found many boys between the ages of 10 and 12 years who reported experiencing erections during a variety of non-sexual but arousing situations, many of which were frightening (e.g. being chased by a policeman). It seemed that at that stage of development there was relatively undiscriminated genital response to any form of arousing stimulus. This raises the issue of how early sexual experience, particularly of an abusive kind that elicits negative emotions, may influence the development of mood-sexuality relations. It is a researchable question whether individuals with a paradoxical mood and sexuality pattern are more likely to have a history of sexual abuse or trauma during childhood. This issue will be revisited in the chapter on sexual development.

With anger, we have much less evidence to work with, but similar mediating mechanisms as suggested for anxiety can be proposed, and development of a simple questionnaire like the MSQ should be pursued to investigate the relationship between anger and sexual interest and response. We can postulate a variety of possible relationships: (i) anger may facilitate sexual response, (ii) anger may reduce sexual response (some individuals appear to find it difficult to be angry and sexually aroused at the same time), (iii) avoidance or rejection of sexual activity may be a way of expressing anger, (iv) sexual arousal may facilitate anger, (v) sexual response may reduce anger (i.e. sexual interaction may be used to defuse an angry situation) and (vi) failure to respond sexually may cause anger (either in the subject or in the partner).

In general, we are at a very early stage in grappling with the complex but profoundly important relationships between negative moods and sexuality. The MSQ, while helping us get started, is a simple and crude measure. More sophisticated plus prospective studies (e.g. using daily diaries) are needed, plus research into early and relevant developmental patterns. An example of the use of daily diaries in assessing the relations between mood and sexual risk taking (Mustanski 2007) is considered in Chapter 14 (p. 433). There is a need to distinguish between different types of sexual activity. It would be of particular interest, for example, to explore the association between depression and masturbation reported by Frohlich & Meston (2002) and Cyranowski et al (2004), using a mood and sexuality scale that distinguished between masturbation and activity with a partner. There is also a need to examine the mixture of different negative affects. The coexistence of anxiety and depression has already been shown to complicate the picture (Nofzinger et al 1993).

The role of hormones in sexual arousal and response

The fundamental role of hormones in the reproductive system and in the crucial process of sexual differentiation was considered in Chapter 3. Here we consider their role in sexual arousal and genital response, with a particular focus on gonadal steroids (T and oestradiol, E) and certain peptides. At the time of writing we have entered a phase of uncertainty about the conventional views of hormone action as they apply to gonadal steroids. This has resulted from two developments: the new focus on intracrine processes, which throw into question many traditional assumptions about the physiological relevance of circulating levels of gonadal steroids (see p. 116), and the discovery of two E receptors and findings of their functional relevance in males and females (Grumbach & Auchus 1999). These issues will be considered in more detail later in the section. First, the conventional literature on the effects of gonadal steroids on sexual behaviour in men and women will be reviewed.

Gonadal steroids – androgens in the male

A good starting point is the effect of T replacement in hypogonadal men. Most controlled studies in the literature start with hypogonadal men already on T replacement for at least several months, who have their exogenous T withdrawn. The effects of this withdrawal on sexual parameters are assessed. This is then followed by the administration of T and placebo, using a double-blind crossover design (for more detailed review, see Bancroft 2003). Such studies predictably show a reduction in the level of sexual interest during T withdrawal, usually evident within 3–4 weeks, consistent with T being necessary for normal levels of sexual interest (and arousability). If T withdrawal lasts long enough, seminal emission will eventually be impaired (Fig. 4.11). Typically, in

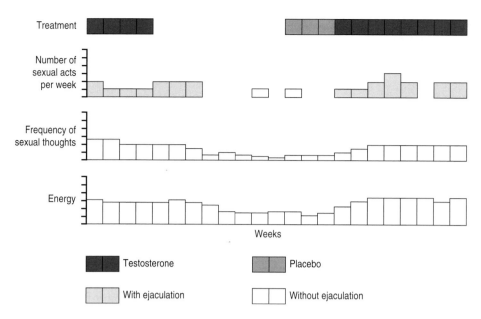

Fig. 4.11 The effects of T replacement in a hypogonadal man aged 40 years, castrated 1 year earlier for testicular neoplasm. Sexual activity, ejaculation, sexual thoughts and energy all declined about 3 weeks after stopping T replacement. There is no response to placebo, but a rapid response within 1 or 2 weeks of restarting T (Skakkebaek et al 1981).

male studies of this kind, placebo has little effect, but T replacement restores sexual interest, showing a dose–response relationship (Fig. 4.12). Effects on sexual activity with a partner are less consistent, partly because they depend on partner and relationship characteristics. Frequency of masturbation tends to follow level of sexual interest, although cultural factors may influence this pattern of sexual expression (Anderson et al 1999).

A few studies have used psychophysiological assessment of response to sexual stimuli to assess the effects of T withdrawal and replacement on genital response (erection) as well as subjective aspects of sexual arousal. Earlier studies, which were based on the maximum change in penile circumference as a measure of erectile response, found little difference between hypogonadal men with and without T replacement. This was interpreted as indicating that the genital response component of sexual arousal was not T dependent. More recently, however, this assessment has been carried out by measuring, in addition to changes in penile circumference, increases in penile rigidity as well as duration of erectile response. This showed significantly more rigid erectile response with T replacement, and a longer duration of erectile response. Without T, the erectile response was 'stimulus bound'. i.e. would recede as soon as the stimulus was switched off. With T replacement, the response would not only show greater rigidity, but would also last beyond the sexual stimulus (Carani et al 1995).

Unfortunately, the more limited evidence of the effects of sexual fantasy in hypogonadal men with and without T replacement has been inconsistent, and as yet the relevance of T to sexual fantasy or imagery (or sexual information processing) remains uncertain.

An interesting and potentially important aspect of sexual arousability to consider is NPT, the occurrence of spontaneous erections during REM sleep. As waking typically occurs from REM sleep, such erections are commonly found on waking. The occurrence of full waking erections, or normal NPT, in men with ED, is conventionally regarded as an indication that the basic mechanisms of erection are intact, and thus the ED is more likely to be 'psychogenic'. The explanation for normal occurrence of NPT is still disputed, but one plausible explanation is that REM sleep is associated with a 'switching off' of the NA cells in the l.c. (Parmeggiana & Morrison 1990), which, via their spinal projections, are probably associated with the inhibitory tone in the penis. Thus, the reduction of inhibitory tone during REM permits what can be called 'excitatory tone' to be expressed as erection. NPT is clearly impaired in hypogonadal men, and restored to normal with T replacement (Fig. 4.13). The l.c. has T receptors (Parmeggiana & Morrison 1990), and this putative 'excitatory tone' can be regarded as T-dependent.

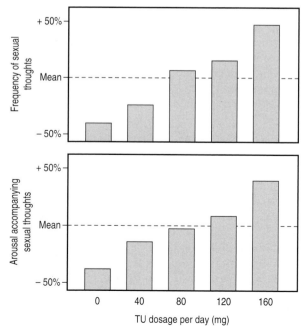

Fig. 4.12 Dose–response relationship between T undecanoate (TU) and median standardized visual analogue ratings of frequency of sexual thoughts (top) and arousal accompanying sexual thoughts (bottom). Both relationships are significant ($p < 0.01$) according to Page's test for ordered alternatives (O'Carroll et al 1985).

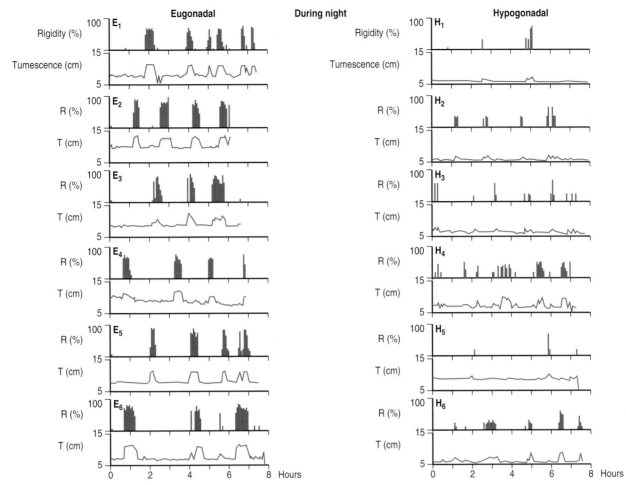

Fig. 4.13 NPT recordings, using Rigiscan, showing tumescence (circumference increase) and rigidity through the night, in six eugonadal men (E1-6) and six hypogonadal men (H1-6). (From Carani et al 1992.)

Recent studies of T manipulation in eugonadal men have produced results consistent with the earlier hypogonadal studies. An experimental study used the GnRH antagonist, NalGlu, to suppress T levels in eugonadal men over a 6-week period (Bagatell et al 1994a). This resulted in lowered sexual interest and associated sexual activity. An additional feature of this study was the administration of varying doses of exogenous T or placebo during the NalGlu administration. This suggested that the plasma level of T needed to avoid the sexual effects of T withdrawal was substantially lower than the pretreatment, baseline level. This is consistent with the idea that most men have more circulating T than they need for the maintenance of normal sexual function.

The exploration of T as a method of male contraception has led to further studies of the effects of increasing circulating T above normal baseline levels by means of exogenous T administration. Bagatell et al (1994b) and Yates et al (1999) found that increasing T in eugonadal men had no effect on frequency of sexual activity, or in the latter study, daily measures of sexual interest. Similar negative findings were reported by O'Connor et al (2004) in a study using intramuscular T undecanoate. Buena et al (1993) explored the effect of varying T levels within the normal range. They first suppressed testicular function with a GnRH agonist (Lupron) and then administered exogenous T in either high or low dosage, to produce T levels that were either at the high end or at the low end of the normal range. They found no difference in sexual activity or sexual interest. These various studies are consistent in finding no effect of increased T levels on simple measures of sexual activity or interest in eugonadal men. However, Anderson et al (1992), using weekly injections of either placebo or T enanthate 200 mg, over 8 weeks, while finding no effect of the exogenous T on sexual activity, either with partner or as masturbation, did find a significant increase in a measure of sexual interest that was independent of sexual interaction with the partner (subscale 2 of the Sexual Experience Scale — Frenken & Vennix 1981). Also Alexander et al (1997) found that T administration to eugonadal men produced an increased attention to auditory sexual stimuli. These two last studies suggest that subtle effects on sexuality may occur by increasing T levels in eugonadal men, without the basic parameters of sexual activity and interest being obviously affected.

Carani et al (1995) evaluated the effects of exogenous T on NPT in eugonadal men. Intramuscular T enanthate had no effect on sleep parameters and did not affect frequency, degree or duration of NPT, when assessed as penile circumference, but did increase, modestly but significantly, penile rigidity during NPT. Buena et al (1993) included NPT assessment in their study and found no effect of increased T, but they did not measure penile rigidity.

The timing of androgen effects in men remains uncertain. In replacement studies of hypogonadal men, positive effects of T replacement are apparent within 7–14 days (Fig. 4.11). In a study of eugonadal men, Su et al (1993) compared methyltestosterone with placebo for only 3-day periods and found an effect on 'sexual arousal'. Carani et al (1995), in their study of NPT, found the effects mentioned above after 2 days. In hypogonadal men it is possible that longer is needed to establish receptor responsiveness.

Androgens in male sexual development

While the importance of T to sexual differentiation, both in early development and around puberty, is beyond dispute (see Chapter 3), the impact of T on the emergence of sexual arousability is less clear. Udry and colleagues carried out two studies in teenage boys in which T levels were related to various aspects of sexuality. In the first (Udry et al 1985), a cross-sectional study, the free T index was found to be a strong predictor of 'sexual motivation', whereas stage of pubertal development was not predictive. In the second, a longitudinal study over 3 years, with six monthly assessments (Halpern et al 1993), they found the reverse; the stage of pubertal development was much more predictive of sexual interest and behaviour than the free T index. One possible explanation for this apparent contradiction, which resulted from a comparison of inter- and intra-individual data, is that the impact of T on sexual arousability (and hence behaviour) has to go through stages of development, which may involve changes in receptor numbers or sensitivity, a process that will also be influenced by individual differences in receptor sensitivity. Gooren (1988), in a study of hypogonadal teenage males, found that boys with primary hypogonadism showed less response to T replacement than boys with secondary hypogonadism. Other studies comparing hypergonadotrophic and hypogonadotrophic hypogonadism have not shown such clear differences, but have all involved males well beyond the age of normal puberty (see Bancroft 2003 for review). More research is required on this important aspect of sexual development.

Androgens and aging in men

Schiavi and his colleagues, in a study of healthy, medication-free men aged 45–74, found a clear decline in sexual interest, arousability and activity with age (Schiavi et al 1990). The relatively predictable effects of T withdrawal and replacement in younger adult men give way to a more complex, or at least less well-understood picture in older men. Here we have to take into account a number of age-related changes, including altered negative feedback of T and hence less increase in LH with falling T levels, increased SHBG and hence relatively reduced

free T, and the likelihood of an age-related decline in T receptor sensitivity. Schiavi et al (1990) also found an age-related decline in NPT to levels that, in younger men, would be regarded as indicative of organic ED, but which in this older age group was associated with relatively normal erectile function, providing there was sufficient tactile stimulation. This suggested an age-related decline in T-dependent central arousability. This will be considered further in Chapter 7.

Conclusions about the role of T in the male

The evidence is fairly clear that in men who have gone through normal puberty, and who have not yet been affected by aging, T plays an important role in their sexual interest and associated sexual arousability. As yet, the evidence is consistent that T affects central arousal mechanisms. The peripheral effects of T on genital response have been well established in lower mammals, and there is a recent shift towards seeing T as also having direct effects on the erectile response in men, possibly by facilitating nitrergic mechanisms in the penis (Lewis & Mills 2004; Montorsi & Oettel 2005; Gooren & Saad 2006). It is also apparent that, in adult eugonadal men, the levels of T in the circulation are substantially higher than required to maintain sexual arousability, suggesting that other T effects, most probably in the periphery, require higher levels than are needed in the CNS. The limited evidence from studies of sexual development suggests that, whereas T plays an important role in the young male's emerging sexual arousability, its effects are not as straightforward as in adult males, possibly reflecting changing patterns of receptor sensitivity and other aspects of brain development, as well as associated learning processes, which serve to provide the T effects with a sexual direction. In addition, as discussed earlier in the section on orgasm (p. 91) we have to consider the possibility that peripubertal increases in T may have an organizing effect on the development of post-ejaculatory refractoriness. In the older male, the picture is complicated by various aging effects, including altered hypothalamo-pituitary feedback, increased T binding and reduced receptor sensitivity.

Androgens in the female

While for the male we find consistent and replicable findings for the key role of T for sexual arousability, at least in young and middle-aged adult men, in the female we find inconsistent and often contradictory evidence. And this is in spite of the fact that we have many more studies of women, usually involving larger samples, than are found in the male literature. This may in part result from the greater complexity of the reproductive endocrine system in women, who experience menstrual cycles, pregnancy and lactation, and a clearly identifiable menopause. At the same time, these endocrine variations offer more opportunities for studying hormone/sexual arousal relationships than is the case with men. Another possible explanation for this inconsistency in the female evidence is that women are more variable than men in their responsiveness to T, although what is clear is that in so far as women do respond to T, they respond to levels of T or increases in T that would be totally ineffective in males. Thus, contrary to some conventional wisdom that sees early exposure to T in the male as sensitizing the individual to later increases in T, it would appear that females, without this early exposure, are much more sensitive to the central nervous system effects of T, or at least some females are. This apparent paradox will be revisited in the final section of this chapter when a 'desensitization hypothesis' will be presented as a possible explanation for this potentially crucial gender difference.

Developmental aspects

Increasing levels of T occur in the development of girls as they approach and go through puberty. However, the changes are much less substantial than in the male. T starts at a lower level in the infant girl and effectively doubles through pubertal maturation, compared with an 18-fold increase in T for boys. The most substantial evidence of the relationship between T and emerging sexual arousability in females comes again from Udry and his colleagues. As with their studies of adolescent boys, they found discrepant results. In a cross-sectional study of eighth to tenth grade girls, they found a relation between T levels and measures of sexual interest and masturbation, but not with the likelihood of having experienced sexual intercourse (Udry et al 1986). In a longitudinal study of girls post menarche, the reverse relations to T were found (Halpern et al 1997). Similar explanations to those discussed for their male studies could apply here, but in addition there is a crucial methodological issue of timing of blood sampling for T in relation to the ovarian cycle (for fuller discussion of these issues, see Bancroft 2003).

Masturbation is an interesting marker of sexual development. In a study of students recalling their masturbation histories, from a recent sample and an age-matched sample from Kinsey's original study, the age of onset was considered in relation to age at puberty (Bancroft et al 2003a). These findings are considered further in Chapter 5 (see p. 151), but they show a clear relation in boys, the large majority reporting onset of masturbation within a window 2 years either side of puberty onset, suggesting that puberty in some sense has an organizing effect on this as well as other aspects of male sexual development. No such clear relation was found between onset of masturbation and age at menarche in girls, who showed a much wider variation in age of onset (see Fig. 5.2). This pattern could be partially explained by a more variable behavioural sensitivity to androgens in females. The early onset of masturbation in girls with high sensitivity to androgens might reflect the increase in androgens at adrenarche. Those with more moderate sensitivity might show their response with the more substantial increase at puberty, whereas those with low sensitivity may not start masturbating till much later. This is a testable hypothesis that warrants further research.

From post-puberty onwards

In recent years there has been a dramatic increase in interest in the role of androgens in women's sexuality. A conference was held in Princeton in 2001 focusing on 'androgen insufficiency in women'. A consensus paper (Bachman et al 2002) and all the individual papers (Supplement No.4) were published in Fertility & Sterility (2002; Volume 77). There was agreement that the clinical features of the postulated 'androgen deficiency syndrome' were relatively non-specific and that assays for free T were currently inadequate for establishing the lower part of the normal range. In the circumstances it was clear that much further research was needed. The proposed algorithm for making a clinical diagnosis will be considered in Chapter 12.

In an attempt to reduce the confusion in the available literature, the role of androgens in the sexuality of women will be looked at in three different ways: (i) relations between sexuality and endogenous levels of androgens, and their natural variations (e.g. menstrual cycle, lactation and menopause), (ii) iatrogenic reductions in endogenous androgen levels or activity (e.g. effects of steroidal contraceptives, antiandrogens and oophorectomy) and (iii) effects of exogenous androgen administration (e.g. hormone replacement therapy, HRT).

Endogenous androgen levels

The most substantial study of the relations between circulating levels of androgens and sexual function in women was reported by Davis et al (2005). In a community-based sample of 1021 women, aged 18–75 years, each woman completed the Profile of Female Sexual Function (PFSF; Derogatis et al 2004) and gave one fasting morning blood sample, which for premenopausal women was collected between the eighth cycle day and onset of next menses. Blood was assayed for T (total and free), androstenedione (A) and DHEA-S. The PFSF provides seven domain scores ('desire', 'arousal', 'orgasm', 'pleasure', 'sexual concerns', 'responsiveness' and 'self-image'), but no total score. The domain scores were not normally distributed and, because of age differences in the scores, the sample was divided into two age groups ('younger', 18–44 years, $n = 339$, and 'older', 45–75 years, $n = 646$). For each domain these two age groups were divided into those with low scores (zero for the older, the lowest 5% for the younger group) and the rest. The low scorers and the rest for each domain were then compared for plasma levels of androgens. Taking a p value of <0.01 as the cutoff, neither total nor free T discriminated for any domain in either age group. DHEA-S, however, was significantly lower in the 'low' scorers in three domains (younger group: 'desire', 'arousal' and 'responsiveness'; older group: 'arousal', 'responsiveness' and 'pleasure'). In addition, androstenedione was significantly lower for the older 'low' responders in the 'pleasure' domain.

This is the most important study to date on androgens and women's sexuality because of the sample size, even allowing for the fact that they achieved a low response rate (9.1%). The use of timed blood sampling is bound to restrict participation. The wide section of the menstrual cycle used for sampling (day 8 onwards) obscures the modest but significant mid-cycle rise in T that typically occurs, which may have introduced relevant 'noise' to their data. Their sample also completed a measure of general well-being. In a separate paper, Bell et al (2005) reported, in the younger age group, a significant association between DHEA-S and 'vitality'. For reasons that were not given, this research group has not reported the relationship between 'vitality' and their measure of sexual function. Given the increasingly recognized relationship between well-being, mood and sexuality, particularly in women, it is distinctly possible that their findings of an association between DHEA-S and sexuality were secondary to a more direct relationship with well-being. Cawood & Bancroft (1996) in a study of women aged 40–60 years found no association between DHEA, DHEA-S, A or T and measures of sexuality, whereas the best predictors of quality of sexual life were the quality of the relationship with the partner and the woman's state of well-being. The only hormonal variable to predict well-being was DHEA.

The comparison in the Davis et al (2005) study of the low scorers on the PFSF with the rest, which may have been necessary because of the non-normal distribution of the scores, raises another potential confound. Many of the women in the 'low' scorer groups may have considered themselves as having a 'problem'. In relation to oral contraceptive use, discussed in Chapter 15, there has been some indication that women in a self-defined 'problem' category do not show correlations between T levels and sexuality, whereas women who do not regard themselves as having a problem do show correlations. One possible explanation for this is that the establishment of a 'sexual problem', with its various repercussions in the relationship, may serve to obscure subtle hormone–behaviour relationships. It would therefore be interesting to know, if the data allow, whether there is any correlation between T levels and PFSF scores across the sample. The PFSF had not been used in this type of sample before and hence the authors were not expecting a skewed distribution of scores. Certainly, if any other large-scale study of this kind is carried out, it would be good to use relevant measures of sexuality that do show close to normal distributions in non-clinical samples (e.g. the SIS-SES, Janssen et al 2002).

Given Davis's earlier commitment to the importance of T in women's sexuality, and the value of T administration in women with sexual problems, these results must have come as a challenge. Davis and her colleagues have reacted by resorting to the intracrine perspective of Labrie et al (2003), which claims that only 10% of the androgens active in women are measurable in the circulation, and that sources of T, in particular DHEA, are converted to T intracellularly (for further discussion of this perspective, see p. 23). The effects of administration of DHEA to women will be considered later in this section.

Van Anders & Hampson (2005) also found no correlation between salivary T levels (which approximate to free T) and levels of sexual desire, as measured by the Sexual Desire Inventory, in 76 healthy women.

Few studies have investigated T levels in women presenting specifically with problems of low sexual desire. Stuart et al (1987) and Schreiner-Engel et al (1989) found no difference in T levels between women with low sexual interest and controls; on the other hand, Riley & Riley (2000) found lower FAI index in women complaining of lifelong absence of sexual drive than in controls.

The menstrual cycle

There is a lack of evidence of T levels during the early cycles of post-menarcheal adolescents, which tend to be irregular and not predictably ovulatory. However, once a woman settles into a pattern of regular ovulatory cycles, T levels typically rise during the follicular phase and are at a maximum approximately for the middle third of the cycle, declining during the final third of the cycle to reach a nadir during the first few days of the next follicular phase (see Fig. 3.23). Within the middle third of the cycle, T levels may be relatively sustained (Backstrom et al 1983) or, as reported in some studies, show more discrete peri-ovulatory peaks. Although there is reasonable consistency across such studies, there is obviously some individual variability. Given this pattern, if T is important for sexual arousability in women, we should expect to find related temporal patterns of arousability through the cycle.

There is a substantial literature on the pattern of sexual interest and behaviour through the menstrual cycle (see Hedricks 1994 for review), although there are many inconsistencies, and Hedricks (1994) has discussed various methodological explanations for them. There is a relatively consistent finding that sexual activity is lowest during the menstrual phase. However, this does not necessarily mean that sexual *arousability* is at its lowest at that stage; there are a number of other non-hormonal explanations for the drop in sexual activity during menstruation. There is also a tendency across studies for indices of sexual interest to be highest during the follicular phase or around ovulation, though with considerable individual variability in this respect (Figs. 4.14 and 4.15). This mid to late follicular pattern is compatible with an effect of the rising T during the follicular phase, although one might have expected a continuation of this T effect into the first part of the luteal phase. Clearly, other hormonal explanations have to be considered.

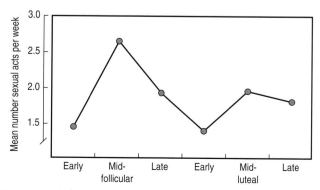

Fig. 4.14 Distribution of sexual activity in six phases of the cycle in 40 women with normal menstrual cycles. Analysis of variance showed a significant cycle effect, with peak in the mid-follicular phase (Bancroft et al 1983).

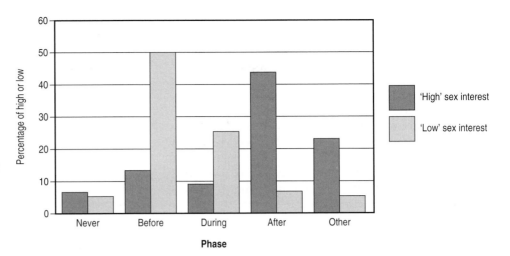

Fig. 4.15 The timing of 'highs' and 'lows' of sexual interest in 3252 women. They were asked to indicate whether the highs and lows occurred in the week before menses, during menses, the week after, other times of the cycle or never. Seventy-six per cent of these women reported their trough of well-being to be the week before, 13% during menses and 52% reported their peak of well-being the week after menses, 37% at other times (Warner & Bancroft 1988).

A much more limited literature looks at the correlation between T level and sexuality as they change through the cycle, and it is very inconsistent (see Bancroft 2003 for review). In part, there may be methodological reasons for this, especially variability in the aspects of sexuality measured. But these inconsistent findings, involving studies with relatively small numbers of participants, could result from substantial individual variability in relation between T and sexuality. Until such research incorporates markers of relevant individual variability that would allow appropriate selection of participants and comparison across studies, we should expect such confounds to continue.

The effects of lactation on androgens and sexuality are considered in Chapter 15, and of menopause and ageing in Chapter 7.

Iatrogenic lowering of androgen levels

Of the various iatrogenic methods of lowering androgen levels in women, the most common is the use of steroidal contraception. This is looked at closely in Chapter 15. Of the other methods, use of antiandrogens and ovariectomy will be considered.

Effects of antiandrogens

Antiandrogens are mainly active by blocking androgenic effects at the receptor, but they also produce reduction in T levels because of negative feedback effects. Cyproterone acetate (CPA) is an antiandrogen with both negative feedback and direct androgen receptor (AR) antagonism, which has been used for the treatment of androgen-dependent conditions such as acne and hirsutism in women. Little attention has been given to the possible sexual side effects of such treatment. Appelt & Strauss (1986) studied 36 women who had not had sexual problems before starting on CPA and of these, 16 (44%) reported negative effects on their sex life; this rose to 61% when women not in sexual relationships were excluded. Such negative effects could result from reduction of androgen effects (either by reduced T levels or antagonism at T receptors) or by some other direct progestagenic effect less well understood.

The effects of ovariectomy

With surgical removal of the ovaries there is an immediate and substantial drop in circulating androgens. The impact on E will obviously depend on whether the ovaries are pre- or post-menopausal at the time of surgery. However, we should keep in mind the possibility that androgen production by the interstitial cells of the post-menopausal ovary, stimulated by post-menopausal levels of LH, is an important source of E from peripheral conversion (see Chapter 7, p. 244). Whether pre- or post-menopausal, therefore, the woman with both ovaries removed is in a state of relative gonadal steroid deficiency. Although there have been a number of studies evaluating the effects of hormone replacement on oophorectomized women with sexual problems, less attention has been paid to what proportion of women who have their ovaries removed experience sexual problems as a consequence. This is in part because ovariectomy is usually carried out together with hysterectomy, and the surgery is usually indicated to relieve a range of health problems (e.g. menorrhagia or pain). In the past, ovaries were often removed during the course of hysterectomy as a precautionary measure to eliminate the risk of later ovarian cancer, based on the assumption that as women approach or pass through menopause their ovaries are no longer of much value. More recently, this has changed as the post-menopausal function of the ovary has become better understood. Now the indication for associated ovariectomy is most often pain associated with endometriosis, which is to some extent E-dependent.

Nathorst-Böös et al (1993) compared women who had had bilateral oophorectomy and hysterectomy without any hormone replacement, with two groups of age-matched hysterectomized women, one having received ovariectomy plus hormone replacement (i.e. E replacement) the other hysterectomy alone. They found little difference between the ovariectomized women with and without hormone replacement, about a half of whom reported a decrease in sexual interest. In contrast, 82% of those with intact ovaries reported an increase in sexual interest post-operatively. Comparable findings were reported by Bellerose & Binik (1993).

Rhodes et al (1999) assessed 1299 women before surgery and again at 12 and 24 months post-operatively. Forty-four percent of the women had both ovaries removed. Overall, this study found more improvement in sexual functioning, sexual desire and dyspareunia post-operatively than worsening, but the report does not make any explicit comparison between those who had both ovaries removed and those who did not. The only indication given was that women who had both ovaries removed were less likely to be experiencing orgasm at 12 months post-operatively. It is not stated what proportion of women received hormone replacement following ovariectomy, and in general the impact of removal of the ovaries remains obscure in this paper, although it seems unlikely that a majority of women had adverse sexual effects from the removal of both ovaries. Farquhar et al (2002) compared 57 women who had hysterectomy with both ovaries removed ('O&H') and 266 women who had hysterectomy alone ('H only'). They found no deterioration sexually in either group at 6 months post-operatively. However, the 'hysterectomy alone' group reported a significant increase in sexual interest and frequency of sexual intercourse, presumably reflecting the health benefits of the surgery. The women who had both ovaries removed showed no such benefits.

Aziz et al (2005) compared 217 women who had 'H only' and 106 women who had 'O&H'. Oestrogen replacement therapy was recommended for all the ovariectomized women and those in the 'H only' group who had menopausal symptoms. Sexuality and well-being was assessed pre-operatively and at 1 year post-operatively. The 'O&H' group showed no change in sexuality or well-being, whereas the 'H only' group showed some worsening in 3 of the 14 sexuality variables. None of the group comparisons was significant. Both groups showed improvement in well-being. There were no correlations between the observed changes pre- to 1 year post operation in androgen levels or any aspect of sexuality or well-being.

Teplin et al (2007) compared 49 women who had 'O&H' with 112 women who had 'H only'. The 'H only' group was significantly younger at the time of surgery (40 vs 45 years; $p < 0.001$). Assessment was carried out at 6 months and 2 years post-operatively. There were no differences in sexual functioning between the two groups.

Removal of both ovaries, in producing a substantial reduction of ovarian androgens in most women, should provide us with a test of the importance of androgens in women, at least at the normal levels found in the circulation, allowing for the age-related decline mentioned earlier. The evidence reviewed above, however, gives us no clear or consistent answer. One reasonable conclusion, however, is that there is no predictable decline in sexual functioning as a result of ovariectomy, and that a substantial proportion of women can experience a reduction in androgens without obvious adverse effects on sexuality or well-being. There are, however, a number of limitations to this source of evidence.

1. Women undergoing such surgery, whether involving bilateral ovariectomy or only hysterectomy, are having the surgery because of some gynaecological problem likely to have an adverse effect on both their sexuality and well-being. Taking the immediate pre-operative period as the baseline, the expected outcome of the surgery is an improvement. None of the studies cited made any attempt to assess the woman's level of sexual functioning before the gynaecological problem became established, and it may in fact be difficult to do so in many cases. In contrast with a woman starting on a steroidal contraceptive, therefore, there is the problem of a lack of a suitable baseline to evaluate the effects of androgen reduction.

2. Women are not randomly assigned to 'H only' or 'O&H', and the decision is made partly on clinical indications and partly on the woman's personal preference. This introduces the potential for confounding individual differences.

3. Studies vary in the extent to which HRT is involved following surgery, and in only one of the cited studies (Bellerose & Binik 1993) is there comparison of HRT involving E only and a combination of E and T.

4. With the exception of the first two studies cited, results are analysed and presented as group averages. As is the case when assessing the effects of oral contraceptives (see p. 446), a group average indicating no change may conceal the fact that some women have experienced improvement and some worsening.

We will return to these points after considering the evidence from T administration, in an attempt to reach some evidence-based conclusions.

The effects of androgen administration on the sexuality of women

Pre-menopausal women with sexual problems

Evidence of the effects of administration of exogenous T on the sexuality of pre-menopausal women is largely restricted to studies of those with sexual problems or endocrine abnormalities. There was an early phase of interest in such treatment which, because it resulted in largely negative findings, was followed by a long period when interest in T as a form of treatment for women waned. Carney et al (1978) assessed the combination of sexual counselling with either T administration or diazepam, for couples in which the woman was sexually unresponsive. The T group showed significantly greater improvement than the diazepam group in satisfaction with sexual intercourse, frequency of orgasm, sexual arousal and frequency of sexual thoughts. These results raised the question of whether this was a positive result of T or a negative effect of diazepam on the effectiveness of the counselling. Mathews et al (1983) attempted to replicate these findings with a similar design, but using placebo rather than diazepam. They found no difference between T and placebo. Dow & Gallagher (1989) questioned whether the combination of T therapy with counselling may have obscured the effects of T therapy alone. They therefore carried out a further replication, adding a third group who received T therapy alone. They found significant improvement in both of the combined groups (i.e. sex therapy plus T or placebo) at the end of treatment and at 4 months follow-up, with no difference between them, and significantly less improvement with T alone. Although there were some changes with T alone (vaginal lubrication, sexual interest and coital pleasure), these were no greater than those in the two combined groups and were not sustained at follow-up. Their conclusion was that there were no advantages in using T therapy alone. In each of these three studies 10 mg of T was administered sublingually (Testoral; Organon) once daily. Unpublished tests in two women confirmed that this method resulted in substantial increases in T above the physiological range for women, for 4–5 hours after administration (Bancroft 1989, Fig. 2. 46).

It is noteworthy that in each of the three above studies, around half of the women were using oral contraceptives, and care was taken to ensure that they were equally distributed across treatments. Bancroft et al (1980) explored androgen administration in 15 oral contraceptive users with sexual problems. Androstenedione was the androgen used. This has the advantage of being well absorbed when taken orally, and producing increases in plasma T as well as androstenedione (A). A double-blind placebo-controlled crossover design was used, with each subject taking A and placebo, each for 2 months. Daily diary and interview ratings were used to assess behavioural change. A significant increase in plasma T occurred in the A treated group, but no significant differences in sexuality variables resulted. One woman, however, showed a clear benefit from the A administration, which was subsequently replicated, with A administration and withdrawal, on three occasions following the study. It is noteworthy that hormonally she differed from the other 14 women, not in terms of increased levels of T as a result of treatment, but of E and of the E:T ratio.

The next comparable study in pre-menopausal women was not published until 2003 (Goldstat et al 2003). Thirty-one women with low libido (mean age, 39.7 ± 4.2 years; mean serum T, 1.07 ± 0.5 nMol/L) used T cream (10 mg/day) and placebo each for 12 weeks (with a 4 week washout period between) in a double-blind crossover study. T administration was associated with significant improvements in general well-being and measures of sexuality (Sabbatsberg Sexual Self-Rating Scale).

Pre-menopausal women with endocrine disease

Miller et al (2001) reported on the abnormally low androgen levels in women with hypopituitarism and went on to assess the effects of T administration in the same group of women, using a placebo-controlled randomized design with 24 women receiving 300 μg T daily in a transdermal patch, and 27 women receiving placebo, each group for 12 months (Miller et al 2006). In comparison with the placebo group, women in the T group showed significant improvement in mood, measured by the BDI, and in sexuality, as measured by the combined score from the Derogatis Interview for Sexual Function, and the subscales for 'arousal' and 'behaviour/experience'.

In a more experimental study, Tuiten et al (1996) studied eight young amenorrhoeic women with low weight, although none had the diagnosis of anorexia nervosa. They showed lower levels of sexual interest and activity, and lower T levels than a comparison group of normally menstruating age-matched women. The amenorrhoeic group was given T undecanoate, 40 mg daily for 8 weeks, and placebo for 8 weeks in a double-blind crossover study. The two treatments did not differ in terms of daily ratings of sexuality or mood. They were also evaluated in a psychophysiology laboratory with measurement of VPA in response to erotic fantasies and erotic films. VPA was significantly greater in response to film in the T condition. However, this effect was not reflected in subjective ratings of arousal. This experiment therefore demonstrated an effect of increasing T on physiological response to erotic stimulation that was not apparent in any subjective or mood measures.

Healthy pre-menopausal women

Tuiten et al (2000) explored the timing of effects of an increase in T on sexual arousal. Eight healthy women without sexual problems, half of whom were using oral contraceptives, were given a single sublingual dose of T in a placebo-controlled experiment. On each of the two occasions, subjective and VPA responses to erotic films were measured just before T administration, 15 min after and on four further occasions 90 min apart. An enhanced VPA response to erotic stimuli was observed 3–4 h after the peak increase in plasma T, significantly correlated with an increase in subjective reports of 'sexual lust' and 'genital sensations'. No difference was found in these respects between the OC and non-OC users.

Post-menopausal women

The more gradual reduction in ovarian androgens, starting some time in the mid-30s and not dependent on the menopause per se (see Chapter 7, p. 244) is in contrast to the more sudden reduction following oophorectomy or the 'surgical menopause'. It is important to consider separately the effects of hormone administration in these two types of menopause. However, in spite of the limited impact of the natural menopause on androgen levels, the inclusion of T in HRT for symptoms of the natural menopause is of potential importance. The administration of exogenous E in HRT increases SHBG and consequently reduces free T. Conversely, T administration will reduce SHBG levels and also, because of competitive binding with SHBG, increase the amount of free E2.

The natural menopause

Unfortunately, in several earlier studies of HRT, women with natural and surgical menopause were combined. Only those with a majority of naturally menopausal women will be considered here.

Burger et al (1987) reported on 20 post-menopausal women whose lack of libido had persisted on 'adequate oral E replacement', but whose 'other main symptoms, such as hot flushes and vaginal dryness', had been relieved. Fourteen of these women had gone through natural menopause. They were randomly assigned to either E implant or E plus T implant. On average, the combined implant group showed improvement in libido and sexual enjoyment within the first 6 weeks, whereas the 'E-only' group did not. They were therefore given an additional T implant and proceeded to show the same improvement as the combined group. It is noteworthy that no other symptoms were reported, and no indication was given of whether these women were suffering from tiredness, lack of concentration or depression before starting the implants.

Myers et al (1990) studied 40 naturally post-menopausal women, who were randomly assigned to four groups of 10 subjects each, P (Premarin only), PP (Premarin plus Provera), PT (Premarin plus methyltestosterone) and PL (placebo), and assessed over a 10-week period. Subjects were assessed with both self-ratings and laboratory measurement of VPA response to erotic stimuli. There were no group differences in treatment effects on any of the sexuality variables, including VPA, except for masturbation. This showed a trend towards higher frequency and a significant increase in enjoyment of masturbation in the PT group. There was a trend ($p = 0.06$) towards group differences in mood but, unfortunately, no further details were given of this measure. This study illustrates well the complex effects of exogenous hormone administration, in particular an increase in SHBG in the P and PP groups and a significantly lower level of SHBG in the PT group. Given that the three treatment groups did not differ in their plasma total E2 levels, this demonstrates the likely increase of free E2 as well as T in the PT group.

Davis et al (1995) studied 34 women, two of whom had had their ovaries removed. All had shown intolerance of, or inadequate response to, oral HRT. They were randomly assigned to either E implant or E+T implants, administered three monthly for 2 years. Women with specific complaints of low sexual desire were excluded (it was considered unethical to randomly assign them to E only!). Women in both groups showed significant improvement in sexuality measures, and, for most of the variables, the E+T group improved significantly more than the E group, except that towards the end of the 2-year study period there was a decline in the measures of sexuality. This was attributed to a reduced frequency of implants because of continuing supraphysiological levels of T. This is a potentially interesting phenomenon that, as we will see, recurs in other studies using supraphysiological doses. This study is limited by having no measures of mood or well-being, and behavioural measures only relating to sex.

More recently, Shifren et al (2006) reported a large placebo-controlled trial of T patches (300 μg) in naturally post-menopausal women meeting the DSM IV criteria for HSDD; 273 women received placebo and 276 T. The average age was around 54 years. This showed significant benefits from the T administration. An important difference from earlier studies, apart from the size of the sample, was that, with the patches, plasma levels of free T and bioactive T remained within the physiological range for women. In addition, modest but significant correlations were found between increase in free T and improvements in several aspects of sexual function. These correlations ranged from 0.1 to 0.23 depending on the behavioural measure. Comparable correlations have been reported in some previous studies but usually the sample sizes were not large enough to establish significance.

Surgical menopause

Two studies will be considered closely. (For a more comprehensive review of the earlier literature see Bancroft 2003.) In the first study, Sherwin et al (1985) investigated women who were about to undergo hysterectomy and bilateral ovariectomy. A 1-month baseline assessment preceded the surgery. Post-operatively, women were assigned randomly to one of four treatment groups: E only, T only, oestrogen plus testosterone (E + T), or placebo. These were given in monthly injections for 3 months. All subjects then received 1 month of placebo following which they were crossed over to one of the other three treatment groups. A fifth group of younger women who had undergone hysterectomy only were assessed in the same way as a control for the effects of surgery. The E+T and T only conditions showed significantly higher levels of sexual interest, fantasy and arousal than either the E-only or the placebo conditions. They did not differ in measures of sexual activity with partner, or orgasm. This is the only study in which T administration on its own has been evaluated in ovariectomized women. It is also noteworthy because it focused on the immediate post-operative period in women who were not reporting significant sexual or mood problems pre-operatively.

In a separate paper, Sherwin & Gelfand (1985a) reported that mood was significantly better with all three hormone regimes (T, E+T and E) compared to placebo. The T-only group also had significantly higher hostility scores than the other three groups. In a third paper from this study (Sherwin & Gelfand 1985b), it was reported that energy level, well-being and appetite were significantly higher in the two groups receiving T than in the E-only or placebo groups.

In the second study, Shifren et al (2000) studied women who had undergone hysterectomy and bilateral ovariectomy from 1 to 10 years previously. In contrast to the previous study, all had impaired sexual function and all had been on Premarin, at least 0.625 mg daily for at least 2 months when recruited for the study. All subjects continued on the same dose of oral E through the study. After a 4 weeks' baseline assessment, they were all given daily transdermal patches with placebo (P), 150 μg, or 300 μg of T as the daily dose, each for 12 weeks with the order of presentation randomized. Sexuality was assessed using the Brief Inventory of Sexual Function (BSFIW). There was a substantial placebo response; however, there was significantly more improvement with the higher T dose than with placebo on measures of frequency of sexual activity, and pleasure/orgasm, though not for sexual desire or arousal (the opposite pattern reported by Sherwin et al 1985).

Mood was significantly improved with the higher T dose for ratings of both depression and 'positive well-being'. The transdermal route used in this study has the advantage of producing more physiological and more stable serum T levels than the intramuscular routes used in most other studies, where supraphysiological peaks soon after injection are followed by gradual decline.

Although one has to be cautious making direct comparisons, there appeared to be a more substantial placebo effect reported by Shifren et al (2000), than by Sherwin et al (1985). The placebo response in Shifren et al's study was more marked in the younger women; for those under 48 years there was no difference between placebo and active treatment on any variable; the overall significant effects depended on the older women. The explanation for this age effect is not clear. It may reflect that for younger women loss of sexual interest or enjoyment is more problematic (see p. 246) and hence the expectation of, or need for, improvement is greater. In Sherwin et al's (1985) study, the less striking placebo effect may reflect the fact that women were recruited before they had established any post-operative decline in sexual interest, whereas such decline was an inclusion criterion in the Shifren et al study. This perhaps emphasizes the importance of placebo control in studies where subjects are seeking a therapeutic effect.

Since Shifren et al's (2000) report, there has been a further study of similar size involving European and Australian women (Davis et al 2006), and three large-scale replications in the USA. They have been similar in design, except for use of parallel groups rather than cross over. Braunstein et al (2005) reported on 318 surgically menopausal women, around 8–9 years following ovariectomy, who were assigned to one of three transdermal T dosage groups (150, 300 and 450 µg/day) or placebo. In comparison to the placebo group, women using 300 µg/day reported significantly higher frequency of satisfying sexual activity, as measured by the 'Sexual Activity Log', and increases in sexual desire and arousal, as measured by the PFSF. The effects of the higher, 450 µg dose came midway between placebo and 300 µg, and were not significantly different to either. Broadly similar results, using the same methods of assessment, but comparing only 300 µg/day T to placebo, were reported by Buster et al (2005; $n = 417$) and Simon et al (2005; $n = 519$). A somewhat different profile of specific changes in sexuality were shown in these three studies (sexual interest and arousal) than found by Shifren et al (2000) (pleasure and orgasm), which may reflect the different instruments used (BISFW vs PFSF) and points to a need for consistency as well as validity in the use of outcome measures. Here again, in all these studies the results are presented only as mean change per treatment group. Thus, for example, Buster et al (2005) report their outcome measure, frequency of satisfactory sexual activity, as increasing by a mean of 1.56 episodes per month (also presented as a 51% increase over the baseline frequency), compared with an increase of 0.73 episodes per month for the placebo group. This effectively obscures the proportion of women who showed a therapeutic response. It is conceivable that most women showed a small response, but more likely, given the other evidence reviewed above, that there was a significant minority who showed no response, and others who showed a substantial improvement. There is no way of knowing from these reports. This reflects an interesting commercial and political scenario. First, the FDA has made it clear that frequency of satisfactory sexual activity is the required criterion of efficacy, a questionable position. In addition, the pharmaceutical industry (and in all five of these transdermal T patch studies, Procter & Gamble were involved) dislikes reporting efficacy in terms of those who respond and those who do not. Consequently, they ended up reporting mean levels of change, which the FDA regarded as too modest to warrant licensing, given uncertainties about long-term risks. It is of crucial importance to the field, both from a theoretical and from a clinical perspective, to identify those women who respond to T therapy and establish in what ways they differ from those women who do not respond.

Hormone replacement of adrenal androgens
Androstenedione has a substantial capacity for conversion to both E and T; DHEA can also be converted to E and T, but the extent of this, and its importance for the availability of T in women are, as discussed earlier, disputed. Studies of exogenous DHEA administration have mainly involved women. In a placebo-controlled study of women between 40 and 70 years of age (Morales et al 1994), DHEA was associated with significant improvement in a somewhat crude measure of well-being, but no effect on 'libido'. In a placebo-controlled study of women with adrenal insufficiency, the addition of DHEA to the corticosteroid replacement improved measures of sexual interest and responsiveness as well as mood and general well-being, although the effects on mood were more substantial. The sexual effects could therefore have been secondary to improvements in general well-being and energy. A number of other comparable studies have been reported and the most consistent benefit is to energy and well-being, with less consistent effects on sexuality (for review see Buvat 2003). Increasing attention has been paid to the use of DHEA in the treatment of depression. Schmidt et al (2005) reported a double-blind, placebo-controlled crossover study of DHEA (for 6 weeks) in the treatment of 23 women and 23 men aged 45–65 years presenting with mid-life onset of depression. In comparison to placebo, there was a significant improvement in mood and sexuality in both women and men. Interestingly, there was a 17% increase in free T in the men, and a five-fold increase in the women. Given the assumed greater sensitivity of women to the behavioural effects of T, and the similar response of men and women in this study, these findings are consistent with a direct effect on mood of DHEA rather than T, and with sexual improvements secondary to the mood change. The uncertainty about the role of DHEA continues.

Inborn errors of metabolism
Two conditions, considered in Chapter 3, are of particular relevance to the role of androgens in women's sexuality.

Complete androgen insensitivity syndrome (CAIS)

Six of the 10 women reported by Money & Ehrhardt (1972) rated themselves as having 'an average level of libido', having orgasms most of the time, and being reserved and passive in coitus. Two women rated themselves as above average in libido, always having orgasms, and predominantly initiating sex. The remaining two were still sexually inexperienced. Vague (1983) reported on seven women with complete or 'more or less complete' testicular feminization (androgen insensitivity) syndrome, who were asked detailed questions about their sexual experiences. All showed normal labial response and vaginal lubrication during sexual stimulation. However, five had a small 'atrophic' clitoris, apparently unresponsive sexually, whereas the other two had a normal-sized and responsive clitoris. All women experienced orgasm; however, this lacked the involuntary spasm component. Vague (1983) made the interesting suggestion that the main part of the sexual response in these women was E dependent and as found in normal women, but the clitoral component may be T dependent and hence lacking. The apparent difference in orgasmic experience was not interpreted. Wisniewski et al (2000), in a study of 14 women with CAIS, reported that 11 women were satisfied with their genitalia in terms of sexual functioning, whereas 3 were dissatisfied. Ten women were satisfied with their sexual function overall, and four women were dissatisfied. Ten women reported libido of 'average strength or stronger', and 10 women reported an ability to experience orgasm.

In a recent study of women with CAIS (Minto et al 2003), 59 completed the Golombok-Rust Inventory of Sexual Satisfaction (GRISS; Rust & Golombok 1986). This instrument yields one global score for sexual function, and seven subscales: sexual frequency, communication about sex, dissatisfaction, avoidance, sensuality, vaginal penetration problems and orgasm. Only 13% of the women indicated dissatisfaction, a subscale that covers time spent on foreplay and on intercourse, general satisfaction with the sexual relationship, and lack of love and affection. However, 90% of the women had one or more of the other subscale scores in the problem range: infrequency 66%, vaginal penetration difficulties 58%, noncommunication 51%, avoidance 49% and orgasm difficulty 34%.

In my unpublished study of 15 women with CAIS (see Chapter 3, p. 47) all subjects were clearly sexually attracted to men. One woman (subject L; aged 21) gave a very restricted account of her sexual experiences, probably because her mother was in and out of the room during the interview. She will not be considered further in this section. Eleven women recalled their age when first attracted to males; these ages ranged from 8 to 22, with an average age of 14.3 years. Ten women recalled their age when first aware of sexual arousal; this ranged from 9 to 18, with an average of 13.6 years. One woman (age 19) had experienced only one attempt at vaginal intercourse, which was difficult because of her small vagina, though not painful. She had avoided sexual contact since that experience. Of the remaining 12 women, 9 had experienced no difficulty or pain initially, and except

for 1, who occasionally experienced slight pain, they continued without any problems. Three women had difficulty and pain initially: in two, this disappeared with continued sexual activity; the remaining woman experienced recurrent cystitis associated with sexual intercourse, which continued intermittently for several years until she started E replacement, when the problem ceased. Seven women reported no difficulty with vaginal lubrication, which did not seem to be dependent on E replacement. Of the remainder, one described her vaginal response as slow, but present; one said she did lubricate but preferred to use jelly; one said she usually lubricated sufficiently but was occasionally dry; one woman tended to be dry and used jelly; and one woman had lubrication problems unless she was taking HRT.

All of the women who were or had been sexually active with a partner, or who masturbated, were orgasmic on occasions; in two, this was most of the time; in five, around 50% of the time; and in the remainder, less frequently. Two women commented that they needed clitoral stimulation for orgasm, and for one, this had been a problem because of her difficulty in asking her partner to stimulate her appropriately. Seven women said they initiated sexual activity some of the time, four said rarely and one, most of the time. Asked whether they preferred to be passive during lovemaking and simply receive caresses and stimulation from their partner, two said most of the time; three, some of the time; and six, rarely.

Seven women had never masturbated. Of the remainder, one did when she was a teenager but then stopped (because of guilt); the others did so when not in a relationship, except for one who masturbated whether or not she had a sexual partner.

The reported level of spontaneous sexual interest varied considerably. In four women it was low (less than once a week), in five it was moderate (at least once a week) and in four it was high (alternate days or more often). Each woman was asked whether she would become sexually excited while fantasizing about sexual activity: six women said 'never', six 'sometimes' and one 'often'. Asked whether this would happen when reading sexual episodes in books, four said 'never', six 'sometimes' and three 'often'. And in response to sexual scenes in films or on television, six said 'never', six said 'sometimes' and one said 'often'.

Apart from an increased likelihood of experiencing difficulties with a small or tight vagina early in their first sexual relationship, this small sample presents a varied picture of female sexuality that is not clearly different from what one would expect in a 'normal' sample of similar age, although possibly shifted towards the less responsive end of the range.

As far as sexual development is concerned, these findings are compatible with those from other studies, given that there does seem to be considerable variability in CAIS women, as there is in women in general. But that raises the key question of what role androgens play in female sexuality. One possibility is that relevant androgen effects in the female brain are dependent on aromatization to oestradiol (see p. 124), in which case women with CAIS would not differ. Another possibility is that certain aspects of sexuality in women are not androgen-dependent. If that is the case, which aspects are they? Level of sexual interest, while it has not been carefully assessed in most of the above studies, nevertheless shows variability, indicating that at least some women with CAIS have high levels, which are presumably not dependent on androgens. Vague (1983) suggested a distinction between an E-dependent component of female sexuality and an androgen-dependent component.

A further explanation is that women with CAIS vary in the precise genetic anomaly involved, and perhaps in some cases the androgen insensitivity is more relevant to the masculinization of the external genitalia than to the brain. CAIS remains a fascinating 'experiment of nature', which deserves continuing research attention.

Congenital adrenal hyperplasia (CAH)

The effect of CAH on the sexuality of women is also of considerable theoretical interest as well as clinical importance, because of the increased levels of androgens involved. The best evidence in this respect comes from the study by Meyer-Bahlburg et al (2003) considered in Chapter 3 (see p. 50). Romantic involvement was lower in the 'salt-wasting' (SW) group than the other three groups. Fewer SW women had experienced heterosexual love, and those who had, experienced it later in their life. The SW group was more likely to show sexual orientation in the bi-homosexual direction and were less likely to have had experience of heterosexual intercourse (61% vs 90% of the remainder), and those who had reported fewer sexual experiences. The level of sexual drive was significantly lower in the SW group compared to each of the other three groups, which did not differ from each other. Meyer-Bahlburg et al (2003) comment that 'the prenatal and postnatal hormonal milieu, genital surgeries and resulting genital status are all likely contributors to this outcome' (p. 231). Clitoral surgery had been carried out in 26 of the 28 women with SW CAH, in six of the nine women with SV CAH, but none of the non-classical (NC or later-onset) group. On the other hand, women in the SW group were much less likely to regard their vaginal width as adequate (32% compared with 78% of SV and 83% of NC groups). Concerns about their genitalia or loss of clitoral sensitivity may therefore be responsible to some extent. There is, however, an interesting comparison to be made with women with CAH who had not been treated until late childhood or adulthood. Ehrhardt et al (1968) reported on 23 such women, who had started treatment from 8 years 6 months, to 47 years of age, with a median of 18 years. The fact that they were late-treated would suggest that they had the SV form of CAH, as the SW form, untreated, is likely to be fatal. However, these women described themselves as relatively sexual. Eleven women rated their sexual drive as higher than other women, eight thought they were average and only one felt she was below average in this respect. This was based on their assessment of sexual interest while on cortisone treatment. Most of the women said that their sexual drive had been somewhat higher before treatment, in some cases to a troublesome extent. Yet most of these women had undergone clitoral and vaginal surgery and had other stigmata of the condition, including short stature. We do not know what their androgen levels were once treatment was established, and it is possible that, while reduced compared to pretreatment, they may still have been relatively high because of a degree of hyperplasia of the adrenal cortex. DHEA and DHEAS production becomes relatively dissociated from corticosteroid production as we get older. It would be of interest to compare the androgen levels of late- and early-treated women with CAH. Is it possible that early pre-natal exposure to high levels of androgens in women with CAH results in a degree of desensitization of the brain to the effects of androgens? Consequently, when they reach adulthood and experience levels of T in the normal range for women, these levels are insufficient to produce normal androgen effects.

Summary of androgen effects in women

Overall, we have an inconsistent picture of the role of androgens in women's sexuality, but with enough pieces of positive evidence to necessitate taking this role seriously. In the studies relating endogenous androgens to sexuality we find inconsistent evidence. One possible explanation is that there is a 'threshold effect' as in men (see p. 127), with the threshold in the lower part of the physiological range (and hence much lower than the male threshold). Limited support for this is considered in Chapter 15 in relation to the effects of oral contraceptives on androgen levels (see p. 451). As with men, we may be failing to find correlations between plasma androgen levels and sexuality measures because for most women their levels of androgens are above the critical threshold. It would be valuable to have comparable evidence from women following ovariectomy; do those women who do not have adverse effects show higher levels of plasma androgens? If the 'threshold' concept proves to be valid it will require a fundamental rethinking of the role of androgens in women.

However, the most substantial evidence of an impact of androgens on women's sexuality comes from studies of administration of exogenous androgens. Here much of the evidence results from induction of supraphysiological levels of androgens. What does this mean? And is it reconcilable with a 'threshold' at levels low in the normal physiological range? This raises the question of whether supraphysiological levels of androgens are influencing sexuality indirectly, in ways that would not be relevant to physiological androgen effects. The possibility that such non-physiological effects may be secondary to pharmacological effects on mood and vitality has been raised. It is particularly important that future research in this area looks carefully at the relationship between mood change and change in sexuality. In very few studies to date has this been looked at, even though in several cases results have been published on mood effects and sexual effects from the same women, but in separate papers.

The confounding effects of psychological reactions to sexual difficulties serving to obscure subtle hormone behaviour relationships has also been raised, and needs to be taken seriously in future research. The substantial placebo effect observed in studies of women seeking help for sexual difficulties underlines this point. The crucial question of whether sexual effects of androgens depend on conversion to oestradiol will be considered further below.

The uncertainties about the role of androgens in women's sexuality remain. An attempt to provide an explanation will be made in the final section of this chapter.

Oestrogens

Oestrogens and female sexuality

There is long-standing and consistent evidence of the importance of E for normal vaginal lubrication, with post-menopausal decline in E commonly resulting in vaginal dryness. However, whether E has a direct effect on sexual interest and arousability has been less certain. In a recent review of the literature, Dennerstein et al (2003) concluded that there is a dramatic decline in sexual functioning with the natural menopausal transition, with changes in most aspects of sexual function correlating with levels of oestradiol but not androgens.

A number of studies of the symptoms of either natural or surgical menopause, reviewed above, have either taken women on E replacement, who continue to have loss of sexual interest or response, and evaluated the effect of adding T, or have compared E replacement with a combination of E and T, or T alone. Much less attention has focused on the effects of E itself on sexual interest and arousal in post-menopausal women.

Dennerstein et al (1980) studied 49 surgically menopausal women, all of whom had stable, satisfying sexual relationships, using a double-blind crossover design in which they spent 3 months on each of four treatments: ethinylestradiol (EE), l-norgestrel, combination of EE and l-norgestrel, and placebo. The EE only regime was significantly better than the others in improving sexual interest, enjoyment, orgasmic frequency and mood. Also found were correlations between measures of sexual desire and of mood, particularly 'feelings of well-being'.

Nathorst-Böös et al (1993b) compared transdermal E (Estraderm 50 μg/24 h) with placebo in 242 naturally menopausal women seeking treatment for menopausal symptoms who had not previously received hormone replacement. After 12 weeks, in comparison with the placebo group, the E group reported significantly more sexual fantasies, better lubrication, less coital pain and more sexual enjoyment.

Only one study of hormone replacement has incorporated different doses of E. Sherwin (1991) randomly assigned 'perimenopausal' women to four treatment regimes, involving either a low (0.625 mg) or high (1.25 mg) dose of Premarin for 25 days out of each month, and either Provera (5 mg) or placebo for days 15–25 of each month. Each woman took the assigned regime for 12 months and was assessed with daily ratings during the 3rd, 6th, 9th and 12th months. The main purpose of the study was to evaluate the effects of the progestagen on mood and sexuality and to assess whether the dose of E would modify any mood effect. Results showed that the progestagen had a negative effect on mood, but not on sexuality. The mood effect was attenuated by the higher E dose. However, it is the comparison of the low and high E dose (combined with placebo), which is of most relevance here. Apparent from the graphed sexual interest data (Figure 3, Sherwin 1991), women in the high E+ placebo group had substantially lower levels of sexual interest during the pre-treatment month than the low E+ placebo group, yet by the 6th month of treatment, and continuing through the 12th month, were showing noticeably higher levels of sexual interest. The results were analyzed using a four groups × five time periods ANOVA, so the implicit assumption is that the comparison of the two E groups was not significant. But this was not commented on in the paper.

The need to establish with more certainty the role of E in women's sexuality is reinforced by uncertainties about the ways the T effects, reviewed above, are mediated. Wallen has strongly advocated that the sexual effects of T in women result from the consequent increase in free E, supporting this conclusion with experimental data from Rhesus monkeys (Wallen & Parsons 1998).

Oestrogens and male sexuality

The effects of E on the sexuality of the human male confronts us with another paradox. There is substantial evidence that administration of exogenous E has a negative effect on men's sexuality. In the past, E was used as a treatment for prostatic carcinoma, based on its assumed antiandrogenic effect, and reduction of sexual interest and response was a typical side effect. Oestrogens have also been used as a treatment of male sexual offenders. Bancroft et al (1974) compared the effects of EE and CPA, an antiandrogen, in 12 incarcerated sexual offenders. Both compounds reduced sexual interest, masturbatory activity and erectile response to erotic fantasies and slides, producing a pattern very similar to that found in hypogonadal men. However, although CPA substantially reduced total T, with no change in SHBG, EE substantially increased both total T and SHBG (Murray et al 1975).

As we shall see in the following section, there is considerable evidence of conversion of T to E in the male brain, hence the paradox.

Mode of action of androgens and oestrogens in the brain

The conventional view is that androgens act in the brain via genomic effects (Rommerts 1990). It has been known for some time, however, that E and progesterone can, in addition, have much more rapid effects directly on the cell membrane (Dufy & Vincent 1980), with E activation having an excitatory and progesterone activation an inhibitory effect. As yet we have little directly relevant data on the speed of action of androgens in the human, although one study in women, discussed earlier (Tuiten et al 2000), showed an effect on genital response within 3–4 h, and limited data from men, considered above, indicate an effect within 2–3 days. Caldwell (2002) has proposed a model of steroid-influenced sexual arousability, which depends on membrane-associated receptors linked to a more enduring change in G-protein coupling. However, the evidence he cites is largely restricted to E and progesterone. It remains a possibility that androgens may produce a relatively rapid membrane-mediated effect by means of aromatization. On the other hand, if T does not have similar rapid membrane activating effects to E, yet is converted to E intracellularly, may there be some advantages in using T for inducing genomic E effects? Is this relevant, for example, to hormone replacement in ovariectomized women, who might need substantial increase in genomic E effects in the brain, but would not benefit from the increased membrane activation (e.g. excitation) that could result from substantial increases in E dosage?

Brain receptors for gonadal steroids

The current evidence indicates one type of AR in the brain activated by either T or DHT. Recent research in mice has shown two E receptors, ERα and ERβ. Development of 'knockout' (KO) mice that are deficient in specific gene functions has given some indication of the functions of these two receptors (reviewed by Simpson & Davis 2006). ERα KO male mice have slightly impaired sexual behaviour but, more strikingly, are unable to ejaculate and are infertile. ERβ KO male mice show little impairment. However, ERα and -β KO male mice (i.e. lacking both ERs) show major disruption of sexual behaviour, with no mounts, intromissions or ejaculations. This has been taken to mean that the two ERs can substitute for each other, but at least one has to be present for normal male sexual behaviour. A similar pattern is found in mice lacking the aromatase gene (ArKO) responsible for aromatization of T to E. Taken together, these findings suggest activation of E receptors is necessary for normal male sexual behaviour, at least in mice. The relevance of the E receptors to female sexuality remains obscure, though likely to be important.

In the human we have very little comparable data. E appears to play a key role in the negative feedback control of T. In long-term castrated male rhesus monkeys, physiological doses of T do not reduce LH unless a small amount of E is also given (Resko et al 1977). Grumbach & Auchus (1999) reviewed the evidence from a rare condition of aromatase deficiency in humans, most of them female. The very low E levels found in such cases, and the consequent high levels of LH, FSH and T, have substantial effects on the sexual differentiation of females, resulting in a degree of genital masculinization and a tendency for polycystic ovaries in adults. In both males and females with this condition, there are substantial effects on bone growth, pointing to the importance of E in normal bone development, but no evidence of abnormalities of psychosexual development. However, the evidence presented was limited to gender identity and sexual orientation. We do not know what impact this rare condition has on sexual arousability, and this limited evidence, while of considerable interest, does not allow firm conclusions about the relative importance of T and E to human sexuality. Grumbach & Auchus (1999) advised restraint in extrapolating from animal evidence to humans in this respect.

We are nevertheless left with the fact that conversion of T to E is evident in brains of men and women. What does this mean? One approach to whether the effects of T are dependent on aromatization to E is to explore the effects of aromatase inhibitors in humans. Gooren (1985) found that, in eugonadal men, the E receptor antagonist, tamoxifen, and the aromatase inhibitor, testolactone, had no adverse sexual effects and that dihydrotestosterone (DHT), which cannot be aromatized to E, was as effective as T in maintaining sexuality in hypogonadal men. He took this to mean that the sexual effects of T within the human male CNS are mediated by DHT but not by E. In a more recent study, Davis et al (2006b) used the opportunity of treating post-menopausal women with low sexual desire with transdermal T to assess the effect of adding letrozole, an aromatase inhibitor, in comparison with placebo. Using the Sabbatsberg Sexual Self-Rating Scale, which assesses seven domains of sexual experience, they found significantly lower scores with the letrozole in only one of the domains, 'sexual activity'. They attributed this to chance. Shifren (2006), who had earlier shown substantial placebo effects in a treatment study of this kind (Shifren et al 2000), commented, in an editorial on this paper, that lack of a placebo control for the T was a potential problem. An effect of the aromatase inhibitor may have been obscured by a placebo effect. This study, with a placebo control, would be worth repeating. But so far we have no direct evidence that blocking the conversion of T to E has a negative impact on the hormonal control of sexual behaviour in either men or women.

Localization of androgen receptors in the brain

Research on the site of action of T in the non-human primate brain has been ongoing for more than 30 years, during which time there have been major changes in the technologies used, and these have to be kept in mind when comparing findings across studies.

Michael et al (1989), using autoradiography in male rhesus monkeys, looked at aspects of both androgenic and oestrogenic activity. They found 5α-reductase activity to be fairly evenly distributed in the brain, whereas, in contrast, aromatase activity was much more localized. They assumed that in areas of high aromatase activity, T was acting by conversion to E. By identifying brain areas where there was overlap in androgen- and E-concentrating neurons, they concluded that the medial preoptic and ventromedial hypothalamic nuclei, the BNST, and the cortical, medial and accessory amygdaloid nuclei were the main sites at which the effects of T are mediated, predominantly by E. In contrast, T activity was thought to be mediated by ARs in the lateral septal, premamillary and intercalated mamillary nuclei.

Roselli et al (2001) used in situ hybridization histochemistry to locate cytochrome P450 aromatase mRNA ($P450_{AROM}$) and androgen receptor RNA (AR mRNA) in the hypothalamus and amygdala of cynomolgus monkeys. Their findings were broadly similar to those of Michael et al (1989). They concluded that T acts through signalling pathways that differ either in specific brain areas or within different cells from the same area.

Abdelgadir et al (1999) studied the distribution of AR mRNA, using a ribonuclease protection assay, in male rhesus monkeys. Their localization of the ARmRNA was again broadly similar to the distribution of androgen activity reported by Michael et al (1989). In this study, intact animals were compared with castrated animals, with and without T replacement. They found little difference between these three groups in the distribution or concentration of ARmRNA and concluded that in the monkey brain this AR is not regulated at the transcriptional level by androgen.

The limited evidence of AR distribution in humans includes two studies of the temporal cortex, both of which found substantial amounts of AR protein (Sarrieau et al 1990; Puy et al 1995). Both studies involved male temporal cortex tissue because it was available from surgical interventions in men with intractable epilepsy, not because the temporal cortex was regarded as a particularly likely site for ARs.

So far, for both non-human primates and humans, the majority of evidence is from males. However, Finley & Kritzer (1999), reporting the presence of AR protein in the prefrontal cortex of rhesus monkeys, found no differences between their male and female monkeys in this respect. Fernandez-Guasti et al (2000) used immunochemical methods to examine the distribution of ARs in the human hypothalamus, involving post-mortem samples from five men and five women. In men, intense AR immunoreactivity (AR-ir) was found in neurons of the horizontal limb of the diagonal band of Broca, and of the lateral mamillary (LMN) and medial mamillary (MMN) nuclei. Intermediate staining was found in other parts of the diagonal band of Broca, the SDN of the POA, paraventricular, suprachiasmatic, ventromedial and infundibular nuclei. Weaker staining was found in the BNST, MPOA, dorsal and ventral zones of the periventricular nucleus, supraoptic nucleus and nucleus basalis of Meynert. In most areas, women revealed less staining of receptor protein. This gender difference was particularly marked in the lateral and medial mammillary nuclei. There was also staining in the paraventricular and supraoptic nuclei in the males, which was apparently absent in the females. Overall, there was greater individual variability in the intensity of receptor staining in the women than in the men.

Bixo et al (1995) measured the concentration of E and T in 17 brain areas as well as in the general circulation in post-mortem samples from six pre-menopausal and five post-menopausal women. There were variations in the concentrations of both steroids across the various brain areas, with highest levels of T and E found in the hypothalamus, POA and substantia nigra. They found that E levels were significantly higher in the brains of pre-menopausal women, reflecting their higher serum levels. This points to the relevance of circulating levels.

As yet, there are no comparative data on the distribution of aromatase activity in women or female primates, though in the rat, greater amounts of aromatase activity are found in the male than the female, in all areas examined except the medial preoptic nucleus (Roselli & Resko 1993). Furthermore, Roselli & Klosterman (1998) concluded from their findings that this male pattern of aromatization is established perinatally and probably forms a fundamental component of masculinization.

While much of the reported localization is consistent with androgenic effects on sexual and reproductive behaviour, it is important to keep in mind that much of the research has been restricted to the hypothalamus, and where more extensive studies have been done, ARs appear to be widespread in the primate and human brain, including various cortical areas (e.g. prefrontal cortex, Finley & Kritzer 1999; temporal cortex, Sarrieau et al 1990; Puy et al 1995). What specific role androgens have in these areas is not yet clear, but in addition to more specifically reproductive actions, other relatively non-specific androgen-mediated brain functions need to be considered, including activation or general arousal as well as stimulation of neuronal growth and gender differentiation of brain function (Kelly 1991).

Brain imaging

Functional brain imaging has considerable potential for studying gonadal steroidal activity in the brain. So far, only two studies provide evidence of direct relevance. Park et al (2001) reported on two hypogonadal men, assessed with functional MRI in their response to sexual stimuli, with and without T replacement. In both men, activation of the inferior frontal lobe, cingulate gyrus, insula and corpus callosum was greater with T replacement. Redoute et al (2005) compared PET scan evidence of brain activity during response to sexual stimuli in nine hypogonadal men with and without T replacement, and eight eugonadal men. They found greater activation in the controls and the treated hypogonadal men than the untreated, in the right orbitofrontal cortex, insula and claustrum. They also found deactivation of the left inferior frontal gyrus, suggestive of reduced inhibition of sexual arousal, but only in the controls and treated patients. There is some consistency across these two studies, and ARs have been reported in the orbitofrontal cortex of primates (Finley & Kritzer 1999) and to a limited extent, in the cingulate cortex (Abdelgadir et al 1999). As yet, however, there is no evidence of ARs in the insula or claustrum of primates or humans.

At the time of writing we can reasonably conclude that both T and E are involved in brain activity, probably including that mediating sexual response and behaviour. Although there is less evidence for females, this would appear to be the case for both males and females. However, we are left with more questions than answers.

Comparison of gonadal steroid effects in men and women

Oestrogens

1. While E in the male may play a fundamental role in the mechanisms underlying sexuality in the brain, this may be restricted to E produced intracellularly from conversion of androgens. The impact of exogenous E on male sexuality suggests that circulating E activates negative mechanisms (e.g. reduction of T levels by enhanced negative feedback). In the female, E probably plays a fundamental role in various aspects of a woman's sexuality, as reflected in the decline of circulating E following menopause, and the sexual benefits of exogenous E for post-menopausal women. A clear benefit of E administration to the post-menopausal woman is improved vaginal lubrication. To what extent the more general improvements in sexual function and enjoyment associated with E replacement are secondary to the specific effect on vaginal lubrication, or involve direct effects in the brain, remains uncertain. If the latter is the case, then the extent to which positive consequences depend on the cell membrane excitatory effects of extracellular E or on intracellular genomic effects remains unclear.

Androgens

2. In the male, the evidence points to a threshold, below or at the lower level of the normal physiological range, above which increased T levels have only subtle behavioural effects, and below which signs of androgen deficiency, with reduced sexual desire and sexual arousability, are likely to occur. The fact that normal levels are clearly well above this threshold in men suggests that other, probably peripheral actions of androgens are required for other aspects of health.

3. Women have circulating levels of T on average around a tenth of those found in men. Their adrenal androgens levels are more similar. Whether there is a threshold for the normal effects of T on women's sexuality is uncertain. The evidence from the effects of steroidal contraceptives is consistent with that possibility (see Chapter 15, p. 451). In general, however, women, while responding to levels of T that would be well below the threshold for men, appear to be much more variable in their responsiveness. Thus some women can experience substantial reductions in T without obvious adverse sexual or mood effects. Other women are affected by such reductions. A major problem in this field is the difficulty in accurately measuring T at the lower end of the female physiological range. It remains possible that all women would experience adverse sexual effects if their T level was reduced sufficiently, the critical level depending on a particular woman's sensitivity. But if that is the case, this indicates a responsiveness to very low levels of T in even more striking contrast to the male.

4. The most convincing behavioural effects of T on women's sexuality have resulted from the administration of exogenous androgens. In most such studies, this has involved supraphysiological levels of T, and in a number of studies sensitivity to these levels appears to decrease over time. The apparent paradox of a possible threshold at very low levels and pharmacological effects at supraphysiological levels, could be explained by two different types of T effect (e.g. a direct androgenic effect around the threshold and an oestrogenic effect dependent on conversion of T to E at higher levels of T).

5. Considerable uncertainty remains about the role of DHEA. DHEA-S, which is generally regarded as a storage form of DHEA, is present in very large amounts in the blood, in comparison with any other steroid. The extent to which DHEA is a supply of T intracellularly is a matter of dispute. It is possible that DHEA is more important for the sexuality of women, and if that is the case, then women may require much more T than is apparent from their circulating levels, depending on intracellular or 'intracrine' conversion of DHEA. Once again we have more questions than answers.

6. The likelihood remains, however, that men are much less sensitive to the behavioural effects of T than are women. A 'desensitization hypothesis' has been proposed to account for this (Bancroft 2002), which postulates that, as men need more T to achieve and maintain peripheral masculinization, desensitization of the brain to the behavioural effects of T occurs during early development in the male (prenatally and during the post-natal T surge). This effectively reduces the manifestations of genetically determined variations in T responsiveness, which remain more manifest in women at lower levels of T. This hypothesis is testable in various ways (see Bancroft 2003 for further discussion). Evidence of possible desensitizing effects of high T levels in early development in women with congenital adrenal hyperplasia has been considered (p. 123). The finding, in several studies inducing supraphysiological levels of T in hormone replacement of post-menopausal women, that symptoms return at increasingly high plasma levels of T is an example of desensitization. The fact that this occurs in women relatively late in life suggests that such desensitization is not restricted to a critical developmental period. In the absence of such desensitization, the hypothesis predicts that women are not only sensitive to much lower amounts of T than are men but also show considerable interindividual variability in their responsiveness to T, probably genetically determined. If valid, this could account for much of the confusion in the literature on androgens and sexuality in women. The main approach to exploring and testing this hypothesis is to look for markers of T sensitivity among women. Such markers would then enable us to predict which women would experience negative effects from androgen reduction (e.g. following ovariectomy or oral contraceptive use) and which

women are most likely to benefit from exogenous T administration. This hypothesis also carries substantial clinical implications for the use of exogenous T in women. If, as appears to be the case, supraphysiological doses of T result in desensitization or habituation, this may prove to be irreversible, hence requiring the continuation of much higher levels of T to maintain the behavioural benefits. The consequences in terms of other, unwanted androgenic effects, together with the implications of aromatization of the high T levels to E, need to be appraised. Clearly it is important to establish whether exogenous T administration should produce plasma levels within the physiological range.

7. A key factor to keep in mind is that androgens and E can influence mood and vitality and that deficiencies in either can be associated with low mood and low vitality. There is increasing evidence, particularly in women (e.g. Bancroft et al 2003d), that normal sexuality depends on 'normal' mood and energy. Hence, effects of gonadal steroids on sexuality could, in some circumstances, be mediated via direct effects on mood and well-being. This emphasizes the importance of looking at both mood and sexuality in hormone behaviour studies and, in particular, examining their relationships with each other. As suggested earlier, there may be two types of effect of exogenous T administration, a direct physiological T effect on sexuality, which would require reinstatement of the appropriate threshold level, and a pharmacological effect, which may result from the increased levels of E and which may be most evident in its effect of mood, energy and well-being.

Peptides

The varied roles of peptides were considered in Chapter 3 (p. 21). In this chapter attention will be restricted to OT, β-endorphin, PRL and melanocortin as representatives of the main types of peptides relevant to sexual arousal.

Oxytocin

It is generally accepted that oxytocin (OT) plays a key role during lactation, facilitating the milk ejection reflex. It may also play a role in facilitating uterine contraction during parturition. For such purposes, OT is produced in the magnocellular neurons of the PVN of the hypothalamus, which project axons into the posterior pituitary and thence into the peripheral circulation (Kupfermann 1991). OT has also been proposed as a key factor in affiliative behaviour or pair bonding (Insel 1992). The evidence for OT being important in sexual arousal, response and behaviour is, however, less consistent. In animal studies, centrally administered OT has induced erection, an effect apparently T dependent, and OT receptor antagonists can prevent non-contact erections, considered an index of sexual arousal (Argiolas 1999). Dopamine agonists may enhance sexual response by increasing central oxytocinergic transmission (Argiolas 1999). In female rats,

studies with OT antagonists indicate that OT facilitates lordosis, an effect apparently dependent on progesterone priming. Less striking effects on proceptive female behaviour (hopping and darting) were also reported. There was also an increase in vocalizations when mounted, consistent with the tactile stimulation leading to lordosis and mounting becoming aversive (Insel 1992). This may be related to the effects of VCS, which has been shown to induce analgesia in rats and in women (see p. 83). Komisaruk & Sansone (2003) have proposed that this analgesic mechanism, which may have a fundamental role in reproduction by making mounting and intromission less noxious for the female, in part involves OT. They also present evidence that VCS results in a release of OT from PVN neurons, which project to the brain stem and spinal cord, activating the sympathetic division of the autonomic nervous system in the process.

Cantor et al (1999) examined the interaction of OT and serotonin. Having demonstrated that fluoxetine, a selective SSRI, impaired ejaculation in male rats and also reduced appetitive behaviours (level changing), they found that OT administration reversed the effect of fluoxetine on ejaculation but not on appetitive behaviour. The authors concluded that serotonin suppresses ejaculation by interrupting the action of OT. They suggested that the effects of OT administration could have been mediated by a central stimulation of sympathetic outflow, or peripherally by facilitating smooth muscle contraction in the reproductive tract.

There is evidence from rat studies that OT facilitates PRL release (e.g. Egli et al 2004), and this will be considered further in the section on PRL.

Thus, so far, the animal evidence is consistent with both a peripheral and central role for OT, the most obvious peripheral effect being facilitation of smooth muscle relaxation and the central role being more as a neuromodulator in a variety of response systems. Both peripheral and central mechanisms, however, appear to be steroid hormone dependent. The enhancement of erections is unlikely to result from the peripheral effects of OT, given that these most obviously facilitate muscle contraction (necessary for ejaculation) whereas erection is dependent on muscle relaxation. However, whereas the central role of OT in lactation remains unchallenged, its fundamental role in sexual behaviour is questioned by the effects of OT gene ablation studies. OT KO mice show clear impairment of milk let-down, but no apparent impairment of either mating or parturition (Nishimori et al 1996; Young et al 1996).

What evidence do we have for humans? Carmichael et al (1987) found that plasma OT increased around the time of orgasm in men and women, remaining raised for at least 5 min after orgasm. The authors postulated that OT has a facilitatory role on sperm and egg transport by increasing smooth muscle contractility in the reproductive tracts. In a recent study of men, OT increased in some subjects following ejaculation, but the individual variability was such that the group effect was not significant (Krüger et al 2003a). Murphy et al (1987) reported an increase in OT in men during sexual arousal, which persisted beyond ejaculation, but with no obvious increase at ejaculation. In a study of women, Blaicher et al (1999) found an increase in OT 1 min after orgasm, but levels were close to baseline by 5 min post orgasm.

It is difficult to draw clear conclusions from this literature on OT and sexual arousal. Whether the increase of OT around orgasm, which has been somewhat inconsistently observed in the human literature, has any specific function, rather than being an epiphenomenon of other changes, remains uncertain. It is possible that this OT rise will affect the experience of orgasm by influencing uterine and other reproductive tract smooth musculature. The possibility that a peri-orgasmic increase in OT contributes to the post-orgasmic refractory period, at least in males, should also be considered. Caldwell (2002) has proposed that OT is a satiety hormone that acts by decoupling the G-protein (see p. 125) and hence reducing sexual arousability. The reader is entitled to feel confused.

The role of OT in pair-bonding or affiliation, while of apparent relevance in some species studied (Carter 1998), is of less certain relevance in the human, given its complex role as a central neuromodulator. This has not, however, stopped some from identifying it as 'the love hormone'.

β-Endorphin

There has been, for many years, widespread awareness of the negative effects of exogenous opiates such as morphine and heroin on the sexuality of male and female drug addicts, reducing sexual interest, impairing genital response and blocking ejaculation and orgasm, with active and spontaneous reversal of such effects often occurring during opiate withdrawal (see Pfaus & Gorzalka 1987 for review). In general, the subsequent animal research has shown similar negative effects of both exogenous and endogenous opiate administration, in male and female animals, with confirmatory evidence from blocking such effects with opiate antagonists such as naloxone, as well as withdrawal effects comparable to those in humans. The picture is complicated by the fact that opiates inhibit LHRH, and hence reduce LH and T. However, the animal evidence shows that the sexually inhibiting effects are predominantly independent of this reduction of T.

β-Endorphin is the endogenous opiate that has received the most research attention. Apart from the anterior pituitary, the synthesis of β-endorphin is limited to two cell groups in the brain, one in the arcuate nucleus of the hypothalamus and the other in the nucleus of the solitary tract in the brainstem. The relevant neurons in the arcuate nucleus project anteriorly to other parts of the hypothalamus, including the MPOA, and also to the amygdala. Dorsally, neurons run to the PVN of the hypothalamus and then on to the brainstem to structures involved in the autonomic nervous system (Herbert 1995). The sexual inhibiting effects of β-endorphin, and related opiate peptides, are believed to occur mainly through their action on the MPOA and the amygdala, the precise inhibiting effect depending on the site of infusion. Thus β-endorphin infused into the MPOA inhibits consummatory mounting and intromission, providing that mounting has not already started with a particular female; in other words, inhibition is of the activation of the consummatory sequence rather than its completion. On the other hand, infusion of β-endorphin into the medial amygdala inhibits the initial appetitive phase (Herbert 1995). According to Argiolas (1999) the inhibitory effect is dose-dependent, with low doses of opiate having facilitatory and high doses inhibitory effects. β-Endorphin may facilitate appetitive behaviour by acting on the VTA to activate the mesolimbic DA system. This raises a crucial question, at least about exogenous opiates, which remains largely unanswered. Exogenous opiates can induce an intense feeling of pleasure, which has been likened to an orgasm, followed by a state of relaxation and calm. What are the mechanisms underlying this? This was considered earlier, in the section on orgasm (see p. 89).

Prolactin

Prolactin (PRL) is secreted by the anterior pituitary into the general circulation, with a diurnal episodic pattern, maximal during sleep. Like OT, it is a peptide hormone with one very clearly established physiological and classically hormonal function: promotion of lactation. There are less well understood, but possibly important effects on ovarian function, in particular maintaining corpus luteum production of progesterone in the early stages of pregnancy until the placenta takes over. With PRL receptors being found in most parts of the body, PRL has been reported as having more than 300 functions across vertebrates, a substantial majority of which relate to reproduction. However, in homozygous PRL receptor KO mice, the female is infertile, lactation is to some extent impaired, the male shows delayed fertility in a minority of animals but other aspects of male and female reproductive behaviour are apparently unaffected (Bole-Feysot et al 1998). Consistent with its reproductive function, plasma PRL levels remain low in the female rat except for a prominent surge during proestrus, which accompanies the LH surge. Also PRL levels remain raised during the first 10 days of pregnancy (Freeman et al 2000).

In the human, low sexual desire is a common symptom of hyperprolactinaemia often associated, in men, with erectile problems (Franks & Jacobs 1983). Although hyperprolactinaemia is also commonly associated with T deficiency in men, and ovarian dysfunction in women, impaired sexual desire can occur in hyperprolactinaemia without obvious gonadal steroid deficiency. This has focused attention on possible negative sexual effects of PRL, and these were discussed earlier.

Studies of PRL and sexual arousal in response to erotic stimuli, not involving direct tactile stimulation or orgasm, have been few, restricted to men and have shown inconsistent results. Rowland et al (1987) reported some increase in PRL while watching erotic videos; Carani et al (1990) found no increase. In contrast, in a recent series of studies in which masturbation or sexual activity with a partner led to orgasm or ejaculation, a clear increase in PRL was observed following orgasm in both men (Krüger et al 1998, 2003a,b) and women (Exton et al 1999), with levels still raised after 60 min (Fig. 4.8). This pattern was not found in a parallel study of men who masturbated without ejaculating (Krüger et al 2003a,b). These findings were considered in the section on orgasm and the refractory period (p. 92). OT plays an important role in PRL production in rats, with both direct stimulation of the lactotrophs in the anterior pituitary by OT from the PVN, and control of the PRL secretory rhythm. It is thus conceivable that the relatively brief increase in OT associated with sexual arousal and orgasm in humans may be contributing to the post-orgasmic increase in PRL in preparation for subsequent conception. Further research on this in the human is required.

Melanocortins

There has been an explosion of interest in the melanocortins in the last few years, sparked by the identification of five melanocortin receptors. Melanocortins have the same origin as β-endorphin and ACTH, all derived from pro-opiomelanocortin (POMC). A wide range of effects of α-melanocyte-stimulating hormone (α-MSH), beyond melanocyte stimulation, have been identified, including effects on feeding and sexual behaviour (Wikberg et al 2000). In male laboratory animals, sex-related effects include grooming, stretching, yawning and penile erection, believed to be an α-MSH effect downstream from dopamine and OT in hypothalamic centres adjacent to the third ventricle at the melanocortin 4 receptor (Van der Ploeg et al 2002). The effects of an analogue of α-MH, PT 141, increase appetitive sexual behaviour (solicitation) in female rats (Pfaus et al 2004). So far there is limited evidence of the effects of PT 141 in humans. Diamond et al (2004) showed an increase in spontaneous erections in sexually functional men, suggesting that the effects on erection are not dependent on sexual stimulation, as with PDE-5 inhibitors. In a placebo-controlled study of PT-141 in women with sexual arousal disorder, the neuropeptide produced significantly more sexual desire than placebo, but no effect on VPA response to erotic films (Diamond et al 2006). It remains to be seen where this new line of research takes us, but we should be prepared for a major increase in complexity of our understanding of the effects of neuropeptides on sexuality.

Hormones and passionate love

One study has explored possible endocrine characteristics of 'passionate love', comparing 24 men and women who had recently fallen in love and 24 who were single or part of a long established relationship (Marazziti & Canale 2004). They found no differences between the male groups and female groups in oestradiol, progesterone, DHEAS or androstenedione. Cortisol levels were significantly higher in those who had recently 'fallen in love'. FSH and T were lower in the men and higher in the women who had 'fallen in love'. These differences had disappeared when subjects were re-tested 12–24 months later. The increased cortisol pattern suggests

a non-specific 'stress' pattern. The authors suggested a 'love-related' gender difference in relation to T. However, a more likely explanation is that this is a non-specific gender pattern, reflecting the much greater contribution of adrenal androgens to plasma T in women than in men.

Making sense of gender differences

Differences in the sexuality of men and women are considered at various places in this book. Given the sexual basis of gender, it is of obvious importance to understand in what ways male and female sexuality are similar and different, and, if possible, why. In this chapter we focused on psychobiological factors and brain mechanisms, and a number of intriguing gender differences emerged. Although the evidence is as yet insufficient to draw conclusions, we found a suggestion of gender differences in some aspects of brain activity during sexual response, as shown in brain-imaging studies (p. 72). Activation of the thalamus and hypothalamus was only apparent in men, with the amygdala being more strongly activated in men. This contrasted with an observed gender difference in brain activity during orgasm, with deactivation of the amygdala being reported in men, and activation in women (p. 89). Are we seeing evidence of gender differences in basic neurophysiological mechanisms involved in sexual response and orgasm, or are we seeing 'noise' from as yet inadequately controlled methodologies and individual variability across gender?

The vagina is a uniquely female organ, and questions can be asked about how changes in VBF relate physiologically to genital or pelvic response in men. This is particularly noteworthy because of the gender difference in the correlations between subjective sexual arousal and genital response (p. 80); men typically show higher correlations. It would not be surprising, however, if men were more aware of what was happening in their penis, compared to women's perception of what is happening in their vagina. This goes someway to explaining why men tend to incorporate genital response into their experience of sexual arousal and sexual desire more than women do. Whether women are more aware of what is happening in their clitoris than their vagina remains to be seen with further research, but it would not be surprising if a woman had less awareness of clitoral tumescence than a man's awareness of penile erection.

Information processing research so far shows some gender similarities and some differences. A greater variability among women is noteworthy, but as yet the research is at an early stage.

The paradoxical relationship between negative mood and sexuality has so far been more commonly reported by men, particularly in relation to depressed mood. However, such paradoxical patterns are far from rare among women. The intriguing relationship between depression and masturbation reported in women (p. 106) has not yet been explored to the same extent in men, so we do not yet know whether this is a gender difference.

The Dual Control model is helping us to see that inhibitory processes are more evident among women, and it remains to be seen whether this reflects different neurophysiological inhibitory mechanisms, a wider range of inhibitory contexts or simply greater propensity for inhibition in women. So there are more questions than answers at this stage. But let us speculate how the basic function of sexuality might differ in men and women, in the hope that this might generate some testable hypotheses.

In Chapter 2 (p. 11) we cited Gagnon & Simon (1973): 'Undeniably, what we conventionally describe as sexual behaviour is rooted in biological capacities and processes, but no more than other forms of behaviour. The sexual area may be precisely that realm wherein the superordinate position of the socio-cultural over the biological level is most complete' (p. 15). The closest this book gets to Gagnon & Simon's position is to suggest that the sexual dimension of the human condition has received the greatest amount of sociocultural control. The history of human sexuality is one of varying degrees of social suppression, particularly of women's sexuality, reflecting the patriarchal systems that have often dominated. In other words, it is because of the essentially biological nature of human sexuality that there has been this sociocultural reaction. It is difficult to think of any other fundamental aspect of the human condition as incongruent with the sociocultural identities that humans aspire to. Even eating behaviour can be and often is channelled into a peculiarly human, 'civilized' context. But compare copulation between a man and a woman, two gorillas, two rats and two elephants, and apart from a greater tendency for the humans to adopt a face-to-face position, there is a striking similarity in what is a basic and not exactly elegant biological function. From one perspective, this can be seen as an advantage to the human race because it reduces the likelihood of us becoming insufferably pompous. On the other hand, those who strive for pomposity have to find ways to conceal, suppress or deny this embarrassing characteristic.

The extent to which we have been able to use evidence from animals, most often rats, to understand how the human brain deals with sexuality points to the existence of basic brain mechanisms that are common, across many, particularly mammalian, species (Pfaus et al 2003). Obviously the precise behavioural manifestations, particularly when considering what animal researchers call 'appetitive' behaviours, are determined by the nature of social structure in a species and the extent to which it is hierarchical. Barry Everitt, an expert in the neurophysiology of rat sexual behaviour, and I compared the sexuality of rats and men (Everitt & Bancroft 1991), and concluded:

'Information processing is crucial to both species. Clearly, the role of cognition in the human will be at a fundamentally different level of complexity. However, it is not unreasonable to postulate that the interface between cognitive processes and both arousal and motor responses share a common anatomical, and probably biochemical basis in the two species, with the amygdala, striatum and hypothalamus involved in both cases. (On the other hand) the uniquely human form of cognition, with its labeling, attribution and expectation may well result in the self-perpetuation of maladaptive responses in a way that would not be relevant to the rat.'

(p. 109)

Recently, Pfaus (2006) published a comparable review for females ('of rats and women'). Here he describes the solicitation and pacing by which the female controls the initiation and rate of copulatory contact as key components of the female pattern, the rewarding nature of which is evident in their capacity to condition place preferences. It has now been shown that the melanocortin agonist bremelanotide enhances female solicitations in the rat, and, as mentioned earlier, preliminary research suggests that the same compound enhances sexual desire in women (Diamond et al 2006). A noteworthy question about human sexual desire, which will be revisited in Chapter 6 (p. 220) is what it is that is actually desired? Until recently, particularly for women, this question has received little attention. To what extent, or in what proportion of women, does bremelanotide enhance sexual desire for 'solicitation and pacing'. i.e. having control over an attractive man who desires you, rather than desire for 'sexual pleasure' per se?

Towards an explanatory model of gender differences in sexuality

Let us consider what are likely to be the key reinforcers or rewards of sexual behaviour and how they might differ between men and women. At the risk of allegations of 'political incorrectness', let us compare and contrast the 'solicitation and pacing' pattern and its associated rewards, with the rewards of 'sexual pleasure' that results from genital stimulation.

It can be argued that women's sexuality has been determined and shaped at three levels. First is a basic component of female sexuality, essential for reproduction, evident, in various respects, across species, as Everitt & Bancroft (1991) argued for male sexuality. Second, there are superadded effects of sexual responsiveness and associated sexual pleasure, which have the same developmental origins as in the male, and which are either 'adaptations' or 'by-products'. as considered earlier in relation to female orgasm (p. 95). Third is the impact of socio-cultural influences, shaping how women in different societies experience, interpret and come to terms with their sexuality. Let us consider each level more closely.

The basic pattern

What is the basic pattern of male sexuality and how does female sexuality compare? In this respect, the male is comparatively straightforward. There is a biological urge or incentive in the male to seek penile stimulation towards the achievement of orgasm and ejaculation. This has crucial hormonal determinants similar across species. Given that vaginal penetration is particularly effective at providing the appropriate penile stimulation, this typically results in a basic pattern leading to deposition of semen in the female reproductive tract, a prerequisite for reproduction. One can recognize this theme in male rats, men and the males of most other mammalian species. Obviously, other types of reward may be involved, including the male version of 'solicitation and pacing', yet they are less directly relevant to reproduction and more variable in importance among men.

What of the female? The basic pattern in the female rat, which is restricted to the oestrous phase of her hormonal cycle, could be described as 'allowing vaginal penetration to occur'. When one considers that the female is mounted and penetrated, it is relevant to ask how such a process, which in other circumstances would be noxious, is permitted. Does it depend on associated sexual pleasure in the female? There are two components of the female rat's sexual behaviour: 'proceptive' and 'receptive'. In the proceptive phase, the female is not passive but 'darting and hopping' around the male, and in the process, pacing the male's mounts. She, in other words, is in control. She will only be activated in this way if the male is showing sexual interest in her. Gilman & Westbrook (1978) came to the conclusion that sexual contacts during oestrus are rewarding for females if they are allowed to pace those contacts. Parades & Alonso (1997) showed that such reward from pacing effectively conditioned place preferences.

The receptive phase involves intromission and hence penetration, with its aversive potential. In the female rat, appropriate tactile stimulation from the male during mounting elicits lordosis, a reflex mechanism that occurs in a number of mammalian species (e.g. rodents and cats) making intromission by the male possible. This complex response has been extensively studied in rodents (Pfaff 1999). Does the female rat enjoy the mounting and intromission, or is her reward the pacing and control of the male's behaviour by her 'darting and hopping', with her involvement then moving to a reflexive pattern, lordosis? McClintock & Adler (1978) showed, some time ago, that if the pacing of intromissions produced specific intervals between them, the likelihood of conception was increased. Ongoing research by Pfaus and his colleagues (personal communication) is suggesting that intermittent VS of the oestrous female rat, if given at these 'reproductively correct' intervals, conditions place preference in the female. Thus, we are beginning to piece together a picture in which the basic reproductive pattern of the female rat, both proceptive and receptive, is rewarding.

Has this any relevance to women? In subhuman primates there are a range of proceptive behaviours in the female. Dixson (1998) listed 28 different behaviours, across many primate species. Examples are lip smacking, tongue protrusion, eye contact and vocalizations, many of which were not confined to proceptive sexuality. Sexual presentation postures by the female were reported in 20 species, including Rhesus macaques, chimpanzees, bonobos and gorillas. Proceptive behaviours in women have received some attention. Moore (1985) identified 52 separate behaviours contributing to what can be called 'flirting' in women. Some of these were similar to the primates, e.g. lip licking, pouting and eye contact of various kinds. Sexual presentation

postures, needless to say, were not included, although a variety of postures, which could be seen as invitational, were listed. How do they compare with the 'pacing' of female rats? Moore (1995) commented '... these subtle indicators of interest allow women to pace the course of a relationship' (p. 327). There is evidence that for women it is important to 'be desired' (e.g. Graham et al 2003), and it would not be surprising if a woman found that her ability to both attract and, in the process, control the behaviour of a male partner was rewarding and indeed arousing.

There is no equivalent of lordosis in the human female, and in non-human primates, a form of lordosis is only found in the prosimian suborder (e.g. lemurs) where there is clear hormonal control of female sexual behaviour, i.e. oestrus (Dixson 1998). But there are some interesting parallels to the receptive phase that have been considered earlier in this chapter. There is, in women, evidence of a preparatory response in the vaginal wall, as shown by the VPA evidence, which is not correlated with subjective arousal or pleasure, and which has been identified in women reacting to stimuli which may even be aversive (see p. 80), leading Laan & Everaerd (1995) to wonder if this was an automatic response. We do not have directly comparable data from other species. However, there is an additional mechanism of relevance: the reduction in pain sensitivity that is elicited by vaginal or cervical pressure, which was considered at some length earlier (p. 83) and which was first identified in female rats, and subsequently in women. If females engage in copulation because it is pleasurable, why is there a need for specialized pain reduction mechanisms?

Yet again, we have more questions than answers here, but we can speculate, as we await further evidence, that the basic female pattern, which exists to make reproduction possible, includes mechanisms to reduce or eliminate noxious consequences of vaginal penetration. There is 'automatic' lubrication of the vagina, which, the evidence from women suggests, occurs to some extent in the presence of any potential sexual stimulus, whether appealing or not. And there is the existence of specialized pain reduction mechanisms that are elicited by vaginal penetration. It is not clear whether VS per se contributes to this pattern. In addition there is a 'solicitation and pacing' component. The process of engaging in a 'non-noxious' act of sexual intimacy, which may involve vaginal penetration by the partner's erect penis, in which the woman feels in control, is rewarding for her. What is more difficult is to be sure about the nature of the reward.

The fact that vaginal erotic sensitivity, particularly in the anterior vaginal wall, is only evident in a proportion of women suggests that it is not an essential part of the reproductive basic pattern. The assumption is that this basic pattern, because of its role in reproduction, is to be found in the large majority of women and that it involves sufficient reward to ensure that its reproductive role is expressed. But, as with the rat, we should be striving to understand in what way this pattern is rewarding.

The superadded component

In addition to the basic pattern, this model recognizes various types of 'sexual pleasure' that are not required for a woman to be reproductive. Sexual pleasure, in its own right, is clearly important for many women. But a reasonable conclusion from the available evidence, much of which is reviewed in various parts of this book, is that women are much more variable in the importance they attach to the experience of sexual pleasure or orgasm, than are men.

Clearly many, if not most, women have erotic sensory mechanisms, stimulation of which results in sexual pleasure and associated sexual arousal. Some women experience such pleasure as a result of VS, and these women may be those who have Levin's 'anterior wall erogenous complex' (see p. 83), which mostly depends on local distribution of clitoral tissue near the vaginal wall. An additional source of pleasure is the orgasm. We have already considered the possible functions of the female orgasm and have failed to find any evidence that, as claimed by evolutionary 'adaptionists'. it increases the likelihood of conception. In any case, the available evidence indicates that for the majority of women vaginal penetration alone is not sufficient to elicit orgasm; some form of additional clitoral stimulation is required. Yet the anatomy of the female does not appear to be designed to lead to clitoral stimulation from vaginal penetration.

There is also no evidence that the experience of clitoral erotic pleasure enhances fertility. But both clitoral pleasure and the anticipation of orgasm may well motivate a woman to engage in sexual activity, and there is a range of potential consequences of such motivation, including reproduction, though not all positive. However, we are left uncertain what motivates a woman to engage in penile vaginal insertion. To what extent is it because of the direct pleasurable stimulation involved? Is it because she enjoys giving her partner pleasure? Is there something of symbolic importance to his being inside her? Does this interaction enhance a feeling of emotional closeness?

While recognizing the need to keep an open mind on this issue, the variability of the importance of sexual pleasure and orgasm among women, and the lack of any clear connection between such pleasures and reproduction, support the idea that they are by-products of male development, essential to enable the basic pattern to be manifested in the male, and not in need of suppression in the female (see discussion of the by-product debate on the female orgasm, p. 94).

A further candidate for inclusion at the 'superadded' level is the effect of T on women's sexuality. As discussed earlier, it is likely that women vary considerably in the extent to which T affects their sexuality. Around half of women can experience substantial reduction of T following ovariectomy without any obvious negative impact on their sexuality. A similar picture relates to the effects of steroidal contraceptives (see Chapter 15). There is further evidence that the impact of T, when it occurs, is more on the woman's spontaneous sexual interest or desire than on her capacity for sexual response and pleasure. As shown by Garde & Lunde (1980) in 40-year-old Danish women, more than 30% reported little or no spontaneous sexual desire, yet most of them had no difficulty enjoying and becoming aroused during sexual interaction with their partner. Thus, spontaneous sexual desire can be regarded as another component at the superadded level, reflecting mechanisms more crucial to the male basic pattern. When we start to collect relevant evidence about the markers of T sensitivity in women we may well find that such markers are associated with specific manifestations of sexual expression, such as certain types of 'desire' or certain objects of sexual desire, which are not generally found in women.

The socio-cultural dimension

The third level, the impact of socio-cultural influences, is considered at various places in this book (in particular, Chapter 6). At this point it is appropriate to suggest that biological mechanisms that may be relatively gender specific, may result in women being more susceptible than men to socio-cultural factors. One obvious example, is the greater propensity for inhibition of sexual response in women, and a wider range of inhibiting situations that affect them, as demonstrated by our studies based on the Dual Control model discussed earlier in this chapter (see also Chapters 2 and 6). The greater importance of inhibitory mechanisms for women has been argued well by Bjorklund & Kipp (1996). At this stage, it remains a possibility that different neurophysiological mechanisms are involved in the inhibitory mechanisms of women compared to men, and as yet the evidence from brain imaging does not allow us to reach any conclusions on this point. However, we can consider at one level, inhibition of the basic pattern, if the need is to avoid inappropriate reproduction. And at another level, inhibition of the sexual pleasure, the superadded component, has been the target of sexual repression through much of history, reflecting male concerns about women's sexual pleasure. What was apparent in the unfolding of our knowledge about sexuality during the 20th century was a progressive lifting of socio-cultural repression of women's sexuality, at least in the Western world (see Chapter 6). As this socio-cultural lid has been taken off women's sexual expression, it has increasingly revealed the fundamental variability of women's sexuality, which this model has attempted to explain.

Conclusion

In a recent pilot study for a new Kinsey Institute survey, 180 women and 175 men were asked to rate how important sex was for a variety of purposes. Men reported significantly higher ratings for sex as a source of pleasure ($p < 0.0001$), as a means of giving pleasure to one's partner ($p = 0.004$) and for experiencing orgasm ($p < 0.0001$). Men and women did not differ in the importance of sex for 'feeling close to their partner' and 'for having children'.

More research of this kind, looking in increasing detail at the specific components of the sexual interaction, is needed before we can feel confident about the differences and similarities of the male and female 'basic sexual experience'. But it remains possible that the super-added component of women's sexuality, as described here, is an important source of variance in female sexuality.

REFERENCES

Abdelgadir SE, Roselli CE, Choate JVA, Resko JA 1999 Androgen receptor messenger ribonucleic acid in brains and pituitaries of male Rhesus monkeys: studies on distribution, hormonal control, and relationship to luteinizing hormone secretion. Biology of Reproduction 60: 1251–1256.

Abrahamson DJ, Barlow DH, Beck JG, Sakheim D 1985 The effects of attentional focus and partner responsiveness on sexual responding: replication and extension. Archives of Sexual Behavior 14: 361–372.

Alexander GM, Swerdloff RS, Wang C, Davidson T, McDonald V, Steiner B, Hines M 1997 Androgen-behavior correlations in hypogonadal men and eugonadal men I. Mood and response to auditory sexual stimuli. Hormones and Behavior 31: 110–119.

Allen LS, Gorski RA 1990 Sex difference in the bed nucleus of the stria terminalis of the human brain. Journal of Comparative Neurology 302: 697–706.

Amaral DG 2000 The anatomical organization of the central nervous system. In Kandel ER, Schwartz JH, Jessell TM (eds) Principles of Neuroscience, 4th edition. McGraw-Hill, New York, pp. 317–336.

Anderson RA, Bancroft J, Wu FCW 1992 The effects of exogenous testosterone on sexuality and mood of normal men. Journal of Clinical Endocrinology and Metabolism 75: 1503–1507.

Anderson RA, Martin CW, Kung A, Everington D, Pun TC, Tan KCB, Bancroft J, Sundaram K, Moo-Young AJ, Baird DT 1999 7α-Methyl-19-Nortestosterone (MENT) maintains sexual behavior and mood in hypogonadal men. Journal of Clinical Endocrinology and Metabolism 84: 3556–3562.

Andersson KE 1995 Discussion. In Bancroft J (ed) The Pharmacology of Sexual Function and Dysfunction. Elsevier Science, Amsterdam, p. 222.

Angst J 1998 Sexual problems in healthy and depressed persons. International Clinical Psychopharmacology 13(suppl 6): S1–S4.

Appelt H, Strauss B 1986 The psychoendocrinology of female sexuality: a research project. The German Journal of Psychology 10: 143–156.

Argiolas A 1999 Neuropeptides and sexual behaviour. Neuroscience and Biobehavioral Reviews 23: 1127–1142.

Arnold MB 1960 Emotion and Personality. Columbia University Press, New York.

Aron A, Fisher H, Mashek DJ, Strong G, Li H, Brown LL 2005 Reward, motivation and emotion systems associated with early stage intense romantic love. Journal of Neurophysiology 94: 327–337.

Aziz A, Bramstrom M, Bergquist C, Silverstolpe G 2005 Perimenopausal androgen decline after oophorectomy does not influence sexuality or psychological wellbeing. Fertility and Sterility 83: 1021–1028.

Bach AK, Brown TA, Barlow DH 1999 The effects of false negative feedback on efficacy expectancies and sexual arousal in sexually functional males. Behavior Therapy 30: 79–95.

Bachman G, Bancroft J, Braunstein G, Burger H, Davis S, Dennerstein L, Goldstein I, Guay A, Leiblum S, Lobo R, Notelovitz M, Rosen R, Sarrel P, Sherwin B, Simon J, Simpson E, Shifren J, Spark R, Traish A 2002 Female androgen insufficiency: the Princeton consensus statement on definition, classification, and assessment. Fertility and Sterility 77: 660–665.

Backstrom T, Sanders D, Leask R, Davidson D, Warner P, Bancroft J 1983 Mood, sexuality, hormones and the menstrual cycle II. Hormone levels and their relationships to the premenstrual syndrome. Psychosomatic Medicine 45: 503–507.

Bagatell CJ, Heiman JR, Rivier JE, Bremner WJ 1994a Effects of endogenous testosterone and estradiol on sexual behavior in normal young men. Journal of Clinical Endocrinology and Metabolism 78: 711–716.

Bagatell CJ, Heiman JR, Matsumoto AM, Rivier JE, Bremner WJ 1994b Metabolic and behavioral effects of high-dose, exogenous testosterone in healthy men. Journal of Clinical Endocrinology and Metabolism 79: 561–567.

Baird AA, Gruber SA, Cohen BM, Renshaw PF, Steingard, RJ, Yurgelen-Todd DA 1999 fMRI of the amygdala in children and adolescents. Journal of the American Academy of Child and Adolescent Psychiatry 38: 195–199.

Baker RR, Bellis MA 1993 Human sperm competition: ejaculation manipulation by females and a function for the female orgasm. Animal Behaviour 46: 887–909.

Bancroft J 1970 Disorders of sexual potency. In: Hill OW (ed) Modern Trends in Psychosomatic Medicine. Butterworths, London, pp. 246–261.

Bancroft J 1974 Deviant Sexual Behaviour: Modification and Assessment. Clarendon Press, Oxford.

Bancroft J 1978 Psychological and physiological responses to sexual stimuli in men and women. In Levi L (ed) Society, Stress and Disease, Vol. 3. The Productive and Reproductive Age. Oxford University Press, Oxford, pp. 154–163.

Bancroft J 1989 Human Sexuality and Its Problems, 2nd edn. Churchill Livingstone, Edinburgh.

Bancroft J 1994 Sexual motivation and behaviour. In Colman AM (ed) Companion Encyclopedia of Psychology, Vol I. Routledge, London, pp. 542–559.

Bancroft J 1995 Are the effects of androgens on male sexuality noradrenergically mediated? Some consideration of the human. Neuroscience and Biobehavioral Reviews 19: 325–330.

Bancroft J 1998 Alfred Kinsey's work 50 years later. Introduction. In Kinsey AC, Pomeroy WB, Martin CE, Gebhard PH (eds) Sexual Behavior in the Human Female. Indiana University Press, Bloomington, pp. a–r. (Originally published in 1953.)

Bancroft J 2002 Sexual effects of androgens in women: some theoretical considerations. Fertility and Sterility 77(Suppl 4): S55–S59.

Bancroft J 2003 Androgens and sexual function in men and women. In Bagatell CJ, Bremner WJ (eds) Androgens in Health and Disease. Humana Press, Totowa, pp. 258–290.

Bancroft J 2004 Kinsey and the politics of sex research. Annual Review of Sex Research 15: 1–39.

Bancroft J, Bell C 1985 Simultaneous recording of penile diameter and penile arterial pulse during laboratory-based erotic stimulation in normal subjects. Journal of Psychosomatic Research 29: 303–313.

Bancroft J, Mathews A 1971 Autonomic correlates of penile erection. Journal of Psychosomatic Research 15: 159–167.

Bancroft J, Tennent TG, Loucas K, Cass J 1974 Control of deviant sexual behaviour by drugs: behavioural effects of oestrogens and antiandrogens. British Journal of Psychiatry 125: 310–315.

Bancroft J, Davidson DW, Warner P, Tyrer G 1980 Androgens and sexual behaviour in women using oral contraceptives. Clinical Endocrinology 12: 327–340.

Bancroft J, Sanders D, Davison DW, Warner P 1983 Mood, sexuality, hormones and the menstrual cycle. III Sexuality and the role of androgens. Psychosomatic Medicine 45: 509–516.

Bancroft J, Munoz M, Beard M, Shapiro C 1995 The effects of a new alpha-2 adrenoceptor antagonist on sleep and nocturnal penile tumescence in normal male volunteers and men with erectile dysfunction. Psychosomatic Medicine 57: 345–356.

Bancroft J, Herbenick D, Reynolds M 2003a Masturbation as a marker of sexual development. In Bancroft J (ed) Sexual Development in Childhood. Indiana University Press, Bloomington.

Bancroft J, Janssen E, Strong D, Vukadinovic Z, Long JS 2003b The relation between mood and sexuality in heterosexual men. Archives of Sexual Behavior 32: 217–230.

Bancroft J, Janssen E, Strong D, Vukadinovic Z 2003c The relation between mood and sexuality in gay men. Archives of Sexual Behavior 32: 231–242.

Bancroft J, Loftus J, Long JS 2003d Distress about sex: a national survey of women in heterosexual relationships. Archives of Sexual Behavior 32: 193–208.

Barclay AM 1969 The effect of hostility on physiological and fantasy responses. Journal of Personality 37: 651–667.

Barclay AM, Haber RN 1965 The relation of aggression to sexual motivation. Journal of Personality 33: 462–475.

Barlow DH 1986 The causes of sexual dysfunction: the role of anxiety and cognitive interference. Journal of Consulting and Clinical Psychology 54: 140–148.

Bartels A, Zeki S 2000 The neural basis of romantic love. NeuroReport 11: 3829–3834.

Bartels A, Zeki S 2004 The neural correlates of maternal and romantic love. Neuroimage 21: 1155–1166.

Baum MJ 1995 Reassessing the role of medial preoptic area/anterior hypothalamic neurons in appetitive aspects of masculine sexual behavior. In Bancroft J (ed) The Pharmacology of Sexual Function and Dysfunction. Elsevier Science, Amsterdam, pp. 133–139.

Beach FA 1967 Cerebral and hormonal control of reflexive mechanisms involved in copulatory behavior. Physiological Reviews 47: 289–316.

Beach FA, Westbrook WH, Clemens LG 1966 Comparison of the ejaculatory response in men and animals. Psychosomatic Medicine 28: 749–763.

Bechara A, Damasio H, Damasio AR 2000 Emotion, decision making and the orbito-frontal cortex. Cerebral Cortex 10: 295–307.

Beck JG, Bozman AW 1995 Gender differences in sexual desire: the effects of anger and anxiety. Archives of Sexual Behavior 24: 595–612.

Beck JG, Barlow DH, Sakheim DK 1983 The effects of attentional focus and partner arousal on sexual responding in functional and dysfunctional men. Behaviour Research and Therapy 21: 1–8.

Becker MA, Byrne D 1988 Type A behavior, distraction and sexual arousal. Journal of Social & Clinical Psychology 6: 472–481.

Beggs VE, Calhoun KS, Wolchik SA 1987 Sexual anxiety and female sexual arousal: a comparison of arousal during sexual anxiety stimuli and sexual pleasure stimuli. Archives of Sexual Behavior 16: 311–319.

Bell RJ, Donath S, Davison SL, Davis SR 2005 Endogenous androgen levels and wellbeing: differences between pre- and post-menopausal women. Menopause 13: 65–71.

Bellerose SB, Binik YM 1993 Body image and sexuality in oophorectomized women. Archives of Sexual Behavior 22: 435–460.

Benson GS 1983 Penile erection: in search of a neurotransmitter. World Journal of Urology 1: 209–212.

Benson GS, McConnell JA, Lipshultz LI, Corriere J 1980 Neuromorphology and neuropharmacology of the human penis. Journal of Clinical Investigation 65: 506.

Bentler PM, Peeler WH 1979 Models of female orgasm. Archives of Sexual Behavior 8: 405–424.

Berman JR, Berman LA, Werbin TJ, Flaherty EE, Leahy NM, Goldstein I 1999 Clinical evaluation of female sexual function: effects of age and estrogen status on subjective and physiological sexual responses. International Journal of Impotence Research 11(Suppl 1): S31–S38.

Bitran D, Hull EM 1987 Pharmacological analysis of male rat sexual behavior. Neuroscience and Biobehavioral Reviews 11: 365–389.

Bitran D, Miller SA, McQuade DB, Leipheimer RE, Sachs BD 1989 Inhibition of sexual reflexes by lumbosacral injection of a GABA_B agonist in the male rat. Pharmacology Biochemistry & Behavior 31: 657–666.

Bixo M, Backstrom T, Winblad B, Andersson A 1995 Estradiol and testosterone in specific regions of the human female brain in different endocrine states. Journal of Steroid Biochemistry and Molecular Biology 55: 297–303.

Bjorklund DF, Kipp K 1996 Parental investment theory and gender differences in the evolution of inhibition mechanisms. Psychological Bulletin 120: 163–188.

Black SL, Biron C 1982 Androstenol as a human pheromone: no effect on perceived physical attractiveness. Behavioural and Neurological Biology 34: 326–330.

Black DW, Kehrberg LLD, Flumerfelt DL, Schlosser SS 1997 Characteristics of 36 subjects reporting compulsive sexual behavior. American Journal of Psychiatry 154: 243–249.

Blaicher W, Gruber D, Bieglmayer C, Blaicher AM, Knogler W, Huber JC 1999 The role of oxytocin in relation to female sexual arousal. Gynecologic and Obstetric Investigation 47: 125–126.

Bocher M, Chisin R, Parag Y, Freedman N, Meir Weil Y, Lester H, Mishani E, Bonne O 2001 Cerebral activation associated with sexual arousal in response to a pornographic clip: a 15O-H20 PET study in heterosexual men. Neuroimage 14: 105–117.

Bochinski D, Brock GB 2001 Medications affecting sexual function. In Mulcahay JJ (ed) Male Sexual Function: a Guide to Clinical Management. Humana, Totowa, pp. 91–108.

Bohlen JG, Held JP, Sanderson MO, Ahlgren A 1982 The female orgasm: pelvic contractions. Archives of Sexual Behavior 11: 367–386.

Bole-Feysot C, Goffin V, Edery M, Binart N, Kelly PA 1998 Prolactin (PRL) and its receptor: actions, signal transduction pathways and phenotypes observed in PRL receptor knockout mice. Endocrine Reviews 19: 225–268.

Boolell M, Gepi-Attee S, Gingell JC, Allen MJ 1996 Sildenafil, a novel effective oral therapy for male erectile dysfunction. British Journal of Urology 78: 257–261.

Bors E, Comarr AE 1960 Neurological disturbances of sexual function with special reference to 529 patients with spinal cord injuries. Urological Survey 10: 191–222.

Both S, Everaerd W, Laan E 2003 Modulation of spinal reflexes by aversive and sexually appetitive stimuli. Psychophysiology 40: 174–183.

Brauer M, Laan E, ter Kuile MM 2006 Sexual arousal in women with superficial dyspareunia. Archives of Sexual Behavior 35: 191–200.

Braunstein GD, Sundwall DA, Katz M, Shifren JL, Buster JE, Simon JA, Bachman G, Aguire OA, Lucas JD, Rodenberg C, Buch A, Watts NB 2005 Safety and efficacy of a testosterone patch for the treatment of hypoactive sexual desire disorder in surgically menopausal women. Archives of Internal Medicine 165: 1582–1589.

Breiter HC, Gollub RL, Weisskoff RM, Kennedy DN, Makris N, Berke JD, Goodman JM, Kantor HL, Gastfriend DR, Riorden JP, Mathew RT, Rosen BR, Hyman SE 1997 Acute effects of cocaine on human brain activity and emotion. Neuron 19: 591–611.

Brindley GS 1983 Cavernosal alpha-blockade: a new treatment for investigating and treating erectile impotence. British Journal of Psychiatry 143: 332–337.

Brindley GS 1984 Pharmacology of erection. Paper presented at 10th annual meeting of International Academy of Sex Research, Cambridge, England.

Brody S, Kruger THC 2006 The post-orgasmic prolactin increase following intercourse is greater than following masturbation and suggests greater satiety. Biological Psychology 71: 312–315.

Brotto LA, Gorzalka BB 2002 Genital and subjective sexual arousal in post-menopausal women: influence of laboratory-induced hyperventilation. Journal of Sex and Marital Therapy 28(Suppl 1): 39–54.

Buena F, Swerdloff RS, Steiner BS, Lutchmansingh P, Peterson MA, Pandian MR, Galmarini M, Bhasin S 1993 Sexual function does not change when serum testosterone levels are pharmacologically varied within the normal male range. Fertility and Sterility 59: 1118–1123.

Burger H, Hailes J, Nelson J, Menelaus M 1987 Effect of combined implants of oestradiol and testosterone on libido in postmenopausal women. British Medical Journal 294: 936–937.

Buster JE, Kingsberg SA, Aguirre O, Brown C, Breaux JG, Buch A, Rodenberg CAS, Wekselman K, Casson P 2005 Testosterone patch for low sexual desire in surgically menopausal women: a randomized trial. Obstetrics & Gynecology 105: 944–952.

Buvat J 2003 Androgen therapy with dehydroepiandrosterone. World Journal of Urology 21: 346–355.

Cacioppo JT, Bernston GG, Lorig TS, Norris CJ, Rickett E, Nusbaum H 2003 Just because you're imaging the brain doesn't mean you can stop using your head: a primer and set of first principles. Journal of Personalitty and Social Psychology 85: 650–661.

Caldwell JD 2002 A sexual arousability model involving steroid effects at the plasma membrane. Neuroscience and Biobehavioral Reviews 26: 13–20.

Cantor JR, Zillmann D, Bryant J 1975 Enhancement of experienced sexual arousal in response to erotic stimuli through misattribution of unrelated residual excitation. Journal of Personality and Social Psychology 32: 69–75.

Cantor JM, Binik YM, Pfaus JG 1999 Chronic fluoxetine inhibits sexual behavior in the male rat: reversal with oxytocin. Psychopharmacology 144: 355–362.

Carani C, Bancroft J, Del Rio G, Granata ARM, Facchinetti HF, Marrama F 1990 The endocrine effects of visual erotic stimuli in normal men. Psychoneuroendocrinology 15: 207–216.

Carani C, Bancroft J, Granata ARM, Del Rio G, Marrama F 1992 Testosterone and erectile function. Nocturnal penile tumescence and rigidity, and erectile response to visual erotic stimuli in hypogonadal and eugonadal men. Psychoneuroendocrinology 17: 647–654.

Carani C, Granata ARM, Bancroft J, Marrama P 1995 The effects of testosterone replacement on nocturnal penile tumescence and rigidity and erectile response to visual erotic stimuli in hypogonadal men. Psychoneuroendocrinology 20: 743–753.

Carmichael MS, Humbert R, Dixen J, Palmisano G, Greenleaf W, Davidson JM 1987 Plasma oxytocin increases in the human sexual response. Journal of Clinical Endocrinology and Metabolism 64: 27–31.

Carney A, Bancroft J, Mathews A 1978 Combination of hormonal and psychological treatment for female sexual unresponsiveness: a comparative study. British Journal Psychiatry 132: 339–356.

Carter CS 1998 Neuroendocrine perspectives of social attachment and love. Psychoneuroendocrinology 23: 779–818.

Cawood EHH, Bancroft J 1996 Steroid hormones, the menopause, sexuality and well-being of women. Psychological Medicine 26: 925–936.

Chahl LA 1995 Modulation of neurotransmitter release by some therapeutic and socially used drugs: exogenous opiates. In Powis DA, Bunn SJ (eds) Neurotransmitter Release and Its Modulation. Cambridge University Press, Cambridge, pp. 305–313.

Chambless DL, Stern T, Sultan FF, Williams AJ, Goldstein AJ, Lineberger MH, Lifshitz JL, Kelly L 1982 The pubococcygeus and female orgasm: a correlational study in normal subjects. Archives of Sexual Behavior 11: 479–490.

Charney DS, Heninger GR 1986 Alpha2-adrenergic and opiate receptor blockade. Synergistic effects on anxiety in health subjects. Archives of General Psychiatry 43: 1037–1041.

Charney DS, Heninger GR, Redmond DE 1983 Yohimbine induces anxiety and increases noradrenergic function in humans: effect of diazepam and clonidine. Life Science 33: 19–29.

Christian JJ 1970 Social subordination, population density, and mammalian evolution. Science 168: 84–90.

Chung WC, DeVries GJ, Swaab DF 2002 Sexual differentiation of the bed nucleus of the stria terminalis in humans may extend into adulthood. Journal of Neuroscience 22: 1027–1033.

Clark RA 1953 The effects of sexual motivation on fantasy. Journal of Experimental Psychology 44: 3–11.

Cohen HD, Rosen RC, Goldstein L 1976 Electroencephalographic laterality changes during human sexual orgasm. Archives of Sexual Behavior 5: 189–199.

Costa M, Braun C, Birbaumer N 2003 Gender differences in response to pictures of nudes:a magnetoencephalographic study. Biological Psychology 63: 129–147.

Cranston-Cuebas MA, Barlow DH 1990 Cognitive and affective contributions to sexual functioning. Annual Review of Sex Research 1: 119–161.

Crenshaw TL, Goldberg JP 1996 Sexual Pharmacology: Drugs That Affect Sexual Function. Norton, New York.

Csillag ER 1976 Modification of penile erectile response. Journal of Behavioral Therapy and Experimental Psychiatry 7: 27–29.

Cuthbert BN, Schupp HT, Bradley MM, Birbaumer N, Lang PJ 2000 Brain potentials in affective picture processing: covariation with autonomic arousal and affective report. Biological Psychology 52: 95–111.

Cutler WB, Preti G, Krieger AM, Huggins GR, Garcia CR, Lawley HJ 1986 Human axillary secretion influences women's menstrual cycles. The role of donor extract from men. Hormones and Behavior 20: 463–473.

Cutler WB, Friedmann E, McCoy NL 1998a Pheromonal influences on sociosexual behavior in men. Archives of Sexual Behavior 27: 1–13.

Cutler WB, Friedmann E, McCoy NL 1998b Response to Wysocki & Preti. Archives of Sexual Behavior 27: 629–634.

Cyranowski JM, Bromberger J, Youk A, Matthews K, Kravitz HM, Powell LH 2004 Lifetime depression history and sexual function in women at midlife. Archives of Sexual Behavior 33: 539–548.

Davis SR, McCloud P, Strauss BJG, Burger H 1995 Testosterone enhances estradiol's effects on postmenopausal bone density and sexuality. Maturitas 21: 227–236.

Davis SR, Davison SL, Donath S, Bell RJ 2005 Circulating androgen levels and self-reported sexual function in women. Journal of the American Medical Association 294: 91–96.

Davis SR, van der Mooren MJ, van Lunsen RHW, Lopes P, Ribot J, Rees M, Moufarege A, Rodenburg C, Buch A, Purdie DW 2006a Efficacy and safety of a testosterone patch for the treatment of hypoactive sexual desire disorder in surgically menopausal women: a randomized, placebo-controlled trial. Menopause 13: 387–396.

Davis SR, Goldstat R, Papalia M-A, Shah S, Kulkarni J, Donath S, Bell RJ 2006b Effects of aromatase inhibition on sexual function and well-being in post-menopausal women treated with testosterone: a randomized, placebo-controlled trial. Menopause 13: 37–45.

Dekker J, Everaerd W, Verhelst N 1984 Attending to stimuli or to images of sexual feelings: effects on sexual arousal. Behaviour Research and Therapy 22: 139–149.

Deliganis AV, Maravilla KR, Heiman JR, Carter WO, Garland PA, Peterson BT, Hackbert L, Cao Y, Weiskoff RM 2002 Female genitalia:dynamic MR imaging with use of MS-325. Initial experiences evaluating female sexual response. Radiology 225: 791–799.

Dennerstein L, Burrows GD, Wood C, Hyman G 1980 Hormones and sexuality: effect of estrogen and progestogen. Obstetrics & Gynecology 56: 316–322.

Dennerstein L, Alexander JL, Kotz K 2003 The menopause and sexual functioning: a review of population based studies. Annual Review of Sex Research 14: 64–82.

Derogatis L, Rust J, Golombok S, Bouchard C, Nachtigall L. Rodenberg C, Kuznicki J, McHorney CA 2004 Validation of the profile of female sexual function (PFSF) in surgically and naturally menopausal women. Journal of Sex & Marital Therapy 30: 25–36.

Deysach LJ 1939 The comparative morphology of the erectile tissue of the penis with special emphasis on the probable mechanisms of erection. American Journal of Anatomy 64: 111–132.

Diamond LE, Earle DC, Rosen RC, Willett MS, Molinoff PB 2004 Double-blind, placebo-controlled evaluation of the safety, pharmacokinetic properties and pharmacodynamic effects of intranasal PT-141, a melanocortin receptor agonist, in healthy males and patients with mild-to-moderate erectile dysfunction. International Journal of Impotence Research 16: 51–59.

Diamond LE, Earle DC, Heiman JR, Rosen RC, Perelman MA, Harning R 2006 An effect on the subjective sexual response in premenopausal women with sexual arousal disorder by bremelanotide (PT-141), a melanocortin receptor agonist. Journal of Sexual Medicine 3: 628–638.

Dickinson RL 1933 Human Sexual Anatomy. Bailiiere, Tindall & Cox, London.

Dixson AF 1998 Primate Sexuality: Comparative Studies of the Prosimians, Monkeys, Apes and Human Beings. Oxford University Press, Oxford.

Dixson AF, Kendrick KM, Blank MA, Bloom SR 1984 Effects of tactile and electrical stimuli upon release of vasoactive intestinal polypeptide in the mammalian penis. Journal of Endocrinology 100: 249–252.

Doty RL, Snyuder PJ, Huggins GR, Lowry RA 1981 Endocrine, cardiovascular and psychological correlates of olfactory sensitivity changes during the human menstrual cycle. Journal of Comparative & Physiological Psychology 95: 45–60.

Dow MGT, Gallagher J 1989 A controlled study of combined hormonal and psychological treatment for sexual unresponsiveness in women. British Journal of Clinical Psychology 28: 201–212.

Dufy B, Vincent JD 1980 Effects of sex steroids on cell membrane excitability: a new concept for the action of steroids on the brain. In de Wied D, van Keep PA (eds) Hormones and the Brain. MTP Press, Lancaster, pp. 29–42.

Dunn ME, Trost JE 1989 Male multiple orgasm: a descriptive study. Archives of Sexual Behavior 18: 377–388.

Dunn KM, Cherkas LF, Spector TD 2005 Genetic influences on variation in female orgasmic function: a twin study. Biology Letters 1: 260–263.

Egli M, Bertram R, Sellix MT, Freeman ME 2004 Rhythmic secretion of prolactin in rats: action of oxytocin coordinated by vasoactive intestinal polypeptide of suprachiasmatic nucleus origin. Endocrinology 145: 3386–3394.

Ehrhardt AA, Evers K, Money J 1968 Influence of androgen and some aspects of sexually dimorphic behavior in women with late-treated adrenogenital syndrome. Johns Hopkins Medical Journal 123: 115–122.

Everitt BJ 1995 Neuroendocrine mechanisms underlying appetitive and consummatory elements of masculine sexual behaviour. In Bancroft J (ed) The Pharmacology of Sexual Function and Dysfunction. Elsevier Science, Amsterdam, pp. 15–31.

Everitt BJ, Bancroft J 1991 Of rats and men: the comparative approach to male sexuality. Annual Review of Sex Research 2: 77–118.

Exton MS, Bindert A, Kruger T, Scheller F, Hartmann U, Schedlowski M 1999 Cardiovascular and endocrine alterations after masturbation-induced orgasm in women. Psychosomatic Medicine 61: 280–289.

Eysenck HJ, Eysenck SBG 1968 Manual of the Personality Inventory. Educational and Industrial Testing Service, San Diego, CA.

Farkas GM, Sine LF, Evans IM 1979 The effects of distraction, performance demand, stimulus explicitness, and personality on objective and subjective measures of male sexual arousal. Behaviour Research & Therapy 17: 25–32.

Farquhar CM, Sadler L, Harvey S, McDougall J, Yazdi G, Meuli K 2002 A prospective study of the short-term outcomes of hysterectomy with and without oophorectomy. Australia & New Zealand Journal of Obstetrics & Gynaecology 42: 197–204.

Fausto-Sterling A 2000 Sexing the Body. Basic Books, New York.

Fergusson DM, Horwood JL, Beautrais AL 1999 Is sexual orientation related to mental health problems and suicidality in young people? Archives of General Psychiatry 56: 876–880.

Fernandez-Guasti A, Kruijver FPM, Fodor M, Swaab DF 2000 Sex differences in the distribution of androgen receptors in the human hypothalamus. Journal of Comparative Neurology 425: 422–435.

Finley SK, Kritzer MF 1999 Immunoreactivity for intracellular androgen receptors in identified subpopulations of neurons, astrocytes and oligodendrocytes in primate prefrontal cortex. Journal of Neurobiology 40: 446–457.

Fiorino DF, Coury A, Phillips AG 1997 Dynamic changes in nucleus accumbens dopamine efflux during the coolidge effect in male rats. Journal of Neuroscience 17:4849–4855.

Fisher S 1973 The Female Orgasm. Basic Books, New York.

Fisher WA, White LA, Byrne D, Kelley K 1988 Erotophobia-erotophilia as a dimension of personality. Journal of Sex Research 25: 123–151.

Franks S, Jacobs HS 1983 Hyperprolactinaemia. Clinics in Endocrinology and Metabolism 12: 641–668.

Freedman JL 1998 The effects of population density on humans. In: Freedman JL (ed) Psychological Perspectives on Population. Basic Books, New York, pp. 209–238.

Freeman ME, Kanyicska B, Lerant A, Nagy G 2000 Prolactin: structure, function and regulation of secretion. Physiological Reviews 80: 1523–1631.

Frenken J, Vennix P 1981 Sexuality Experience Scales Manual. Swets and Zeitlinger B.V., Zeist, The Netherlands.

Freud S 1935 A General Introduction to Psychoanalysis (translated by J Riviere). Perma Giants, New York.

Frohlich P, Meston C 2002 Sexual functioning and self-reported depressive symptoms among college women. Journal of Sex Research 39: 321–325.

Fournier GR, Juenemann K-P, Lue TF, Tanagho EA 1987 Mechanism of venous occlusion during canine penile erection: an anatomic demonstration. Journal of Urology 137:163–167.

Fox CA, Fox B 1969 Blood pressure and respiratory patterns during human coitus. Journal of Reproduction and Fertility 19: 405–415.

Gagnon J, Simon W 1973 Sexual Conduct: The Social Sources of Human Sexuality. Aldine, Chicago.

Garcia-Velasco J, Mondragon M 1991 The incidence of the vomero-nasal organ in 1000 human subjects and its possible clinical significance. Journal of Steroid Biochemistry 39: 561–563.

Garde K, Lunde I 1980 Female sexual behaviour. A study in a random sample of 40 year old women. Maturitas 2: 225–240.

Gebhard PH, Johnson AB 1979 The Kinsey Data: Marginal Tabulations of the 1935–1965 Interviews Conducted by the Institute for Sex Research. Saunders, Philadelphia.

Geer JH, Bellard HS 1996 Sexual content induced delays in unprimed lexical decisions: gender and context effects. Archives of Sexual Behavior 25: 379–395.

Geer JH, Fuhr R 1976 Cognitive factors in sexual arousal. The role of distraction. Journal of Consulting and Clinical Psychology 44: 238–243.

Geer JH, Melton JS 1997 Sexual content-induced delay with double-entendre words. Archives of Sexual Behavior 26: 295–316.

Geer JH, Judice S, Jackson S 1994 Reading time for erotic material; the pause to reflect. Journal of General Psychology 121: 345–352.

Gillman M, Lichtigfield F 1983 The effects of nitrous oxide and naloxone on orgasm in human females: a preliminary report. Journal of Sex Research 19: 49–57.

Gilman DP, Westbrook WH 1978 Mating preference and sexual reinforcement in female rats. Physiology and Behavior 20: 11–14.

Giraldi A, Levin R 2005 Vascular physiology of female sexual function. In Goldstein I, Meston CM, Davis SR, Traish AM (eds) Women's Sexual Function and Dysfunction; Study, Diagnosis and Treatment. Taylor & Francis, London, pp. 174–180.

Giuliano F, Rampin O, Allard J 2002 Neurophysiology and pharmacology of female genital response. Journal of Sex & Marital Therapy 28(Suppl 1): 101–121.

Goldstat R, Briganti E, Tran J, Wolfe R, Davis SR 2003 Transdermal testosterone therapy improves well-being, mood and sexual function in premenopausal women. Menopause 10: 390–398.

Goodall J 1986 The Chimpanzees of Gombe: Patterns of Behavior. Belknap Press, Harvard.

Gooren LJG 1985 Human male sexual functions do not require aromatization of testosterone: a study of tamoxifen, testolactone, and dihydrotestosterone. Archives of Sexual Behavior 14: 539–548.

Gooren LJG 1986 The neuroendocrine response of lutcinizing hormone to estrogen administration in heterosexual, homosexual and transsexual subjects. Journal of Clinical Endocrinilogy and Metabolism 63: 583–588.

Gooren LJG 1988 Hypogonadotropic hypogonadal men respond less well to androgen substitution treatment than hypergonadotropic hypogonadal men. Archives of Sexual Behavior 17: 265–270.

Gooren LJG, Saad F 2006 Recent insights into androgen action on the anatomical and physiological substrate of penile erection. Asian Journal of Andrology 8: 3–9.

Gorski RA 2000 Sexual differentiation of the nervous system. In Kandel ER, Schwartz JH, Jesell TM (eds) Principles of Neural Science. McGraw-Hill, New York, pp. 1131–1148.

Graber B, Kline-Graber G 1979 Female orgasm — role of pubococcygeus. Journal of Clinical Psychiatry 40: 34–39.

Graber B, Rohrbaugh JW, Newlin DB, Varner JL, Ellingson RJ 1985 EEG during masturbation and ejaculation. Archives of Sexual Behavior 14: 491–504.

Grafenberg E 1950 The role of the urethra in female orgasm. International Journal of Sexology 3: 145–148.

Graham CA, McGrew WC 1980 Menstrual synchrony in female undergraduates living on a coeducational campus. Psychoneuroendocrinology 5: 245–252.

Graham CA, Janssen E, Sanders SA 2000 Effects of fragrance on female sexual arousal and mood across the menstrual cycle. Psychophysiology 37: 76–84.

Graham CA, Sanders SA, Milhausen RR, McBride KR 2003 Turning on and turning off: a focus group study of the factors that affect women's sexual arousal. Archives of Sexual Behavior 33: 527–538.

Gray JA 1987 The Psychology of Fear and Stress. Cambridge University Press: Cambridge.

Gray JA 1994 Three fundamental emotion systems. In Eckman P, Davidson RJ (eds) The Nature of Emotion: Fundamental Questions. Oxford University Press, Oxford, pp. 243–247.

Grumbach MM, Auchus RJ 1999 Estrogen: consequences and implications of mutations in synthesis and action. Journal of Clinical Endocrinology & Metabolism 84: 4677–4694.

Halbreich U, Kinon BJ, Gilmore JA, Kahn LS 2003 Elevated prolactin levels in patients with schizophrenia: mechanisms and related adverse effects. Psychoneuroendocrinology 28: 53–67.

Hale VE, Strassberg DS 1990 The role of anxiety in sexual arousal. Archives of Sexual Behavior 19: 569–581.

Halpern CJT, Udry JR, Campbell B, Suchindran C 1993 Testosterone and pubertal development as predictors of sexual activity: a panel analysis of adolescent males. Psychosomatic Medicine 55: 436–447.

Halpern CJT, Udry JR, Suchindran C 1997 Testosterone predicts initiation of coitus in adolescent females. Psychosomatic Medicine 59: 161–171.

Hamann S, Herman RA, Nolan CL, Wallen K 2004 Men and women differ in amygdala response to visual sexual stimuli. Nature Neuroscience 7: 411–416.

Hansen CH, Hansen RD 1988 Finding the face in the crowd: an anger superiority effect. Journal of Personality and Social Psychology 54: 917–924.

Hart BL, Leedy MG 1985 Neurological bases of male sexual behavior: a comparative analysis. In: Adler N, Goy RW, Pfaff DW (eds) Handbook of Behavioral Neurobiology, vol. 7. Plenum, New York, pp. 373–342.

Hatfield E, Rapson RL 1993 Love, Sex and Intimacy: Their Psychology, Biology and History. Harper Collins, New York.

Heath RG 1972 Pleasure and brain activity in man. Journal of Nervous and Mental Diseases 154: 3–18.

Heaton JPW 2000 Central neuropharmacological agents and mechanisms in erectile dysfunction: the role of dopamine. Neuroscience and Biobehavioral Reviews 24: 561–570.

Hedricks CA 1994 Female sexual activity across the human menstrual cycle: a biopsychosocial approach. Annual Review of Sex Research 5: 122–172.

Heiman J 1977 A psychophysiological exploration of sexual arousal patterns in females and mates. Psychophysiology 14: 266–273.

Heiman JR, Maravilla KR 2007 Female sexual arousal response using serial magnetic resonance imaging with initial comparisons to vaginal photo-plethysmography: overview and evaluation. In Janssen E (ed) Sexual Psychophysiology. Indiana University Press, Bloomington, pp. 103–128.

Heiman JR, Rowland DL 1983 Affective and physiological sexual response patterns: the effects of instructions on sexually functional and dysfunctional men. Journal of Psychosomatic Research 27: 105–116.

Henson DE, Rubin HB 1971 Voluntary control of eroticism. Journal of Applied Behavioral Analysis 4: 37–47.

Herbert J 1993 Peptides in the limbic system: neurochemical codes for co-ordinated adaptive responses to behavioural and physiological demand. Progress in Neurobiology 41: 723–791.

Herbert J 1995 Neuropeptides, stress and sexuality: towards a new psychopharmacology. In Bancroft J (Ed), The Pharmacology of Sexual Function and Dysfunction. Excerpta Medica International Congress Series 1075, Amsterdam, pp. 77–92.

Higgins GE 1979 Sexual response in spinal cord injured adults: a review. Archives of Sexual Behavior 8: 173–196.

Hilliges M, Falconer C, Ekman-Ordeberg G, Johansson O 1995 Innervation of the human vaginal mucosa as revealed by PGP9.5 immunohistochemistry. Acta Anat (Basel) 153: 119–126.

Hines TM 2001 The G-Spot: a modern gynecological myth. American Journal of Obstetrics and Gynecology 185: 359–362.

Hines M 2004 Brain Gender. Oxford University Press, Oxford.

Hite S 1976 The Hite Report. Talmy Franklin, London.

Hoffmann H, Janssen E, Turner SL 2004 Classical conditioning of sexual arousal in women and men: effects of varying awareness and biological relevance of the conditioned stimulus. Archives of Sexual Behavior 33: 45–53.

Holstege G, Georgiadis JR, Paans AMJ, Meiners LC, van der Graaf FHCE, Reinders AATS 2003 Brain activation during human male ejaculation. The Journal of Neuroscience 23: 9185–9193.

Hoon PW, Wincze JP, Hoon EF 1977 The effects of biofeedback and cognitive mediation upon vaginal blood volume. Behaviour Research and Therapy 8: 694–702.

Hoyt RF 2006 Innervation of the vagina and vulva. In Goldstein I, Meston CM, Davis SR, Traish AM (eds) Women's Sexual Function and Dysfunction; Study, Diagnosis And Treatment. Taylor & Francis, London, pp. 113–124.

Huffman JW 1948 The detailed anatomy of the periurethral ducts in the adult human female. American Journal of Obstetrics and Gynecology 55: 86–100.

Hull EM, Du J, Lorrain DS, Matuszewich L 1995 Extracellular dopamine in the medial preoptic area: implications for sexual motivation and hormonal control of copulation. Journal of Neuroscience 15: 7465–7471.

Hull EM, Lorrain DS, Du J, Matuszewich L, Bitran D, Nishita JK, Scaletta LL. 1998 Organizational and activational effects of dopamine on male sexual behavior. In Ellis L, Eberty L (Eds). Male/female differences in behavior: Toward biological understanding. Greenwood Press, New York NY, pp. 79–96.

Ignarro LJ, Bush PA, Buga GM, Wood KS, Fukuto JM, Rajfer J 1990 Nitric oxide and cyclic GMP formation upon electrical field stimulation cause relaxation of corpus cavernosum smooth muscle. Biochemistry & Biophysics Research Communications 170: 843–850.

Insel TR 1992 Oxytocin: a neuropeptide for affiliation: evidence from behavioral, receptor autoradiographic, and comparative studies. Psychoneuroendocrinology 17: 3–35.

Iversen S, Kupfermann I, Kandell ER 2000 Emotional states and feelings. In Kandel ER, Schwartz JH, Jessell TM (eds) Principles of Neuroscience, 4th edition. McGraw-Hill, New York, pp. 982–997.

Jaffe Y, Malamuth N, Feingold J, Feshback I 1974 Sexual arousal and behavioural aggression. Journal of Personality and Social Psychology 30: 759–764.

Jannini EA, d'Amati G, Lenzi A 2006 Histology and immunohistochemical studies of female genital tissue. In Goldstein I, Meston CM, Davis SR, Traish AM (eds) Women's Sexual Function and Dysfunction; Study, Diagnosis and Treatment. Taylor & Francis, London, pp. 125–133.

Janssen E (ed) 2007 The Psychophysiology of Sex. Indiana University Press, Bloomington.

Janssen E, Everaerd W 1993 Determinants of male sexual arousal. Annual Review of Sex Research 4: 211–245.

Janssen E, Everaerd W, Spiering M, Janssen J 2000 Automatic processes and the appraisal of sexual stimuli: toward an information processing model of sexual arousal. Journal of Sex Research 37: 8–23.

Janssen E, Vorst H, Finn P, Bancroft J 2002 The Sexual Inhibition (SIS) and Sexual Excitation (SES) Scales: I. Measuring sexual inhibition and excitation proneness in men. Journal of Sex Research 39: 114–126.

Kahn F 1931 Das leben des menschen:eine volstumliche anatomie, biologie, physiologie und entwicklungsgeschichte des menschen. Kosmos, Stuttgart.

Kalichman SC, Kelly JA, Morgan M, Rompa D 1997 Fatalism, current life satisfaction, and risk for HIV infection among gay and bisexual men. Journal of Consulting & Clinical Psychology 65: 542–546.

Kandel ER 2000 The brain and behavior. In Kandel ER, Schwartz JH, Jessell TM (eds) Principles of Neuroscience, 4th edition. McGraw-Hill, New York, pp. 5–18.

Karama S, Lecours AR, Leroux JM, Bourgouin P, Beaudoin G, Joubert S, Beauregard M 2002 Areas of brain activation in males and females during viewing of erotic film excerpts. Human Brain Mapping 16:1–13.

Katzenstein L 2001 Viagra (Sildenafil Citrate): the Remarkable Story of the Discovery and Launch. Medical Information Press, New York.

Kelly DD 1991 Sexual differentiation of the nervous system. In Kandel ER, Schwartz JH, Jessell TM (eds) Principles of Neural Science. Appleton & Lange, Norwalk, pp. 959–973.

Kenney MJ, Seals DR 1993 Postexercise hypotension. Key features, mechanisms, and clinical significance. Hypertension 22: 653–664.

Keverne EB 1978 Olfactory cues in mammalian sexual behaviour. In: Hutchison JB (ed) Biological Determinants of Sexual Behaviour. Wiley, Chichester, pp. 727–763.

Keverne EB, Velluci SV 1988 Social, endocrine and pharmacological influences on primate behavior. In Sitsen JMA (ed) Handbook of Sexology, the Pharmacology and Endocrinology of Sexual Function. Elsevier Science, Amsterdam, pp. 265–296.

Kinsey AC, Pomeroy WB, Martin CF 1948 Sexual Behavior in the Human Male. Saunders, Philadelphia.

Kinsey AC, Pomeroy WB, Martin CF, Gebhard PH 1953 Sexual Behavior in the Human Female. Saunders, Philadelphia.

Kolodny RC, Masters WH, Johnson VE 1979 Textbook of Sexual Medicine. Little, Brown, Boston.

Komisaruk BR 1971 Induction of lordosis in ovariectomized rats by stimulation of the vaginal cervix: hormonal and neural interrelationships. In Sawyer CH, Gorski RA (eds) Steroid Hormones and Brain Function. University of California Press, Berkeley, pp. 127–135.

Komisaruk BR, Sansone G 2003 Neural pathways mediating vaginal function: the vagus nerves and spinal cord oxytocin. Scandinavian Journal of Psychology 44: 241–250.

Komisaruk BR, Whipple B 1995 The suppression of pain by genital stimulation in females. Annual Review of Sex Research 6: 151–186.

Komisaruk BR, Whipple B 2005 Functional MRI of the brain during orgasm in women. Annual Review of Sex Research 15: 1–25.

Komisaruk BR, Beyer-Flores C, Whipple B 2007 The Science of Orgasm. The Johns Hopkins University Press, Baltimore.

Korenchevsky V 1937 The female prostatic gland and its reaction to male sexual compounds. Journal of Physiology 90: 371–376.

Kuffel SW, Heiman JR 2006 Effect of depressive symptoms and experimentally adopted schemas on sexual arousal and affect in sexually healthy women. Archives of Sexual Behavior 35: 163–178.

Kupfermann I 1991 Hypothalamus and limbic system: peptidergic neurons, homeostasis, and emotional behavior. In Kandel ER, Schwartz JH, Jessell TM (eds) Principles of Neural Science, 3rd edition. Appleton & Lange, Norwalk, pp. 735–760.

Krantz KE 1958 Innervation of the human vulva and vagina. Obstetrics and Gynecology 12: 382.

Krüger T, Exton MS, Pawlak C, von zur Muhlen A, Hartmann U, Schedlowski M 1998 Neuroendocrine and cardiovascular response to sexual arousal and orgasm in men. Psychoneuroendocrinology 23: 401–411.

Krüger THC, Haake P, Hartmann U, Schedlowski M, Exton MS 2002 Orgasm-induced prolactin secretion: feedback control of sexual drive? Neuroscience and Biobehavioral Reviews 26: 31–44.

Krüger THC, Haake P, Chereath D, Knapp W, Janssen OE, Exton MS, Schedlowski M, Hartmann U 2003a Specificity of the neuroendocrine response to orgasm during sexual arousal in men. Journal of Endocrinology 177: 57–64.

Krüger THC, Exton MS, Pawlak C, von zur Muhlen A, Hartmann U, Schedlowski M 2003b Neuroendocrine and cardiovascular response to sexual arousal and orgasm in men. Psychoneuroendocrinology 23: 401–411.

Krüger THC, Schledowski M, Exton MS 2007 Neuroendocrine processes during sexual arousal and orgasm. In Janssen E (ed) Sexual Psychophysiology. Indiana University Press, Bloomington, pp. 83–102.

Kuhn RA 1950 Functional capacity of the isolated human spinal cord. Brain 73: 1.

Kurtz RG, Adler NT 1973 Electrophysiological correlates of copulatory behavior in the male rat: evidence for a sexual inhibitory process. Journal of Comparative and Physiological Psychology 84: 225–239.

Laan E, Everaerd W 1995 Determinants of sexual arousal: psychophysiological theory and data. Annual Review of Sex Research 6: 32–76.

Labrie F, Luu-The V, Labrie C, Belanger A, Simard J, Lin S-X, Pelletier G 2003 Endocrine and intracrine sources of androgens in women; inhibition of breast cancer and other roles of androgens and their precursor dehydroepiandrosterone. Endocrine Reviews 24: 152–182.

Lalumiere ML, Quinsey VL 1998 Pavlovian conditioning of sexual interests in human males. Archives of Sexual Behavior 27: 241–252.

Lang PJ, Bradley MM, Cuthbert BN 1990 Emotion, attention and the startle reflex. Psychological Review 97: 377–395.

Laumann EO, Gagnon JH, Michael RT, Michaels S 1994 The Social Organization of Sexuality: Sexual Practices in the United States. University of Chicago Press, Chicago.

Laws DR, Rubin HB 1969 Instructional control of an autonomic sexual response. Journal of Applied Behavioral Analysis 2: 93–99.

LeDoux J 1996 The Emotional Brain. Simon & Schuster, New York.

Letourneau EJ, O'Donohue W 1997 Classical conditioning of female sexual arousal. Archives of Sexual Behavior 26: 63–78.

Levi L 1969 Sympatho-adreno-medullary activity, diuresis and emotional reactions during visual sexual stimulation in human females and males. Psychosomatic Medicine 31: 251–268.

Levin RM 1992 The mechanisms of human female sexual arousal. Annual Review of Sex Research 3: 1–48.

Levin RM 2001 Sexual desire and the deconstruction and reconstruction of the human female sexual response model of Masters & Johnson.

In Everaerd W, Laan E, Both S (eds) Sexual Appetite, Desire and Motivation: Energetics of the Sexual System. Royal Netherlands Academy of Arts & Sciences, Amsterdam, pp. 63–93.

Levin RM 2003a The ins and outs of vaginal lubrication. Sexual & Relationship Therapy 18: 509–513.

Levin RM 2003b The G-spot — reality or illusion? Sexual & Relationship Therapy 18: 117–119.

Levin RJ 2005a The mechanisms of human ejaculation — a critical analysis. Sexual & Relationship Therapy 20: 123–131.

Levin RJ 2005b Sexual arousal –its physiological roles in human reproduction. Annual Review of Sex Research 16: 154–189.

Levin RM 2007 Discussant. In Janssen E (ed) Sexual Psychophysiology. Indiana University Press, Bloomington, pp. 129–136.

Levin RJ, Wagner G 1985 Orgasm in women in the laboratory — quantitative studies on duration, intensity, latency and vaginal blood flow. Archives of Sexual Behavior 14: 439–450.

Levin RM, Wagner G 1997 Human vaginal blood flow — absolute assessment by a new quantitative heat wash-out method. Journal of Physiology London 504P: 188P–189P.

Levin RM, Wein AJ 1980 Adrenergic alpha receptors outnumber beta receptors in human penile corpus cavernosum. Investigative Urology 18: 225.

Lewis RW, Mills TM 2004 Effect of androgens on penile tissue. Endocrine 23: 101–105.

Littler WA, Honour AJ, Sleight P 1974 Direct arterial pressure, heart rate and electrocardiogram during human coitus. Journal of Reproduction and Fertility 40: 321–331.

Lloyd EA 2005 The Case of the Female Orgasm: Bias in the Science of Evolution. Harvard University Press, Cambridge.

Lockhart AB, Thrall PH, Antonovics J 1996 Sexually transmitted diseases in animals: ecological and evolutionary implications. Biological Reviews 71: 415–471.

Lorrain DS, Matuszewich L, Hull EM 1997 Extracellular serotonin in the lateral hypothalamic area increases during postejaculatory interval and impairs copulation in male rats. Journal of Neuroscience 17: 9361–9366.

Lorrain DS, Matuszewich L, Hull EM 1998 8-OH-DPAT influences extracellular levels of serotonin and dopamine in the medial preoptic area of male rats. Brain Research 790: 217–223.

Lundberg PO 1992 Sexual dysfunction in patients with neurological disorders. Annual Review of Sex Research 3: 121–150.

Lykins AD, Janssen E, Graham CA 2006 The relationship between negative mood and sexuality in heterosexual college women and men. Journal of Sex Research 43: 136–143.

Mah K, Binik YM 2001 The nature of human orgasm; a critical review of major trends. Clinical Psycology Review 21: 823–856.

Mancia G 1993 Autonomic modulation of the cardiovascular system during sleep. New England Journal of Medicine 328: 347–349.

Maravilla KR 2006 Blood flow: magnetic resonance imaging and brain imaging for evaluating sexual arousal in women. In Goldstein I, Meston CM, Davis SR, Traish AM (eds) Women's Sexual Function and Dysfunction: Study, Diagnosis and Treatment. Taylor & Francis, London, pp. 368–382.

Maravilla KR, Cao Y, Heiman JR, Yang C, Garland PA, Peterson BT, Carter WO 2005 Noncontrast dynamic magnetic resonance imaging for quantitative assessment of female sexual arousal. Journal of Urology 173: 162–166.

Marazziti D, Canale D 2004 Hormonal changes when falling in love. Psychoneuroendocrinology 29: 931–936.

Marks I, Gelder MG, Bancroft J 1970 Sexual deviants two years after electric aversion. British Journal of Psychiatry 117: 173–186.

Marson L, McKenna KE 1992 A role for 5-hydroxytryptamine in descending inhibition of spinal sexual reflexes. Experimental Brain Research 88: 313–320.

Martin-Alguacil N, Schober J, Kow L-M, Pfaff D 2006 Arousing properties of the vulvar epithelium. Journal of Urology 176: 456–462.

Mas M, Fumero B, Perez-Rodriguez I, Gonzalez-Mora JL 1995 The neurochemistry of sexual satiety. An experimental model of inhibited desire. In Bancroft J (ed) The Pharmacology of Sexual Function and Dysfunction. Excerpta Medica, Amsterdam, pp. 115–126.

Masters WH, Johnson VE 1966 Human Sexual Response. Churchill, London.

Masters WH, Johnson VE 1970 Human Sexual Inadequacy. Churchill, London.

Mathew RJ, Weinman ML 1982 Sexual dysfunction in depression. Archives of Sexual Behavior 11: 323–328.

Mathews A, Whitehead A, Kellett J 1983 Psychological and hormona: factors in the treatment of female sexual dysfunction. Psychological Medicine 13: 83–92.

McClintock M 1971 Menstrual synchrony and suppression. Nature 229: 244–245.

McClintock MK, Adler NT 1978 The role of the female during copulation in wild and domestic Norway rats (Rattus norvegicus). Behaviour 67: 67–96.

McIntosh TK, Barfield RJ 1984 Brain monoaminergic control of male reproductive behavior. III. Norepinephrine and the post-ejaculatory refractory period. Behavior & Brain Research 12: 275–281.

McKenna KE 1999 Central nervous system pathways involved in the control of penile erection. Annual Review of Sex Research 10: 157–183.

McKenna KE 2000 Some proposals regarding the organization of the central nervous system control of penile erection. Neuroscience and Biobehavioral Reviews 24: 535–540.

Meisel RL, Sachs BD 1994 The physiology of male sexual behavior. In Knobil E, Neill JD (eds) The Physiology of Reproduction, 2nd edition. Raven Press, New York, pp. 3–105.

Meisler AW, Carey MP 1991 Depressed affect and male sexual arousal. Archives of Sexual Behavior 20: 541–554.

Melis MR, Argiolas A 1995 Dopamine and sexual behavior. Neuroscience and Biobehavioral Reviews 19, 19–38.

Meston CM, Bradford A 2007 Autonomic nervous system influences: the role of the sympathetic nervous system in female sexual arousal. In Janssen E (ed) Sexual Psychophysiology. Indiana University Press, Bloomington, pp. 66–82.

Meston CM, Gorzalka BB 1996a The differential effects of sympathetic activation on sexual arousal in sexually functional and dysfunctional women. Journal of Abnormal Psychology 105: 582–591.

Meston CM, Gorzalka BB 1996b The effects of immediate, delayed and residual sympathetic activation on sexual arousal in women. Behaviour Research & Therapy, 34: 143–148.

Meston CM, Heiman J 1998 Ephedrine activated physiological sexual arousal in women. Archives of General Psychiatry 55: 652–656.

Meston CM, Worcel M 2002 The effects of yohimbine plus l-arginine glutamate on sexual arousal in postmenopausal women with sexual arousal disorder. Archives of Sexual Behavior 31: 323–332.

Meston CM, Gorzalka BB, Wright JM 1997 Inhibition of subjective and physiological sexual arousal in women by clonidine. Journal of Psychosomatic Medicine 59: 399–407.

Meston CM, Levin RJ, Sipski ML, Hull EM, Heiman JR 2004 Women's orgasm. Annual Review of Sex Research 15: 173–258.

Meyer-Bahlburg HFL, Baker SW, Dolezal C, Carlson AD, Obeid JS, New MI 2003 Long-term outcome in congenital adrenal hyperplasia: gender and sexuality. The Endocrinologist 13: 227–232.

Michael RP, Bonsall RW, Warner P 1974 Human vaginal secretions: volatile fatty acid content. Science 186: 1217–1219.

Michael RP, Rees HD, Bonsall RW 1989 Sites in the male primate brain at which testosterone acts as an androgen. Brain Research 502: 11–20.

Miller K, Biller BMK, Beauregard C, Lipman JG, Jones J, Schoenfeld D, Sherman JC, Swearingen B, LoefflerJ, Klibanski A 2001 Androgen deficiency in women with hypopituitarism. Journal of Clinical Endocrinology & Metabolism 86: 1683.

Miller K, Sesmilo G, Schiller A, Schoenfeld D, Burton S, Klibanski A 2006 Effects of testosterone replacement in androgen deficient women with hypopituitarism: a randomized, double-blind, placebo-controlled study. Journal of Clinical Endocrinology & Metabolism 91: 561–567.

Minto CL, Liao KL-M, Conway GS, Creighton SM 2003 Sexual function in women with complete androgen insensitivity syndrome. Fertility & Sterility 80: 157–164.

Mitchell WB, Marten PA, Williams DM, Barlow DH 1998 Effects of positive and negative mood on sexual arousal in sexually functional males. Archives of Sexual Behavior 27: 197–207.

Money J, Ehrhardt AA 1972 Man & Woman, Boy & Girl: Differentiation and Dimorphism of Gender Identity from Conception to Maturity. Johns Hopkins University Press, Baltimore.

Money J, Yankowitz R 1967 The sympathetic inhibiting effects of the drug Ismelin on human male eroticism, with a note on Melleril. Journal of Sex Research 3: 69–82.

Montgomery SA, Baldwin DS, Riley A 2002 Antidepressant medications: a review of the evidence for drug-induced sexual dysfunction. Journal of Affective Disorders 69: 119–140.

Montorsi F, Oettel M 2005 Testosterone and sleep-related erections: an overview. Journal of Sexual Medicine 2: 771–784.

Moore MM 1985 Nonverbal courtship patterns in women: context and consequences. Ethology & Sociobiology 6: 237–247.

Moore MM 1995 Courtship signaling and adolescents: "Girls just wanna have fun"? Journal of Sex Research 32: 319–328.

Morales AJ, Nolan JJ, Nelson JC, Yen SSC 1994 Effects of replacement dose of dehydroepiandrosterone in men and women of advancing age. Journal of Clinical Endocrinology & Metabolism 78: 1360–1367.

Morris NM, Udry JR 1978 Pheromonal influences on human sexual behavior: an experimental search. Journal of Biosocial Science 10: 147–157.

Morokoff PJ, Heiman JR 1980 Effects if erotic stimuli on sexually functional and dysfunctional women: multiple measures before and after sex therapy. Behaviour Research & Therapy, 18: 127–137.

Mosovich A, Tallafero A 1954 Studies on EEG and sex function at orgasm. Diseases of the Nervous System 15: 218–220.

Moulier VG, Mouras H, Pelegrini-Issac M, Glutron D, Rouxel R, Grandjean B, Bittoun J, Stoleru S 2006 Neuroanatomical correlates of penile erection evoked by photographic stimuli in human males. Neuroimage 33: 689–699.

Mouras H, Stoleru S 2007 Functional neuroanatomy of sexual arousal. In: Kandeel F, Lue T, Pryor J, Swerdloff R (eds) Male Sexual Dysfunction: Pathophysiology and Treatment. Marcel Dekker, New York.

Mouras H, Stoleru S, Moulier VG, Pelegrini-Issac M, Rouxel R, Grandjean B, Glutron D, Bittoun J 2007 Activation of mirror-neuron system by erotic vide-clips predicts degree of induced erection. Neuroimage.

Munoz M, Bancroft J, Turner M 1994a Evaluating the effects of an alpha-2 adrenoceptor antagonist on erectile function in the human male. I. The erectile response to erotic stimuli in volunteers. Psychopharmacology 115: 463–470.

Munoz M, Bancroft J, Beard M 1994b Evaluating the effects of an alpha-2 adrenoceptor antagonist on erectile function in the human male. II. The erectile response to erotic stimuli in men with erectile dysfunction, in relation to age and in comparison with normal volunteers. Psychopharmacology 115: 471–477.

Murphy MR, Seckl JR, Burton S, Checkley SA, Lightman SL 1987 Changes in oxytocin and vasopressin secretion during sexual activity in men. Journal of Clinical Endocrinology & Metabolism 65: 738–741.

Murray MAF, Bancroft JHJ, Anderson DC, Tennent TG, Carr PJ 1975 Endocrine changes in male sexual deviants after treatment with anti-androgens, oestrogens or tranquillizers. Journal of Endocrinology 67: 179–188.

Mustanski B 2007 The influence of state and trait affect on HIV risk behaviours: a daily diary study of MSM. Health Psychology 26: 618–626.

Mustanski B, Bancroft J 2006 Sexual dysfunction: neurobiological, pharmacological and genetic consideration. In Gorwood P, Hamon M (eds) Psychopharmacogenetics. Springer, New York, pp 479–494.

Myers LS, Dixen J, Morrissette D, Carmichael M, Davidson JM 1990 Effects of estrogen, androgen, and progestin on sexual psychophysiology and behavior in postmenopausal women. J Clinical Endocrinology & Metabolism 70: 1124–1131.

Nakamura Y, Yamamoto Y, Muraoka I 1993 Autonomic control of heart rate during physical exercise and fractal dimension of heart rate variability. Journal of Applied Physiology 74: 875–881.

Nathorst-Böös J, von Schoultz B, Carlström K 1993a Elective ovarian removal and estrogen replacement therapy — effects on sexual life, psychological wellbeing and androgen status. Journal of Psychosomatic Obstetrics & Gynaecology 14: 283–293.

Nathorst-Böös J, Wiklund I, Mattson LA, Sandin K, von Schoultz B 1993b Is sexual life influenced by transdermal estrogen therapy? A double blind placebo controlled study in postmenopausal women. Acta Obstetrica & Gynecologica Scandinavica 72: 656–660.

Nishimori K, Young LJ, Guo Q, Wang Z, Insel TR, Matzuk MM 1996 Oxytocin is required for nursing but not essential for parturition or reproductive behavior. Proceedings of the National Academy of Science USA 93: 1699–1704.

Nofzinger EA, Thase ME, Reynolds CF III, Frank E, Jennings JR, Garamoni GL, Fasiczka AL, Kupfer DJ 1993 Sexual function in depressed men: assessment by self-report, behavioral, and nocturnal penile tumescence measures before and after treatment with cognitive behavior therapy. Archives of General Psychiatry 50: 24–30.

O'Carroll RE, Shapiro C, Bancroft J 1985 Androgens, behaviour and nocturnal erections in hypogonadal men: the effect of varying the replacement dose. Clinical Endocrinology 23: 527–538.

O'Connell HE, Sanjeevan KV 2006 Anatomy of female genitalia. In Goldstein I, Meston CM, Davis SR, Traish AM (eds) Women's Sexual Function and Dysfunction; Study, Diagnosis and Treatment. Taylor & Francis, London, pp. 105–112.

O'Connor DB, Archer J, Wu FCW 2004 Effects of testosterone on mood, aggression, and sexual behavior in young men: a double-blind, placebo-controlled, cross-over study. Journal of Clinical Endocrinology & Metabolism 89: 2837–2845.

O'Donohue W, Plaud JJ 1994 The conditioning of human sexual arousal. Archives of Sexual Behavior 23: 321–344.

Oriel JD, Hayward AHS 1974 Sexually-transmitted diseases in animals. British Journal of Venereal Diseases 50: 412–420.

Ottesen B, Wagner G, Virag R, Fahrenkrug J 1984 Penile erection: a possible role for vasoactive intestinal polypeptide as a neurotransmitter. British Medical Journal 288: 9–11.

Ottesen B, Pedersen B, Nielsen J, Dalgaard D, Wagner G, Farhenkrug J 1987 Vasoactive intestinal polypeptide provokes vaginal lubrication in women. Peptides 8: 797–800.

Over R, Koukounas E 1995 Habituation of sexual arousal: product and process. Annual Review of Sex Research 6: 187–223.

Palace EM, Gorzalka BB 1990 The enhancing effects of anxiety on arousal in sexually dysfunctional and functional women. Journal of Abnormal Psychology 99: 403–411.

Parades RG, Alonso A 1997 Sexual behavior regulated (paced) by the female induces conditioned place preference. Behavioural Neuroscience 111: 123–128.

Park K, Kang HK, Seo JJ, Kim HJ, Ryu SB Jeong GW 2001 Blood-oxygenation-level-dependent functional magnetic resonance imaging for evaluating cerebral regions of female sexual arousal response. Urology 57: 1189–1194.

Parmeggiana PL, Morrison AR 1990 Alterations in autonomic functions during sleep. In Loewy AD, Spyer KM (eds) Central Regulation of Autonomic Functions. Oxford University Press, New York, pp. 367–386.

Paton JFR, Boscan P, Pickering AE, Nalivaiko E 2005 The yin and yang of cardiac autonomic control: vago-sympathetic interactions revisited. Brain Research Reviews 49: 555–565.

Perry JD, Whipple B 1981 Pelvic muscle strength of female ejaculators: evidence in support of a new theory of orgasm. Journal of Sex Research 17: 22–39.

Pfaff DW 1999 Drive: Neurobiological and Molecular Mechanisms of Sexual Motivation. MIT Press, Cambridge, MA.

Pfaus JG 2006 Of rats and women: preclinical insights into the nature of female sexual desire. Sexual and Relationship Therapy 21: 463–476.

Pfaus JG, Gorzalka BB 1987 Opioids and sexual behavior. Neuroscience and Biobehavioral Reviews 11: 1–34.

Pfaus, JG, Kippin TE, Coria-Avila G 2003 What can animal models tell us about human sexual response. Annual Review of Sex Research 14: 1–63.

Pfaus JG, Shadiak A, Van Soest T, Tse M, Molino P 2004 Selective facilitation of sexual solicitation in the female rat by a melanocortin receptor agonist. Proceedings of the National Academy of Science 101: 10201–10204.

Pollen JJ, Dreilinger A 1984 Immunohistochemical identification of prostatic acid phosphatase and prostate specific antigens in female periurethral glands. Urology 23:303–304.

Posner MI 1994 Attention: the mechanisms of consciousness. Proceedings of the National Academy of Sciences of the United States of America 91, 7398–7403.

Powell K 2006 Neurodevelopment: how does the teenage brain work? Nature 442: 865–867.

Price KP 1973 Feedback effects of penile tumescence. Paper presented at Eastern Psychological Association, Washington, DC, May 1973.

Przybyla DPJ, Byrne D 1984 The mediating role of cognitive processes in self-reported sexual arousal. Journal of Research in Personality 18: 54–63.

Puts DA 2006 Review of the case of the female orgasm by Lloyd EA. Archives of Sexual Behavior 35: 103–108.

Puy L, MacLusky NJ, Becker L, Karsan N, Trachtenberg J, Brown TJ 1995 Immuno-cytochemical detection of androgen receptor in human temporal cortex: characterization and application of polyclonal androgen receptor antibodies in frozen and paraffin-embedded tissues. Journal of Steroid Biochemistry & Molecular Biology 55: 197–209.

Rachman S 1966 Sexual fetishism: an experimental analogue. Psychological Record 16: 293–296.

Ramsey GV 1943 The sexual development of boys. American Journal of Psychology 56: 217–234.

Rao SP, Collins HL, DiCarlo SE 2002 Postexercise alpha-adrenergic receptor hyporesponsiveness in hypertensive rats due to nitric oxide. American Journal Physiology Regulatory Integrative Comparative Physiology 282: R960–R968.

Rechtschaffen A, Siegel J 2000 Sleep and dreaming. In Kandel ER, Schwartz JH, Jessell TM (eds) Principles of Neuroscience, 4th edition. McGraw-Hill, New York. pp. 936–947.

Redoute J, Stoleru S, Grégoire MC, Costes N, Cinotti L, Lavenne F, Le Bars D, Forest MG, Pujol J-F 2000 Brain processing of visual sexual stimuli in human males. Human Brain Mapping 11: 162–177.

Redoute J, Stoleru S, Pugeat M, Costes N, Lavenne F, Le Bars D, Dechaud H, Cinotti L, Pujol J-F 2005 Brain processing of visual sexual stimuli in treated and untreated hypogonadal patients. Psychoneuroendocrinology 30: 461–482.

Rehman J, Melman A 2001 Normal anatomy and physiology. In Mulcahy JJ (ed) Male Sexual Function: a Guide to Clinical Management. Humana Press, Totowa, pp. 1–46.

Resko JA, Quadri SK, Spies HG 1977 Negative feedback control of gonadotrophins in male rhesus monkeys: effects of time after castration and interactions of testosterone and estradiol-17ß. Endocrinology 101: 215–224.

Rhodes JC, Kjerulff KH, Langenberg PW, Gusinski GM 1999 Hysterectomy and sexual functioning. Journal of the American Medical Association 282: 1934–1941.

Richfield EK, Twyman R, Berent S 1987 Neurological syndrome following bilateral damage to the head of the caudate nuclei. Annals of Neurology 22: 768–771.

Riley AJ 1994 Yohimbine in the treatment of erectile disorder. British Journal of Clinical Practice 48: 133–136.

Riley A, Riley E 2000 Controlled studies on women presenting with sexual drive disorder: I. Endocrine status. Journal of Sex & Marital Therapy 26: 269–283.

Robbins TW, Everitt BJ 1996 Neurobehavioural mechanisms of reward and motivation. Current Opinion in Neurobiology 6: 228–236.

Robbins TW, Everitt BJ 2002 Limbic-striatal memory systems and drug addiction. Neurobiology of Learning & Memory 78: 625–636.

Robbins MB, Jensen GD 1978 Multiple orgasm in males. In Gemme R, Wheeler CC (eds) Progress in Sexology. Plenum, New York.

Robinson TE, Berridge KC 2000 The psychology and neurobiology of addiction: an incentive-sensitization view. Addiction 95: 91–117.

Robinson BW, Mishkin M 1968 Penile erection evoked from forebrain structures in Macaca mulatta. Archives of Neurology 19: 184–198.

Rodriguez-Manzo G, Fernandez-Guasti A 1994 Reversal of sexual exhaustion by serotonergic and noradrenergic agents. Behavior & Brain Research 62: 127–134.

Rodriguez-Manzo G, Fernandez-Guasti A 1995a Opioid antagonists and the sexual satiation phenomenon. Psychopharmacology 122: 131–136.

Rodriguez-Manzo G, Fernandez-Guasti A 1995b Participation of the central noradrenergic system in the reestablishment of copulatory behavior of sexually exhausted rats by yohimbine, naloxone, and 8-OH-DPAT. Brain Research Bulletin 38: 399–404.

Role LW, Kelly JP 1991 The brain stem: cranial nerve nuclei and the monoaminergic systems. In Kandel ER, Schwartz JH, Jessell TM (eds) Principles of Neural Science, 3rd edition. McGraw-Hill, New York, pp. 683–699.

Rommerts FFG 1990 Testosterone: an overview of biosynthesis, transport, metabolism and action. In Nieschlag E, Behre HM (eds),Testosterone: Action, Deficiency, Substitution. Springer-Verlag, Berlin, pp. 1–22.

Roose SP, Glassman AH, Walsh BT, Cullen K 1982 Reversible loss of nocturnal penile tumescence during depression: a preliminary report. Neuropsychobiology 8: 284–288.

Root WS, Bard P 1947 The mediation of feline erections through sympathetic pathways with some remarks on sexual behavior after deafferentiation of the genitalia. American Journal of Physiology 151: 80–89.

Roselli CE, Klosterman S 1998 Sexual differentiation of aromatase activity in the rat brain: effects of perinatal steroid exposure. Endocrinology 139: 3193–3201.

Roselli CE, Resko JA 1993 Aromatase activity in the rat brain: hormonal regulation and sex differences. Journal of Steroid Biochemistry and Molecular Biology 44: 499–508.

Roselli CE, Klosterman S, Resko JA 2001 Anatomic relationships between aromatase and androgen receptor mRNA expression in the hypothalamus and amygdala of adult male Cynomolgus monkeys. Journal of Comparative Neurology 439: 208–223.

Rosen RC 1995 Pharmacological effects on nocturnal penile tumescence (NPT) In Bancroft J (ed) The Pharmacology of Sexual Function and Dysfunction. Excerpta Medica International Congress Series 1075, Amsterdam, pp. 295–301.

Rosen RC, Beck JG 1988 Patterns of Sexual Arousal: Psychophysiological Processes and Clinical Applications. Guilford Press, New York.

Rosen RC, Shapiro D, Schwartz GE 1975 Voluntary control of penile tumescence. Psychosomatic Medicine 37: 479–483.

Rowland DL, Heiman JR, Gladue BA, Hatch JP, Doering CH, Weiler SJ 1987 Endocrine, psychological and genital response to sexual arousal in men. Psychoneuroendocrinology 12: 149–158.

Rust J, Golombok S 1986 The GRISS: a psychometric instrument for the assessment of sexual dysfunction. Archives of Sexual Behavior 15: 153–165.

Sachs BD 1995 Discussion. In Bancroft J (ed) The Pharmacology of Sexual Function and Dysfunction. Excerpta Medica International Congress Series 1075, Amsterdam, pp. 130–131.

Sachs BD, Barfield RJ 1976 Functional analysis of masculine copulatory behavior in the rat. Advances in the Study of Behavior 7: 91–154.

Saenz de Tejada IS, Kim N, Lagan I, Krane RJ, Goldstein I 1989 Regulation of adrenergic activity in penile corpus cavernosum. Journal of Urology 142: 1117–1121.

Sakheim DK, Barlow DH, Gayle Beck J, Abrahamson DJ 1984 The effect of an increased awareness of erectile cues on sexual arousal. Behaviour Research and Therapy 22: 151–158.

Sala M, Braida D, Leone MP, Calcaterra P, Monti S, Gori 1990 Central effect of yohimbine on sexual behavior in the rat. Physiology & Behavior 47: 165–173.

Salamone JD, Correa M 2002 Motivational views of reinforcement: implications for understanding the behavioral functions of nucleus accumbens dopamine. Behavioural Brain Research 137: 3–25.

Salemink E, van Lankveld JDM 2006 The effects of increasing neutral distraction on sexual responding of women with and without sexual problems. Archives of Sexual Behavior 35: 179–190.

Sanders D, Warner P, Backström T, Bancroft J 1983 Mood, sexuality, hormones and the menstrual cycle. I. Changes in mood and physical state: description of subjects and method. Psychosomatic Medicine 45: 487–501.

Sandfort TGM, de Graaf R, Bijl RV, Schnabel P 2001 Same-sex sexual behavior and psychiatric disorders. Archives of General Psychiatry 58: 85–91.

Saper CB 2000 Brain stem, reflexive behavior, and the cranial nerves. In Kandel ER, Schwartz JH, Jessell TM (eds) Principles of Neuroscience, 4th edition. McGraw-Hill, New York, pp. 873–888.

Sarrieau A, Mitchell JB, Lal S, Olivier A, Quirion R, Meaney MJ 1990 Androgen binding sites in human temporal cortex. Neuroendocrinology 51: 713–716.

Schiavi RC, Schreiner-Engel P, Mandeli J, Schanzer H, Cohen E 1990 Healthy aging and male sexual function. American Journal of Psychiatry 147: 766–771.

Schmidt PJ, Daly RC, Bloch M, Smith MJ, Danaceau MA, Simpson St Clair L, Murphy JH, Haq N, Rubinow DR 2005 Dehydroepiandrosterone monotherapy in midlife-onset major and minor depression. Archives of General Psychiatry 62: 154–162.

Schreiner-Engel P, Schiavi RC, White D, Ghizzani A 1989 Low sexual desire in women: the role of reproductive hormones. Hormones & Behavior 23: 221–234.

Schupp HT, Cuthbert BN, Bradley MM, Birbaumer N, Lang PJ 1997 Probe P3 and blinks: two measures of affective startle modulation. Psychophysiology 34: 1–6.

Sell LA, Morris J, Bearn J, Frackowiak RSJ, Friston KJ, Dolan RJ 1999 Activation of reward circuitry in human opiate addicts. European Journal of Neuroscience 11: 1042–1048.

Semans JH, Langworthy OR 1938 Observations on the neurophysiology of sexual function in the male cat. Journal of Urology 40: 836–846.

Sherwin BB 1991 The impact of different doses of estrogen and progestin on mood and sexual behavior in postmenopausal women. Journal of Clinical Endocrinology & Metabolism 72: 336–343.

Sherwin BB, Gelfand MM 1985a Sex steroids and affect in the surgical menopause: a double-blind, cross-over study. Psychoneuroendocrinology 10: 325–335.

Sherwin BB, Gelfand MM 1985b Differential symptom response to parenteral estrogen and/or androgen administration in the surgical menopause. American Journal of Obstetrics & Gynecology 151: 153–160.

Sherwin BB, Gelfand MM, Brender W 1985 Androgen enhances sexual motivation in females: a prospective, crossover study of sex steroid administration in the surgical menopause. Psychosomatic Medicine 47: 339–351.

Shifren JL 2006 Is testosterone or estradiol the hormone of desire? A novel study of the effects of testosterone treatment and aromatase inhibition in postmenopausal women. Menopause 13: 8–9.

Shifren JL, Braunstein GD, Simon JA, Casson PR, Buster JE, Redmond GP, Burki RE, Ginsburg ES, Rosen RC, Leiblum SR, , et al 2000 Transdermal testosterone treatment in women with impaired sexual function after oophorectomy. New England Journal of Medicine 343: 682–688.

Shifren JL, Davis SR, Moreau M, Waldbaum A, Bouchard C, Derogatis L, Derzko C, Bearnson P, Kakos N, O' Neill S, Levine S, Wekselman K,

Buch A, Rodenburg C, Kroll R 2006 Testosterone patch for the treatment of hypoactive sexual desire disorder in naturally menopausal women: results from the INTIMATE NM1 Study. Menopause 13: 770–779.

Simon J, Braunstein G, Nachtigall L, Utian W, Katz M, Miller SS, Waldbaum AS, Bouchard C, Derzko C, Buch A, Rodenberg C, Lucas J, Davis S 2005 Testosterone patch increases sexual activity and desire in surgically menopausal women with hypoactive sexual desire disorder. Journal of Clinical Endocrinology and Metabolism 90: 5226–5233.

Simonsen U, Prieto D, Hernandez M, Saenz de Tejada I, Garcia-Sacristan A 1997 Prejunctional alpha-2-adrenoreceptors inhibit nitrergic neurotransmission in horse penile resistance arteries. Journal of Urology 157: 2356–2360.

Simpson ER, Davis SR 2006 Another role highlighted for estrogens in the male: sexual behavior. Proceedings of the National Academy of Sciences 97: 14038–14040.

Singer I 1973 The Goals of Human Sexuality. Wildwood House, London.

Sipski ML, Alexander CJ, Rosen RC 2001 Sexual arousal and orgasm in women: effects of spinal cord injury. Annals of Neurology 49: 35–44.

Sisk CL 2006 New insights into the neurobiology of sexual maturation. Sexual & Relationship Therapy 21: 5–14.

Skakkebaek NE, Bancroft J, Davidson DW, Warner P 1981 Androgen replacement with oral testosterone undecanoate in hypogonadal men: a double-blind controlled study. Clinical Endocrinology 14: 49–67.

Somers VK, Dyken ME, Mark AL, Abboud FM 1993 Sympathetic-nerve activity during sleep in normal subjects. New England Journal of Medicine 328: 303–307.

Spiering M, Everaerd W 2007 The sexual unconscious. In Janssen E (ed) Sexual Psychophysiology. Indiana University Press, Bloomington, pp. 166–184.

Spiering M, Everaerd W, Elzinga E 2002 Conscious processing of sexual information: interference caused by sexual primes. Archives of Sexual Behavior 31: 159–164.

Spiering M, Everaerd W, Janssen E 2003 Priming the sexual system: Implicit versus explicit activation. Journal of Sex Research 40: 134–145.

Spiering M, Everaerd W, Laan E 2004 Conscious processing of sexual information: mechanisms of appraisal. Archives of Sexual Behavior 33: 369–380.

Stahl SM 1996 Essential Psychopharmacology. Cambridge University Press, Boston.

Steers WD 2000 Neural pathways and central sites involved in penile erection: neuroanatomy and clinical implications. Neuroscience & Biobehavioral Reviews 24: 5078–516.

Stein EA, Pankiewiscz J, Harsch HH, Cho J-K, Fuller SA, Hoffmann RG, Hawkins M, Rao SM, Bandettini PA, Bloom AS 1998 Nicotine-induced limbic cortical activation in the human brain: a functional MRI study. American Journal of Psychiatry 155: 1009–1015.

Steinman JL, Hoffman, SW, Banas C, Komisaruk BR 1994 Vaginocervical stimulation attenuates hind paw shock-induced substance P release into spinal cord superfusates in rats. Brain Research 647: 204–208.

Stock WE, Geer JH 1982 A study of fantasy-based sexual arousal in women. Archives of Sexual Behavior 11: 33–47.

Stoléru S, Mouras H 2007 Brain functional imaging studies of sexual desire and arousal in human males. In Janssen E (ed) The Psychophysiology of Sex. Indiana University Press, Bloomington, pp. 3–34.

Stoléru S, Redouté J, Costes N, Lavenne F, Le Bars DF, Dechaud H, Forest MG, Pugeat M, Cinotti L, Pujol J-F 2003 Brain processing of visual sexual stimuli in men with hypoactive sexual desire disorder. Psychiatry Research: Neuroimaging 124: 67–86.

Stuart FM, Hammond DC, Pett MA 1987 Inhibited sexual desire in women. Archives of Sexual Behavior 16: 91–106.

Su TP, Pagliaro M, Schmidt P, Pickar D, Wolkowitz G, Rubinow D 1993 Neuropsychiatric effects of anabolic steroids in male normal volunteers. Journal of the American Medical Association 269: 2760–2764.

Symons D 1979 The Evolution of Human Sexuality. Oxford University Press, Oxford.

Teplin V, Vittinghoff E, Lin F, Learman LA, Richter HE, Kuppermann M 2007 Oophorectomy in premenopausal women. Health-related quality of life and sexual functioning. Obstetrics & Gynecology, 109: 347–354.

Thase ME, Reynolds CF, Glanz LM, Jennings JR, Sewitch DE, Kupfer DJ, Frank E 1987 Nocturnal penile tumescence in depressed men. American Journal of Psychiatry 144: 89–92.

Tiihonen J, Kuikka J, Kupila J, Partanen K, Vainio P, Airaksinen J, Eronen M, Hallikainen T, Paanila J, Kinnunen I, Huttunen J 1994 Increase in cerebral blood flow of right prefrontal cortex in man during orgasm. Neuroscience Letters 170: 241–243.

Truitt WA, Coolen LM 2002 Identification of a potential ejaculation generator in the spinal cord. Science 297: 1566–1569.

Tuiten A, Laan E, Panhuysen G, Everaerd W, de Haan E, Koppeschaar H, Vroon P 1996 Discrepancies between genital responses and subjective sexual function during testosterone substitution in women with hypothalamic amenorrhea. Psychosomatic Medicine 58: 234–241.

Tuiten A, Van Honk J, Koppeschaar H, Bernaards C, Thijssen J, Verbaten R 2000 Time course of effects of testosterone administration on sexual arousal in women. Archives of General Psychiatry 57: 149–153.

Udry JR, Billy JOG, Morris NM, Groff TR, Raj MH 1985 Serum androgenic hormones motivate sexual behavior in adolescent boys. Fertility and Sterility 43: 90–94.

Udry JR, Talbert LM, Morris NM 1986 Biosocial foundations of adolescent female sexuality. Demography 23: 217–229.

Vague J 1983 Testicular feminization syndrome: an experimental model for the study of hormone action on sexual behavior. Hormone Research 18: 62–68.

Van Anders SM, Hampson E 2005 Waist-to-hip ratio is positively associated with bioavailable testosterone but negatively associated with sexual desire in healthy premenopausal women. Psychosomatic Medicine 67: 246–250.

Vance EB, Wagner NN 1976 Written descriptions of orgasms — a study of sex differences. Archives of Sexual Behavior 5: 87–89.

Van der Ploeg LHT, Martin WJ, Howard AD, Nargund RP, et al 2002 A role for the melanocortin 4 receptor in sexual function. Proceedings of the National Academy of Science USA 99: 11381–11386.

Van Lankveld JJDM, van den Houte MA 2004 Increasing neutral distraction inhibits genital but not subjective sexual arousal of sexually fictional and dysfunctional men. Archives of Sexual Behavior 33: 559–570.

Veith J, Buck M, Getzlaf S, Van Dalfsen P, Slade A 1983 Exposure to men influences the occurrence of ovulation in women. Physiology and Behavior 31: 313–315.

Virag R 1982 Intracavernous injection of papaverine for erectile failure. Lancet ii: 938.

Virag R, Ottesen B, Fahrenkrug J, Levy C, Wagner G 1982 Vasoactive intestinal polypeptide release during penile erection in man. Lancet, 4: 1166.

Wagner G, Brindley G 1980 The effect of atropine and beta blockers upon human penile erection — a controlled pilot study. In: Zorgniotti A (ed) First International Conference on Vascular Impotence. Charles C Thomas, New York.

Wagner G, Bro-Rasmussen F, Willis EA, Nielsen MH 1982 New theory on the mechanism of erection involving hitherto undescribed vessels. Lancet ii: 416–418.

Wallen K, Parsons WA 1998 Androgen may increase sexual motivation in estrogen-treated ovariectomized rhesus monkeys by increasing estrogen availability. Serono International Symposium on Biology of Menopause. Newport Beach, CA, USA.

Warner P, Bancroft J 1988 Mood, sexuality, oral contraceptives and the menstrual cycle. Journal of Psychosomatic Research 32: 417–427.

Weinberger DR, Elvevag B, Giedd JN 2005 The adolescent brain: a work in progress. The National Campaign to Prevent Teen Pregnancy. http://www.teenpregnancy.org/resources/reading/pdf/BRAIN.pdf.

Weisberg RB, Brown TA, Wincze JP, Barlow DH 2001 Causal attributions and male sexual arousal: the impact of attributions for a bogus erectile difficulty on sexual arousal, cognitions, and affect. Journal of Abnormal Psychology 110: 324–334.

West-Eberhard MJ 1992 Adaptation. In Keller EF, Lloyd EA (eds) Keywords in Evolutionary Biology. Harvard University Press, Cambridge, pp. 13–18.

Whitelaw GP, Smithwick RH 1951 Some secondary effects of sympathectomy: with particular reference to disturbance of sexual function. New England Journal of Medicine 245: 121–130.

Wiegel M, Scepkowski LA, Barlow DH 2007 Cognitive-affective processes in sexual arousal and sexual dysfunction. In Janssen E (ed), Sexual Psychophysiology. Indiana University Press, Bloomington, pp. 143–165.

Wikberg JES, Muceniece R, Mandrika I, Prusis P, Lindblom J, Post C, Skottner A 2000 New aspects of melanocortins and their receptors. Pharmacological Research 42: 393–420.

Wilson EO 1975 Sociobiology. Belknap/Harvard University Press, Cambridge, MA.

Wilson CA 1993 Pharmacological targets for the control of male and female sexual behaviour. In Riley AJ, Peet M, Wilson C (eds) Sexual Pharmacology. Clarendon Press, Oxford, pp. 1–58.

Wisniewski AB, Migeon CJ, Meyer-Bahlburg HFL, Gearhart JP, Berkowitz GD, Brown TR 2000 Complete androgen insensitivity syndrome: long-term medical, surgical and psychosexual outcome. Journal of Clinical Endocrinology & Metabolism 85: 2664–2669.

Wolchick SA, Beggs VE, Wincze JP, Sakheim DK, Barlow DH, Mavissakalian M 1980 The effect of emotional arousal on subsequent sexual arousal in men. Journal of Abnormal Psychology 89: 595–598.

Wonnacott S 1995 Modulation of neurotransmitter release by some therapeutic and socially used drugs: Nicotine. In Powis DA, Bunn SJ (eds) Neurotransmitter Release and Its Modulation. Cambridge University Press, Cambridge, pp. 293–299.

Wouda J, Hartman PM, Bakker RM, Bakker, JO, van de Wiel HBM, Weeijmar Schultz WCM 1998 Vaginal photoplethysmography in women with dyspareunia. Journal of Sex Research 35: 141–147.

Wynne-Edwards VC 1964 Population control in animals. Scientific American 211: 68–74.

Wysocki CJ, Preti G 1998 Pheromonal influences. Archives of Sexual Behavior 27: 627–629.

Yates WR, Perry PJ, MacIndoe J, Holman T, Ellingrod V 1999 Psychosexual effects of three doses of testosterone cycling in normal men — a controlled personality study. Biological Psychiatry 45: 254–260.

Young WS, Shepard E, Amico J, Henninghousen L, LaMarca ME, McKinney C, Ginns EI 1996 Deficiency in mouse oxytocin prevents milk ejection, but not fertility or parturition. Journal of Neuroendocrinology 8: 847–854.

Zhou J, Hofman MA, Gooren LJG, Swaab DF 1995 A sex difference in the human brain and its relation to transexuality. Nature 378: 68–70.

Zillmann D 1972 The role of excitation in aggressive behavior. Proceedings of the Seventeeth International Congress of Applied Psychology, 1971, Editest, Brussels.

Zillman D 1983 Transfer of excitation in emotional behavior. In Cacioppo JT, Petty RE (eds) Social Psychophysiology: A Sourcebook. Guilford Press, New York.

5 Sexual development

The developmental process 144
An eclectic interactional model of sexual development............. 145
The functions of sexual behaviour 146
Sexual preferences.. 146

The development of sexual behaviour and sexual
relationships.. 146
Sources of evidence.. 146
Sexual development in the pre-pubertal child 148

The transition from childhood to adolescence........................... 154

Sexual preferences and the development of sexual
identity 159
Sexual identities in men and women 159
Sexual preferences in animals 165
The interactive processes leading to sexual identity 166

Conclusions 169

People may differ in what they regard as mature sexual behaviour; such judgement inevitably involves values. But few would disagree that the route to sexual maturity is complicated, with many points of possible and untoward departure. In this chapter we consider how various strands of development during childhood and early adolescence eventually combine to produce the sexual adult. We also need to keep in mind that the adult continues to develop sexually well into the latter part of his or her life.

The developmental process

When considering an individual's development from the early embryonic stage to the mature sexual adult, we are faced with a dynamic process shaped by a multitude of influences. Our understanding of the process of sexual differentiation of the genitalia has progressed substantially, largely due to what we have learnt from abnormalities, and together with the development of gender identity, this was looked at closely in Chapter 3. In this chapter, we focus on development as it affects our capacity for sexual response and behaviour, and the development of our sexual identities. The challenge is to formulate in a useful way the continuing interaction between inborn, including genetic determinants (traditionally regarded as nature) and environmental influences (nurture). In the process we have to take into account substantial development of brain structure and activity during childhood, and most particularly around puberty and during adolescence. This is considered more closely in Chapter 4 (p. 60). But the role of learning remains crucially important.

There are two models of learning to consider: social learning (Mischel 1966) and cognitive learning (Kohlberg 1966). Social learning is the process by which behaviour is shaped by its consequences, encouraged and discouraged by reward and punishment, its effects facilitated by modelling or the example of others. This type of learning has equal relevance to animal and human development, and we will be drawing parallels between sexual learning of this kind in primates and humans.

Cognitive learning is perhaps uniquely human. In this case the stimuli that impinge upon the individual, and the responses elicited, are cognitively organized according to categories. This has an added and often crucial effect on the basic social learning process. Consequences become rewarding or punishing according to the category they are assigned.

Kohlberg (1966) drew the distinction between these two paradigms with the following illustration. 'In social learning, "I want reward, I am rewarded for doing boys' things, therefore I want to be a boy". In cognitive learning "I am a boy, therefore I want to do boys' things, therefore the opportunity to do boys' things is rewarding". To take this illustration further, any reward given for behaving like a boy will, through cognitive processes, strengthen the concept 'I am a boy'. Failure to be rewarded, or to be punished for such behaviour, will challenge and possibly weaken the concept 'I am a boy'.

Thus, these two types of learning process interact, raising learning to a much more complex plane than that of social learning alone. We assume that cognitive learning is unique to humans because it depends on the use of language, which animals do not have, except perhaps in a most rudimentary form.

How we conceptualize and categorize our environment and our experiences must also develop. Piaget has elegantly shown how this ability goes through crucial stages of development in a stepwise rather than continuous fashion, analogous to the development of the motor nervous system. Curiously, the Piagetian school has almost totally ignored the development of thinking as it applies to sexuality and reproduction. We will return to this later. As we considered in Chapter 3, cognitive learning is of particular significance for the gender development of the child, who at some time between the ages of 18 months and 3 years becomes able to categorize people in simple ways and assigns itself to the category of boy or girl. It is possible that this same process of 'either–or' categorization or labelling plays an important part much later in development when the young adolescent is responding to socially prescribed categories such as homosexual or heterosexual.

The best-known and most influential model of sexual development is the psychoanalytic model. I have not found psychoanalytic theory or concepts helpful in this respect, though undoubtedly psychoanalysts have drawn our attention to some crucially important aspects of development. Some of the major modifications of psychoanalytic theory have been more useful, in particular those of the ego analysts such as Erikson (1950). This may be because the ego analysts have concerned themselves with explaining the normal rather than extrapolating from the abnormal, as is typical of orthodox psychoanalysis.

Miller & Simon (1980) usefully compared various models of sexual development. They pointed out that, in the Freudian view, the child enters adolescence with 'an articulated set of erotic meanings that seek appropriate objects and behaviour', whereas Erikson (1950) sees the child making this entry with a number of skills, which are relevant to the sexual encounters of adolescence but not confined to them, e.g. the capacity for intimacy and trust. Erikson also proposes useful ways of recognizing and describing different stages of identity development, which allow us to see childhood experiences as crucially important to later sexual development without requiring the assumption of the degree of early sexual organization central to the Freudian view.

Sociologists such as Gagnons & Simon, whose theoretical ideas were examined in Chapter 2, talk of scripts, or prescriptions of how people can or should behave in certain situations, which is entirely consistent with the cognitive learning model playing a fundamental part in the unfolding of our sexuality. Such scripts, which we acquire from our social group, in particular the peer group of the adolescent, help us to attribute meaning to internal states, organize sequences of specific sexual acts, decode novel situations, set the limits for sexual response and link meanings from non-sexual aspects of life to specifically sexual experience (Gagnon & Simon 1973). Such a view attaches major importance to social and cultural factors in determining our sexuality but, as discussed in Chapter 2, neglects, in the process, the importance of biological factors.

Heiman et al (2003) reviewed theoretical approaches to understanding the developmental sequence from childhood experience to adult sexuality. They emphasized the unfolding nature of the developmental process by which, at each stage, the child's experiences are given meaning and value by the family and socio-cultural context. This also involves reviewing and reinterpreting earlier experiences in the light of more recent influences, a process that has received little research attention. Childhood sexual experiences, from this perspective, are more likely to be incorporated into a learnt 'sexual script', if they originally involved intense emotional reactions, either positive or negative, and if they are repeated. Attachment theory (Bowlby 1969, 1973, 1980) may be useful in conceptualizing early experiences with significant others, including physical closeness, touch and learning emotional regulation, and how they might impact on sexual development.

Browning & Laumann (2003) discussed theoretical models of the impact of child sexual abuse (CSA). They contrasted psychogenic models, which have dominated the literature on the effects of CSA, with the life course approach involving a cumulative series of behavioural transitions. Whereas the psychogenic approach sees the long-term consequences of CSA as the lingering presence of the initial traumatic effects, the life course approach sees the sexual abuse as influencing the next stages of sexual and personal development, which in turn influence subsequent behavioural patterns. Thus, if the CSA experience establishes a link between sexual feelings and negative mood, then this will influence how subsequent sexual relationships are negotiated, often with an early onset of sexual activity, leading to other consequences, including increased number of sexual partners, risk of sexually transmitted infections and associations with relatively delinquent peer groups. In both the psychogenic and life course approaches, it is recognized that the sexual outcomes can be polarized, in some cases leading to avoidance of sexual encounters, and in others increased confrontation with sexual situations. The mediating mechanisms that determine which of these contrasting trajectories is followed remain obscure. Finkelhor's (1988) traumagenic dynamics model does provide some degree of integration of psychogenic and life course factors. The effects of CSA, according to this model, are affected by the presence or absence of four key factors: powerlessness, betrayal, traumatic sexualization and stigmatization.

An eclectic interactional model of sexual development

Borrowing from these various theoretical approaches, the following model attempts to integrate both biological and socio-cultural factors.

First are two dimensions: strands and stages. There are three main *strands*:

1. sexual differentiation into male or female and the development of gender identity
2. sexual responsiveness
3. the capacity for close, dyadic relationships.

Stages can be defined in varying degrees of detail but are summarized as six basic stages:

1. pre-natal stage
2. childhood
3. adolescence and early adulthood
4. marriage (or the establishment of a stable sexual relationship)
5. early and late parenthood
6. mid-life.

At the pre-natal stage, sexual differentiation is taking place most obviously in anatomical terms. But the organization of brain function along male or female lines probably begins before birth, carrying on into childhood and possibly into adolescence. Little can be said, at the present time, about the other two strands, sexual

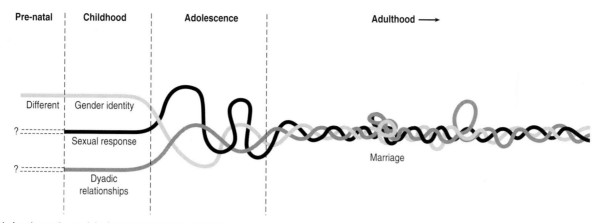

Fig. 5.1 A schematic model of sexual development showing three strands of development: gender identity, sexual response and the capacity for close, dyadic relationships, at different stages of the life cycle. During childhood these three strands are relatively independent of each other. During adolescence they start to integrate to form the sexual adult.

responsiveness and capacity for dyadic relationship, at the pre-natal stage.

During most of childhood, the three strands are developing in relative independence of one another. During late childhood and early adolescence the strands begin to be woven together or integrated to form the young sexual adult. Further periods of integration or reorganization, though less fundamental than that during adolescence, do occur at a number of important transitional phases during adult life and account for many of the crises we see in marriage and families. This varying interaction of strands of sexual development over time is shown schematically in Figure 5.1.

There are two other aspects of this interactional model to consider:

1. The variety of *functions* or consequences of sexual behaviour, which influence the interactional process at each stage, as a result of both social and cognitive learning.
2. *Sexual preferences* for certain types of sexual partner or activity, which first result from these interactions and then influence our subsequent sexual behaviour as labels or parts of sexual scripts, and ultimately our sexual identity.

The functions of sexual behaviour

In addition to the basic function of reproduction, many other functions or purposes of sexual behaviour can be recognized:

1. assertion of masculinity or femininity
2. bolstering or maintenance of self-esteem
3. exertion of power or dominance
4. bonding dyadic relationships and fostering intimacy
5. source of pleasure
6. reduction of tension
7. expression of hostility
8. risk-taking as a source of excitement
9. material gain.

Many of these functions are not peculiarly human and can be recognized in the behaviour of non-human primates. They provide the variety of rewards that affect

sexual learning, with some functions being more in evidence than others at certain stages of development. Many of the problems of human sexual relationships stem from the two participants using sex to fulfil different functions at any one time. We will consider these functions and the problems they may generate at various points in this book.

Sexual preferences

The concept of sexual preference is an uneasy one. It indicates the type of person (or thing) and/or type of activity with that person that is most likely to provoke sexual interest and arousal. It is an uneasy concept partly because it is interpreted by some people as implying choice, when in fact we do not choose what we find most sexually arousing. But also the choice of partner (e.g. as in marriage) may reflect other needs of equal or greater importance than the experience of sexual pleasure. And yet, as we shall see, the sexual preference we recognize in ourselves plays an important part in the cognitive learning process. The most important dimension of sexual preference is the sex of the preferred partner: whether the preference is heterosexual or homosexual. This development will be considered in more detail later in this chapter. The possible origins of other variations of preference (e.g. fetishism or sadomasochism) will be considered in Chapter 9.

The first strand and its various stages we considered in Chapter 3. Now let us look more closely at the second and third strands and their stages.

The development of sexual behaviour and sexual relationships

Sources of evidence

What are the available sources of evidence of early sexual development? The large majority of research on sexuality at any age relies on self-report, which is clearly limited by problems of recall error and bias, depending on the time period being recalled. When recalling as adults, or even adolescents, our sexual experiences during childhood, there is the further problem of recalling events that occurred at a time in our development when the sexual significance of them may not have been apparent to us. Empirical studies of the validity and reliability of adults' recall of childhood sexual experiences are almost entirely confined to recall of CSA (Graham 2003). A number of studies have assessed the consistency of recall of CSA by asking adults on more than one occasion, finding variable degrees of inconsistency, and other studies have asked adults who recalled such childhood experiences whether they had gone through phases of not remembering these experiences, and many had. Fortenberry & Aalsma (2003) found inconsistency among mid-adolescents when asked, on two occasions 7 months apart, to recall CSA experienced before age 12. There have been two prospective studies in which individuals with previously documented histories of sexual abuse as children have been followed up in adulthood (Williams 1994; Widom & Morris 1997). These found from 32% to 60% under-reporting of CSA at follow-up, depending on the particular measure of CSA. These findings have generated considerable debate about whether repression or simply forgetting was responsible. Overall, women have been found to be more likely to forget (or repress) earlier CSA experiences than men.

This restructuring of childhood by adult recall can also have a validating effect: attributing sexual meaning to a childhood experience with the wisdom of hindsight. Also, whether the sexual meaning is understood at the time or not, there are other developmental factors that may influence and possibly distort how a child or adolescent would report experiences, making later adult recall more valid. A good example of this was reported by Halpern et al (2000), who found that young adults recalled masturbation during early adolescence as substantially more frequent than was reported by those same adults 8–9 years earlier when they were around age 13. Although it could be argued that the adults were over-reporting this behaviour, it is more likely that the adolescents were reluctant to acknowledge this behaviour and, hence, under-reported it. In support of this, Halpern et al (2000) had shown that the under-reporting was more likely in those with negative attitudes towards masturbation.

Use of parental reports is the next most widely used method, although this has mainly been used for parental observations of young preschool children. Most studies have used questionnaires or checklists completed by a parent (usually the mother) (e.g. Sex Problem Scale of the Child Behavior Checklist, Achenbach 1991; Child Sexual Behavior Inventory (CSBI), Friedrich 2003; Meyer-Bahlburg & Steel 2003). There are two major limitations to this approach; first, its value is largely restricted to observations of children young enough not to have learnt that sexuality related behaviours are taboo and therefore not to be enacted in front of adults; second, there is scope for observation bias in the mothers (see below).

Another approach to parental observation involves training the parent to observe the child over a period of time (e.g. Schuhrke 2000). This has been used to a very limited extent, and whereas it has considerable potential value, partly because the parent is helped to interpret behaviours they might observe, it will always be limited by a participation-bias factor; it will not be the 'average parent' who agrees to participate in such a study.

Obtaining information directly from the child has been tried to a limited extent, and the methodological issues involved have been reviewed by O'Sullivan (2003). Most research of this kind has focused on the child's sexual knowledge and how this varies with stage of cognitive development. The pioneering studies of Goldman & Goldman (1982), for example, used interviews in their study of children aged from 5 to 15 years. Their questions were to some extent nested, so that use of more advanced questions, about sexual behaviour in particular, would depend on the child's answer to earlier questions. Kinsey and his colleagues interviewed 305 boys and 127 girls aged 4–14 years. The only report of this data is a brief account by Elias & Gebhard (1970). A detailed description of the method is given in Kinsey et al (1948, p. 58). For children aged 12 or older, the regular interview was adapted with appropriate vocabulary. For younger children, especially those under 8, a totally different approach was used. One parent was always present. The interviewer interacted with the child in a range of activities that children generally enjoy, involving toys, dolls, puzzles, romps, telling stories, getting the child to draw pictures, etc. Questions were inserted at appropriate points during these activities and followed no set sequence. Volbert (2000) interviewed children between the ages of 2 and 6, the interviews being carried out at the child's kindergarten school. Drawings were used to lead into discussions about various topics, including genital differences, gender identity, sexual body parts, pregnancy, birth, procreation and sexual behaviour of adults. In another recent study, Rademakers et al (2003) used a semistructured interview with 8- and 9-year-old children. The children were asked to talk about 'romping' (as a non-intimate form of physical contact), cuddling and 'being in love'. The children were also invited to mark on a drawing of a same-sex child's body, which parts they considered pleasant and which exciting, and to tell stories in reaction to drawings portraying scenes such as 'playing doctor' or having a bath with an adult. The children's reactions were compared with comments from their parents. Such projective methods with children are of interest, but their validity and meaning need further methodological research. O'Sullivan et al (2000) interviewed boys aged 7–13. Although the boys were not upset by their participation, considerable reticence was expressed by some of them when responding to questions about sexual knowledge, which seemed to be the result of both a limited sexual vocabulary and, in this group of inner city, mainly African American and Hispanic boys, a clearly evident taboo against talking openly with adults about sex. In an early study, Ramsey (1943) found that boys, aged 10–12 years, had a reasonable knowledge of sexual matters, but very little socially acceptable vocabulary to communicate this knowledge. Schoof-Tams et al (1976) studied the sexual attitudes, values, and meanings of school children aged 11–16. They used a questionnaire approach, in which three or four response options were presented in cartoon form. Other methods, which have appeared in the literature and are of interest, include direct observation of children through one-way screens (i.e. without the child's knowledge; e.g. Langfeldt 1990) and using older children as 'interviewers' (Borneman 1990).

Studying normal sexual development in adolescence also presents methodological challenges. Recent studies have shown that adolescents are more likely to reveal sensitive information about their behaviour to a computer than in a face-to-face interview or pencil and paper questionnaire (Turner et al 1997), and that it may be easier for a teenager to reveal delinquent behaviour than sexually sensitive behaviour such as masturbation. Fortenberry and his colleagues (Fortenberry et al 1997; Fortenberry & Aalsma 2003) have used daily diaries to explore the relationship between the sexual activity of male and female adolescents and such ongoing factors as interaction with the partner and mood, providing a rare example of research into what might be regarded as the basic fundamentals of adolescent sexual behaviour.

The crucial importance of longitudinal studies is fairly clear. As yet, no such study has been designed to look specifically at sexual development, but a number of studies (e.g. Kagan & Moss 1962; Caspi et al 1997; Fergusson et al 1997; Bates et al 2003) have included questions about sexual development in a more general developmental project.

In the case of CSA, a considerable amount of data based on retrospective recall has been collected, but much of it is inconsistent. Current social attitudes to CSA are likely to influence how people recall such experiences, and the relatively recent social trend towards 'survivor movements' is likely to influence how people interpret their childhoods when searching for explanations for their current problems.

Overall, there is no escaping the fact that those of us who seek to study normal sexual development in childhood and adolescence face substantial methodological challenges, and for the present time we must rely to a considerable extent on informed speculation. The issues at stake, however, are sufficiently important that it must be hoped that research into improving relevant methods will be given high priority.

Sexual development in the pre-pubertal child

Early sexually relevant behaviours — observations by parents and other adults

Although erections in little boys can occur spontaneously, they commonly result from genital handling, and it is clear from observations of both boys and girls that genital stimulation is a source of pleasure. One of

the first to describe this was Moll (1912), who wrote: 'When we see a child lying with moist, widely opened eyes, and exhibiting all the other signs of sexual excitement as we are accustomed to observe in adults, we are justified in assuming that the child is experiencing a voluptuous sensation'. Freud regarded various types of non-genital self-stimulation such as thumb sucking as forms of sexual activity. Moll preferred to restrict sexual significance to genital stimulation.

Galenson & Roiphe (1974), observing infants and small children in a nursery, reported that boys usually begin genital play at about 6–7 months of age, whereas girls start a little later at 10 or 11 months. They found boys continued with this form of stimulation until more obvious masturbation became established at 15–16 months of age. The girls showed more intermittent genital play. There is also a tendency for girls to transfer to less direct methods of stimulation, such as thigh pressure or rocking. Both boys and girls may use direct genital contact with an inanimate object such as a doll or toy, as if mounting it.

Masturbation to the point of obvious orgasm has been observed in children of both sexes as young as 6 months (Bakwin 1973). Behaviour of this kind in the young child, unassociated with any embarrassment or self-consciousness, can be observed and is occasionally reported by parents and others in contact with small children.

Friedrich (2003) came to the study of normative sexual behaviour in childhood from his earlier studies of sexually abused children. Starting with the assumption that sexual behaviours in a child are indicative of previous sexual abuse, he was confronted by the fact that most such behaviours were ubiquitous from ages 2 to 12 years. Friedrich had first used the Child Behavior Checklist (CBCL; Achenbach 1991) which has six questions of sexual relevance and which was carefully reviewed by Meyer-Bahlburg & Steel (2003). Friedrich went on to develop the CSBI as a more comprehensive standardized method of asking parents about sexually relevant behaviours observed in their children. The most recent version has 38 items (Friedrich 1997). Examples are 'touches sex parts in public', 'masturbates with a toy or object', 'touches another child's sex parts', 'rubs body against people or furniture', 'puts objects in vagina or rectum', 'pretends that dolls or stuffed animals are having sex', 'talks about sexual acts' and 'is very interested in the opposite sex'. Parents are asked to indicate whether each behaviour occurs 'never' (0) to 'at least once a week' (3). In order to show age relatedness of such behaviours, Friedrich identified behaviours endorsed by at least 20% of parents in each age group. These are listed in Table 5.1.

Many of the behaviours in the CSBI are endorsed by parents of children with no history of sexual abuse or behavioural problems. However, in a study comparing such children with a sample of sexually abused children, and a sample of psychiatric outpatient attenders, Friedrich found the behaviours most common in the sexually abused group. They were, however, also more common in the psychiatric outpatient children than in the non-clinical, non-abused group (Friedrich et al

TABLE 5.1	Items from Child Behavior Check List endorsed by at least 20% of parents, by age group and gender (Table 1 from Friedrich 2003)		
Age group	Item	Boys	Girls
2–5 years	Stands too close to people	29.3	25.8
	Touches sex parts when in public places	26.5	
	Touches/tries to touch mother's or other woman's breasts	42.4	43.7
	Touches sex parts at home	60.2	43.8
	Tries to look at people when they are nude or undressing	26.8	26.9
6–9 years	Touches sex parts at home	39.8	20.7
	Tries to look at people when they are nude or undressing	20.2	20.5
10–12 years	Is very interested in the opposite sex	24.1	28.7

2001). Meyer-Bahlburg et al (2000) used the CBCL of Achenbach (1991) with parents of 6- to 10-year-old children in a community sample. The data were collected from 1986 to 1988. Sexual behaviour, as described in the CBCL, was reported by the parents of one in six boys and one in seven girls. An association with 'externalizing' behaviours (i.e. hyperactivity, attention problems, rule breaking and aggression) was found, particularly in boys.

Friedrich (2003) also reviewed three studies in which cross-cultural comparisons of the CSBI were involved, comparing children from the USA with Dutch, Belgian and Swedish children. In each study, the European children, most notably the Dutch children, were reported as showing more of these sexual behaviours than the American children. These cultural differences may be to some extent explainable by more relaxed sexual attitudes in the European mothers, leaving us with the question of whether European children show more of such behaviours, or whether their mothers are more comfortable reporting them — probably a combination of the two.

In general, therefore, evidence based on parental observations indicates sexually relevant behaviour as most likely to be observed in younger children, confronting us with the older child's retreat as a reaction to sexual taboos. Whereas children clearly vary in the age at which this shift towards 'concealed' sexuality occurs, it appears to occur somewhere between the ages of 6 and 10.

The development of 'sexual meaning', 'sexual behaviour' and 'sexual response'

The first conceptual step is to distinguish between the physiological responses that are the basis of a sexual experience, and the 'sexual' meanings attributed to such response patterns. It is conceivable, though as yet not demonstrated, that the impact of the physiological response may be altered, and possibly intensified, by the attribution of sexual meaning to it. It is also possible that the occurrence of an experience involving a sexual response may activate a child's need to seek and comprehend a 'meaning' for this response. It is nevertheless appropriate to assume that the acquisition of 'sexual meaning' and the experience of a response, such as orgasm or erotic sensation, which become central to the adult's sexual experience, can be disconnected during childhood. Furthermore, some children may develop concepts of sexual meaning before they have any physiological experiences that can be regarded as sexual, and vice versa. What evidence do we therefore have of the 'normal' development of sexual meaning, on the one hand, and sexually relevant physiological response patterns on the other hand? And how do they interact to lead to a 'sexual experience'?

Sexual meaning

Goldman & Goldman (1982) interviewed children from ages 5 to 15, in four countries: Australia, Britain, North America and Sweden. Overall, sexual learning and understanding was behind other aspects of cognitive development, except for the Swedish children, who had received more sex education from an earlier age. Children from larger families, particularly those with opposite sex siblings, tended to show more advanced sexual thinking, and to some extent boys were more advanced than girls. Boys attached more importance to companionship and girls to romantic love. Given the gradual progression of sexual thinking through the age range studied, Goldman & Goldman (1982) concluded that there was no support for the psychoanalytic concept of a latency period. However, their evidence also indicated the children's growing awareness of social taboos about sexuality, particularly in relation to the sexuality of their parents. They found that children perceived a special relationship between men and women early in development, but took much longer to recognize or comprehend the sexuality of such relationships. The sexual taboos additionally compound children's delay in understanding sex by depriving them of an appropriate vocabulary.

Volbert (2000) interviewed 147 children, aged 2–6. While these children had knowledge of gender identity, genital differences and sexual body parts, they had little understanding of pregnancy, birth and procreation, and almost no knowledge of adult sexual behaviour. While 73.5% mentioned kissing and cuddling, only 8% of 6-year-olds and 3% of 5-year-olds gave a description of adult sexual behaviour. Rademakers et al (2003), in a study of 8- and 9-year-old Dutch children (15 girls and 16 boys), asked the children to talk about cuddling and being in love. Not surprisingly, cuddling was familiar to almost all the children as a positive experience, though not one to which they appeared to attribute any sexual meaning. Falling in love, while familiar to most of them, and half of them said they were 'in love' at that time or previously, was interestingly a cause of some embarrassment. Most regarded being in love as a positive experience, but one that made them vulnerable to teasing. Again, it was not apparent that this vulnerability was linked to any sexual meaning. Schoof-Tams et al (1976) noted a shift from understanding sex as a means to procreate, at age 11, to seeing it, by mid-adolescence, as central to affectionate relationships. For many years, young children have been confronted with numerous scenarios of romantic love on movies and television. While these are often based on traditional fairy tales (e.g. Cinderella or Beauty and the Beast), the 'love' component is conveyed more intensely and graphically than has been the case in traditional written versions. Yet, there is typically an innocent quality to the romance, which does not require any sexual meaning to be conveyed, beyond the fact that the love is between a man and a woman.

Gebhard (1977) asked young adults to recall the age at which they learnt sexual meanings. He compared a small group of current students at his university with comparable data from Kinsey's original study, which had not been previously reported. This showed a progression of knowledge about sexual behaviour, which accelerated around puberty, and also earlier acquisition of such knowledge in his recent sample, compared with the Kinsey sample interviewed about 25 years earlier.

The evidence is consistent in showing that children learn, first, about gender differences and body parts, somewhat later about procreation, and later still about sexual behaviour. The earlier and more extensive knowledge shown by Swedish children in Goldman & Goldman's (1982) study, compared with Australian, British and North American children, all of whom had received less sex education, plus Gebhard's (1977) evidence of earlier learning in children over a 25-year period, during which both sex education and general dissemination of information about sex had increased, demonstrate that not only the stage of cognitive development but also the environment and culture determines the learning of sexual meaning, with such learning occurring earlier than in the past.

Sexual behaviours and taboos

A crucial and culturally determined phase in this learning process is when a child first learns that sexual issues are taboo, at least in the adult world. To begin with, taboos about sexual and excretory functions are somewhat linked (a linkage that does not always disappear), and the issue is one of 'bathroom' language. What they have in common, apart from the challenging overlap of excretory and sexual anatomy, is the issue of privacy and the need for the child to learn when and how to maintain privacy. With excretory function, the child may retain some embarrassment, not infrequently reflecting parental awkwardness with this topic, but at least there is a general acceptance that excretory function should happen in private. With sexual activities, it is a different matter, although how different is, once again, determined by the family's cultural context and the parents' degree of comfort with the topic of sex. The child is either explicitly encouraged to keep sexual acts, such as touching one's genitals, private or concludes that this is necessary to avoid censure. An important consequence

is that whereas prior to the recognition of the sexual taboo many children display such behaviours as touching their own genitals and those of other people and, in some cases, overtly displaying pleasure from touching themselves, such behaviours either stop or are concealed from adult view, a stage of development mistakenly interpreted by psychoanalysts, at least until recently, as the latency period.

One study involved direct questioning of children. This was carried out by Kinsey and his colleagues in the 1940s and early 1950s; the methodology used was described above (Elias & Gebhard 1970). The sample included 305 boys and 127 girls, all pre-pubescent, ranging in age from 4 to 14 years. Reported behaviour was only considered sexual if it involved self-manipulation of genitalia, the exhibition of genitalia or the manual or oral exploration of the genitalia of or by other children. Among the boys, 52% reported sexual activity with other boys and 34% with girls. Among the girls, 35% reported sexual activity with other girls and 37% with boys (Elias & Gebhard 1970).

Apart from this unique study, we have to depend mainly on recall by adults of their own childhood experiences. Elias & Gebhard (1970) commented on the 'surprising agreement' between these findings from children and the percentages given by adults recalling their childhoods in the main Kinsey survey.

Reynolds et al (2003) recruited a sample of university students, aged 18–22 years, 154 females and 149 males, who answered an extensive series of questions about sexual experiences during different stages of their childhood, as well as questions about their current sexual adjustment. Data were collected during 1998 and 1999 using computer-assisted self-interviewing. A further age-matched and much larger sample of university students was taken from Kinsey's original study: 1913 women and 1770 men. Thus, there were two samples studied approximately 50 years apart. Although there were limitations to direct comparison of the two data sets, some interesting comparisons were drawn.

In the earlier sample, 68% of males and 42% of females reported childhood sexual experiences with peers (CSEP). Of those with such experiences a similar proportion of males and females had experiences (not exclusively) with the same sex (75% of the boys and 71% of the girls). In the more recent sample, 87% of males and 84% of females reported CSEP. Not only does this suggest an increase in CSEP over the past 50 years, but also a much greater increase for the females, effectively eliminating the earlier gender difference. As expected, CSEP was more common during elementary school years than pre-elementary, and CSEP involving genital touching or more advanced sexual behaviour increased substantially with age, especially among the males. Although at each stage of schooling the majority of males and females reported CSEP only with opposite sex peers, during pre-elementary and elementary years girls were more likely than boys to have CSEP with same sex peers. During junior high school, it was the other way round. The most frequently stated reason for CSEP at each stage was curiosity about sexual matters.

Physical or sexual pleasure as a reason was more common during junior high school, particularly for the boys.

Using the same two samples, Bancroft et al (2003) reported on the age at first masturbation. Here there were some striking similarities as well as differences over the 50 years. In the recent sample, 98% of men and 83% of women indicated they had masturbated prior to the study, and 38% of men and 40% of women reported first masturbation before puberty. This compares with 95% of men and 39% of women having masturbated in the earlier sample, with 27% and 13%, respectively, reporting a pre-pubertal onset. Thus, we see relatively little change in masturbation histories for the males, but a major change for the females. When those who had masturbated in each study were compared for the age of onset of masturbation in relation to the age at puberty, there was a striking similarity across the two samples both for males and for females. Eighty per cent of the males had started to masturbate within 2 years either side of the age at puberty (i.e. spermarche). For women, the age of onset was much more widely spread, and in both samples, for those with a pre-pubertal onset, the females on average started 2 years earlier than the males. What this reflects is a relatively marked organizing effect of puberty on masturbation onset in males, which is not apparent in females (see Fig. 5.2).

Both of these papers (Bancroft et al 2003; Reynolds et al 2003) reported subtle relations between childhood experiences (CSEP and pre-pubertal masturbation) and earlier, more frequent or more enjoyable sexual experiences during teenage years. This raises the crucial question of whether the childhood experiences, along the lines of the life course perspective, influenced later sexual development, or whether they indicated a greater inherent 'sexuality' in those children, which was also manifested in their adolescent development. One must be cautious in generalizing from these student studies to other socio-economic and ethnic groups. Thigpen et al (2003) reported the negative consequences of having even less normative data for African American than for white children. Their study was driven by concern that young African American children in foster care were being labelled as 'sexually aggressive' because of sexual behaviours that may well have been within the norm for their age and culture. Their concerns reflect two potentially important aspects of sexual development, consistent and close parenting and the experience of privacy; the lack of both typifies the child brought up in foster care. Whether or not the lack of consistent, positive parenting directly influences behavioural development, it is likely that in such circumstances adult reactions to observed sexual behaviours of the child are different, with possibly long-term adverse consequences. This underlines a fairly obvious but important point about sexual development during childhood: how parents or other adults react to a child's emerging sexuality can have major effects on that child's subsequent development, either positively or negatively.

An earlier, comparable study of students recalling their childhoods was reported by Leitenberg et al (1989). They divided childhood experiences into 'pre-adolescent' (aged 12 and under) and 'early adolescent' (age 13–15). Their sample was 526 students, 188 male and 388 female. However, they reported pre-adolescent and early adolescent experiences for males and females combined. In pre-adolescence 75% had sexual experience with an opposite sex child, and 25% a same sex child. The average age for these experiences was 9.5 ($\pm$ 2.3) years, with age of partner only slightly older (10 $\pm$ 2.7 years). In early adolescence 96% had a sexual experience with an opposite sex, and only 4% with a same sex partner. The average age for these experiences was 14.2 ($\pm$ 0.8) years. These experiences involved genital stimulation in 41% of cases in pre-adolescence and 69% in early adolescence.

Other examples of studies using adult recall of childhood sexual experiences include Finkelhor (1980), Green (1985), Haugaard & Tilly (1988), Kilpatrick (1992) and Lamb & Coakley (1993). Estimates of child sexual experiences with peers range from 39% to 85% depending on several factors: how 'childhood' is defined (e.g. prior to age 6, prior to age 13, inclusive of adolescence), and the type of memory elicited by the researchers (e.g. 'sexual games' or 'most memorable experience').

Sexual response in childhood

Penile erections occur in infants and children. Whether pre-pubertal boys vary in the likelihood of experiencing erections is not known, and we should not assume that all pre-pubertal boys are capable of erections. The relevance of erections during childhood to erectile function post-puberty is not clear; anatomically, the pre-pubertal penis is not fully developed, and the hormonal component of erectile function in the adult is not present before puberty.

An interesting 'window' into the development of erectile function is nocturnal penile tumescence (NPT or sleep erection). Although the evidence from pre-pubertal boys is limited, it suggests that NPT does occur before puberty, but the erections are less frequent, and of shorter duration. Obviously the amount of tumescence will be smaller, due to the smaller size of the penis. The frequency, duration and rigidity of NPT peak round the age of 13, and thereafter slowly decline with age (Karacan et al 1976). This association between NPT and puberty is a good illustration of the role of testosterone in male sexual function (see p. 112). Adult men who are deficient in testosterone have NPT episodes, but they involve substantially less tumescence and rigidity and are of shorter duration than those in eugonadal men, a difference that is readily eliminated by testosterone replacement (Bancroft 2003). NPT in hypogonadal men is probably similar to that of pre-pubertal boys, although their comparability is limited by the developmental differences in size of the penis and erectile tissues.

Genital response in female children, i.e. vasocongestion of the vaginal wall, vulva and clitoris, is obviously much less likely to be observed by adults if it occurs, and we consequently have little evidence of this. Some children, both boys and girls, do stimulate their genitalia in ways that indicate arousal and pleasure and sometimes orgasm. There are striking case reports in the literature of such masturbation in very young children

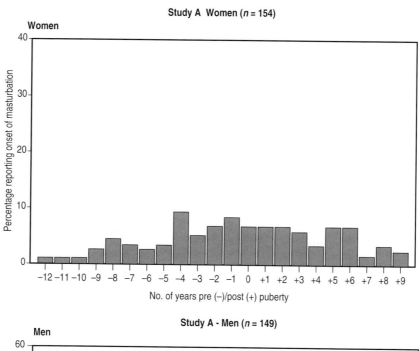

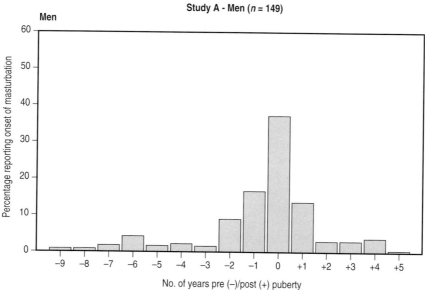

Fig. 5.2 Onset of masturbation in relation to puberty (0). Study A: 154 female and 149 male college students, interviewed 1998–99. Study B: 1875 female and 1722 male college students from original Kinsey studies. (From Bancroft et al 2003).

(Continued)

who, because of their age, are oblivious of being observed by their parents (e.g. Kinsey et al 1948, 1953). We also have clear reports of young adults recalling orgasmic experiences prior to puberty, most often as a result of masturbation. In our recent study (Bancroft et al 2003) 12% of women and 13.5% of men reported their first orgasm before onset of puberty (i.e. menarche, or age at first menstruation for females, or spermarche for males). For women the mean age was 8.5 years, ranging from 4 to 13, and for men 9.6 years, ranging from 5 to 13.

In the adult female, multiple orgasms are possible, although they are not part of typical sexual experience for most women. Men are clearly different in having a post-ejaculatory refractory period in which sexual

arousal and orgasm is inhibited for a period of time. It is possible that these refractory mechanisms in the male are established around puberty as part of the organizing effects of androgens (Sachs 1995), which may be interacting with new functional brain developments at that stage. This then raises the question of whether some boys (and girls) are capable of repeated orgasm before puberty, with boys losing this ability around puberty.

We can conclude that some children are capable of genital response and orgasm prior to puberty, possibly in infancy, but we have no idea of how many children this applies to. It is possible that the large majority of children have this capability, but only a few have the relevant experiences or circumstances to realize it.

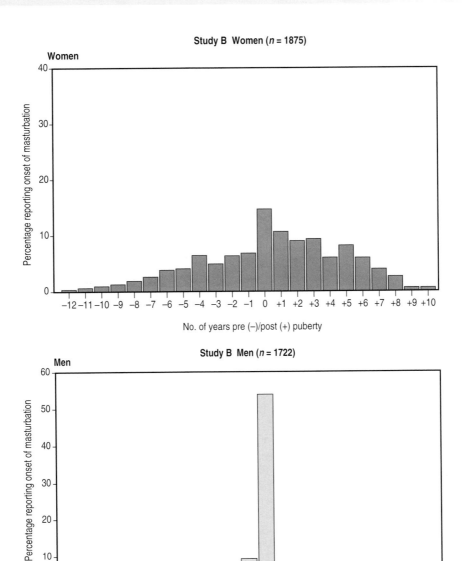

Fig. 5.2 Cont'd

Alternatively, some children may be more sexually responsive, and others relatively unresponsive prior to puberty. In either case, we are left uncertain of whether variability across children in either the capability or its expression depends on variable learning experiences, or is genetically determined. Such genetic variability may be expressed as variable responsiveness to hormonal changes that occur at adrenarche (i.e. increase in adrenal androgens) as well as puberty.

The issue of individual variability is particularly relevant to girls. As indicated earlier, data from both a recent study and Kinsey's original study (Bancroft et al 2003) show the age of onset of masturbation, which can be regarded as a useful marker of sexual development, to be close to the age at puberty in the large majority of boys, but not so in girls. One possible explanation of this greater variability in girls is greater individual variability in the behavioural effects of

androgens from adrenarche onwards (Bancroft 2003). Thus, those girls who are highly sensitive to the behavioural effects of androgens may experience onset of sexual interest, and possibly masturbation in association with the increases in androgens at adrenarche. Those who are more moderately sensitive may be activated around puberty, while those who are relatively insensitive to such hormonal effects, develop their sexual arousability more gradually, some quite late in adolescence or early adulthood.

With the male, the small proportion of boys who first experience orgasm and sexual arousal more than 2 years before puberty may be more responsive to androgens than normal and hence are activated by hormonal changes at adrenarche, at a time when they are unrestrained by the peri-pubertal development of refractory inhibition. At this stage of our knowledge, we can only speculate on such matters.

The transition from childhood to adolescence

Sexually relevant behaviours

While the awareness of sexual taboos leads to most sexual activity of the child being contained within his or her private non-adult world, there emerges a more open phase of interest, usually in the opposite sex, and the onset of dating behaviour in a proportion of children. Here we see the impact of socially sanctioned scripts for interactions between boys and girls, acceptable providing that they retain a childlike innocence. It is quite possible that at this developmental stage, in the minds of many boys and girls, such scripts remain disconnected from their earlier or even current childhood sexual experiences.

Table 5.2 shows findings from our recent study of young adults (Reynolds et al 2003) in relation to first experience of sexual arousal, sexual attraction to another person and sexual fantasy. Sexual arousal, comparable for boys and girls, first occurs before puberty for the majority, with an average age of onset of 9.7 years for boys and 10.8 years for girls. However, it is not clear how this was assessed by the participants. The males may have relied on memories of penile erections. It is less likely that girls recognized sexual arousal because of awareness of genital response. In further studies of this kind, this aspect should be examined more closely, though this will be limited by problems of recall. First sexual attraction shows a gender difference, with the majority of boys reporting it occurring before puberty, with an overall average age of 11.4 years, and a majority of girls reporting it post-puberty, with an overall average age of 12.4 years. The onset of sexual fantasies shows the gender difference more strongly (average for boys 11.6, for girls 13.3 years). To some extent this reflects the greater variability of timing of sexual development in girls, as discussed earlier in relation to onset of masturbation (Bancroft et al 2003). However, it also points to gender differences of wider relevance, which are as yet not well understood.

TABLE 5.2	Sex differences in first intrapsychic sexual experience in relation to puberty onset (Table A4 from Reynolds et al 2003)	
	Pre-pubertal	**Post-pubertal**
SEXUAL AROUSAL (MEAN AGE)		
Male	70% (8.8 years)	30% (12.0 years)
Female	63% (9.2 years)	37% (13.6 years)
SEXUAL ATTRACTION (MEAN AGE)		
Male	67%* (11.0 years)	33%* (12.1 years)
Female	38%[†] (10.2 years)	62%[†] (13.7 years)
SEXUAL FANTASY (MEAN AGE)		
Male	55%* (10.8 years)	45%* (12.6 years)
Female	29%[†] (10.5 years)	71%[†] (14.4 years)

*Significantly different from
[†]For gender difference comparisons ($p < 0.05$)

Dating

Kagan and Moss (1962), in a unique longitudinal study from birth to early adulthood, commented that although dating may start from age 10, 'it is not until 11 or 12 years of age that interactions between boys and girls acquire a sexual connotation'. They also found some interesting relations between early behavioural patterns and late adolescent and adult behaviours, although only in boys. Thus boys who did not adopt conventional masculine behaviours between the ages of 3 and 10 years were more likely to report high sexual anxiety, less likely to engage in early dating, and more likely to show avoidance of erotic behaviour in adolescence. Boys who avoided dating between 10 and 14 years were less likely to establish intimate heterosexual relationships, or engage in erotic activity during late adolescence and adulthood. Their inability to identify similar predictors in girls is noteworthy.

Broderick (1966) characterized three developmental phases. First, 10–11-year-olds showed predominantly same-sex social interactions but were expressing some heterosexual interest; around 25% had had their first date, and 'kissing games' were common at parties. Second, 12–13-year-olds showed little inclination to form close attachments with the opposite sex, but they were increasingly likely to identify 'objects of romantic attraction'. Third, 14–15 years was 'an age of transition' with increasing cross-gender social interactions, previously 'secret loves' being more openly acknowledged, and dating increasingly popular. In Schofield's (1965) study of English teenagers, a quarter of the boys and nearly a third of the girls had their first date by the age of 13; this changed rapidly over the next 2 years of age, and by age 16, over 70% of boys and 85% of girls had experienced dating. Broderick (1966) regarded 10–13 years as a period of rehearsal of skills and feelings appropriate for later heterosexual relationships. Schoof-Tams et al (1976) found that two-thirds of 11-year-old German children reported having been in 'in love', about a half had kissed, and yet only 7–8% had experienced first ejaculation or menarche. One might have expected changes in these patterns over the last 40 years, but there is no clear evidence that is the case.

Reynolds et al (2003) found the average age for experiencing a first 'crush' was 8–9 years, first girlfriend or boyfriend was 12–13 years and first date, between 14 and 15 years. Phinney et al (1990), in a nationally representative sample of adolescent females, found that dating started, on average, 2.5 years after menarche. The average age at menarche in our study (Reynolds et al 2003) was 12.6 years. According to Montgomery & Sorell (1998), dating typically progresses through a group dating phase before couple dating is established. They found more adolescent boys than girls saying that they were or had been 'in love', although clearly an adolescent's concept of what being 'in love' means evolves. Montgomery and Sorell (1998) comment '... adolescent girls, as well as boys, utilize adolescence (a time of sanctioned delay of adult functioning), to experiment with attracting and being attracted to others while continuing to sort who one is' (p. 686).

Zimmer-Gembeck et al (2001) reported on a longitudinal study in which development was compared at ages 12 and 16 years. The average age at initiation of dating and first romantic relationships was around 14 years. Adolescents who were over-involved in dating at age 16 were more likely to have shown psychosocial and behavioural problems at age 12. However, dating, in what these authors regarded as more appropriate ways, was associated with positive consequences including greater competence in the peer social domain.

Sexual activity

An interesting and potentially important example of the void in our knowledge is the recent focus within the media on oral sex as an increasingly common substitute for vaginal intercourse among teenagers. According to Remez (2000), we have little clear evidence of whether such behaviour has actually increased among teenagers. Remez (2000) attributes this to the barriers that exist against asking adolescents for details of their sexual experiences. She goes on to describe the impact of such barriers in the abstinence only movement, in which there is ongoing disagreement about whether educators should avoid going into details about what 'having sex' actually means, for fear of shattering the teenager's innocence, or whether they should be specific about which behaviours are covered by 'abstention' (which usually means anything beyond perhaps kissing on the lips). Oral sex is an interesting issue. In earlier studies of adolescent sexual behaviour, it was unusual for teenagers to have experienced oral sex before they had experienced vaginal intercourse, oral sex being seen, in some way, as a more advanced type of sexual activity (e.g. Kinsey et al 1948, 1953; Schofield 1965). Studies in the 1980s suggested that oral sex was more frequent among adolescents than previously, but still predominantly seen in those who had already experienced vaginal intercourse (Gagnon & Simon 1987; Newcomer & Udry 1985). More recently, Schwartz (1999) found a majority of males and females had had experience of oral sex before intercourse, although this was a small convenience sample of students. The question of whether oral sex was an example of 'having sex' became a public issue with the attempts to impeach President Clinton, and it was soon apparent that many students, like President Clinton, did not make the connection (Bogart et al 2000; Sanders & Reinisch 1999). Teenagers in the USA are entitled to feel confused about what *is* acceptable for them to do with their romantic partners, particularly in an age when young people, as well as every one else, are bombarded with sexual images and messages.

Keeping in mind that we know little about non-intercourse expressions of sexuality in adolescent relationships, what have we learnt about sexual intercourse per se? Perhaps not surprisingly, there has been far more research on teenage girls than boys, reflecting the societal attachment to the double standard, but also, according to Sonenstein et al (1997), the belief that teenage males are more difficult to survey. A number of surveys of adolescent females, starting in 1971, and repeated every few years, showed a substantial increase in the proportion engaging in sexual intercourse, and a reduction in age at first intercourse, during the 1970s and early 1980s. This trend was accompanied by an increase in the average number of sexual partners. During the late 1980s and 1990s this pattern for teenage girls levelled out, although the number of girls with experience of sexual intercourse before age 15 has continued to increase (Abma & Sonenstein 2001). The National Survey of Adolescent Males (NSAM), the first systematic survey to assess teenage males (ages 15–19), started in 1988 (Sonenstein et al 1989). Santelli et al (2000) compared four national surveys that had been repeated over time: National Survey of Family Growth (NSFG), NSAM, Youth Risk Behavior Survey (YRSB) and National Longitudinal Study of Adolescent Health (Add Health). All four surveys covered high school students, aged 15–17, and between them covered the period from 1988 to 1997. There was a consistent finding across the surveys that the proportion of males who had ever experienced sexual intercourse had fallen significantly. Santelli et al (2000) warned, however, that survey data on adolescent sexual behaviour should be treated with caution. Other trends were not consistent across surveys, reminding us of the methodological difficulties of obtaining sensitive information from adolescents. Overall, however, male adolescents tend to initiate sexual experience earlier and to have more sexual partners than female adolescents. (See Chapter 6 for further details.)

Given the emphasis that has been placed on the age at first intercourse, we understand surprisingly little about how the timing of this seemingly pivotal event impacts on the developmental process (Graber et al 1998).

What is 'appropriate' sexual development?

Distinguishing between, and understanding the determinants of, 'appropriate' and 'inappropriate' sexual development as the child enters and proceeds through adolescence presents us with a formidable challenge. We have at least three patterns of influence to consider. First, there is the emerging sexual responsiveness, which may have a substantial hormonal as well as neurophysiological basis, which needs to be incorporated into the young persons evolving sexual meanings and should be regarded as central to normal sexual development. Let us call this the 'peri-pubertal' pattern. Although the timing of puberty can be affected by a variety of environmental factors, we are dealing here principally with individual variability, relatively independent of the child's social and family context at this age.

Second, we need to recognize that adolescence involves a process of developing a separate identity, which in part is achieved by rejecting, often transiently, some of the values or norms or expectations that one's parents uphold. This process has been amplified by the emergence of a youth culture (Hobsbawm 1994). This relatively new social phenomenon thrives in many respects on modern technology, which allows music and television, for example, and the various messages conveyed by such media, to be shared widely among teenagers, often crossing cultural as well as geographic boundaries. Identification with a peer group therefore takes on an 'institutionalized' form, at least for many teenagers. A substantial part of the 'scripts' of such youth culture are sexual. Along with drug use and other behaviours that worry parents, sex is a vehicle, albeit a problematic one, for asserting one's emerging autonomy and independence. Schoof-Tams et al (1976), in their study of German adolescents, commented that attitudes towards sexuality change dramatically between the ages of 11 and 16. Their 11-year-olds were representing a more traditional morality, presumably consistent with that of their parents, whereas by 16, attitudes and morals about sex were more permissive. These authors considered this a shift to more gender equal roles in sexuality, and 'an abandonment of the double standard'. There is evidence that in some parts of Europe there has been a move towards a 'single standard' (e.g. Haavio-Mannila & Kontula 2003). In the USA, however, the 'double standard' seems to remain very much alive (Crawford & Popp 2003), particularly for adolescents, with teenage girls needing to guard their reputations, in ways that do not apply to boys (Orenstein 1994; Tolman 2002). We therefore need to understand the balance between parental influences, which tend to predominate during pre-pubertal childhood, and peer group influences, which are increasingly important during adolescence. Let us call this the parent vs peer group pattern.

Third, and this overlaps with the second, we see sexual behaviour as one of the adolescent externalizing behaviours which are often part of a pattern of maladaptive behaviour beginning in childhood and associated with a range of negative developmental influences. Sexual 'acting out' gets added to the list of such behaviours as the child enters adolescence; let us call this the maladaptive pattern.

The peri-pubertal pattern is thus intrinsically about normal sexual development, although individuals clearly vary in how they experience this process, reflecting the interaction between hormonal changes and evolving brain function. The parent vs peer group pattern involves a normative developmental process, but one which is very susceptible to socio-cultural influences, with the youth culture being, in various respects, reactive to the current adult world. Here the outcomes are uncertain, as adolescents grapple with their emerging capacity for decision-making. For most adolescents, this period of rebellion is formative in the long term; for others, particularly where sex is concerned, the consequences can be disastrous, so inevitably the adult world looks on with apprehension. The maladaptive pattern, by definition, recognizes certain types of adolescent sexual behaviour as symptoms of a more long-standing problematic development, in which other forms of acting out may be equally or more disastrous in their long-term effects. The challenge is to distinguish between these three patterns.

What have we learnt from the research that has been done about the peri-pubertal and parent vs peer group patterns of development in adolescents? A few pieces of the jigsaw puzzle are beginning to emerge.

The peri-pubertal pattern

The changes that occur in association with puberty represent probably the most discontinuous phase in human development. Puberty is considered closely in Chapter 3. There are major changes in body shape and function. It is not simply a matter of growing more or more quickly. Body shape changes, particularly for females, who also have to contend with the onset of menstruation. Males grow hair where they did not have it before, their voices change substantially, and they have to come to terms with an associated increase in genital responsiveness as well as size. All of these changes impact on the individual's gender identity, requiring re-establishment and revalidation. As discussed in Chapter 4, there are substantial changes in brain function, moving towards a more adult pattern, but obviously to a variable extent across individual adolescents. Alongside these major individually oriented shifts, the young person's social scripts change, with sexual scripts taking on a new importance.

The challenge in understanding the peri-pubertal pattern, which clearly shows considerable individual variability in timing, is to assess the relative importance of cognitive development, the availability of social scripts and the impact of hormonal changes. McClintock & Herdt (1996; Herdt 2000) point to evidence that in both gay and heterosexual males, sexual attraction starts around age 10, and they link this to the hormonal changes associated with adrenarche. This idea will be considered more closely below. This developmental stage in adrenal function, which is associated with an increase in adrenal androgens in both boys and girls, occurs, on average, around 8 years. The extent to which adrenal androgens can account for this stage of development in both boys and girls is questionable. The principal adrenal androgen is dehydroepiandrosterone (DHEA), and whereas a small amount of this steroid is converted into testosterone, the resulting levels, compared to those associated with puberty in the male, are very low. On the other hand, DHEA receptors have recently been identified (see p. 24), and it is a possibility that these direct DHEA effects are important for both male and female sexual development at this stage. It is conceivable that boys are more responsive to androgens when adrenarche begins and become less responsive as the levels increase dramatically with puberty, whereas girls' responsivity to androgens might remain unchanged. But apart from the fact that males are exposed to androgens in utero whereas female are not, there is a substantial rise in testosterone for a period of 2–3 months shortly after birth in the male but not in the female (Forest et al 1976). I have postulated elsewhere (see Chapter 4, p. 127) that early exposure to androgens desensitizes the male to the central nervous system effects of testosterone, so that when puberty occurs, high levels of androgens necessary for the peripheral secondary sexual differentiation of the male can occur without over-stimulation of the brain (Bancroft 2002). Females, on the other hand, remain, in general, much more sensitive to the behavioural effects of testosterone, although there is substantial inter-individual variability in this responsiveness, and quite possibly intra-individual variability across different stages of the reproductive life span. As discussed earlier, the substantial difference between males and females in age of onset of masturbation, which can be regarded as a useful marker of sexual development, suggests on the one hand that male sexuality is substantially organized around as well as activated by pubertal changes, whereas the impact of puberty, and here we should also consider adrenarche, will be much less predictable in the female. Those women who are highly responsive to androgens may be activated at adrenarche, with those who have lower responsiveness showing an onset either around puberty or even much later. In other words, the impact of hormonal changes on sexual development in pre-adolescence and adolescence will be variable in males, but substantially more variable in females.

What relevance does the timing of puberty have on sexual development? Kinsey et al (1948) found that boys going through puberty earlier (i.e. earlier age of first ejaculation) showed earlier onset and higher frequency of sexual activity subsequently, including masturbation and partnered sexual activity, suggesting a higher level of sexual desire or arousability. This association was not found in women (Kinsey et al 1953). Ostovich & Sabini (2005) explored these relationships further. Their timing of puberty was based on age of onset of body hair growth and not first ejaculation. They found that men with earlier age at puberty reported higher sexual drive, but this association was only borderline significant. Their measure of sexual drive consisted of four questions covering typical frequencies of sexual desire, orgasm and masturbation, and a comparison 'with that of the average person'. They also found a correlation between age at first sexual arousal and age at puberty, and between age of first sexual arousal and current sex drive. Their 'age at first sexual arousal' was based on one question: 'How old were you when you first experienced sexual desire?' Given the uncertain relation between sexual arousal and sexual desire (see p. 64), particularly at this age, their results should be interpreted as 'age at first sexual desire'. In particular, it is possible that children at this age experience sexual arousal before they have felt any specific attractions that would lead to 'sexual desire'. This variable was a stronger predictor of current sexual drive than age at puberty. In women, they found no association between 'age at puberty' (which included menarche) and current sexual drive. They did find, however, a clear correlation between age at first sexual desire and current sexual drive.

Little research has looked directly at the relation between hormonal levels and behavioural change in early adolescence, and most of the research that has been done has been by Udry and his colleagues. Their earlier studies were cross-sectional. From a study of 102 boys in 9th or 10th grade, using questionnaires and blood sampling, they concluded that free testosterone was a strong predictor of sexual motivation, with stage of pubertal development otherwise having little effect (Udry et al 1985). In a later longitudinal study of boys over a 3-year period, they were unable to replicate these findings; stage of pubertal development was now a much stronger predictor of sexual interest and behaviour (Halpern et al 1993). In a cross-sectional study of white girls in 8th, 9th or 10th grades, testosterone level was correlated with sexual interest and frequency of masturbation but was not predictive of sexual intercourse, which seemed to be more determined by peer group influences (Udry et al 1986). In a later longitudinal study, testosterone levels were related to transition to first sexual intercourse, but not to sexual interest or masturbation (Halpern et al 1997). It is difficult to understand these conflicting results, although I have discussed the possible implications more fully elsewhere (Bancroft 2003).

However, whereas the effects of sex steroids, such as testosterone and oestradiol on the physical changes of puberty are by comparison straightforward, we should not expect simple relationships between hormones and aspects of sexual arousal and response, particularly at this stage of development. Changing hormone levels at this stage do activate sexual responses, resulting in a new phase of sexual arousability. However, such effects are also dependent on other changes, probably involving brain development. If an individual goes through normal puberty and then experiences hormone deficiency, hormone administration restores sexual arousability to its previous level. The other necessary developmental changes had already occurred. On the other hand, in hypogonadal adolescents or young adults who have not gone through normal puberty, exogenous hormones have an incomplete effect on sexual arousability (Gooren 1988; Finkelstein et al 1998), although they can result in increased aggression (Finkelstein et al 1997).

Some attempts have been made to explore the role of genetic factors in determining the age of first sexual intercourse. Dunne et al (1997) used the Australian Twin Registry and found higher correlation between age at first intercourse for monozygotic (MZ) than for dizygotic (DZ) twins. An interesting finding was that the genetic contribution was more apparent in twins aged 40 years or less, compared with older twins. Their interpretation of this finding was that in the older group, social factors controlling adolescent sexual behaviour were more powerful, obscuring the genetic influences. In more recent years, with a less repressive sexual environment for young people, genetic effects are more apparent. Rodgers et al (1999) reported a behavioural genetic analysis of age at first intercourse, assessing genetic, shared environmental and selected non-shared environmental influences. They found some evidence of a genetic influence most evident in white males. Mustanski et al (2007), using the Finnish Twin Register, found both genetic and non-shared environmental factors were related to age at first sexual intercourse and number of sexual partners. Miller et al (1999) found a relationship between dopamine receptor genes and age at first sexual intercourse in white Americans, more evident in men than women. It is not yet clear whether such genetically mediated effects are manifestations of what we have here called the peri-pubertal pattern or whether their effects are more relevant to adolescents' reaction to the parent vs peer group phase. The interesting cohort effect reported by Dunne et al (1997), with genetic influences being more evident in those who have gone through adolescence more recently, is of relevance in that respect.

Clearly, more research is needed on these issues, but we should not expect the interaction between biological factors, cognitive development and socio-cultural influences to be simple.

The parent vs peer group pattern

There is limited evidence directly addressing the relative importance of parents and peers on adolescent development. Kinsman et al (1998) assessed 1389 6th graders, with a mean age of 11.7 years, at the beginning (time 1) and at the end of the school year (time 2). At time 1, 30% had already experienced sexual intercourse; 5% had first experience between time 1 and time 2. These 'initiators' were more likely to be male, African American, attending a poor school and living in an area with many single-parent families. The strongest predictor of initiation was the belief that most friends had already experienced sexual intercourse, indicating a significant peer group effect. Ramirez-Valles et al (1998) found, in their predominantly African American high-school students, that those engaging in risky sexual behaviour were more likely to live in poor neighbourhoods and less likely to engage in 'prosocial activities' (e.g. church programmes, youth programmes and organized sports).

Several studies have looked at parental influences, mainly those of mothers. Parental communication about sex and birth control is seen as important for reducing adolescent sexual risk behaviour (Jaccard & Dittus 1991; Jaccard et al 2000). Perceived maternal disapproval of sexual intercourse in mother–child relationships characterized by high levels of warmth and closeness may be important protective factors related to delay of first sexual intercourse (Sieving et al 2000), although the mother's values and beliefs appear to influence daughters more than sons (McNeely et al 2002).

The impact of religion on the sexual experiences of 3356 adolescent girls (mean age 16 years), in the Add Health study, was reported by Miller & Gur (2002). Personal devotion (i.e. a sense of personal connection to God) and frequent attendance at church activities was associated with greater sexual responsibility, i.e. less likely to have partners outside of a romantic, loving relationship, and more likely to use contraception within such relationships. 'Personal conservatism', which meant a rigid adherence to one's religious creed, was associated with more exposure to unprotected sex, including forced sex, and greater tendency to leave birth control to their male partners. This religious 'personality style' was regarded as leading to fewer coping resources in sexual situations.

Bearman & Brückner (2001) found that 'pledging virginity' was associated with a substantial delay in initiating sexual intercourse, but this effect was not apparent at all ages of adolescence, and was more effective when the pledge was not the norm for one's group. They concluded that the pledge worked because it was part of establishing one's identity, for which pledging needed to be at least partially non-normative. Pledgers who broke their promise were less likely to use contraception at first sexual intercourse.

Halpern et al (2000) used data from the Add Health study, in which 100 white boys were assessed over 3 years, and 200 white and black girls over 2 years. Controlling for age, physical maturity and mother's education, they found a curvilinear relationship between intelligence and experience of sexual intercourse; the upper and lower ends of the intelligence range were less likely to have experienced sexual intercourse. Furthermore, those with higher intelligence were more likely to have postponed initiation of the full range of partnered sexual activities. It was postulated that intelligence might be associated with a greater ability to consider the consequences of sexual activity and to weigh up the pros and cons. It was acknowledged that further research was needed to fully understand this effect of intelligence, and it may well be relevant to the effects of adolescent brain development considered earlier (p. 60).

These and other studies reinforce the idea that adolescents who feel positive about their future, look forward to a successful career or who have relatively high self-esteem are more likely to delay sexual intercourse. Maybe such positive self-esteem factors make the adolescent less dependent on peer group influences.

What is strikingly missing, in the modern discourse on adolescent sexuality, is the idea of helping teenagers to become more responsible in this emerging part of their life which, if only because of the potential for creating new life, carries huge responsibilities from the time they are fertile. These responsibilities are, or should be, as great for the teenage boy as for the girl. The policy of advocating sexual abstinence until marriage, with no consideration of how to implement abstinence at the stage of life when, at least for boys, sexual arousability is at its maximum, is a disturbing form of denial. How the young adolescent negotiates this developmental phase to move towards a stable and rewarding sexual life as an adult receives scant attention.[1] As Weinberger et al (2005) commented in the conclusion to their review of adolescent brain development, 'If teens are not the full neurological equivalent of adults, what specific systems and practices will help them grow and mature in appropriate ways? ...Under what circumstances should teens be allowed to make their own choices and under what circumstances should directed guidance be offered and options limited?' (p. 19). These are not trivial questions.

The maladaptive pattern

There is now an extensive literature showing that during adolescence, sexual behaviour, particularly in terms of early age at first sexual intercourse, number of sexual partners and sexual risk taking, is associated with other types of maladaptive or 'delinquent' behaviour, such as drug and alcohol use. There is much more limited evidence from longitudinal studies, indicating that

---

[1]Many interesting and informative narratives by young adults of their adolescent sexual development can be found in Martinson (1994).

maladaptive behaviour in childhood is predictive of later, sexual patterns in adolescence. Thus Caspi et al (1997) found that 'under-controlled' behaviour at age 3 predicted high 'negative emotionality' and low 'constraint', from the Tellegen personality profile (Tellegen & Waller 1985), at age 18, which in turn predicted a range of high-risk behaviours, including sexual behaviour, at the age of 21. Bates et al (2003) showed that personality factors, such as a tendency to 'externalizing behaviour' in kindergarten-age children, are predictive of number of sexual partners in late adolescence.

There is also an extensive literature on the relationship between CSA and maladaptive patterns of sexual behaviour and function in adolescence and adulthood. This is covered in Chapter 16.

There is one particular aspect of the maladaptive pattern which warrants closer scrutiny: the relation between negative mood and sexuality. A paradoxical relationship between negative mood and sexuality was discussed in Chapter 4. As this relationship is more likely in younger adults, the question arises of when this pattern, which may lessen as one gets older, first becomes established. Is it in childhood or around the peri-pubertal transition? Could there be a stage of sexual development when the arousing effects of negative mood, such as anxiety, become associated with the arousal response to sexual stimuli, at least in some people, what might be described as age-dependent 'excitation transfer' (Zillman 1983). This brings to mind Ramsey's (1943) early study in which boys aged 10–12 years reported erections occurring to a variety of 'arousing' but non-sexual situations, such as being chased by a policeman, flying in an airplane or wrestling with a friend. This transitional phase of non-specific genital responsiveness soon gave way, at least in most of the boys he interviewed, to a more discriminatory sexual response pattern. Could that type of sexual learning process be disrupted by the effects of CSA, leading to the establishment of a paradoxical relation between negative mood and sexual interest and response? How does this relate to the developmental stages of brain function outlined by Weinberger et al (2005)?

Sexual preferences and the development of sexual identity

As the three strands, sexual responsiveness, gender identity and dyadic relationships, start to integrate in this transitional stage between childhood and adolescence, a key element among the evolving sexual meanings is an emerging sexual identity – initially, 'What type of person am I sexually attracted to?' and, subsequently, 'What kind of sexual person am I?' Perhaps the most important aspect of this question in Western culture is, 'Am I heterosexual or homosexual?' The nature–nurture issue, mentioned at the start of this chapter, is particularly controversial in relation to the origins of homosexuality. It is noteworthy that, in most such debates, the origins of heterosexuality are not an issue; they are a 'given'. The issue is what makes it happen differently. However, we know little about normal heterosexual development, and we know even less about normal homosexual development (Savin-Williams 1995). The nature–nurture divide takes on an added moral significance in this context. There is a long-standing pattern of seeing homosexuality at best as abnormal and at worst, sinful, with pathological coming midway. Because of this, homosexuality resulting from natural causes has been defended as not the responsibility of the individual. On the other hand, homosexuality that is 'learnt' is more readily regarded as sinful. The history of this struggle will be considered in Chapter 8. It impacts on the terms we use. Should we talk of sexual preference, sexual orientation or sexual identity? This question led to an interesting discussion in a Kinsey Institute workshop on the Role of Theory in Sex Research, held in 1998 (Bancroft 2000; pp. 133–139). 'Sexual preference' was considered by Ehrhardt (p. 137) to imply a choice, with the implication that the object of our sexual attraction is not integral to our lives. She preferred 'sexual orientation' as a descriptive term based on the Kinsey scale, allowing consideration of sexual attractions and behaviours on a continuum, rather than as a dichotomy. Gagnon had problems with both words. 'It seems that sexual orientation is such a historically embedded and politicized word...we may want to use (it) because it connotes a phenomenon that appears to be deeper in the organism, harder to change, and more profound than "preference"...' (p. 137). To put it briefly, 'preference' implies 'acquired' or 'chosen', the result of 'nurture' and hence morally vulnerable; 'orientation' implies innate or determined by 'nature'. As I remain committed to the idea that our sexual attractions result from an interaction between nature and nurture (Bancroft 1983, 1990), I will strive to avoid both terms, and use 'sexual identity' instead. How an individual identifies him or herself in sexual terms may well reflect the sexual scripts that individual has encountered, but does not inform us about the factors that influence the choice of script.

Sexual identities in men and women

In Chapter 8 we will look more closely at the concept of sexual identity and how different sexual identities prevail in different cultures. At this stage it is sufficient to recognize that, in our culture, the proportion of individuals who identify as exclusively homosexual or 'gay' is small, around 2–3% for males and 1–2% for females (e.g. Laumann et al 1994). But there is more variability among women, with less certainty about a specific identity being relatively common and bisexual identity being somewhat more prevalent than among men, although often changing over time (Schreurs 1993; Peplau et al 1999; Diamond 2003a, b; Kinnish et al 2005). By comparison, a larger majority of men in our culture arrive at a clear sexual identity, either 'straight ' or 'gay', which remains relatively fixed. Bisexuality, particularly for adult men, is much less often acknowledged. We should conclude, however, that once a sexual identity is established it determines the gender of subsequent sexual partners, and we will consider this issue more closely in Chapter 8.

As Peplau et al (1998) point out, it has been frequently asserted in the literature that the essential ingredients of sexual attraction are different for men and women. Thus Symons (1979) concluded that 'heterosexual men tend to see women as sex objects and to desire young, beautiful women; homosexual men tend to see men as sex objects and to desire young, handsome men; but women whether heterosexual or homosexual, are much less likely to be sexually aroused primarily on the basis of cosmetic qualities' (p. 301). Blumstein & Schwartz (1983), in their study of couples, both heterosexual and homosexual, concluded that for women, whether lesbian or heterosexual, emotional attraction more often precedes erotic attraction, whereas the reverse applies for men. Weinrich (1987) described two types of erotic attraction: 'lust' and 'limerence'. 'Lust', according to his definition, is directed at a particular class of object. 'Limerence' is erotic attraction that follows emotional attachment to a particular person. Both men and women may experience both lust and limerence, but men are more likely to experience lust and women limerence. According to these views, there are some fundamental differences in the way that we organize our sexual identities. In men, sexual identity is most predictably related to the gender of those found sexually attractive: 'Am I sexually attracted to men or women?' In women, the emphasis is on emotional involvement and closeness, which is not something that one can recognize before establishing some form of relationship, sexual or otherwise. If a woman has consistently found herself experiencing the ingredients of sexual attractiveness in a series of relationships with women, then she is likely to regard herself as a lesbian. But then, at a later stage, she may find herself in a comparable relationship with a man, or vice versa. Hence, there is the contrast between relative certainty about sexual identity in men, and relative openness in women.

We might therefore expect different trajectories of sexual identity development, and quite possibly different timing between men and women.

Possible explanatory mechanisms

Let us now consider the range of explanatory models relevant to this developmental process, at each stage keeping in mind that the relevant mechanisms may be different for males and females. We will find a variety of mechanisms or factors that are potentially relevant, but none sufficient as an explanation. We will then consider the various ways that such mechanisms might interact. We start with the three strands from our interactive model and move on to a variety of other explanatory mechanisms that have been postulated or explored.

Gender identity

One of the must robust associations in developmental psychology of males is an association between gender non-conformity during childhood and subsequent homosexual identity. A limited amount of prospective data, mainly reported by Green (1974, 1987), shows that 75–80% of boys diagnosed as having gender identity disorder (GID) in childhood report bisexual or homosexual identities in late adolescence (Zucker 1990). There is no comparable data for girls with GID. There is, however, a substantial literature based on retrospective recall of childhood gender identity by adults. Bailey & Zucker (1995) reported a meta-analysis of 48 studies, showing a substantial connection between childhood gender non-conformity and later homosexual identity, significant in both men and women, but much more so in men. They estimated that 51% of boys but only about 6% of girls, with the requisite degree of cross-sex-typed behaviour, will become homosexual.

Thus we have strong evidence that gender identity either influences the developmental process directly or is associated with other factors that directly influence sexual identity development. However, such influences, it would seem, are not necessary as many men and women with homosexual identities do not report gender non-conformity in childhood.

Sexual responsiveness

In the childhood stage we found evidence of sexual play between children, common for both boys and girls, more so than 50 years earlier, particularly for girls. A substantial minority of such children had same-sex sexual play experiences, more so for girls when younger and more so for boys at junior high school level (see p. 154). What remains unclear is the significance of such play to later sexual identity.

Moving on to the sexually relevant stage, we recognized the emergence of a more open phase of interest, followed before long by the onset of dating. In our recent Kinsey Institute study (Reynolds et al 2003; see Table 5.3), recall of first sexual arousal was at a similar age for boys and girls (9.7 and 10.8 years, respectively, not significantly different). First sexual attraction, however, came later (average age 11.4 and 12.4 years, respectively), with boys being significantly more likely to experience this before puberty than girls (67% vs 38%, $p < 0.05$). Age at first sexual fantasy was also significantly younger for boys (11.6 vs 13.3 years). Ostovich & Sabini (2005) asked 'How old were you when you first experienced sexual desire?'. Males reported an average age of 11.2 (± 2.9) years, and females 12.6 (± 3.0) years, a significant difference ($p < 0.001$). These ages for first sexual attraction and first sexual desire are very similar, reinforcing the idea that, at this age, sexual desire, as such, is dependent on their being someone to desire.

How does this compare in males and females who subsequently develop a homosexual identity? Herdt & Boxer (1993), in an interview study of 147 gay-identified male and 55 lesbian-identified female youths (aged 14–20 years), recruited from a community support group for gay and lesbian youth, found an average age of first same-sex attraction of 9.6 years for males and 10.1 years for females. They did not comment on age at first sexual arousal. The average age for first same-sex sexual fantasy was somewhat later (11.2 and 11.9 years, respectively, not significantly different), and their first same sex sexual activity later still (13.1 years for males and 15.2 years for females, a significant gender difference). D'Augelli & Hershberger (1993) also studied gay, lesbian and bisexual youths in a community setting. They found first awareness of homosexual orientation typically at age 10, with first disclosure to others on average around age 16. Remafedi et al (1991), in a study of gay and bisexual male youth, found a mean age for first same-sex attraction to be 10.2 years, with a standard deviation around 3.5 years. First same-sex sexual activity was at a mean age of 15.6 years. Hamer et al (1993), in their genetic linkage study, asked their gay respondents at what age they were first attracted to another male. The results, reported in Figure 2 of their paper, showed a wide range from age 4 to 17, with an average around 10 years. Self-acknowledgement of their sexual orientation was reported at an average age around 15. Acknowledging their orientation to others occurred on average about 5–6 years later (early 20s). The respondents in this study were much older (mean age 36 ± 9 years) than in the previous three studies, and also clearly 'came out' at a later age. We should keep in mind that different methods of recruiting gay and lesbian respondents may reflect different developmental trajectories. In particular, those who identify sufficiently early to join gay and lesbian teenage groups may have experienced same-sex attraction earlier than average.

Pattatucci & Hamer (1995) found that lesbian and heterosexual women reported similar average ages for experiencing sexual attraction to their preferred gender (10.6 ± 3.1 years for heterosexual, 10.6 ± 4.7 years for lesbian). Ostovich & Sabini (2005) reported significantly younger age for first experience of sexual desire by lesbian women (11.5 ± 2.4 years) than by heterosexual women (12.8 ± 3.1 years; $p = 0.03$).

As considered earlier (p. 156) Herdt & McClintock (2000) proposed that the age of 10 was a key developmental stage for the emergence of sexual attraction, whether or not the individual proceeded to establish a heterosexual or homosexual identity. However, the limited evidence reviewed here points to considerable variability, with an average age around 10 years (i.e. before puberty for the majority), but with a tendency for sexual attraction to emerge slightly earlier in pre-homosexual males, and possibly in pre-homosexual females. In any case, it appears that something of importance to the development of sexual identity is happening in the period from about age 8 or 9 until the onset of puberty. Is it possible that an earlier age for experiencing sexual attraction would increase the likelihood of developing same-sex attraction?

Capacity for dyadic relationships

To what extent does a young individual's ability to establish and maintain close dyadic relationships relate to his or her sexual identity? As yet we have little directly relevant evidence. In an earlier phase of the literature, particular types of parent–child relationship were implicated in the causation of homosexuality (e.g. Bieber et al 1962). Studies have varied, some showing particular types of mother–son relationships (in particular, the so-called 'closed binding intimate' mother), others the father–son relationship (in particular, detached, absent or hostile father). Most of these observations, however, involved psychiatric patient populations. It subsequently became clear that such relationships are more obviously related to personality characteristics than to homosexual preferences per se. In a series of studies of non-clinical populations, Siegelman (1974, 1978) found that homosexual men did report more disturbed relationships with their parents than did the heterosexual controls. However, men in the homosexual group were on average more neurotic and when low-neuroticism groups were compared, these differences in parental relationships disappeared. The relevance of neuroticism or other personality attributes to sexual identity formation is discussed later. Given the possibility that in many such cases gender non-conformity shows itself quite early, it becomes difficult to sort out what parent–child problematic patterns of interaction are cause or effect. More research on this potentially important aspect of development is required.

Abnormal masculinization of the brain

Compatible with the gender identity evidence are long-standing ideas that homosexuality is a consequence of an abnormality of masculinization of the brain, deficient in male homosexuals, excessive in lesbians, and a wide variety of attempts to pinpoint the relevant mechanism (s) have been reported. However, a crucial and often overlooked point here is the need to distinguish between effects on gender identity (which then may secondarily influence sexual identity), and direct hormonal effects on sexual identity development per se.

In the early part of the 20th century, Hirschfeld (1913) put forward the view that homosexuality was a form of hormonal intersex. Evidence obtained during the 1940s countered this view. But with the development of modern hormone assay techniques, interest in this possibility returned, leading to a number of studies looking for endocrine differences between adult homosexuals and heterosexuals. Most of these studies were notable for their naivety in assuming that relative androgen deficiency during early development would be evident in adult levels of androgens. A reasonable conclusion from this research is that adult male homosexuals and heterosexuals do not differ in circulating levels of androgens (Meyer-Bahlburg 2000). A slightly less naïve idea was pursued by Dörner et al (1975), who compared groups of exclusively homosexual and heterosexual men in their responses to oestrogen provocation. In a normal female ovarian cycle, oestrogen produces a positive feedback effect late in the follicular phase which leads to the surge of luteinizing hormone (LH) that precedes ovulation (p. 40). The homosexual group showed a pattern of LH response that was closer to the normal female positive feedback response than that found in the heterosexual group. Dörner's conclusion was that the brains of the homosexual men had been inadequately defeminized and this was evidence of the biological basis of their homosexuality. These findings have always been controversial and the comparability of this so-called positive feedback response to that in the female seriously questioned. This idea was explored further by Gladue et al (1984) with the crucial difference that, in addition to including a heterosexual female comparison group, they also assessed the effects of oestrogen provocation on the testis. They found an LH response to the oestrogen provocation, which in the male homosexual group was midway between the heterosexual women and men, similar to that reported by Dörner et al (1975). However, they also found less testicular response (i.e. less increase in testosterone) to the increase in LH in the homosexual group. Hence less negative feedback of testosterone on the pituitary in the homosexual men is therefore the most likely explanation for the more pronounced rise in LH in that group. In other words, the difference in hypothalamic response was really a difference in testicular response, and as such was probably unrelated to defeminization of the brain. There are various ways in which the lifestyle that prevailed among homosexual men at that time could have impacted testicular function, e.g. marijuana use. For some reason, Gladue and his colleagues rejected this interpretation of their findings, which they took to reinforce Dörner's conclusions. But the testicular explanation is the more likely.

Perhaps the final nail in the coffin of Dörner's model was provided by Gooren (1986). He showed, in both male and female transsexuals, that the hypothalamic response to oestrogen provocation was consistent with the prevailing hormonal milieu at the time. Thus, before sex reassignment surgery the hypothalamic response was consistent with the genetic sex. After surgery (and castration) it was in the opposite direction. The response was therefore not a fixed product of early organization of the brain but a function of the dynamic organizing effects of the prevailing hormonal milieu (see Bancroft 1990 for fuller discussion).

Comparison of adult androgen levels in heterosexual and lesbian women gives a less clearly negative result; some studies have found higher androgen levels in lesbian women, others have not (reviewed by Mustanski et al 2002). Overall, there is no consistent support for early masculinization of the brain by androgens as being relevant to female homosexuality (Peplau et al 1999). The effects of pre-natal DES, considered in Chapter 3 (p. 51), are of interest, resulting in bisexual or same-sex interests in a minority of women. It is not clear how this worked or why in only some women. However, such evidence in women, but not in men, is compatible with the greater fluidity of female sexual identity.

Two studies have compared 'butch' (i.e. relatively masculine) and 'femme' lesbians and found that the 'butch' women had higher salivary testosterone than the 'femme' (Pearcey et al 1996; Singh et al 1999). However, here we are seeing a possible relationship between androgens and gender identity, not sexual identity. Interestingly, no one has attempted to compare more masculine and more feminine homosexual men in this way.

If differences in androgen effects on the brain cannot be found between homosexual and heterosexual men and women, perhaps other brain indicators of defeminization in male homosexuals or masculinization in lesbians are apparent. As new technologies have emerged, they have been used to pursue this question. Functional cerebral asymmetry refers to the degree of lateralization of function between the two hemispheres. There is somewhat inconsistent evidence that men show more lateralization than women, and a suggestion from limited data that homosexual men may come midway between heterosexual men and women in this respect (Mustanski et al 2002). Handedness is another aspect of cerebral lateralization. Are homosexual men more like heterosexual women and lesbian women more like heterosexual men in their likelihood of being left-handed? The conclusion from the inconsistent literature so far is that this may be the case with lesbian women, but not, apparently, for homosexual men (Mustanski et al 2002).

The search for neuroanatomical differences in brain structure of men and women has been closely followed by a search for differences relevant to sexual identity. Gender differences in brain structure were considered in Chapter 4 (p. 60). There is some evidence that INAH 3, one of the nuclei in the pre-optic-anterior hypothalamic region, which is smaller and contains fewer neurons in women than in men, is smaller in homosexual than heterosexual men, though the numbers of neurons do not differ (Hines 2002). However, this is based on one small sample and remains to be replicated.

Attempts to identify differences in brain activity related to sexual identity have recently started. Brain processing of olfactory cues has shown differences related to gender and sexual orientation. Savic et al (2006) used positron emission tomography to assess brain activation to a typically male pheromone (4,16-androstadien-3-one or AND), found mainly in male sweat, and a typically female pheromone, an oestrogen-like steroid (EST), typically found in female urine. Brain activation depended on sexual identity. Thus in women, AND produced maximal activation in the medial pre-optic area (MPOA)/anterior hypothalamus, which is central to sexual response, whereas EST was treated like a common odour and processed by the olfactory brain. In heterosexual men, the reverse was found: EST produced maximal activation in the MPOA/anterior hypothalamus. Homosexual men were similar to heterosexual women in showing the MPOA/anterior hypothalamus activation to AND. In a further study, using the same methodology, Berglund et al (2006) found lesbian women to be more like men than heterosexual women. These findings demonstrate a link between pheromonal stimuli and sexual orientation, but as yet we cannot say to what extent this is a learnt pattern that reflects the development of sexual identity or is an intrinsic mechanism that influences that development. Preliminary evidence from a functional magnetic resonance imaging study of brain activity in response to preferred sexual stimuli showed similar patterns of brain activity in homosexual and heterosexual men when the stimulus was in the preferred category, except that the homosexual men showed greater activity in the amygdala in response to their preferred stimuli (Bailey et al 2006).

In men the length of the index finger is shorter than the ring finger, particularly in the right hand. In women these two fingers are close to equal in length. It has been assumed that this gender difference, which is apparent by 2 years of age, is in some way a consequence of different androgen effects during early development. Do homosexual men have finger length ratios closer to women and lesbian women closer to men? The results are so far inconsistent and inconclusive (Mustanski et al 2002). A similarly inconsistent and inconclusive picture has emerged for a number of other variables possibly affected by androgens, including dermatoglyphics, weight and height, body morphology, penis length and oto-acoustic emissions, the evidence for which has been reviewed by Mustanski et al (2002).

Genetic factors

The possibility that factors determining sexual identity may be inherited has been studied in three ways: (i) Does homosexuality run in families? If so, then a distinction needs to be made between genetic factors and the influence of shared environment. (ii) Do MZ twins show greater concordance for homosexuality than DZ? (iii) Are there specific genetic markers of homosexuality?

Bailey & Pillard (1995), in reviewing the family studies, found the rate of homosexuality among brothers to be around 9%, higher than the prevalence estimates for male homosexuality in population samples. Lesbian women were more likely to have lesbian sisters than heterosexual women, but the familiality estimates varied widely across studies (from 6% to 25%). It remains unclear whether male and female homosexuality runs in families, or whether family effects are gender specific.

Twin studies have consistently shown higher concordance in MZ than DZ twins since the early reports of Kallmann (1952) and Heston & Shields (1968). The most recent studies have used better samples, and multivariate modelling with sexual orientation as the dependent variable and childhood gender non-conformity and continuous measures of gender identity as covariates (Bailey et al 2000; Kirk et al 2000). The results point to both genetic and non-shared environmental influences on sexual identity development, with a suggestion that genetic influences are stronger in males than females (Mustanski et al 2002).

The recent history of research on genetic mechanisms influencing sexual orientation is evolving and, at this stage, is not easy for the non-geneticist to understand. It combines family pedigree study with the search for genetic linkages. In 1993 Hamer et al reported on the families of 114 homosexual men. They found an increased rate of homosexuality in maternal uncles and cousins, but not in paternal relatives, suggesting an X-linked transmission on the maternal side. They went on to explore DNA linkage in 40 pairs of homosexual brothers and found such linkage to markers on Xq28, on the long arm of the X chromosome in 64% of the brother-pairs tested, significantly more than the 50% expected by chance. They postulated that at least in some homosexuals there is a gene involved in determining sexual orientation in the Xq28 region of the X chromosome, which in males is inherited from the mother. There have so far been three attempts to replicate this finding. Hamer's group reported a successful replication, including assessment of brother pairs discordant for sexual identity, which showed 22% sharing Xq28, significantly less than expected by chance (Hu et al 1995). In this same report, Xq28 was investigated for linkage in pairs of lesbian sisters; no linkage was found. The other two studies failed to replicate the Xq28 finding, but it is not clear to what extent methodological differences accounted for these inconsistencies (Mustanski et al 2002). Pattatucci & Hamer (1995) studied family pedigrees in women and found no similar evidence of maternal transmission as in men.

Turner (1995) reported further family pedigree evidence showing a significantly lower proportion of male relatives in the maternal lineage in male but not female homosexuals. He concluded that this resulted from wastage of male fetuses due to early death manifested as miscarriages or infertility. He estimated a 36% excess of death of male over female fetuses. He drew parallels with the evidence from the families with each of nine distinct 'semilethal' disorders resulting from genes in the Xq28 region (e.g. Addison's disease, nephrogenic diabetes insipidus and fragile X syndrome), likening, in a somewhat disturbing way, homosexual inheritance to such pathologies.

Women have two X chromosomes, one inherited from the father and one from the mother. Men, for obvious reasons, inherit their one X chromosome from their mother. Normally, in women, one X in each cell is randomly inactivated, so that usually any tissue consists of approximately 50% each of cells with maternal and paternal X chromosomes. Bocklandt et al (2006) examined this distribution in 97 mothers of homosexual sons and 103 age-matched control women. Significantly more of the mothers of homosexual men had extreme skewing of X inactivation (i.e. more than 90% of cells of a particular type having the same X chromosome): 23% in mothers of two or more homosexual sons, 13% in mothers of one or more homosexual sons and 4% in control women. This was taken to be evidence that the X chromosome is regulating sexual orientation, at least in some men, possibly as a result of an as yet unidentified imprinted gene on the X chromosome (i.e. a gene the expression of which depends on the parent of its origin).

Green & Keverne (2000) found a disparate maternal aunt–uncle ratio, similar to that found in homosexual men, in male to female transsexuals, but not in female to male transsexuals. They hypothesized that imprinted genes on the X chromosome, which had escaped inactivation, may be involved. They also cited evidence from Turner's syndrome (XO) (see p. 45), in which the child may have inherited either a paternal X (Xp) or a maternal X (Xm). The ratio of Xm to Xp in Turner individuals is 70:30, showing evidence of fetal wastage of the Xp fetuses. Furthermore, Skuse et al (1997) reported that Turner syndrome girls differ in their social disposition according to the origin of their one X; those with Xm had more social problems, associated with a range of behavioural characteristics more typical of boys than girls. Hence the Xm had, in some way, a masculinizing and Xp a feminizing effect. This led Green & Keverne (2000) to comment: 'normal boys always inherit the maternal X, but if they were to inherit the paternal X then a possibility arises for their social behaviour to be feminized' (p. 60). These ideas from studies of both homosexual and transsexual men, while speculative, and requiring further supportive evidence, point to a genetic influence, although it is not clear whether it is gender identity, sexual identity or both which are being influenced.

There have now been two attempts to identify specific genes involved in sexual identity development, both related to the androgenization model. Macke et al (1993) looked for DNA sequence variation in the androgen receptor gene. DuPree et al (2004) looked for variations in CYP19, the gene for aromatase cytochrome P450, an enzyme necessary for conversion of androgens to oestrogens, on the basis that, at least in non-human mammals, aromatization is a crucial step in the early masculinization of the brain. Neither study found positive evidence.

The most recent genetic study involved a full genome scan of 456 individuals from 146 families with two or more gay brothers (Mustanski et al 2005). With the goal of extending previous research that only focused on the X chromosome, the authors commented, 'Given the complexity of sexual orientation, numerous genes are likely to be involved, many of which are expected to be autosomal rather than sex-linked. Indeed, the modest levels of linkage that have been reported for the X chromosome can account for, at most, only a fraction of the overall heritability of male sexual orientation as deduced from twin studies'. They went on to report three new regions of the genome of possible interest; one, on chromosome 7 'falls just short of ... criteria for genome-wide significance'. The other two, on chromosomes 8 and 10, 'approached the criteria for suggestive linkage'. As with all first reports, it would seem prudent to await further replication before becoming involved in interpreting the numerous mechanisms with genetic linkages to those three regions and extrapolating to sexual identity. In any case, we are probably looking at genotypic mechanisms involved in a wide range of developmental factors, which may be of only indirect relevance to sexual identity development. It remains to be seen whether a genotype exists directly related to same-sex or opposite-sex sexual attraction.

Given the extraordinary similarity of the genomes of mice, chimpanzees and humans, there is a need for further mechanisms to explain the very different phenotypes across such species. Genetic explanation of sexual identity development is not going to be easy!

Early learning

Coming midway between prenatal determination and the effects of culture at a later stage is the idea of 'preparedness for learning' (Seligman & Hager 1972),

something in our constitution which makes us particularly reactive to certain types of environmental influence. Most psychoanalytic theorists have emphasized the importance of early experience in determining later sexual preference. Some, more biologically oriented, such as Money (1980) and Perper (1985), talked of templates. For Perper this is a 'prefigured gestalt' of an ideal (woman) sexual partner. 'It is not', he suggested, "encoded" in the genes, but is created by a slow developmental process involving genetic regulation of neural development and later neurophysiological construction of an increasingly detailed and recognizably female image of a woman' (p. 16–17). Money called his templates 'lovemaps' and talked of 'schemes implanted in the brain'. Like a native language, a lovemap is not completed on the day of birth. It requires input from the social environment. The critical period for its development is not puberty, Money proposed, but before the age of 8 years. The implication of the template concept is that, whilst it is influenced by environmental factors, it is formed fairly early and thereafter is relatively fixed. It is not clear on what evidence such ideas are based or, as theoretical models, how they could be tested. However, with recent developments in our understanding of brain development during adolescence, such a mechanism has become more feasible. The challenge is to find ways to identify its presence.

Another aspect of learning of possible relevance is conditioning. To what extent do our sexual responses become conditioned to certain types of sexual stimuli? This was considered earlier in Chapter 4 (p. 104), and overall the evidence is inconclusive. However, there is one striking gender difference that is of relevance in this context. The more unusual forms of sexual preference, such as fetishes, are almost exclusively found in men. Sadomasochism shows a less striking gender difference; it is less unusual in women than fetishism (see Chapter 9). However, sado-masochism, compared to fetishism, is less about the nature of the desired sexual object and more about the type of interaction (relationship) with the sexual object. Something is happening in the sexual development of some men that results in their developing predictable sexual arousal to very specific types of stimulus. This is consistent with the idea that sexual attraction in men is stimulus specific whereas in women it is more determined by relationship factors. But as yet we do not know what this gender difference means in terms of learning.

Cultural factors

How sexual identity is organized and expressed across different cultures and within the same culture at different time periods is a large subject, which will be visited at various points in this book. In this section, we will briefly consider how culture may influence the development of sexual identity. Herdt (1990) divides patterns of sexual development into linear or continuous and sequential or discontinuous.

Linear development implies a steady, continuous progression from childhood, through adolescence to adulthood, with those involved in child rearing having clear and continuous expectations of how the child's sexuality should emerge, which they presumably communicate to the child. Herdt (1990) gives examples of non-industrial societies of this type (e.g. the !Kung bushmen, the Trobriand Islanders and Tahitians). Maybe some industrial societies, which promote a predominantly positive set of values in relation to sex, also come into this category (e.g. The Netherlands and Sweden), although the history of Western societies indicates variability in such patterns over time.

Discontinuous development involves a series of stages which, although they follow a particular sequence, differ in substantial ways from each other, with varying degrees of awareness or involvement by family or society. Most relevant to our current consideration is a discontinuous pattern in which the individual passes through a phase of homosexual activity on to a later heterosexual and reproductive phase. Such discontinuous patterns vary in the extent to which the homosexual phase is institutionalized in the culture, in contrast to being relatively recognized but unacknowledged, or 'covert'.

These examples show us how cultural factors might predispose to adoption of an exclusively homosexual or heterosexual identity in some cultural contexts, and a more flexible or bisexual identity in other contexts which do not require such a distinction and which therefore accept, explicitly or implicitly, various types of sexual interaction at different times in a person's life. We see this distinction within Western society in the contrast between male and female sexual identities.

Sexual preferences in animals

Before we attempt to integrate these various influences in the human let us briefly consider the evidence for sexual preference in other species and see if this throws light on the human enigma.

The clearest examples of sexual preferences in animals are in birds. Some species show sexual imprinting at an early stage; this is a form of learning during a critical period of development. For example, the polymorphous snowgoose tends to mate with geese the same colour as those it was exposed to early in its life (usually its parents). The mechanism of such imprinting is not understood and its relevance to mammals or man is very uncertain (Bateson 1978).

Beagle bitches, when in heat, show a preference for male dogs even when they have had no previous mating experience (Beach & LeBoeuf 1967). Similar evidence has been reported in some female rodents (Larsson 1978). It may be relevant that this limited evidence appears to be confined to female animals.

Beach (1979) emphasized the importance of complementarity of sexual behaviour. This is the tendency for an animal to adopt a receptive posture when being mounted or to mount an animal presenting in a receptive posture. It so happens that males are more likely to show mounting and females to be receptive, and this tendency can be influenced by hormones during development. However, the fact that a male animal mounts another male does not mean that either animal has a homosexual preference. Beach (1979) made a pungent critique of studies that used such animal interaction as a model for human homosexuality.

The extent of same-sex behaviour, or at least that which is observed, varies considerably across species (Tyler 1984; Bagemihl 1999; Vasey 2002). Goy & Goldfoot (1975) pointed out that for mammals the main variable is the extent of bisexuality. Not only do species vary in this respect, but within species the sexes usually differ, i.e. in species where the male shows a lot of bisexual behaviour, the female tends to show little and vice versa. In most species it is the female who shows more bisexual behaviour (i.e. mounting other females as well as adopting the characteristic posture for being mounted — lordosis in rodents, presenting in primates).

In the case of primates the early organizational effects of hormones are more related to the degree of later bisexuality than whether sexual behaviour is either heterosexual or homosexual. Thus, a female given large amounts of testosterone may show increased mounting behaviour as a result, but not a decrease in her presenting behaviour.

Evidence from primate species is likely to be the most relevant for understanding human sexuality. According to Goy & Goldfoot (1975), the male rhesus monkey shows much more bisexual behaviour than the female, particularly during the pre-pubertal years. During its first year of life the male rhesus mounts other males and females in its peer group with more or less equal frequency. Mounting of the mother is also common. If separated from the mother but left with its peer group, the male initially shows more mounting of females, though this appears to be part of the assertion of dominance in the motherless group. After a while there is a return to a more equal ratio of male to female mounts. When the male reaches adolescence any mount of a female that results in intromission is usually followed by more exclusively heterosexual mounting behaviour (Goy 1979). This pattern suggests that early mounting by males is more an expression of dominance or masculinity than an erotic response. Once puberty is reached, however, and erotic responses become enhanced by hormonal effects, the dominance function is superseded by the sexual.

Akers & Conoway (1979), somewhat in contrast to Goy, reported relatively frequent homosexual interactions between adult female rhesus monkeys living in a heterosexual group. The mounting female was usually in the follicular phase of her oestrous cycle, while the female being mounted was in her periovulatory phase. Little activity of this kind occurred during the luteal phase. These authors did not see this behaviour as a substitute for heterosexual activity. These homosexual pairs tended to spend much more time soliciting than in actual physical contact and affectional ties may have been important. They suggested that 'sexual gratification may be a fringe benefit of a relationship that develops for a variety of reasons', a possibility that crops up frequently in our attempts to understand many human relationships.

In a more recent review of the primate evidence, Wallen & Parsons (1997) concluded that same-sex sexual behaviour was common among juvenile male primates but typically decreased or ceased with the establishment of puberty. By contrast, same-sex sexual behaviour among female primates is unusual before puberty but increases once females have reached reproductive age. This is a striking across-species gender difference.

Field studies of troops of rhesus monkeys have identified a predictable pattern with a group of leader or alpha males in the centre surrounded by the females. The subordinate males are not admitted to the central group and are progressively forced to the periphery of the troop where they show a considerable amount of homosexual behaviour (Goy & Goldfoot 1975).

Goldfoot et al (1984) have also demonstrated that the extent of bisexual behaviour can be influenced by manipulating environmental factors. At the age of 3 months, infant rhesus monkeys were assigned either to heterosexual groups (i.e. with both male and female infants) or to isosexual groups (i.e. all infants of the same sex). The isosexual condition increased the likelihood of homosexual behaviour (i.e. presenting by males and mounting by females), though this effect was more marked in the males than the females. The authors concluded from this evidence that 'presenting behaviour is extremely responsive to social conditions, mounting behaviour is intermediate in this regard and rough and tumble play seems to be only mildly influenced by the social environment'.

Early experience in same-sex peer groups is one form of environmental manipulation. There is also a considerable amount of evidence of the effects of more extreme forms of social deprivation on later adult sexual behaviour. In all species of mammals studied so far, including the rat, guinea-pig, cat, dog and rhesus monkey, being deprived of tactile contact with either the mother or the peer group during infancy and early childhood results in abnormal or disrupted adult sexual behaviour in male animals. The same disruptive effect has not been demonstrated in females. In the rat such disruption can be easily treated by subsequent sexual experience, i.e. the rat readily learns to overcome this disability. In the rhesus monkey, on the other hand, the disability is relatively intractable, suggesting that there may be a critical period during the first 6 or so months for this crucial learning to take place (Larsson 1978). Such disruption results in a failure of normal copulation in the older animal, but the precise reason for this failure is not entirely clear. It is unlikely to be due to an impaired sexual appetite as such animals show fairly frequent masturbation. Some workers have suggested that the primary deficit is a problem of motor coordination, making successful mounting (a fairly acrobatic performance in many species) and intromission impossible. Others, such as Harlow (1971) and Goy (1979), saw this as a failure in the formation of affectional bonds, both homophilic and heterophilic. Mounting behaviour, in their view, is a way of establishing such bonds, which in the heterophilic case become more obviously erotic with the onset of puberty. The female's development in this respect seems obscure or at least passive.

Since the last edition of this book there has been renewed interest in animal models of homosexuality.

The prevailing view, however, has been that long-lasting exclusive homosexual preference is extremely rare in other primates (Wallen & Parsons 1997; Dixson 1998). A specific case of a primate choosing a same-sex partner in preference to an available and receptive heterosexual partner has been cited often as the exception that proves the rule (Erwin & Maple 1976). However, Bagemihl (1999), in a book dedicated to reviewing homosexual behaviour in the animal kingdom, claimed exclusive homosexuality in a variety of species including some primates. Vasey (2002) considered that Bagemihl's (1999) criteria of sexual behaviour were too broad and went on to apply much more stringent criteria. On that basis, he concluded that there was evidence of exclusive sexual preference in five species, one of which was a primate, the Japanese macaque. The other species were pukakos, a bird, the Ugandan kobs, an ungulate, domestic sheep and domestic cattle. Interestingly, with the exception of the sheep, where the same-sex behaviour was observed among rams, the other four examples were confined to females.

How relevant are these observations, particularly of primates, to the establishment of sexual identity in humans? We have seen sexual behaviour serving more than one function (e.g. mounting being used to establish and maintain dominance, and female same-sex interactions often part of an affiliative pattern), early relationships with both parents and peers affecting later sexual behaviour (though not sexual preference per se) and facultative homosexuality occurring among males denied access to females. In general, we have seen how innate factors (e.g. hormonally mediated mechanisms) and social learning interact during the course of childhood development to determine the pattern of post-pubertal sexual behaviour. Of particular interest are the differences between male and female primates in relation to pre-pubertal same-sex interactions (Wallen & Parsons 1997) and the one example of exclusive same-sex preference being confined to females (Japanese macaques). These instances point to a fundamental gender difference in sexual development in non-human primates. Exclusive male homosexual preference is perhaps a uniquely human phenomenon, but one which is likely to result from an interaction between socio-cultural (or cognitive learning) influence and some more biological, possibly genetically determined set of characteristics.

The interactive processes leading to sexual identity

We have considered a range of mechanisms of potential relevance to the development of sexual identity, but none appears to be sufficient as an explanation for sexual identity in general. Let us now consider the various ways in which such mechanisms might interact, perhaps resulting in a multifactorial process of identity development, varying considerably across individuals in the relative importance of specific factors.

For those children who find themselves attracted to the same sex, what follows will probably depend to a considerable extent on two related factors: firstly, the child's self-confidence and self-esteem, and secondly, involvement in and acceptance by the peer group. What seems to be happening in the transition from childhood to adolescence, at least in part, is an investment in exploring the meanings of sexuality and sexual relationships. In the Western world, it becomes increasingly difficult for children to ignore the bombardment of sexual messages that pervades modern society, even when their parents or teachers choose to evade the subject. Pre-pubertal children therefore become intrigued by the idea of dating or a having a boy or girl friend. Kagan & Moss (1962) showed in their longitudinal study that boys who had shown gender non-conformity and who would, as a consequence, have been less accepted by their male peer group, were more likely to show anxiety about sexuality and less likely to engage in dating. As we have already seen, many such boys, showing gender non-conformity during childhood, will develop homosexual identity, although there will be many others who develop such identity who did not show this gender non-conformity. This confronts us with a crucial question that cannot yet be answered. Do the gender non-conforming boys distance themselves from this normal heterosexual developmental stage because they have difficulty integrating with their peer group, or because they are in some way aware that they are destined to develop homosexual identities (by recognizing attraction to other males)?

Meyer-Bahlburg (1999), on the basis of his clinical experience with boys diagnosed with GID, has recognized a 'temperamental syndrome' that includes low interest in rough-and-tumble play and sports, low aggressiveness with other boys, aesthetic sensibility and high emotionality. Others have suggested that GID boys meet the criteria for 'inhibited child syndrome' (Coates & Wolfe 1995) or have 'largely insecure attachments' (Bradley & Zucker 1997). Is it such personality problems associated with GID that account for the eventual homosexual identity in the majority of cases? In an earlier study of adults, Siegelman (1978) found that high femininity, in both homosexual and heterosexual males was associated with neuroticism. However, when he compared the homosexual and heterosexual males with high femininity, the only significant difference was a higher score for 'tender mindedness' in the homosexual group. The low femininity homosexual and heterosexual men did not differ on any personality measure, except that the homosexual men scored higher for nurturance. Thus, there may be relatively non-specific personality factors, by no means restricted to boys with gender non-conformity, that make involvement in the peer group and participation in these early presexual involvements less likely. However, such factors do not appear to have direct relevance to the establishment of a homosexual identity and are often associated with development of a heterosexual identity.

Is there any way that being distanced from one's peer group increases the likelihood of attraction to the same sex? One concerted attempt at such an explanation is Bem's Exotic-Becomes-Erotic theory (Bem 1996, 2000).

This postulates that sexual attraction develops, at a time in the developmental sequence not specified, to others who are 'unfamiliar' (hence exotic). In particular, the unfamiliarity is with others of the same gender in individuals who are gender atypical. Thus the feminine, unmasculine boy who feels more familiar with girls will find other boys unfamiliar, 'exotic', and by a proposed mechanism comparable to 'excitation transfer' (see p. 111), sexually arousing. Similarly, girls with masculine, unfeminine gender identities, more familiar with boys, will become attracted to other girls. While Bem's idea is an interesting one, he has not so far offered any supportive evidence, beyond the common association between gender non-conformity and homosexual identity, and it is not difficult to find evidence inconsistent with his theory (Peplau et al 1998; Meyer-Bahlburg 2000). Peplau et al (1998) also point to the inappropriateness of this theory in accounting for sexual identity development in women.

How does all this fit into the peri-pubertal pattern discussed earlier? Bogaert et al (2002), in a secondary analysis of the NHSLS survey (Laumann et al 1994), found age at puberty to be significantly younger in men identifying as homosexual/bisexual ($n = 38$; mean age, 12.6 ± 1.3 SD) than heterosexual ($n = 1449$; mean age, 13.1 ± 1.4; $p = 0.02$). Puberty onset was defined as 'when your voice changed or you began growing pubic hair' (neither criterion precise in time). No significant difference was found for women, homosexual/bisexual ($n = 22$, mean age 12.2 ± 1.6) and heterosexual ($n = 1860$, mean age 12.7 ± 1.6). The authors also reviewed a number of earlier studies consistent with these findings. In attempting to explain this mechanism, Bogaert et al (2002) looked at the earlier age of puberty in women and therefore saw this earlier pattern in homosexual males as evidence of feminization, supporting the feminization hypothesis considered earlier. It is noteworthy, however, that boys who go through puberty earlier, whether homosexual or heterosexual, tend to show higher levels of sexual arousability and drive, as considered above, an association not found in females. Feminization could, at best, only account for part of this picture. More recently, Ostovich & Sabini (2005) found no difference in pubertal age between lesbian and heterosexual women. Savin-Williams & Ream (2006) reported a secondary analysis of adolescents in the Add Health study, based on questions about pubertal development and romantic attraction, asked during the first two waves of the study (mean ages 15.8 and 16.7 years, respectively), and about sexual identity, asked during the third wave (mean age 21.7 years). They found that males identifying as homosexual were more likely to report a later rather than earlier onset of puberty, and homosexual females tended to have an earlier onset. The report on this study, however, was difficult to follow.

How does age at puberty relate to peer group composition? Storms (1981) suggested if an individual enters puberty early, he or she is more likely to be associated with a peer group of the same sex. Given that the pubertal process, particularly in boys, is associated with an increased sexual arousability, this could result in sexual arousal in response to same-sex members of the peer group. However, as Ostovich & Sabini (2005) point out, the differences in age at puberty between homosexual and heterosexual males is small, as well as reflecting substantial individual variability, and no consistent difference has been found in females. The extent to which peer groups around peri-pubertal age have involved both boys and girls has possibly changed over the past 50 years. There is, for example, less single-sex education. But for those peri-pubertal boys who do not have ready access to a mixed-sex peer group (e.g. the classic example of the British single-sex boarding school), this phase may well involve same-sex interactions which, at an earlier age, could be regarded as 'play' but now, with the emergence of sexual arousal and before long orgasm and ejaculation, takes on an additional reinforcer, sexual pleasure. As considered earlier, in relation to cultural influences, this most often is a 'discontinuous' developmental phase, determined more by sexual pleasure and the availability of other boys as a stimulus for that pleasure than by the sexual attractiveness of those other boys (although an interesting possibility is that those other boys, around peri-pubertal age, may be more female like than older, post-pubertal boys). But what is the impact of these same-sex experiences on the development of sexual identity? To what extent is this impact, and indeed the child's participation in same-sex sexual activity in the first place, influenced by awareness of culturally imposed distinction between heterosexual and homosexual? Has the decline in prevalence of these sexual interactions between peri-pubertal boys resulted from their greater awareness of how the adult world might interpret this behaviour? In any case, it is clear that the majority of boys who engage in peri-pubertal sexual activity with other boys do not develop homosexual identities. How does this majority differ from the minority who move on to homosexual identity? As yet, we cannot answer these questions.

Puberty is a gradual process and, as we have seen, is associated with key changes in brain function and structure. It is not clear when recognizable sexual attraction to a particular gender or type of individual becomes established in the developmental sequence. It is reasonable to assume that the basic developmental mechanisms will be the same for those who end up with heterosexual and homosexual identities, although there may be differences in timing. We can consider a pre-labelling stage, when childhood and early adolescent sexual experiences occur, including feelings of attraction, without the need to categorize them as either heterosexual or homosexual. As Herdt & McClintock (2000) suggest, sexual attraction may not be the same for a child as an adult: 'a child's diffuse, more emergent properties of liking, friendship, and emotional closeness or intimacy have meanings different to those of an adult that is sexually aroused' (p. 590). As discussed earlier, it is also possible that sexual arousal can be experienced before, or separate from any specific sexual attractions. Hence early sexual arousal may occur without an identified 'attractive person' as the 'object of desire'. The impact of puberty, with its associated increase in hormones, particularly androgens, is likely to alter and intensify the experience of sexual arousal.

But does it have any direct effect on the recognition of an 'attractive person'? Earlier, we briefly considered the role of sexual conditioning (p. 104) and its apparently greater relevance to male sexuality. Do the changes in brain function associated with puberty result in a new phase of conditionability, which leads, at least in the male, to the linkage of sexual arousal and 'objects of desire', resulting in sexualized attraction?

In our three-strand model we move on from the peri-pubertal stage, to the parent vs peer group stage. This is likely to be crucial in terms of cultural influences on identity development. The parental factor may well play a part, reinforcing conventional views about acceptable sexuality. But in many families the parents evade the issue of how the early adolescent interprets his or her sexuality, by basically denying its existence, or at least its acceptability (until after he or she gets married). The peer group, on the other hand, may be more crucial. This distinguishes between the young person who can identify with the adolescent culture norm, which in most respects will be promoting heterosexuality, and the uncertain or homosexually inclined individual who is going to feel excluded. (There have, however, been some interesting recent examples of teen culture promoting alternative identities, which obscure the hetero/homosexual dichotomy.) Whereas the individual may have been privately asking the question, 'Am I straight or gay?' as part of the self-labelling stage, the teenage cultural world starts asking the same questions about the individual, the social labelling stage, typically reinforcing the idea that 'you are either one thing or the other'. The normalizing influence of the social labelling process, particularly as it is expressed through the peer group, is clearly going to have very different effects on the adolescent experiencing cross-gender attraction, who will progress, almost without consideration, into a heterosexual identity. In contrast, one who is experiencing same-gender attraction will be either struggling in a sociocultural vacuum or, more likely, experiencing the impact of social stigmatization. It is therefore to be expected that the integration of our three developmental strands will take substantially longer in those who emerge with a homosexual identity, rendering them more psychologically vulnerable in the process.

What can we conclude about sexual identity development? We find no simple explanation for why some people develop homosexual or bisexual identities and the large majority identify as heterosexual. But there are indications of either innate or early developmental mechanisms being involved. The main support from this comes from the evidence of heritability. Of obvious relevance is the influence of culture, and in European and North American culture, for which we have the most evidence, there are strong cultural determinants of dichotomous sexual identities, either hetero or homosexual, with bisexuality having no apparent cultural recognition. This is most clearly relevant to male sexuality, and there has been an interesting lack of cultural attention to female sexual identity, consistent with a more widespread denial of the importance of female sexuality beyond the need for it to be contained. But lack of containment of sexual activity between women poses no threat of 'cuckoldry' to men!

There have been indications of a discontinuous pattern of male sexuality in the Western world, with same-sex activity being relatively common but concealed among early adolescent boys, and this pattern has apparently lessened over the past 50 years. We can speculate that if there was no cultural control of the gender of sexual partners, but rather an acceptance of diverse types of sexual relationship, we would, by nature, have a widespread capacity for sexual interaction with either same or opposite sex partners, until the time that we chose to settle into a reproductive phase and rear a family. However, it would also be likely that a minority would end up with exclusively same-sex partners, and another minority would have opposite-sex partners from the start. What determines membership of those minorities remains obscure. We can find some cultures close to this bisexual potential pattern. In our own culture, it is the sexuality of women that comes closest.

The differences between men and women in the impact of sexual identity are striking. Let us return to the comparison of male and female sexuality discussed in Chapter 4 (p. 131). I proposed that there is a male and a female basic pattern, each one designed for the purpose of reproduction. The postulated male basic pattern is comparatively simple and is based on incentive for penile stimulation leading to orgasm, which because it is effectively achieved by vaginal penetration and ends in ejaculation, serves the fundamental reproductive function of sex. How, then, could this pattern end up with a preference for sexual interaction with men? A key component of the male basic pattern is the association between specific sexual stimuli (e.g. the 'attractive' female) and penile insertion. A further key component to male sexual development, as we have seen, is a capacity for conditioning of sexual arousal and associated incentive motivation, to specific sexual stimuli, with the possibility that such conditioning may occur at critical periods of development and be influenced by male-type brain mechanisms. On that basis, all that is required to direct the male to same-sex sexual activity is the conditioning to male sexual stimuli, a selective process that may be determined genetically or by some other as yet innate or early acquired learning process. The long-term consequences of such a pattern will then be further determined by socio-cultural factors, reinforcing the either/or sexual identity.

According to this model, the female basic pattern is not only different and in several respects more complex, but is accompanied, to a very variable extent across women, by a 'superadded' component, similar in various ways to the male basic pattern. The female basic pattern has to do with interaction with a partner, the reward associated with an accompanying sense of control, or intimacy or 'being desired'. It does not depend on conditioned sexual attraction to particular types of men, although as an effective sexual relationship becomes established, sexual attraction to the partner may emerge. Basic physiological mechanisms of vaginal lubrication and pain regulation render vaginal penetration non-aversive, and quite possibly rewarding in specific ways. If we accept this basic pattern for women, we can see how this would lead to a very different developmental history as far as sexual identity is concerned. However, we have to add in the consequences of the superadded component. This, which varies in importance across women, probably for genetic reasons, adds a component of sexual arousability, genital pleasure and orgasm to a woman's sexual experience. Part of this, it is postulated, results from the superadded genetically determined sexual impact of testosterone, which in women is most evident in its effects on sexual desire rather than genital response or orgasm. We therefore have the combination of a basic pattern of female sexuality, necessary for reproduction and likely to be evident in most women, and a superadded component, varying considerably in importance across women, which will further motivate sexual behaviour, comparable to the male pattern in some respects, regarded in evolutionary terms as a by-product of male sexuality, but without the peculiarly male capacity for conditioning to specific sexual stimuli. Hence, we have not only the impact of the female basic pattern on sexual identity development, but also an added major source of variance from the superadded component, and a less influential socio-cultural component, together accounting for the much greater variability of sexual identity in women than in men.

Conclusions

The three strands, gender identity, dyadic relationships and sexual response, can be usefully considered as relatively independent during childhood. The factors that influence a child's emerging sense of gender identity have, as far we as know, relatively little effect on the emerging ability to establish and maintain close dyadic relationships, and vice versa. While the child's gender identity may influence whether peer relationships are same sex or not, important learning, relevant to the dyadic strand, is occurring in interactions with both mother and father, and older siblings, relatives and friends. The intervening impact of personality characteristics requires further study. Both gender identity and the capacity for close dyadic relationships are fundamental to childhood development in a more general sense. In contrast, the sexual response strand has a much more variable role during childhood, with some children having clear sexual awareness and associated experiences, such as masturbation, and other children remaining relatively unaware. We remain uncertain of the extent to which these individual differences result from early learning and family environment or are genetically or pre-natally determined. As the child approaches adolescence, however, all three strands become increasingly interactive and interdependent. Gender identity is thrown into a transient state of confusion; whereas the pre-pubertal child is likely to have established a secure understanding of what it means to be a boy or a girl, the physical changes that occur around puberty produce a new phase of considerable uncertainty: 'What shape am I going to end up?' 'How much like a "normal male" (or female) am I going to be?' and, as a relatively new concern, 'How sexually attractive am I going to be?'. Hierarchies of relationships between peers can be disrupted. Previously dominant boys and girls can find themselves left behind by the earlier pubertal development of their peers. In turn, the newly organizing sense of masculinity or femininity will influence how dyadic relationships, both sexual and non-sexual, are formed and experienced. The emerging adolescent scripts for male and female behaviour will now have a clearer sexual component, and sexual response will impact on new relationships, leading to an emerging distinction between sexual and non-sexual relationships. The sexual response strand may make an early entry in the developmental process for some, and a late entry for others, neither having clear implications for eventual normal sexual development. Important developments in brain function occur and the resulting change in the cognitive processing of acquired meanings, and other brain functions, interact with the key biological factors associated with adrenarche and puberty. There is a crucial shift from predominantly parental influence early in this integrative process to a greater peer group influence during adolescence. We have also considered various ways in which this integrative developmental process can be derailed, either as a result of early negative sexual experiences or because of the establishment of non-sexual maladaptive patterns during childhood, evolving into adolescent maladaptive patterns, which include sexual 'acting out'. In addition, problems in relating to the peer group may result in a relatively isolated stage of discriminative sexual learning when inappropriate or paraphilic response patterns are more likely to become established. At a later stage, problems in establishing intimate dyadic relationships may present a further barrier to the development of a 'mature' sexuality, in which we incorporate our sexuality into the primary relationship in our lives, leading typically to new family formation.

We have strived to understand how the emergence of sexual identity fits into this picture, but we remain with considerable uncertainty about the relative importance of genetically determined mechanisms, family and peer group experiences, and the impact of culture on this process. We have, however, seen how the striking difference between sexual identity development in men and women fit into the previously proposed model of basic reproductive patterns and superadded components.

Overall, this chapter has asked more questions than it has provided answers. We are left with many gaps in our knowledge and understanding of normal sexual development, and significant methodological as well as political constraints on our ability to fill them. We must hope for more substantial progress in the future.

REFERENCES

Abma JC, Sonenstein FL 2001 Sexual activity and contraceptive practice among teenagers in the United States, 1988 and 1995 (DHHS Publication No.2001-1997). Government Printing Office, Washington, DC.

Achenbach TM 1991 Manual for the Child Behavior Checklist/4-18 and the 1991 profile. University of Vermont, Department of Psychiatry, Burlington.

Akers JS, Conoway CH 1979 Female homosexual behavior in *Macacca mulatto*. Archives of Sexual Behavior 8: 63–80

Bagemihl B 1999 Biological Exuberance: Animal Homosexuality and Natural Diversity. St Martin's Press, New York.

Bailey JM, Pillard RC 1995 Genetics of human sexual orientation. Annual Review of Sex Research 6: 126–150.

Bailey JM, Zucker KJ 1995 Childhood sex-typed behavior and sexual orientation: a conceptual analysis and quantitative review. Developmental Psychology 31: 43–55.

Bailey JM, Dunne MP, Martin NG 2000 Genetic and environmental influences on sexual orientation and its correlates in an Australian twin sample. Journal of Personality and Social Psychology 78: 524–536.

Bailey JM, Safron A, Reber PJ 2006 Neural correlates of sexual arousal in heterosexual and homosexual men. Presented at the International Academy of Sex Research, Amsterdam.

Bakwin H 1973 Erotic feelings in infants and young children. American Journal of Diseases of Childhood 126: 52–54.

Bancroft J 1983 Human Sexuality and Its Problems, 1st edn. Churchill Livingstone, Edinburgh.

Bancroft J 1990 Biological determinants of sexual orientation. In McWhirter D, Sanders SM Reinisch JM (eds) Homosexuality/Heterosexuality: Concepts of Sexual Orientation. Oxford University Press, New York.

Bancroft J (ed) 2000 The Role of Theory in Sex Research. Indiana University Press, Bloomington.

Bancroft J 2002 Sexual effects of androgens in women: some theoretical considerations. Fertility and Sterility 77(Suppl 4): S55–S59.

Bancroft J 2003 Androgens and sexual function in men and women. In Bagatell CJ, Bremner WJ (eds) Androgens in Health and Disease. Humana, Totowa, NJ, pp. 259–290.

Bancroft J, Herbenick D, Reynolds M 2003 Masturbation as a marker of sexual development. In Bancroft J (ed) Sexual Development in Childhood. Indiana University Press, Bloomington.

Bates JE, Alexander DB, Oberlander SE, Dodge KA, Pettit GS 2003 Antecedents of sexual activity at ages 16 and 17 in a community sample followed from age 5. In Bancroft J (ed) Sexual Development in Childhood. Indiana University Press, Bloomington, pp. 206–238.

Bateson PPG 1978 Early experience and sexual preferences. In: Hutchison J (ed) The Biological Determinants of Sexual Behaviour. Wiley, Chichester.

Beach FA 1979 Animal models for human sexuality. In: Sex, Hormones and Behaviour. Ciba Foundation Symposium 62. Excerpta Medica, Amsterdam.

Beach FA, LeBoeuf BJ 1967 Coital behavior in dogs I. Preferential mating in the bitch. Animal Behavior 15: 546–558.

Bearman PS, Brückner H 2001 Promising the future: virginity pledges and first intercourse. American Journal of Sociology 106: 859–912.

Bem DJ 1996 Exotic becomes erotic: a developmental theory of sexual orientation. Psychological Review 103: 320–335.

Bem DJ 2000 The exotic-becomes-erotic theory of sexual orientation. In Bancroft J (ed) The Role of Theory in Sex Research. Indiana University Press, Bloomington, pp. 67–81.

Berglund H, Lindstrom P, Savic I 2006 Brain responses to putative pheromones in lesbian women. PNAS 103: 8269–8274.

Bieber I, Dain HJ, Dince PR, 1962 Homosexuality: a Psychoanalytic Study. Basic Books, New York.

Blumstein P, Schwartz P 1983 American Couples. Morrow, New York.

Bocklandt S, Horvath S, Vilain E, Hamer DH 2006 Extreme skewing of X chromosome inactivation in mothers of homosexual men. Human Genetics 118: 691–694.

Bogaert AF, Friesen C, Klentrou P 2002 Age at puberty and sexual orientation in a national probability sample. Archives of Sexual Behavior 31: 67–75.

Bogart LM, Cecil H, Wagstaff DA, Pinkerton SD, Abramson Pr 2000 Is it 'sex'? College students' interpretations of sexual behavior terminology. Journal of Sex Research 37: 108–116.

Borneman E 1990 Progress in empirical research on children's sexuality. In Money J, Musaph H (series eds), Perry ME (vol. ed) Handbook of Sexology, vol. VII. Childhood and Adolescent Sexology. Elsevier, Amsterdam, pp. 201–210.

Bowlby J 1969 Attachment and Loss, vol. 1. Attachment. Basic Books, New York.

Bowlby J 1973 Attachment and Loss, vol. 2. Separation. Hogarth Press, London.

Bowlby J 1980 Attachment and Loss, vol. 3. Loss, Sadness and Depression. Basic Books, New York.

Bradley SJ, Zucker KJ 1997 Gender identity disorder: a review of the past 10 years. Journal of the American Academy of Child & Adolescent Psychiatry 36: 872–880.

Broderick CB 1966 Socio-sexual development in a suburban community. Journal of Sex Research 2: 1–24.

Browning CR, Laumann EO 2003 The social context of adaptation to childhood sexual maltreatment: a life course perspective. In Bancroft J (ed) Sexual Development in Childhood. Indiana University Press, Bloomington, pp. 383–403.

Caspi A, Begg D, Dickson N, Harrington HL, Langley J, Moffitt TE, Silva Pa 1997 Personality differences predict health-risk behaviors in young adulthood: evidence from a longitudinal study. Journal of Personality & Social Psychology 73: 1052–1063.

Coates SW, Wolfe SM 1995 Gender identity disorder in boys: the interface of constitution and early experience. Psychoanalytic Inquiry 15: 6–38.

Crawford M, Popp D 2003 Sexual double standards: a review and methodological critique of two decades of research. Journal of Sex Research 40: 27–35.

D'Augelli AR, Hershberger SL 1993 Lesbian, gay, and bisexual youth in community settings: personal challenges and mental health problems. American Journal of Community Psychology 21: 421–448.

Diamond LM 2003a What does sexual orientation orient? A biobehavioral model distinguishing romantic love and sexual desire. Psychological Review 110: 173–192.

Diamond LM 2003b Was it a phase? Young women's relinquishment of lesbian/bisexual identities over a 5-year period. Journal of Personality & Social Psychology 84: 352–364.

Dixson AF 1998 Primate Sexuality: Comparative Study of the Prosimians, Monkeys, Apes and Human Beings. Oxford University Press, Oxford.

Dörner G, Rohde W, Stahl F, Krell L, Masius Wg 1975 A neuroendocrine predisposition for homosexuality in men. Archives of Sexual Behavior 4: 1–8.

Dunne MP, Martin NG, Statham DJ, Slutske WS, Dinwiddie SH, Bucholz KK, Madden PA, Heath AC 1997 Genetic and environmental contributions to variance in age at first sexual intercourse. Psychological Science 8: 211–216.

DuPree MG, Mustanski BS, Bocklandt S, Nievergelt C, Hamer DH 2004 A candidate gene study of CYP19 (Aromatase) and male sexual orientation. Behavior Geneticsa 34: 243–250.

Elias J, Gebhard P 1970 Sexuality and sexual learning in childhood. In Taylor DL (ed) Human Sexual Development: Perspectives in Sex Education. Davis, Philadelphia, pp. 16–27.

Erikson EH 1950 Childhood and Society. Norton, New York.

Erwin J, Maple T 1976 Ambisexual behavior with male–male anal penetration in male rhesus monkeys. Archives of Sexual Behavior 5: 9–14.

Fergusson DM, Horwood LJ, Lynskey M 1997 Childhood sexual abuse, adolescent behaviors, and sexual revictimization. Child Abuse & Neglect 21: 789–803.

Finkelhor D 1980 Sex among siblings: a survey on prevalence, variety, and effects. Archives of Sexual Behavior 9: 171–194.

Finkelhor D 1988 The trauma of child sexual abuse: two models. In Wyatt G, Powell E (eds) Lasting Effects of Child Sexual Abuse. Sage, Newbury Park, pp. 61–84.

Finkelstein JW, Susmanm EJ, Chinchilli VC, Kunselman SJ, D'Arcangelo MR, Schwab J, Demers LM, Liben LS, Kulin HE 1997 Estrogen or testosterone increases self-reported aggressive behaviors in hypogonadal adolescents. Journal of Clinical Endocrinology & Metabolism 82: 2433–2438.

Finkelstein JW, Susmanm EJ, Chinchilli VC, D'Arcangelo MR, Kunselman SJ, Schwab J, Demers LM, Liben LS, Kulin He 1998 Effects of estrogen or testosterone on self-reported sexual responses and behaviors in hypogonadal adolescents. Journal of Clinical Endocrinology & Metabolism 83: 2281–2285.

Forest HG, Deperetti E, Bertrand J 1976 Hypothalamic-pituitary-gonadal relationships from birth to puberty. Clinical Endocrinology 5: 551–569.

Fortenberry JD, Aalsma MC 2003 Abusive sexual experiences before age 12 and adolescent sexual behaviors. In Bancroft J (ed) Sexual Development in Childhood. Indiana University Press, Bloomington, pp. 359–369.

Fortenberry JD, Cecil H, Zimet GD, Orr DP 1997 Concordance between self-report questionnaires and coital diaries for sexual behaviors of adolescent women with sexually transmitted infections. In Bancroft J (ed) Researching Sexual Behavior: Methodological Issues. Indiana University Press, Bloomington, pp. 237–249.

Friedrich WN 1997 Child Sexual Behavior Inventory: Professional Manual. Psychological Assessment Resources, Odessa, FL.

Friedrich WN 2003 Studies of sexuality of nonabused children. In Bancroft J (ed) Sexual Development in Childhood. Indiana University Press, Bloomington, pp. 107–120.

Friedrich WN, Fisher J, Dittner CA, Acton R, Berliner L, Butler J, 2001 Child sexual behavior inventory: normative, psychiatric, and sexual abuse comparisons. Child Maltreatment 6: 37–49.

Gagnon J, Simon W 1973 Sexual Conduct: the Social Sources of Human Sexuality. Aldine, Chicago.

Gagnon J, Simon W 1987 The scripting of oral-genital conduct. Archives of Sexual Behavior 16: 1–25.

Galenson E, Roiphe H 1974 The emergence of genital awareness during the second year of life. In: Friedman RC, Richart RM, Van de Wiele RL (eds) Sex Differences in Behavior. Wiley, New York, pp. 233–258.

Gebhard PH 1977 The acquisition of basic sex information. Journal of Sex Research 13: 148–169.

Gladue BA, Green R, Heilman RE 1984 Neuroendocrine response to estrogen and sexual orientation. Science 225: 1496–1499.

Goldfoot DA, Wallen K, Neff DA, McBrair MC, Goy RW 1984 Social influences on the display of sexually dimorphic behavior in rhesus monkeys: isosexual rearing. Archives of Sexual Behavior 13: 395–412.

Goldman R, Goldman J 1982 Children's Sexual Thinking: a Comparative Study of Children Aged 5 to 15 Years in Australia, North America, Britain and Sweden. Routledge and Kegan Paul, London.

Gooren LJG 1986 The neuroendocrine response of luteinizing hormone to estrogen administration in the human is not sex specific but dependent on the hormonal environment. Journal of Clinical Endocrinology & Metabolism 63: 589–593.

Gooren LJG 1988 Hypogonadotropic hypogonadal men respond less well to androgen substitution treatment than hypergonadotropic hypogonadal men. Archives of Sexual Behavior 17: 265–270.

Goy RW 1979 Discussion. In: Sex, hormones and behaviour. Ciba Foundation Symposium 62. Excerpta Medica, Amsterdam, pp. 141–142, 264–265.

Goy RW, Goldfoot D 1975 Neuroendocrinology: animal models and problems of human sexuality. Archives of Sexual Behavior 4: 405–420.

Graber JA, Brooks-Gunn J, Galen BR 1998 Betwixt and between: sexuality in the context of adolescent transitions. In Jessor R (ed) New Perspectives on Adolescent Risk Behavior. Cambridge University Press, Cambridge, UK, pp. 270–316.

Graham CA 2003 Methodological issues involved in adult recall of childhood sexual experiences. In Bancroft J (ed) Sexual Development in Childhood. Indiana University Press, Bloomington, pp. 67–76.

Green R 1974 Sexual Identity Conflict in Children and Adults. Basic Books, New York.

Green R 1987 The 'Sissy Boy Syndrome' and the Development of Homosexuality. Yale University Press, New Haven, CT.

Green V 1985 Experiential factors in childhood and adolescent sexual behavior: family interactions and previous sexual experiences. Journal of Sex Research 21: 157–182.

Green R, Keverne EB 2000 The disparate maternal aunt-uncle ratio in male transsexuals: an explanation invoking genomic imprinting. Journal of Theoretical Biology 202: 55–63.

Haavio-Mannila E, Kontula O 2003 Single and double standards in Finland, Estonia and St.Petersburg. Journal of Sex Research 40: 36–49.

Halpern CJT, Udry JR, Campbell B, Suchindran C 1993 Testosterone and pubertal development as predictors of sexual activity: a panel analysis of adolescent males. Psychosomatic Medicine 55: 436–447.

Halpern CJT, Udry JR, Suchindran C 1997 Testosterone predicts initiation of coitus in adolescent females. Psychosomatic Medicine 59: 161–171.

Halpern CT, Joyner K, Udry JR, Suchindran C 2000 Smart teens don't have sex (or kiss much either). Journal of Adolescent Health 26: 213–225.

Hamer DH, Hu SH, Magnuson VL, Hu N, Pattatucci AML 1993 A linkage between DNA markers on the X chromosome and male sexual orientation. Science 261: 321–327.

Harlow HF 1971 Learning to Love. Albion, San Francisco.

Haugaard JJ, Tilly C 1988 Characteristics predicting children's responses to sexual encounters with other children. Child Abuse and Neglect 12: 209–218.

Heiman JR, Verhulst J, Heard-Davison AR 2003 Childhood sexuality and adult sexual relationships: How are they connected by data and by theory? In Bancroft J (ed) Sexual Development in Childhood. Indiana University Press, Bloomington, pp. 404–420.

Herdt G 1990 Developmental continuity as a dimension of sexual orientation across cultures. In McWhirter D, Sanders SA, Reinisch JM (eds) Homosexuality/Heterosexuality: Concepts of Sexual Orientation. Oxford University Press, New York.

Herdt G 2000 Why the Sambia initiate boys before age 10. In Bancroft J (ed) The Role of Theory in Sex Research. Indiana University Press, Bloomington, pp. 82–104.

Herdt G, Boxer A 1993 Children of Horizons: How Gay and Lesbian Teens are Leading a New Way Out of the Closet. Beacon Press, Boston.

Herdt G, McClintock M 2000 The magical age of 10. Archives of Sexual Behavior 29:587–606.

Heston LL, Shields J 1968 Homosexuality in twins: a family study and a register study. Archives of General Psychiatry 18: 149–160.

Hines M 2002 Sexual differentiation of human brain and behavior. In Pfaff DW, Arnold AP, Etgen AM, Fahrbach SE, Rubin RT (eds) Hormones, Brain & Behavior, vol. 4. Academic Press, San Diego, pp. 425–462.

Hirschfeld 1913 Die Homosexualität des Mannes und des Weibes. In: Bloch I (ed) Handbuch der Sexualwissenschaft in Einzeldarstellungen, vol. III. Marcus, Berlin.

Hobsbawm E 1994 Age of Extremes: the Short Twentieth Century 1914–1991. Abacus, London.

Hu S, Pattatucci A, Patterson C, Li L, Fulker D, Cherny S 1995 Linkage between sexual orientation and chromosome Xq28 in males but not females. Nature Genetics 11: 248–256.

Jaccard J, Dittus PJ 1991 Parent–teen Communication: Toward the Prevention of Unintended Pregnancies. Springer-Verlag, New York.

Jaccard J, Dittus PJ, Gordon VV 2000 Parent–teen communication about premarital sex: factors associated with the extent of communication. Journal of Adolescent Research 15: 187–208.

Kagan J, Moss HA 1962 Birth to Maturity: a Study in Psychological Development. Wiley, New York.

Kallmann FJ 1952 Twin and sibship study of overt male homosexuality. American Journal of Human Genetics 4: 136–146.

Karacan I, Salis PJ, Thornby JI, Williams RL 1976 The ontogeny of nocturnal penile tumescence. Waking & Sleeping 1: 27–44.

Kilpatrick A 1992 Long-Range Effects of child and Adolescent Sexual Experiences: Myths, Mores, Menaces. Erlbaum, Hillsdale.

Kinnish KK, Strassberg DS, Turner CW 2005 Sex differences in the flexibility of sexual orientation: a multidimensional retrospective assessment. Archives of Sexual Behavior 34: 173–184.

Kinsey AC, Pomeroy WB, Martin CE 1948 Sexual Behavior in the Human Male. Saunders: Philadelphia.

Kinsey AC, Pomeroy WB, Martin CE, Gebhard PH 1953 Sexual Behavior in the Human Female. Saunders: Philadelphia.

Kinsman SB, Romer D, Furstenberg F, Schwartz DF 1998 Early sexual initiation: the role of peer norms. Pediatrics 102: 1185–1192.

Kirk KM, Bailey JM, Dunne MP, Martin NG 2000 Measurement models for sexual orientation in a community twin sample. Behavior Genetics 30: 345–356.

Kohlberg L 1966 A cognitive–developmental analysis of children's sex role concepts and attitudes. In: Maccoby EE (ed) The Development of Sex Differences. Stanford University Press, Stanford.

Lamb S, Coakley M 1993 'Normal' childhood sexual play and games: differentiating play from abuse. Child Abuse and Neglect 17: 515–526.

Langfeldt T 1990 Early childhood and juvenile sexuality, development and problems. In: Money J, Musaph H (series eds), Perry ME (vol. ed) Handbook of Sexology, vol. VII. Childhood and Adolescent Sexology. Elsevier, Amsterdam, pp. 179–200.

Larsson K 1978 Experimental factors in the development of sexual behaviour. In: Hutchison J (ed) Biological Determinants of Sexual Behaviour. Wiley, Chichester.

Laumann EO, Gagnon JH, Michael RT, Michaels S 1994 The Social Organization of Sexuality: Sexual Practices in the United States. University of Chicago Press, Chicago.

Leitenberg H, Greenwald E, Tarran M 1989 The relation between sexual activity among children during preadolescence and/or early adolescence and sexual behavior and sexual adjustment in young adulthood. Archives of Sexual Behavior 18: 299–313.

Macke JP, Hu N, Hu S, Baiely M, King VL, Brown T, Hamer D, Nathans J 1993 Sequence variation in the androgen receptor gene is not a common determinant of male sexual orientation. American Journal of Human Genetics 53: 844–852.

Martinson FM 1994 The Sexual Life of Children. Bergin & Garvey, Westport, CT.

McClintock M, Herdt G 1996 Rethinking puberty: the development of sexual attraction. Current Directions in Psychological Science 5: 178–183.

McNeely C, Shew ML, Beuhring T, Sieving R, Miller BC, Blum RW 2002 Mothers' influence on the timing of first sex among 14- and 15-year-olds. Journal of Adolescent Health 31: 256–265.

Meyer-Bahlburg HFL 1999 Psychosexual disorders: variants of gender differentiation. In Steinhausen H-C, Verhulst F (eds) Risks and Outcomes in Developmental Psychopathology. Oxford University Press, Oxford, pp. 298–313.

Meyer-Bahlburg HFL 2000 Sexual orientation-discussion of Bem and Herdt from a psychobiological perspective. In Bancroft J (ed) The Role of Theory in Sex Research. Indiana University Press, Bloomington, pp. 110–124.

Meyer-Bahlburg HFL, Steel JL 2003 Using the parents as a source of information about the child with special emphasis on the sex problems scale of the child behavior checklist. In Bancroft J (ed) Sexual Development in Childhood. Indiana University Press, Bloomington, pp. 34–53.

Meyer-Bahlburg HFL, Dolezal C, Sandberg DE 2000 The association of sexual behavior with externalizing behaviors in a community sample of prepubertal children. In Sandfort TGM, Rademakers J (eds) Childhood Sexuality: Normal Sexual Behavior and Development. Haworth, New York, pp. 61–79.

Miller PY, Simon W 1980 The development of sexuality in adolescence. In Adelson J (ed) Handbook of Adolescent Psychology. Wiley, Chichester.

Miller L, Gur M 2002 Religiousness and sexual responsibility in adolescent girls. Journal of Adolescent Health 31: 401–406.

Miller WB, Pasta DJ, Macmurray J, Chui C, Wu H, Comings DE 1999 Dopamine receptor genes are associated with age at first sexual intercourse. Journal of Biosocial Science 31: 43–54.

Mischel W 1966 A social-learning view of sex differences in behavior. In Maccoby EE (ed) The Development of Sex Differences. Stanford University Press, Stanford.

Moll A 1912 The Sexual Life of the Child. Translated by Paul E. McMillan, New York.

Money J 1980 Love and Love Sickness: the Science, Gender Difference, and Pair Bonding. Johns Hopkins University Press, Baltimore.

Montgomery MJ, Sorell GT 1998 Love and dating experience in early and middle adolescence: Grade and gender comparisons. Journal of Adolescence 21: 677–689.

Mustanski BS, Chivers ML, Bailey JM 2002 A critical review of recent biological research on human sexual orientation. Annual Review of Sex Research 13: 89–140.

Mustanski BS, DuPree MG, Nievergelt CM, Bocklandt S, Schork NJ, Hamer DH 2005 A genomewide scan of male sexual orientation. Human Genetics 116: 272–278.

Mustanski B, Viken RJ, Kaprio J, Winter T, Rose RJ 2007 Sexual behavior in young adulthood: a population-based twin study. Health Psychology 26: 610–617.

Newcomer SF, Udry JR 1985 Oral sex in an adolescent population. Archives of Sexual Behavior 14: 4146.

Orenstein P 1994 School Girls: Young Women, Self-Esteem, and the Confidence Gap. Doubleday, New York.

Ostovich JM, Sabini J 2005 Timing of puberty and sexuality in men and women. Archives of Sexual Behavior 34: 197–206.

O'Sullivan LF 2003 Methodological issues associated with studies of child sexual behavior. In Bancroft J (ed) Sexual Development in Childhood. Indiana University Press, Bloomington, pp. 23–33.

O'Sullivan LF, Meyer-Bahlburg HFL, Wasserman G 2000 Reactions of inner-city boys and their mothers to research interviews about sex. In Sandfort TGM, Rademakers J (eds) Childhood Sexuality: Normal Sexual Behavior and Development. Haworth, New York, pp. 81–103.

Pattatucci AML, Hamer D 1995 Development and familiality of sexual orientation in females. Behavior Genetics 25: 407–421.

Pearcey SM, Docherty KJ, Dabbs JM Jr 1996 Testosterone and sex role identification in lesbian couples. Physiology & Behavior 60: 1033–1035.

Peplau LA, Garnets LD, Spalding LR, Conley TD, Veniegas RC 1998 A critique of Bem's 'Exotic Becomes Erotic' theory of sexual orientation. Psychological Review 105: 387–394.

Peplau LA, Spalding LR, Conley TD, Veniegas RC 1999 The development of sexual orientation in women. Annual Review of Sex Research 10: 70–99.

Perper T 1985 Sex Signals. The Biology of Love. ISI Press, Philadelphia.

Phinney VG, Jensen LC, Olsen JA, Cundick B 1990 The relationship between early development and ps:chosexual behaviors in adolescent females. Adolescence 25: 321–332.

Rademakers J, Laan MJC, Straver CJ 2003 Body awareness and physical intimacy: an exploratory study. In Bancroft J (ed) Sexual Development in Childhood. Indiana University Press, Bloomington, pp. 121–125.

Ramirez-Valles J, Zimmerman MA, Newcomb MD 1998 Sexual risk behavior among youth: modeling the influence of pro-social activities and socioeconomic factors. Journal of Health and Social Behavior 39: 237–253.

Ramsey GV 1943 The sex information of younger boys. American Journal of Orthopsychiatry 8: 347–352.

Remafedi G, Farrow JA, Deisher RW 1991 Risk factors for attempted suicide in gay and bisexual youth. Pediatrics 87: 869–875.

Remez L 2000 Oral sex among adolescents: is it sex or is it abstinence? Family Planning Perspectives 32: 298–304.

Reynolds MA, Herbenick DL, Bancroft J 2003 The nature of childhood sexual experiences: two studies 50 years apart. In Bancroft J (ed) Sexual Development in Childhood. Indiana University Press, Bloomington, pp. 134–155.

Rodgers JL, Rowe DC, Buster M 1999 Nature, nurture and first sexual intercourse in the USA: fitting behavioural genetic models to NLSY kinship data. Journal of Biosocial Science 31: 29–41.

Sachs BD 1995 Discussion. In Bancroft J (ed) The Pharmacology of Sexual Function and Dysfunction. Excerpta Medica, Amsterdam, p. 130.

Sanders SA, Reinisch JM 1999 Would you say you 'had sex' if…? Journal of the American Medical Association 281: 275–277.

Santelli J, Lindberg LD, Abma J, McNeely CS, Resnick M 2000 Adolescent sexual behavior: estimates and trends from four nationally representative surveys. Family Planning Perspectives 32: 156–166.

Savic I, Berglund H, Lindstrom P 2006 Brain response to putative pheromones in homosexual men. PNAS 102: 7356–7361.

Savin-Williams RC 1995 An exploratory study of pubertal maturation timing and self-esteem among gay and bisexual male youths. Developmental Psychology 31: 56–64.

Savin-Williams RC, Ream GL 2006. Pubertal onset and sexual orientation in an adolescent national probability sample. Archives of Sexual Behavior 35: 279–286.

Schofield M 1965 The Sexual Behaviour of Young People. Little, Brown, Boston.

Schoof-Tams K, Schlaegel J, Walczak L 1976 Differentiation of sexual morality between 11 and 16 years. Archives of Sexual Behavior 5: 353–370.

Schreurs KMG 1993 Sexuality in lesbian couples: the importance of gender. Annual Review of Sex Research 4: 49–66.

Schuhrke B 2000 Young children's curiosity about other people's genitals. In Sandfort TGM, Rademakers J (eds) Childhood Sexuality: Normal Sexual Behavior and Development. Haworth, New York, pp. 27–48.

Schwartz IM 1999 Sexual activity prior to coital initiation: a comparison between males and females. Archives of Sexual Behavior 28: 63–69.

Seligman MEP, Hager JL 1972 Biological Boundaries of Learning. Appleton-Century-Crofts, New York, pp. 1–6.

Siegelman M 1974 Parental background of male homosexuals and heterosexuals. Archives of Sexual Behavior 3: 3–18.

Siegelman M 1978 Psychological adjustment of homosexual and heterosexual men: a cross-national replication. Archives of Sexual Behavior 7: 1–12.

Sieving R, McNeely CS, Blum RW 2000 Maternal expectations, mother–child connectedness, and adolescent sexual debut. Archives of Pediatrics & Adolescent Medicine 154: 809–816.

Singh D, Vidaurri M, Zambarano RJ, Dabbs JM Jr 1999 Lesbian erotic role identification: behavioral, morphological and hormonal correlates. Journal of Personality and Social Psychology 76: 1035–1049.

Skuse DH, James RS, Bishop Dvm, Coppins B, Dalton P, Aamodt-Leeper G, Bacarese-Hamilton M, Cresswell C, McGurk R, Jacobs PA 1997 Evidence from Turner's syndrome of an impaired X-linked locus affecting cognitive function. Nature 387: 705–708.

Sonenstein FL, Ku L, Pleck JH 1997 Measuring sexual behavior among teenage males in the United States. In Bancroft J (ed) Researching Sexual Behavior: Methodological Issues. Indiana University Press, Bloomington, pp. 87–105.

Sonenstein FL, Pleck JH, Ku LC 1989 Sexual activity, condom use, and AIDS awareness among adolescent males. Family Planning Perspectives 21: 152.

Storms MD 1981 A theory of erotic orientation development. Psychological Review 88: 340–353.

Symons D 1979 The Evolution of Human Sexuality. Oxford University Press, Oxford.

Tellegen A, Waller NG 1985 Exploring personality through test construction: development of a multidimensional personality questionnaire. In Briggs SR, Cheek JM (eds) Personality Measures: Development and Evaluation, vol. 1. Jai Press, Greenwich, CT.

Thigpen JW, Pinkston EM, Mayefsky JH 2003 Normative sexual behavior of African American children: preliminary findings. In Bancroft J (ed) Sexual Development in Childhood. Indiana University Press, Bloomington, pp. 241–254.

Tolman DL 2002 Dilemmas of Desire: Teenage Girls Talk about Sexuality. Harvard University Press, Cambridge, MA.

Turner WJ 1995 Homosexuality, Type 1: an Xq28 phenomenon. Archives of Sexual Behavior 24: 109–134.

Turner CF, Miller HG, Rogers SM 1997 Survey measurement of sexual behavior: problems and progress. In Bancroft J (ed), Researching Sexual Behavior: Methodological Issues. Indiana University Press, Bloomington, pp. 37–60.

Tyler PA 1984 Homosexual behaviour in animals. In: Howells K (ed) The Psychology of Sexual Diversity. Blackwell, Oxford.

Udry JR, Billy JOG, Morris NM, Groff TR, Raj MH 1985 Serum androgenic hormones motivate sexual behavior in adolescent boys. Fertility and Sterility 43: 90–94.

Udry JR, Talbert LM, Morris NM 1986 Biosocial foundations of adolescent female sexuality. Demography 23: 217–229.

Vasey PL 2002 Same-sex sexual partner preference in hormonally and neurologically unmanipulated animals. Annual Review of Sex Research 13: 141–179.

Volbert R 2000 Sexual knowledge of preschool children. In Sandfort TGM, Rademakers J (eds) Childhood Sexuality: Normal Sexual Behavior and Development. Haworth, New York, pp. 5–26.

Wallen K, Parsons WA 1997 Sexual behavior in same-sexed nonhuman primates: is it relevant to understanding human homosexuality? Annual Review of Sex Research 8: 195–223.

Weinberger DR, Elvevag B, Giedd JN 2005 The adolescent brain: a work in progress. The National Campaign to Prevent Teen Pregnancy. http://www.teenpregnancy.org/resources/reading/pdf/BRAIN.pdf.

Weinrich JD 1987 Sexual Landscapes: Why We Are What We Are, Why We Love Whom We Love. Scribner's, New York.

Widom CS, Morris S 1997 Accuracy of adult recollections of childhood victimization: Part 2. Childhood sexual abuse. Psychological Assessment 9: 34–46.

Williams LM 1994 Recall of childhood trauma: a prospective study of women's memories of child sexual abuse. Journal of Consulting and Clinical Psychology 62: 1166–1176.

Zillman D 1983 Transfer of excitation in emotional behavior. In Cacioppo JT, Petty RE (eds) Social Psychophysiology: A Sourcebook. Guilford Press, New York, pp. 215–240.

Zimmer-Gembeck MJ, Siebenbruner J, Collins WA 2001 Diverse aspects of dating: Associations with psychosocial functioning from early to middle adolescence. Journal of Adolescence 24: 313–336.

Zucker KJ 1990 Gender identity disorders in children: clinical descriptions and natural history. In Blanchard R, Steiner BW (eds) Clinical Management of Gender Identity Disorders in Children and Adults. American Psychiatric Press, Washington DC, pp. 1–23.

6 Heterosexuality

The history of sex surveys... 174
The methodology of sex surveys 179
Theoretical bases of sex surveys.. 182
Cross-cultural comparisons 183

Masturbation... 183
Social attitudes to masturbation 183
The prevalence of masturbation.. 184
Techniques of masturbation... 186
Conclusions 186

Sex and the unmarried... 186
Cross-cultural and historical aspects...................................... 186
The reduction in age at first intercourse in Europe and
North America during the 20th century.................................... 191
Non-coital sexual activity 197
Teenage pregnancies 197
The influence of the family 199

Marriage and co-habitation... 200
Sexual attraction, falling in love and mate selection................ 200
Incidence of marriage and co-habitation 205
Age at marriage.. 205
Sexual activity within marriage and co-habitation 207

Sexual well-being and the importance of sex in marriage
and relationships 210
The fate of marriage 212

The impact of social class... 213

The impact of culture.. 214
Cultural contrasts within North America and Europe................ 214
The black American... 215
Acculturation... 217
Immigrant groups in North America 218
An example of an indigenous culture: China 219

Sexual desire and sexual fantasy 220
Sexual desire.. 220
Sexual fantasy 223

Response to erotica... 225

Sex and the Internet... 226

Personality and individual differences in sexuality 228
Measures of sexual attitudes 228
The Dual Control model 229

Comparison of men and women... 231

The preceding chapters have considered the psychobiological basis of human sexuality and how it interacts with culture during sexual development. We will now look at how human sexuality is experienced and expressed. In this chapter, we consider these aspects of heterosexuality.

There are three important sources of information: historical evidence of changing patterns of sexual behaviour, cross-cultural anthropological studies of mainly primitive societies, and surveys of sexual attitudes and behaviour in modern societies.

The study of social history as it applies to sexuality and marriage is an expanding field, and a proper review is beyond the scope of this book. Here attention will be limited and mainly focused on historical aspects of the 20th century, with particular emphasis on sex survey research.

Anthropological data are also a rich, appealing and intrinsically important source. Anthropological studies of pre-industrial or primitive societies focusing specifically on sexuality are still limited (Malinowski 1929; Mead 1929, 1931; Marshall & Suggs 1971; Herdt 1981; Ortner & Whitehead 1981) Much of the writing on cross-cultural comparisons of primitive societies has relied on the Human Relations Area File (e.g. Ford & Beach 1952; Barry & Schlegel 1980), a collection of information about 186 cultures which varies considerably in the amount of attention paid to sexual behaviour in each culture, and which has been gathered by a motley collection of observers whose sexual values and prejudices were probably highly influential (Broude & Greene 1980). In 1991, Vance (cited in Parker & Easton 1998) distinguished between the 'cultural influence' model in which sexuality is conceptualized as a universal immutable state, mediated to a variable extent by cultural context, and 'social construction theory' which sees sexuality as constructed differently across cultures and over time. The cultural influence approach prevailed in anthropological studies of human sexuality until the early 1990s, since when social constructionism has been more influential. Hopefully, this will prove to be a dialectic process with a synthesis resulting in a more balanced appraisal of the importance of both biology and culture. There is now a considerable amount of literature on cross-cultural comparisons of more industrialized societies and some of this will be briefly reviewed in this and following chapters.

The history of sex surveys

Our main sources of information are the various surveys of modern Western societies. This history of sex surveys during the 20th century, at least of those carried out in the USA, has been tellingly chronicled by Ericksen (1999). Her account confronts us with the need to understand our own motives for carrying out sex research, and the various ways that our personal values can bias both the methods we use and how we interpret the results. But it also confronts us with an intriguing cyclical pattern; although the way we think does change with the passage of time, many of the basic ideas seem to recur and then become reburied, as we will see. Much of the following summary is based on Ericksen's account.

A series of themes have driven sex surveys during the 20th century, reflecting prevailing concerns at the time, and usually aimed at solving a problem of one kind or another. No such research, with the exception of Kinsey's, has been primarily driven by a need to know more about or to better understand human sexuality. The relevant concerns, which have overlapped and interacted to varying degrees, have included (i) concern about male masturbation, (ii) the declining birth rate, (iii) the need for good sex education to counter bad influences, (iv) the need to improve marital sex and hence improve marriage, (v) concern that the lower social classes were having more children and the middle classes fewer, (vi) the 'sexual revolution' and subsequent increase in premarital sex, (vii) the harmful effects of premarital sex on marriage, (viii) teenage pregnancies, (ix) sexually transmitted diseases and (x) AIDS.

The first sex survey in the 20th century, by Brockman (1902), was driven by concern about precocious male sexual development, manifested as adolescent males masturbating themselves to degeneracy. This survey of boys in early adolescence confirmed Brockman's fears; 57% reported masturbation to be their severest temptation, and all but one of them had succumbed. At that stage, there was less concern about women's sexuality because, it was assumed, they had less sexual drive and hence less need for self-control, a belief which paved the way for the assumption that, therefore, women should be responsible for containing sexual activity.

This was followed by concern that young men were ill-informed about sex, confirmed by Exner's (1915) survey, showing that 90% of respondents learnt about sex from 'unwholesome sources', with 79% believing this had bad consequences. Thus sex education was seen to be the solution. But this opened up another problem: this would make sex, a private affair, more public. For that reason, those carrying out surveys to better inform sex education, in spite of asserting strong moral justifications, were strongly criticized. Robie (1916), a 'radical conservative', surveyed the middle classes, seeing them as the 'normal' section of society. He supported sex education on the grounds of the high prevalence of venereal disease in men, and to some extent in women, by the time they married. He believed that women could experience strong sexual desire, particularly around menstruation, regarded at that time as the fertile phase of the menstrual cycle. Furthermore, he defended masturbation as a safer, and hence preferable, alternative to premarital and extramarital sex.

World War I, perhaps not surprisingly, was followed by a lessening of male dominance, consideration of the 'new woman' and increasing attention to women's sexuality. Davis (1929), one of the very few women to carry out sex surveys in the first half of the century, studied 2200 upper-middle-class married and single women. Women, she concluded, were sexual beings, whether or not they were married. Sixty per cent of her unmarried subjects had masturbated, and she found no difference in marital satisfaction between those women who had and had not masturbated before marriage. She also asked about sexual activity with other women. Half of her unmarried and a third of the married respondents reported erotic feelings for other women; half of these were romantic crushes, the others more overtly sexual.

A Census report had shown a 31% increase in divorce between 1916 and 1922, and this was predominantly apparent among the middle class. This resulted in major concern about the future of marriage, and a new focus on sex as the main hope for marital happiness; 'the new ideology of sexual pleasure was celebrated in magazines, newspapers and movies. Advertisers used sexual desire to sell products and sexual freedom itself became a commodity' (Ericksen 1999, p. 37). The 'companionate marriage' was born, based on 'equality' between men and women, but with differences in their sexuality which should be complimentary. In 1931 came a major work by Dickinson, a gynaecologist, and Beam, a female professional writer, with their report, *A Thousand Marriages* (Dickinson & Beam 1931). Their focus was on marital adjustment, and around 30% of the women reported difficulties adjusting to marital sex, because of either pain or 'frigidity'. Dickinson & Beam considered the husbands to be partly responsible because of inadequate or inappropriate sexual technique. Attention continued to focus on marital adjustment, with a new wave of surveys aimed principally at providing relevant information for the married. The era of the marriage course was born, and by 1949 almost half of the nation's universities had courses designed to prepare students for marriage, although in most cases these were attended more by women than men. One message was that sexual pleasure for women meant orgasm, shown in surveys to be a difficulty for some women. This was compounded by the prevalent Freudian view that 'mature' women experienced orgasm from vaginal intercourse. This resulted in performance anxiety, not only in women but also in men concerned to ensure that their wives experienced sexual pleasure. The need for many men to have their female partner experience orgasm, perhaps as an indication of their effectiveness as lovers, has been apparent for a long time, and often contributes to difficulties in the sexual relationship (see Chapter 11). Burgess, a sociologist, and Terman, a psychologist, used surveys to look for predictors of marital happiness (Terman 1938; Burgess & Cottrell 1939; Burgess & Wallin 1953) and reassured women that sexual happiness was not dependent on their experiencing orgasm.

And then came Kinsey, a biologist. His long-standing research on one insect species, the gall wasp, was driven by his interest in intra-species individual variability. The 'official' explanation for Kinsey's transition from entomology to human sexology was that he was asked to teach a marriage course for students and was confronted by the lack of scientific evidence. That is not a sufficient explanation, however. He apparently grew up in a very sex-negative family, common in that era, suffered guilt about his adolescent masturbation and experienced the trauma of being, with his wife, unable to consummate their sexual relationship when first married (Gathorne-Hardy 1998). He was therefore painfully aware of the consequences of a repressive sexual upbringing, and it is probable that in the course of collecting the scientific evidence, he felt an increasing need to counter-act the prevailing 'sex-negativism' by exposing its consequences.

Kinsey's primary scientific objective, however, was to demonstrate the extraordinary individual variability in human sexuality; no two people were the same, and when one looked at the distribution of sexual character-istics, there were no obvious cut-offs that would justify the concept of 'normal' versus 'abnormal'. In many respects this was his most fundamental challenge to both scientific and public opinion, particularly in relation to premarital and extra-marital sex, and to homosexuality. We will return to this issue. Kinsey, however, considered marriage to be important in both personal and social terms, and sex to be an important factor in determining marital well-being and stability. In the female volume he addressed the frequency of sexual problems within marriage, focusing on the differences between male and female sexuality, and the resulting lack of mutual understanding that accounted for many of these pro-blems. It is noteworthy that in the male volume he used 'orgasm', whether derived from heterosexual intercourse and petting, masturbation, nocturnal emissions, homo-sexual activity or sexual contact with animals, as the criterion of 'sexual outlet', and reported frequencies of 'total sexual outlet' as a measure of the man's sexual drive; not an unreasonable concept, if somewhat sim-plistic, but one that certainly challenged the prevailing sexual mores. By the time he came to write the female volume he had been confronted by the variability in orgasmic capacity among women, leading him to con-clude that 'orgasm cannot be taken as the sole criterion for determining the degree of satisfaction which a female may derive from sexual activity ... Whether or not she herself reaches orgasm, many a female finds satisfaction in knowing that her ... partner has enjoyed the contact, and in realizing that she has contributed to the male's pleasure' (Kinsey et al 1953, p. 371).

But the most immediate and obvious impact of Kinsey's work on public opinion had little to do with the scientific detail or merit of his research. *Sexual Behav-ior in the Human Male* was published in 1948 (Kinsey et al 1948). *Sexual Behavior in the Human Female* followed in 1953 (Kinsey et al 1953). The male volume, an extremely dry book filled with dense tables, sold more than 200 000 copies in the first 6 weeks. Within 4 months, it was top of the *New York Times* bestseller list. Within the first year, there were translations in French, Spanish, Italian and Swedish. By 1950, the attention of the public and media turned to anticipating the female volume. Although at the outset this also received a massive response in the media (most of it in the 3 weeks before it was officially published), the reaction was brief by comparison with the male volume. Overall, reactions to both books ranged from outrage to admiration. For examples of out-rage, Roman Catholic Archbishop Paul Schulte (from the diocese in which Kinsey lived) commented 'There can be no valid objections to a scientific investigation of sexual behaviour, that would assist lawmakers, educators, cler-gymen, physicians and other professional people ... but Dr Kinsey has degraded science. Instead of circulating

the findings among those competent to weigh and apply them to the betterment of mankind, he publicizes them like a cheap charlatan.' This points to the importance of keeping information about sex away from ordinary folk. Representative Heller, Democrat from New York, urged that the book be banned from the mail. 'He (Kinsey) is contributing to the depravity of a whole gen-eration, to the loss of faith in human dignity and human decency...' In other words, any open discussion of sex, particularly in reference to women, is degrading. Heller had not even read the book! Nor had the Reverend Billy Graham when he declared that Dr Kinsey '... certainly could not have interviewed any of the millions of born-again Christian women in this country who put the highest price on virtue, decency and modesty'. This idea that sex surveys are flawed because decent people do not participate in them has, as we shall see, recurred (for a review of the media reactions see Brinkman 1971). It is noteworthy that more outrage was provoked by the female volume than the male volume.

Kinsey's books had 'taken the lid off'. As never before, the details of the sexual experiences of ordinary men and women, at least in terms of physiological responses and behaviours, were out in the open for all to read about. The initial, extraordinary worldwide impact indicated two things. Many people were amazed and excited that they could read about such things, other than as the subject of humour or gossip, or as the setting of moral standards, and yet with the stamp of apparent scientific authority. Others, who believed that sex should be confined to the bedroom and not be talked about, were alarmed that control of information about this fun-damental aspect had been lost. The question remains why Kinsey had such a large impact compared, for example, to the earlier provocative studies of women's sexuality by Davis (1929) and Robert Latou Dickinson (Dickinson & Beam 1931, 1934). Would Kinsey's work have had the same impact if it had appeared before World War II?

However, ever since Kinsey's two books, there has been no shortage of information on sex available to the general public, admittedly of mixed quality. 'The sex survey' has become a popular format in the media, where large numbers of readers of magazines, such as *Redbook* (Tavris & Sadd 1977), provide material for arti-cles in those magazines, based on samples, which are, of course, far from representative. Most of these have come and gone without much impact, with some excep-tions (e.g. *The Hite Report* 1976; plus Hite 1978, 1991). One of the lessons from Kinsey's research is that, typi-cally, there is, or has been, a discrepancy between what people do sexually and what society assumes, and expects them to do. Whereas before Kinsey the assump-tion was more restrictive than the reality, with the com-mercialization of sex, particularly to sell magazines, there has been an increasing tendency to 'sell' the idea that people are more sexual than they are in reality.

In the reactions to Kinsey we see the first explicit political opposition to sex research. Kinsey's research was funded by the National Research Council with money from the Rockefeller Foundation. In 1953, in the wake of the outrage caused by the female volume, a House Committee, chaired by Tennessee Congressman Carrol Reece, was set up to assess the tax exempt status of private foundations, but with the clear primary aim of challenging the Rockefeller Foundation funding of Kinsey. As a result, this funding was withdrawn, a serious blow to Kinsey who spent the next and last 3 years of his life desperately and unsuccessfully trying to obtain alternative funding (Bancroft 2004).

Whereas discomfort about research on what people do in their bedrooms prevailed, by the late 1930s concern about the most fundamental consequence of such activity, fertility, was growing. There was a declining birth rate in the USA, particularly among the middle class. A survey by Riley & White (1940) found that almost all non-sterile women used birth control, the assumption being that women alone were responsible for this. The Birth Control Federation of America changed its name to the Planned Parenthood Federation of America, encouraging families to plan for the number of children they could afford (i.e. mainly the middle classes). Then followed the post-war 'baby boom', initially expected to be brief but which persisted. Freedman et al (1959), from the sociology department at Michigan University, conducted the first Growth of American Families study, seeking to establish women's intentions about having children. Ericksen (1999) describes the cautious approach used, as well as new and improved survey methods. There was concern that this new survey should avoid the sensationalism attributed to Kinsey, with the university requiring approval from the Detroit Archdiocese, as well as advisory committees of physicians and lay people. While avoiding questions about sex, the survey found widespread use of contraception, with family size typically from two to four children, and the lower educated tending to have more children than they wanted because of their difficulties in obtaining or using effective contraception. The success of this survey, with a 91% response rate, placed survey research at the centre of social science (Ericksen 1999), and the Survey Research Center at the University of Michigan has remained in the forefront of the field ever since.

In the 1960s we see increasing involvement of the National Institutes of Health, government agencies for funding research, in surveys of various consequences of sexual behaviour. In 1965, the first National Fertility Study (NFS) was carried out, funded by the National Institute of Child Health and Human Development (NICHD). This tentatively inquired about the frequency of sexual behaviour in order to assess the relation between sexual activity and fertility, but avoided using the word 'sex', (e.g. 'In the past 4 weeks, how many times have you had intercourse?'), (Ryder & Westoff 1971). With subsequent repeats of the NFS, in 1970 and 1975, a steady increase in the frequency of intercourse within marriage was reported, with the startling finding that as women felt more secure in their ability to avoid conception, their interest in sex increased. Hitherto, women's relatively low level of sexual desire had been attributed to either their upbringing or their constitution.

This led to increased attention to the fertility of the lower socio-economic groups (previously studied by Rainwater 1966) and, inevitably, black women, who were found to have more unplanned children than white women. However, as one-third of black women were not married when they became pregnant, there was a reluctant inclusion of the unmarried in such surveys. But at least, by this stage, sex of a potentially reproductive kind, whether within or without marriage, became one of the key issues in fertility surveys (Ericksen 1999).

The 1960s and 1970s are often described as the era of 'sexual liberation', or for those who were deeply concerned about the challenge to moral standards, the 'sexual revolution'. It is not, therefore, surprising that the previous restriction of research attention to sex as an aspect of marriage, changed with mounting concern about the impact of the sexual revolution on the behaviour of the unmarried, particularly the adolescent. The concept of premarital sex prevailed, reflecting a needful assumption that sex among the unmarried was hopefully in preparation for sex after marriage. Attention was paid to whether premarital sex had a negative impact on marital sexual adjustment. Numerous surveys of young college students were carried out, reflecting, in part, the focus on the middle classes, who were regarded by the moral establishment as the most crucial section of society as far as sex and reproduction were concerned. This emphasis on student samples has, in fact, continued to this day, now more a reflection of the convenience of students as research subjects, particularly for sex research, which is generally very difficult to get funded.

Reiss carried out a series of studies of sexual attitudes, rather than behaviour, among the unmarried (e.g. Reiss 1967), and found evidence of a shift towards 'permissiveness with affection', i.e. it is acceptable to be sexual with someone with whom you have an affectionate relationship. Whereas previously most women experienced sex before they married, but not until they were engaged to be married, now there was greater acceptance of sexual activity without an explicit commitment to marriage. Whereas numerous unrepresentative student surveys pointed to an increase in sexual activity among the unmarried during the 1960s, Simon et al (1972), using representative samples of college students in 1967 and of 14- to 18-year-olds in 1972 concluded that the increase in premarital sex since the findings of the Kinsey surveys in the 1940s was small in comparison with increases around the beginning of the 20th century. On the other hand, DeLamater & MacCorquodale (1979), in a representative survey of both students and non-students, reported substantial increases in sexual permissiveness since Simon et al's (1972) survey 6 years previously; this is a somewhat conflicting picture, perhaps reflecting the vagaries of survey research at that time, as well as it being a period of change.

An increasing acceptance that sex occurred before marriage was countered by a growing concern that young adolescent girls were not only having sex, but also getting pregnant. By this time the National Institutes of Health were funding sex surveys not only focused on teenage pregnancies, but also other sex-related problems, such as sexually transmitted diseases, and sexual assault and rape. Results from these studies will be considered later in this chapter and elsewhere in the book. Noteworthy was a phase of interest in homosexuality, which probably reflected the growing unrest among the homosexual community. A National Institute of Mental Health (NIMH) Task Force on Homosexuality was established in 1967 by Stanley Yolles when he was Director of NIMH, and chaired by Evelyn Hooker. Although the final report of this task force was not published until 1972 (NIMH 1972), the main conclusions were made public in 1969, just 6 months after the Stonewall riots which heralded the start of the Gay Liberation Movement in New York City. The principal recommendation of the Task Force was for the establishment of an NIMH Center for the Study of Sexual Behavior, which would enable research into homosexuality to be placed 'within the context of the study of the broad range of sexuality, both normal and deviant'. Such a centre was never established, and the more specific recommendations of the report received a mixed reception by the gay and lesbian community. Soon to follow, however, was NIMH funding of two major grants to the Kinsey Institute. One led to a series of new surveys on male homosexuality (Williams & Weinberg 1971; Weinberg & Williams 1974; Bell & Weinberg 1978; Bell et al 1981). The other grant was aimed at a national survey of public attitudes to homosexuality. This project, which came to cover attitudes and values about sex more generally, had a long and painful history. The data, collected in 1970 but not published until 1989, indicated that moral values about sex had not changed as much by 1970 as was widely assumed to be the case (Klassen et al 1989).

In 1977, NIMH hosted a conference entitled the Methodology of Sex Research (Green & Wiener 1980). This covered research topics such as sexual differentiation, neurobiological basis of sexual behaviour, heterosexual relationships, sex and ageing, sexual dysfunction, rape and homosexuality, and was further evidence of NIMH's commitment to sex research.

By the mid-1980s, concern about AIDS dominated the scene, and a number of surveys relevant to HIV transmission were supported by NIH. Most notable was the series of National AIDS Behavioral Surveys, funded by NIMH, the first sample collected in 1990, with more than 10 000 respondents (Catania et al 1992). While such surveys, specifically focusing on AIDS transmission, survived political scrutiny, others with a more general relevance did not. This takes us to an exceptional period in this history, which lasted from 1988 to 1991. The NICHD was funding a number of modest-sized surveys relevant to reproductive health and sexually transmitted diseases, including HIV/AIDS (e.g. Billy et al 1993; Ku et al 1993). But, responding to calls for additional data from the Institute of Medicine, they invited bids to design two larger scale national surveys, one covering the full adult age range for both men and women, the other to study adolescent sexuality more comprehensively than

before. Edward Laumann, Robert Michael and John Gagnon were successful in the competition for designing the adult survey. Ronald Rindfuss and Richard Udry were the successful bidders for designing what became known as the American Teenage Study (ATS). However, NICHD encountered political resistance both inside and outside Congress. As a result the adult survey did not get funded beyond the planning stage, and funding for the ATS, which had been approved and awarded, was subsequently withdrawn.

The two politicians mainly responsible for the opposition to these two surveys were Representative William Dannemeyer of Orange County, California, and Senator Jesse Helms of North Carolina. Dannemeyer charged that the plan was to spend large amounts of tax money under the pretext of containing the spread of AIDS, and in the process reduce the social stigma associated with sexual deviance. He indicated that this outcome would be made more likely because of the unreliability of sex surveys, the crucial point being that 'upstanding Americans' would not agree to participate. He went on, at a later stage, to reveal that his particular concern was about the lessening of social stigma associated with homosexuality. Helms, who believed that the intent of the surveys was to convince Americans that homosexuality was normal and acceptable, introduced an amendment to the budget bill in the Senate. In this, he proposed taking the money committed to the two big surveys and using it for abstinence education. His amendment, asking Congress to choose between educating the young to restrain themselves sexually on the one hand and promoting sexual decadence on the other, was passed. Interestingly, although several people spoke against his amendment, they were seemingly at a loss to know how to deal with the sexual aspect of it. In general, it can be said, American politicians do not find sex an easy topic to discuss, other than negatively.

In spite of these obstacles, both groups were eventually able to carry out surveys, which were, however, very different to those originally planned or approved. Laumann, Michael and Gagnon, together with Stuart Michaels, obtained funding from private foundations for what became The National Health & Social Life Survey (NHSLS; Laumann et al 1994), but whereas the original survey had aimed at a sample of around 20 000, the NHSLS involved around 3500. In 1993, Congress, having preventing funding of the ATS, called on NICHD to conduct a comprehensive study of adolescent health. Udry then submitted a new grant application which was more broadly aimed at adolescent health, but which also included, discretely, a fair amount about adolescent sexuality. This was funded and became known as the Add Health survey.

In 2002, another political campaign against sex research started, this time aimed at psychophysiological sex research, what the *Washington Times* described as the 'use of tax payers money to show women pornography'. This was followed by 20 House Republicans sending a letter to NIH, questioning this 'bizarre spending decision'. It became apparent that the Republican Study Committee was scrutinizing carefully the federal funding of sex research. In 2003, an amendment to the HHS Appropriations Bill was introduced into the House of Representatives, by Representative Toomey (R-PA). calling for withdrawal of funding from four grants that had been approved by NICHD, one on age-related changes in sexual behaviour in older men, one on drug- and HIV-related factors among Asian prostitutes and masseurs in San Francisco, another on transgender issues among Native Americans, and the fourth a Kinsey Institute psychophysiological study of the effects of mood on sexual arousal. The amendment was defeated by only two votes. Within the next month, the House Energy and Commerce Committee faxed to NIH a list (HHS Grant Projects) of 180 researchers and around 200 peer-reviewed NIH-funded research grants, all related in some way to research on sex, sexually transmitted diseases or related risk-taking behaviours. The list had been developed by the Traditional Values Coalition, an organization claiming to represent more than 43 000 churches, ostensibly as part of an ongoing investigation of NIH grants. This caused a stir in Congress, leading to pressure on NIH to defend its peer-review system in this area of funding. There was a heartening reaction from the scientific community, with 37 professional organizations, including the American Association for the Advancement of Science, American Psychological Association, American Sociological Association and the National Campaign to Prevent Teen Pregnancy, writing letters to express their support of NIH funding of sex research, and of the peer-review process (Leshner 2003). In January 2004, Elias Zerhouni, Director of NIH responded. He had asked the directors of the relevant institutes within NIH to conduct a comprehensive review of the human sexuality research funded by NIH, particularly that included in the list of grants. On the basis of their reviews, he strongly endorsed NIH involvement in this research (Zerhouni 2004). NIH and the academic community were standing firm (for a more detailed review of political opposition to sex research, see Bancroft 2004).

The above short history of sex surveys and the various types of opposition to them relates to the USA. The situation in Europe, though not well chronicled, shows a somewhat less troubling story. However, while NICHD was contending with the political opposition to its funding of the national survey by Laumann and colleagues, a strikingly similar story was unfolding in the UK. In 1987, interest emerged in carrying out a large-scale British survey to allow estimation of the possible spread of HIV within the UK. This involved a number of epidemiologists, together with members of the Health Education Authority, the Department of Health and Social Security (DHSS) and the Economic and Social Research Council (ESRC), all Governmental bodies. The idea was approved by the DHSS, and a feasibility study was carried out, followed by submission of an application to the ESRC for funding the main study. Then the previously smooth-running process became stuck. The researchers remained in the dark until a newspaper article in 1989 revealed that the Prime Minister, Margaret Thatcher, had personally vetoed the study, on the grounds of its 'intrusiveness and unacceptability to the British people'. This was quickly followed by a successful submission to the Wellcome Foundation, who agreed to fund the same size survey as originally intended, which ended with a sample of 18 876 (Johnson et al 1994). A comparable large-scale French survey, also aimed at assessing sexual behaviour relevant to the AIDS epidemic, met no such governmental opposition (Spira et al 1994). The British survey was repeated in 1999/2001, this time funded by the Medical Research Council, a Government funding agency.

A number of issues have emerged in this brief history of sex survey research. Why is the research being done? This is not always clearly apparent. Given the societal and political constraints on funding as well as allowing such surveys, objectives are often stated which may have more to do with making the study acceptable than describing what the researcher is actually interested in. This is particularly relevant to large surveys. Whereas the primary aim, e.g. to assess degree of risk of HIV transmission, may be clear, the researchers may feel that in obtaining a large sample, particularly if representative, opportunities for exploring other issues or answering other questions should not be missed. It is therefore not altogether surprising that the motives of survey researchers are sometimes misconstrued. How is the objective of the survey being addressed? Here there is often uncertainty reflecting a relative absence of any clear hypothesis testing. This will be considered more closely below. In what ways have the methods of data collection influenced the results? What are the ethical issues in such research? This is of particular importance considering the extent of public or at least political opposition to sex research. Let us look at some of these issues more closely.

The methodology of sex surveys

Survey design

Most community-based surveys have been and will continue to be cross-sectional. Longitudinal studies have obvious and considerable advantages, but because of their long-term nature, are exceptionally difficult to implement. Examples are the Melbourne Women's Midlife Health Project (Dennerstein et al 1999), a prospective, population-based study of Australian-born women, assessed annually for 8 years, as they progressed through the menopausal transition. The purpose of this study was to assess factors that affect women's sexual functioning and how these change over time. Another longitudinal study that, while principally focused on issues of mental health, assessed sexual problems, is the Zurich cohort study (Ernst et al 1993). A sample of men and women were interviewed on four occasions over a 10-year period, between the ages of 20 and 30 years.

Longitudinal studies involving repeated assessment over a relatively short period (e.g. 2 or 3 years) are becoming increasingly feasible with the development of established survey panels (see below).

Obtaining a sample

Surveys that aim to establish prevalence of sexual problems and associated factors clearly need to be representative, if any generalization to the general population is to be made. This presents a challenge. Currently, the only feasible way to generate a representative national sample is to employ one of the survey organizations that have the mechanisms for sampling in place (e.g. Laumann et al 1994; Johnson et al 1994; Bancroft et al 2003a). This is extremely costly. Whereas a few years ago, random digit dialing (RDD) was the most commonly used method for generating a sample, this is no longer considered acceptable due to problems with telephone surveys in general (discussed further below). Obtaining a sample of a known but limited population, e.g. general practitioner's lists (e.g. Nazareth et al 2003) is more feasible, but problems of generalizability and participation biases remain.

When selecting a representative sample, the specific aims of the project should be taken into consideration. Thus, if age is an important factor, the use of probability-based over-sampling of otherwise under-represented age groups will allow sufficient power to test the age-related hypotheses. Other examples of groups that, if a focus of the study, may require over-sampling, are gay men and lesbian women, celibate individuals and various ethnic groups.

Participation biases have to be taken into consideration. The most relevant evidence on this point comes from an Australian longitudinal twin study ($n = 9112$) in which a substantial amount of information about all participants had been obtained before asking them to participate in a study about their sexual behaviour and attitudes (Dunne et al 1997). Twenty-seven per cent explicitly refused, 52% explicitly consented and 19% agreed to receive the questionnaire but did not return it. Those explicitly consenting had higher levels of education, attended church less often, and had less conservative sexual attitudes and voting preferences. In their response to personality measures, they were more novelty seeking and reward dependent, and less harm avoidant than refusers. Responders had higher lifetime prevalence of major depression, alcohol dependence and childhood conduct disorder, and also reported an earlier age at first sexual intercourse and higher rates of sexual abuse. Those who did not return the questionnaires were more like the responders than the refusers. Other evidence of participation bias in sex research has been reported by Catania et al (1986) and Strassberg & Lowe (1996).

There are other research objectives for which representative samples are not essential. This particularly applies to studies that are focusing on relationships between factors of possible causal relevance, rather than prevalence rates. For this purpose a sample is required which has sufficient variance in each of the factors of interest to allow assessment of their inter-relationships. Eysenck's (1976) study of sex and personality is a good early example of this principle. His prime purpose was to study the relationship between aspects of sexuality assessed by his questionnaire and his own measures of personality, in particular neuroticism, extroversion and psychoticism. The validity of associations observed in this way then needs to be established with replication using further samples. He studiously avoided drawing any inferences about the population incidence of these aspects of his data.

It is noticeable how few surveys of sexual behaviour, representative or not, have built-in hypothesis testing of this kind. This reflects the relative lack of theory, and a prevailing empiricism in this aspect of sex research.

Methods of data collection

Surveys conventionally have used self-report questionnaires, interview methods, or a combination of the two. There are advantages and disadvantages with each of these methods. In face-to-face interviews, the interviewer can clarify the meaning of questions and probe for more detailed responses if necessary, but this also can result in greater variance in how questions are asked and meanings conveyed. The training of the interviewer is of crucial importance here as are possible biases related to gender, age and ethnic background of the interviewer (Catania et al 1996). A disadvantage of interviews, particularly for large-scale surveys, is that they are expensive and labour intensive. Problems of under-reporting of sexual problems due to concerns about stigmatization may also be more likely if interviews are used, particularly when conditions of privacy cannot be assured. In the Laumann et al (1994) survey, 21% of the face-to-face interviews were conducted with a third person present (most often children or stepchildren, but in some cases spouses or sexual partners). Whereas for many survey topics this may not be a problem, asking questions about sensitive issues such as sex requires confidentiality if not anonymity.

Telephone surveys have been used in several of the large-scale AIDS behavioural surveys, such as the survey carried out in France (Spira et al 1994). In a direct comparison of telephone survey and face-to-face interviewing, although questions were more easily answered on the telephone, they were more likely to be influenced by social desirability, compared to the interview method (ACSF 1992). Although telephone surveys are less expensive than interviews, it has become increasingly difficult to recruit participants by telephone.

The use of various kinds of computer-assisted interviews in surveys has increased. There are a number of advantages of these methods; use of 'branching' and 'skip' questions, checks for inconsistencies, automatic data entry and time stamping, as well as the increased confidentiality and anonymity that they provide respondents. Some studies have found that computerized methods elicit more accurate reports of sensitive behaviours such as same-sex sexual activity (Turner et al 1997). In a comparative study of different methods, Erens et al (1997) found computer-assisted self-interview (CASI) to produce more consistent data and lower non-response rate, although no difference in the likelihood of reporting sensitive behaviours. If a method such as audio-computer-assisted self-interview (A-CASI) is used in a respondent's home, then an interviewer might be present to answer questions about the survey, although this adds to the expense. Such methods have been incorporated into recent telephone surveys, either with the interviewer entering the participant's responses directly into a computer (i.e. computer-assisted telephone interview) or with the respondent entering responses directly into the computer using touch-tone telephones (telephone-audio-computer-assisted self-interview (T-ACASI; Bancroft et al 2003a) Such methods do not, however, solve the participation problems with telephone surveys.

A newly emerging method, which has not as yet been used to collect sexuality-related information, but is being increasingly used for health-related surveys, and which has considerable potential, is the use of Internet panels. An example of this is the Knowledge Networks panel[1] involving approximately 40 000 individuals aged over 18 years. In return for receiving cable connections and computer facilities, an individual agrees to complete a short survey every few weeks. This is a fairly representative sample demographically, although its representativeness is limited by the original use of RDD for establishing the panel. There are a number of distinct advantages to this approach. Firstly, all of the advantages of computerized interviewing are present. Secondly, a substantial amount of information about the panelists is already available, which not only can be used to augment the data collected in a specific survey, but also allows better description of those who decline to participate. Thirdly, screening of a large number of individuals can be used before selecting probability-based subsamples and a substantial number of questions can be asked by using a series of short surveys. Lastly, repeated surveying allows assessment of stability of responses and change over time. In a recent comparative study of this Internet approach and telephone interviewing, Chang & Krosnik (unpublished data) found the Internet method to have some advantages in terms of data quality. It remains to be seen whether this approach is effective in collecting sexuality-related data.

Survey questions

Surveys assessing prevalence of factors relevant to sexual dysfunction need to carefully address issues such as question wording and comprehension. Items should be as clear and specific as possible (Fenton et al 2001). Pre-testing of items, with either individuals or focus groups, should be carried out (Catania et al 1993), and checked in pilot surveys with subjects being asked, after completing the survey, how they interpreted the questions.

Assessing the frequency of sexual activity or sexual problems raises important methodological issues, mainly because of recall error; accuracy of retrospective recall of sexual behaviour declines significantly with longer recall periods (Catania et al 1990; Graham et al 2003). At the same time, assessing the duration of a problem is clearly important, and often requires reporting over relatively long time periods. Assessment of

a short and recent time period allows reasonably accurate assessment of the current situation (e.g. Dunn et al 1998; Bancroft et al 2003a; Nazareth et al 2003). Care should be taken, however, with how such frequency is recorded. With a short time interval, such as a month, the number of occasions of sexual activity can be realistically recorded, followed by the proportion of those occasions in which a particular response (e.g. orgasm, vaginal lubrication) did or did not occur (e.g. Bancroft et al 2003a). Asking for approximate frequencies — e.g. How often do you have sexual intercourse? Once or twice a month, once or twice a week? — invites 'normative' answers; people will be more likely to choose which answer they think it should be (Bozon 2001). Asking approximations of frequency ('often', 'occasionally', 'rarely' or 'never', e.g. Eplov et al 2007) are even more questionable as it is impossible to know how much people vary in their interpretation of such concepts.

In addition to the recent time period, it is clearly important to establish how long a particular pattern has been evident. A combination of a relatively precise frequency for a recent time period, and a more realistic estimate of duration or intermittence, is therefore appropriate.

Comprehensive reviews of the methodological issues involved in sex surveys have been provided by Catania et al (1995) and Fenton et al (2001).

The nature of the questions has ethical implications. This was central to the controversy surrounding Kinsey's research. Kinsey attached great importance to presenting himself to his research subjects as non-judgemental. No matter what behaviour they revealed to him, he would not convey any moral judgement. This was of particular importance at that time and had a powerful effect on many of his subjects in enabling them to speak openly about their sexual lives. We should keep in mind that, at that point in history, the majority of types of sexual expression, including some within marriage, were against the law. Whether previous sex surveys had been similarly non-judgemental is unclear, but given the moral agenda of many of the earlier studies, it seems unlikely.

This non-judgemental approach remains a requirement for any effective research in this area — and herein lies a problem for many critics. Persuading someone to describe the full range of his or her sexual experiences, devoid of moral judgement, is seen by the critics as, in some sense, giving that person implicit permission to engage in such behaviours. Thus sex research, according to this view, is undermining the prevailing moral values — the subject leaves the interview feeling, 'maybe I'm not so bad after all'. The answer to this is to inform research subjects that the research they have agreed to participate in, aims to find out what people do in their sexual lives, and is not intended to convey any message about what they should or should not do.

There have been a substantial number of surveys assessing the age of onset of sexual activity in teenagers, as well as the prevalence of sexually transmitted

---

[1]Knowledge Networks, Inc. 1350 Willow Rd, Menlo Park, CA 94025 www.knowledgenetworks.com/ganp.

infections and unplanned pregnancies in that age group (e.g. Santelli et al 2000a). By comparison, these have encountered little political opposition. But, beyond these bald statistics, concern is expressed about asking teenagers what they do sexually, particularly when asked in a non-judgemental fashion, because by doing so the researcher is 'putting ideas into teenagers' heads', leading to behaviours that would not otherwise have occurred. One cannot entirely rule this out, but the implication of this criticism is that it is better to remain in ignorance of what they are doing, the costs of which are likely to greatly outweigh any such risks of influencing their behaviour. In addition, the weight of evidence from studies of the effects of sex education, which is often opposed for the same reason — e.g. teaching about contraception will encourage sexual behaviour — is that the benefits outweigh any such costs (Kirby 1997).

Hence the fate of the ATS, which, as discussed above, was looking at what could be considered normal adolescent sexual development. It was okay to study adolescent sexual behaviour as long as the focus was on the negative consequences. Although such negative statistics might be reacted to in various ways (e.g. Alan Guttmacher Institute (AGI) 1976), which wanted to promote the availability of contraception for teenagers; and see Nathanson 2000, for broader discussion), the figures in general were fuel for those wanting to eliminate adolescent sexuality, and foster abstinence until marriage. It is striking how little research has been done on 'normal' adolescent sexuality, and on how adolescents learn to be sexual and acquire sexual responsibility (Bancroft 2005).

Confidentiality is obviously a key ethical issue in sex research, and with surveys, which collect and document extensive details about the participant, is of particular importance. Kinsey dealt with this by memorizing a code for all the answers, and recording the data on cards, only interpretable by someone who knows the code. Obviously this admirable method is not generally usable, so particular care has to be taken in making the data secure. This can be achieved by eliminating any identifying information, such as name, once the data collection is complete. An additional challenge arises, however, if there are plans to carry out repeat assessments over time. Clearly the participant should know about and agree to such use.

Theoretical bases of sex surveys

As mentioned earlier, the bulk of sex research has, until recently, been atheoretical, and descriptive rather than hypothesis testing. This can be considered a weakness in the field, which was considered more closely in Chapter 2. A comprehensive review of theoretical issues across the field of sex surveys is beyond the scope of this chapter, but brief consideration will be given to two of the principal surveys, the data from which will be used extensively in the rest of this chapter, the British NATSAL (Johnson et al 1994) and the American NHSLS (Laumann et al 1994).

Johnson et al (1994) state the rationale for their survey. 'Without doubt the emergence of the HIV epidemic provided the impetus, the legitimation and the funding opportunities for this study, and the public health implications of the growing epidemic guided the direction of the research' (p. 5). Their theoretical approach, however, is briefly described as 'one that accepts the influence of social factors and the importance of human agency in sexual expression and changing sexual lifestyles, but which at the same time recognizes the potentially harmful effects of repressive social engineering'. If 'human agency' refers to the capacity of the individual to make decisions, there can be little argument with this statement, yet it does not exactly generate testable hypotheses, and none are apparent in the ensuing report.

Laumann et al (1994) have a substantial section on the theoretical basis of their survey, which is in three parts: scripting theory, choice theory and social network theory. 'Together, these theories allow us to move toward the construction of a more comprehensive theory of the social dimensions of sexuality' (p. 5). However, the impact of these theories on the design of the survey and how the data were analysed is not clear. The difficulties in using script theory as a basis for research methodology, particularly quantitative research, was considered in Chapter 2 (p. 11). Economic 'choice' theory is about how people utilize the resources available to them in pursuit of a specific goal. We are told: 'securing partners is not without cost; one must expend time, money, emotional energy, and social resources in order to meet people and negotiate a sexual relationship. Solely on the basis of this consideration, it would seem to be more cost effective to fulfil one's sexual needs by remaining in a long-term relationship than by constantly searching for new partners' (p. 9); not the most romantic rationale for a long-term relationship! Once again it is difficult to find indications of how this theory has shaped the survey or influenced interpretation of results. Social network theory is, on the face of it, more obviously relevant, but it depends on complex analyses of particular types of data. Laumann et al (1994) struggled in the report of this survey to demonstrate evidence of 'sexual networks', but because of the nature of their survey data they were restricted to demonstrating that most relationships involved two people who had met within a social group or family network and that such groups were typically distinguished by socio-economic, racial and/or religious criteria. The reader is left with the impression that this large, and inherently valuable, data set was being used post hoc to justify the researchers' theoretical orientations rather than vice versa. However, they apparently learnt from this experience, and moved on to design and implement a very different type of survey, the Chicago Health and Social Life Study (CHSLS), much smaller in sample size, focusing on four specific communities within the area of Chicago, and combining qualitative and quantitative methods of data collection to allow more direct access to the study of sexual networks (Michaels 1997). In a subsequent book, Laumann et al (2004) presented some of the results and, by using the concept of 'sex market', were able to combine their network and economic choice theoretical ideas. Their findings will be considered later in this chapter.

It is easy to be critical of the theoretical approaches, or lack of them, used by sex researchers, but as discussed in Chapter 2, few sex researchers can escape such criticisms, the present author included. It is, however, becoming increasingly clear that large-scale surveys would benefit by the inclusion of clearly-defined theoretically-based hypotheses central to the main objectives of the survey. It may be the case that only a limited number of such testable hypotheses can realistically be addressed in any one survey, and this does not preclude the collection of other potentially useful data.

Cross-cultural comparisons

Throughout this chapter, although emphasis will be placed on data from English language surveys, cross-cultural comparisons will be made when the evidence allows it. Methodologically, we should be aware of the difficulties inherent in such comparisons because of cultural differences in the way sexuality is conceived. The WHO Global Program on AIDS, which aimed to collect cross-cultural sexuality data relevant to AIDS transmission (Carballo et al 1989) ran into difficulty because of the tendency to use concepts of sexuality which were derived from the developed countries in Europe and North America. Comparative evidence of this kind has to be interpreted cautiously (Parker 1997).

The value of qualitative data

The challenge of cross-cultural survey research confronts us with the importance of understanding the socio-cultural meanings applied to sexuality. How masturbation, for example, is conceptualized in very different cultures emphasizes the need to find out about those meanings before formulating the precise questions for a survey. And the best way to find this out is by talking to people. The value of this is, however, not restricted to cross-cultural research. There is a strong case for using qualitative studies before designing any survey research. I learnt this lesson rather late in my career. In the Kinsey Institute research on sexual risk taking, covered in Chapter 14, we carried out quantitative (non-representative) survey research and qualitative research in a proportion of our survey participants, in parallel. Clearly, we would have improved the quantitative component if we had carried out the qualitative component first. Conversely, one can often throw light on a finding from survey data by asking individuals what it means to them.

With the predominantly quantitative sources of evidence available, let us consider patterns of heterosexual behaviour in adolescence and adulthood under the following headings:

1. masturbation
2. sex in the unmarried
3. sexual attraction, falling in love and partner choice
4. marriage.

Masturbation

Social attitudes to masturbation

Self-stimulation to achieve sexual pleasure and orgasm is so effective and so widespread that one is tempted to ask why we bother with sexual partners. At least part of the answer lies in the negative attitudes to masturbation and other forms of non-procreative sex, which have universally prevailed. Even though it is well established that almost all men and a substantial majority of women masturbate, at least occasionally, the extent to which negative attitudes towards this behaviour still prevail is noteworthy. In the NHSLS (Laumann et al 1994), whereas the rest of the survey was carried out by face-to-face interview, questions about masturbation were asked in a pencil-and-paper questionnaire, which the participant completed and sealed in an envelope so that the interviewer did not see it, a technique which had been shown in previous studies to produce higher rates of reporting of 'socially disapproved behaviours'. They chose this method because interviewers had expressed anxiety about asking about masturbation, and government officials reviewing the method of a pre-test version, insisted that questions on masturbation be removed from the study (p. 81). In the first British NAT-SAL survey, carried out at around the same time as the American survey, no questions were asked about masturbation. In qualitative studies which preceded the survey design, discussion of masturbation 'had met with both distaste and embarrassment' and 'it appeared unwise to prejudice response to questions of greater relevance to public health policy' (Johnson et al 1994). In the same year as these two national surveys were published, Jocelyn Elders, the US Surgeon General, was dismissed by President Clinton because of a remark about masturbation. At a World AIDS day held at the United Nations, Elders was asked, in reference to recommending less risky sexual behaviours, 'What are the prospects of a more explicit discussion and promotion of masturbation?' She replied 'I think (masturbation) is a part of human sexuality and it's part of something that perhaps should be taught. But we've not even taught our children the very basics ....' Elders can be criticized for her choice of words, which could be interpreted as meaning that we should teach children to masturbate. As we shall see, the large majority learn to masturbate without being taught; what is needed is that they should feel less guilty about it. Clinton's reaction can be criticized for reinforcing unwarranted negative attitudes about masturbation. At a time when sexual behaviour of young people is causing so much concern, the low risk of masturbation as a way of dealing with one's sexual appetite is something to be taken seriously. Ironically, the media reaction to the Elders incident has probably brought the topic of masturbation out into the open with some positive benefits. We now have a well-researched and sensible book for the general public called *The Big Book of Masturbation* (Cornog 2003). As with most aspects of human sexuality there are benefits and costs, and we will consider negative aspects of masturbation later. But it is clearly an example of a behaviour which is almost universal, which plays an important part in normal sexual development for many of us, is a source of pleasure without risks, is used constructively by sex therapists to help men and women deal with sexual problems, and in no way warrants its negative reputation. But let us look more closely at the long history of this reputation.

Since the time of the Old Testament, people have argued as to whether the sin of Onan, for which he was severely punished, was masturbation or coitus interruptus (Genesis 38: 8–10). The attitudes to masturbation in different cultures and at different periods have usually reflected the general attitudes to sex at the time. Thus in ancient China, with its poetic mysticism, life was seen as a balancing act between the active and passive forces of yin and yang. Sex was an important example of this harmonious balance. The essence of sexual yang in the male was the man's semen, and that of yin was the woman's vaginal fluids. Whereas the latter were thought to be inexhaustible, the former was by contrast precious, needing to be maintained by a regular supply of yin (Tannahill 1980). Thus coitus reservatus, where the man strives to avoid ejaculation, was widespread and masturbation regarded as a waste of vital yang essence. Female masturbation was more or less ignored (Bullough 1976). In the Middle Ages, when venereal pleasure was only tolerated when associated with procreation, lust was regarded as a vice because, according to St Thomas Aquinas, 'it exceeded the order and mode of reason'. In Aquinas's league of sins against nature (i.e. non-procreative and hence sins against God), masturbation was the least serious, but it nevertheless carried heavier penalties than sexual sins against the person, such as adultery or even rape.

These two examples illustrate the two themes that have recurred in social attitudes to masturbation; first a threat to health and secondly a form of immorality. As religion gave way to medical science as the main influence on sexual standards in the late 18th and 19th century, these two themes became combined. Tissot's *Onanism*, or *A Treatise upon the Disorder of Masturbation*, written in 1766, used medical authority to declare that masturbation was a serious danger to be avoided. The threat to health appeared to be used to reinforce the traditional moral message. The idea of immorality in non-procreative sex has obvious biological implications for a social group struggling to maintain population size, as was undoubtedly the case during the Middle Ages. But it is impossible to judge the extent to which such basic biological advantages determine such social attitudes in the first place. More apparent has been the moral threat stemming from lack of sexual control. Procreative sex is tolerated because it would be difficult to do otherwise without offending God's plan, but perhaps it is the dignity and civilized status of man that is being primarily protected by such moral strictures, rather than the population size. Bullough (1976) has made the interesting suggestion that the reinforcement of repressive sexual attitudes which occurred in the late 18th century was a reaction not only to the period of

sexual permissiveness that had preceded it, but also the anxieties engendered by the French Revolution: 'the emerging middle classes of the 19th century seized upon sexual purity as a way of distinguishing themselves from the sexual promiscuity of the noble and the lower-classes'. Sex, he suggested, is a manifestation of the beast in man that appeared to surface in the bloodier aspects of the French Revolution. We will return to this theme later when considering changing attitudes to premarital sexuality.

The social significance of this fear of sexual excess and the uncontrolled aspect of human nature underlying it remains an issue of some importance. Now, when the biological advantages of discouraging non-procreative sex have not only disappeared, but also have been put into reverse, the conventional sexual taboos remain resistant to change in most cultures.

Masturbation is often regarded as 'unnatural'. However, it occurs in many subhuman mammals. Ellis (1942) described autoeroticism in horses and stags, and male primates have been observed to induce ejaculation by such means, even in circumstances when coitus would have been possible. Until recently, this was considered to be restricted to male animals, but there is now evidence that some female primates masturbate (Dixson 1998).

The prevalence of masturbation

Cross-cultural evidence of masturbation is limited, partly reflecting varying degrees of reluctance to report or ask about it. But there does seem to be variability. In some primitive societies studied, masturbation is expected and accepted as normal among children, but should not be needed by adults. In others it is unacceptable in children as well as adults, and in yet other societies there is a more accepting view of masturbation even among adults. A useful summary of the limited evidence is provided by Cornog (2003). There is relative consistency across modern societies in the finding that masturbation occurs in most men but a smaller proportion of women. The precise numbers are no doubt affected by varying degrees of reporting bias. There is a general consistency between acceptance of premarital sex and of masturbation in those countries with more 'sex-positive' value systems (e.g. Scandinavian countries, Germany, Australia).

Fortunately, one question about masturbation was asked in the second British NATSAL (2000) survey ($n = 4762$ men; 6399 women; aged 16–44 years) and, based on this, a useful analysis of the associations between masturbation and other psychosocial variables has been reported by Gerressu et al (2008). The one question was, 'When, if ever, was the last occasion you masturbated, that is aroused yourself sexually?' Answers ranged from 'within the last 7 days' to 'never'. Ninety-five per cent of men and 71.2% of women indicated that they had masturbated at some point in their lives; 73% of men and 36.8% of women in the past 4 weeks, a highly significant gender difference. With weighting applied, binary logistic regression was used to assess the relations between 'having masturbated in the past 4 weeks' and other variables, after adjusting for age, marital status, children, social class, education, ethnicity and religiosity, in men and women separately. Recent masturbation was most likely in the 25- to 34-year-age group for men and the 35- to 44-year group for women, less likely in the married, most likely in the previously married and less likely in those with children. It was more likely in social class I/II than lower classes, but this was only significant for men, more likely in the higher educated groups, for both men and women, more likely in whites than other ethnic groups and less likely in those for whom religion was important, though this was only significant for women. A further interesting gender difference was observed: masturbation in the past 4 weeks was associated with frequency of partnered sexual activity, but in the opposite direction for men and women. For men, the more partner activity, the less likelihood they had masturbated; for women the other way round, and this was mainly in those women who did not have difficulty with orgasm.

In the NHSLS (Laumann et al 1994) the frequency of masturbation during the past year was assessed. Direct comparison with the NATSAL findings is not therefore possible. However, 63% of men and 42% of women had masturbated during the past year, 27% of men and 8% of women indicated they did so at least once a week. The associations with age, education and race were similar to those from the NATSAL data. The striking gender difference in the association between masturbation and frequency of partnered activity, found in the NATSAL data, is not apparent here, but the same analyses were not carried out. The NHSLS participants were asked to give their reasons for masturbating; of those who had masturbated in the past year, 73% of men and 63% of women indicated 'to relieve sex tension', 32% of men and women because 'partner was unavailable', and 40% of men and 42% of women 'for physical pleasure'.

In the Sex in Australia survey (Richters et al 2003) 65% of men and 35% of women reported masturbating during the past year, with 48% of the men and 25% of the women having done so in the past 4 weeks, with men reporting an average frequency of 5.8 times and women 3.3 times in the month.

In the re-analysis of the Kinsey data (Gebhard & Johnson 1979), 94% of men and 40% of women had masturbated to orgasm at some time in their lives. This is a somewhat lower proportion for women than had been originally reported (58%), presumably due to the 'cleaning' of the data described above. Neither the NATSAL nor the NHSLS established to what extent those who had masturbated had experienced orgasm. In the original Kinsey report about 4% of women had masturbated without experiencing orgasm, whereas less than 1% of men came into this category.

In a recent Kinsey Institute study (Bancroft et al 2003b) a new sample of male and female college students were compared to an age-matched sample of college students from the original Kinsey study, about 50 years earlier. This showed striking increase in the proportion of women reporting having masturbated in the more recent sample, and differences in the age of onset of masturbation between males and females which were very similar across the two samples. Because of their relevance to sexual development, these findings are discussed in more detail in Chapter 5 (p. 151).

Dekker & Schmidt (2002) report findings about masturbation from three studies of German students carried out in 1966, 1981 and 1996. Whilst the most marked changes in heterosexual behaviour occurred between 1966 and 1981, the changes in masturbation were most marked between 1981 and 1996. These changes included a greater proportion who masturbated, particularly among the women, whether or not they were in a relationship, more frequent masturbation and an earlier age of onset of masturbation. However, they do not report ages younger than 13 years so it is not possible to assess whether there was an increase in pre-pubertal onset. In 1996, 94% of the males and 74% of the females reported masturbating during the previous month. A limited comparison can be made with the NATSAL data (Gerressu et al 2008). Student status was not given in that study, but for those with degrees, controlling for other variables, 82% of men and 50% of women reported masturbating in the past month. Dekker & Schmidt's (2002) findings also suggested signs of a new attitude; that masturbation 'is a form of sexual activity in its own right', and does not serve as a form of compensation for lack of satisfying partner sex. This contrasts with a recent US survey of black and white women in established heterosexual relationships: the frequency of the woman's masturbation during the preceding month was negatively predictive of her satisfaction with her sexual relationship, and this effect was more marked in the white than the black women (Bancroft et al in press). Thus, we see here a possible difference between German and American culture, as well as difference between cultural groups within the USA. This comparison of black and white women will be considered further later in this chapter.

Kontula & Haavio-Mannila (2002) report a comparison of the national studies carried out in Finland in 1971, 1992 and 1999. They analysed prevalence of masturbation by generation rather than simply by age, and found that each new generation has masturbated more than previous generations, showing relatively little change as they increase in age. They concluded that 'the masturbation habits that each generation had internalized in adolescence seemed to remain unchanged through the course of their lives' (p. 49). They found little effect of relationship status or duration of relationship on the prevalence of masturbation. They compared the Finnish data with two 1996 surveys in Sweden, and St Petersburg (previously Leningrad), and a 2000 survey in Estonia, then part of the Soviet Union, between 1944 and 1991. In spite of the close proximity of these four areas, there was a marked difference between the Russian and Estonian data, on the one hand, and the Finnish and Swedish on the other. The Soviet-influenced culture of the first two areas was associated with much more sex negativism, reflected in a lower prevalence of masturbation. The sexual revolution in Russia came much later than in Northern Europe (Kon 1995).

Techniques of masturbation

For the male by far the commonest method is manual stimulation. Other methods are used occasionally by many men and predominantly by a few. These include lying face down, making pelvic thrusts against a bed or pillow, use of a vibrator, holes in objects or water jets (Gebhard & Johnson 1979). For women, the principal method is direct stimulation of the clitoris, sometimes associated with insertion of something into the vagina; 73% of Hite's women came into this category (Hite 1976). Vibrators are now commonly used for this purpose. Other techniques, such as squeezing the thighs together, are used predominantly by a small proportion of women, although only 1–3% rely on inserting objects into their vaginas (Hite 1976; Gebhard & Johnson 1979).

Conclusions

The evidence across studies shows a lessening of stigma associated with masturbation, and an associated increase in the likelihood of young people starting to masturbate, a lessening of the assumption that one should not masturbate when in a relationship, but continuing evidence of the differential effects of social class and other aspects of culture in these respects.

Although it is becoming increasingly apparent that masturbation is compatible with sexual health, and can play a positive role in our sexual development, we should also consider how it might contribute to negative outcomes. Because it is an individual activity, it is not determined or restrained by the dynamics of a relationship. As considered in Chapter 5, one pattern of sexual responsiveness is potentially problematic: the use of sex as a mood regulator. As we shall see in Chapter 11, this pattern is frequently found in those who develop 'out of control' sexual behaviour. Such problematic patterns are not 'caused' by masturbation, but the use of masturbation may serve to reinforce them (see p. 330). Also, the trend among German students, reported by Dekker & Schmidt (2002), towards seeing masturbation as a sexual activity 'in its own right', has been considered by Schmidt (1998) as possibly indicating a 'retreat from intimacy', particularly in males who find modern expectations of intimate sexuality challenging. There is an added factor which may well compound any such trend, the impact of the Internet; this will be considered further later in this chapter. The need for responsibility in our sexual lives, so well articulated by the Surgeon-General who followed Jocelyn Elders, David Satcher (2001), to avoid causing harm to others or ourselves by our sexual behaviour, applies also to masturbation.

The gender difference in masturbation is clearly persisting, and is of considerable interest. Whereas the difference in prevalence of masturbation among men and women has lessened, it has not and may not disappear. The pattern of gender differences postulated in Chapter 4 (p. 131) may be relevant here: the distinction between the 'basic pattern', which is of general relevance to women and does not involve masturbation, and various 'superadded' components, similar to the male basic pattern, and involving a need for clitoral stimulation and orgasm, which vary in importance across women. It is perhaps those women with the superadded component who, once they are freed from socio-cultural constraints, use masturbation as a more efficient method of meeting their superadded sexual needs. The women who show only the basic pattern will have little need for masturbation. Hopefully, such possibilities will become clarified when research looks for evidence of these different types of sexual women.

Sex and the unmarried

Cross-cultural and historical aspects

In their review of sexual behaviour in primitive societies, Ford & Beach (1952) divided their societies into three types:

1. Restrictive societies in which sexuality outside marriage was generally discouraged.
2. Semi-restrictive societies with formal prohibitions but not enforced with any vigour. Sexual behaviour amongst the unmarried was accepted provided it was in secret, but if pregnancy ensued marriage was expected.
3. Permissive societies; in some cases the permissiveness applied to early childhood only, but often continued at least until marriage. Sexual activity between young people was expected, but once again, the occurrence of pregnancy was seen as an indication for marriage.

In a later anthropological analysis of the Human Relations Area File (HRAF), Broude & Greene (1980) examined 141 societies for which adequate information on premarital sexuality was available. They reported attitudes to premarital female sexuality (Table 6.1). Premarital sexual activity was regarded as uncommon for females in 43%, and for males in 31% of societies. According to Whyte (1980) a double standard for premarital sexuality was evident in 44% of cultures.

Societies also vary in their view of adolescence. In some cultures, such as our own, adolescence is a long period involving different expectations and responsibilities from both childhood and full adulthood. In other societies this period may be very short or only recognized as the occurrence of puberty, often marked by some puberty ritual, so that the child passes suddenly into adulthood.

TABLE 6.1 Attitudes to premarital female sexuality (from Broude & Greene 1980)	
Attitude to premarital sex	**Percentage**
Expected and approved; virginity has no value	24
Accepted if discreet	21
Mildly or moderately disapproved; virginity is valued	26
Disallowed except with bridegroom	4
Strongly disapproved; virginity is required (virginity tests, severe reprisals for non-virginity)	26

Schlegel & Barry (1980) reviewed the HRAF data from 183 societies for cross-cultural evidence of adolescent initiation ceremonies. These occurred in a minority of the societies, at ages usually close to puberty, though ranging from 8 to 18 years. In 25% there were ceremonies for both sexes, in 21% only for girls and in 9% only for boys. For both sexes the major themes were fertility–sexuality and responsibility, but responsibility was more important for boys, and for girls fertility–sexuality clearly predominated. Same-sex bonding was a characteristic of 37% of boys' ceremonies, but of only 8% of girls' ceremonies, supporting the widely held assumption that men form same-sex bonds outside the kin circle much more than women do. Genital operations (e.g. circumcision and clitoridectomy) were involved in 32% of boys' and only 8% of girls' ceremonies, although other unpleasant or painful experiences were involved in 32% and 25%, respectively.

Another form of institution for regulating and influencing adolescent sexuality in some pre-industrial societies was the dormitory, where older children and teenagers were segregated as a group from their nuclear families. The form and influence of such dormitories varied considerably however. Hotvedt (1988) contrasted the Sambian model (described by Herdt 1981 and discussed in Chapter 5) with that of the Munda of northeast India (described by Elwin 1968). The Sambian dormitory represented sexual segregation in an extreme form, with homosexual initiation of younger boys by older youths as a method of reinforcing masculinity and male bonding, in a society in which heterosexual relationships were somewhat antagonistic (see p. 266). The Munda, on the other hand, had mixed-sex dormitories; they were similar in the respect that it was the older adolescents who were the sex educators, but in this case the education was in heterosexual behaviour and relationships.

So we find a rich variety of patterns of attitudes and behaviour in relation to premarital sexuality. Hotvedt (1988) reviewed attempts to account for these cultural variations. The important dimensions include the importance of wealth and inheritance, the degree of differentiation of sexual roles, sexual segregation and sexual stratification (i.e. when one gender group has greater access to rewards, prestige and power), and the complexity of social structure. Drawing from cultural materialism, Hotvedt explained how much of this variability can be accounted for by the level of social development. The contrast is between the hunter–gatherer society, now largely extinct (the !Kung of the Kalahari desert remain as one of the few surviving examples, much researched by anthropologists), and the pre-industrial agricultural society (i.e. with mechanized food production), with pastoral and horticultural societies falling in between. The hunter–gatherer society was characterized by nuclear families combining and cooperating as small residential groups. These were classless societies with egalitarian decision making and restrictions on personal wealth and power. Horticultural and pastoral systems introduced the important component of wealth (either land or domestic animals). This dimension became of much greater importance in the agricultural societies, where because of relatively efficient food production by a minority, other productive roles could be developed, resulting in the elaboration of more complex social systems; this process was greatly amplified by the industrial revolution.

Thus the hunter–gatherer society was most likely to be permissive towards premarital sexuality and the class-ridden agricultural society restrictive, as the need to protect lineage and the inheritance of wealth became more relevant.

This analysis combines an overview of relatively recent and existing pre-industrial societies with a historical perspective of human societies in general. It therefore provides us with a bridge to the ever-growing social history of western European society, as well as a relevant model for interpreting some of the changes and variations we see there.

When considering the social history of sexual behaviour and marriage in Europe we have two dimensions to consider: one geographical, the other temporal. We find repeated indications that north (or perhaps more correctly north-western) and south (or south-eastern) Europe have different early sources of influence on this aspect of behaviour, perhaps exemplified by the Viking culture in the north, with its hunter–gatherer origins, and the Christian and Islamic cultures in the Mediterranean south, with predominantly agricultural origins. This divide became compounded by the religious divide after the Reformation, which in itself probably reflected this basic geographical difference.

Temporally, there is a turning point, which by general agreement appears to be the latter part of the 18th century, in the early stages of the Industrial Revolution. Figure 6.1. shows the demographic evidence of a dramatic rise in both prenuptial pregnancy and illegitimacy *and* an associated fall in the age at marriage; this combination led to the extraordinary increase in birth rate, which continued until the 1930s. Both Stone (1979) and Gillis (1985) have documented the associated changes in behaviour in Britain over this period, with Gillis focusing more on the contrasts between the social classes. In pre-industrial Britain there was not only late marriage, but also predominant chastity amongst the unmarried. This was facilitated by the tendency for young people to 'live in' with the families of their rural employers. Early heterosexual experience was dominated by what Gillis called 'polygamous play': the innocent sexuality of the group that protects the young person from premature pairing. Courtship, once started, was highly ritualized, with betrothal the most important event. Sexual license was given once betrothal was established, on the understanding that pregnancy would lead to marriage. This was a time of relatively high prenuptial pregnancy. Courting in rural Britain was of the 'bundling' or night-visiting variety, where it was assumed that the courting couple would spend time together at night, often in the girl's sleeping quarters. But sexual activity would usually be limited, especially in the early stages of courtship. Hertoft (1977) described this courtship pattern as typical of peasant communities in

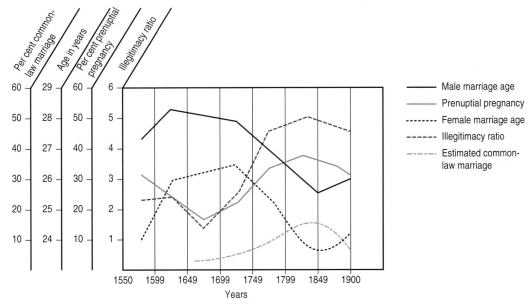

Fig. 6.1 Age of marriage, prenuptial pregnancy, illegitimacy, and common-law marriage in Britain 1550–1900. (Collected by Gillis (1985) from various sources.)

Scandinavia and northern Europe, also spreading to New England colonies in North America. According to his description, girls invited boys of their choice to spend the night with them. A traditional set of rules required them to keep all their clothes on initially, but if the relationship flourished in other ways and familiarity increased, sexual activity would progress until full intercourse occurred. At this stage (though it is not clear whether this was usually before or after first intercourse) the couple would announce their betrothal, often marrying once pregnancy resulted. This custom was still widespread in Nordic countries in the mid-19th century and may still be found occasionally in remote rural areas. Although there may have been variations on this theme, the important element was the graduated process of mate selection, which preceded coitus and pregnancy, and the commitment associated with coitus. There was a single standard of premarital sexuality (i.e. equal for boys and girls), applied within a clear set of rules and linked to betrothal and marriage. Such a society would be regarded as permissive according to Ford & Beach's definition, but clearly very different to our 'permissive' society today.

Then came the sexual revolution between 1750 and 1850, with its dramatic changes apparent in almost every region of Europe and the USA. Shorter (1973) considered various possible explanations for this change, concluding that there had been a dramatic increase in premarital sexual behaviour, a trend in his view predominantly amongst the urban working class. Gillis (1985) attributed a large part of the increase in illegitimacy in Britain to a simultaneous increase in the number of common-law unions, whose offspring would be recorded as illegitimate, rather than to desertion of the pregnant woman. These were times of important changes in attitudes to marriage in Britain, which can be seen as part of the complex evolution of both individual and religious values. Stone (1979) summarized this evolutionary

process as follows. In the 16th century and earlier, the purpose of life was to assure continuity of the family, the class, the village or the state. Personal preference should always be subordinated to the common good. In the 16th and 17th centuries there was an increasing tendency to recognize the uniqueness of the individual, leading to competition, which required control by the power of the stern patriarchal family or the state. In the late 17th and 18th centuries the sense of individual uniqueness and pursuit of personal happiness was tempered by respect for the rights of others. Stone discussed the socio-economic changes associated with this evolution of the human spirit. One crucial aspect was the growth of the wealthy bourgeoisie or middle class, who shared some of the political and social as well as economic power that had previously been in the hands of the landed gentry. It was this emerging class that espoused the new religious attitude, starting with Puritanism, that led to greater emphasis on holy matrimony and hence the importance of personal choice in selecting one's spouse. This resulted in conflict with the continuing importance of patriarchal authority over marriage and a state of relative confusion over attitudes to mate selection, which we will consider in more detail later in the chapter.

Around that time there were other factors encouraging early marriage, particularly amongst the poor. Relief for the poor discriminated against single men and women and employment was easier to obtain for the married or co-habiting couple, seen more or less as two for the price of one. The agricultural workers, who previously had lived in at the employers' household in circumstances favouring celibacy, were now expected to fend for themselves in the community, with various resulting encouragements to sexual activity.

The married couple, whilst benefiting from the work input of younger teenage children, would nevertheless need to encourage them to leave the home once they were of marriageable age. A pregnancy became a means of securing a marriage or parish maintenance. From Gillis's (1985) account we see clearly the separation of sexual values; for the poor working class, who had no property to protect or pass on to their children, for whom fertility was important for several reasons; and for the propertied classes who were still intent on protecting lineage and appropriate inheritance of wealth, and eventually the bourgeoisie who strove to establish a foundation for the family based on the work ethic and Puritan values. Thus we see the origins of the profound influence of social class on sexual behaviour, still very much in evidence when Kinsey carried out his surveys. Furthermore, from the mid-18th century we see the affluent classes attempting to impose their standards on the rest of society with varying degrees of success. Gillis (1985), somewhat contrary to Shorter (1975), saw the vanguard of this changing sexual morality in the countryside rather than the city. In his view the more traditional objectives of marriage, with the couple waiting until they had accumulated enough material possessions and income to provide a secure basis for family life, prevailed for longer in the city where perhaps the opportunities for such self-improvement were greater. Prostitution, on the other hand, flourished in the cities.

By the early Victorian era the cities had changed places with rural areas in terms of early marriage. By then the full impact of the Industrial Revolution and of the new middle class could be seen. Somehow during this period the double standard of sexual morality became established not only across Europe but also across the social classes.

Schmidt (1977) drew an interesting comparison between the views of Shorter, an American, and van Ussell, a Belgian historian of Marxist persuasion. Industrialization, according to van Ussell, resulted in small social groups becoming less self-sufficient and more dependent on each other, an extension of the process described earlier, as societies developed from the hunter–gatherer to the agricultural model. Discipline as a guarantee for complicated social interaction became the value of the emerging bourgeoisie: 'The body was transformed from an organ of pleasure to an organ of achievement'. Body function, including sex, became something to be concealed. Nudity became unacceptable. Expressions of feelings became inhibited, and keeping oneself under control was regarded as a moral virtue. A parallel with these changes was the breakdown of large family groups, with people becoming more private in their habits, particularly when affluent. Premarital sex became forbidden, a taboo that was almost certainly effective amongst bourgeois girls. However, the more people struggled against sexuality, the more the environment became sexualized. The combination of sexual preoccupation and taboo led to dissociation between love and sexuality that previously had been combined so effectively in the 'bundling' scene. Men started to exploit female partners from a lower social class or increasingly through prostitution. The double standard and all the negative consequences of human

sexuality for the role of women had arrived — or at least returned. Schmidt concluded that whereas the bourgeois girl was protected by strict parental control, the working-class girl was, as a result of industrialization and urbanization and the relative collapse of the family as a close community, deprived of the security of the 'bundling' system. At the same time, she fell victim to the uncaring, exploitative sexuality of the dominant double standard male.

This analysis has however assumed that, prior to industrialization and urbanization, the relatively permissive Nordic system was the norm. Schmidt, based in West Germany, is perhaps more familiar with the northern European pattern where the double standard has been less entrenched. Mediterranean societies probably had a repressive system of much longer standing; the tradition of the virgin bride (enforced by strict chaperonage) and the dowry dates back to ancient Chaldean, Jewish and other codes (Kinsey et al 1953) and was still evident in rural Italy in recent times (Littlewood 1978). In such systems, the importance of virginity and the associated dowry places the woman as a form of property, handed over from one man (i.e. the father) to another. Such a double standard, which is also evident in many modern machismo cultures in the Latin American world, is less easily attributable to industrialization and more to the deep-rooted dominance of the male. We are therefore left with an important gap in our understanding of this aspect of European history. Did the virginity ethic spread to northern Europe, at least as far as the propertied classes were concerned, becoming more socially spread as industrialization took its toll? Or have such values always been present when wealth and property are involved, as our earlier anthropological summary had hinted? As far as Britain is concerned we must take into account its peculiarly deep class divisions. And in the USA we are now seeing the results of a mixture of very different cultural backgrounds in which the Nordic, Mediterranean and African American all play a part.

Goody (1971) proposed a Eurasian model that he contrasted with an African model. Eurasia he defined as the area from the Mediterranean region to the Ganges plain. According to the Eurasian model the inheritance of landed property was the principal focus of marriage. Such societies upheld strict codes of sexual morality, restricting sex to within marriage. The African model, Goody suggested, was based on a more egalitarian distribution of landed property. Here the emphasis was on reproduction, and much more relaxed attitudes and mores about sexual behaviour. This can be seen as a contrast between the 'virginity ethic' and the 'fertility' patterns considered earlier. However, Goody has been criticized for underestimating the variability and contrasts amongst African societies, and hence oversimplifying his African model (Njikam Savage & Tchombe 1994).

When we consider modernization in other parts of the world, an even more varied historical background influences the situation. In Africa, where there has been considerable variability across cultures (Njikam Savage & Tchombe 1994), many of the old traditional values prevail but migration and urbanization have led to a weakening of their effects (Sai 1978). Muslim countries typically maintain powerful restrictions on premarital sexuality. To a large extent this has been possible because of early marriage for girls. The disadvantages of such early marriage, both in terms of over-population and reduction in women's status, are considerable. Many countries have combated this by raising the minimum legal age for marriage (Farman-Farmaian 1978) but the taboos on premarital sex remain strong. Sexual norms in Russia since the Revolution changed to a more modern, permissive pattern much later than the rest of Northern Europe (Kon 1995). China has a long history of suppressing explicit sexual expression. Public expression of affection, even holding hands, has been discouraged. Within relationships, affection was expressed verbally or by eye contact, not physical contact (Renaud et al 1997). In the past 20 years, however, there have been substantial changes, and China can be seen in transition as far as sexual life is concerned (Pan 1993) and is considered more closely later in this chapter.

We must therefore avoid any tendency to over-simplify the historical and sociological antecedents of the present situation. But we have no difficulty in recognizing the historical precedents for the association between premarital (and marital) sexuality and social class.

A recent review of survey data from 56 countries around the world, largely based on demographic and health surveys (Measure DHS 2006) provides us with an over-view of premarital sexuality across cultures (Wellings et al 2006). The median ages at first sexual intercourse and at first marriage across these countries are shown in Table 6.2. For age at first sexual intercourse, the six industrialized countries are fairly similar, with little gender difference, averaging 17.5 years for men and 17.8 years for women. For the 29 African countries there is more variability, but with the overall average being older for males, 18.5 years, than for females, 16.7 years. The median age for individual African countries ranged from 15.5 years in 11 countries to 20.5 years in Rwanda. Latin American countries showed a somewhat younger age for males, 16.9 years, than females, 18.6 years, with Asian and transitional countries showing more similar ages for males and females. Age at first marriage is older for males than females in the industrial countries, 27 years for males and 23.6 years for females, and with an average age gap of around 2 years. This difference is greater in the African countries, on average 24.4 years and 18.8 years, respectively, with an even larger age gap averaging 9.2 years, and ranging from 7.2 years in Zambia to 14.7 years in Burkina Faso. Latin America and Asia come midway in these respects, although there is considerable variability in the median age at first marriage for females across the Asian countries, with Bangladesh having a median age of 14 years and the Philippines 22 years.

This cross-cultural overview suggests a global tendency towards earlier onset of sexual activity, and with age at first marriage tending to get older, an increasing likelihood of first sexual intercourse preceding marriage. However, the regional differences indicate a persistence of varied socio-cultural patterns.

TABLE 6.2　Median age at first sexual intercourse, at first marriage, and age gap at marriage in men and women from 54 countries (from Wellings et al 2006)*

Countries	Men		Women		
	Age at first sexual intercourse	Age at first marriage	Age at first sexual intercourse	Age at first marriage	Age gap at marriage
Industrialized countries					
Britain	16.5	24	17.5	22	—
Australia	17.5	29	17.5	24	1.9
USA	17.3	27.9	17.5	24.8	2.2
France	17.5	—	18.5	—	—
Italy	17.5	—	18.5	—	—
Norway	18.5	—	17.5	—	—
Africa					
Central Africa (n = 6)[‡]	18[†] (17.5–18.5)	23.5 (22–25)	15.5	18.2 (15–22)	10.5 (10.3–10.8)
West Africa (n = 10)	19.3 (17.5–20.5)	25.2 (22–29)	16.5 (15.5–17.5)	16.9 (15–19)	11.5 (8–14.7)
East and South Africa (n = 13)	18 (16.5–19.5)	24 (21–29)	17.3 (15.5–20.5)	20.6 (15–26)	7.8 (6.3–9.4)
Lating America and the Caribbean (n = 9)	16.9 (16.5–17.5)	23.8 (23–26)	18.6 (17.5–20.2)	19.75 (18–21)	4.8 (3.2–6.3)
Asia (n = 6)	19.0 (18.5–24.5)	22.75 (20–24)	18.8 (16.5–21.5)	17.7 (14–22)	3.9 (3.2–4.6)
Countries in transition (n = 4)	19.8 (18.5–20.5)	23.7 (23–24)	20.5	20.25 (20–21)	3.5 (2.7–4.3)

*Countries included from *Central Africa*: Central African Republic, Cameroon, Chad, Egypt, Gabon, Morocco; *West Africa*: Benin, Burkina Faso, Cote d'Ivoire, Ghana, Guinea, Mali, Niger, Nigeria, Senegal, Togo; *East and South Africa*: Comoros, Ethiopia, Kenya Madagascar, Malawi, Mozambique, Namibia, Rwanda, South Africa, Tanzania, Uganda, Zambia: *Latin America and the Caribbean*: Bolivia, Brazil, Chile, Colombia, Dominican Republic, Guatemala, Haiti, Nicaragua, Peru; *Asia*: Bangladesh, India, Indonesia, Nepal, Philippines,Vietnam; *Countries in transition*: Armenia, Kazakhstan, Turkey, Uzbekistan
[†]For the groups of countries figures shown are the average of medians for each country, with the range of medians in brackets
[‡]The *n* for each region is the number of countries included. Not all countries had data available for all variables

The reduction in age at first intercourse in Europe and North America during the 20th century

From the above historical background we can identify two themes which have presumably contributed to the present picture, but which have both varied in importance according to the cultural background. We can call these themes (i) the virginity ethic, with its origins in early agricultural societies, and (ii) the role of fertility, originating in earlier hunter–gatherer societies.

The virginity ethic

The importance of virginity of the woman at marriage has been linked to the property rights of men over women, a pattern with a long tradition in Mediterranean countries in particular (Kinsey et al 1953). The socio-biological view is that men prefer chaste women in order to ensure their paternity (Daly & Wilson 1978). Whereas the basic economic implications of the bride price and dowry may have largely disappeared except in ritualistic form, the importance of 'owning' the woman for the self-esteem of many men is still evident. By the same token, 'scoring' with women represents a method of asserting dominance over other men, what Gagnon & Simon (1973) described as 'homosocial' sexuality. Such methods of bolstering the self-esteem of men may have been used less frequently as alternative sources of self-esteem gain in importance. At least until recently, in modern urban societies both the virginity ethic and the 'homosocial' exploitation of women have been somewhat more marked amongst the lower socio-economic groups (Gagnon & Simon 1973). This will be considered further in the later section on social class.

The role of fertility

In the early northern European pattern of premarital sexuality, the so-called 'bundling' system, pregnancy was expected to lead to marriage and in many respects was required in order to demonstrate the young woman's fertility. To what extent does fertility, or the need to demonstrate it, influence modern premarital sexual behaviour?

The first issue to be considered is the relevance of adolescent infertility. Humans and some of the higher primates are typically infertile for a period of time following puberty. According to Hrdy (2000) a young female chimpanzee mates an average of 3600 times before her first conception. Ford & Beach (1952) mentioned several permissive societies where premarital intercourse was usual for periods of 2–3 years, but pregnancy unusual. In the !Kung, hunter–gatherers of the Kalahari desert, Kolata (1974) found that menarche and marriage occurred at the age of 15.2 years, whereas the average age for bearing the first child was 19.2 years. Short (1976) suggested that in humans and other primates who rely on pair-bonding, a period of adolescent sterility may be important for allowing proper sexual learning and mate selection to occur, free from the complications of early pregnancy. Short also commented that

the human female is the only primate in which full breast development occurs at puberty, rather than at the time of first pregnancy. This, he suggested, is to allow sexual attractiveness to develop in advance of fertility. Thus, one way of looking at adolescent sexuality is that it is a biologically important stage of sexual development protected by adolescent sterility. This may then lead to the need to prove fertility after a period of infertile sexual activity. That is the background.

An added factor to consider, however, is the age at menarche, relevant to the age at fertility. In the past 100 years or so, age at menarche has declined steadily in most developed countries, from around 14 years, until the 1970s since when it has levelled at around 12.5 years, but with some manifestations of puberty, such as breast development, starting even earlier (see Chapter 5). This has been associated with a reduction in the age when first fertile, though it is important to remember that there is, and always has been, considerable individual variability in the interval between menarche and fertility. In 1970 it was calculated that 94% of girls were fully fertile by 17.5 years. By contrast, it has been estimated that in 1870 only 13% would have been fully fertile at that age (Bury 1983). Earlier menarche may also mean earlier onset of sexual responsiveness and sexual activity, as we shall see. However, the factors that determine onset of puberty, as discussed in Chapter 5, are not well understood. But there has been a well-documented difference across ethnic groups. In general, young people who come from Mediterranean countries, or countries relatively close to the Equator, tend to have earlier age at puberty than those from more Northern or Southern societies. Within the USA, this is reflected in earlier age at puberty in African Americans than in white Americans of European origin, with Mexican Americans coming between (Witchel & Plant 2004). It is generally assumed that the overall trend towards earlier age at puberty reflects improvement in nutrition, and there is even evidence that females who are too well nourished and overweight have an even earlier age at puberty. The racial differences, however, cannot be explained simply in terms of nourishment, raising the possibility that there are genetic differences that reflect earlier patterns of food acquisition and availability. It is interesting to speculate whether those from Northern Europe, with a hunter–gatherer heritage, have a genetic predisposition which reduces the likelihood of early puberty, whereas those from Mediterranean countries, which predominantly have an agricultural heritage, are genetically predisposed to early puberty, providing food supply is adequate, fitting more readily into the 'virginity ethic' pattern with early marriage and early childbearing. To take this speculation further, is it possible that adolescent infertility had a greater adaptive significance when food supply was less readily available, avoiding the demands of early fertility, not only in terms of infant feeding, but also the reduction of the female's role in food collection as a result of maternity? Have women from agricultural societies evolved with less reliance on adolescent infertility?

Adolescent infertility, or the lack of it, remains a potentially highly relevant issue when striving to understand modern trends in adolescent sexuality and fertility. The concept, however, that today's teenagers are deprived of the advantages of adolescent infertility for their sexual development, is strikingly missing from public debates about adolescent sexuality. The relevance of contraception, as well as sex education, to normal sexual development takes on an added significance when viewed from that perspective.

We should also keep in mind that whereas sexual success may be an important source of self-esteem for the young male, fertility can have comparable importance for the young female, particularly in societies where falling population is a problem and pro-natalism prevails. In most modern Western societies where there is not only a problem with over-population, but also substantial changes in women's roles, there are many more alternative ways for the young girl to gain status and bolster her self-esteem. Nevertheless, for the underprivileged, socially deprived girl of today, confronted with high levels of youth unemployment, fertility and parenthood may be one of the very few forms of achievement open to her. It should therefore not be surprising that such girls get themselves pregnant in spite of the many major long-term disadvantages that often follow. Bury (1983) considered the balance of advantages and disadvantages of motherhood for the British teenager and how this might influence the decision to proceed with a pregnancy once conceived. She doubted that teenagers choose to get pregnant for such reasons. But on the other hand, in a social climate where alternative roles and opportunities are so palpably lacking, awareness of such deficiencies may well influence the level of contraceptive risk taking.

The issue of teenage pregnancy has become something of a political minefield. Right-wing politicians have alleged that provision of welfare to teenage unmarried mothers has encouraged them to get pregnant, leading to political decisions to withdraw such support. The reaction to this has been to state that the cause of teenage motherhood is poverty, not the other way round, as has been widely assumed (Nathanson 1991; Luker 1996; for a lively debate on this issue see Nathanson 2000, followed by discussion pp. 294–304). This reaction is one example of a current version of political correctness, which sees the responsibility for problems to be with society rather than with the individual, and hence disapproves of focus on the individual and how that individual might change. This issue will recur at various points in this book. From my perspective, I have no doubts about the role of poverty in relation to teenage motherhood, and the USA is especially problematic in this respect. However, in addition to the need to reduce poverty, and distribute wealth more equitably, I firmly believe in the need to help individuals look after themselves, and if we are to do that as sexual scientists then we need to understand how and why individuals react to their socio-sexual context in the way that they do.

Let us keep both themes, of virginity and fertility, in mind as we attempt to understand the major changes in premarital sexual behaviour that occurred in the second-half of the 20th century.

It so happens that the last edition of this book was published in 1989 at a pivotal time in the recent history of attitudes to sex in the unmarried, particularly the adolescent and young adult. In the 1960s there was concern about the extent of premarital intercourse, and the associated threat to moral standards and the institution of marriage, resulting in what has been called a 'virginity census' (Clement 1990). In the 1970s there was concern about the alarming rate of teenage pregnancies, particularly within the USA. Both of these phases were seen as a consequence of the sexual revolution in the late 1960s and 1970s, and in both decades, the research emphasis was on the young female. By the late 1980s the new concern about HIV and AIDS had shifted because of a growing awareness that this was a pandemic of relevance to heterosexual men and women, not only homosexual men and intravenous drug users. As mentioned earlier, this fuelled a new and continuing need for more surveys, including attention to the sexuality of teenage boys as well as girls. The evidence relating to teenage sexual behaviour will therefore be reviewed in two sections, pre-1989 and post-1989. More detailed consideration of the developmental aspects of adolescent sexuality is to be found in Chapter 5.

What is striking about this extensive literature is the focus on age at first sexual intercourse. Much less attention has been paid to other aspects of sexual activity in young people, except use of condoms and number of partners, emphasizing the pre-occupation with the negative consequences, rather than any interest in understanding the normal and appropriate developmental process in this age group.

Pre-1989

Evidence from early studies indicated a significant increase in premarital sexuality in the 1920s followed by a period of relative stability until the 1960s (e.g Bell 1966; Reiss 1969). Caplow et al (2001) estimated from various sources that in 1900 6% of white unmarried 19-year-old American women had experienced sexual intercourse, and by 1991 this had risen to 74%. Throughout this time period rates were higher for men than women and for blacks than whites.

Kinsey divided his sample into two halves according to the year of birth, the 'older' and 'younger' generations. In the men, this showed little difference, with the younger generation first having premarital intercourse a year or two earlier (Kinsey et al 1948, p. 396, Table 99). However, among the women born before 1900, less than half as many had had premarital intercourse than among the women born in subsequent decades, although there was not much difference between the 1900–1909 and the 1920–1929 cohorts (Kinsey et al 1953, p. 299, Table 83).

Schofield's (1965) survey of British teenagers in the early 1960s found an incidence comparable to that of the whites in Kinsey's study (Fig. 6.2). Farrell (1978), in a further British survey approximately 10 years later,

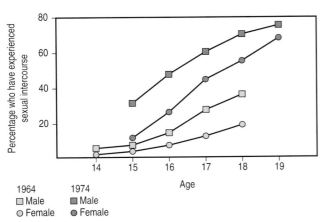

Fig. 6.2 Cumulative incidence of experience of sexual intercourse, by age, amongst UK teenagers for 1964 and 1974. (From Schofield 1965 and Farrell 1978.)

reported a dramatic change (Fig. 6.2), so that by 18 years of age, 69% of boys and 55% of girls had experienced intercourse as compared with 34% and 17% in Schofield's study 18 years earlier. In contrast, the proportion of single 16- to 19-year-old women in Scotland in 1982 who had experienced sexual intercourse was 26%, compared with 42% in England and Wales 7 years earlier (Bone 1986). The explanation for this apparent discrepancy is not clear.

In the USA a series of studies of teenage girls by Zelnick & Kantner (1977, 1980; Zelnick & Shah 1983) and the 1982 National Survey of Family Growth (NSFG) (reviewed by Hofferth 1990) followed trends over the 1970s and early 1980s. A pattern comparable to that in England and Wales, between 1971 and 1976, is shown in Figure 6.3, with the additional demonstration of a striking difference between white and black women in the USA. Figure 6.4 shows the percentage of unmarried

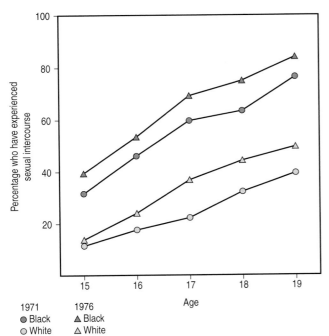

Fig. 6.3 Cumulative incidence of experience of sexual intercourse amongst US unmarried teenage girls by age and colour, for 1971 and 1976. (Zelnick & Kantner 1977.)

females who were sexually active at three different ages in five birth cohorts of white and black women. This showed a substantial increase in the percentage of 17- and 20-year-old sexually active white women during the 1970s. In the black women there had been less change in the 20-year-old group, but increases in the 17-year-olds indicated a comparable though less dramatic shift towards earlier onset of sexual activity.

Earlier surveys repeated at intervals were carried out in American school children (Vener & Stewart 1974) and university students (Bell & Chaskes 1970; Christensen & Gregg 1970) with generally consistent results.

Clement et al (1984) documented comparable increases amongst West German students between 1966 and 1981, with differences between males and females becoming less marked. A comparable trend was reported in Japanese students (Asayama 1976), although the increase was to a low level by European or American standards (14% of males and 7% of females had experienced intercourse by 18 years of age). An important cross-cultural comparison was reported by Jones et al (1985), and will be considered more closely in the section on teenage pregnancies. The comparable figures for premarital sexual experience in six countries are shown in Figure 6.5.

Thus, a universal trend among women towards earlier age at first sexual intercourse has been noticeable since the mid-1960s, accelerating most rapidly during the 1970s and levelling off during the 1980s. Males, who have shown on average younger age at first intercourse than females throughout the 20th century, showed less obvious dramatic increase during the 1960s and 1970s, with a reduction in the gender difference by the late 1980s.

Frequency of premarital sex and number of partners

Schofield (1965) found that although fewer British girls than boys were sexually experienced, those who were had intercourse more frequently but with fewer partners than boys. In other words, the pattern of female teenage sexuality was more linked to stable relationships than it was for boys. In the USA, Bell & Chaskes (1970) found that engagement (i.e. betrothal) was becoming less of a prerequisite for premarital intercourse in their female subjects. But in a later study in the USA half of women were going steady with or engaged to their first sexual partner, compared with only two-fifths of white men and one-fifth of black men. Although there was an apparent shift from premarital monogamy to serial premarital monogamy, there was no evidence of any major increase in the number of casual sexual relationship amongst teenage girls.

Zelnick & Shah (1983), comparing data from 1971, 1976 and 1979, found that the frequency of intercourse was generally low amongst teenagers, and in spite of earlier onset, lower for black than white girls. Furthermore, there was little evidence of increased frequency during the period under study. Frequency of sexual activity during the previous 3 months was assessed in the 1982 NSFG, as shown in Table 6.3 (Hofferth 1990).

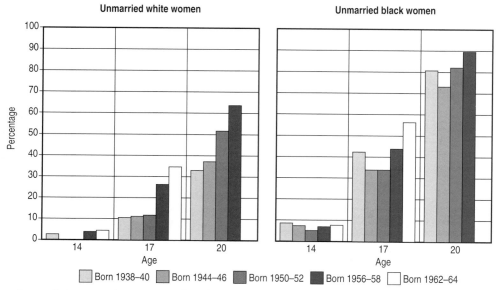

Fig. 6.4 Percentage of unmarried women who were sexually active at ages 14, 17 and 20 years for five cohorts born in 1938–1940, 1944–1946, 1950–1952, 1956–1958 and 1962–1964. (From Hofferth 1990.)

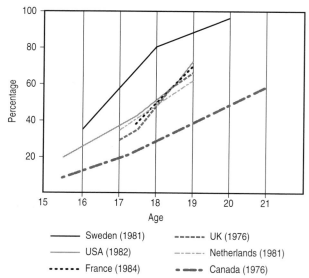

Fig. 6.5 Percentage of women who ever had intercourse, by age, for six countries. The year of the most recent information available for each country is given in brackets. (From Jones et al 1985, reprinted with permission from Family Planning Perspectives, The Alan Guttmacher Institute.)

TABLE 6.3	Frequency of sexual activity in the previous 3 months in unmarried white and black women (from the 1982 National Survey of Family Growth; Hofferth 1990)			
	White		**Black**	
	Age 15–19	Age 20–24	Age 15–19	Age 20–24
No sexual intercourse in past 3 months	20.7	27.8	9.5	15.0
Once a month	12.4	14.5	30.8	12.6
Two to three times a month	24.1	20.5	27.2	29.8
Once a week	21.6	17.0	17.4	21.3
More than twice a week	17.6	19.3	12.3	18.8
Daily	3.6	0.9	2.7	2.5

Clement et al (1984) found a modest increase in frequency in their German students. The mean monthly frequency for males was 6.6 in 1966 and 9.4 in 1981; for females it was 2.4 and 3.5, respectively.

As far as number of partners is concerned, Zelnick & Shah (1983) found that of 15- to 19-year-old sexually experienced women in 1979, half of the white and two-fifths of the black women had only had one partner, whilst 9% of the white and 5% of the black women had had six or more partners. This represented a fall in the number with only one partner, an increase in the number with two or three partners, and no real change in the proportion with many partners.

The West German students reported more partners. In 1981, 42% of both men and women had had more than six partners, compared with 27% for men and 14% for women in 1966. There was also an increased tendency to engage at least occasionally in sexual relations outside the steady relationship — with women in 1981 showing as much if not more infidelity than men — a further example of the disappearing sex differences in the sexuality of West German students. Clement et al (1984) interpreted this trend as a reduction in the double standard and in the importance of virginity in West Germany.

Post-1989

Santelli et al (2000a) reported trends from three nationally representative samples of teenagers collected in the late 1980s and 1990s. These were the NSFG for 1988 and 1995, which as indicated earlier, only assessed females, the National Survey of Adolescent Males (NSAM) for 1988 and 1995, and the Youth Risk Behavior Survey (YRBS) for 1991, 1993, 1995 and 1997, assessing both females and males. The principle objectives were assessment of fertility in females (NSFG), sexual and reproductive behaviour in males (NSAM) and health risk behaviours (YRBS). The NSAM has not been repeated since 1995. The NSFG included males for the first time in their 2002 survey.

Santelli et al (2000a) extracted the data from these various surveys for 15- to 17-year-olds who had experienced sexual intercourse. These are shown for the YRBS in Table 6.4, for NSAM in Table 6.5 and for NSFG in Table 6.6. Santelli et al comment on the substantial differences across these three surveys over time, most likely reflecting differences in samples and data collection methods used. Hence they stressed the need for methodological caution when comparing different surveys. All three surveys covered 1995. Of the three surveys, YRBS reported the highest rates for both males and females in that year. However, none of the surveys indicated an increase during the time period covered. The data for females are relatively stable, only the black teenagers in the YRBS showing a significant change, which was a decrease. For males, there was more consistent evidence of decline. YRBS data for 2005 have been reported (Eaton et al 2006), and rates for 2005 are added to Table 6.5. However, comparisons with the earlier years are of limited value because these rates are for high school attenders, Grades 9–12, and are not restricted to 15- to 17-year-olds.

Data from the 2002 NSFG has been reported by Mosher et al (2005). The graph of the percentage of females who have experienced sexual intercourse by age shows a substantial jump between 17 and 18 years, with a more gradual rise thereafter, consistent with a median age of first intercourse around 17.5 years (Fig. 6.6).

Joyner & Laumann (2001) explored possible predictors or determinants of onset of sexual intercourse before age 18 in the NHSLS (Laumann et al 1994). In this sample, 50% of white and 77% of black men, 42% of white and 61% of black women reported onset before 18. They compared subjects who had reached adolescence before and after the sexual revolution (those born between 1933 and 1952 versus those born 1953–74). In the pre-revolution group, 47% of males and 31% of females had first sexual intercourse before 18; for the post-revolution group, it was 60% of males and 53% of females, a 28% increase for males and a 71% increase for females, demonstrating the partial closure of this gender gap. For males, the younger the age at puberty, the greater the odds of a pre-18 onset (see Chapter 5 for further discussion). Being Catholic reduced the odds among the pre-revolution group, but had the opposite (though non-significant) effect for the post-revolution group. For females, earlier puberty was also associated with increased odds of pre-18 onset, as was sexual contact during childhood (see Chapter 16). Joyner & Laumann (2001) had predicted that adolescent behaviour was now less influenced by membership in social groups and more influenced by personal biography. They found partial support for this; they found less influence of gender, social class and religion in the post-revolution group. They failed to find increased effect of their measures of personal biography, but these were limited; both age at puberty and sexual contact before puberty remained relatively constant in their effects. What they were unable to assess was the impact of the youth culture which, with the emergence of the media and information technology, was a powerful new factor evolving during the 1960s and 1970s, and has remained influential across traditional cultures ever since (see Chapter 5).

Wellings et al (2001) reported on early onset of sexual intercourse in the UK, using data from the NATSAL 2000 (4762 men and 6399 women aged 16–44 years). In order to explore a possible cohort effect, they compared the proportions of those with first sexual intercourse before the age of 16 across 5-year age groups between 16 and 44. This showed no significant difference across

TABLE 6.4	Youth Risk Behavior Survey. Percentage of high school adolescents who had experienced sexual intercourse (i) aged 15–17 1991–1997 (Santelli et al 2000) and (ii) grades 9–12, 2005 (Eaton et al 2006)				
	1991	1993	1995	1997	2005
FEMALE					
Total	50.6	50.7	52.1	48.4	45.7
White	47.3	48.1	48.9	44.7	43.7
Black*	75.1	68.8	66.8	67.2	61.2
Hispanic	44.5	50.0	55.0	48.1	44.4
MALE					
Total[†]	55.5	54.5	52.9	46.8	47.9
White[†]	50.1	47.8	47.5	41.0	42.2
Black[†]	87.3	89.5	80.8	78.9	74.6
Hispanic*	66.1	63.8	62.6	56.8	57.6

Significant trend over time:
*p < 0.05
[†]p < 0.001

TABLE 6.5	National Survey of Adolescent Males. Percentage of male high school adolescents aged 15–17 who had experienced sexual intercourse (Santelli et al 2000)	
	1988	1995
Total*	49.5	41.3
White[†]	44.3	32.8
Black	77.8	76.8
Hispanic	53.5	47.4

Significant trend over time:
*p < 0.05
[†]p < 0.01

TABLE 6.6	National Survey of Family Growth. Percentage of female high school adolescents aged 15–17 who had experienced sexual intercourse (Santelli et al 2000)	
	1988	1995
Total	34.3	36.5
White	32.2	34.3
Black	49.1	45.4
Hispanic	—	47.8

No trends significant over time

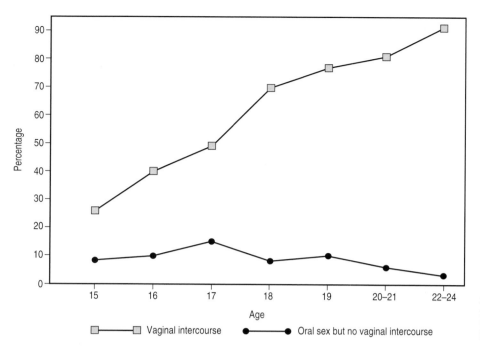

Fig. 6.6 National Survey of Family Growth 2002 Percentage of females aged 15–24 years who had experienced vaginal intercourse or oral sex but no vaginal intercourse. (Mosher et al 2005.)

age groups among the men, and 29.9% of the 16–19 age group were in this early onset category. For the women there was a significant difference, with 25.6% in the 16–19 age group, peaking in the 20–24 group, at 28.4%, and falling to 13.8% in the 40–44 age group. The authors concluded tentatively that the trend towards earlier onset of sexual activity in females had continued somewhat longer in the UK than in the USA but had probably now levelled out.

Although there was convergence of the gender difference in age at first sexual intercourse, gender differences remained in how the first occasion was experienced. Women were twice as likely as men to regret the first occasion, and three times more likely to say that they were the less willing partner. Of the other variables examined, level of education was strikingly relevant. Compared with those who left school after 17, the odds ratio (OR) for likelihood of early onset was 3.0 for those leaving school at 16 with qualifications, and 4.5 for those leaving at 16 without qualifications. The main source of information about sex also proved to be relevant. Compared with those whose main source was from lessons at school, the OR for early onset, for those learning mainly from friends, was 3.1, with those learning mainly from parents coming midway. After controlling for other variables, onset of sexual intercourse before 16 was not associated with increased likelihood of sexually transmitted infection.

Wellings et al (2001) concluded that whereas there had been an increase in early onset of sexual intercourse, it had been accompanied by an encouraging increase in use of risk reduction (i.e. condoms; see below), and with signs that sex education in schools was having a positive effect.

Number of partners

The proportions of 15- to 17-year-olds in the YRBS (from 1991 to 1997) reporting four or more sexual partners in

their lifetime are shown in Table 6.7. This shows no significant change for females, but a modest decrease in the males, significant for the combined groups and for the white males. Similar patterns were reported by NSFG and NSAM. Comparing the 2001 YRBS with 1991, the percentage of school children who had had sexual intercourse with more than four partners decreased significantly: 18.7% in 1991 and 14.2% in 2001 (Grunbaum et al 2002). Laumann et al (1994) found in the NHSLS that both men and women who reached the age of 20 during or after the sexual revolution reported more sexual partners by that age than those born earlier, though there was no evidence of a sustained increase after that shift. The numbers of lifetime sexual partners in those aged 16–24 years in 1990 and 2000 from the NATSAL surveys (Johnson et al 1994, 2001) are shown in Table 6.8. This shows a slight increase in number of partners over this 10-year period, more striking in the women and almost removing the earlier gender difference.

TABLE 6.7	Youth Risk Behavior Survey. Percentage of sexually experienced high school adolescents aged 15–17 who reported having had four or more sexual partners in their lifetime (Santelli et al 2000)			
	1991	**1993**	**1995**	**1997**
FEMALE				
Total	26.1	29.3	25.1	29.7
White	25.3	26.9	22.9	27.3
Black	32.5	38.6	32.1	38.2
Hispanic	20.2	23.3	19.4	21.2
MALE				
Total*	39.2	39.1	38.4	35.1
White*	30.1	28.9	29.1	24.2
Black	69.4	67.3	66.0	64.1
Hispanic	36.1	39.5	39.4	33.0

Significant trend over time:
*p < 0.05

TABLE 6.8 Number of lifetime partners for 16–24 year old men and women in the NATSAL 1990 (Johnson et al 1994) and NATSAL 2000 (Johnson et al 2001)

	None	1	2	3-4	5-9	10+
NATSAL 1990						
Men (%)	20.4	16.3	9.8	19.4	17.9	16.2
Median 3						
Women (%)	20.7	27.0	14.7	18.8	14.1	8.5
Median 2						
NATSAL 2000						
Men (%)	19.6	14.9	8.2	16.6	21.0	19.7
Median 3						
Women (%)	17.7	18.1	11.1	17.1	21.5	14.6
Median 3						

Frequency of sexual intercourse among unmarried teenagers is more difficult to assess from these recent national surveys.

Non-coital sexual activity

Prior to 1989, most teenagers engaged in 'necking' (i.e. kissing and caressing of breasts and above) and 'petting' (i.e. including genital caressing with or without orgasm) before they first experienced intercourse. In Kinsey's sample 46% of the women first experienced orgasm in a heterosexual relationship whilst petting (Kinsey et al 1953). This may well be still the case. However, more recent surveys have largely ignored non-coital sexual activity, apart from oral (and anal) sex because of their relevance to HIV transmission.

The changing trends amongst the unmarried in oral sex (i.e. fellatio (oral stimulation of the penis) and cunnilingus (oral stimulation of the vulva)) are of some interest, however. In the Kinsey surveys oral sex was more or less confined to males and females who were already coitally active — and the more coitally active, the more likely they were to engage in oral sex. In 1967, some 20 years later, Gagnon & Simon (1987) found a doubling in the proportion of coitally active unmarried males and females who had experienced oral sex (from 45% to 80% for females), but still it remained a behaviour that occurred after regular coitus had been established. By 1982, in a survey of schoolchildren (Newcomer & Udry 1985), there was an appreciable minority of boys (25%) and girls (15%) without experience of sexual intercourse who had given or received oral–genital stimulation, though in this study cunnilingus was more frequently reported than fellatio. Thus, not only was oral sex becoming more accepted as a form of premarital sexual interaction, but it was also beginning to occur as a precursor of coital sex (see Chapter 5). Mosher et al (2005), from the NSFG for 2002, reported on the percentage of each age group who had experienced oral sex but not sexual intercourse. This is shown in Figure 6.6, and indicates that substantially less come into this category than the sexual intercourse category, the highest being 15% among 17-year-olds. These data do not clearly indicate,

however, how many teenagers experience oral sex before sexual intercourse, as the time interval between starting oral sex and starting intercourse might be quite short. Nevertheless, these figures do not indicate that a substantial proportion of teenagers are using oral sex as an alternative to vaginal intercourse.

Overall, we saw evidence of substantial reduction in age of first intercourse in the pre-1989 data, and a levelling off, with a slight trend in the opposite direction among males, in the teenage data since 1989. The impact of the sexual revolution appears to have passed its peak, at least in the Western world.

Teenage pregnancies

In Britain, following 1938, when statistics of the age of mothers at birth started to be recorded, the birth rate amongst teenagers rose, reaching a peak in the early 1970s and then showing an unsteady decline since. Trends in abortion were substantially altered by the legal availability of the procedure, and meaningful statistics have only been available since 1968, when the Abortion Act was implemented.

The incidence of teenage pregnancies is impossible to establish precisely because of the unknown number of spontaneous abortions, which are probably more frequent in this age group. However, a combination of births and abortions gives us a fairly close estimate.

When Dryfoos (1978) compared the birth and abortion rates in 1966 and 1975 for unmarried teenagers in the USA, he found a decrease in births in the 18- to 19-year-age group, but an increase in the 15- to 17-year group. Abortion rates increased and by 1975 nearly one in three pregnant adolescents elected to have their pregnancy terminated. This prompted the AGI in the USA to carry out a cross-cultural study of teenage pregnancy (Jones et al 1985). A number of socio-economic indices and their relationship to adolescent fertility were explored in 37 developed countries. Teenage childbearing was positively associated with a measure of low socio-economic status (i.e. the proportion of the workforce employed in agriculture) and with the level of maternity benefit. In addition, birth rates were lower in countries with more liberal attitudes to sex, and with more equitable distribution of income.

This contrast was studied further in a more detailed comparison of six countries, all highly developed socio-economically: the USA, Canada, England and Wales, France, Sweden and The Netherlands. Teenage pregnancy rates (births plus abortions), by age, for the six countries in 1981 are shown in Figure 6.7; the US rates were dramatically higher, especially for the younger teenagers, while The Netherlands showed noticeably lower rates for all ages. Sweden had higher teenage abortion rates than the other countries, with the notable exception of the USA, where the teenage abortion rate alone was as high or higher than the overall teenage pregnancy rate in any of the other countries.

In 2001, Darroch and colleagues from the AGI published a further report in which they compared changes in teenage birthrate from 1970 to 2000 in five developed

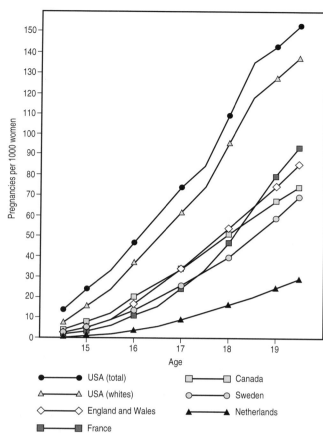

Fig. 6.7 Teenage pregnancies in seven countries in 1981. (From Jones et al 1985, reprinted with permission from Family Planning Perspectives, The Alan Guttmacher Institute.)

In the British NATSAL 2000, motherhood before the age of 18 years was reported by 4.9% of women and this did not vary significantly across the age groups interviewed (Wellings et al 2001). There were two predictors of early motherhood, first intercourse before the age of 16 years, not surprisingly, and educational level. Compared with those who left school at 17 or later, those who left at 16 (i) with qualifications and (ii) without qualifications had adjusted ORs of 12.2 and 41.5, respectively. However, this strong finding must be to some extent confounded by the impact of early pregnancy on education. More recent figures from the UK show rates of abortion for under 18s to be 18.2 per thousand in 2003 and 17.8 in 2004 (Department of Health 2005).

The US teen abortion rate, after rising in the 1970s and remaining fairly constant through the 1980s, then started to decline. In 1997, there were 28 abortions per 1000 15- to 19-year-old women, 33% less than 10 years earlier (Boonstra 2002). A comparison of the rates of unintended pregnancy, abortion and unintended birth in young women in the USA for 1994 and 2001 is shown in Table 6.9 (Finer & Henshaw 2006), indicating slight reduction in all three variables, most marked in the 15- to 17-year group.

Contraceptive and condom use

In 1999, the AGI examined the teenage pregnancy rates for 1988 and 1995, using data from the NSFG. They concluded that 25% of the decline in pregnancy rates over that 7-year period was attributable to increased abstinence, and the remainder to changes in teenager's sexual behaviour. There had been only slight increase in overall contraceptive use, but a more relevant increase in more effective methods, such as long acting hormonal contraceptives, e.g. Depo-Provera and Norplant, which became available in the early 1990s (Boonstra 2002).

The YRBS showed a non-significant reduction in the percentage of sexually active 15- to 17-year-old girls using oral contraceptives (23.6% in 1991; 17.6% in 1997). This was counterbalanced by a substantial increase in the proportion who used condoms (39.7% in 1991; 51.9% in 1997; $p < 0.001$). In the males a similar pattern was found: reliance on oral contraception declined slightly from 13.9% in 1991 to 11.3% in 1997 (not significant), whereas condom use increased from 57.4% in 1991 to 63.8% in

countries: the USA, England and Wales, Canada, France and Sweden. Figure 6.8 shows that the decline has been less in the USA than the other four countries. The adolescent pregnancy rate for the USA, based on a combination of births and abortions, was still nearly twice that in Canada and Great Britain, and approximately four times that in Sweden and France (Boonstra 2002).

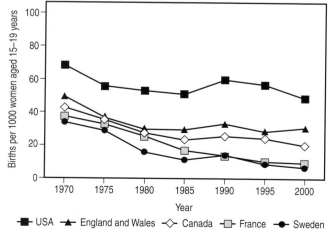

Fig. 6.8 Teenage birthrates in the USA and four other countries between 1970 and 2000. Data are for 1997 in Canada, 1998 in France and 1999 in England, Wales and Sweden. (Darroch et al 2001; with permission of the Alan Guttmacher Institute.)

TABLE 6.9	Unintended pregnancy, abortion and birth rates in young women in the USA for 1994 and 2001 (Finer & Henshaw 2006)					
	Unintended pregnancy rate		Abortion rate		Unintended birth rate	
	1994	2001	1994	2001	1994	2001
<15	4	3	2	1	1	1
15–17	61	40	24	14	27	21
18–19	115	108	48	37	54	53
20–24	105	104	52	45	43	46
All women	51	51	24	21	20	22

1997 ($p < 0.05$) (Santelli et al 2000a). This trend in condom use had levelled off by 2001 (Grunbaum et al 2002).

In the UK, the NATSAL 2000 showed a striking increase in use of condoms on the first occasion of sexual intercourse in the younger age groups; 82.5% of men and 80% of women who were 16–19 years when interviewed compared to 30% and 37%, respectively, in those 40–44 years when interviewed. Of the women, around 26% had started on oral contraception before first sexual intercourse, and this did not vary much across the age groups (22.5–29.5%). Men who had discussed sex with their parents were significantly more likely to use a condom on the first occasion. This was not apparent in women. Educational level, however, had a strong effect on contraceptive use. Compared with those who left school after the age of 17, the OR for non-use of contraception on the first occasion for those who left at 16 without qualifications, was 3.94 for men and 5.22 for women (Wellings et al 2001).

Comparison of the USA with other countries with lower teenage pregnancy rates has shown little difference in age of onset or frequency of sexual activity. The higher pregnancy and birth rates in the USA have presumably resulted from less use of contraception, and less choice of abortion by American teenagers. This reflects a generally more negative attitude to the provision of contraception for teenagers in the USA, which continues to differ from European countries both in terms of more restrictions on sex education and of contraception being less accessible, particularly at low cost. The cross-cultural evidence certainly undermines the view that the provision of contraception or access to abortion increases the likelihood of teenage sexual behaviour. The changes over time show that the important increase in teenage sexuality preceded the availability of contraception (in particular oral contraception). Initially, this trend in behaviour resulted in an increase in teenage pregnancies. Once teenagers started to use contraception, teenage pregnancies and abortions started to decline (Bury 1983).

The influence of the family

Social historians have described vividly how changes in the family have influenced premarital sexual behaviour over the last few centuries (Shorter 1975; Stone 1979; Gillis 1985). To what extent have changes in the family contributed to the more recent changes in teenage sexuality in the second half of the 20th century? According to Shorter (1975), 'In the 1960s and 1970s the entire structure of the family began to shift'. Certainly increasing numbers of families were being affected by marital breakdown. But our knowledge of the impact of the family on teenage sexuality remains limited and fragmentary. The most straightforward evidence relates the effects of the number and consistency of parents in the home to the age of onset of female sexual activity. Kantner & Zelnick (1972) found that the lowest incidence of premarital sexuality occurred in girls living in families headed by their natural fathers. Whereas 70% of the white teenagers came into this category, only 41% of the black girls did so. However, whereas the incidence of sexual activity was 60% higher if a white girl's family was headed by her mother rather than her father, the effect was less marked with the black girls (i.e. 15% higher). It is therefore difficult to know to what extent this factor could account for the ethnic differences. Wyatt (1990) found that the presence of both biological parents and a more consistent pattern of parenting (i.e. without change of parental figures) were associated with later onset of sexual activity in both black and white Californian women.

Schofield (1965) found that sexual experience was more likely in teenagers subjected to less parental discipline. Single parents offered more information about sex whilst tending to be more permissive (Fox 1981). Teenagers whose parents were more open about sex were more likely to use contraception (Bury 1983). Fox & Inazu (1980) assessed a large group of mothers and daughters and found that daughters who discussed birth control with their mothers had more knowledgeable and responsible attitudes and were more likely to use contraception.

More recent evidence is largely consistent with these earlier findings. Santelli et al (2000b), looking at 14- to 17-year-olds in the 1992 YRBS, found that having neither parent or only a single parent were predictive of early onset of sexual intercourse ($p < 0.05$ neither parent; $p < 0.01$ mother only; $p < 0.05$ father only). For the males, low parental educational attainment was strongly predictive ($p < 0.001$ for less than high school, and $p < 0.01$ for 'some college'). Family income was not predictive for either males or females. Joyner & Laumann (2001), in exploring predictors or determinants of onset of sexual intercourse before the age of 18 years in the NHSLS (Laumann et al 1994), found that living with a single parent increased the odds; living with a step-parent increased the odds even more. Joyner & Laumann suggested that this may reflect greater instability associated with two family transitions rather than one. If neither parent had completed high school the odds were increased by 75%. Having parents with college education reduced the odds, but this effect was stronger in those who reached adolescence before the sexual revolution. In the British NATSAL 2000 (Wellings et al 2001), onset of sexual activity before the age of 16 was significantly less likely in those living with both parents compared with those with only one or neither parent.

However, precisely what accounts for the link between parental presence and sexual development is another matter. Some of the evidence points to specific guidance by the parent (e.g. Fox & Inazu 1980), and this limited evidence is discussed in Chapter 5. But an alternative possibility is that parents who are more likely to have short duration marriages started their own sexual lives earlier, and passed this on, to some extent in genetic terms, to their offspring. Hrdy (2000) makes a reasoned case for not being simplistic about genetic explanations, but we nevertheless need to take into account the sexual histories of the parents in explaining those of their children. As yet that has not been addressed.

Marriage and co-habitation

Human beings are unusual amongst mammals in maintaining an alliance between a sexual pair that persists through gestation and lactation. Although the form of this alliance varies enormously, it is in the general sense a 'universal' amongst human societies, which institutionalize it as marriage. In Murdock's (1967) survey of more than 800 human societies, 83% were polygamous, 16% monogamous and 0.5% polyandrous. In most polygamous societies, however, the majority of men are monogamously married because they cannot afford more than one wife. In Whyte's (1980) analysis of 93 societies, 57 were polygamous but in 35 (38%), polygamous unions formed less than 20% of all marriages. The relative status of women in these societies varied considerably. For example, women in one society may have had important property rights whilst being excluded from key religious posts; they may have had important roles in political life whilst suffering from a severe sexual double standard. However, there is little doubt that for more or less all the variables Whyte examined, if there was a preference for one sex in terms of power, privilege or opportunity it would be in favour of men. In 70% of societies there was an explicit view that men should dominate their wives, although in only 29% was there a clearly stated belief that women were generally inferior to men.

The relative weakness of the position of women is to some extent amplified by the age difference between husband and wife. In only 13% of societies were women likely to be of the same age or older than their husbands, whereas in 44% the men were usually more than 4 years older than their wives (Whyte 1980). The marriage of girls soon after puberty, or even before, maximizes their reproductive potential whilst at the same time reducing, if not eliminating, their opportunities for alternative forms of status. Age at marriage and the age gap between husband and wife still varies considerably across societies, as shown in the recent survey (see Table 6.2; Wellings et al 2006); possibly the most striking example is Bangladesh, where currently the median age for women when first married is 14.

The emphasis on monogamy in the Western world has been strongly reinforced by the Christian church. Until relatively recently, divorce and remarriage was difficult, if not impossible. The major increase in both during the 20th century indicates that when the social constraints are lessened, lifelong monogamy gives way to serial monogamy in an increasing number of people. This raises the difference between arranged marriages and freedom of choice of one's spouse. Here cultural differences are fundamental. We are familiar with arranged marriages in Asian and Jewish communities; the pattern in rural Ireland, reflecting the economic constraints on marriage, is probably less well known (Mullan 1984). Arranged marriages are also common in some African countries and other parts of the world. There is a gradual tendency in most such countries towards free choice. In 1950, the People's Republic of China (PRC) legislated against the previous tradition of arranged marriages. The general tendency has been for parental control to remain strongest where parental affluence and hence the importance of inheritance is greater, or where ethnic communities are alienated within a culture and therefore need to intermarry to maintain their ethnic identity, as in the Jewish example. According to Rosenblatt & Anderson (1981), movement towards freedom of choice is not without difficulties. In comparison with the rate of marital breakdown in societies where such free choice is well established, the arranged marriage has quite a good record.

Sexual attraction, falling in love and mate selection

What are the characteristics of a sexually attractive person? Which factors lead from sexual attraction to the establishment of a sexual relationship and possibly marriage? And what part does falling in love play in this process?

Sexual attraction

This involves visual signals of how a person looks and how he or she behaves. Smell may also be important, at least for some people; this factor could operate without their knowledge, and is not well understood (Graham et al 2000). Once two people begin to interact, personality factors will also operate. It is nevertheless difficult to go much beyond this rather obvious statement in our attempts to explain what is often referred to as the 'chemistry' of sexual attraction.

Most research and writing on the characteristics of a sexually attractive person comes from socio-biologists and evolutionary psychologists. The conventional evolutionary perspective was well described by Symons (1995). In this view, selection favoured men who perceived cues of 'nubility' and of good health and 'design' as sexually attractive. A 'nubile' female, according to Symons, is one who is just beginning to ovulate and has not yet become pregnant (the dictionary definition of 'nubile' is 'marriageable'!). Good 'design' overlaps with good health and includes bilateral symmetry and lack of fluctuating asymmetry, which biologists attribute to low pathogen resistance, among other things (Symons 1995). Age, it is postulated, has a negative impact on these cues for various reasons. Considering the widely held view among evolutionary psychologists that males have evolved to mate with as many females as possible to increase their likelihood of offspring and continuation of their genes, Symons recognized a snag in the emphasis on nubility. He pointed out that, particularly in the period of early human history when these adaptations are assumed to have occurred, the environment of evolutionary adaptedness (EEA), there would have been quite a time between a woman appearing nubile and her being likely to conceive (see the discussion of adolescent infertility on p. 191). So he concluded that this adaptation was more to do with detecting a good wife than being attracted to a short-term mate.

The best documented cues of nubility, in Symons' terms, are low waist-to-hip ratio (WHR) and lighter than average skin colour. A low WHR indicates substantial oestrogenic effects, as manifested in increased fat deposits on the hips, and also less directly is an indicator of good health. The lighter skin colour is a characteristic of a reproductive phase female who has not yet conceived.

Facial attraction in women has been studied quite extensively, starting with Galton (1883) who produced an 'average' face by photographically combining the face of a number of individuals, eliminating the irregularities and peculiarities in the process. He was surprised to find that the average or composite face was more attractive than any of the individual faces that contributed to it. This finding has been replicated in many studies, with some non-composite faces being rated as equally or more attractive to a limited extent. Symons (1995) saw the average or composite face as an 'attractiveness default position'. Buss (1989) studied men and women in 37 cultures. Assessment of visual images, however, was not used. Subjects were asked to rate the importance of various characteristics in choosing a husband or wife. Men across cultures attached more importance to a wife being physically attractive and younger than the male. Women were universal in wanting a man who was older and with good financial prospects! A range of explanations could be presented to account for these findings.

The last decade has seen an increase in related research not based on evolutionary biology assumptions. In particular, Tovee et al (1999) found that body mass index (BMI, which is a ratio of height to weight) was a much stronger predictor of a woman's body shape being regarded as sexually attractive than her WHR, a finding that has now been replicated extensively. Although, BMI is relevant to a woman's reproductive potential, it is less predictive than WHR. In their review of the literature, Weeden & Sabini (2005) concluded that, whereas WHR and BMI are predictive of both attractiveness and health, symmetry and other sex-typical hormonal markers were not.

Sexual attractiveness of the male has been less studied and less clearly described. Dixson et al (2003) asked women from Britain and Sri Lanka to rate different body profiles of men for sexual attractiveness. They compared four somatotypes: endomorph (heavily built, typically overweight profile), mesomorph (muscular body with broader shoulders than hips), ectomorph (generally thin profile) and an average of the first three. Women from both cultures found the mesomorph profile the most attractive, followed by the average, then ectomorph, with endomorph least attractive. Attractiveness was enhanced by evidence of body hair. Similar findings were reported by Dixson et al (2007) from the African community of Bakossiland, a region of Cameroon, although the preference for body hair was less evident. However, in their review, Weeden & Sabini (2005) concluded that there were no indicators of male attractiveness that related positively to male health (e.g. the mesomorph male has less positive health prospects than the ectomorph).

Cultural differences in what is regarded as sexually attractive are of obvious interest. The available cross-cultural evidence, which is limited, suggests that facial attractiveness is broadly similar across cultures, with some exceptions (e.g. size of cheek bones or lips; Symons 1995). Attractiveness in terms of body shape and size may be a different matter. Ford & Beach (1952), in their overview of a large number of preliterate societies, reported that for the majority of societies with relevant evidence, a plump woman was more attractive than a slim one. There were relatively few of the societies where slim women were considered more attractive. The sexual attractiveness of African American women is less dependent on low weight than it is for white American women. This is considered more closely on p. 216 and points to a need for better understanding of cultural influences in this respect. Interestingly, Tovee et al (2006) have shown that whereas Zulu men and women living in South Africa rate heavier women more attractive than do white Caucasians in Britain, Zulus who had emigrated recently to Britain, and those with Zulu origins who had grown up in Britain, did not differ from the white Caucasians in this respect. In other words, these apparent cultural differences can be modified by a change in the cultural context. African Americans can be seen differently in this respect, as they have a long heritage of institutionalized segregation in the USA, not exactly the conditions for acculturation. Nevertheless, the impact of acculturation indicates that these cultural differences are not constitutionally determined.

Ford & Beach (1952) commented that 'in most societies the physical beauty of the female receives more explicit consideration than does the handsomeness of the male. The attractiveness of the man usually depends predominantly upon his skills and prowess rather than upon his physical appearance' (p. 91). Dion (1981), in reviewing the available evidence, came to a similar conclusion. This is also reflected in the recent Sexual Excitation (SE)/Sexual Inhibition (SI) Scale for Women (SESII-W; Graham et al 2006) in which two partner characteristics that many women find sexually arousing are 'seeing a partner doing something that shows his talent' and 'someone doing something that shows he is intelligent'.

Two earlier studies in which I was involved remain of interest. Mathews et al (1972), asked men to rate photographs of women for sexual attractiveness, and found an attractiveness factor relevant to all the male respondents. A further factor, however, which appeared to relate to the sexiness or sexual availability of the woman, showed much more variation of ratings amongst the men. This points to a distinction between 'beauty' and 'sexiness'. In a parallel study, we showed photographs of men to women from various occupational groups. This also revealed a general factor of attractiveness, though the women's ratings of this factor were generally lower than the men's in the earlier study. Furthermore, social class differences were much more evident; women preferred men who appeared to belong to the same social class as themselves (Bancroft 1978).

In Chapter 5 we considered the development of sexual preferences and sexual identity. It was there proposed that the establishment of who or what is sexually attractive in terms of visual appearance, occurs during a relatively critical period of development in the male, (whether or not he develops opposite sex or same sex preferences) but not apparently in the female, who is more concerned about relationship issues, and whose sexual identity is less fixed, emerging over a much more variable period of time across women, and not as stable. On the other hand her own attractiveness influences her self-esteem; being sexually desired and desirable is of fundamental importance. Obviously, in today's society in which we are all bombarded with visual images, women will not be indifferent to how men look, but it is reasonable to conclude that such factors are of secondary importance in their selection of a sexual partner, at least of a long-term sexual partner.

Where does all this leave Symon's evolutionary perspective? Although more evidence is needed on this point, the impact of acculturation, demonstrated by Tovee et al (2006), undermines the idea that our criteria of sexual attractiveness were established in the EEA. There is an alternative explanatory model proposed some time ago by Eysenck & Wilson (1979). The essence of sexual attractiveness, they suggested, is the difference between male and female features. In other words, an attractive woman is one who is clearly non-male and vice versa, hence the importance of facial structure, breasts, hips, body hair, physique, etc. This is basic to sexual reproduction; whether we are a human or an insect, we are programmed to be attracted to the opposite sex (in most cases), a mechanism that preceded adaptations in the EEA! The intriguing question of the determinants of sexual attraction for gay men and lesbian women will be addressed in Chapter 8, but they are certainly not going to be explained as adaptations from the EEA! How we recognize the opposite sex is influenced by cultural factors, allowing for some variability in the extent to which individuals are attracted to the 'typical' opposite sex, with some, for other reasons, preferring various degrees of atypicality. What of Symons' focus on healthiness? Tovee et al (2006) proposed an explanation for the changeability of preference for high or low body weight; in the Zulu homeland where food was in short supply the heavier woman was not only likely to be wealthier, but also healthier. In that social context ill-health is predominantly manifested as wasting and low body weight. In Britain, health problems are more commonly associated with being overweight. One's reactions to these contrasting contexts does not need to have been established as an adaptation in our ancestors. On the other hand, the possibility that different cultural patterns in the past influenced reproductive fitness, resulting in some ethnic differences, which are in part genetically determined, is worth keeping in mind. Returning to the hunter–gatherer/agricultural contrast as an example, is it possible that in agricultural societies, where food supply was different, with more emphasis on carbohydrates, and associated effects on weight, relatively overweight young females may have been both attractive and fertile at a young age, fitting in well with the virginity ethic and an early marriage scenario? In the typical fishing community of Northern Europe, conforming to the hunter–gatherer pattern, and with food collection shared among men and women, marriage delayed by adolescent infertility, and allowing for some premarital activity and more involvement of the female in food production, may have fitted in with attraction to the more slender young female with a more protein-dominant diet. These are speculations, but not beyond scientific evaluation.

Given the increasing importance of free choice in marriage, let us now consider how this is enacted.

Mate selection

Sexual attraction, it would seem, is not a passive process; in addition to the impact of culture, the response of the individual to the subject may influence how attractive that individual appears. Perhaps the most interesting evidence of this involves the eyes. Eye contact is an important part of the courting process. Our pupils dilate when we look at something that interests us, and women with dilated pupils are judged more attractive by male observers (Hess 1965).

Perper (1985) described the typical behaviour of two people meeting and establishing a sexual contact in a singles bar in the USA. He calls this the 'courtship sequence'. When two people are strangers, courtship begins when one approaches or moves next to the other. After initial conversation, the next step is when the two people turn to face each other (a step which can take from 10 minutes to 2 hours or more!) The next step involves touching — one person touches the other. As the sequence develops further, eye contact becomes prolonged. Then the couple start to move or gesture in a synchronized manner. By then the courtship sequence is well on its way. Turning to face or touching the other person are examples of what Perper calls 'escalation points' — what happens next depends on how the other person responds; if he or she responds positively the sequence 'escalates'.

Perhaps the most interesting conclusion drawn by Perper is that it is women who tend to control these sequences, showing proceptive behaviour in a variety of subtle ways. Although it could be said that Perper goes beyond his data, he develops the interesting idea that selection of a mate is a process that is principally under the woman's control. She decides when to let the sequence develop; she feels entitled to stop it at any stage and, as considered in Chapter 4, she is more likely to feel sexual interest when she feels that the male is desiring her but she remains in control of the interaction.

Being sexually attracted to someone, and 'escalating' in a singles bar is one thing; choosing that person as a partner for a more permanent relationship, possibly leading to marriage, is another. What happens when there is freedom of choice? The available evidence presents rather a dull picture. In general, there is a tendency for like to marry like, which has been evident for some time. This applies to living in the same neighbourhood (Ineichen 1979), the same degree of physical attractiveness (Dion 1981), the same ethnic or religious group, social class and level of education (Udry 1974). When these boundaries are crossed there is a higher rate of marital breakdown. In the USA, the NHSLS (Laumann et al 1994) showed that not only married relationships but also short-term relationships were embedded in social networks. The authors commented that it was 'misleading to speak of a person *choosing* on the basis of specific racial/ethnic, educational or religious characteristics' (p. 266) — it was more a matter of which social network an individual found him or herself in, and such networks become organized around these social attributes. The NHSLS data, however, allowed only limited assessment of social networks. In a subsequent survey, CHSLS, four distinct neighbourhoods in Chicago were studied, using a combination of conventional survey and qualitative methods (Laumann et al 2004). The concept of 'sex market' was used; a 'spatially and culturally bounded arena in which searches for sex partners and a variety of exchanges or transactions are conducted' (p. 8). The four neighbourhoods or 'sex markets' differed in various ways. Traditional cultures in two of them encouraged some 'market' activities to take place in church or church-sponsored activities, and these 'markets' also accorded the family a central role, structuring who one meets, determining the types of people one might have a relationship with, and acting as a stakeholder in any emerging relationship. In a third neighbourhood, family or church had little impact, and work or school were more important. The impact of such 'sex markets' on same-sex relationships probably have more explanatory value and will be considered further in Chapter 8.

Laumann et al (1994) found that of those who ended up marrying, 10% had their first sex with each other within a month of first meeting. For those who co-habited, it was 35% and for short-term partnerships, 37%. The percentages who had known each other for more than a year before they first had sex were 47% for the married, 22% for those co-habiting and 26% for short-term partners. In the NATSAL 2000 survey from Britain, of those who had started a new relationship within the past year, 56.5% of men and 42.8% of women had first sex with the new partner within the first month of meeting (Johnson et al 2001).

Where does love fit in?

Sitting awkwardly in the midst of all this is the concept of love. Kinsey did not attempt to assess love. In a secondary analysis of data from the NHSLS (Waite & Joyner 2001), men and women who said they last had sex to express love also reported more emotional satisfaction with their sexual relationship. But what it meant to 'express love' was not considered further. The NATSAL 1990 and 2000 surveys in Britain did not ask about love. The French national survey (Spira et al 1994) asked one question: Were you in love when you first had sexual intercourse? Two-thirds of women said they were very much in love with their first partner but only one-third of men.

Falling in love remains an enigma, and not one easily studied in surveys. Tennov (1979), who coined the word 'limerence' to describe the state of being in love, struggled in her attempts to study it. Limerence, she decided, was not an emotion, a perception, a form of learning, a cognitive process or a behaviour, although it included components of all of them. 'Linguistically invisible under ordinary circumstances, limerence was clearly present when present and fully absent when absent' (Tennov 1980). There has been some progress since.

The nature of love was considered from a neurophysiological perspective in Chapter 4 (p. 73). The distinction, as defined by Hatfield & Rapson (1993), between 'passionate' (or 'romantic') and 'companionate' was adopted (see p. 65). Not surprisingly, brain imaging studies have indicated that what we call 'passionate love', at least in the manifestations of it studied, involves activity in various regions of the brain, which overlap with activity elicited by maternal love but also, in other ways, with activity during sexual arousal. Amongst other things, there is activation of the incentive motivation system and deactivation of some aspects of critical appraisal!

It is often assumed that women are more romantic than men. The evidence, such as it is, suggests the opposite; men more readily fall in love; women show more caution before becoming involved and are more likely to decide when an affair ends, while men take longer to get over a love affair (Hatfield & Walster 1981).

Various attempts have been made to measure love with questionnaires. One of the best established is the Passionate Love Scale (PLS; Hatfield & Sprecher 1986), recently used in the brain imaging studies described in Chapter 4. Behavioural characteristics of people in love have also been studied. Probably the most convincing is the tendency to engage in prolonged eye contact and also to stand close to one another (Hatfield & Walster 1981).

How important is romantic love when choosing a partner for marriage? According to Burgess & Wallin (1953), 'The expected, approved, and sanctioned precondition to marriage in American society is falling in love.' However, romantic love as the basis for marriage is a relatively new phenomenon, leading to expectations of marriage difficult to realize. Margaret Mead (1950), considering the modern American style of marriage, said: 'It is one of the most difficult marriage forms that the human race has ever attempted and the casualties are surprisingly few, considering the complexities of the task.'

Prior to the 19th century, according to Stone (1979), it was the accepted wisdom that marriage based on romantic love or sexual attraction was less likely to lead to lasting happiness than one based on common sense considerations. 'Almost everyone agreed that both physical desire and romantic love were unsafe bases for an enduring marriage since both were violent mental disturbances which would inevitably be of only short duration.' Gillis (1985) paints a rather different and, to me, more attractive historical picture: 'As we turn to the 16th and 17th century it is not the capacity for love but the *form* of affection that separates their world from ours.' 'Direct and personal expressions of love were inhibited and in their place we find highly ritualized forms of courtship, whose actions and symbols seem to us strangely impersonal.' In other words, we should be not be surprised to find that romantic love has been expressed in different ways at different times in history and in different cultures, whilst involving some basic neuropsychological mechanisms in common. Gillis saw romantic love and its associated passion as an important part of the courtship process, which was 'exorcised at the time of the wedding' as 'too much affection was perceived as unnatural and a threat to the broader social obligations that come with the establishment of a household'. Gillis dealt more with ordinary working people than Stone. Such people had negligible property or possessions and hence were generally freer to make their own choice of partner. They nevertheless saw marriage as a long-term serious business of coping and rearing a family — the adult phase of life. Romantic love, whilst important for the bonding process, was perhaps too couple-centred, too light-hearted for the serious business of living. In the more affluent families, who provided much more of the evidence reported by Stone, the need for arranged marriages was stronger. It is not difficult to see how in such circumstances romantic love would seem to the parents of the aspiring bride or groom a threat to the orderly choice of suitable partner, whilst for the young person the inevitability of major parental influence would discourage the development of emotional attachments which could so easily be thwarted. In these accounts, we see the impact of social class and affluence and the power of social control over mate selection. Udry (1974), having reviewed the evidence, concluded that 'the emotion of love has probably existed as a natural social phenomenon wherever young people were allowed to associate with the opposite sex. Wherever it has existed it has had as much influence on mate selection as the society would let it'. He was also unable to find any evidence that marriages based on romantic love have a worse outcome — which might reassure the romantics amongst us.

However, we have to consider a more recent change, pervasive in its effects; the emergence of 'individualism' from the more traditional 'collectivism'. In individualistic societies, the main concern is with one's own interests and those of one's immediate family. In collectivist societies, people identify with and conform to the expectations of more extended groups who look after one's interests in return for loyalty. The modern USA is often regarded as a good example of an individualistic culture. Whereas most societies have remained traditional in this respect for longer than the USA, there is evidence of a more pervasive change, which can be seen as one manifestation of 'Westernization' throughout the world. A number of studies have compared different cultures in this respect.

The largest cross-cultural study, reported by Buss (1989) and involving samples from 37 countries, focused on characteristics of a desirable mate but did not consider the role of love (see p. 201). Sprecher et al (1994) assessed male and female students in three countries: the USA, Russia and Japan. They assessed attachment types originally described for children, but adapted by Hazan & Shaver (1987) to describe attachment in romantic love relationships. There are three such types: 'secure', characterized by trust, friendship and positive emotions, 'avoidant', in which there is fear of closeness and lack of trust, and 'anxious/ambivalent', in which love is a 'pre-occupying, almost painfully exciting struggle to merge with another person' (Hazan & Shaver 1987). They also assessed type of love, as defined by Lee (1976). There are three such types: 'eros' (physical attraction, sensuality, close intimacy and rapport), 'ludus' (playful, hedonistic and uncommitted) and 'storge' (affectionate, compassionate). These three types can combine in various ways with three other dimensions: 'pragma' (practical, realistic), 'mania' (feverish, obsessive and jealous) and 'agape' (selfless). In all three countries, the majority indicated they had been in love at least once, that love should be the basis for marriage, and that personality, visual appearance and reciprocal liking were important requirements for falling in love. There were, however, several cultural differences. Americans were more likely to report a 'secure' attachment style (rather than 'avoidant' or 'anxious/ambivalent'); they scored higher on 'eros', and attached more importance to the partner's appearance when falling in love. The Russians reported more 'avoidant' attachment style, and were more willing to marry without love. The Japanese came midway between the other two in terms of attachment style and requiring love before marriage. They also rated themselves as less romantic than the other two samples. In comparing men and women, there were more similarities than differences. Women were more likely to report 'anxious/ambivalent' attachments, and scored lower on 'agape'. Overall, gender differences were more marked in the US sample than the Japanese or Russian. For example, American men scored higher on 'ludus' than the women; and American women scored higher on 'storge' than the men. Neither gender difference was apparent with the Japanese or Russians.

Levine et al (1995) compared students from 11 countries: England, the USA, Australia, Brazil, Mexico, India, Pakistan, Japan, Thailand, Philippines and Hong Kong. There were clear differences across cultures in the extent to which people would be willing to get married without being in love. This was most likely in India, Pakistan and Thailand, and least likely in Brazil, Hong Kong, Australia, the USA and England, which were all very similar in this respect. Japan and Philippines were midway, with more respondents being undecided. These cultural differences were less evident when asking about the importance of love for the maintenance and stability of marriage. To a reasonable extent, one can regard the second, largest group of countries to be individualistic, and the first group of three to be collectivist, with Japan and Philippines being in transition. However, this was a study of students, and the findings may have been very different with, for example, rural working class subjects, or affluent city dwellers.

Kim & Hatfield (2004) compared male and female students from the USA and Korea. They measured passionate love with the PLS (Hatfield & Sprecher 1986), companionate love with the Companionate Love Scale (CLS; Sternberg 1986) and used measures of satisfaction with life (SWLS) and positive and negative affect (PANAS). As they predicted, they found the CLS to be predictive of SWLS, and PLS to be predictive of PANAS. The association between companionate love and satisfaction with life was stronger in the women than the men. The association between passionate love and positive and negative mood was stronger in men than women. Interestingly, they found no differences in these respects between the two cultures. They had predicted that, as members of a more collectivist culture, the Koreans would show stronger correlations between companionate love and life satisfaction, whereas Americans, as members of a more individualistic society, would show stronger correlations between passionate love and positive and negative mood. These predictions were based on the assumption that in a collectivist society, where kinship networks are more important, and marriages more determined by family choice of partner, passionate love would have more negative connotations. They did not find this and attributed this to the substantial amount of Westernization in Korean culture, which is likely to be particularly evident among Korean university students. If this explanation is valid it is a further example of how cultural change can influence key components of our sexuality.

Diamond (2004) proposed that there are two evolutionarily distinct phenomena: sexual mating, on the one hand, and pair bonding, which evolved in order to establish mother–infant pair bonds. Pair-bonding between lovers, she suggests, is an exaptation, i.e. it evolved for one reason but came to serve another. However, it is not yet clear to what extent pair-bonding of the type that occurs between mother and infant is a component of passionate love. It is perhaps more relevant to companionate love. As shown by Bartels & Zeki (2004) in their brain imaging studies of maternal and romantic love, there are some things in common and some differences, which are not as yet clearly interpretable. It is therefore possible that whatever is involved in pair-bonding may be involved in passionate or romantic love but continues to be involved as the relationship moves to companionate love, whereas other things change.

Some progress has been made in studying love, as it relates to sexual relationships and mate choice. However, as with sexual arousal and desire, we should not assume that we are dealing with any unitary neuropsychological process, but rather a combination of mechanisms, which will vary according to the circumstances as well as to characteristics of the individual. The information processing involved, which results in us attributing meaning to the emotional responses involved, are likely be influenced and shaped by culture. We should be cautious, however, in generalizing from these cross-cultural studies, most of which have involved students.

Incidence of marriage and co-habitation

The incidence of marriage rose from the early years of the century, reaching a peak in the late 1960s and early 1970s. Since then it has declined steadily. The major increase in remarriages in Britain in the early 1970s followed the Divorce Reform Act of 1969 that allowed many separated individuals to divorce and remarry (Fig. 6.9). The percentage of the British population aged 18–49 years who were married, and the percentage who were unmarried but co-habiting in 1979–2002 are shown in Figure 6.10. This shows the steady decline in marriage, from 74% to 49% and the steady increase in co-habitation, from 3% to 15%. Combining the two, however, shows a decline in the percentage either married or co-habiting. Marriage, co-habitation and divorce rates by age group are shown in Table 6.10.

In the USA the marriage rate, expressed as the number of marriages per year, per 1000 unmarried women aged 15 years or over, was 92 in 1920. It peaked at 118 in 1946 when the post-war baby-boom started, and declined thereafter, reaching 50 in 1996. Married couples headed 80% of US households in 1910, 71% in 1970 and 53% in 1998. Co-habitation has increased. In 1960, 0.2% of all American couples were co-habiting; by 1998 it was 7.1% (Caplow et al 2001). Comparable patterns of change have been evident in most European countries.

Age at marriage

The so-called European marriage pattern, with a relatively late age of marriage and a relatively high proportion of unmarried women reaching the menopause, has been a characteristic of Western Europe (i.e. west of an imaginary line drawn between Trieste and Leningrad). In Eastern Europe, age at marriage tended to be

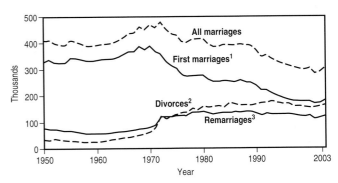

Fig. 6.9 The numbers of marriages and divorces in the UK, from 1950 to 2003. [1]For both partners; [2]includes annulments (data for 1950 to 1970 for Great Britain only; [3]for one or both partners. (Social Trends No 36, 2006). Source: Office for National Statistics, General Register Office for Scotland, Northern Ireland Statistics and Research Agency.

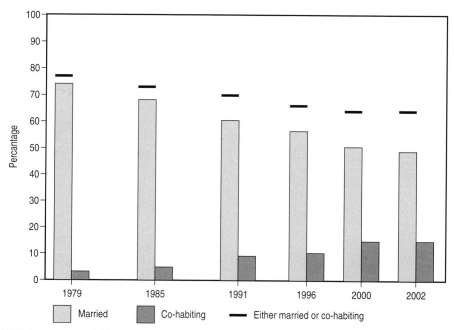

Fig. 6.10 Percentage of British women aged 18–49 years who were married or co-habiting: 1979–2002. (General Household Survey 2004/5.)

TABLE 6.10 Percentage of each age group who are married, cohabiting, single or divorced/separated * for Great Britain 2002 (General Household Survey 2002)

Age	Married		Co-habiting[†]		Single		Divorced/separated	
	Men	Women	Men	Women	Men	Women	Men	Women
16–24	2	7	10	16	87	76	0	1
25–34	37	44	22	20	38	30	3	6
35–44	64	64	12	10	16	12	7	13
45–54	70	71	7	6	10	6	12	14
55–64	77	71	4	3	6	4	11	13
65–74	76	58	2	1	5	4	7	9
75+	63	28	1	1	4	5	4	5

*100 minus the sum of each row for each gender is the percentage who are widowed
[†]Divorced or separated who are co-habiting are included in the co-habiting group

younger and the proportion remaining unmarried to be lower (Glass 1974). However, there was a universal decline in age at first marriage in most countries after World War II. In 1931, 26% of women in the UK in the 20- to 24-year age group were married; in 1963 it was 60%. In 1931 the average age at marriage for women was 25.5 years. In 1971 the average age was 23 years for women and 25 years for men. By 2003, this had increased to 29 years for women and 31 years for men. There has been a similar trend across Europe. Between 1971 and 2002, the average age at first marriage in the European Union (the EU-15) increased from 26 to 30 years for men and 23 to 28 years for women. When 10 other countries, mainly from Eastern Europe, joined the EU in 2004 this resulted in more variability. In 2003, the country with youngest age at first marriage was Lithuania, with 24 years for women and 27 years for men. This contrasted with Sweden, with the oldest ages; 31 years for women and 33 years for men. The average age difference between husband and wife ranged from just under

2 years in Ireland and Portugal to just under 4 years in Greece (Babb et al 2006). These figures can be compared with those from the recent global study (Wellings et al 2006) shown in Table 6.2. Note, however, that the figures in this table are based on medians rather than means.

In the USA in 1900 the average age at first marriage was 22 years for women and 26 years for men. These ages declined until 1960, when they were about 20.5 years for women and 23 years for men. From around 1970 the trend reversed, and by 1996 the figures were 25 years for women and 27 years for men (Caplow et al 2001). These patterns showed differences between white and black Americans, which will be considered later in the chapter.

An important factor in the general tendency for later age at first marriage and fewer marriages is the increase in co-habitation (se Fig. 6.10), particularly among the never married. Thus, increasingly, couples are co-habiting when previously they would have married.

Sexual activity within marriage and co-habitation

One of the most relevant changes in marriage in the second half of the 20th century has been in its relevance to sexual activity. The traditional concept of marriage, across cultures and religions, has involved the legitimization of sexual activity. As discussed earlier, there was an increasing acceptance, in the last 100 years, of premarital sex as preparation for the marriage to follow, reflecting the establishment of the romantic norm for mate selection. But that change has now gone much further. Marriage, increasingly, is a formal arrangement, which may be pursued by two people once they have established a sexual relationship. This may reflect partial acceptance of traditional moral values and a wish to conform in the long term or, alternatively, the various legal implications of marriage, particularly in relation to having children. The following section on sexual activity is therefore more to do with couples in an established relationship, living together, than with marriage per se. This is reflected in how sexual activity is now reported by survey researchers, particularly European researchers (Bozon 2001). In fact, until recently, apart from Kinsey, little research attention was paid to marital sex.

Now that more attention is being paid to sex in marriage and in co-habiting couples, it is noteworthy that most of the attention is focused on frequency of sexual intercourse, with very little attention to other aspects of sexual interaction, apart from oral and anal sex because of their potential for transmitting infection.

Bozon (2001) emphasized that the frequency of sexual activity in an established sexual relationship, whether marriage or co-habitation, does not show a continuous downward trend, but rather goes through stages in the development or evolution of the relationship. 'In the early phase of the relationship, sexual activity is entirely dedicated to the construction of the couple' (Bozon 2001, p. 16). After this initial phase, which quite often is brought to an end by the first childbirth, there is a more stable pattern of gradual decline.

How does the frequency of sexual intercourse within marriage or co-habiting relationships today compare with relationships during Kinsey's time, around 50 years ago? This often asked question remains difficult to answer with certainty because of variations in how 'frequency' questions are worded (see p. 181) and because of uncertain validity of recall of frequencies for earlier periods in one's life (of particular relevance to the Kinsey data). Figure 6.11 shows the frequency of sexual intercourse in the past month for married couples and co-habitors from the 1988 National Survey of Families and Households ($n = 13\ 008$), reported by Call et al (1995). One can speculate that with the range of distractions that have emerged in modern life outside one's work commitments (e.g. television and the Internet), frequencies may have declined further since 1988. However, until we have new studies employing the same questions as earlier ones, we should be cautious in interpreting such evidence.

This study showed higher frequencies of sexual intercourse in co-habiting couples than married couples, and this is consistent with other studies (e.g. Blumstein & Schwartz 1983; Johnson et al 1994). This probably reflects a tendency for those with higher levels of sexual interest to be more permissive in their sexual attitudes, hence increasing their likelihood of co-habiting before marrying.

In the British NATSAL 1990, Johnson et al (1994) reported frequencies of sexual activity (including vaginal, oral and anal sex) in the married and co-habiting. However, because of the skewed distributions, these were given as medians rather than means, making it

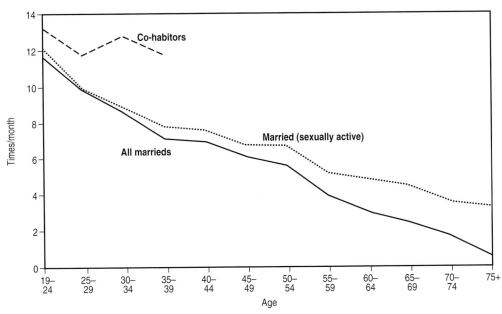

Fig. 6.11 Frequency of sexual intercourse in the past month for married couples and co-habitors from the 1988 National Survey of Families and Households ($n = 13\ 008$). (Reported by Call et al (1995).)

difficult to compare with the earlier studies. The median frequency during the past 4 weeks reported by married men was 4 (ranging from 7 in the 16- to 24-year group to 3 in the 45- to 59-year group) and by co-habiting men was 6 (ranging from 8–3). Similar frequencies were reported by women.

Consistent across studies is considerable variability across couples. Some attempts have been made to assess determinants of this variability. Call et al (1995) used logistic regression to assess the impact of a range of variables on the decline in frequency of sexual activity in marriage over time. Age, not surprisingly, was the strongest predictor, and the impact of age on sexual activity is discussed more fully in Chapter 7. Other significant negative predictors, in order of importance, were unhappy marriage, educational level (a curvilinear effect; lowest and highest levels of education had a negative effect), poor health, having a young child, being Catholic and wife pregnant. The first year of the marriage had a significantly positive effect, and second year was less positive but still significant. After these first 2 years the duration of the marriage did not predict the frequency when controlling for the other variables. This substantiates Bozon's (2001) point that frequency stabilizes after the first 2 years, apart from the impact of other factors such as age and health. The analysis by Call et al (1995), however, only accounted for 22% of the variance in marital frequency, leaving us with the need to identify other determinants.

Johnson et al (1994), in the British NATSAL 1990, found that duration of the relationship and age of partner were significant negative predictors of frequency of sexual activity (including vaginal, oral and anal sex) in the married and co-habiting, though the effects of age were small under 45 years. In a comparison of NATSAL 1990 and 2000, frequency of sexual intercourse during the past month was not given, but the percentages of all respondents, single married or co-habiting, who had experienced sexual intercourse in the past month did not differ significantly (Johnson et al 2001).

It is likely that there are individual differences in sexual desire and arousability that both men and women bring into their relationships, accounting for much of the variance in these frequencies across studies. We will consider such factors further later in this chapter, in the section on personality.

Initiation of sex

Men have traditionally been the initiators in love-making (although according to Perper (1985) not in socio-sexual interactions). In Blumstein & Schwartz's (1983) study of American couples, only 12% of wives said they were more likely to initiate love-making and only 16% of the men said their wives were more likely to do so. In contrast, 51% of husbands usually initiated sex. This study found that many men often felt uncomfortable when their partner initiated, and by the same token men may feel guilty for failing in their duty to initiate sex. Not surprisingly, women found it more difficult than men to cope with refusal. This traditional

pattern appears to be deeply rooted. Of interest was the finding that couples who were more equal in their initiation and refusal of sex were more likely to report a happy sex life (Blumstein & Schwartz 1983). Gray (1984) using the cross-cultural evidence from the HRAF, found that societies with high female power within marriage exhibited better, or certainly no worse, adjustment than societies with a low degree of female power. Societies with high female power tended to have open discussion of sexual matters, attach importance to foreplay, show less disapproval of female premarital sexual activity and allow women to initiate sex. They also tended to show less male fear of impotence and less evidence of male homosexual behaviour (though greater acceptance of it). It is an interesting idea that men would be sexually more functional if they were not expected to be sexually dominant.

Bozon (2001) emphasized the importance of the degree of gender equality in the relationship for how the sexual relationship evolves over time, in particular the continuation of mutual desire, and shared initiation. In the more traditional marriage, the dominance of the male becomes more clearly manifested as the relationship continues, and associated with this is what Bozon (2001) calls 'gradual female disinvestment' in the sexual relationship. This is an interesting perspective, and relates to the discussion on the impact of the menopause in Chapter 7.

Non-coital activities

Kissing

Kissing is seen by many couples as the height of intimacy, especially by women. Blumstein & Schwartz (1983) found that people kiss less during sex when they feel somewhat removed emotionally but still want physical release. The Kinsey surveys assessed how often it occurred both premaritally and maritally (Gebhard & Johnson 1979) and reported it to be more frequent in higher educated groups. Ford & Beach (1952) described some primitive societies in which kissing was not a normal part of love-making, and others in which modified forms of kissing were used. Something akin to kissing has also been observed in primates. What is lacking is information on how people vary in their attitudes to and acceptance of kissing. It is remarkable how little attention has been paid to kissing in recent surveys of sexual behaviour, presumably because it is not seen as relevant to HIV transmission.

Oral sex

The relevance of oral sex as a component of premarital sex was considered earlier in the chapter, with evidence that it has increased to some extent as a substitute for vaginal intercourse in teenagers (see p. 197). What part does oral sex play in married and co- habiting relationships? Kinsey found that 51% of their college-educated and 70% of their non-college-educated subjects reported no cunnilingus (oral stimulation of the female genitalia) during their first marriage and 15% and 11%, respectively, reported cunnilingus as frequent. For fellatio (oral stimulation of the penis) the percentages were very similar for no experience (49.5% and 70%, respectively) with

TABLE 6. 11	Prevalence (%) of oral and anal sex during the last year by sex, age and marital status (NATSAL 1990; Johnson et al 1994)			
	Oral sex		Anal sex	
Age	Men	Women	Men	Women
16–17	30.5	32.1	7.4	5.4
18–24	69.6	69.8	8.1	8.6
25–34	77.0	73.3	6.6	6.6
35–44	68.1	59.0	6.2	4.8
45–59	41.7	29.8	5.1	4.3
MARITAL STATUS (ALL AGES)				
Married	63.7	58.0	5.5	5.4
Co-habiting	88.7	79.6	9.8	10.1
Single	83.3	80.9	10.3	9.6

12% of college and 9% of non-college-educated reporting it as frequent (Gebhard & Johnson 1979).

In the British NATSAL 1990, the proportions who had experience of oral sex were much higher (Table 6.11). Furthermore, comparison with the NATSAL 2000, 10 years later, shows a significant further increase (OR adjusted for age, 1.5 for men and 1.8 for women; Johnson et al 2001). The higher prevalence in the younger age and single groups is consistent with there being an increase in this behaviour in recent years. The higher frequency in co-habiting than in married couples is consistent with co-habiters having less traditional sexual attitudes.

Anal sex

Kinsey found that 89% of college and 93% of non-college males had no experience of anal sex in their first marriage, with similar percentages for females (89% and 87%, respectively). In heterosexual relationships this remains a relatively unusual form of sexual activity (see Table 6.11). However, as with oral sex, a significant increase was reported in the NATSAL 2000 compared to the NATSAL 1990 (OR 1.9 for men and women; Johnson et al 2001).

Orgasm and ejaculation

It is generally assumed that men ejaculate and experience orgasm with appropriate stimulation, and that this occurs with most forms of sexual activity, particularly vaginal intercourse and masturbation. On that basis, Kinsey defined 'total sexual outlet' in males as the frequency of ejaculation/orgasm, from whatever type of stimulation. Of his male sample, 2.1% had a zero frequency of total sexual outlet (Kinsey et al 1948; Table 40). Inability to ejaculate, or delayed ejaculation, is the least common form of male sexual dysfunction, which will be considered more closely in Chapter 11. However, there is a tendency for ejaculation to become more difficult as men age (see Chapter 7). In the NHSLS (Laumann et al 1994), the question asked was, 'When you and your partner had sex during the past 12 months, did you always/ usually/sometimes/rarely/never have an orgasm, that is come to climax?'. Of the men, 72% answered 'always', 21.8 'usually', 3.7%

'sometimes' and 2.6% 'rarely' or 'never'. In the French ACSF (Spira et al 1994) men reported achieving orgasm most easily through vaginal penetration (47% 'always' and 49% 'rather easily'); for manual stimulation by their partner the figures were 22% and 53%, and for fellatio 22% and 43%.

Orgasm in the female is a different story. As discussed in Chapter 4 (p. 86) women vary in the types of stimulation that are most likely to lead to orgasm, and for many such stimulation does not result from vaginal penetration per se. In any case, women are much more variable than men in their likelihood of experiencing orgasm during sexual activity, and in the type of stimulation required to achieve orgasm. Lloyd (2005) scrutinized the literature that reports on women's orgasmic experiences, and summarized data from 32 studies. Most of these were not based on representative samples, and many of them did not make clear whether or not orgasm during intercourse involved additional clitoral stimulation. From the studies indicating the proportion of women who 'always' experienced orgasm during intercourse, the mean was 25.3%. For the 'sometimes' or 'rarely' categories, the mean was 19.7% (Lloyd 2005). Kinsey et al (1953) reported on the wide age range for when women first experience orgasm, from any type of stimulation (see p. 85), and concluded that '9 percent … would probably not reach orgasm in the course of their lives' (p. 513). Lloyd (2005) found that this figure ranged from 5% to 10% across studies.

In the NHSLS (Laumann et al 1994), to the question cited above for the male, 27.1% of women answered 'always', 41.3% 'usually', 21.6% 'sometimes' and 10% 'rarely' or 'never'. This does not distinguish between different types of stimulation during sexual activity. In the French survey (ACSF, Spira et al 1994), which was not included in Lloyd's review, women, rather surprisingly, reported achieving orgasm most easily through vaginal penetration (23% 'always' and 55% 'rather easily'), when masturbated by their partner the figures were 15% and 53%, with cunnilingus 15% and 42%. This is somewhat inconsistent with evidence reviewed by Lloyd, raising the question whether there is a cultural difference here either in the actual sexual experiences, or in what women are comfortable reporting. The evidence is nevertheless clear that the capacity for orgasm is much more variable in women than in men.

How important is orgasm and/or ejaculation for sexual satisfaction? In the NATSAL 1990 (Johnson et al 1994) questions about personal experience of orgasm were considered too intrusive. But reactions to the following general statement were requested: 'sex without orgasm, or climax, cannot be really satisfying for a man'; 49% of men agreed and 34% disagreed, 43% of women agreed and 29% disagreed. The same statement was made for a woman; 29% of women agreed and 50% disagreed, 37% of men agreed and 35% disagreed.

In a recent Kinsey Institute survey of women in a heterosexual relationship (Bancroft et al 2003a; Bancroft et al in press), frequency of orgasm during sexual

TABLE 6.12 Reponses of 987 women (%) in established heterosexual relationships to four questions: 'How important to your sexual happiness is it…?'. (Bancroft et al, in press)

	Not at all	Somewhat	Moderately	Very	Extremely
…to have an orgasm	10.6	32.4	27.4	24.7	4.9
…to fell emotionally close to your partner	2.4	6.5	7.5	46.7	36.8
…that your partner be sexually satisfied	1.7	6.9	12.4	52.1	26.8
…to fell comfortable talking to your partner about sexual acts	4.1	10.1	24.3	37.5	24.0

activity with their partners was not predictive of how women evaluated their sexual relationship or their own sexuality. Women were also asked, 'How important to your sexual happiness is it to have an orgasm?'. The results, together with those from three other related questions, are given in Table 6.12. Only 29.6% of the women answered that having an orgasm was 'very' or 'extremely' important.

Impact of menstruation

The restriction of sexual activity during menstruation has been widespread in human societies. In the majority of societies, the menstruating woman is considered unsuitable as a sexual partner, and in some cases there may be general rejection of the woman as 'unclean' during this phase of her cycle. Islamic religion regards the menstruating woman as impure, requiring ritual cleaning. Apart from not having intercourse, she is forbidden to touch the Koran, repeat a verse from it or enter a mosque (Bullough 1976). Hindu women are similarly ostracized when menstruating. Orthodox Jewish women still require a ritual bath after menstruation. In a WHO-sponsored study of patterns of menstruation in 10 countries, Snowden & Christian (1983) found that almost all respondents believed that sexual intercourse should be avoided during menstruation. The UK, the only Western country in the study, was an exception; just over half interviewed held that view, though the authors believed that in terms of actual practice the proportion would have been higher. In Whyte's (1980) cross-cultural study, only 10 of the 93 societies were free from menstrual taboos.

A woman's sexual interest and arousability does tend to vary across the menstrual cycle, although women vary substantially in how this is experienced (see Chapter 4). Hedricks (1994) reviewed the relevant literature which, though quite extensive, is largely restricted to white college-educated heterosexual women in the USA. A consistent finding was that all aspects of women's sexuality, including their sexual interaction with their partner, is lowest during menstruation, and a variety of factors, including psychoendocrine (see Chapter 4, p. 116) and cultural, could account for that. For those women who report a predictable peak in sexual interest during the cycle, the commonest time for the peak is approximately a week before or around the likely time of ovulation. There is a smaller proportion of women who report a pre-menstrual peak. Interestingly, Kinsey found that the pre-menstrual peak was most commonly reported in his sample (34% of white college women; Gebhard & Johnson 1979).

It would be interesting to know if attitudes to sex during menstruation are changing and whether women feel differently to men about sex at this time. Pietropinto & Simenauer (1977) asked their male subjects how they felt about sex during menstruation. About a third said they enjoyed it as usual; for the remainder it presented varying degrees of 'turn off' with 11% avoiding the partner completely at that time. Little attention has been paid to this in recent sex surveys, which is noteworthy given the potential relevance of menstruation and phases of the menstrual cycle to sexual transmission of infection (Ehrhardt & Wasserheit 1991). The French ACSF asked about attitudes towards body fluids; 67% of men found contact with their partner's menstrual blood unpleasant, with 16% finding it neither pleasant nor unpleasant (Spira et al 1994).

Sexual well-being and the importance of sex in marriage and relationships

In the NHSLS (Laumann et al 1994), the associations between degree of current happiness and various aspects of the individual's sexual life were assessed. People with only one sexual partner tended to be happier than those with more than one or none. The physical pleasure and emotional satisfaction from a sexual relationship was greater in those with only one partner than in those with more than one. Those with a higher frequency of sexual activity with the partner tended to be happier, whereas frequency of masturbation showed the opposite association. Frequency of orgasm, while unrelated in men, was associated with happiness in women. Interestingly, those women reporting never having orgasms were somewhat happier than those reporting orgasm rarely. Laumann et al (1994) stressed the uncertainties in knowing what is cause or effect in such associations. Does a couple have more frequent sex when they are happier, or does the more frequent sex make them feel happier? Does more frequent masturbation reduce one's happiness, or is masturbation used by some people to improve mood when they are feeling unhappy? It is likely that both directions of causality are relevant and it would require more detailed study to assess the relative importance of each.

The French ACSF survey (Spira et al 1994) considered sexual satisfaction briefly. Participants were asked whether they were satisfied with their current sex life. Of men, 45% were 'very satisfied' and 44% 'quite satisfied'; for women, the percentages were 48% and 36%, respectively. Young women, aged 20–34 years, were somewhat more likely than men of that age group to be very satisfied, and overall, the degree of satisfaction dropped after the age of 45 years. The number of sexual partners in the past year was relevant; thus the percentage who were very satisfied who had had no partner was 15%, for those with only one partner it was 50%, and for those with more than one partner it was 38%.

A recent Kinsey Institute survey of 987 women in a heterosexual relationship focused on predictors and possible determinants of sexual well-being and distress or concern about sex. The survey was restricted to those with English as their first language, and black women were over-sampled. Comparisons of the white and black women will be considered in the section on culture later in this chapter. Women were asked to evaluate two aspects of their sexual lives, their sexual relationship and their own sexuality, by rating each aspect as 'excellent', 'very good', 'good', 'fair' or 'poor', and also indicating how much distress or worry each aspect had caused them during the past 4 weeks, rating 'no distress', 'slight distress', 'moderate distress' or 'a great deal of distress'. As the last two categories were indicated infrequently, they were combined as 'marked distress'. The distributions of these evaluations of sexual relationship and own sexuality are shown in Table 6.13a (Bancroft et al in press) and Table 6.13b (Bancroft et al 2003a).

A range of potential predictors were assessed, covering demographic factors (age, education, income and number of children), health (BMI, menopausal status, mental health and physical health) and aspects of sexual activity in the past month (frequency of sexual activity with partner, masturbation, orgasm, vaginal lubrication, rapid ejaculation or erectile problems in the partner, and two composite scales covering the woman's own response during sexual activity (physical response and subjective response scales).

Using logistic regression, the following variables were significant predictors of an excellent/very good sexual relationship: mental health (positive, as measured by the MCS12; $p < 0.01$), frequency of sexual activity (positive, $p < 0.01$), frequency of masturbation (negative, $p < 0.01$), partner's sexual attractiveness (positive, $p < 0.01$) and subjective response scale (positive, $p < 0.01$). This scale covers the proportion of occasions of sexual activity when the woman felt 'pleasure', 'emotionally close', 'not indifferent' and 'no unpleasant feelings'. The following were significant predictors of excellent/very good own sexuality: mental health (positive, $p < 0.01$), orgasm frequency (positive, $p < 0.01$), self-ratings of sexual attractiveness (positive, $p < 0.01$) and income (negative, $p < 0.05$). It is noteworthy that the physical response scale, which assesses the proportion of sexual acts when the

woman felt sexually aroused, felt pleasant tingling in genitals and enjoyed genitals being touched, was not predictive of their evaluation of either their sexual relationship or their own sexuality.

Using multinomial logit, the following were significant positive predictors of distress about the sexual relationship: low ratings on the subjective response scale ($p < 0.01$), low scores for mental health (MCS; $p < 0.01$), low frequency of sexual activity ($p = 0.01$), rapid ejaculation in the partner ($p = 0.01$), thinking about sex daily ($p = 0.04$), impaired physical response (physical response scale; $p = 0.04$) and age ($p = 0.05$). For distress about own sexuality, low mental health (MCS12) was the strongest predictor ($p < 0.01$), but poor physical health (PCS 12) was also significant ($p = 0.01$). Subjective response scale and partner's rapid ejaculation were less strongly predictive ($p = 0.03$ in each case), than of sexual relationship. Neither impaired physical response nor frequency of sexual thoughts were predictive.

These findings emphasize the importance of frequency of sexual activity to sexual well-being for many women, though it is not clear whether it is the sexual activity per se or the fact that their partner wants sex (i.e. the woman is 'desired') that is important, and this may vary across women. The weak though interesting association between frequency of sexual thoughts and distress about the relationship suggests that women who are thinking about sex with interest, but are infrequently engaging in sexual activity with their partner, are more likely to be distressed about the relationship. The importance of mental health is also clear. The occurrence of sexual arousal appears to be of limited importance to women's sexual well-being. Frequency of orgasm was predictive of positive ratings of the woman's own sexuality, but not of her relationship, and not of distress or worry in either respect. In contrast, the more subjective aspects of the sexual experience were more important to her sexual relationship. This is consistent with the other findings from this study, shown in Table 6.12. Feeling emotionally close to one's partner was very important for the sexual happiness of 83.5% of the women, knowing that your partner is sexually satisfied, very important for 78.9%, and feeling comfortable talking to one's partner about sexual activity, very important for 61.8%. In contrast, having an orgasm herself was very important for the sexual happiness of only 29.6% of the women. These findings suggest that sexual happiness is more dependent on the relationship than the woman's own sexuality. It would be interesting to have directly comparable evidence from men. These findings in relation to distress about sex and their relevance to sexual problems will be considered further in Chapter 11.

TABLE 6.13a Evaluations of 'sexual relationship' and 'own sexuality' in women in heterosexual relationships (n = 987; age 20–65); Bancroft et al in press	Fair/poor	Good	Very good	Excellent
Sexual relationship	24.3%	24.4%	31.9%	19.4%
Own sexuality	18.5%	29.0%	37.0%	15.5%

TABLE 6.13b	Ratings of distress or worry about the sexual relationship and the woman's own sexuality during the past month (Bancroft et al 2003a)		
	None	Slight	Marked
1. Sexual relationship	53.1%	27.1%	19.8%
2. Own sexuality	57.7%	27.5%	14.7%
3. 1 and/or 2	44.2%	31.4%	24.4%

Johnson et al (1994), in the NATSAL 1990, obtained responses to two statements about the importance of sex within a marriage or relationship: (i) 'Companionship and affection are more important than sex', 67% of men and 68% of women agreed, 11% of men and 10% of women disagreed; (ii) 'Sex is the most important part of any marriage or relationship', 17% of men and 16% of agreed, 62% of men and 68% of women disagreed. Of various factors, faithfulness and mutual respect ranked the highest in importance, sex came third, followed by having children, shared interests, shared chores, adequate income and shared religious beliefs.

When participants, aged 16–44 years, in the NATSAL 2000 survey were asked to choose what would be the ideal relationship 'now', 40.9% of the men chose 'married with no other sex partners', 17.6% chose 'not married, but living with a partner, and no other sex partners', 21.1%, 'one regular partner but not living together'. For the women, the percentages for these choices were 48.5, 19.0 and 21.7, respectively. Comparable figures from the NATSAL 1990 showed greater preference for monogamous marriage (47.1% for men and 54.3% for women) and less preference for monogamous co-habiting (10% of men and 14.4% of women), further evidence of a shift from marriage to co-habiting. These percentages in the NATSAL 2000 data varied considerably by age, as one would expect. For example, of those 16–19 years, only 3.9% of men and 5.4% of women saw marriage as the ideal 'now', whereas 45.5% of men and 50.4% of women in that age group chose 'one regular partner, but not living together' (Erens et al 2003).

The fate of marriage

The increase in marital breakdown and divorce is an international phenomenon, occurring in just about every country in which it has been studied. Most countries showed a rise after World War II, presumably reflecting the unstable nature of many wartime marriages; this was followed by a decline in the 1950s. However, the number of divorces each year in the UK doubled between 1958 and 1969. In England and Wales divorce became legally easier to obtain in 1971 with the divorce law reform. This was followed by a further rise in the divorce rate (Fig. 6.9). Further legislation in 1976 led to a similar increase in Scotland.

Divorce rates are expressed in various ways (e.g. absolute numbers, rates per 100 married, rates per 1000 per capita), making comparisons in the literature difficult. According to Crouch et al (2007), divorce rates in 1999, expressed as number of divorces per 1000 per capita,

ranged in European countries from 0.6 in Italy to 3.65 in Russia, with the UK fourth highest with 2.66. About 20% of the general increase has been attributed to legal reforms making divorce easier, which have taken place in most European countries (Gonzalez & Viitanen 2006).

In the USA there is considerable variability across states in the divorce rates, partly due to the variations in divorce laws from state to state. For the USA overall, Crouch et al (2007) reported rates of 2.6 per 1000 capita in 1950 peaking at 5.3 in 1979 and reducing steadily to 4.0 in 2001. These rates still remain higher than in any European countries.

Divorce is most likely in the early years of marriage. After 5 years, around 10% of marriages have ended in divorce, by 10 years of marriage another 10% (20% total). However, it is not until about the 18th year that the total reaches 30%, and the 40% level not until around the 50th year of marriage (Kreider & Fields 2002). The average age at time of divorce in the UK rose from 39 in 1991 to 43 in 2004 for husbands, and from 36 to 40 for wives in the same time period (Babb et al 2006).

The explanations for these universal trends are likely to be complex. Changes in the role of women, resulting in their having more independence, are likely to be relevant, as are changes in the emphasis on marriage as the only acceptable status for sexual activity.

Extramarital sex

Clearly the relationship between sexual satisfaction and marital happiness is likely to be a two-way process and it is thus very difficult to establish to what extent marital breakdown actually results from sexual incompatibility. Similarly, it is not easy to decide to what extent extra-marital sexuality is a result or a cause of marital disharmony. Extramarital sex may be tried by someone in an unhappy marriage to see if an alternative relationship is preferable (Walster et al 1978) and in this sense commonly occurs in the period preceding divorce. The available evidence certainly suggests that women are more likely to experience extramarital sex if they are unhappy in their marriage (Bell et al 1975) and this may be less obvious for men.

Social sanctions against extramarital sex are found in the majority of societies. In some, such as modern Islam, the punishment for offenders can be severe. In certain states of the USA adultery, to use the legal term, is still a criminal offence, though rarely prosecuted as such. Most primitive societies restrict extramarital sex and in the exceptions limits are usually set as to who can be involved (Ford & Beach 1952). In general, the taboo against extramarital sex is greater than that against premarital sex. Another manifestation of the 'double standard' is that extramarital activity by husbands tends to be more accepted than that by wives. Broude & Greene (1980), in their analysis of 116 societies, found 43% in which extramarital sex was accepted for men but not for women, and only 11% where it was accepted for both men and women. The related aspect, which is probably important for the married man who is expected to take responsibility for the fathering and material welfare of his children, is the threat of cuckoldry, of being deceived by another man into rearing his child. This is an intriguing issue. There is an inescapable and fundamental sex difference in the reproductive consequences of extramarital sexuality. The male may see the surreptitious introduction of another man's child into his 'nest' as a serious attack on his honour or he may see it as a threat to the existence of his own offspring. How can he be sure that any of his children are his own? These two reactions may be different versions of the same thing, the first being a humanized version of a basic biological mechanism. The idea of one man deceiving another man into bringing up his child raises some questions. This concept obviously derives from evolutionary psychology, where male sexual behaviour is seen as determined by a need to father as many children as possible, and hence assure that one's genes thrive. An alternative view is that men's sexuality is driven by a need for sexual pleasure which may be unaccompanied by a sense of responsibility for the consequences. 'Cuckoldry' may well capture a genuine male concern, but this may be more to do with passing on one's assets to a child who is not one's own, possibly compounded by a sense of being deceived by one's wife.

Whereas there has been a substantial reduction in the stigma associated with premarital sex, this is not the case with extramarital sex, or even 'extra-relationship' sex in the case of co-habiting couples. In the British NATSAL 1990 and 2000 surveys (Johnson et al 1994; Erens et al 2003) the negative attitudes to such 'infidelity' actually increased. In 1990, 77.6% of men and 83.2% of women considered extramarital sex wrong. In 2000, the figures were 84.4% and 88.7%, respectively. Intolerance of infidelity in co-habiting relationships was not much less, and showed a similar increase. Even with non-co-habiting but 'regular' relationships, 70.3% of men and 81.1% of women in 2000 considered sex outside the relationship to be wrong, and this had increased from 59.2% of men and 70% of women in 1990. There is comparable evidence from the General Social Survey (GSS) in the USA (GSS 1972–2000). Between 1972, when the GSS started and 1982, 70.5% of the respondents indicated that extramarital sex was always wrong. This proportion increased gradually and by 1998 was 77.9%. Thus there seems to be a strengthening of the importance of fidelity and commitment whether married, co-habiting or not. However, we do not have comparable data from surveys before the 1970s and it is possible that we are seeing a return to earlier values after a period, around the 1960s and 1970s when the stigma associated with extramarital sex lessened.

Apart from attitudes about extramarital sex, to what extent does it occur? In Kinsey's study, 28.7% of white college-educated males in his sample and 21% of the white college-educated females reported engaging in extramarital sexual intercourse during their first marriage. According to the NHSLS, in 1991 25.2% of males and 14.5% of females reported extramarital sex, similar to the figures from the 1991 GSS, 21.7% and 13.4%, respectively (Laumann et al 1994). Thus in the USA, the behaviour appears to have changed along with the attitudes, particularly among women. However, we should keep in mind that Kinsey's sample was college educated and not representative. Unfortunately, neither the British NATSAL nor the French ACSF established the incidence of extramarital sex.

The impact of social class

Kinsey's data indicated a striking social class difference for teenage sexuality, also apparent in the sexual play of children. Working-class adolescents were more likely to experience sexual intercourse and at an earlier age than those from the middle classes. Conversely, middle-class adolescents were more likely to participate in sexual activity other than coitus (e.g. heavy petting, mutual masturbation and oral sex). However, Kinsey's findings in this respect were probably amplified by the problems with his sample, particularly for the lower socio-economic groups. Schofield (1965) found broadly similar associations in the UK, particularly for the boys. His middle-class girls were much more likely to have experienced genital stimulation short of intercourse than the working-class girls, though the proportions with experience of intercourse were similar.

Schmidt & Sigusch (1971) compared young workers with students in West Germany. In their first study of 20-year-olds carried out between 1966 and 1968, they found a striking social class difference in sexual experience. Whereas 81% of the male workers had experienced coitus by the age of 20, only 44% of the male students had done so. This difference was evident from the age of 13 onwards, the workers showing two to four times higher incidence at each age. Similarly, for the females, 83% of the workers and 33% of the students had experienced coitus, a difference also maintained throughout adolescence. On average, the workers, both male and female, started their sexual careers about 4 years earlier than the students (though they also married earlier so the duration of the premarital sexual activity was not so different). There was also a social class effect on the gender difference in number of sexual partners. The male workers had experienced sex with more partners than the female workers. This gender difference was not marked for the students. The pattern of sexual activity other than coitus also showed class differences similar to those reported by Kinsey. The students were more likely to report manual-genital and oral-genital contact as well as nudity during love-making than were the workers, who were more likely to limit their activities to coitus proper.

Schmidt & Sigusch (1972) went on to reveal striking changes in this pattern between 1962 and 1970. This was mainly in the higher education group. By the age of 17, male and female schoolchildren in the Gymnasium stream (i.e. pre-university) had had as much sexual experience as students born 8 years earlier had had by the age of 20 years. Thus, the striking social class difference in age of onset of sexual activity had largely disappeared. Conversely, the lower educational group was now experiencing more non-coital forms of sexual activity.

In 1981, Fisher and Byrne reviewed the evidence, and summarized it as follows: compared with the lower classes, middle-class men and women had more permissive sexual attitudes, were more likely to masturbate, starting earlier, more likely to experience orgasm during petting (for males), had first premarital sexual intercourse at a later age, used more varied techniques during marital sexual activity, had less extramarital sexual activity early in marriage, but more later in marriage, and reported more subjective satisfaction with marital sex. Overall, the generational changes that were moving towards more permissive sexuality were occurring across the social classes and were, in some societies more than others, reducing the social class differences. In Australia, for example, McCabe & Collins (1983) found no effect of social class on the dating behaviour of adolescents.

The impact of social class end educational level on teenage pregnancies was emphasized earlier in this chapter (see p. 197). The reasons for this, as discussed, are likely to be complex, but some consideration has been given to contraceptive use. In the British NATSAL 1990, the minority of men and women not using any form of contraception were more likely to come from the lower classes. However, for the remainder there were no clear class differences in which contraceptive methods were used.

In the NHSLS, Laumann et al (1994) concluded that oral sex had increased in 'nearly all sections of society, not just the better educated or middle class groups' (p. 102). 'Social class', however, is not used as one of the 'master statuses' in their analyses, reflecting a different approach to socio-economic stratification in the USA compared to Britain. Instead, level of education and, to a limited extent, income were used. More conservative sexual attitudes were more likely in the lower educational groups, whereas masturbation was more likely and more frequent in the higher educated.

The British NATSAL 1990 (Johnson et al 1994), suggested that these social class differences were also lessening in Britain, but more slowly. The age at first sexual intercourse showed a similar social class difference in the age cohorts from 16 to 44 years, though it was more marked in those aged 45 years and above. These data also suggest that the convergence of males and females in their age at first intercourse started earlier in the higher social class groups. The substantial increase in recent years in non-coital behaviours, such as oral sex, was apparent across social classes, while the extent of the class differences remained much as before.

The impact of culture

Cultural contrasts within North America and Europe

Kinsey was struck by the gender difference in the apparent impact of socio-cultural factors. He found marked social class differences in patterns of sexual behaviour among his male subjects, which he did not find with women. He interpreted this as indicating that male sexuality was more socio-culturally determined and female sexuality more biologically determined. His own evidence, however, goes against this explanation. Comparison of cohorts of women in his study, born in the late 19th century with those born mid 20th century shows substantial changes in patterns of sexual behaviour, which can only be the result of changes in the impact of socio-cultural factors. An alternative explanation for this gender difference is therefore that the sexuality of men gets shaped but not suppressed by social influences, whereas the sexuality of women can be suppressed across the socio-cultural spectrum (Bancroft 1998). The past 50 years have seen further major changes in the role of women, and in their ability to control their reproductive lives, changes likely to be associated with further reduction of social suppression of female sexuality. And indeed, the most recent evidence shows further change in women's sexuality, with further reduction in some of the gender differences. This raises questions about the impact of culture on sexuality.

The USA is a multi-cultured society, as increasingly are most European societies, and involves three types of culture. First, the indigenous Native Americans; unfortunately, as yet we have little evidence of their sexuality. Secondly, immigrant cultures; the predominant group in this category have been the whites of European origin. More recently there has been a substantial increase in Hispanics with various Latin American origins and to a lesser extent, Asians, mainly from West Asia (e.g. China, Japan or Korea), but also from East Asia (e.g. India). Third, there are African Americans, who are not immigrants; their ancestors were brought to the USA as slaves. There are no equivalent subcultures in Europe with this origin. In the case of native cultures, we need to focus on countries where there is a clearly dominant ethnic group. With immigrant groups we have the impact of acculturation, which obscures to varying degrees how their original culture shapes their sexuality. With African Americans we have convincing evidence of a specific subculture in the USA (Weinberg & Williams 1988), with different attitudes, norms and beliefs compared to whites (Sterk-Elifson 1994), argued by Staples (1981) to have resulted from the African past, the impact of slavery and the continuing oppression and exploitation. This involves a long history of socio-economic deprivation in comparison with white Americans, making it important to disentangle cultural from socio-economic effects. However, this long history enables us to make comparisons between a relatively discreet subculture and the main culture, and over a longer period. We will therefore consider them first. We will then look at the process of acculturation before making comparisons among immigrant groups. Finally, we will look at a society with a predominantly 'native' culture. In recent years the literature on the sexuality of such cultures has increased substantially. Here attention will be restricted to one important example, China.

The black American

In 2002, 13% of the population in the USA were black (US Census Bureau 2003). Although differences in the early sexual experiences and sexual attitudes of white and black American men and women have been documented for some time, until relatively recently there has been little survey research focusing on these racial differences.[2] Kinsey, in his two volumes (Kinsey et al 1948, 1953) did not report on his black sample as he did not consider it large enough. His findings, however, were presented by Gebhard & Johnson (1979). The black sample (177 men and 223 women) were all college educated, and are compared with the large sample of college-educated whites in Table 6.14. This shows gender as well as racial differences. The black males were much more likely to report early onset of sexual activity than the whites. A similar racial difference is apparent for the females, but at a much lower level. Those reporting three or more premarital partners show a similar pattern, with the gender difference being less marked. The black females had almost twice the incidence of premarital pregnancy. The numbers who had experience of oral sex were not only low by recent standards, but also showed the reverse racial pattern, more marked in the females. Of interest are the numbers who had masturbated before the age of 13 years; they show more white than black males, but for the females the racial difference, while not as large, is in the opposite direction. We will return to this point later.

This pattern of earlier onset of coital sex in blacks than whites but more non-coital sex in whites than blacks has persisted, although in recent years both the gender and the racial gaps have been narrowing. The higher rates of premarital pregnancy in black women has been associated with an even greater racial difference in the rates of teenage childbirth, a sensitive issue in the political controversy about teenage pregnancy, considered earlier. But again the racial gap has narrowed. Between 1970 and 1996 the non-marital birth rate for white teenagers rose from 10.9 to 34.5 per 1000. Among black teenagers it increased from 96.9 in 1970 to 108.5 per 1000 in 1991, and then declined to 89.2 per 1000 in 1996. The racial difference is still large, but less so (Nathanson 2000).

The earlier age at first sexual intercourse is still evident. Santelli et al (2000b), using logistic regression, assessed predictors of sexual intercourse experience among 14- to 17-year-olds in the 1992 Youth Risk Behaviour Survey. Being black was predictive though more strongly for males than females. Joyner & Laumann (2001) explored possible predictors or determinants of onset of sexual intercourse before age 18 in the NHSLS (Laumann et al 1994). To assess how this had changed over time they divided their respondents into those who reached adolescence before and those after the sexual revolution. For males, being black increased the odds almost threefold, but this did not change from pre to post revolution. For females, being black increased the odds, but this effect was greater in the post-revolution group. Joyner & Laumann (2001) had predicted it would be greater in females in the pre-revolution group, but pointed out that this group difference was only a trend ($p < 0.10$).

The greater likelihood of vaginal intercourse in black, and heavy petting and oral sex in white, relationships raises the question of which is 'conventional' or 'traditional'. This was a manifestation of social class difference in the past (e.g. Kinsey et al 1948), but such differences between black and white women persisted (Weinberg & Williams 1988), or became even more marked (Mahay et al 2001) when controlling for socio-economic factors.

Age at puberty is a factor in determining age at first sexual activity, and racial differences in this respect have to be taken into consideration. Average age at puberty is earlier in African Americans than white Americans, with Mexican Americans coming midway. These differences apply to both males and females (Witchel & Plant 2004). The reasons for such racial differences are likely to be complex, with dietary factors being of possible relevance. This is reflected in the tendency to higher body weight in African American than white American women (see below). We should keep in mind, however, that genetic factors, in addition to cultural influences, may be involved, reflecting different patterns of adaptation to contrasting environments in earlier human development (e.g. Mediterranean versus Northern European; see p. 191 for further discussion).

Racial differences are found in relation to marriage and divorce. Between the 1950s and late 1970s, the mean age of white women at first marriage rose from 21.4 to 23.0 years; for black women the increase was from 21.9 to 26.1 (Hofferth 1990). By 1996, for men aged 25–29 years, 45% of white and 62% of black men had never married; for women of that age, it was 31% and 58%, respectively. Also by 1996, 40% of white and 48% of black marriages had ended in divorce (Kreider & Fields 2002).

TABLE 6.14	Sexual experiences in white and black college-educated Americans (The Kinsey Data; Gebhard & Johnson 1979)			
	Males		**Females**	
	White	**Black**	**White**	**Black**
$n =$	4694	177	4358	223
First sexual intercourse by age 16	20.9%	55.8%	6.0%	16.1%
3 or more premarital partners	61.2%	88.4%	34.9%	49.6%
Experience of oral sex				
Fellatio	21.0%	10.2%	37.8%	8.9%
Cunnilingus	11.8%	7.6%	41.4%	13.8%
First masturbated before age 13	30.7%	17.2%	16.7%	21.0%
Premarital pregnancy	—	—	13.4%	24.3%

[2]The terminology in this context is a sensitive issue. In this book I will use 'race' when referring to a group with common origins, and 'ethnicity' when referring to a racially distinct nation. The USA is not a racially distinct nation.

Given our particular interest in the major changes in women's sexuality during the 20th century, how do black and white American women compare in the role that sexuality plays in their lives and their relationships? Orbuch et al (2002) compared white and black marriages over their first 14 years. They found substantially more of the black marriages had ended in divorce during the 14 years (50.3% versus 29.3%). Interestingly, relationship problems were less predictive of divorce in the black compared to the white marriages. Oggins et al (1993a,b) studied white and black newly married couples; they were all aged 35 years or younger, and were assessed between the fifth and eighth month of their marriage. White women were more likely than black women to link sexual enjoyment with affirmation of their marriage. Black wives gave greater weight to positive sexual relations per se. This led Oggins et al (1993a) to suggest that 'white culture is relatively puritanical about people — and particularly women — enjoying sexual experience in its own right' (p. 158). Other evidence is consistent with this suggestion. For example, in an earlier study of college women (Houston 1981), greater interest in one's own sexual satisfaction than that of one's partner was more often indicated by black than white women.

In the recent Kinsey Institute survey of women in heterosexual relationships, black women were oversampled to allow racial comparisons with white women (Bancroft et al, in press). As described earlier (see p. 211; and Table 6.13a) women in this study were asked to evaluate their 'sexual relationship' and their 'own sexuality'. Controlling for socio-economic factors, black women were significantly more positive than white women about their own sexuality. This is consistent with the evidence, discussed above, that black women are more likely to value their sexual pleasure for its own sake. It is also consistent with the conclusion by Mahay et al (2001) that for white women sex is more relationship dependent. Another clear finding was that a woman's rating of her own sexual attractiveness was strongly predictive of her evaluation of her own sexuality, emphasizing how important feeling attractive is to a woman's sexual well-being. Black women were significantly more likely to rate themselves as sexually attractive than were white women, accounting for around one-third of the racial difference in ratings of own sexuality. We therefore explored predictors of sexual attractiveness. Of particular interest was body weight. Women with BMI scores in the ideal range were more likely to regard themselves as sexually attractive. However, black women clearly have a different concept of 'ideal' weight, at least as far as its relevance to sexual attractiveness is concerned. For each category of BMI, black women were more likely than white women to rate themselves as sexually attractive. These findings are consistent with the literature in two particular respects. Black women tend to have higher self-esteem than white women (Twenge & Crocker 2002). Self-esteem may be further enhanced in those with established sexual relationships, given that usually there are more women than men in African American communities. In addition, black women have more positive body images than white

women, and this applies to both weight-related and non-weight-related aspects of body image (Roberts et al 2006). Our findings suggested that black women's higher self-esteem and more positive body image translate into feeling more sexually attractive than white women feel.

White and black women did not differ in their evaluations of their sexual relationships. However, the predictors of these evaluations did differ for the two groups in several respects, and two of these differences are of particular interest. A tendency for their partners to ejaculate rapidly was associated with more negative evaluations of their sexual relationship by black women. This is consistent with their attaching more importance to their own sexual pleasure than white women. A partner's rapid ejaculation may lead to early termination of the sexual interaction, with the potential for leaving the woman frustrated. On the other hand, the frequency of the woman's masturbation had a negative impact on white women's evaluations of their relationship. This may be because they see the need for masturbation as resulting from insufficient sexual activity with the partner, possibly indicating that the partner is not sufficiently attracted to them. But it may also reflect the white woman's need to justify her sexuality in terms of her relationship. In the NHSLS, black women masturbated more often than white women, and felt less guilty about it, though the significance of these differences was not addressed (Laumann et al 1994). If black women feel more comfortable with their sexual pleasure in its own right, this could result in masturbation being a more positive experience for them. It is therefore of interest that, in the original Kinsey data from college-educated women, shown in Table 6.14, a higher proportion of black women than white women reported masturbating.

The importance of four factors to the woman's sexual happiness were also assessed in Bancroft et al (in press), and the responses for the whole sample are shown in Table 6.12. In comparing white and black women in this sample, there were two significant differences. White women attached more importance to feeling emotionally close to their partner (38.9% rating this 'extremely important' compared to 24% of black women, $p = 0.002$). Black women attached more importance to being able to talk to their partner about sex (59.4% of white women rating this 'very important' or 'extremely important' compared with 74.4% of black women; $p < 0.05$).

The findings of this and other studies clearly point to cultural differences in how black and white women experience their sexuality and sexual relationships, differences not explainable by socio-economic factors. The apparently greater comfort of black women with their own sexual pleasure, independent of their partner's pleasure, may in part result from black women's greater self-reliance and autonomy. Given the predominant African American culture in the USA, black women have less opportunity to rely on male partners for financial security and, as a consequence, are taught to value and pursue financial as well as emotional independence more than white women (e.g. Dugger 1988; Berkowitz and Padavic 1999). This cultural fostering of individualism may well contribute to their having higher self-esteem than white women.

The impact of religion also needs to be considered. The Protestant background of most white women in the USA may well account for their being more 'puritanical' about sex, as Oggins et al (1993a) commented, and their resulting need to justify their sexuality as a way of strengthening their marriages. Mahay et al (2001) found that black women were more likely to say that their religious beliefs shaped their sexuality, but even though most of them were Protestant and many of them were devout, it would seem that religion has shaped their sexuality differently. This was suggested sometime ago by Reiss (1967). Having found significantly greater permissiveness about premarital sex in black women compared to white (Reiss 1964), he went on to show that this ethnic difference was mainly found in 'high church attenders', with the black church attenders being more permissive. Furthermore, the black church attenders combined greater sexual permissiveness with high importance of romantic love; in white women these two were negatively correlated. Mahay et al (2001) concluded that black women preferred vaginal intercourse because they were more conservative in their sexual attitudes. An alternative view is that black women prefer vaginal intercourse because it is the 'natural' form of sexual expression, linked to reproduction, whereas white women (and men) have turned to non-coital forms of sexual expression as a way of coping with their more 'puritanical' constraints.

It is tempting to revisit the distinction between the virginity ethic and the fertility factor considered earlier in this chapter, and in particular the contrast between the Eurasian and African patterns of sexuality proposed by Goody (1971). Although probably an over-simplification, the difference we have been considering between black and white Americans fits this distinction. There is little evidence that virginity has held any importance in the African American culture, whereas there are indicators of a fertility factor. Visotsky (1969) described the attitudes to adolescent sexuality amongst blacks in a deprived area of Chicago. It was assumed that every girl would have sexual relations, whether married or not, and if this did not happen by the age of 18 or 19 years then there was something wrong with her. Boys not only gained in status by demonstrating their potency, but also by fathering children. 'Girls seek to please boys by having babies' was the attitude, even though the girl was expected to take responsibility for the offspring. Although lip service was paid to the undesirability of pregnancies out of wedlock, the resulting children were usually accepted by the girls' mothers.

To what extent can these differences between black and white women in the USA help us understand the substantial changes in women's sexuality through the 20th century? Such changes have occurred in the black community, but to a lesser extent than among whites, resulting in a narrowing of the racial gap. This points to the sexual revolution, with its move towards greater sexual permissiveness, as more relevant to the white community, and underlines the fundamental importance of culture to this major change.

Acculturation

When we consider the other racial minorities in the USA, in particular the Hispanic and Asian minorities, we are not only faced with much less evidence, but also the complicating effect of acculturation (Brotto et al 2005). In comparing, for example, white Americans and Asian Americans, we have to weigh up both the continuing impact of the culture of origin and the extent to which there has been acculturation to the new culture. This will depend in part on the extent to which the family lives in a relatively discrete ethnic community within the USA, and it is not simply a result of the length of time lived in the USA. There is also the issue of age and stage of development. Acculturation may be more evident in a young person who grows up in the new culture, whereas the impact on a couple who married in their country of origin and then immigrated may be different. Brotto et al (2005) explored the effects of acculturation in Asian Canadian female college students (average age 19.8 years). There were clear differences in various aspects of sexuality between Asian Canadian and European Canadian women, which will be considered further below. But by using a method developed by Ryder et al (2000) to measure separately the impact of (i) the 'heritage' culture (i.e. the culture of origin) and (ii) the 'mainstream' culture, they accounted for more of the variance in sexual attitudes, behaviours and responses than by simply comparing racial group or length of residency. We should also keep in mind that immigrants who go to college are more likely to experience acculturation than those who remain predominantly within their racial group.

An interesting example of acculturation was considered earlier (see p. 201). Whereas Zulu men living in their country of origin find heavier women more sexually attractive than white men do, Zulus who had emigrated to the UK, even quite recently, were similar to white British men in preferring slimmer women (Tovee et al 2006). The migration of Iranians to Sweden, two very contrasting cultures, is also of interest. The Islamic culture as found in Iran promotes two strikingly different aspects of sexuality. On the one hand, the Islamic principle of 'unity', by which the body and soul are seen as one, leads to a celebration of sexual pleasure, rather than the guilt that pervades Christian cultures. On the other hand, there is a powerful patriarchy, not in itself attributable to Islamic religious texts, which leads to objectification and subordination of women. The combination of these two factors leads to Iranian men believing themselves to have the right to demand sexual pleasure from their wives whenever they feel the urge. Female genitalia relate to cultural symbols of passiveness and submissiveness, whereas male genitalia relate to cultural symbols of action and dominance (Ahmadi 2003). In many Iranian couples who emigrate to Sweden there is a shift to more equity in the relationship, and a tendency to separation and divorce, with the women not infrequently finding it easier to adapt and integrate to the Swedish culture than the men (Darvishpour 1999). In a qualitative study, Ahmadi (2003) gave examples of how Iranian women resented their patriarchal suppression in Iran, and welcomed the chance to be more independent in Sweden, both sexually and financially. The Iranian men, on the other hand, were more likely to strive to maintain the original status quo in their marital relationship. This raises the point that different individuals, in this case different genders, may obtain different benefits from a new culture. It also confronts us with the possibility that those who emigrate are different in important ways to those who stay at home. Thus, the USA, as a supreme example of this, has evolved by the interaction of immigrant groups, who rejected their traditional cultures for something new. So we have to keep in mind not only the impact of a culture, but also varying individual sensitivities to that impact.

Immigrant groups in North America

With this complicating impact of acculturation in mind, let us consider the limited evidence comparing immigrant groups within North America. The European white group will be used for comparison, but we should not forget its heterogeneous origins, Germany, the UK and Ireland being the most common, and no more than 20% coming from any one European country (Mahay et al 2001).

Hispanic Americans

In 2002, 13.3% of the population of the USA were Hispanic (US Census Bureau 2003), now the largest and most quickly growing racial minority. The term 'Hispanic' is used differently by different people, making demographic research difficult. According to Sabogal et al (1997), the terms 'Hispanic' and 'Latino' denote current residents of the USA who trace their background to a Latin American country, Spain or Portugal. By far the largest subgroup of Hispanics in the USA are Mexican Americans (66.9%); 14.3% are from Central and South America, 8.6% from Puerto Rico and 3.7% from Cuba (US Census Bureau 2003).

Mahay et al (2001) focused on the Mexican Americans in the NHSLS sample. They were predominantly and strongly Catholic, younger on average than the other racial groups, though with the same proportion married, and less educated. They held more traditional sexual values than European Americans and were more likely to believe that their religion shaped their sexuality. They showed little difference, however, in their likelihood of experiencing premarital sex. Mexican American women were more likely than white women to say they were in love the first time they had sexual intercourse. Mexican Americans' frequency of sexual activity with their partner was similar, though they were less likely to report engaging in oral sex, coming midway between whites and blacks in that respect. The other Hispanics

in this sample did not differ to any extent from the Mexican American group.

Acculturation and education play a significant role in determining the extent to which the traditional Hispanic pattern persists. This pattern shows traditional family attitudes, more conservative sexual values, but also patriarchal relationships between men and women, with men proving their virility by having multiple sex partners (Sabogal et al 1997).

Asian Americans

In 2002, 4.4% of the population of the USA were Asian or Pacific Islanders (US Census Bureau 2003). As yet, however, we have little research on the sexuality of American Asians, and more on Canadian Asians, particularly those who have emigrated to the west of Canada.

Meston et al (1996) compared Asian and non-Asian undergraduate students at a university in the west of Canada. Asian students were significantly more conservative than non-Asian on all measures of interpersonal sexual behaviour; their sexual fantasies were conservative and they were less likely to masturbate. There were no significant differences between Asians who were born in Canada and those who immigrated. In a later report on the same data, Meston et al (1998) reported that the number of years of residence was predictive of the change to more permissive sexual attitudes in the Asian immigrants.

Brotto et al (2005) compared Asian and white Euro-Canadian women college students in Canada. The Euro-Canadians reported significantly more sexual knowledge and experiences, more liberal sexual attitudes, and higher rates of sexual desire, arousal, sexual receptivity and sexual pleasure than the Asian women, who reported significantly more anxiety in anticipation of sexual activity.

Comparison of white, black, Hispanic and Asian women

An important new longitudinal study of middle-aged women is the Study of Women's Health Across the Nation. While not a nationally representative sample, women were recruited in the late pre-menopause phase or early peri-menopausal transition in order to follow them through to post-menopause. This study is considered in Chapter 7, in relation to the impact of the menopause on sexuality (Avis et al 2005). The sample of 3262 women, aged 42–52 years, included 47% white, 28.2% black, 8.8% Hispanic (mainly Puerto Rican), 7.5% Chinese and 8.5% Japanese, providing several racial groups large enough to permit statistical comparisons of sexuality variables from the baseline assessment, as reported by Cain et al (2003). The importance of sex was greatest for the black women, and least for the Japanese and Chinese women, with the white and Hispanic similar in this respect and between the others. Involvement in sexual activity did not differ across racial groups for those who were married, but unmarried black women were more likely to be active than unmarried whites. The most common reason for lack of sexual activity was lack of a sexual partner, except for the Japanese for whom lack of sexual interest was the most frequent reason. Lack of sexual interest was reported by around a third of women, and the racial groups did not differ significantly in this respect. Frequency of sexual desire, however, was lower in the Chinese and Japanese women compared to the other three groups. Amongst those who were sexually active, frequency of sexual intercourse, in comparison with white women, was significantly higher in black (OR 1.43) and lower in Japanese (OR 0.56) women. Oral sex was significantly less frequent in black, Chinese and Japanese, than in white and Hispanic. In comparison with whites, masturbation was significantly less frequent in all other racial groups. The percentages in each group who reported masturbating, at least occasionally, were 63.4% white, 37.9% black, 20.4% Hispanic, 35.9% Chinese and 49.6% Japanese. There was little difference across racial groups for emotional satisfaction or physical pleasure associated with sex. Overall, these findings for whites, blacks and Hispanics were consistent with those from the NHSLS (Mahay et al 2001); the number of Asian women in the NHSLS was insufficient for statistical analysis. We should be cautious in generalizing from this study however, because of the lack of representativeness of the samples, and the exclusion, because of the primary goals of the study, of women who had been hysterectomized or were using steroidal contraceptives or hormone replacement therapy. We should also keep in mind the possibility of cultural differences in how questions about sex are interpreted.

An example of an indigenous culture: China

China has the largest population of any country in the world. In 1995 this was 1.2 billion. Although 92% of the population are ethnic Chinese (Han Chinese) there are 55 racial groups represented in the remaining 8%. The long history of Chinese culture is mainly one of patriarchal domination of women, particularly since the Neo-Confucianists of the 12th Century. Chinese women were expected to be obedient to the father and elder brothers when young, to the husband when married, and to the sons when widowed. For more than 2000 years, for the vast majority of Chinese women, marriage was arranged by their parents, with emphasis on bearing male children and running an efficient household. The wife's acceptance within her husband's family remained uncertain until she had a male child. Belonging to a home was her only means of subsistence.

This changed to some extent with the establishment of the communist regime in 1949, the PRC. The Marriage Law of 1950 asserted equal rights for women but, while explicitly countering the traditional institutionalization of male dominance, did not address how this equality should be achieved, beyond enabling women to pursue careers outside the home. The expectation that women would also run the home persisted. To some extent this may have resulted from the political emphasis on collectivism; the husband and wife should be acting together

in support of the revolution. Since the end of the revolutionary period in the 1980s there has been a shift to individualism, with evidence of Westernization in various respects, the consequences of which are not all positive for women (Evans 2002). The repression of sexual expression, on the other hand, has had a very long history, was reinforced during the cultural revolution, and only started to lessen during this recent phase.

Although Buddhism, Islam and Christianity (both Catholic and Protestant) have all entered Chinese culture, the religious and spiritual heritage of China has principally been determined by Taoism and Confucianism. Taoism promotes the more joyful and carefree, whereas Confucianism promotes the more austere, purposeful and moral aspects of Chinese culture. The ancient concepts of yin and yang pervade Chinese ways of conceptualizing the world. Among other things, yin is conceived of as earth, female, dark, passive and absorbing; yang as heaven, male, light, active and penetrating (*Encyclopaedia Britannica* 2001). These quintessentially Chinese concepts have also been used to describe female (yin) and male (yang) genitalia for several thousand years. When yin and yang combine 'all things become harmony' (Ruan & Lau 2001). This underlines a crucial issue when making cross-cultural comparisons; here is a fundamentally different way of thinking about one's world, with a common theme applied to a wide range of issues. From an English language perspective, this may be reflected in the use of gender in many other languages (e.g. French or Italian), where inanimate objects are either male or female. Certainly in Chinese culture, gender is linked to many other things; there is no clear and discrete conceptualization of 'male' and 'female', and sex is derived from this way of thinking about gender. This confronts us with the likelihood of considerable differences in the ways that ethnic Chinese and ethnic English think about sex, and the challenge of drawing meaningful comparisons of sexual experience.

In several respects, however, we are seeing a sociocultural change in Chinese sexuality that parallels earlier changes in Europe and North America. But even today, the prevailing sexual morality is that sexual expression should be restricted to heterosexual intercourse within monogamous marriage. A wide variety of sexual behaviours are explicitly proscribed: prostitution, premarital and extramarital sex (including co-habitation arrangements); homosexuality, and paraphilias are still against the law, although are less and less likely to be prosecuted (Ruan & Lau 2001). Non-coital activity such as oral sex and masturbation remain stigmatized, and the belief that masturbation damages one's health is still prevalent. Officially both men and women are meant to be monogamous; however, responsibility for this is still seen to lie with the woman (Evans 2002), a feature of most patriarchal societies, and a basis of the 'double standard'.

A particular problem for the Chinese in recent times, which has promoted change in their 'official' approach to sex, has been over-population. As in the West, there were also increases in rates of teenage pregnancy, juvenile sex crime and sexually transmitted diseases. A birth control programme was instituted in the 1970s and there have been limited attempts to provide sex education for young people since (Ruan & Lau 2001). In addition, there are clear demographic indications of change in the 'Westerly' direction; an increase in the proportion of the population who are unmarried, a substantial increase in the number of divorces, mainly initiated by women on the grounds of infidelity by their husbands, and an increase in the proportion of women who have a career outside the home.

In 1992, the results of a large survey of sexuality in China were reported (Liu et al 1992). The following is based on a summary of the findings included in Ruan & Lau (2001). The typical adolescent female was described as 15.5 years old, with menarche at 13 years (older than in many parts of the world, but younger than it used to be in China), with interest in sex starting around 14–15. By age of 15.5 years, 11% were dating and 6% were 'in love'. Only 5% reported having ever masturbated although nearly 40% 'did not understand the question'. Less than 2% had engaged in kissing or non-coital sexual touching and 1% had experienced sexual intercourse. The typical male teenager was 15.5 years old and his average age at spermarche 14.5 years — again this is older than in most other societies but younger than in China previously. At that age he started to show sexual interest and was attracted to girls, but was too shy or busy to act on his feelings. About one-third of adolescent boys desired sexual contact, and 43% had been sexually aroused enough to want sexual intercourse. Only 13% were dating and 8% were 'in love'. Less than 5% of secondary school boys had engaged in kissing or sexual touching, and 0.9% had experienced sexual intercourse. These figures for both girls and boys are strikingly different to those from Western countries.

The typical female college student in this sample had received little sex education, accepted romantic love if it is 'properly guided', saw sex as being primarily for reproduction, but accepted that the female can be an active partner during sexual intercourse. Premarital sex was acceptable if there was mutual love, but extramarital sex was not. Seventy per cent did not feel good about their bodies, for various reasons, including being overweight, or their breasts being too small, and 43% said they would prefer to be male if they had the choice. Only 6% had had a sexual relationship and sexual activity of any kind was unusual until after the age of 17 years. Masturbation was reported by 16.5% at some stage, with 8% continuing to masturbate. Most thought it 'harmless' or 'normal'. The typical male college student was similar in most respects, although only 8% wished they were female. Masturbation was reported by 59%, starting between 14 and 16 years. Only 12.5% had had a sexual relationship, and seldom more than one.

The typical urban married couple, aged around 36 years, and married on average about 11 years, considered 'love ' and 'understanding' more important than material well-being or their social standing. They had sex four to five times a month on average, and regarded marital sex as primarily for satisfying emotional and physical needs. Foreplay was usually brief, and gave less pleasure to the woman. Those urban wives with more independence and higher self-esteem felt less compelled to have sex when they did not want it. They had an equal wish to have a boy or girl child. Premarital sex was reported by 25% of husbands and 16% of wives.

The typical rural couple reported a slightly higher frequency of sexual intercourse, on average five to six times a month. Premarital sex was reported by 7% of husbands and 17% of wives.

Overall, these recent findings, together with those from other smaller Chinese surveys, indicate a substantial shift from traditional patterns of sexuality and gender relationships, consistent with the influence of Western standards through the media and advertising (Evans 2002).

Sexual desire and sexual fantasy

Sexual desire

The concept of sexual desire was considered in Chapter 4 and its conceptual limitations recognized (p. 131). The crucial issue is the distinction between sexual 'desire' and sexual 'arousal', and in the earlier chapter I proposed that we see these two constructs as 'windows' into the complexity of sexual arousal, one focusing on the incentive motivation component (desire), the other on the arousal component (excitement). In any case we are dealing with an aspect of human sexuality of fundamental importance. 'Appetite' for sex varies across time, dependent on a range of factors, varies across individuals and across genders. Some individuals have strong and some weak appetites for sex. On average men have stronger appetites for sex than women (for review see Baumeister et al 2001). However, as with most aspects of sexuality there is more variability in this respect in women than in men. Part of our problem is that this issue has mainly been considered in relation to sexual problems, or 'dysfunctions', and this literature will be considered more closely in Chapter 11. But whereas attention has been paid to those who complain of low sexual desire, designated in the DSM-IV as hypoactive sexual desire disorder (HSDD), we have little understanding of 'normal' sexual desire, and how individuals vary in this respect, nor how many individuals have lived most of their lives with little or no sexual desire, and are not troubled by it; this relates to the concept of 'asexuality' which will be considered later. Once again we are confronted by some crucial questions about gender differences.

Kinsey and colleagues did not directly attempt to assess sexual desire, sexual interest or sexual appetite. They focused on behaviours and responses, and took orgasm to be the marker of relevant sexual activity, and the frequency of orgasm, from whatever cause, a measure of 'total sexual outlet'. Based on the assumption that if a male becomes sexually aroused he will do something to achieve orgasm, they used total sexual outlet as a measure of an individual's sexual drive (Kinsey et al 1948). In their male sample they found a mean total outlet of 2.7 orgasms per week (SD 0.02), and a median of 2.0. To illustrate the possible range, they described one male who had ejaculated once in 30 years and another, a lawyer, who had averaged 30 per week for 30 years! However, they recognized that this concept did not fit so well for women; in the female volume they commented that 'a considerable portion of the female's sexual activity does not result in orgasm' (Kinsey et al 1953, p. 45). They retained interest in the concept, however, seeing it as a useful measure of a woman's interest in or need for sex, and they presented their findings for total sexual outlet as the last chapter of results in the female volume. Their findings were very different for women; not only was the average total sexual outlet much lower, the variability was much greater, varying substantially not only by age and year of birth, but by marital status, socio-economic status and religion. Among those born after 1910, the average male had experienced more than 1500 orgasms before first marriage, the average female, 223. The median frequency per week by age, for single males and females, is shown in Fig. 6.12.

In recent surveys, even less attention has been paid to sexual desire or sexual interest. Laumann et al (1994) had one question; 'On the average, how often do you think about sex?' The possible answers were 'several times a day', 'every day', 'one to a few times a week', 'one to a few times a month', 'less than once a month' and 'I never think about sex'. 'Every day' or 'several times a day' was reported by 54% of men and 19% of women, 'a few times a month' to 'a few times a week' by 43% of men and 67% of women and 'less than once a month' or 'never' by 4% of men and 14% of women. Relevant questions were not asked in the British NATSAL, in either 1990 or 2000, nor in the French ACSF. More attention has been paid to assessing sexual interest in surveys focusing on ageing, and these are considered more closely in the next chapter (e.g. Table 7.2).

Assessing the level of sexual desire or interest in surveys of this kind raises methodological challenges. The approach used by Laumann et al (1994) was reasonable in that estimates of actual frequency were asked for. However, with this single question one is left with no idea

about the time period covered by the response or how stable the reported frequency is. Some studies have been even less informative in that no attempt to assess frequency was made, but rather some judgement about whether the frequency was low or not (see p. 181). Thus, Fugl-Meyer & Fugl-Meyer (1999), in a Swedish survey of men and women, asked whether there was 'decreased sexual interest' or a 'low level of desire'. While such questions enabled them to report that positive answers to both questions increased with age, one is left with no idea of what level of sexual interest is involved. In a recent large Danish survey (Eplov et al 2007), participants were asked 'How often do you have sexual desire?'. Not an unreasonable question, but the respondent was given the following response options: 'often', 'occasionally', 'rarely' or 'never'. Such choices are determined by what the respondent understands 'often' or 'occasionally' to mean, and it is highly likely that there will be considerable variability in such meanings. They also asked 'If you compare your sexual desire with your sexual desire 5 years ago, is it higher or lower now?'. This enabled them to report an association between reduced sexual desire and older age. However, they also concluded that men had significantly higher levels of sexual desire than women. All they can say is that men are more likely to report 'often' than women are. Given the potential for gender differences as well as individual differences in what such terms mean, their conclusion, while supported by other studies, is not justified on the basis of their data.

Asking someone how often they think about sex does not necessarily reveal how interested they are or how much desire they experience. In our research we have used 'frequency of sexual thoughts' as our way of assessing sexual interest or desire, but have always described what type of thoughts we are referring to, i.e. 'During the past 4 weeks, about how often did you think about sex with interest or desire? This includes times of just being interested, daydreaming and fantasizing, as well as times when you wanted to have sex' (Bancroft et al 2003a). The response options were 'not at all', 'once or twice', 'once a week', 'several times a week' and 'at least once a day'.

The relevant data from this survey, for frequency of sexual thoughts in the past month, are shown in Table 6.15 by age group. We have no comparable data

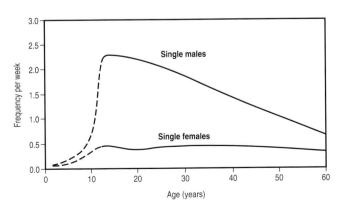

Fig. 6.12 Comparison of ageing patterns of frequency of orgasm (total outlet) in single women and men; median frequency per week. (From Kinsey et al 1953; Figure 143, p. 714.)

TABLE 6.15 Frequency of thinking about sex in the past month in women in heterosexual relationships (% of weighted sample, $n = 853$; Bancroft et al 2003a)

	Age groups			
	20–35	36–50	51–65	Total
Not at all	3.2	7.0	13.5	7.2
Once or twice	19.1	18.6	31.9	21.8
Once a week	30.4	31.5	31.2	31.0
Several times a week	27.8	29.9	16.0	26.0
Daily	19.5	13.0	7.3	14.0
Total	35.0	42.0	23.0	100

The full question was, 'How often did you think about sex with interest or desire? This includes times of just being interested, daydreaming or fantasizing, as well as times when you wanted to have sex' for men, although data for older men and women in the AARP study are shown in Table 7.2 (Chapter 7), indicating a much higher frequency of sexual thoughts for men than for women in these older age groups.

As mentioned earlier (see p. 211), we found in these women an association between higher frequency of sexual thoughts and distress about the sexual relationship (Bancroft et al 2003a). Was this because the woman with high frequency of sexual thoughts and more sexual desire was more likely to be dissatisfied with her relationship because her needs were not being met, or did she think more about sex because she was not happy about her sexual relationship? We cannot make a certain distinction between these two interpretations; many women in this study with high and low frequency of sexual thoughts were satisfied with their relationship.

Beck et al (1991) pointed out that without clear evidence of the level of experienced desire in the non-clinical population, it is problematic to make a diagnosis of hypoactive or inhibited desire. Only limited progress has been made since then. There has been a lack of clear focus on what it is that is being desired. Whereas for men this may be relatively predictable, it is not so in the case of women, and even with men we should not make assumptions on this point. There are two studies of particular relevance. Regan & Berscheid (1996), in a qualitative study, asked male and female college students, 'What is sexual desire?'. The majority of both men and women regarded it as a motivational state (e.g. a longing, urge, drive or craving), but men and women differed in how they described the goals and the objects of sexual desire. Women were more likely than men to see the goal of desire as love or emotional intimacy, whereas men were more likely to see sexual activity as the goal. Men were more likely than women to define the object of sexual desire in terms of the physical or sexual attractiveness of the desired person. Spector et al (1996) developed the Sexual Desire Inventory(SDI), which distinguishes between desire for sexual activity involving a partner (Dyadic scale) and desire for 'behaving sexually by yourself' (i.e. masturbating or self-stimulation; Solitary scale). In the Dyadic scale a range of possible interactions could be involved. But the Solitary scale excludes the partner, at least in real terms, as the object of desire. It is important to keep in mind that both of these studies were based on responses from young students, and different responses may have been obtained from older men and women. In a recent focus group study of women asked to describe what had excitatory and inhibitory effects on their arousal (Graham et al 2004), the younger women (18–24 years) were more likely to cite partner-related themes as important influences on their sexual arousal than were older women. As yet no studies involving representative community samples of men and women have used the SDI. It would be interesting to know what the normal ranges are for the Dyadic and Solitary scales for men and women. It would be particularly interesting to take women who scored high on the Solitary scale and those who scored low, and compare them in other aspects of their sexual lives. Given the discussion of this issue in Chapter 4 (see p. 132) this may be more relevant to understanding sexual desire in women than in men. For example, in how many women is 'desire to be desired' more important than desire for specific types of physical stimulation. Such women would be expected to score low on the Solitary scale.

An increasing number of questionnaires for assessing sexual dysfunction have been published in recent years, almost as many as there are pharmaceutical companies developing medical treatments for such dysfunctions! Some have focused on sexual desire, though their use has been largely restricted to clinical studies of HSDD. The following are some of the more relevant examples.

The Sexual Interest and Desire Inventory-Female (SIDI-F) was designed to measure severity of female HSDD (Clayton et al 2006). In this questionnaire the meaning of 'sexual desire' is defined before the relevant questions are asked: 'By sexual desire, I mean your interest in having a sexual experience whether alone or with a partner. Sexual interest involves thoughts, feelings and/or a willingness to become involved in some sort of way'. One interesting item on this scale was called 'receptivity': 'Over the past month, did your partner approach you for sex?'. If yes, 'How often did you accept and when you accepted, what was your level of enthusiasm?'. If the answer to the first question was no, this was followed by 'If your partner *had* approached you during the last month for sex how often would you have accepted and how enthusiastic would you have been?'. This questionnaire item is of interest because it taps into the impact of the partner's desire on the woman's desire. It is noteworthy that the introductory definition of 'sexual desire' concluded with '. . . and/or a willingness to become involved in some sort of sexual activity'. This raises the important issue of whether such willingness is an indicator of desire or rather an indicator that the woman is willing to meet her partner's needs; the assessment of her enthusiasm may in part answer this. On the other hand, the question remains whether the enthusiasm is for the consequent sexual stimulation or the consequent emotional closeness and intimacy. All of these are aspects of women's sexual interest which may be important, which may vary substantially in importance from woman to woman, or from occasion to occasion in the same woman (e.g. menstrual cyclicity), yet so far have received little research attention, reflecting the prevailing unitary concept of sexual desire.

Toledano & Pfaus (2006) developed a Sexual Arousal and Desire Inventory (SADI). They started by asking around 500 men and women, in person or via the Internet, how they would describe their experiences of sexual arousal and desire, both positively and negatively. They obtained 86 descriptor terms and asked a further sample of men and women to rate how well each term described their experience of sexual arousal and of sexual desire. Interestingly, several participants asked why they were being asked to do the same thing twice (i.e. rate arousal and desire), and as a result the authors combined the two experiences. They then carried out factor analysis and four factors emerged, accounting for 42% of the variance: 'evaluative', 'motivational', 'physiological' and 'negative/aversive'. They correlated the four factor scores with scores from the SDI (Spector et al 1996). Only the motivational scale correlated significantly, reflecting the extent to which the other three factors were descriptive of arousal as well as or instead of desire. The items on the motivational scale were 'anticipatory', 'driven', 'urge to satisfy', 'frustrated', 'lustful', 'tempted', 'impatient', 'naughty', 'alluring' and 'horny'. Men and women's scores on the motivational and physiological scales were not significantly different, whereas men scored higher on the evaluative scale and women higher on the negative/aversive scale. However, it is important to keep in mind that these scores reflected the extent to which the factor items described the individual's experience of arousal and desire, not its frequency or strength. Once again, this instrument does not help us to identify what it is that is being desired.

Breaking new ground in this respect, McCall & Meston (2006) explored the cues that stimulate sexual desire. Using a similar approach to Toledano & Pfaus (2006) they had an initial item generating stage, but their request differed in an important way. The open-ended question was, 'What makes you desire sexual activity?' (not, 'How do you experience sexual desire?'). This resulted in 125 items, or cues, which were then given to 874 females to rate the likelihood that each cue would make them desire sexual activity. The final number of items retained was 40, which combined to produce four factors: emotional bonding cues, erotic/explicit cues, visual/proximity cues and romantic/implicit cues. The three highest loading items on each of these factors were as follows:

1. emotional bonding cues: feeling a sense of:
   a. love with a partner
   b. security in a relationship
   c. one's partner being supportive of you
2. erotic/explicit cues:
   a. watching an erotic movie
   b. reading about sexual activity
   c. watching or listening to others engaging in sex
3. visual/proximity cues: seeing or talking to:
   a. someone powerful
   b. someone famous
   c. someone wealthy
4. romantic/implicit cues:
   a. partner whispering in your ear (or vice versa)
   b. dancing closely
   c. having a romantic dinner with your partner.

Women with HSDD ($n = 30$) scored lower than controls ($n = 63$) on all four factors. McCall & Meston (2006) concluded from these findings that whereas the relevant cues may remain similar, a woman's responsiveness to them may wax and wane. Thus their emphasis was on the receptivity of the woman to external cues as the determinant of her sexual desire, with women with HSDD being unable to 'trigger or access sexual desire when relevant cues are present'. However, it has not yet been established to what extent women vary in the cues that are important to them, and whether, for example, there are some women who are mainly affected by emotional/bonding cues and other women for whom erotic/explicit cues are equally or more important.

This raises the question of the extent to which sexual desire is 'spontaneous', i.e. not responsive to some external cue. Garde & Lunde (1980) in a survey of 40-year-old Danish women, found that more than 30% reported little or no spontaneous sexual desire, yet most of them had no difficulty enjoying and becoming aroused during sexual interaction with their partner. This indicates that to some extent the remaining majority did at least occasionally experience 'spontaneous' desire, although it is likely that on many if not most occasions their desire is 'receptive' or reactive to their partner's interest or initiation. Although there are no clear gender comparisons on this issue, it is probable that 'spontaneous' sexual desire is more commonly experienced by men.

Recently, some attention has been paid to the concept of 'asexuality' — the idea of a person who has no interest in sex, or at least in sexual interactions with another person. This is another sexual minority which is establishing itself via the Internet — there are now websites for asexuals who want to connect with each other (e.g. asexuality.meetup.com). Asexuals are now 'coming out' and asserting their asexual identities (Westphal 2004). This minority is considered more closely in Chapter 9.

Our knowledge and evidence of 'normal' sexual desire is therefore patchy and incomplete. It is a crucial aspect of human sexuality, and requires better understanding before we can deal effectively with 'problems' of low sexual desire or HSDD.

Sexual fantasy

As discussed above, fantasizing about sex may be one manifestation of what we have been struggling to conceptualize as 'sexual desire'. However, fantasies represent a complex manifestation of the information-processing component of sexual arousal, considered closely in Chapter 4. Dwelling on a sexual fantasy may lead to incentive motivation for sexual activity, and may result in sexual arousal. However, sexual fantasy may be a reaction to awareness of incentive motivation cues or sexual arousal. Hence fantasy has the potential for being both stimulus and response, and in a manner characteristic of sexual experience there is likely to be an interaction of both. However, sexual fantasies provide a whole new level of information about what an individual 'desires' or finds arousing, and in that sense are potentially much more informative than simply assessing the frequency of sexual thoughts.

We discussed in Chapter 5 the possible relevance of early sexual fantasies in determining our sexual identities. In some individuals, the fantasies which were used early in that person's sexual life retain some special erotic effect long after the content of the fantasy has any other current relevance. It is an intriguing but as yet unanswered question why in some individuals these specific fantasies retain their potency as conditioned erotic stimuli whilst in others the erotic fantasies change to reflect current sexual activities and interest. The scope that is possible in fantasy for an imaginative person may lead to imagery frightening in its effects or implications. The possibility that one may act out a fantasy can cause considerable anxiety. Fantasies of socially unacceptable or immoral sexual behaviour can cause guilt. In some people, their early sexual fantasies developed at a time when their comprehension of sexuality was undeveloped and was influenced by immature anxieties or needs. These fantasies, retaining their erotic effect into adulthood, may later cause concern, suggesting to their user that he or she is seriously disturbed. Because fantasies can, and usually do, remain concealed, their frightening significance may continue unchallenged. Fantasies may be used to enhance or otherwise make more acceptable 'real' sexuality. As discussed in Chapter 12, identifying the discrepancies between an individual's real world and his or her fantasized, ideal world can be invaluable in helping people with sexual problems. Fantasies in their frequency, form or content may reveal interesting differences between males and females. There are therefore many reasons for taking sexual fantasies seriously.

The literature on sexual fantasies, until the early 1990s, was comprehensively reviewed by Leitenberg & Henning (1995). The following are some of their conclusions. Contrary to the Freudian view that sexual fantasies compensate for what is lacking in reality, they tend to be more frequent in those who are more sexually active. But they become less frequent in both men and women as they age. Around 25% of men and women are guilty about their sexual fantasies. Men fantasize more than women during non-sexual activity and masturbation, but not during sexual intercourse. Factor analytic studies have identified four principal categories of sexual fantasy for both men and women: (i) 'conventional' heterosexual imagery involving past, present or imaginary lovers, (ii) scenes indicating sexual power and irresistibility, (iii) variations in settings, practices and positions adopted and (iv) submission or dominance, with some level of coercion or physical force implied. However, the content of such sexual fantasies shows some striking gender differences. Men more than women imagine doing something to their partner; women more than men imagine having something done to them. Men are more likely to report sexually explicit and visual imagery, women more emotional and romantic imagery. Men are more likely to involve more than one partner in their fantasies. Women are more likely to imagine themselves in a submissive role, whereas men are more likely to see themselves in a dominant role. Leitenberg & Henning (1995) suggest that both the female submission and the male dominance pattern can be explained as manifestations of sexual attractiveness and irresistibility, i.e. the woman submits because in her fantasy the man finds her irresistible and the man dominates because the woman in his fantasy finds him irresistible.

Since Leitenberg & Henning's (1995) review further research on sexual fantasy has been limited. One of the contentious issues in this literature is that many women report fantasies in which they are forced to have sex. A possible connection between force fantasies and childhood sexual abuse has been reported. Briere et al (1994) found that women, but not men, who had been sexually abused during childhood, were more likely to report 'force' fantasies as adults, and this association was stronger in those whose sexual abuse occurred earlier in childhood. No such association has been found following sexual assault as an adult (Leitenberg & Henning 1995), and there has been no evidence to suggest that women with such fantasies would enjoy similar experiences in reality. An alternative explanation from earlier studies was that such fantasies enabled the woman to 'experience' such sexual interaction, at least in fantasy, without feeling guilty, because, as it was 'forced', she could not be held responsible (e.g. Moreault & Follingstad 1978). In a more recent study, Strassberg & Lockerd (1998) found no support for this explanation. In fact they found such fantasies to be more frequently reported by women who were not guilty about sex, were more 'erotophilic' and more open to sexual experimentation. Furthermore, 'force' fantasies of this kind, while reported by many of their women subjects, were seldom among their favourite fantasies. Hicks & Leitenberg (2001) explored the predictors of extradyadic sexual fantasies, i.e. being unfaithful to one's current partner in one's fantasies. They cited a *New York Times* poll in which 48% of respondents considered such fantasies unacceptable, even if the infidelity was confined to fantasy. In their mainly college student sample, 98% of men and 80% of women reported such fantasies in the past 2 months. Although this pattern was more likely in men, for both genders such fantasies increased in frequency as the length of the current relationship increased.

Zurbriggen & Yost (2004), in one of the few studies in this area not using college students, focused on issues of power, desire and pleasure in men and women's sexual fantasies. Using a qualitative approach, participants were asked to describe their favourite or most frequent fantasies. These accounts were then coded on a number of themes, including dominance and submission, and desire and pleasure experienced by the self or by another person. Attitudes were also measured, including the Rape Myth Acceptance Scale, to assess stereotypical and false beliefs about rape, and Attitude Towards Women Scale, to assess traditional beliefs about the place of women in society. In most respects the findings were similar to previous research. Men were equally likely to describe fantasies in which they were dominant or submissive; in women submissive fantasies were more common than dominant. For men, desire and pleasure were strongly correlated; for women they comprised two distinct factors. Somewhat surprisingly, the men were more likely to focus on the partner's desire and pleasure whereas the women were more likely to focus on their own pleasure. Zurbriggen & Yost (2004) suggested that this reflected men's need to feel that they were giving pleasure to their partner, whereas women felt more comfortable focusing on their own pleasure in their fantasy than in reality. Men who described fantasies in which they were dominant were more likely to express stereotypical beliefs in 'rape myths' (e.g. that a woman invites rape by her behaviour or dress; women could avoid being raped if they really wanted to). Given the relationship between rape myth acceptance and increased likelihood of being sexually aggressive (e.g. Dean & Malamuth 1997), this type of fantasy in men may be potentially problematic.

Zurbriggen & Yost's (2004) study is unusual in relating sexual fantasy content to other aspects of the individual's personality and sexuality. An early study in this category, involving married women, is also noteworthy. Hariton & Singer (1974) used factor analysis to identify four factors and associated types of women. Women scoring high on factor I tended to fantasize a great deal in general, using many sexual fantasies as well as other types of fantasy. These women showed personality features of aggression, exhibition, impulsivity, autonomy and dominance whilst scoring low on measures of nurturance and affiliation, two traditionally feminine traits. Their exploratory approach to sex was reflected in high frequencies of premarital and extramarital affairs, with the latter being apparently motivated more by curiosity than marital unhappiness. One is tempted to see these women as showing less typically feminine characteristics, at least as far as sex role stereotypes would indicate. The second group of women experienced sexual dissatisfaction or guilt and tended not to use enjoyable sexual fantasies. The third group were somewhat older, and reared in a more traditional background of sexual repression. They were generally satisfied with their sexual relations in marriage but used fantasies of sexual submission to enhance their enjoyment in some way.

In 2007, Kahr, a psychoanalytic psychotherapist, published a 622-page book on sexual fantasies. This was largely based on an Internet survey of more than 13 000 men and women, recruited from an Internet panel (YouGov), mainly used for surveying political opinions. The response rate was nearly 40%, but the panel itself cannot be regarded as representative. This is nevertheless a potentially valuable data set. Unfortunately, the evidence is not presented in this book in a scientific manner. It does, however, provide a rich source of examples of less common sexual fantasies.

More research is needed in which fantasy content is related to other characteristics of men and women's sexuality and personality. It is of particular importance to examine these associations across the age range as they could well change. And even in the younger age groups we should not confine our attention to university students.

Response to erotica

Somewhere between overt sexual activity and sexual fantasy come the various forms of visual or literary erotica as sources of erotic stimulation. Their very tangible existence and considerable commercial exploitation has resulted in phases of concern about possible harmful effects and the need for control or censorship. In the USA this led to the Commission on Obscenity and Pornography, which started in 1968 to direct and fund a series of research studies (Technical Reports of the Commission on Obscenity and Pornography 1970). The general findings were reassuring as far as they went, but were rejected outright by the US government, presumably because the results were not in the desired direction. In the UK, Lord Longford, on his own initiative, set up a private enquiry into pornography in 1971 which, it could be said, was predestined to reach opposing conclusions to the US commission (Longford 1972). Later, a government-sponsored committee delivered its report, perhaps less biased than either of the previous two, but none the less controversial in its conclusions (Williams 1979). The main concern of such inquiries is the possibility that pornography may have an undesirable effect on morals or, to put it more practically, on the behaviour of members of society, particularly the young. We are now in a new phase as a result of the Internet which has had a huge impact on the accessibility and variability of sexual stimuli. This will be considered further below. The possible relationship between explicit sexual stimuli and sexual crime will be considered further in Chapter 16. The term 'pornography', originally referring to the activities of prostitutes and their clients, is now a more generally pejorative term for sexually explicit material, visual images or text, which is considered offensive or 'obscene', judgements which vary across cultures and individuals; as the *Encyclopaedia Britannica* (2007) put it, 'pornography is in the eye of the beholder'. The term 'erotica', meaning material intended to be sexually stimulating, at least to some people, will be generally used in this book.

The psychophysiological aspects of response to erotica in men and women were considered in Chapter 4. In studies relying on self-report, most of which involve university students, what are the short-term effects of exposure to erotica? How do males and females compare in their responses? How do different types of erotica compare in their effects?

The short-term effects are much as one might expect. Erotica tends to induce a degree of sexual arousal, often followed by a temporary increase in sexual activity, either masturbation or sex with the usual partner, and the effect is noticeable for no more than 1 or 2 days. There has been little evidence that new types of sexual activity, as depicted in erotica, have resulted, though they may have done so in fantasy (Yaffe 1972; Schmidt 1975; Bancroft 1978). It nevertheless seems inherently likely that exposure to a novel kind of sexual stimulation, if it is found to hold appeal for the observer and does not generate anxiety or guilt, may result in it being tried out eventually when the circumstances are right.

Of more interest is the comparison of male and female responses. It has been conventional wisdom for some time that men are interested in explicit depictions of sexual activity, and women in more romantic accounts, as reflected in the predominant use of erotica by men and the predominant use of romantic fiction by women (Leitenberg & Henning 1995). Kinsey et al (1953) found a greater proportion of males than females reporting erotic responses to a variety of types of stimuli, though the differences were most marked for erotic images. Gender differences of this kind have been less marked in later studies, and there are various factors that could contribute to this change. Murnen & Stockton (1997) carried out a meta-analysis of 46 studies in which self-reported arousal to visual sexual stimuli were assessed in men and women. Overall there was significantly more sexual arousal reported by men than women, but the difference was small. A number of factors contributed to the variability in this gender difference. Stimuli used in the studies were categorized as either 'erotica' or 'pornography', but this was based solely on which term was used in the individual report. Fifteen studies used 'pornography' and 31 'erotica' and the gender difference was significantly greater in those using pornography ($p < 0.02$). This probably reflects a tendency for the pornographic stimuli to involve objectification or exploitation of women, whereas the erotica may have presented a more 'gender equal' scenario. All but seven of the studies involved college students. The non-student participants were older and the gender difference was significantly less with these older samples ($p < 0.01$). This apparent age effect requires further study, but may indicate that the conventional gender difference is more marked in younger age groups, with women becoming more comfortable and tuned-in to their own sexual pleasure as they get older (Graham et al 2004). Non-visual sexual stimuli were used in 19 of the studies, the remainder using visual stimuli. Interestingly, there was no significant difference in gender effect between these two types of stimuli, which challenges the assumption, made much of by evolutionary psychologists (e.g. Buss 1994), that females are less influenced by visual stimuli to avoid impairing their judgement of likely parental investment by a potential male partner.

In considering these differences, and the variables influencing gender difference as summarized by Murnen & Stockton (1997), we need to consider how social attitudes may have changed, allowing women to feel less inhibited in their reactions to erotica, and also how the content of erotica may have changed to become more appealing to women. A number of studies have now shown that, whereas men tend to respond with more sexual arousal than women to erotic films, when films are used which are designed for women, the difference is less (Laan et al 1994; Mosher & MacIan 1994; Janssen et al 2003).

Sex and the Internet

At various points in this chapter we have considered the changes in human sexuality through the 20th century, particularly the reduction in social suppression of women's sexuality. To a considerable extent the earlier imposition of social control of sexuality depended on control of information about sex. It was much easier to persuade people to feel guilty about engaging in premarital sex, or same sex activity, if they at the same time thought such behaviours were unusual, abnormal or weird. A major part of Kinsey's impact was uncovering what was happening — releasing information that people were up to much more

than was assumed to be the case. The opening up of discussion about sex and hence the spread of ideas about sexual behaviour that followed, took root in the media which ever since have bombarded the public with a variety of 'norm-setting' information, much of it misleading. But by now, such information, correct or otherwise, is out of control. This process escalated dramatically with the advent of the Internet.

The Internet presents us with the latest, and in many respects, most powerful form of new technology to impact on sexuality. In the 19th century one of the earliest uses of the new daguerreotype technology was to capture sexually explicit images. There are many examples of early photography of this kind in the Kinsey Institute. Whereas initially such images were available to relatively few, accessibility of erotic images produced by emerging technologies has gradually widened. There were the early stag films and their subsequent developments. By the time sexually explicit videos were on the scene there was much wider accessibility. Over the relatively short history of the erotic video we saw some striking changes. Whereas in the 1970s many such videos were telling erotic stories, those of the 1990s were zooming in to genital sexuality with minimum delay. The impression is that the earlier videos were used more by couples, for whom the erotic content would impact their sexual relationship. By contrast, later videos seem more designed for the individual viewer, presumably male, who was pursuing the uncomplicated, uninvolved release of masturbatory sexual pleasure. As if to compensate for this change, we have seen the development of erotic videos designed for women, by women, where the erotic story regains importance. The technology and the accessibility were probably not responsible for the 'triumph of the individual' but they undoubtedly fostered it.

The Internet has revolutionized communications more dramatically than any other technological development since the widespread household use of the telephone. Growth in the use of the Internet is explosive. In 1998, 39% of the American public was going online; in 2001 the proportion was 63%. Whereas in 1994, in the USA, the male-to-female ratio for use of the Internet was 20:1, now it is very close to that of the US population. According to a survey in 2001, Internet users were becoming similar to all Americans in terms of race, ethnicity and gender; they tended to be younger — 46% were under the age of 40 years — compared to 26% of non-users (Markle Foundation 2001).

Like the telephone, but unlike radio and television, the Internet is an interactive medium and many people use it for sexual purposes. For example, searches on the web are predominantly sex related. In 2001, 33 of the top 40 websites visited by males aged 18–24 years, were 'adult' websites (Mustanski 2001). This represents an astounding increase in accessibility of sexual materials and sexual information of all kinds in the last few years. However, access to explicit sexual images or material is only one way the Internet is used. Interaction with one or more individuals via the Internet is now known as 'cyber sex'. Various types of interaction may result, but frequently it involves at least one of the participants masturbating during the interaction.

Other uses involve 'chatting', discussion forums and arranging 'off line' meetings (possibly the most problematic). It is noteworthy that men use the Internet more for access to sexually explicit material, whereas women use it more for interactions or cybersex (Daneback et al 2005). Internet interactions are free of the risk of pregnancy, STDs or physical assault, allowing women the opportunity to explore their sexuality in ways that have not existed previously (Leiblum 2001).

The implications of this dramatic change for the social determinants of sexuality and sexual relationships are not yet known. We can expect some obvious benefits. Most aspects of the Internet have the potential for interactive use, which can be educational, informative, therapeutic or otherwise positive. The Internet has exceptional potential for disseminating information and guidance about safe and responsible sex as well as other health-related behaviours. The potential for developing online counselling or therapy is considerable, but as yet in an early stage of development.

The potential for Internet sex to cause harm is, however, alarming. Each aspect of the Internet has its own potential for producing problems in the sexual lives of its users. We are seeing an explosion of availability of sexually explicit material over which it is extremely difficult to exercise any kind of social control. Already there is convincing evidence that large numbers of individuals, both men and women, and quite possibly young adolescents, are becoming involved in web sex of one kind or another to an extent which is out of their control, or at least problematic in use of time or money or in its effects on relationships. This ready access to a seemingly endless supply of sexually explicit material could produce significant social changes in patterns of sexual responsiveness, with consequent unpredictable but probably negative effects on patterns of social interactions and relationships. In addition, there is increasing use of the Internet to find 'real space' sexual partners, adding a new dimension to high-risk sexual behaviour and the sexual transmission of disease. 'Out of control' Internet use for sexual purposes is considered further in Chapter 11.

At this stage, we do not know how socially dangerous these new and escalating developments are, but it is an urgent priority that they are monitored carefully. It is reasonable to assume, however, that for the substantial majority, sexual use of the Internet will either not happen, or, if it does, will not escalate into a problem.

One large survey of sexual use of the web (Cooper et al 1999) indicated that the majority of people, both men and women, who visit sexual websites or chat rooms do so occasionally and without obvious problems resulting. This sample of 9265 was obtained from a link to a MSNBC site over 2 months in spring 1998. Forty-seven per cent used the Internet for sexual purposes less than 1 hour a week or not at all; 45% from 1 to 10 hours a week; 5.6% from 11 to 20 hours and 2.8% 21 hours+ a week. There was a 6:1 male-to-female ratio; men preferred visual erotic material (50%:23%) whereas women preferred chat rooms (49%:23%). For the large majority of this sample, sexual use of the web was not problematic. Although 2.8% reporting excessive use is a small

proportion, in terms of users of the Internet, this translates into large numbers. One would not expect high rates with this particular sample obtained from a news site. Also of interest was the finding that the only over-represented occupational group among the excessive users was students.

In February 2002, Public Broadcasting Service aired a Frontline documentary on American porn. The Kinsey Institute designed a survey that was posted on the programme's companion website and which, over a period of 4 months, was completed by 10 017 website visitors (8275 men and 1742 women) (Janssen, unpublished data). Most of the men (62%) and women (65%) were between ages 21 and 40 years, with 27% and 22%, respectively, above the age of 40 years. Eighty-eight per cent of the men and 77% of the women were heterosexual, 5% of the men and 2.5% of the women were homosexual, and 5% of the men and 15% of the women were bisexual. Eighty-five per cent of the men indicated that they had viewed sexual images on the Internet during the past month; 34% of the men had done this a few times a week; 25% at least once a day. Of the women, 50% had viewed sexual images on the Internet during the past month. Twelve per cent had done this a few times a week, and 9% at least once a day. Of the participants who had used the Internet to access porn during the past month, 5% (men 8.5%, women 7%) had done this for 26–50 hours a week, and an additional 4% (men 4%, women 5%) had spent more than 50 hours weekly doing this. Forty-two per cent of the men and 28% of the women indicated that they felt bad either during or after using porn, and 11% of the men and 4% of the women indicated that they had tried but could not stop themselves from using porn. The differences between Cooper et al's (1999) survey and this Kinsey Institute survey may be because both used convenience samples. Representative samples are needed to enable us to assess properly the prevalence of these behaviours and their consequences. The GSS is a large-scale survey of the US population conducted every 2 years since 1966. In the 2000 survey (GSS 2000), for the first time, 668 participants were asked, 'In the past 30 days, how often have you visited a website for sexually explicit material?' Of the 90% who answered, 76.1% of the men answered 'never', 16.6% 'once or twice', 2.7% 3–5 times and 4.5% more than 5 times. Of the women, 95.8% answered 'never', 1.8% 'once or twice', 1.5% 3–5 times and 0.9% more than 5 times. The amount of use was higher in gay/lesbian/bisexual men and women than in heterosexuals. As is to be expected, the use reported in the GSS appears to be less than in the convenience samples.

Richters et al (2003) reported on a representative sample of Australian men and women, aged 16–59 years, using computer-assisted telephone interviews. More than 9000 men and a similar number of women answered questions about Internet use. Intentional visiting of Internet sex sites was reported by 16.5% of men and 2.4% of women. The likelihood of men doing so was significantly associated with the following variables: less in the older men, particularly over 50 years and greater among gay and bisexual men, men with higher levels of education, living in major cities, in white-collar or managerial/

professional jobs, who had no regular partner and more than one partner in the past year. The likelihood of women visiting such sites was greater in younger women, in lesbian or bisexual women, or in those with more than one sexual partner.

We have no evidence from representative samples of the prevalence of using the Internet to find partners for offline sex or of 'out of control' use of the Internet for sexual purposes.

We should, however, be prepared for these patterns, as most other aspects of web use, to be changing substantially over time. Whereas there will be some individuals who respond to the novelty of the web with initially high rates which then decline, others may find themselves steadily increasing their usage. This increase in use is made easy because Internet access is available through the same computer that one uses for work or other ordinary aspects of one's life. And although there are ways in which such use can be tracked down, the user has the strong feeling (somewhat misguided) of privacy and anonymity in the process.

Personality and individual differences in sexuality

Given the fundamental importance of individual variability of human sexuality, and the extensive work that has been carried out in the field of personality measurement, surprisingly little attention has been paid to the influence of personality variables on sexual behaviour. An early exception was Eysenck (1976), who devised a questionnaire covering various aspects of sexual attitudes and behaviours (Eysenck 1971) and related the answers to his usual personality measures of extroversion–introversion (E), neuroticism (N) and tough mindedness (P). His sexuality questionnaire produced two factors that Eysenck called 'libido' (or sexual desire) and 'satisfaction'. He found that extroverts were high on libido and tended to the positive end of the satisfaction factor. Introverts were at the low end of the libido factor, although they showed greater satisfaction at older age levels. High neuroticism scorers complained more of sexual dysfunction of various kinds and reported high anxiety about sex (i.e. low satisfaction) whilst being high on the libido dimension.

Other writers have criticized the strength of Eysenck's claims. Farley et al (1977), using different but comparable measures of personality and sexuality, concluded that there was a 'general lack of contribution of personality variables to sexuality, as measured'. Schenk et al (1981), using Eysenck's measures of E and N, found no support for his conclusions in a study of married couples, concluding that the quality of the marriage was more important than personality variables in determining the sexual relationship. In a later study of single men (Schenk & Pfrang 1986) they found some support for the link between sexuality and extroversion but not neuroticism.

Frenken (1976), in developing his sexual experience scales which measure aspects of sexual attitudes as well as behaviour, drew comparisons with various measures of personality and found the predictive power of personality

characteristics to be weak. Gender, age and frequency of church attendance were the best predictors of sexual behaviour.

Costa et al (1992) measured the five principal factors of personality, neuroticism (N), extraversion (E), openness to experience (O), agreeableness (A) and conscientiousness (C), in 454 adults being evaluated in a sexual problems clinic. High N was correlated with dysphoric symptoms, negative body image and lowered sexual satisfaction. High E was associated with higher sexual drive, more sexual experience, and positive body image. Agreeableness was unrelated to sexual drive and satisfaction but was negatively related to symptomatology. Openness was positively related to amount of information, range of sexual experience, liberal attitudes towards sex, sexual drive and fantasy. Greater conscientiousness was associated with lower sexual drive, better body image and fewer dysphoric symptoms. These findings provide some support for Eysenck's earlier conclusions, though it is not clear to what extent these observed associations would be found in a non-clinical population.

Measures of sexual attitudes

A crucial aspect of individual variability concerns attitudes and values relating to sex. To what extent are individuals 'sex-positive' or 'sex-negative' in their attitudes and values?

Fisher et al (1988) developed a 21-item questionnaire to measure what they call erotophilia–erotophobia. This is known as the Sexual Opinion Survey (SOS). The items combined to form three factors, which were called 'open sexual display' (10 items accounting for 34% of the variance), 'sexual variety' (7 items and 11% of the variance) and 'homoeroticism' (4 items and 7% of variance). Six of the 10 items in the open sexual display factor assess reactions to erotica (or what was called pornography in the first version of the scale). The second factor, sexual variety, factor evaluates attitudes to masturbation, oral sex, sexual intercourse, engaging in 'unusual sexual practices' and daydreaming about sex. The third factor, homoeroticism, assesses attitudes to same-sex attraction, or interest. Most studies using this scale have combined these three factors into one scale, erotophobia–erotophilia.

Fisher et al (1988) described erotophobia–erotophilia, as measured by the SOS, as the 'disposition to respond to sexual cues along a negative–positive dimension of affect and evaluation'. This is perhaps a somewhat over-generalized definition, given the specific items used. Much of typical sexual interaction and responsiveness is not addressed. However, a short form of the scale was developed using just five items that were good predictors of total scores for both men and women. These items were: 'Masturbation can be an exciting experience', 'Almost all erotic (sexually explicit) material is nauseating', 'It would be emotionally upsetting for me to see someone exposing themselves publicly', 'The thought of engaging in unusual sexual practices is highly arousing' and 'The thought of having long-term sexual relations with more than one sex partner is not disgusting to me'. This therefore indicates that the scale assesses positive or negative attitudes to masturbation, erotica, sexual display in public, unconventional sexual practices, and monogamous commitment.

A number of studies have related this dimension to other personality attributes or behaviour patterns (Fisher et al 1988; Byrne & Schulte 1990). Authoritarian individuals tend to be erotophobic. Androgynous men and women (using Bem's (1974) measure of androgyny) tend to be more erotophilic than those who conform to traditional sex roles. Erotophobic men generally tend to adhere more to the work ethic. In women erotophilia was negatively associated with achievement aspirations but positively with understanding. Erotophobia correlates with measures of 'sex guilt' (Mosher 1968). Erotophilia is related to frequency of masturbation, number of sexual partners and the amount of past sexual experience, in both men and women. It is also associated with more consistent use of contraception. Erotophobia is associated with reports of parental strictness during childhood, leading Fisher et al (1988) to speculate that erotophobia–erotophilia is a learned disposition.

The Dual Control model

This theoretical model used in various parts of this book was elaborated in Chapter 2, and given as an example of a theoretical model of potential heuristic value. The model postulates the existence of an excitatory system and an inhibitory system within the brain, which interact to determine whether a sexual response occurs on any particular occasion. The model further postulates that individuals vary in their propensity for sexual excitation (SE) and also for sexual inhibition (SI). Thus, both excitatory and inhibitory systems are considered as fundamental to normal and appropriate or adaptive sexual response. However, the individual variability in each may account for much of the variability in sexual behaviour. The mechanisms involved in excitation and inhibition are examined in Chapter 4. The relevance of high inhibition proneness and low excitation proneness to sexual problems or dysfunctions, and of low inhibition particularly when combined with high excitation proneness, to sexual risk taking, are considered further in Chapters 12 and 14. At this point we will consider the relevance of this model to conceptualizing individual variability.

Two questionnaires have been developed to measure SE and inhibition proneness, one for men (SIS/SES; Janssen et al 2002), the other for women (SESII-W; Graham et al 2006). In contrast to the SOS, all questions in both instruments focus on whether particular situations result in sexual arousal, loss of sexual arousal or make sexual arousal unlikely. The respondent indicates a rating of agreement or disagreement with each statement (e.g. 'When I think about someone I find sexually attractive, I easily become sexually aroused'). Further examples of items, and results of the factor analyses are given in Chapter 2 (p. 16). The SIS/SES has three higher-order factors, called sexual excitation (SES), SI due to threat of performance failure (SIS1) and SI due to threat of performance consequences (SIS2), and a number of lower order factors, or subscales. We have hypothesized that SIS1 may also be a measure of 'inhibitory tone' which needs to be reduced before sexual arousal occurs (Bancroft & Janssen 2000; see p. 105). The SESII-W has two higher-order factors, SE and SI and a number of subscales (see p. 16 for details). The two questionnaires were developed somewhat differently. Items for the male SIS/SES were based on suggestions from a number of sex researchers; items for the SESII-W were based on a series of focus groups for women (Graham et al 2004). Not surprisingly, there are some differences, as well as similarities between the two scales, with some of the items being exactly the same.

As yet neither questionnaire has been used in representative community samples, but they have been completed in a series of large convenience samples, and the data show close to normal distributions. Examples of these data are shown in Figures 6.13 and 6.14.

Both SIS/SES and SESII-W show some degree of correlation with SOS (erotophobia–erotophilia). In men, SOS was positively correlated with SES, $r = .45$, negatively with SIS2, $r = -.29$, both significant, $p < 0.001$. It was not correlated with SIS1. In women, SOS was correlated with SE, $r = .53$, and with SI, $r = -.41$, both significant, $p < 0.01$. Let us consider to what extent these two questionnaires are tapping the same influences. SOS, which is a mixture of sexual attitude and 'response to stimuli' items, does not specifically attempt to assess inhibition of sexual response. As mentioned earlier, Fisher et al (1988) have postulated that erotophilia–erotophobia results from early learning, particularly the degree of sex-negativism or sex-positivism in the individual's family during childhood. The assumption with the two Dual Control instruments is that they are measuring basic neurophysiological propensities, involved in an excitation system and a separate and relatively independent inhibitory system (see p. 65). In view of the inclusion of some items in the SOS measuring sexual arousal response to specific situations (e.g. 'manipulating my genitals would probably be an arousing experience'), there is some conceptual overlap between the two instruments. However, the SOS is more determined by 'sexual attitudes and values' and the two Dual Control instruments, by neurophysiological propensities for sexual arousal and inhibition. But these two conceptual systems may be related. The impact of a 'sex-negative' childhood on subsequent sexuality may be greater in an individual with a relatively high propensity for inhibition and low propensity for SE; conversely the impact of a 'sex-positive' childhood. But these neurophysiological propensities may be in part genetically determined. As yet there is one twin study of males showing evidence of heritability of SI (see Chapter 2, p. 17). The possibility that propensity for SI is heritable is of particular relevance to interpreting the development of 'sex-negative' attitudes.

An earlier instrument for measuring propensity for sexual arousability in women was the Sexual Arousability Inventory (Hoon et al 1976) mentioned earlier. Another interesting and relevant aspect of individual

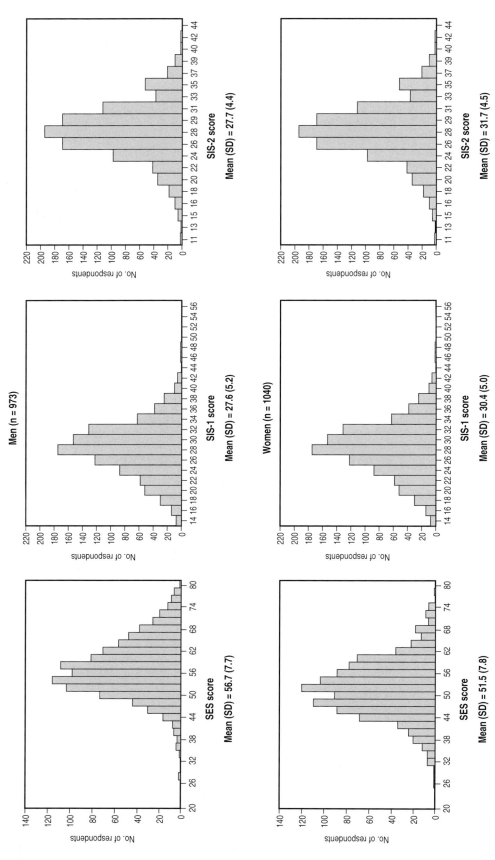

Fig. 6.13 Distribution of SIS/SES scores in a non-clinical sample of men, and using an adaptation of the male SIS/SES suitable for women, in a non-clinical sample of women. SES is sexual excitation scale, SIS-1 is sexual inhibition due to threat of performance failure and SIS-2 is sexual inhibition due to threat of performance consequences. (From Janssen et al 2002 and Carpenter et al 2008.)

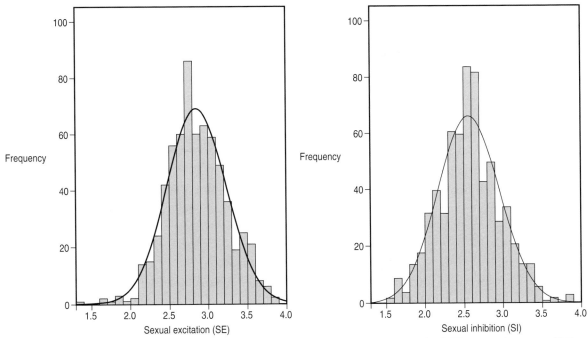

Fig. 6.14 Distributions of the two higher-order factors from the SESII-W scores in a non-clinical sample of 655 women (mean age 33.9 years). (From Graham et al 2006 with permission.)

variability is the association between mood and sexuality. This was considered closely in Chapter 4, and as it is of particular relevance to problematic sexual behaviour it will be revisited in Chapter 11.

The relevance of individual variability to the success of sexual relationships is an important issue that has so far received little research attention. Are relationships in which partners share similar patterns of erotophobia–erotophilia or SE/SI proneness more successful than those where there are differences? Smith et al (1993) showed that married couples were similar in their sexual attitudes. Cupach & Metts (1995) looked at unmarried student couples and compared them with randomized pairing of other male and female students to check that similarities were not just reflective of the student culture. They found that the couples showed more similarities on a measure of sexual attitudes than the random pairings. It would be interesting to explore the similarity of excitation and inhibition proneness in couples.

Comparison of men and women

In this chapter, we have encountered a number of gender differences. The role of orgasm is a notable example. The proportion of individuals who never experience an orgasm is higher in women than men, and for the remainder women are much more variable in their likelihood of experiencing orgasm during a sexual encounter, with many women requiring specific stimulation beyond that resulting from vaginal intercourse. There was an interesting phase in the 1920s and 1930s when orgasm was recognized as the criterion of satisfactory sex for women, resulting in some degree of performance pressure on women, and expectation by men that their partners

should experience orgasm. As the second half of the 20th century progressed, this became less of an issue, and it now seems that women are much more variable than men in the importance they attach to orgasm.

The gender difference in the incidence of masturbation has lessened, but differences remain in its prevalence, its age of onset and the likelihood of masturbating when in a sexual relationship. The recent finding from the NATSAL 2000 survey (Gerressu et al 2008) that women showed a positive relationship between frequency of masturbation and frequency of sexual activity with the partner, and men showed the opposite, warrants further research.

Gender differences in the age at first sexual intercourse lessened between the 1960s and 1980s, but females continue to be more likely to confine their sexual interactions to 'established' relationships. In some respects there has been lessening of the 'double standard' but it has by no means disappeared, particularly in the USA and UK.

Somewhat contrary to stereotypical assumptions, men 'fall in love' more readily; women are more cautious. On the other hand, women are more likely to report being in love on their first experience of sexual intercourse. The type of 'love' experienced differs to some extent, with women being more likely to experience companionate love and men passionate love.

One of the less clearly understood aspects of sexual relationships from a gender perspective is the issue of initiation. In an established sexual relationship, men are more likely to initiate specific sexual interactions. But in the early establishment of a sexual relationship, women seem to exert subtle control over the process, which, given its importance, has not been adequately studied.

Sexual interest or desire, a difficult concept, appears, on average, to be stronger in men than women but probably differs in important ways in what it is that is desired. In general, the level of a woman's sexual interest or desire appears to be more determined by her current circumstances as well as age. There are gender differences in the content of sexual fantasy. Men, in their sexual fantasies, are more likely to be doing something to their partner; women are more likely to fantasize that their partner is doing something to them.

The propensity for inhibition of sexual arousal and response appears to be stronger in women, on average, and induced by a greater variety of circumstances. This is not surprising given the clear biological reasons for women to be more selective in their involvement sexually.

How do these gender differences fit into the theoretical model of basic patterns and superadded effects developed in Chapter 4? The greater variability of sexual expression in women is certainly compatible with the idea that the sexuality of some women conforms and is largely confined to the female basic pattern; the sexual motivation of such a woman is towards engaging the male who 'desires' her, and her main rewards result from the emotional engagement that results, together with her sense of, in some way, being 'in control', rather than from her sexual pleasure per se. In addition, there may be other women for whom sexual pleasure is an important motivator, much as it is for males. This may be reflected not only in their capacity for orgasm, but also the importance they attach to the orgasmic experience. These are testable ideas which need to be researched. Is it possible, for example, to distinguish between the woman whose main rewards are from emotional engagement with her 'loved one' that sexual interaction provides, and the woman who may enjoy this aspect but who in addition is motivated by a desire for sexual pleasure, comparable to that of the male? Is it the second type of woman who is most responsive to testosterone and who experiences a decline in her sexual interest when her testosterone levels are lowered (see p. 127)? One study of possible relevance reported on women aged 40–60 years of age (Cawood & Bancroft 1996), some of whom were pre- and some post-menopausal. Their answers to a number of detailed questions about their recent sexual experiences (basically the same questions used by Bancroft et al (2003a) and considered earlier), were subjected to principal components analysis. Two factors emerged: the first we called 'negative feeling factor' (30.7% of the variance) and the second, 'positive response factor' (16.8% of the variance). For the first factor the two items loading most positively were 'number of occasions suffered pain' and 'number of times woman's advance was rejected'. The two items loading most negatively were 'number of times enjoyed intercourse' and 'number of times felt close to partner'. For the 'positive response factor' the two most positive items were 'frequency of orgasm' and 'number of times sexually aroused'. In addition a significant negative predictor of the first factor was the 'attraction to marriage' (SES4) scale from the Frenken Sexual Experience Scales (Frenken & Vennix 1981), which was not predictive of the second factor. The first factor might be a negative correlate of the female basic pattern and the second factor a positive correlate of the superadded component.

Unfortunately, we did not explore to what extent we could divide the women on the basis of these two factors. However, given the answers to our 'sexual happiness' questions (Table 6.15) we might expect to find that most women fit the basic pattern, whereas a minority fit the superadded pattern. This awaits further research. We will return to this conceptual model in the next chapter, when we consider the impact of the menopause and ageing.

Overall, there have been substantially more changes in the sexuality of women than of men during the 20th century. This is consistent with a reduction in the socio-cultural suppression of women's sexuality. Given the greater potential for inhibition of sexual response and arousal in women, it is not surprising that this reduction has affected women across the socio-economic spectrum. However, one important consequence of this lessening of suppression and increasing acceptance of women's sexuality in its own right is that the greater variability of women's sexuality has become more apparent. Now is the time to explore the origins of this variability.

REFERENCES

ACSF Principal Investigators and their associates 1992 Analysis of sexual behaviour in France. A comparison between two modes of investigation: telephone survey and face-to-face survey. AIDS 6: 315–323.

Ahmadi N 2003 Rocking sexualities: Iranian migrants' views on sexuality. Archives of Sexual Behavior 32: 317–326.

Alan Guttmacher Institute 1976 11 million teenagers. Planned Parenthood Federation of America, New York.

Asayama S 1976 Sexual behaviour in Japanese students: comparisons for 1974, 1960 and 1952. Archives of Sexual Behavior 5: 371–390.

Avis NER, Zhao X, Johannes CB, Ory M, Brockwell S, Greendale Ga 2005 Correlates of sexual function among multi-ethnic middle-aged women: results from the Study of Women's Health Across the Nation (SWAN). Menopause 12: 385–398.

Babb P, Butcher H, Church J, Zealey L 2006 Social trends, No 36. Office for National Statistics, HMSO, London.

Bancroft J 1978 Psychological and physiological responses to sexual stimuli in men and women. In Levi L (ed) Society, Stress and Disease, Vol. 3. The productive and reproductive age. Oxford University Press, Oxford.

Bancroft J 1998 Introduction to Kinsey AC, Pomeroy WB, Martin CF, Gebhard PH 1953 Sexual Behavior in the Human Female. Saunders, Philadelphia (reprinted 1998).

Bancroft J 2004 Kinsey and the politics of sex research. Annual Review of Sex Research 15: 1–39.

Bancroft J 2005 Normal sexual development. In Barbaree HL, Marshall WM (eds) The Juvenile Sex Offender. Guilford, New York, pp. 19–57.

Bancroft J, Janssen E 2000 The dual control model of male sexual response: a theoretical approach to centrally mediated erectile dysfunction. Neuroscience & Biobehavioral Reviews 24: 571–579.

Bancroft J, Loftus J, Long JS 2003a Distress about sex: a national survey of women in heterosexual relationships. Archives of Sexual Behavior 32: 193–208.

Bancroft J, Herbenick D, Reynolds M 2003b Masturbation as a marker of sexual development. In Bancroft J (ed) Sexual Development in Childhood. Indiana University Press, Bloomington, pp. 156–185.

Bancroft J, McCabe J, Loftus J, Long JS (in press) Sexual well-being: comparing the self-assessments of black and white women in heterosexual relationships.

Barry H III, Schlegel A (eds) 1980 Cross-cultural Samples and Codes. University Pittsburgh Press, Pittsburgh.

Bartels A, Zeki S 2004 The neural correlates of maternal and romantic love. Neuroimage 21: 1155–1166.

Baumeister RF, Catanese KR, Vohs KD 2001 Is there a gender difference in strength of sex drive? Theoretical views, conceptual distinctions and a review of relevant evidence. Personality and Social Psychology 5: 242–273.

Beck JG, Bozman AW, Qualtrough T 1991 The experience of sexual desire: psychological correlates in a college sample. Journal of Sex Research 28: 443–456.

Bell RR 1966 Premarital Sex in a Changing Society. Prentice-Hall, Englewood Cliffs, New Jersey.

Bell AP, Weinberg MS 1978 Homosexualities: A Study of Diversity among Men & Women. Simon & Schuster, New York.

Bell RR, Chaskes JB 1970 Premarital sexual experience among coeds, 1958 and 1968. Journal of Marriage and the Family 32: 81–84.

Bell RR, Turner S, Rosen L 1975 A multivariate analysis of female extramarital coitus. Journal of Marriage and the Family 37: 375–384.

Bell AP, Weinberg MS, Hammersmith SK 1981 Sexual Preference: Its Development among Men and Women. Indiana University Press, Bloomington.

Bem SL 1974 The measurement of psychological androgyny. Journal of Consulting and Clinical Psychology 42: 155–162.

Berkowitz A, Padavic I 1999 Getting a man or getting ahead: a comparison of white and black sororities. Journal of Contemporary Ethnography 27: 530–557.

Billy JOG, Tanfer K, Grady WR, Klepinger DH 1993 The sexual behavior of men in the United States. Family Planning Perspectives 25: 52–60.

Blumstein P, Schwartz P 1983 American Couples. Morrow, New York.

Bone M 1986 Trends in single women's sexual behaviour in Scotland. Population Trends 43: 7–14.

Boonstra H 2002 Teen pregnancy: trends and lessons to be learned. The Guttmacher Report on Public Policy 5: 7–10.

Bozon M 2001 Sexuality, gender and the couple: a socio-historical perspective. Annual Review of Sex Research 12: 1–32.

Briere J, Smiljanich K, Henschel D 1994 Sexual fantasies, gender and molestation history. Child Abuse and Neglect 18: 131–137.

Brinkman PD 1971 Dr Alfred C. Kinsey and the press: historical case study of the relationship of the mass media and a pioneering behavioral scientist. Unpublished doctoral dissertation. Indiana University, Bloomington, IN.

Brockman FS 1902 A study of moral and religious life of 251 preparatory school students in the United States. Pedagogical Seminary 9: 267.

Brotto LA, Chik HM, Ryder AG, Gorzalka BB, Seal Bn 2005 Acculturation and sexual function in Asian women. Archives of Sexual Behavior 34: 595–612.

Broude GJ, Greene SJ 1980 Cross-cultural codes on 20 sexual attitudes and practices. In Barry H III, Schlegel A (eds) Cross-cultural Samples and Codes. University of Pittsburgh Press, Pittsburgh, pp. 313–333.

Bullough VL 1976 Sexual Variance in Society and History. Wiley, New York.

Burgess EW, Cottrell LS 1939 Predicting Success and Failure in Marriage. Prentice-Hall, New York.

Burgess EW, Wallin P 1953 Engagement and Marriage. Lippincott, Chicago.

Bury J 1983 Teenage pregnancies in Britain. Birth Control Trust, London.

Buss DM 1989 Sex differences in human mating preferences: evolutionary hypotheses tested in 37 cultures. Behavioral and Brain Science 12: 1–49.

Buss DM 1994 The Evolution of Desire: Strategies of Human Mating. Basic Books, New York.

Byrne D, Schulte L 1990 Personality dispositions as mediators of sexual responses. Annual Review of Sex Research 1: 93–117.

Cain VS, Johannes CB, Avis NE, Mohr B, Schocken M, Skurnick, Ory M 2003 Sexual functioning and practices in a multi-ethnic study of midlife women: baseline results from SWAN. Journal of Sex Research 40: 266–276.

Call V, Sprecher S, Schwartz P 1995 The incidence and frequency of marital sex in a national sample. Journal of Marriage and the Family 57: 639–652.

Caplow T, Hicks L, Wattenberg BJ 2001 The First Measured Century: An Illustrated Guide to Trends in America 1990–2000. AEI Press, Washington.

Carballo M, Cleland J, Carael M, Albrecht G 1989 A cross national study of patterns of sexual behaviour. Journal of Sex Research 26: 287–299.

Carpenter DL, Janssen E, Graham CA 2008 Women's scores on the Sexual Excitation/Sexual Inhibition Scales (SIS/SES): gender similarities and differences. Journal of Sex Research 45: 36–48.

Catania JA, McDermott LJ, Pollack LM 1986 Questionnaire bias and face-to-face interview sample bias in sexuality research. Journal of Sex Research 22: 52–72.

Catania JA, Gibson DR, Chitwood DD, Coates TJ 1990 Methodological problems in AIDS behavioral research: influences on measurement error and participation bias in studies of sexual behavior. Psychological Bulletin 108: 339–362.

Catania JA, Coates TJ, Stall R, Turner H, Peterson J, Hearst N, Dolcini MM, Hudes E, Gagnon J, Wiley J et al 1992 Prevalence of AIDS-related risk factors and condom use in the United States. Science 258: 1101–1106.

Catania JA, Turner H, Pierce RC, Golden E, Stocking C, Binson D, Mast K 1993 Response bias in surveys of AIDS-related sexual behavior. In Ostrow DG, Kessler RC (eds) Methodological issues in AIDS behavioral research. Plenum Press, New York, pp. 133–162.

Catania JA, Binson D, van der Straten A, Stone V 1995 Methodological research on sexual behavior in the AIDS era. Annual Review of Sex Research 6: 77–125.

Catania JA, Binson D, Canchola J, Pollack LM, Hauck W 1996 Effects of interviewer gender, interviewer choice, and item wording on responses to questions concerning sexual behavior. Public Opinion Quarterly 30: 345–75.

Cawood EHH, Bancroft J 1996 Steroid hormones, the menopause, sexuality and well-being of women. Psychological Medicine 26: 925–936.

Christensen HR, Gregg CF 1970 Changing sex norms in America and Scandinavia. Journal of Marriage and the Family 32: 616–627.

Clayton AH, Segraves RT, Leiblum S, Basson R, Pyke R, Cotton D, Lewis-D'Agostino D, Evans KR, Sills TL, Wunderlich GR 2006 Reliability and validity of the Sexual Interest and Desire Inventory–Female (SIDI-F), a scale designed to measure severity of female Hypoactive Sexual Desire Disorder. Journal of Sex & Marital Therapy 32: 115–136.

Clement U 1990 Surveys of sexual behaviour. Annual Review of Sex Research 1: 45–74.

Clement U, Schmidt G, Kruse M 1984 Changes in sex differences in sexual behavior: a replication of a study of West German students (1966–81). Archives of Sexual Behavior 13: 99–120.

Cooper A, Scherer CR, Boies SC, Gordon BL 1999 Sexuality on the Internet: from sexual exploration to pathological expression. Professional Psychology: Research and Practice 30: 154–164.

Cornog M 2003 The Big Book of Masturbation. Down There Press, San Francisco.

Costa PT, Fagan PJ, Piedmont RL, Ponticas Y, Wise TN 1992 The Five-Factor Model of personality and sexual functioning in outpatient men and women. Psychiatric Medicine 10: 199–215.

Crouch J, Scoville M, Beaulieu R, Sharpe A, Thrine K, Dukat S, Williams S 2007 No-fault divorce laws and divorce rates in the United States and Europe. www.divorcereform.org/DivorceLawAbstract.html.

Cupach WR, Metts S 1995 The role of sexual attitude similarity in romantic heterosexual relationships. Personal Relationships 2: 287–300.

Daly M, Wilson M 1978 Sex, Evolution and Behaviour. Wadsworth, Belmont, CA.

Daneback K, Cooper A, Mansson S-A 2005 An Internet study of cybersex participants. Archives of Sexual Behavior 34: 321–328.

Darroch JE, Frost JJ, Singh S, and The Study Team 2001 Teenage sexual and reproductive behavior in developed countries. Can more progress be made? Occasional Report No 3. Alan Guttmacher Institute, New York.

Darvishpour M 1999 Immigrant women challenge the role of men: conflict intensification within Iranian families in Sweden. Nordic Journal of Women's Studies 7: 20–33.

Davis KB 1929 Factors in the Sex Lives of Twenty-Two Hundred Women. Harper, New York.

Dean KE, Malamuth NM 1997 Characteristics of men who aggress sexually and of men who imagine aggressing: risk and moderating variables. Journal of Personality and Social Psychology 72: 449–455.

Dekker A, Schmidt G 2002 Patterns of masturbatory behaviour: changes between the sixties and the nineties. Journal of Psychology & Human Sexuality 14: 35–48.

DeLamater J, MacCorquodale P 1979 Premarital Sexuality: Attitudes, Relationships, Behavior. University of Wisconsin Press, Madison.

Dennerstein L, Lehert P, Burger H, Dudley E 1999 Factors affecting sexual functioning of women in the midlife years. Climacteric 2: 254–262.

Department of Health 2005 Abortion statistics, England & Wales: 2004. Statistical Bulletin, 11. www.dh.gov.uk/en/Publicationsandstatistics/Publications/PublicationsStatistics/DH_4116461.

Diamond LM 2004 Emerging perspectives on distinctions between romantic love and sexual desire. Current Directions in Psychological Science 13: 116–119.

Dickinson RL, Beam L 1931 A Thousand Marriages. Williams & Wilkins, Baltimore.

Dickinson RL, Beam L 1934 The Single Woman: A Medical Study in Sex Education. Williams & Wilkins, Baltimore.

Dion K 1981 Physical attractiveness, sex roles and heterosexual attraction. In Cook M (Ed) The Bases of Human Sexual Attraction. Academic, London, pp. 3–22.

Dixson AF 1998 Primate sexuality: comparative studies of the prosimians, monkeys, apes and human beings. Oxford University Press, Oxford.

Dixson AF, Halliwell G, East R, Wignarajah P, Anderson MJ 2003 Masculine somatotype and hirsuteness as determinants of sexual attractiveness to women. Archives of Sexual Behavior 32: 29–40.

Dixson BJ, Dixson AF, Morgan B, Anderson MJ 2007 Human physique and sexual attractiveness: sexual preferences of men and women in Bakossiland, Cameroon. Archives of Sexual Behavior 36: 369–376.

Dryfoos JG 1978 The incidence and outcome of adolescent pregnancy in the United States. Journal of Biosocial Science Supplement 5: 85–99.

Dugger K 1988 Social location and gender-role attitudes: a comparison of black and white women. Gender & Society 2: 425–428.

Dunn KM, Croft PR, Hackett GI 1998 Sexual problems: a study of the prevalence and need for health care in the general population. Family Practitioner 15: 519–524.

Dunne MP, Martin NG, Bailey JM, Heath AC, Bucholz KK, Madden PAF, Statham DJ 1997 Participation bias in a sexuality survey: psychological and behavioural characteristics of responders and non-responders. International Journal of Epidemiology 26: 844–853.

Eaton DK, Kann L, Kinchen S, Ross J, Hawkins J, Harris WA, Lowry R, McManus T, Chyen D, Shanklin S, Lim C, Grunbaum JA, Wechsler H 2006 Youth Risk Surveillance-United States, 2005. MMWR Surveillance Summaries, June 9, 2006/55(SS05):1–108.

Ehrhardt AA, Wasserheit JN 1991 Age, gender, and sexual risk behaviors for sexually transmitted diseases in the United States. In Wasserheit JN, Aral SO, Holmes KE, Hitchcock PJ (eds) Research Issues in Human Behavior and Sexually Transmitted Diseases in the AIDS Era. American Society for Microbiology, Washington, DC, pp. 97–121.

Ellis H 1942 Studies in the Psychology of Sex. Vol 1, Part 1. Random House, New York.

Elwin V 1968 The Kingdom of the Young. Oxford University Press, Oxford.

Encyclopaedia Britannica 2007 Encyclopaedia Britannica Online: http://www.britannica.com/eb/article-9077972.

Eplov L, Giraldi A, Davidsen M, Garde K, Kamper-Jorgensen F 2007 Sexual desire in a nationally representative Danish population. Journal of Sexual Medicine 4: 47–56.

Erens B, Korovessis C, Field J, Johnson AM, Copas AJ, Fenton K, Wellings K et al 1997 The impact of computer assisted self-interviewing om the national survey of sexual attitudes and lifestyles. CAT.INIST.FR Cat@inist via Google Scholar.

Erens B, McManus S, Prescott Field J, Johnson AM, Wellings K, Fenton K, Mercer C, Macdowell W, Copas AJ, Nanchahal K 2003 National Survey of Sexual Attitudes and Lifestyles II: Reference Tables and Summary Report. National Centre for Social Research, London.

Ericksen JA 1999 Kiss and Tell. Harvard University Press, Cambridge, MA.

Ernst C, Földényi M, Angst J 1993 The Zurich study: XXI. Sexual dysfunctions and disturbances in young adults. European Archives of Psychiatry & Clinical Neuroscience 243: 179–88.

Evans H 2002 Past, perfect or imperfect: changing images of the ideal wife. In Brownell S, Wasserstrom JN (eds) Chinese Femininities/Chinese Masculinities. University of California Press, Berkeley, pp. 335–360.

Exner M 1915 Problems and Principles of Sex Education. Association Press, New York.

Eysenck HJ 1971 Personality and sexual adjustment. British Journal of Psychiatry 118: 593–608.

Eysenck HJ 1976 Sex and Personality. Open Books, London.

Eysenck HJ, Wilson G 1979 The Psychology of Sex. Dent, London.

Farley F, Nelson JG, Knight WC, Garcia-Colberg E 1977 Sex, politics and personality: a multidimensional study of college students. Archives of Sexual Behavior 6: 105–120.

Farman-Farmaian S 1978 Socio-cultural aspects of age at marriage in the middle-east. Journal Biosocial Science Supplement 5: 215–226.

Farrell C 1978 My Mother Said...: the way young people learn about sex and birth control. Routledge & Kegan Paul, London.

Fenton KA, Johnson AM, McManus S, Erens B 2001 Measuring sexual behaviour: methodological challenges in survey research. Sexually Transmitted Infections 77: 84–92.

Finer LB, Henshaw SK 2006 Disparities in rates of unintended pregnancy in the United States, 1994 and 2001. Perspectives on Sexual and Reproductive Health 38: 90–96.

Fisher W, Byrne D 1981 Social background, attitudes and sexual attraction. In Cook M (ed) The Bases of Human Sexual Attraction. Academic Press, London, pp. 23–64.

Fisher W, Byrne D, White LA, Kelley K 1988 Erotophobia–erotophilia as a dimension of personality. Journal of Sex Research 25: 123–151.

Ford CS, Beach FA 1952 Patterns of Sexual Behaviour. Eyre & Spottiswoode, London.

Fox GL 1981 The family role in adolescent sexual behavior. In: Ooms T (ed) Teenage Pregnancy in a Family Context. Temple University Press, Philadelphia.

Fox GL, Inazu JK 1980 Patterns and outcomes of mother–daughter communication about sexuality. Journal of Social Issues 36: 7–29.

Freedman R, Whelpton PK, Campbell AA 1959 Family Planning, Sterility and Population Growth. McGraw-Hill, New York.

Frenken J 1976 Afkeer van seksualiteit. English summary. Van Loghum Staterus, Deventer, pp. 219–225.

Frenken J, Vennix P 1981 Sexuality Experience Scales Manual. Swets and Zeitlinger B.V.: Zeist, The Netherlands.

Fugl-Meyer AR, Fugl-Meyer KS 1999 Sexual disabilities, problems and satisfaction in 18–74 year old Swedes. Scandinavian Journal of Sexology 2: 79–105.

Gagnon J, Simon W 1973 Sexual Conduct: the Social Sources of Human Sexuality. Aldine, Chicago.

Gagnon J, Simon W 1987 The sexual scripting of oral genital contacts. Archives of Sexual Behavior 16: 1–26.

Galton F 1883 Inquiries into Human Faculty and its Development. Macmillan, London.

Garde K, Lunde I 1980 Female sexual behaviour. A study in a random sample of 40 year old women. Maturitas 2: 225–240.

Gathorne-Hardy J 1998 Sex, the Measure of all Things: a life of Alfred C Kinsey. Chatto & Windus, London.

Gebhard PH, Johnson AB 1979 The Kinsey Data. Marginal tabulations of the 1938–63 interviews. Saunders, Philadelphia.

General Household Survey 2004/5. Internet only publication, ONS: www.statistics.gov.uk/ghs/.

Gerressu M, Mercer CH, Graham CA, Wellings K, Johnson Am 2008 Prevalence of masturbation and associated factors from a British national probability survey. Archives of Sexual Behavior 37: 266–278.

Gillis JR 1985 For Better, For Worse. British marriages, 1600 to the present. Oxford University Press, Oxford.

Glass DV 1974 Population growth in developed countries. In: Parry HB (ed) Population and its Problems: a Plain Man's Guide. Clarendon Press, Oxford.

Gonzalez L, Viitanen T 2006 The effect of divorce laws on divorce rates in Europe. Paper presented at Royal Economic Society's Annual Conference.

Goody JR 1971 Class and marriage in Africa & Eurasia. American Journal of Sociology 76: 585–603.

Graham CA, Janssen E, Sanders SA 2000 Effects of fragrance on female sexual arousal and mood across the menstrual cycle. Psychophysiology 37: 76–84.

Graham CA, Catania JA, Brand R, Duong T, Canchola JA 2003 Recalling sexual behavior: a methodological analysis of memory recall bias via interview using the diary as the gold standard. Journal of Sex Research 40: 325–332.

Graham CA, Sanders SA, Milhausen RR, McBride KR 2004 Turning on and turning off: a focus group study of the factors that affect women's sexual arousal. Archives of Sexual Behavior 33: 527–538.

Graham CA, Sanders SA, Milhausen RR 2006 The Sexual Excitation/Sexual Inhibition Inventory for women: psychometric properties. Archives of Sexual Behavior 35: 397–409.

Gray JP 1984 The influence of female power in marriage on sexual behavior and attitudes: a holocultural study. Archives of Sexual Behavior 13: 223–232.

Green R, Wiener J (eds) 1980 Methodology in sex research. Proceedings of the Conference held in Chevy Chase, MD, November 18 and 19 1977. US Department of Health and Human Services, Washington, DC.

Grunbaum JA, Kann L, Kinchen S, Williams B, Ross J, Lowry R, Kolbe L 2002 Youth Risk Surveillance-United States, 2001. MMWR Surveillance Summaries, June 28, 2002/51(SS04): 1–64.

GSS 1972–2000 Cumulative codebook. http//:webapp.icpsr.umich.edu/gss.

GSS 2000 General Social Survey. NORC. http://www.norc.uchicago.edu/projects/gensoc.asp

Hariton EB, Singer JL 1974 Women's fantasies during sexual intercourse: normative and theoretical implications. Journal of Consulting and Clinical Psychology 42: 313–322.

Hatfield E, Rapson R 1993 Love, Sex and Intimacy: the Psychology, Biology and History. Harper Collins. New York.

Hatfield E, Sprecher S 1986 Measuring passionate love in intimate relations. Journal of Adolescence 9: 383–410.

Hatfield E, Walster GW 1981 A New Look at Love. University Press of America, Lanshaw, Maryland.

Hazan C, Shaver P 1987 Romantic love conceptualized as an attachment process. Journal of Personality and Social Psychology 52: 511–524.

Hedricks CA 1994 Sexual behavior across the menstrual cycle: a biopsychosocial approach. Annual Review of Sex Research 5: 122–172.

Herdt GH 1981 Guardians of the Flutes. McGraw-Hill, New York.

Hertoft P 1977 Nordic traditions of marriage: the betrothal system. In Money J, Musaph H (eds) Handbook of Sexology. Excerpta Medica, Amsterdam, pp. 505–510.

Hess EH 1965 Attitudes and pupil size. Scientific American 212: 46–54.

Hicks TV, Leitenberg H 2001 Sexual fantasies about one's partner versus someone else: gender differences in incidence and frequency. Journal of Sex Research 38: 43–50.

Hite S 1976 The Hite Report: A Nationwide Study on Female Sexuality. Talmy Franklin, London.

Hite S 1978 The Hite Report on Male Sexuality. Alfred A. Knopf, New York.

Hite S 1991 The Hite Report on Love, Passion and Emotional Violence. Macdonald Optima, London.

Hofferth SL 1990 Trends in adolescent sexual activity, contraception and pregnancy in the United States. In Bancroft J, Reinisch J (eds) Adolescence and Puberty. Third Kinsey symposium. Oxford University Press, New York, pp. 217–232.

Hoon EF, Hoon PW, Wincze JP 1976 An inventory for the measurement of female sexual arousability: the SAI. Archives of Sexual Behavior 5: 291–300.

Hotvedt ME 1988 Emerging and submerging adolescent sexuality: culture and sexual orientation. In: Bancroft J, Reinisch J (eds) Adolescence and Puberty. Third Kinsey Symposium. Oxford University Press, New York, pp. 157–172.

Houston LN 1981 Romanticism and eroticism among black and white college students. Adolescence 16: 263–272.

Hrdy SB 2000 Sexuality across the life cycle: discussion paper. In Bancroft J (ed) The Role of Theory in Sex Research. Indiana University Press, Bloomington, pp. 33–45.

Ineichen B 1979 The social geography of marriage. In Cook M, Wilson G (eds) Love and Attraction. Pergamon, Oxford.

Janssen E, Vorst H, Finn P, Bancroft J 2002 The Sexual Inhibition (SIS) and Sexual Excitation (SES) Scales: I. Measuring sexual inhibition and excitation proneness in men. Journal of Sex Research 39: 114–126.

Janssen E, Carpenter D, Graham CA 2003 Selecting films for sex research: gender differences in erotic film preference. Archives of Sexual Behavior 32: 243–252.

Johnson AM, Wadsworth J, Wellings K, Field J 1994 Sexual Attitudes and Lifestyles. Blackwell, Oxford.

Johnson AM, Mercer CM, Erens B, Copas AJ, McManus S, Wellings K, Fenton KA, Korovessis C, Macdowall W, Nanchahal K, Purdon S, Field J 2001 Sexual behaviour in Britain: partnerships, practices and HIV risk behaviours. Lancet 358: 1835–1842.

Jones EF, Forrest JD, Goldman N, Henshaw SK, Lincoln R, Rosoff JI, Westoff CF, Wulf D 1985 Teenage pregnancies in developed countries: determinants and policy implications. Family Planning Perspectives 17: 53–63.

Joyner K, Laumann EO 2001 Teenage sex and the sexual revolution. In Laumann EO, Michael RT (eds) Sex, Love, and Health in America: Private Choices and Public Policies. University of Chicago Press, Chicago, pp. 41–71.

Kahr B 2007 Sex and the Psyche. Allen Lane, London.

Kantner JF, Zelnick M 1972 Sexual experience of young unmarried women in the United States. Family Planning Perspectives 4: 9–18.

Kim J, Hatfield E 2004 Love types and subjective well-being: a cross-cultural study. Social Behavior and Personality 32: 173–182.

Kinsey AC, Pomeroy WB, Martin CF 1948 Sexual Behavior in the Human Male. Saunders, Philadelphia.

Kinsey AC, Pomeroy WB, Martin CF, Gebhard PH 1953 Sexual Behavior in the Human Female. Saunders, Philadelphia.

Kirby D 1997 No easy answers: research findings on programs to reduce teen pregnancy. The National Campaign to Prevent Teen Pregnancy, Washington, DC.

Klassen AD, Williams CJ, Levitt EE 1989 Sex and Morality in the US: An Empirical Enquiry under the Auspices of the Kinsey Institute. Wesleyan University Press, New York.

Kolata GB 1974 !Kung hunter-gatherers: feminism, diet and birth control. New York Science 185: 932–934.

Kon IS 1995 The Sexual Revolution in Russia. From the Age of the Czars to Today. The Free Press, New York.

Kontula O, Haavio-Mannila E 2002 Masturbation in a generational perspective. Journal of Psychology & Human Sexuality 14: 49–83.

Kreider RM, Fields JM 2002 Number, Timing, and Duration of Marriages and Divorces: 1996, US Census Bureau Current Population Reports, February 2002, p. 18.

Ku L, Sonenstein FL, Pleck JH 1993 Young men's risk behaviors for HIV and sexually transmitted diseases. American Journal of Public Health 83: 1609–1615.

Laan E, Everaerd W, van Bellen G, Hanewald G 1994 Women's sexual and emotional responses to male- and female-produced erotics. Archives of Sexual Behavior 23: 153–169.

Laumann EO, Gagnon JH, Michael RT, Michaels S 1994 The Social Organization of Sexuality: Sexual Practices in the United States. University of Chicago Press, Chicago.

Laumann EO, Ellingson S, Mahay J, Paik A, Youm Y 2004. The Sexual Organization of the City. University of Chicago Press, Chicago.

Lee JA 1976 Lovestyles. Dent, New York.

Leiblum SR 2001 Women, sex and the Internet. Sexual and Relationship Therapy 16: 398–405.

Leitenberg H, Henning K 1995 Sexual fantasy. Psychological Bulletin 117: 469–496.

Leridon H 1996 Coital frequency: data and consistency analysis. In Bozon M, Leridon H (eds) Sexuality and the Social Sciences: A French Survey on Sexual Behaviour. Dartmouth, Aldershot, pp. 203–228.

Leshner AI 2003 Don't let ideology trump science [editorial]. Science 302: 1479.

Levine R, Sato S, Hashimoto T, Verma J 1995 Love and marriage in eleven cultures. Journal of Cross-cultural Psychology 26: 554–571.

Littlewood B 1978 South Italian couples. In Corbin M (ed) The Couple. Penguin, London.

Liu D, Ng ML, Zhou LP, Haeberle EJ 1992. Sexual Behavior in Modern China: Report on the Nationwide Survey of 20 000 Men and Women. (In Chinese). Shanghai, Joint Publishing Co. English translation published by Continuum, New York, 1997.

Lloyd EA 2005 The Case of the Female Orgasm: Bias in the Science of Evolution. Harvard University Press, Cambridge.

Longford 1972 Pornography: the Longford Report. Coronet, London.

Luker K 1996 Dubious Conceptions. Harvard University Press, Cambridge.

Mahay J, Laumann EO, Michaels S 2001. Race, gender and class in sexual scripts. In Laumann EO, Michael RT (eds) Sex, Love and Health in America. University of Chicago Press, Chicago.

Malinowski B 1929 The Sexual Life of Savages. Routledge, London.

Markle Foundation 2001 Toward a Framework for Internet Accountability. Markle Foundation, New York.

Marshall DS, Suggs RC (eds) 1971 Human Sexual Behavior. Prentice-Hall, Englewood Cliffs, NJ.

Mathews AM, Bancroft J, Slater P 1972 The principal components of sexual preference. British Journal of Social and Clinical Psychology 11: 35–43.

McCabe MP, Collins JK 1983 The sexual and affectional attitudes and experiences of Australian adolescents during dating: the effects of age, church attendance, type of school and socioeconomic class. Archives of Sexual Behavior 12: 525–540.

McCall K, Meston C 2006 Cues resulting in desire for sexual activity in women. Journal of Sexual Medicine 3: 838–852.

Mead M 1929 Coming of Age in Samoa. Jonathan Cape, London.

Mead M 1931 Growing Up in New Guinea. Routledge, London.

Mead M 1950 Male and Female. Pelican, London.

Measure DHS 2006 Demographic and health surveys 1984–present. http://www.measuredhs.com.

Meston CM, Trapnell PDF, Gorzalka BB 1996 Ethnic and gender differences in sexuality: variations in sexual behavior between Asian and non-Asian university students. Archives of Sexual Behavior 25: 33–72.

Meston CM, Trapnell PDF, Gorzalka BB 1998 Ethnic, gender and length of residency influences on sexual knowledge and attitudes. Journal of Sex Research 35: 176–188.

Michaels S 1997 Integrating quantitative and qualitative methods in the study of sexuality. In Bancroft J (ed) Researching Sexual Behavior: methodological issues. Indiana University Press, Indiana, pp. 299–308.

Moreault D, Follingstad DR 1978 Sexual fantasies of females as a function of sex guilt and experimental response cues. Journal of Consulting and Clinical Psychology 46: 1385–1393.

Mosher DL 1968 Measurement of guilt in females by self-report inventories. Journal of Consulting and Clinical Psychology 30: 25–29.

Mosher DL, MacIan P 1994 College men and women respond to X-rated videos intended for male or female audiences: gender and sexual scripts. Journal of Sex Research 31: 99–114.

Mosher WD, Chandra A, Jones J 2005 Sexual behavior and selected health measures: men and women 15–44 years of age, United States, 2002. Advance data from Vital & Health Statistics, 362. September 15, 2005.

Mullan B 1984 The Mating Trade. Routledge & Kegan Paul, London.

Murdock GP 1967 Ethnographic Atlas. University Pittsburgh Press, Pittsburgh.

Murnen SK, Stockton M 1997 Gender and self-reported sexual arousal in response to sexual stimuli: a meta-analytic review. Sex Roles 37: 135–153.

Mustanski BS 2001 Getting wired: exploiting the Internet for the collection of valid sexuality data. Journal of Sex Research 38: 292–301.

Nathanson CA 1991 Dangerous Passage: the Social Control of Sexuality in Women's Adolescence. Temple University Press, Philadelphia.

Nathanson CA 2000 In Bancroft J (ed) The Role of Theory in Sex Research. Indiana University Press, Bloomington, pp. 241–257.

National Institute of Mental Health 1972 National Institute of Mental Health Task Force on homosexuality: final report and background papers (DHEW publication no. 72-9116), Livingood JM (ed). US Government Printing Office, Washington, DC.

Nazareth I, Boynton P, King M 2003 Problems with sexual function in people attending London general practitioners: cross sectional study. British Medical Journal 327:423–429.

Newcomer SF, Udry JR 1985 Oral sex in an adolescent population. Archives of Sexual Behavior 14: 41–46.

Njikam Savage OM, Tchombe TM 1994 Anthropological perspectives on sexual behaviour in Africa. Annual Review of Sex Research 5: 50–72.

Oggins J, Leber D, Veroff J 1993a Race and gender differences in black and white newly wed's perceptions of sexual and marital relations. Journal of Sex Research 30: 152–160.

Oggins J, Veroff J, Leber D 1993b Perceptions of marital interactions among black and white newly weds. Journal of Personality and Social Psychology 65: 494–511.

Orbuch TL, Veroff J, Hassan H, Horrocks J 2002 Who will divorce: a 14 year longitudinal study of black and white couples. Journal of Social & Personal Relationships 19: 179–202.

Ortner SB, Whitehead H (eds) 1981 Sexual Meanings: the Cultural Construction of Gender and Sexuality. Cambridge University Press, Cambridge.

Pan S 1993 A sex revolution in current China. Journal of Psychology & Human Sexuality 6: 1–14.

Parker R 1997 International perspectives on sexuality research. In Bancroft J (ed), Researching Sexual Behavior: Methodological Issues. Indiana University Press, Bloomongton, pp. 9–22.

Parker R, Easton D 1998 Sexuality, culture, and political economy: recent developments in anthropological and cross-cultural sex research. Annual Review of Sex Research 9: 1–19.

Perper T 1985 Sex Signals: the Biology of Love. ISI Press, New York

Pietropinto A, Simenauer J 1977 Beyond the Male Myth. A Nationwide Survey. Times Books, New York.

Rainwater L 1966 Some aspects of lower class sexual behavior. Journal of Social Issues 22: 96–108.

Regan PC, Berscheid E 1996 Beliefs about the state, goals and objects of sexual desire. Journal of Sex & Marital Therapy 22: 110–120.

Reiss IL 1964 Premarital sexual permissiveness among negroes and whites. American Sociological Review 29: 688–698.

Reiss IL 1967 The Social Context of Premarital Sexual Permissiveness. Rinehart & Winston, New York.

Reiss IL 1969 Premarital sexual standards. In Broderick CB, Bernard J (eds) The Individual, Sex and Society: a Siecus Handbook for Teachers and Counselors. Johns Hopkins Press, Baltimore.

Renaud C, Byers ES, Pan S 1997 Sexual and relationship satisfaction in mainland China. Journal of Sex Research 34: 399–410.

Richters J, Grulich AE, de Visser RO, Smith AMA, Rissel CE 2003 Sex in Australia: autoerotic, esoteric and other sexual practices engaged in by a representative sample of adults. Australian and New Zealand Journal of Public Health 27: 180–190.

Riley JW, White M 1940 The uses of various methods of contraception. American Sociological Review 5: 890–903.

Roberts A, Cash TF, Feingold A, Johnson BT 2006. Are black–white differences in females' body dissatisfaction decreasing? A meta-analytic review. Journal of Consulting and Clinical Psychology 74: 1121–1131.

Robie WF 1916 Rational Sex Ethics. Richard G. Badger, Boston.

Rosenblatt P, Anderson R 1981 Human sexuality in cross-cultural perspective. In Cook M (ed) The Bases of Human Sexual Attraction. Academic, London, pp. 215–250.

Ruan F-F, Lau MP 2001 China. In Francoeur RT (ed) The International Encyclopedia of Sexuality 1997–2001, Volumes 1–4, The Continuum Publishing Company, www2.hu-berlin.de/sexology/IES/.html.

Ryder NM, Westoff CF 1971 Reproduction in the United States, 1965. Princeton University Press, Princeton.

Ryder AG, Alden LE, Paulhus DL 2000 Is acculturation unidimensional or bidimensional? A head-to-head comparison in the prediction of personality, self-identity and adjustment. Journal of Personality and Social Psychology 79: 49–65.

Sabogal F, Binson D, Catania JA 1997 Researching sexual behavior: methodological issues for Hispanics. In Bancroft J (ed) Researching Sexual Behavior: Methodological Issues. Indiana University Press, Bloomington, IN, pp. 114–133.

Sai FA 1978 Social and psychosexual problems of African adolescents. Journal of Biosocial Science Supplement 5: 235–247.

Santelli J, Lindberg LD, Abma J, McNeely CS, Resnick M 2000a Adolescent sexual behavior: estimates and trends from four nationally representative surveys. Family Planning Perspectives 32: 156–166.

Santelli JS, Lindberg LD, Abma J, McNeely CS, Resnick M 2000b The association of sexual behaviors with socio-economic status, family structure, and race/ethnicity among US adolescents. American Journal of Public Health 90: 1582–1588.

Satcher D 2001 The surgeon general's call to action to promote sexual health and responsible sexual behavior. http://www.surgeongeneral.gov/library.

Schenk J, Pfrang H 1986 Extraversion, neuroticism and sexual behavior: interrelationships in a sample of young men. Archives of Sexual Behavior 12: 31–42.

Schenk J, Pfrang H, Rausche A 1981 Personality traits versus the quality of the marital relationship as the determinants of marital sexuality. Archives of Sexual Behavior 15: 449–456.

Schlegel A, Barry H III 1980 Adolescent initiation ceremonies. A cross-cultural code. In: Barry H III , Schlegel A 1980 (eds) Cross-cultural Samples and Codes. University of Pittsburgh Press, Pittsburgh, pp. 227–288.

Schmidt G 1975 Male–female differences in sexual arousal and behavior during and after exposure to sexually explicit stimuli. Archives of Sexual Behavior 4: 353–366.

Schmidt G 1977 Introduction, socio-historical perspectives. In Money J, Musaph H (eds) Handbook of Sexology. Excerpta Medica, Amsterdam, pp. 269–282.

Schmidt G 1998 Sexuality and late modernity. Annual Review of Sex Research 9: 224– 241.

Schmidt G, Sigusch V 1971 Patterns of sexual behavior in West German workers and students. Journal of Sex Research 7: 89–106.

Schmidt G, Sigusch V 1972 Changes in sexual behavior among young males and females between 1960 and 1970. Archives of Sexual Behavior 2: 27–45.

Schofield M 1965 The Sexual Behaviour of Young People. Longman, London.

Short RV 1976 The evolution of human reproduction. In: Short RV, Baird DT (eds) Contraceptives of the Future. Royal Society, London.

Shorter E 1973 Female emancipation, birth control and fertility in European history. American Historical Review 78: 605–640.

Shorter E 1975 The Making of the Modern Family. Basic Books, New York.

Simon W, Berger AS, Gagnon JH 1972 Beyond anxiety and fantasy: the coital experiences of college youth. Journal of Youth and Adolescence 1: 203–232.

Smith ER, Becker MA, Byrne D, Pryzbala DPJ 1993 Sexual attitudes of males and females as predictors of interpersonal attraction and marital compatibility. Journal of Applied Social Psychology 23: 1011–1034.

Snowden R, Christian B 1983 Patterns and Perceptions of Menstruation. A WHO International Study. Croom Helm, London.

Social Trends 2006 No 36. Office for National Statistics. www.statistics.gov.uk.

Spector IP, Carey MP, Steinberg L 1996 The Sexual Desire Inventory: development, factor structure and evidence of reliability. Journal of Sex & Marital Therapy 22: 175–190.

Spira A, Bajos N, the ACSF Group 1994 Sexual Behaviour and AIDS. Avebury, Hampshire, UK.

Sprecher S, Aron A, Hatfield E, Cortese A, Potpava E, Levitskaya A 1994 Love: American style, Russian style, and Japanese style. Personal Relationships 1: 349–369.

Staples R 1981 The Black Family: Essays and Studies. Wadsworth, Belmont, CA.

Sterk-Elifson C 1994. Sexuality among African-American Women. In Rossi AS (ed) Sexuality Across the Lifecourse. University of Chicago Press, Chicago, pp. 99–126.

Sternberg RJ 1986 A triangular theory of love. Psychological Review 93: 119–135.

Stone L 1979 The Family, Sex and Marriage in England 1500–1800. Pelican, London.

Strassberg DS, Lowe K 1996 Volunteer bias in sexuality research. Archives of Sexual Behavior 24: 369–382.

Strassberg DS, Lockerd LK 1998 Force in women's sexual fantasies. Archives of Sexual Behavior 27: 403–414.

Symons D 1995 Beauty is in the adaptations of the beholder: the evolutionary psychology of human female sexual attractiveness. In Abramson PR, Pinkerton SD (eds) Sexual Nature, Sexual Culture. University of Chicago Press, Chicago, pp. 80–120.

Tannahill R 1980 Sex in History. Hamish Hamilton, London.

Tavris C, Sadd S 1977 The Redbook Report on Female Sexuality: 100 000 married women disclose the good news about sex. Delacorte, New York.

Technical Reports of the Commission on Obscenity and Pornography, vol I–VII. 1970 US Government Printing Office, Washington.

Tennov D 1979 Love and Limerence: the Experience of Being in Love. Stein & Day, New York.

Tennov D 1980 The clarification of proximate mechanisms. Comment on D Symon's The evolution of human sexuality. Behavioral and Brain Science 3: 200.

Terman L 1938 Psychological Factors in Marital Happiness. McGraw-Hill, New York.

Toledano R, Pfaus J 2006 The Sexual Arousal and Desire Inventory (SADI): a multidimensional scale to assess subjective arousal and desire. Journal of Sexual Medicine 3: 853–877.

Tovee MJ, Maisey DS, Emery JL, Cornelissen PL 1999 Visual clues to female physical attractiveness. Proceedings of the Royal Society of London. Series B, 266: 211–218.

Tovee MJ, Swami V, Furnham A, Mangalparsad R 2006 Changing perceptions of attractiveness as observers are exposed to different cultures. Evolution and Human Behavior 27: 443–456.

Turner CF, Miller HG, Rogers SM 1997 Survey measurement of sexual behavior: problems and progress. In Bancroft J (ed) Researching Sexual Behavior: Methodological Issues. Indiana University Press, Bloomington, pp. 37–60.

Twenge JM, Crocker J 2002 Race and self-esteem: meta-analyses comparing whites, blacks, Asians and American Indians and comment on Gray-Little and Hafdahl (2000). Psychological Bulletin 128: 371–408.

Udry JR 1974 The social context of marriage. 3rd edn. Lippincott, Philadelphia.

US Census Bureau 2003 US Census 2002, Summary Files 1 and 2. Available from US Census Bureau website,http://www.census.gov.

Vener AM, Stewart CS 1974 Adolescent sexual behavior in middle America revisited: 1970–1973. Journal of Marriage and the Family 36: 728–735.

Visotsky HM 1969 A community project for unwed pregnant adolescents. In Pollak O, Friedman AS (eds) Family Dynamics and Female Sexual Delinquency. Science and Behavior Books, Palo Alto.

Waite LJ, Joyner K (2001) Emotional and physical satisfaction with sex in married, cohabiting, and dating sexual unions: do men and women differ? In Laumann EO, Michael RT (eds) Sex, Love and Health in America. University of Chicago Press, Chicago, pp. 239–269.

Walster E, Traupmann J, Walster GW 1978 Equity and extramarital sexuality. Archives of Sexual Behavior 7: 127–142.

Weeden J, Sabini J 2005 Physical attractiveness and health in Western societies: a review. Psychological Bulletin 131: 635–653.

Weinberg MS, Williams CJ 1974 Male Homosexuals: Their Problems and Adaptations. Oxford University Press, New York.

Weinberg MS, Williams C 1988 Black sexuality: a test of two theories. Journal of Sex Research 25:197–218.

Wellings K, Nanchahal K, Macdowall W, McManus S, Erens B, Mercer CH, Johnson AM, Copas AJ, Korovessis C, Fenton KA, Field J 2001 Sexual behaviour in Britain: early heterosexual experience. Lancet 358: 1843–1850.

Wellings K, Collumbien M, Slaymaker E, Singh S, Hodges Z, Patel D, Bajos N 2006 Sexual behaviour in context: a global perspective. Lancet 368: 1706–1728.

Westphal SP 2004 Glad to be asexual. New Scientist 14th October 2004 www.newscientist.com/article.n?id=dn6533.

Whyte MK 1980 Cross-cultural codes dealing with the relative status of women. In Barry H III , Schlegel A (eds) Cross-cultural Samples and Codes. University of Pittsburgh Press, Pittsburgh, pp. 335–361.

Williams B 1979 Report of the Committee on Obscenity and Film Censorship. HMSO, London.

Williams CJ, Weinberg MS 1971 Homosexuals and the Military. Harper & Row, New York.

Witchel SF, Plant TM 2004 Puberty: gonadarche and adrenarche. In Strauss JF, Barbieri RL (eds) Yen & Jaffe's Reproductive Endocrinology, 5th edn. Elsevier, Philadelphia, pp. 463–492.

Wyatt GE 1990 Factors affecting adolescent sexuality. Have they changed in 40 years? In: Bancroft J, Reinisch J (eds) Adolescence and Puberty. Third Kinsey Symposium. Oxford University Press, New York, pp. 182–206.

Yaffe M 1972 Research survey. Appendix V. In Longford F (ed) Pornography: the Longford Report. Coronet, London.

Zelnick M, Kantner JF 1977 Sexual and contraceptive experience of young unmarried women in the United States, 1976 and 1971. Family Planning Perspectives 9: 55–71.

Zelnick M, Kantner JF 1980 Sexual activity, contraceptive use and pregnancy among metropolitan area teenagers 1971–79. Family Planning Perspectives 12: 230–237.

Zelnick M, Shah FK 1983 First intercourse among young Americans. Family Planning Perspectives 15: 64–70.

Zerhouni EA 2004 Letter to The Honorable Judd Gregg, Chairman, Committee on Health, Education, Labor and Pensions, US Senate, January 26.

Zurbriggen EL, Yost MR 2004 Power, desire and pleasure in sexual fantasies. Journal of Sex Research 41: 288–300.

7 Sexuality and ageing

Changes in sexual behaviour with age 238
Surveys of both men and women 238

Ageing and sexual function in men 240
Surveys of older men 240
Ageing mechanisms 241

Ageing and sexual function in women 243
Surveys of older women 243
Age or menopause? 244
The precise nature of the decline in sexuality............................ 245

Conclusions 250

Human beings are living longer and longer as education, the quality of life and medical science reduce the impact of illness. Women tend to live longer than men. Three consequences of these trends are that we have more elderly people who are healthy, more who are in need of care, and more women than men in the older age groups. The part that healthy old people play in our society, and the increasing needs of the very old, continue to pose some of the most crucial questions facing modern societies.

These age and gender patterns are evident throughout the European Union. In 2004, Italy had the highest percentage population aged 65 years or older, 19.2%. Germany had the next highest, 18%, then Greece, with 17.8%. The UK, with 16%, was slightly below the European Union average of 16.5%.

In the USA this percentage is somewhat lower; in 2000, 12.4% were 65 years or older (US Census Bureau 2000).

Table 7.1 shows the percentage of the UK population in the older age groups (55–64, 65–74 and 75+ years) from 1971 to 2004, with projected percentages for 2011 and 2021. This shows little change in the 55–64 age group, but a more substantial increase in the 75+ group. The life expectancy of women has averaged around 6 years longer than for men for some time. In 1971 the percentage of women in the 75+ age group was more than twice that for men. However, as we see in Table 7.1, there has been a slight reduction in this difference. The gender difference increases, however, in the very elderly; in the UK in 2004 at age 89, there were 40 men per 100 women (Babb et al 2006). In the USA in 2000 at age 85, there were 40.7 men per 100 women (US Census Bureau 2000).

Changes in sexual behaviour with age

Kinsey et al (1948), in their volume on the male, concluded that 'from the early and middle years the decline in sexual activity is remarkably steady and there is no point at which old age suddenly enters the picture' (p. 227). In the female volume, a somewhat different picture was painted. 'There is little evidence of any ageing in the sexual capacities of the female until late in life' (Kinsey et al 1953, p. 353). The number of really elderly people in their otherwise large samples was relatively small and the conclusions about the effects of old age were drawn rather tentatively. However, this trend, at least as far as the male is concerned, has been shown to some extent in later studies, several of which will be considered in this chapter. Of particular importance is the extent to which men and women age differently in their sexual lives. Very few of the available surveys of older age groups have asked the same questions of men and women. The few that have will be reviewed first to seek a perspective of gender differences in relation to sex and ageing. We will then consider the evidence of ageing effects in men and women in separate sections.

Surveys of both men and women

In 1999 the AARP (American Association for Retired Persons) carried out a survey of older men and women in the USA (NFO 1999). A reasonably representative sample of 1376 individuals, 45 years and older (636 men and 740 women), were recruited from the National Family Opinion Research panel of 565 000 individuals who had agreed to participate in occasional surveys. The data were made more representative by applying weights. The mean age was 60 years for men and 61 years for women. Three age groups were compared: 45–59 years (341 men and 368 women), 60–74 years (205 men and 253 women) and 75+ years (90 men and 119 women). The percentages who were married or living with a partner at the time of the survey, for the three age groups, were 80.1%, 77% and 69% for men, respectively, and 71.4%, 56% and 25.5% for women. Having a satisfying sexual relationship was considered important or very important for quality of life by 74%, 61% and 50% of men in the three age groups. For women, the equivalent percentages were 66%, 48% and 44%.

The frequency of sexual thoughts, a measure of sexual interest, by age group, in men and women, is shown in Table 7.2. Not only is there a clear decrease in this measure across the age groups, there is a striking gender difference, with women reporting much less frequent sexual thoughts across the age groups. This measure does not differ much between men with and without

TABLE 7.1 Percentage of the total population of the UK in the older age groups since 1971, with projected estimates for 2011 and 2021. (Derived from Babb et al 2006). Percentages for the USA are shown for 2000 only (US Census Bureau)

| | Age group (years) | | | | | |
| | 55–64 | | 65–74 | | 75+ | |
	Male	Female	Male	Female	Male	Female
UK						
Historic						
1971	11.5	12.0	7.4	9.6	3.1	6.3
1981	10.8	11.2	8.3	10.1	3.9	7.7
1991	10.2	10.1	8.1	9.5	4.9	8.9
2001	10.7	10.5	8.0	8.7	5.6	9.3
2004	11.6	11.5	8.1	8.7	5.9	9.3
Projected						
2011	11.8	11.9	8.7	9.2	6.6	9.3
2021	12.6	12.9	9.9	10.5	8.3	10.6
USA						
2000	8.4	8.8	6.5	6.0	4.4	7.3

TABLE 7.2 Frequency of sexual thoughts by age group (years) in men and women (AARP; NFO 1999)

| | Men | | | Women | | |
	45–59	60–74	75+	45–59	60–74	75+
Once a day or more	43.3	18.1	9.1	8.8	0.8	1.2
Once to three times a week	40.9	35.4	26.4	32.6	13.0	4.1
Once to three times a month	8.1	16.7	25.6	19.6	17.1	11.5
Less than once a month	4.0	16.6	14.0	17.8	20.0	17.9
Not at all	2.0	11.0	18.2	16.8	43.6	57.2

TABLE 7.3 Frequency of sexual activities by age group (years) in men and women (AARP; NFO 1999)

| | Men | | | Women | | |
	45–59	60–74	75+	45–59	60–74	75+
SEXUAL TOUCHING WITH PARTNER						
Once a week or more	68.9	61.2	45.2	61.4	36.6	14.9
Not at all	12.4	21.9	35.6	22.4	51.4	78.4
SEXUAL INTERCOURSE						
Once a week or more	54.8	30.9	19.1	49.6	24.2	6.6
Not at all	17.0	31.3	51.4	27.0	53.7	83.8
SELF STIMULATION (MASTURBATION)						
Once a week or more	33.5	14.2	5.2	4.5	2.0	0.6
Not at all	35.8	64.5	73.5	67.5	80.0	90.4

sexual partners, whereas women without sexual partners are much more likely to report no sexual thoughts than women with partners (47.8% and 22.2%, respectively). Frequencies of sexual activity with partner and of masturbation are shown in Table 7.3. Once again we see decreasing frequencies across the age groups, and a marked gender difference. This to some extent reflects the smaller number of women with a sexual partner, but is also apparent with masturbation. The likelihood of reporting dissatisfaction with one's sex life does not follow the same age-related pattern, and in the 75+ age group 46% of men and 49% of women described themselves as 'neither satisfied nor dissatisfied'.

In 2004 the AARP carried out a further survey aimed at assessing changes since 1999 and also to compare racial minorities with the white majority (AARP 2005). Overall, there were few major changes. In 2004 there was greater acceptance of the role that sex plays in relationships, and less opposition to sex for the unmarried. Slightly more men reported masturbating. An increased proportion of men reported erectile problems (31% vs 26% in 1999) and men were more likely to seek information and medical help, and more likely to try the effects of medication to improve their sexual responsiveness. African Americans were less likely to have a sexual partner.

DeLamater & Sill (2005) carried out a secondary analysis of the AARP data, focusing on factors influencing sexual desire. They confirmed the substantially greater link in women than in men between experiencing sexual desire and having a sexual partner. They also explored the impact of attitudes to sexuality, seeing these as reflecting psychosocial rather than biological influences. After a factor analysis of the various attitudinal questions in the survey, they derived two factors; one positive, focusing on the relationship, the other negative, focusing on the self. The positive attitude factor consisted of three items: sexual activity is important to my overall quality of life, sexual activity is a critical part of a good relationship and sexual activity is a duty to one's spouse/partner. The negative factor also consisted of three items: I do not particularly enjoy sex, I would be quite happy never having sex again and sex is only for younger people. They used these two factors and a number of other variables to predict level of sexual desire. In both women and men, age was the strongest predictor of sexual desire, followed by the two 'attitude' measures. However, it is questionable whether these attitude measures are cause or effect in this respect. For the negative factor, the first two items can be regarded as description of a lack of desire and enjoyment rather than an attitude. The third, 'sex is only for younger people', could reflect a socio-cultural belief which has certainly been widespread at least until recently. But this could also reflect a way of coming to terms with a loss of sexual desire or response. The items in the positive factor can be regarded as attitudes but may also reflect the extent to which sex is playing a positive role. Hence, someone with little sexual desire or response may be less likely to agree to the three statements.

The Global Study of Sexual Attitudes and Behaviors (GSSAB) was an international survey of men and women aged 40–80 years, recruited from 29 countries and involving more than 13 000 women and a similar number of men. Predictors of sexual problems, including age, were explored (Laumann et al 2005). When controlling for other variables, such as physical and mental health, education and financial status, increasing age in men was clearly associated with erectile problems, difficulty in reaching orgasm and lack of sexual interest, across all regions studied. In women, on the other hand, age was only associated with lubrication difficulties, in all regions studied except Central/South America, and South-East Asia. Early ejaculation was the commonest sexual problem reported by men (ranging from 12.4% of men in the Middle East to 30.5% in South-East Asia), but tended to be less prevalent in the older age groups, consistent with the age-related difficulty in reaching orgasm. Laumann et al (2005), while pointing out the limitations of this huge study, with an average response rate of only 19%, varying methods of data collection and uncertainty about the equivalence of meaning of the questions across cultures and languages, concluded that sexual problems were more associated with ageing and physical health in men than in women. However, it is important to keep in mind that the focus of this study was sexual problems. As we will see at various points in this chapter, older women are less likely than older men or younger women to regard a decline in sexual function or activity as a problem.

In an early longitudinal study of 261 men and 241 women aged 45–71 years, Pfeiffer and colleagues (Pfeiffer & Davis 1972; Pfeiffer & Verwoerdt 1972) found a much greater decline in both sexual activity and interest among the women, with the most dramatic decline occurring between 50 and 60 years of age. In the 66–71 age group, 50% of women said they had no sexual interest, compared with only 10% of the men.

In looking more closely at the possible mechanisms underlying age-related sexual decline, it is clear that there are important gender differences, and we will consider possible explanations for these in the following sections.

Ageing and sexual function in men

Surveys of older men

A steady decline in the frequency of sexual activity in men was reported by Martin (1977) from the Baltimore Longitudinal Aging Study. Martin (1977) also found that the extent of the decline was a function of the level of sexual activity during early adult life. Those with the highest level of sexual activity when younger showed proportionately the least decline, so that the differences between the high- and low-activity groups became much more marked in the later years. This is an important observation, which has been largely ignored in subsequent research. There is consistent evidence over the now numerous surveys that whereas there is an age-related decline in male sexuality, it is very variable, with some men remaining sexually active well into old age. This variability is also apparent when controlling for the effects of ill-health. This leaves us with the question of why some men show the ageing effect more than others, which has not yet been adequately addressed.

Martin (1981) commented on the association between the duration of a sexual relationship and the level of sexual interest. It is often suggested that lack of novelty and boredom are important factors contributing to the age-related decline, as evidenced by the commonplace increase in interest and activity with a new partner. However, as Martin points out, as it is those men who are most active when younger who show the least decline, boredom is not a sufficient explanation for the overall ageing effect and other sources of individual variability need to be looked for.

Hegeler & Mortensen (1978) reported an age-related decline in several aspects of male sexual function in 1163 Danish men aged 51–95 years. Figure 7.1 shows that sexual interest and morning erections decline in parallel fashion, reflecting the relation of sleep erections to excitatory tone considered in Chapter 4 (p. 110). Frequency of masturbation declined but less markedly than coitus, so that in the over 80s it is the more common sexual outlet.

Longitudinal data on the relation between increasing age and change in sexual function was reported from the Massachusetts Male Aging Study (MMAS). In 1987–1989, 1290 men aged 40–70 years were recruited to the study (a 53% response rate). In the baseline assessment, 52% of men reported some degree of erectile problem (minimal 17.2%, moderate 25.2%, complete 9.6%). Although diabetes, heart disease, hypertension and associated medications were all relevant, age was the variable most strongly associated with reporting of erectile dysfunction (ED). Moderate ED was reported by 17% of the 40 and 34% of the 70-year-olds; complete ED by 5% of the 40 and 15% of the 70-year-olds. In multiple regressions, no other variable diminished the

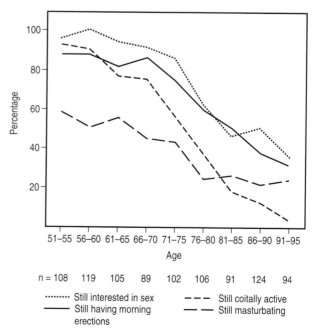

Fig. 7.1 Sexuality and ageing in 936 Danish men aged 51–95. (From Hegeler & Mortensen 1978.)

significance of age in predicting ED ($p < 0.0001$) (Feldman et al 1994). Further analyses were carried out based on subsequent assessments of this cohort, at an average of 8.8 years later. Araujo et al (2004) reported on the extent of change over this follow-up period. There were significant longitudinal declines in sexual desire, and frequencies of erection and sexual intercourse, and increased difficulty in achieving orgasm, and pain during intercourse. Araujo et al (2000) examined the relationship between decline in sexual function and depressive symptoms, anger and dominant/submissive aspects of personality. All of these had been associated with the presence of ED at the baseline assessment, although they were unable to conclude whether the ED was the cause or effect of these psychological factors. In order to look for psychosocial predictors of ED development, they excluded those who had reported ED at baseline. They found that new cases of ED were much more likely to occur in men with submissive personalities. They speculated whether this might be mediated by such personalities having greater difficulty coping with stress.

Bacon et al (2003) used the Health Professionals Follow-up Study, which involves a panel of 43 235 men, aged 53–90 years, who have completed questionnaires every 2 years since 1986, to ask questions about sexual function in the preceding 3 months. They achieved a 79% response rate (34 282 men). There was a substantial decline in sexual function across the age range. In those aged 59 or younger, 74% reported sexual function as good or very good; for those over 80, 10% did so (see Table 7.4). Scores for sexual function, particularly erectile function, were lower in those with other health problems. However, the age patterns were parallel in those with and without chronic ill-health. The age-standardized prevalence of ED was 33%.

These studies and several others in the literature show clearly that there is a decline in sexual function of men as they get older, affecting sexual desire, erectile response and ability to ejaculate, which is not dependent on the presence of chronic illness or medication use. In the next section, we will explore what possible mechanisms may be involved in this age-related process.

Ageing mechanisms

Brain function

We need to take into account a decline in brain function with increasing age, associated with loss of neurons in various parts of the brain. This shows considerable individual variability, with some old individuals retaining high levels of cerebral function, and others showing varying degrees of decline, which in more severe cases leads to dementia (Alzheimer's or senile). The age-related neuronal loss tends to occur more in certain brain areas, and as yet there has been no clear evidence of such loss relating directly to declining sexual function. However, areas most often affected include the frontal cortex, hippocampus, amygdala, thalamus, locus coeruleus and substantia nigra, all of which are involved, in various ways, in sexual function (Creasey & Rapoport, 1985; Goldman et al 1994; Schiavi 1999; see Chapter 4).

Androgens

Recently, attention to the role of androgens in older men has increased substantially, with the concept of PADAM (Partial Androgen Deficiency in Ageing Men) coming into fashion, and while concerns about prostatic risks of exogenous testosterone (T) remain, there is growing evidence of health benefits from androgen administration to older men (e.g. cardiovascular; Malkin et al 2006).

The evidence is now clear that there is a variable but predictable decline in T with increasing age, most evident in levels of bioavailable T (reviewed by Vermeulen 2001; Tenover 2003). In 75-year-old men, the mean total T is about two-thirds whereas the mean free T and bioactive T are only 40% of the mean for 20- to 30-year-olds (Vermeulen 2001). The normal circadian rhythm of young men, with peak T levels in the morning, flattens in older men, and as yet the mechanisms underlying this loss of diurnal variation is not understood (Bremner et al 1983), although a recent study showed a clear relationship between morning T levels and the amount of sleep in older men (Penev 2007), which may be relevant. Changes in the synchronicity of the hypothalamo–pituitary–gonadal axis, with altered sensitivity to negative feedback of T, result in reduced free T levels and increases in lutenizing hormone (LH) that are not as great as they would be in younger men with the same T levels (Veldhuis et al 1999). There is an increase in sex hormone binding globulin (SHBG), possibly due to an age-related increase in estradiol secretion by the Sertoli cells of the testis, resulting in relatively less reduction of total T than free T. However, in contrast to the comparison of oestrogens in pre- and post-menopausal women, there is considerable variation in older men and about 20% of 70-year-old men have T levels in the upper third of the normal 20–40-year range (Vermeulen 2001).

In one of the earlier studies, Tsitouras et al (1982), working with a group of healthy older men with relatively normal levels of T, divided their subjects into three groups according to the level of sexual activity; the high-activity group had significantly higher levels of T than the low-activity group. In contrast, when they divided their subjects into those with and without erectile problems they found no difference in T levels. There is a

| TABLE 7.4 | Mean scores for male sexual function in the Health Professionals Follow-up Study (Bacon et al 2003) |

	Age group (years)			
	≤59	60–69	70–79	≥80
n =	9754	10 573	8690	2725
Sexual desire	4.0	3.7	3.2	2.6
Erectile ability	4.1	3.4	2.4	1.7
Ability to reach orgasm	4.3	3.8	3.0	2.1
Overall ability to function sexually	4.1	3.5	2.6	1.8

A rating scale of 1 (very poor) to 5 (very good) was used. Mean group scores are shown

consistent failure to show a clear relationship between reduced androgens and ED in older men, although there is a minority of such men whose erections improve with T replacement (Buvat & Lemaire 1997). The evidence is more consistent with an effect on sexual interest and arousability. In a recent study, the association between sexual interest and total T levels was only modest (Travison et al 2006), and free or bioavailable T is a better marker. In a careful study of healthy, medication-free men with ages from 45 to 74 years, Schiavi and his colleagues, in a series of papers (reviewed by Schiavi 1999), reported a clear decline in sexual interest, sexual arousability and sexual activity with age. There was also an age-related decline in frequency, duration and degree of nocturnal penile tumescence (NPT), which is known to be T dependent (see Chapter 4, p. 112). The relationship between the age-related decline in free T and these other age-related changes was not straightforward, but could be explained by an age-related alteration in receptor responsiveness to T or a reduction in androgen receptors within the CNS (Vermeulen 2001). To support this hypothesis Schiavi (1999) described three age-related patterns involving free T and NPT. In the younger age group (45–54 years), no relationship was found between free T levels and NPT, after age adjustment, consistent with the idea that at that age T levels are well above the threshold necessary for T effects. In the middle age group (55–64 years), a relationship was found between free T and NPT, consistent with the idea that free T levels are close to the threshold level in that age range, and in the older age group (65–74 years) no relationship was found, suggestive of free T levels falling below the threshold.

Age-related changes in NPT also raise other interesting possibilities about age-related changes in T effects and related brain mechanisms. As Schiavi et al (1990) have demonstrated, NPT is often reduced in older men who have no erectile problems, to an extent which in younger men would be suggestive of organic ED. The older man may maintain acceptable erectile function by means of increased direct tactile stimulation, and the reduced NPT may be a marker of his age-related decline in T-dependent central arousability. As discussed in Chapter 4 (p. 112), this could reflect a reduction in the T-dependent NE system, which underlies central arousal, and which is organized by the locus coeruleus in the brain stem, one of the brain structures susceptible to age-related neuronal loss.

In Chapter 4 (p. 70) we also considered evidence that increased alpha-2 noradrenergic tone may contribute to psychogenic ED. α2 receptors, when activated, increase re-uptake of noradrenaline (NA) at the synapse, thus reducing NA transmission. α-2 antagonists counter this effect and increase NA transmission. Whereas in the periphery this leads to increased inhibitory tone in the penile smooth muscle, in the brain this leads to increased NA-mediated central arousal. Earlier research had shown that α-2 antagonists (yohimbine and idazoxan) could partially restore sexual arousability in castrated male rats, leading to the conclusion that NA mediated at least some of the effects of T on sexual arousability. Experimental studies in men showed that delequamine, an α-2 antagonist, enhanced sexual arousal in response to visual erotic stimuli and increased NPT during non-REM sleep in young men with psychogenic ED, but had no effect in older men (>47 years of age) with psychogenic ED (Munoz et al 1994; Bancroft et al 1995). As yet there is no evidence of the effects of α-2 antagonists in hypogonadal men or in older men without ED. However, the interesting difference between younger and older men with ED suggests that there may be an age-related decline in responsiveness of the NA system which is not dependent on T reduction (Bancroft 1995). We can therefore tentatively conclude that the age-related decline in sexual arousability and sexual desire could be partly explained by falling free T but also by reduced receptor response to T effects in the NA system.

In general, given the complexity of these various age-related processes, we should not expect to find the same clear relationship between androgen withdrawal and replacement and sexual function that has been found in younger hypogonadal men (see Chapter 4). But what happens to sexual function when older men are given testosterone replacement?

In one small placebo-controlled study of two groups of eugonadal men one with the primary complaint of low sexual desire, the other of ED, O'Carroll & Bancroft (1984) found a modest but significant increase in sexual desire with testosterone treatment in the first group, but no improvement in erections in the second group. In studies of men showing some degree of hypogonadism in association with ED, Carani et al (1990) and Morales et al (1994) found improvement in erectile function in a minority of cases. Hajjar et al (1997) reported substantial improvement in libido in older hypogonadal men on T replacement (mean age 72 years), but did not comment on effects on erectile function. Several of these men discontinued treatment after a fairly short time, and this may have been because of no improvement in erectile function. Some men may not find it beneficial to have increased sexual desire if they do not have the erections to go with it. So far it has been difficult to predict which cases of ED are likely to benefit from testosterone, although low baseline levels of testosterone certainly increase the likelihood. On the basis of a large clinical series of such cases, Buvat & Lemaire (1997) recommended that in men with ED under 50 years of age, measurement of serum testosterone should only be done when there was an associated loss of sexual interest, whereas in men over 50 years of age with ED, testosterone should be measured in all cases.

Peripheral response mechanisms

The importance of tactile sensitivity to sexual stimulation was discussed in Chapter 4 (p. 97). Age-related decrease in tactile sensitivity of the penis was reported by Edwards & Husted (1976), and more convincingly demonstrated by Rowland et al (1989) using vibrotactile and electrical stimuli. Although in other species tactile responsiveness of the genitalia is androgen dependent, the relevance of androgens to this mechanism in humans has not yet been clearly established.

It is clear that ED can result from various manifestations of vascular disease as well as its treatment, but there is also evidence of age-related changes in erectile vascular mechanisms in healthy older men. Schiavi (1999) summarizes the evidence as follows: 'At the vascular level, aging is associated with decreased inflow of blood into the cavernosa tissue and prolonged arterial response time following pharmacologically induced erections in physically normal men. At the cavernous smooth muscle level, aging is associated with a reduced response to nitric oxide and other endothelium-derived relaxing factors and with an enhanced effect of endothelin-1, a potent endothelium-generated vasoconstrictor. The level of prostacyclin, an agent secreted from endothelial tissues that mediates relaxation of vascular smooth muscle and inhibits thrombosis formation, decreases with age.... Structurally, endothelial dysfunction appears to promote an age-related subintimal accumulation of collagen, monocytes and smooth muscle cells and a decrease of elastin in the vascular walls. Changes in the extracellular matrix of the fibromuscular frame of the corpora may contribute to deficient penile rigidity in older men' (p. 40).

There is evidence from animal studies that T plays an important part in facilitating the effects of nitrergic (NO) mechanisms in the penis, and androgen receptors have been identified in the penile smooth muscle of most rodent species studied (Mills et al 1996). Recently, evidence of such peripheral effects of T in humans has been reported (reviewed by Montorsi & Oettel 2005). We therefore need to consider age-related changes involving T in both central and peripheral aspects of sexual arousal.

Of particular interest is the finding by Christ et al (1992) that smooth muscle in the erectile tissues becomes more responsive to peripheral inhibitory (NA) stimulation with increasing age (and in men with diabetes). This in vitro observation raises the possibility of an interaction between personality-related trait factors and ageing to increase the likelihood of ED. In particular, our studies based on the Dual Control model (see p. 321), have established a measure of inhibition proneness, SIS1, which is not only strongly related to erectile problems (Bancroft & Janssen 2000; Bancroft et al 2005), but is also positively correlated with age and weakly to neuroticism (Janssen et al 2002). We have postulated that the SIS1 score, which is relatively normally distributed in non-clinical samples, is a measure of erectile inhibitory tone (Bancroft & Janssen 2000). Men with high inhibitory tone, measurable as SIS1, are not only vulnerable to ED when younger, but may also be more vulnerable to the effects of ageing on erectile function. This can be tested in future prospective or longitudinal studies, such as the MMAS. Given the relationship between submissive personality traits and the development of ED in the MMAS study, it will be interesting to see if such submissive trait measures correlate with SIS1.

We have therefore identified a range of factors that could contribute or interact to account for the common age-related decline in male sexual function. We have raised the possibility that a key factor is a decline in the NA central arousal component of sexual arousal, though as yet it is difficult to weigh up the relative importance of lowered T and of reduced neuronal responsiveness, and both are likely to be involved. Other effects of reduced T in the brain and in the periphery have to be taken into account. We also have a hint of an interaction between personality trait mechanisms and age-related increases in peripheral response to inhibitory signals from the brain, which could open up a new research agenda.

Ageing and sexual function in women

Surveys of older women

In the first section of this chapter we saw a more complex, and to some extent less predictable, ageing pattern in women than in men. This partly reflects the fact that the sexuality of women is much more dependent on a current relationship, combined with the much greater likelihood that older women will be without sexual partners.

Studies restricted to women have, however, shown age-related changes. Hallstrom (1977) studied a representative sample of Swedish women from four age bands, 38, 46, 50 and 54 years. He found a decline in both sexual interest and orgasmic capacity over this relatively narrow age range. Hawton et al (1994) studied a randomly selected community sample of 436 women with partners, in five age bands, 35–39, 40–44, 50–54 and 55–59 years. Frequency of sexual intercourse, orgasm and enjoyment of sexual activity were positively related to marital adjustment and negatively related to age, with partner's age also having a negative impact. However, women's satisfaction with their sexual relationship was closely related to marital adjustment, but not to age.

Hayes & Dennerstein (2005) reviewed 18 cross-sectional community-based studies of women's sexuality with ages ranging from 16 (mean youngest age 27.7) to 96 years (mean oldest age 65). They concluded that sexual activities and sexual function decline with age, possibly starting somewhere between the late 20s and late 30s. There is a decline in the number of women who remain sexually active, particularly in the older age groups, and a decline in the frequency of sexual intercourse. There was general agreement that sexual interest or desire decreases with age, though this pattern was variable across women. It was also apparent that the extent to which declining sexual interest is seen as a problem or a cause for distress does not clearly increase with age and may get less. Frequency of orgasm decreases with age, presumably in line with frequency of sexual activity, as there was no clear evidence of an age-related increased difficulty in reaching orgasm. Evidence for changes in sexual arousability were less consistent. Interestingly, most studies reported that problems with pain during intercourse decrease with age or show little change. Hayes & Dennerstein

(2005) emphasized the importance of the relationship in determining women's sexuality as they get older, in terms of whether a relationship exists, and when it does, the emotional quality of the relationship and the partner's sexual function.

There have been a limited number of longitudinal studies most of which, so far, have focused on the menopausal transition. We still lack prospective data from women proceeding through the post-menopausal life span. Koster & Garde (1993) reported on 474 Danish women born in 1936 who were assessed at the ages of 40, 45 and 51 years. In the final assessment, 59.4% said their sexual desire had not changed over the previous 10 years, 10.6% said it had increased and 30% said it had decreased. Hallstrom & Samuelsson (1990) assessed 497 Swedish women at ages 38–54 years and then again 6–7 years later (aged 44–60 years). Sexual desire was unchanged in 63%, increased in 10% and decreased in 27%. There was an increased likelihood of depression in the group with low interest, and several of the women who reported an increase in sexual desire at follow up had been depressed when first assessed. In the Melbourne Women's Midlife Health Project 438 women aged 45–55 years, who were still menstruating, were enrolled and assessed at yearly intervals over the next 8 years (Dennerstein et al 2001). By the late menopausal transition there was a significant decline in sexual responsivity, and an increase in the partner's sexual problems. By post-menopause, there was further decline in sexual responsivity, frequency of sexual activity and sexual desire, and significant increase in pain during intercourse and in partner's sexual problems. The authors concluded that sexual responsivity is adversely affected by both ageing and the menopausal transition, with further negative effects of post-menopausal status.

Two issues remain contentious: (a) the extent to which the menopause rather than age determines this decline and (b) the precise nature of the sexual decline and causal mechanisms involved.

Age or menopause?

There is some inconsistency in the evidence for the specific contribution of the menopause, over and above age. Koster & Garde (1993) concluded that the decline in sexual desire was not related to menopausal status. However, their age range (up to 51 years) limited the extent to which they could address this question. Hawton et al (1994) found little difference in sexual function between age-matched groups of pre- and post-menopausal women, concluding that it was age that was the key factor. However, they acknowledged that, in age matching, they ended up with groups too small to provide adequate power. Cawood & Bancroft (1996) in a study of 141 women aged 40–60 years (50 pre-menopausal, 37 in menopausal transition and 54 post-menopausal) found, using multiple regression, that menopausal status did not predict any of the sexuality variables, and age predicted only one negatively, i.e. the SES2 subscale of the Frenken Sexual Experience Scales (Frenken & Vennix, 1981). This measures the extent to which someone seeks or accepts rather than avoids or rejects sexual stimuli of an auditory–visual or imaginary kind. This is of limited relevance to sexual interaction with one's partner, but is relevant to sexual desire. The most important predictors of sexual function were other aspects of the sexual relationship, sexual attitudes and measures of well-being. Avis et al (2000), in a subset of 200 women from the Massachusetts Women's Health Study, found that satisfaction with one's sex life, frequency of sex and dyspareunia did not vary with menopausal status. Post-menopausal women, however, had lower sex desire and reported less sexual arousal. However, in multiple regression analyses, health, marital status, vaso-motor symptoms, mental health and smoking each had a greater impact on the woman's sexual functioning than menopausal status.

In contrast, Hallstrom (1977), who had selected women at specific ages (38, 46, 50 and 54 years), compared pre-, peri- and post-menopausal women at each age, and concluded that menopausal status was much more relevant to sexual function than age. Dennerstein et al (2003) in reviewing this literature concluded, mainly on the basis of their own longitudinal study, that there is 'a dramatic decline in female sexual functioning with the natural menopausal transition' (p. 64).

Hormonal changes associated with ageing and the menopause

Androgens

Adrenal androgens, in particular DHEA and DHEA-S, have been shown in a number of studies (Orentreich et al 1984; Bancroft & Cawood 1996; Sulcová et al 1997; Burger et al 2000; Davison et al 2005) to decline in women with age over a relatively wide age span. This was most convincingly demonstrated in a study of oophorectomized women where ovarian androgens could not obscure the picture (Crilley et al 1979). The situation with ovarian androgens is more complex. The concept of menopause and its stages are considered in Chapter 3 (p. 42). Decline in T starts a few years before the menopausal transition, probably due to a reduction in the mid-cycle rise of T (Roger et al 1980; Zumoff et al 1995; Mushayandebvu et al 1996). However, contrary to much conventional wisdom, there is no predictable decline in ovarian androgens attributable to the menopause per se. In a longitudinal study of 172 women, all of whom changed from pre-menopausal to post-menopausal during the 7 years of the study (Burger et al 2000), total T did not change, whereas free T *increased* from pre- to post-menopausal. Davison et al (2005), in their large cross-sectional study, also found a steady decline in T (both total and free), androstenedione (A) and DHEA-S, with menopausal status having no influence on the decline. They also found no age-related change in SHBG. Previous findings for SHBG have been inconsistent, with decreases, increases and no change all being reported across studies (see Burger et al 2000).

A crucial change in function of the interstitial cells of the ovary from pre- to post-menopause complicates the picture. Whereas in pre-menopausal women gonadotrophic stimulation of the interstitial cells is regulated by the negative feedback of ovarian steroids, the rise in LH that accompanies the menopausal transition, resulting from the reduction in oestrogen-induced negative feedback, may stimulate the interstitial cells to produce T and A, sometimes excessively. In addition, factors such as body weight and insulin resistance influence this ovarian androgen production (see Bancroft & Cawood 1996 for brief review of the evidence; there has been recent opposition to this view, see Couzinet et al 2001).

Given this somewhat complex picture, what might we reasonably expect to find from studies of androgen/sexual arousability relationships in women as they get older? The relevance of androgens to the sexuality of women was examined closely in Chapter 4, leaving us with an inconsistent picture. The explanation offered was that women vary in the impact that androgens have on their sexuality, and as yet we have no basis on which to identify the T-responsive woman. It is likely, therefore, that the age-related decline in androgens is going to have a negative impact in some women, contributing to the varying pattern of change in women, and contrasting with the more predictable relevance of T decline in ageing men.

Oestrogens

A decline in oestrogens is a fundamental characteristic of the menopause per se, and was described in Chapter 3 (see p. 42). Paradoxically, there has been much less attention paid to the role of oestrogens in women's sexuality than to the role of androgens. Although there is clear evidence of the importance of ostrogens for vaginal response and lubrication, their impact on sexual arousal and interest is much less clear (Chapter 4, p. 124). Dennerstein et al (2003) concluded that there is a dramatic decline in sexual functioning with the natural menopausal transition, with changes in most aspects of sexual function correlating with levels of oestradiol but not androgens. However, we remain uncertain of how changes in oestradiol contribute to this decline. The limited evidence of the effects of oestrogen replacement in vaginal dryness and other aspects of sexual responsiveness is considered below.

The precise nature of the decline in sexuality

We therefore face a crucial issue which is central to much of the debate and controversy about female sexuality: when is a decline in sexual interest or sexual responsiveness a natural change associated with ageing, when is it a consequence of the hormonal changes associated with the menopause, when is it a consequence of the end to a woman's fertility, when is it an understandable reaction to circumstances, such as changes in the relationship, when is it part of a 'depressive reaction' to current circumstances, when is it a symptom of a depressive illness, and when is it a 'sexual dysfunction', i.e. a malfunction of the sexual response system? Some of these questions will be considered closely in Chapter 11 on sexual problems, but they raise conceptual and definitional problems that are highly relevant to our understanding of the ageing process.

As considered in Chapter 6, sexual desire is a difficult concept to define, probably more so for women than for men, and we find widely varying estimates of how often women experience sexual desire, and little understanding of what they desire when they do experience it. This in part reflects variations in the time period during which sexual desire is assessed. What evidence do we have of the levels and changes in levels of sexual desire in women as they get older?

Leiblum et al (2006) reported data from women who had completed the Profile of Female Sexual Function (PFSF; McHorney et al 2004), which measures sexual desire. Given that the authors set out to assess the prevalence of hypoactive sexual desire disorder (HSDD), the DSM-IV definition of which involves not only low sexual desire, but also associated distress, they also used the Personal Distress Scale, which measures the distress caused by low sexual desire. The sample included 414 pre-menopausal (mean age 35 ± 7.6 years) and 252 naturally post-menopausal women (mean age 56 ± 6.7 years). Low sexual desire, according to their criteria, was reported by 24% of the pre-menopausal and 29% of the post-menopausal women; this is not a big difference. When distress was taken into account, 14% of the pre-menopausal and 9% of the post-menopausal women were categorized as HSDD, evidence that older women are less like to regard sexual decline as a problem than younger women. However, the use of HSDD diagnosis in this context is questionable. The PFSF questions about sexual function, including sexual desire, applied to the past month. No clinician would diagnose HSDD on the basis of one month's symptoms. The importance of the time period used was demonstrated by Mercer et al (2003), using the 2000 NATSAL survey of 16- to 44-year-old women and men in the UK. When asked if they had 'lacked interest in sex' for *at least a month* during the past year, 40.6% of women answered yes. When asked if they had lacked interest for at least 6 months in the past year, the positive answers dropped to 15.6% (see Chapter 11).

To consider these conceptual issues further, we will revisit the recent Kinsey Institute study that was reviewed in Chapter 6 (see p. 211) (Bancroft et al 2003). The 987 women, 20–65 years old, were asked about sexual interest and response during sexual activity in the preceding month, in such a way as to minimize implications that any particular frequency was 'problematic'. Thus, women were not asked, 'Do you have a problem with . . .' (except for vaginal lubrication). Instead the proportion of occasions of sexual activity during which a particular response pattern occurred or did not occur was established. Separate from these questions, each woman was asked the extent to which they felt distressed or worried about (a) their sexual relationship and (b) their own sexuality. Marked distress (i.e. moderate or a great deal) was reported by 19.8% of women about their sexual relationship and 14.3% about their own sexuality (24.4% about either or both). Multivariate analysis was then used to assess which aspects of the woman's sexual experience, together with other potentially relevant variables, were predictive of either type of sexual distress.

Older age was weakly predictive of distress about the relationship, holding all other variables constant. Menopausal status (pre-menopausal, menopausal transition or post-menopausal) was not predictive once age was added to the model. Mental health was the strongest predictor of both types of distress, and the only aspect of the woman's sexuality which was predictive was her 'subjective response' (a combination of 'feeling pleasure', 'feeling emotionally close', 'feeling indifferent' or having 'unpleasant feelings' during sexual activity).

Sexual interest was assessed as frequency of sexual thoughts (see Chapter 6, p. 221). 'No sexual thoughts' in the past month was reported by 7.2% of women, and this significantly varied with age: 20–35 age group 3.2%, 36–50 years 7.0%, 51–65 years 13.5% ($p < 0.001$). However, the likelihood of these 'low interest' women reporting sexual distress was higher in the younger age group, though not significantly so ('marked distress' about own sexuality: 20–35 years 35.3%, 36–50 years 19.4%, 51–65 years 21.7%).

Lubrication problems were reported by 31.2% of the women, more in the 51–65 age group (39.2%) than the younger women, but not significantly so. The likelihood of such women reporting distress about their own sexuality was significantly greater in the 36–50 age group (29%) than either the youngest group (12.8%) or the 51–65 years group (22%) ($p = 0.02$). None of the other indicators of impaired sexual response (arousal, orgasm, pain) were associated with age or reporting of distress.

The relevant conclusions from this study were that general health, especially mental health, and the subjective quality of sexual interactions were the most important determinants of sexual distress and they were not age or menopause-status related. Although there was a tendency for more older women to describe impairments of sexual function, it was the younger women with such impairments who were more likely to be worried or distressed about their sexual life. Menopausal status did not appear to explain sexual distress. However, its relationship to specific sexual response variables was not assessed.

One of the most widely cited effects of the menopause is vaginal dryness, a reduction in vaginal lubrication during sexual activity, usually regarded as a consequence of the menopause-related decline in oestrogen levels. As mentioned at the start of this chapter, Laumann et al (2005) in their GSSAB, found lubrication difficulties to be the only sexual problem clearly related to age in women across most countries. In the UK Osborn et al (1988) found lubrication difficulties in 8% of the 35–39 years age group, 12% of the 40–44 groups, 16% of the 45–49 group, 26% of the 50–54 group and 22% of the 55–59 group. In Sweden, Fugl-Meyer & Fugl-Meyer (2006) reported lubrication difficulties in 11% of the 18–24 years group, 10% of the 25–34 group, 6% of the 35–49 group, 24% of the 50–65 group and 26% of the 66–74 group. Variations across studies probably reflect different criteria in terms of frequency or proportion of sexual acts affected. Nevertheless, vaginal dryness is not confined to women in the menopausal transition and later, and many post-menopausal women do not complain of vaginal dryness during sexual activity. Also, given that vaginal lubrication is part of genital response to sexual stimulation (see Chapter 4), we are faced with the problem of distinguishing between impaired vaginal response secondary to loss of sexual interest or impaired arousability, and loss of sexual interest or response secondary to vaginal dryness and the discomfort that often accompanies it.

What is the evidence for oestrogen lack as the cause of vaginal dryness and atrophy? A number of studies have reported correlations between these vaginal problems and levels of circulating oestradiol (e.g. Chakravarti et al 1979; Dennerstein et al 2002). Avis et al (2000), in multivariate analyses of the predictors of sexual function, found that when menopausal status was added, oestradiol level was predictive of pain during sexual intercourse, but not other aspects of sexual functioning. Leiblum et al (1983), on the other hand, found that in 52 post-menopausal women (mean age 57 years), those with more vaginal atrophy had significantly lower blood levels of T and A, and gonadotrophins, in particular LH. They did not differ in levels of oestrogens. However, as discussed above, the age-related decline in androgens is not menopause dependent. Although plasma oestrogen levels decline with the menopausal transition (Dennerstein et al 2002) oestrogen requirements of the post-menopausal woman are met to a substantial extent by aromatization of T and A to oestrogen in the peripheral tissues (including the vagina). Dennerstein et al (2005) used the data from their longitudinal study to assess the relative impact of both hormone levels and relationship factors during the menopausal transition. Using structural equation modelling, they concluded that previous sexual function and relationship factors are more important than hormonal determinants. However, they also estimated that the amount of oestrogen needed to improve sexual response was about twice that required to improve vaginal lubrication and reduce dyspareunia.

What can we learn about the relevance of oestrogen to vaginal dryness and atrophy, and also to sexual interest and response from studies of oestrogen treatment, either systemic or vaginally administered? There is limited evidence from placebo-controlled studies of a positive effect for vaginal dryness (Bachmann & Leiblum 2004; Altman & Deldon-Saltin 2006). However, this does not always help; in a controlled study in which women were randomly assigned to oestrogen/progestagen therapy or non-hormone therapy, after 5 years of treatment there was significant improvement in the hormone-treated group. However, 15% of the hormone-treated group continued to report vaginal dryness compared with 30–40% of the comparison group (Vestergaard et al 2003).

We have some limited evidence of the effects of oestrogen administration on other aspects of women's sexuality. Early studies of the effects of hormone replacement therapy on menopausal symptoms did not focus on sexual problems, and the now quite extensive literature of the effects of T administration on women's sexuality have mainly involved women following surgical menopause, already on oestrogen (E) replacement but with continuing sexual difficulties. In one study, transdermal oestradiol (Estraderm 50 µg/24 h) was compared with placebo in 242 naturally menopausal women seeking treatment for menopausal symptoms who had not previously received hormone replacement. After 12 weeks, in comparison with the placebo group, the oestrogen group reported significantly more sexual fantasies, better lubrication, less coital pain and more sexual enjoyment (Nathorst-Böös et al 1993). Wiklund et al (1993) in a further placebo-controlled study of transdermal oestradiol (50 µg), involving 223 women aged 45–65 years, showed similar improvements. In only one study have different dosages of E been compared (Sherwin 1991), and this was considered in Chapter 4 (p. 124). This literature, and that involving surgically menopausal women, was reviewed by Alexander et al (2004). We need more research on the effects of E replacement, in varying dosage, on the sexuality of post-menopausal women.

Physiological response

There has been little attempt to assess the genital responses of women as they age past the menopause. Masters & Johnson's (1966) observations of older women responding to sexual stimulation therefore remain relatively unique. Despite its limitations, most notably the unrepresentativeness of the sample, particularly for older women, who are willing to participate in such direct observational studies, and the lack of systematically reported data, this account remains of interest and will be briefly summarized. Sixty-one menopausal and post-menopausal women were studied, with the following age distribution: age 41–50 $n = 27$, 51–60 $n = 23$, 61–70 $n = 8$, 71–78 $n = 3$. They were then compared with the younger women also studied. In the case of extragenital reactions to sexual stimulation, nipple erection occurred in older much the same as in younger women. The vasocongestive increase in breast size, however, showed an age-related decline. It was relatively normal in 16 of the 41–50-year group (59%), only 5 of the 51–60-year group (22%) and none of the older women. Clitoral response, as Masters & Johnson's (1966) pointed out, is very variable in extent in younger women, reflecting variable clitoral size (see Chapter 4, p. 83). Visibly obvious swelling of the clitoral glans during sexual arousal, according to Masters & Johnson, is apparent in about 40% of pre-menopausal women. In their older women, it was apparent in 9 of the 41–50 year group (33%), 4 of the 51-60 year group (17%) and one older woman, aged 67. The clitoral retraction response, described by Masters & Johnson as occurring shortly before orgasm, was evident in all of these older women, but the resolution of the various clitoral changes after orgasm was much more rapid than in younger women. Changes in the labia majora, flattening, separation and elevation, most marked in nulliparous women, were not apparent in these older women. The labia majora, they commented, lose fatty tissue deposits and elastic tissue post-menopausally. The labia minora in younger women undergo vasocongestive thickening during sexual arousal that extends the vaginal barrel by approximately 1 cm. This change was still apparent in 18 (67%) of the 41–50 age group, 7 (30%) of the 51-60 age group and none of the older women. The colour change of the minora (from 'cardinal red to burgundy wine color') that predictably precedes orgasm in younger women was observed in all of the 41–50 age group, 19 (83%) of the 51–60 group, but only 3 (27%) of the older women.

Masters & Johnson's (1966) described the post-menopausal vagina as losing the well-corrugated, thickened, reddish-purple appearance of the pre-menopausal vagina, becoming tissue-paper thin, without the rough, corrugated look, and changing to a light pinkish colour. The vagina also becomes shorter and narrower. The 11 women over 60 years in their study had vaginas measuring 4.5–6 cm in length and 1–1.5 cm in width, contrasting with a length of 7–8 cm and a width of approximately 2 cm in their younger subjects. Vaginal lubrication, the production of transudate by the vaginal wall, is the first obvious sign of sexual response in the vagina. Masters & Johnson concluded that once a woman is around 5 years past her last menses, there is an obvious reduction in the speed and amount of vaginal transudate. What takes 10–30 seconds of effective stimulation in the younger woman may take 1–3 minutes in the older woman, despite the fact that the older woman is enjoying and anticipating further pleasure from the stimulation. This pattern is the typical one, but there are exceptions. Three of their women aged over 60 years responded with rapid and substantial vaginal lubrication, typical of a 20- to 30-year-old, and in spite of their clearly thin and atrophic vaginal walls. Their offered explanation for these interesting exceptions was that they had all maintained regular and frequent sexual activity (once or twice a week) throughout their adulthood.

Masters & Johnson's (1966) described the 'orgasmic platform' around the outer third of the vagina (see Chapter 4, p. 79) and its associated contractions, as a characteristic of female orgasm. This pattern continued in their older women, but to a reduced extent and with fewer contractions. The uterus of the post-menopausal women, with low oestrogens, shrinks in size, most obviously in its body, and there is little evidence of uterine vasocongestion that has been observed in pre-menopausal women during sexual arousal. Uterine contractions during orgasm, which occur in many younger women, were not observed in their older women. However, several of their women over 60 years reported severe cramping pain during orgasm, suggestive of a uterine contraction that was now painful. As one woman put it 'almost like labour pains except that they occur more rapidly'. Over all, Masters & Johnson's (1966) concluded that 'steroid starvation' reduced rapidity and intensity of physiological response. They did, however, report individual variations, and we need to keep in mind that this group of 61 women might differ in various ways from this age group in general.

Some validation of Masters & Johnson's anatomical description was found in an MRI study by Suh et al (2003) (see Fig. 7.2.). In a comparison with pre-menopausal

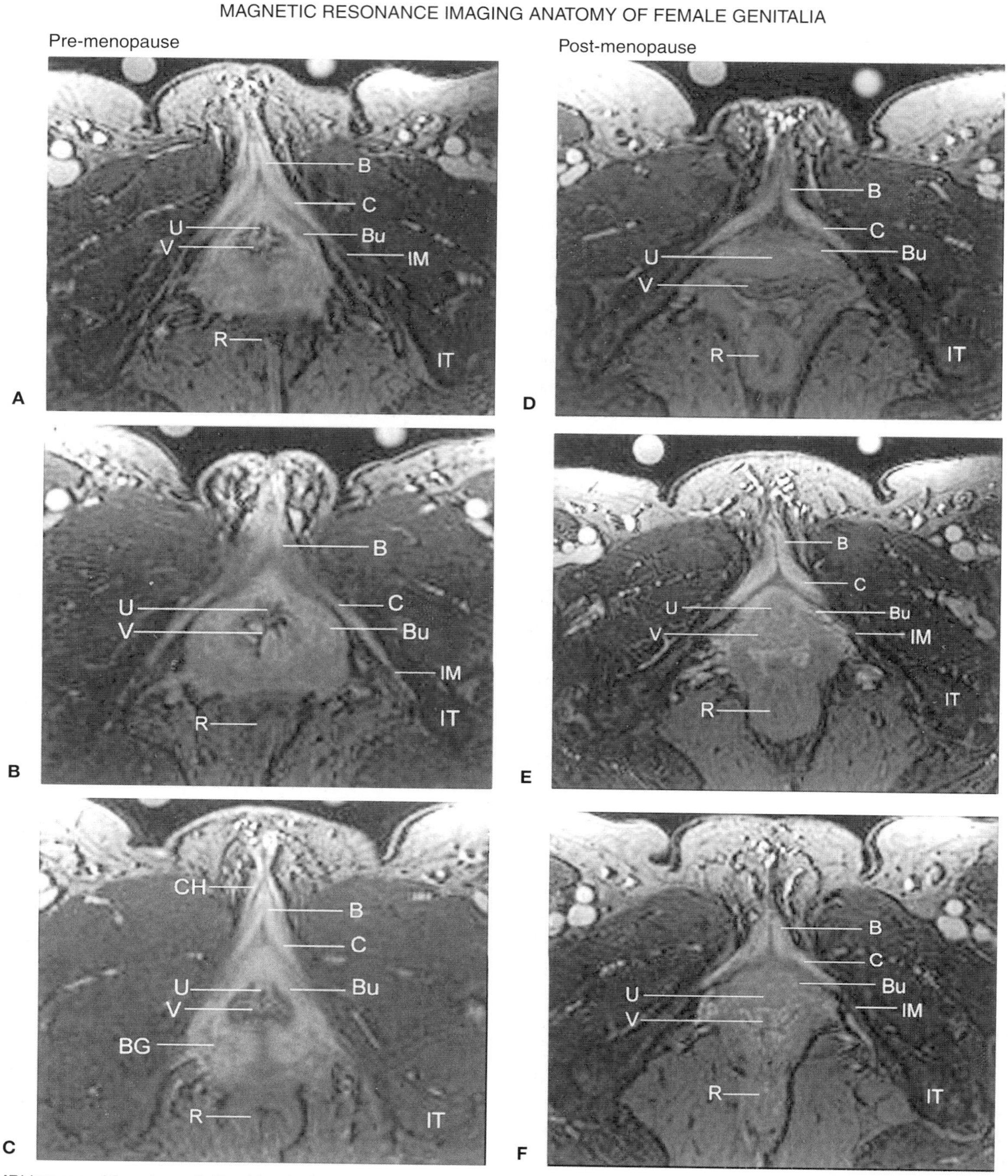

MAGNETIC RESONANCE IMAGING ANATOMY OF FEMALE GENITALIA

Pre-menopause

Post-menopause

Fig. 7.2 MRI images of female genitalia at level of greatest clitoral prominence (i.e. ischial tuberosity level) in 3 pre-menopausal (**A** to **C**) and 3 post-menopausal (**D** to **F**) women, using T1-weighted post-contrast imaging. The clitoris is a wishbone-shaped structure just anterior to inverted V of bulbs surrounding urethra (U) and vagina (V) anterolaterally. Posteriorly, each clitoral crus tapers to become continuous with ischiocavernosus muscle attached to ischial ramus. CH, clitoral hood; B, clitoral body; C, clitoral crus; Bu, vestibular bulb; BG Bartholin's gland; IM, ischiocavernosus muscle; R, rectum; IT, ischial tuberosity. From Su et al 2003, with permission.

women, they found that post-menopausal women (not on hormone treatment) had smaller width of the labia minora, bulb of the clitoris, and vagina, thinner vaginal walls, without the infoldings or rugae of the vaginal lining, and smaller cervical diameter.

Psychophysiological evidence

Given the considerable attention paid to vaginal pulse amplitude measurement (VPA) in women's genital response, reviewed in Chapter 4, what evidence relates to ageing? There is, unfortunately, very little evidence and this is confined to comparison of pre-menopausal and early post-menopausal women. Laan & van Lunsen (1997) found significantly lower baseline VPA in post-menopausal women, with moderate vaginal atrophy and vaginal dryness. VPA, they concluded, discriminates well between an atrophied and a non-atrophied vaginal wall. During subsequent erotic stimulation, however, both groups showed similar increases in VPA. Baseline VPA was correlated with oestrogen level, but the VPA increase in response to sexual stimulation was not. These findings were replicated in a further study (Laan et al 2003) that compared four groups: pre-menopausal and post-menopausal women with and without female sexual arousal disorder (FSAD; diagnosed according to strict DSM-IV criteria, i.e. diminished or absent lubrication-swelling response to sexual stimulation, causing distress, and not attributable to a medical condition). As in the previous study, post-menopausal women had lower levels of VPA at baseline, whether in a FSAD group or not. In response to visual sexual stimuli, VPA levels increased at a similar pace in the pre- and post-menopausal groups. However, of the two non-FSAD groups, VPA increase was significantly less in the post-menopausal than the pre-menopausal women. In both studies, therefore, baseline VPA correlated with estradiol levels and also degree of vaginal atrophy, but increases of VPA to sexual stimuli did not. Although there is a need for caution in comparing VPA across women (see p. 80), van Lunsen & Laan (2004) in reviewing these two studies stressed the consistency of the results.

There is as yet very limited evidence from fMRI studies of sexual arousal in pre- and post-menopausal studies, and the numbers involved are too small to justify statistical comparisons. However, in reviewing their series of studies, Heiman & Maravilla (2007) concluded that whereas the MRI evidence showed relevant structures to be somewhat smaller in post-menopausal women (see above; Suh et al 2003), post-menopausal women not taking hormone replacement showed significant increases in volume during response to visual sexual stimuli, in the same structures as pre-menopausal women. This is consistent with the findings of van Lunsen & Laan (2004) with VPA.

Psychosocial factors

If we accept that some of the change in sexuality that occurs around the menopause is the consequence of hormone- and age-related alterations of physiological function, we also have to acknowledge the considerable impact of other psychological and cultural factors.

Sexual problems are commonly reported by women attending menopause clinics (Sarrel & Whitehead 1985). This contrasts in an interesting way with attendance at sexual problem clinics. In a report on 1194 referrals to sexual problem clinics in Edinburgh between 1981 and 1983, there was a highly significant difference in the age of men and women attending the clinics (Warner et al 1987; see Chapter 11, p. 315). The peak age in the women was 21–25 years, with a decline thereafter. Men showed a generally flatter age distribution, but with the peak being 46–55 years. This is consistent with sexual problems causing more concern in younger, pre-menopausal women, and older women being more likely to reveal their sexual problems, if at all, when attending a clinic for another related issue, such as other menopausal symptoms. Depression is also common in women attending menopause clinics. Hay et al (1994) found that 45% of new menopause clinic attenders were clinically depressed. Of these depressed women, 83% had a history of previous depression. This raises two issues. First, the menopausal transition appears to be a phase of increased vulnerability to depression, for reasons not well understood. Second, depression is an important cause of loss of sexual desire and other forms of sexual impairment, and is therefore likely to be contributing to the increase in sexual problems during the menopausal transition. The idea that menopausal changes might increase vulnerability in women prone to sexual problems for other reasons is worth considering.

Relationship factors have consistently featured as important determinants. They have not been closely studied in relation to ageing, however. Sexual dysfunction in the partner, who in many cases will be older than the woman, is another important factor leading to withdrawal from sexual activity.

Attitudes and expectations may be important. Koster & Garde (1993) found that women who anticipated a negative change sexually with the menopause were more likely to experience one. This raises the question of whether such expectations may reflect negative attitudes towards sexuality. Some women cope with sex because of its importance to their marriage, as well as its obvious reproductive significance. But they may implicitly welcome a retreat from sex when older and the menopause may provide a justification for this. This aspect has not been studied and it is uncertain how many women would fit this description. In general, the non-linearity of the ageing pattern in women compared with men raises the possible importance of the cessation of fertility, which is clearly marked in women with the menopause. With the basic pattern of women's sexuality proposed in Chapter 4 (p. 131), and considered further in Chapter 6, and the very variable extent to which women are influenced by superadded by-products of the male basic pattern, we can postulate that women whose sexuality is relatively restricted to the female basic pattern may experience a more obvious decline post-menopausally, whereas those with more obvious superadded components to their sexuality may show less decline, at least following the menopause. This would help to explain the more variable picture of ageing in the female than the male. To test this hypothesis we will need more detailed study of how women experience sexual desire, and how this varies, and how such variation might fit the basic pattern. Relevant to this is the detailed analysis of the sexuality of older women from the Kinsey study, reported by Christenson & Gagnon (1965). They found the same relation between the extent of decline in late life and level of sexual activity earlier in life that Martin (1981) had reported for males.

Greene (1984) reviewed the limited evidence of socio-economic factors influencing the experience of menopause. He concluded that negative attitudes to the menopause are not as widespread or marked as is often assumed. They are more likely in women of lower socio-economic status, and in younger women compared with women of menopausal age. Hallstrom (1973) found that the decline in sexuality in post-menopausal women was greater in the lower socio-economic groups. Greene (1984) found little support for the idea that menopausal complaints are manifestations of modern industrialized societies. However, the form in which complaints are expressed are likely to be subject to social influences and vary cross-culturally. Lock (1986), in her study of menopause in Japanese women, found 'shoulder stiffness' as a common complaint, probably reflecting stress.

She also found that 'hot flushes' were much less common among Japanese women than Western women. It is questionable whether such a symptom would be culturally determined, and we should keep in mind that there may also be genetic factors, differing across ethnic groups, which influence how the menopause is experienced.

Attitudes to the elderly vary across cultures. Winn & Newton (1982) searched the Human Relations Area Files for relevant evidence from primitive societies. As usual with this source of anthropological data, evidence of sexual behaviour is often very limited, superficial or anecdotal. Nevertheless, Winn & Newton looked at the files on 106 societies. In 20 they found continuing sexual activity amongst old men, together with the shared expectation that this should happen. Not infrequently, anecdotes of sexual interaction between old men and young girls would be cited. There was evidence relating to elderly women from 26 societies, of which 22 revealed continuing sexual activity. There was often evidence of lessening sexual inhibitions in older women, leading them to be more openly expressive of their sexual wishes. Sexual relations between old women and much younger men were not unusual.

More recent cross-cultural studies of the modern world, such as the GSSAB (Laumann et al 2005), which compared different parts of the world, Dennerstein & Lehert (2004), who compared 12 European countries, and SWAN (Avis et al 2005), which compared ethnic groups within the USA, have found many similarities in how ageing and the menopause are experienced sexually, but also some interesting differences which warrant closer study. This may reveal how cultural differences in the role of women influence the impact of ageing on women's sexuality.

Conclusions

There is a clear decline in sexuality in both men and women as they age. In men, as a group, the relation to age is relatively linear, though there is considerable individual variability, with some men showing an early decline, others a late one. A variety of mechanisms related to ageing, including hormonal change, and alteration in responsiveness of the genitalia, account for much of this pattern, with some evidence that it is the men most sexually active when young who show the least decline. The impact of physical health, depression and relationship problems are important; the relevance of socio-cultural factors less well understood.

In women, the pattern is less linear, showing a more marked decline in midlife, and more gradual thereafter, and considerable variation across women. The physiological impact of the menopause is an important factor. But there are many other factors, less dependent on physiological mechanisms, which appear to be important. These include physical health and depression, as in men, but also relationship factors, especially lack of relationship, sexual function of the partner and socio-cultural factors relating to the role of women and women's sexuality. This more variable picture in women

than in men reflects the greater variability of women's sexuality across the life span. However, to explain this we can, as yet, only speculate.

REFERENCES

AARP 2005 Sexuality at midlife and beyond. 2004 Update of attitudes and behaviors. AARP The Magazine. http://www.aarp.org/research/searchResults.html?search_keyword=sexuality+study&x=13&y=12

Alexander JL, Kotz K, Dennerstein L, Kutner SJ, Wallen K, Noelovitz M 2004 The effects of post-menopausal hormone therapies on female sexual functioning: a review of double-blind randomized trials. Menopause 11: 749–765.

Altman AM, Deldon-Saltin DM 2006 Available therapies and outcome results in premenopausal women. In Goldstein I, Meston CM, Davis SR, Traish AM (Eds) Women's Sexual Function and Dysfunction: Study, Diagnosis and Treatment. Taylor & Francis: London, pp. 549–559.

Araujo AB, Johannes CB, Feldman HA, Derby CA, McKinlay JB 2000 Relation between psychosocial risk factors and incident erectile dysfunction: prospective results from the Massachusetts Male Aging Study. American Journal of Epidemiology 152: 533–541.

Araujo AJ, Mohr BA, McKinlay JB 2004 Changes in sexual function in middle-aged and older men: longitudinal data from the Massachusetts Male Aging Study. Journal of the American Geriatric Society 52: 1502–1509.

Avis NE, Stellato R, Crawford S, Johannes C, Longcope C 2000 Is there an association between menopause status and sexual functioning? Menopause 7: 297–309.

Avis NER, Zhao X, Johannes CB, Ory M, Brockwell S, Greendale GA 2005 Correlates of sexual function among multi-ethnic middle-aged women: results from the Study of Women's Health Across the Nation (SWAN). Menopause 12: 385–398.

Babb P, Butcher H, Church J, Zealey L 2006 Social Trends. No 36. Office for National Statistics, Palgrave Macmillan.

Bachmann GA, Leiblum SR 2004 The impact of hormones on menopausal sexuality: a literature review. Menopause 11: 120–130.

Bacon CG, Mittleman MA, Kawachi I, Giovannucci E, Glasser DB, Rimm EB 2003 Sexual function in men older than 50 years of age: Health Professionals Follow-Up Study. Annals of Internal Medicine 139: 161–168.

Bancroft J 1995 Are the effects of androgens on male sexuality noradrenergically mediated? Some consideration of the human. Neuroscience and Biobehavioral Reviews 19: 325–330.

Bancroft J, Cawood EHH 1996 Androgens and the menopause: a study of 40 to 60 year old women. Clinical Endocrinology 45: 577–587.

Bancroft J, Janssen E 2000 The dual control model of male sexual response: a theoretical approach to centrally mediated erectile dysfunction. Neuroscience and Biobehavioral Reviews 24: 571–579.

Bancroft J, Munoz M, Beard M, Shapiro C 1995 The effects of a new alpha-2 adrenoceptor antagonist on sleep and nocturnal penile tumescence in normal male volunteers and men with erectile dysfunction. Psychosomatic Medicine 57: 345–356.

Bancroft J, Loftus J, Long JS 2003 Distress about sex: a national survey of women in heterosexual relationships. Archives of Sexual Behavior, 32:193–208.

Bancroft J, Herbenick D, Barnes T, Hallam-Jones R, Wylie K, Janssen E, and members of BASRT 2005 The relevance of the Dual Control Model to male sexual dysfunction: The Kinsey Institute/BASRT Collaborative Project. Sexual and Relationship Therapy 20: 13–30.

Bremner WJ, Vitiello MV, Prinz PN 1983 Loss of circadian rhythmicity in blood testosterone levels with aging in normal men. Journal of Clinical Endocrinology & Metabolism 56: 1278–1281.

Burger HG, Dudley EC, Cui J, Dennerstein L, Hopper JL 2000 A prospective longitudinal study of serum testosterone, dihydroepiandrosterone sulfate, and sex hormone-binding globulin levels through the menopause transition. Journal of Clinical Endocrinology & Metabolism 85: 2832–2838.

Buvat J, Lemaire A 1997 Endocrine screening in 1022 men with erectile dysfunction: clinical significance and cost-effective strategy. Journal of Urology 158: 1764–1767.

Carani C, Zini D, Baldini A, Casa LD, Ghizzani A, Marrama P 1990 Effects of androgen treatment in impotent men with normal and low levels of free testosterone. Archives of Sexual Behavior 19: 223–234.

Cawood EHH, Bancroft J 1996 Steroid hormones, the menopause, sexuality and well-being of women. Psychological Medicine 26: 925–936.

Chakravarti S, Collins W, Thom M, Studd J 1979 The relation between plasma hormone profile, symptoms and response to oestrogen treatment of women approaching the menopause. British Medical Journal 281: 181–183.

Christ GJ, Schwartz CB, Stone BA, Parker M, Janis M, Gondre M, Valcic M, Melman A 1992 Kinetic characteristics of alpha₁-adrenergic contractions in human corpus cavernosum smooth muscle. American Journal of Physiology 263: H15–H19.

Christenson CV, Gagnon JH 1965 Sexual behavior in a group of older women. Journal of Gerontology 20: 351–356.

Couzinet B, Meduri G, Lecce MG, Young J, Brailly SD, Loosfelt H, Milgrom E Schaison G 2001 The postmenopausal ovary is not a major androgen-producing gland. Journal of Clinical Endocrinology & Metabolism 86: 5060–5066.

Creasey H, Rapoport SI 1985 The aging human brain. Annals of Neurology, 17: 2–10.

Crilley RG, Marshall DH, Nordin BE 1979 The effect of age on plasma androstenedione concentration in oophorectomised women. Clinical Endocrinology 10: 199–201.

Davison SL, Bell R, Donath S, Montalto JG, Davis SR 2005 Androgen levels in adult females: changes with age, menopause and oophorectomy. Journal of Clinical Endocrinology & Metabolism 90: 3847–3853.

DeLamater JD, Sill M 2005 Sexual desire in later life. Journal of Sex Research 42: 138–149.

Dennerstein J, Lehert P 2004 Women's sexual functioning, lifestyle, mid-age, and menopause in 12 European countries. Menopause 11: 778–785.

Dennerstein L, Dudley E, Burger H 2001 Are changes in sexual functioning during the midlife years due to ageing or menopause? Fertility & Sterility 76: 456–60.

Dennerstein L, Randolph J, Taffe J, Dudley E, Burger H 2002 Hormones, mood, sexuality and the menopausal transition. Fertility & Sterility 77(Suppl 4): S42–S54

Dennerstein L, Alexander JL, Kotz K 2003 The menopause and sexual functioning: a review of the population-based studies. Annual Review of Sex Research 14: 64–82.

Dennerstein J, Lehert P, Burger H 2005 The relative effects of hormones and relationship factors on sexual function of women through the natural menopause transition. Fertility and Sterility 84: 174–180

Edwards AE, Husted JR 1976 Penile sensitivity, age and sexual behavior. Journal of Clinical Psychology 32: 697–700.

Feldman HA, Goldstein I, Hatzichristou DG, Krane RJ, McKinlay JB 1994 Impotence and its medical and psychosocial correlates: results of the Massachusetts Male Aging Study. Journal of Urology 161: 54–61.

Frenken J, Vennix P 1981 Sexuality Experience Scales Manual. Swets & Zeitlinger: Lisse, The Netherlands.

Fugl-Meyer AR, Fugl-Meyer KS 2006 Prevalence data in Europe. In Goldstein I, Meston CM, Davis SR, Traish AM (Eds) Women's Sexual Function and Dysfunction: Study, Diagnosis and Treatment. Taylor & Francis: London, pp. 34–41.

Goldman JE, Calingasan NY, Gibson GE 1994 Aging and the brain. Current Opinion in Neurology 7: 287–293.

Greene JG 1984 The Social and Psychological Origins of the Climacteric Syndrome. Gower: Aldershot.

Hajjar RR, Kaiser FE, Morley JE 1997 Outcomes of long-term testosterone replacement in older hypogonadal males: a retrospective analysis. Journal of Clinical Endocrinology & Metabolism 82: 3793–3796.

Hallstrom T 1973 Mental Disorder and Sexuality in the Climacteric. Scandinavian University Books: Stockholm.

Hallstrom T 1977 Sexuality in the climacteric. Clinics in Obstetrics & Gynaecology 4: 227–239.

Hallstrom T, Samuelsson S 1990 Changes in women's sexual desire in middle life: the longitudinal study of women in Gothenburg. Archives of Sexual Behavior 19: 259–268.

Hawton K, Gath D, Day A 1994 Sexual function in a community sample of middle-aged women with partners: effects of age, marital, socioeconomic, psychiatric, gynecological, and menopausal factors. Archives of Sexual Behavior 23: 375–395.

Hay AG, Bancroft J, Johnstone EC 1994 Affective symptoms in women attending a menopause clinic. British Journal of Psychiatry 164: 513–516.

Hayes R, Dennerstein L 2005 The impact of aging on sexual function and sexual dysfunction in women: a review of population based studies. Journal of Sexual Medicine 2: 317–330.

Hegeler S, Mortensen M 1978 Sexuality and ageing. British Journal of Sexual Medicine 5: 16–19.

Heiman JR, Maravilla KR 2007 Female sexual arousal response using serial MR Imaging with initial comparisons to vaginal photoplethysmography: overview and evaluation. In Janssen E (Ed), Sexual Psychophysiology. Indiana University Press: Bloomington, pp 103–128.

Janssen E, Vorst H, Finn P, Bancroft J 2002 The Sexual Inhibition (SIS) and Sexual Excitation (SES) Scales: I. Measuring sexual inhibition and excitation proneness in men. Journal of Sex Research 39: 114–126.

Kinsey AC, Pomeroy WB, Martin CF 1948 Sexual Behavior in the Human Male. Saunders: Philadelphia.

Kinsey AC, Pomeroy WB, Martin CF, Gebhard PH 1953 Sexual Behavior in the Human Female. Saunders: Philadelphia.

Koster A, Garde K 1993 Sexual desire and menopausal development. A prospective study of Danish women born in 1936. Maturitas 16: 49–60.

Laan E, van Lunsen R 1997 Hormones and sexuality in postmenopausal women: a psychophysiological study. Journal of Psychosomatic Obstetrics & Gynecology 18: 126–133.

Laan E, van Driel E, van Lunsen RHW 2003 Sexual responses of women with sexual arousal disorder to visual sexual stimuli [in Dutch]. Tijdschrift Seksuologie 27: 1–13.

Laumann EO, Nicolosi A, Glasser DB, Paik A, Gingell C, Moreira E, Wang T for the GSSAB Investigators Group 2005 Sexual problems among women and men aged 40–80y: prevalence and correlates identified in the Global Study of Sexual Attitudes and Behaviors. International Journal of Impotence Research 17: 39–57.

Leiblum SR, Bachmann G, Kemmann E, Colburn D, Swarzman L 1983 Vaginal atrophy in the postmenopausal woman: the importance of sexual activity and hormones. Journal of the American Medical Association 249: 2195–2198.

Leiblum SR, Koochaki PE, Rodenberg CA, Barton IP, Rosen RC 2006 Hypoactive sexual desire disorder in postmenopausal women: US results from the Women's International Study of Health and Sexuality (WISHeS). Menopause 13: 46–56.

Lock M 1986 Ambiguities of aging: Japanese experience and perceptions of menopause. Culture, Medicine & Psychiatry 10: 23–46.

McHorney CA, Rust J, Golombok S, Davis S, Bouchard C, Brown C 2004 Profile of Female Sexual Function: a patient-based, international, psychometric instrument or the assessment of hypoactive sexual desire in oophorectomized women. Menopause 11: 474–483.

Malkin CJ, Pugh PJ, West JN, van Beek EJR, Jones TH, Channer KS 2006 Testosterone therapy in men with moderate severity heart failure: a double-blind randomized placebo controlled trial. European Heart Journal 27: 57–64.

Martin CE 1977 Sexual Activity in the Ageing Male. In Money J & Musaph H (Eds) Handbook of Sexology. Elsevier/North Holland: Amsterdam, pp. 813–824.

Martin CE 1981 Factors affecting sexual functioning in 60-79 year old married males. Archives of Sexual Behavior 10: 399–420.

Masters WH, Johnson VE 1966 Human Sexual Response. Churchill: London.

Mercer CH, Fenton KA, Johnson AM, Wellings K, Macdowall W, McManus S, Nanchahal K, Erens B 2003 Sexual function problems and help seeking behaviour in Britain: national probability sample survey. British Medical Journal 327: 426–427.

Mills TM, Reilly CM, Lewis RW 1996 Androgens and penile erection. Journal of Andrology 17: 633–638.

Montorsi F, Oettel M 2005 Testosterone and sleep-related erections: an overview. Journal of Sexual Medicine 2: 771–784.

Morales A, Johnston B, Heaton JWP, Clark A 1994 Oral androgens in the treatment of hypogonadal impotent men. Journal of Urology 152: 1115–1118.

Munoz M, Bancroft J, Beard M 1994 Evaluating the effects of an alpha-2 adrenoceptor antagonist on erectile function in the human male. 2. The erectile response to erotic stimuli in men with erectile dysfunction, in relation to age and in comparison with normal volunteers. Psychopharmacology 115: 471–77.

Mushayandebvu T, Castracane VD, Gimpel T, Adel T, Santoro N 1996 Evidence for diminished mid-cycle ovarian androgen production in older reproductive aged women. Fertility & Sterility 65: 721–723.

Nathorst-Böös J, Wiklund I, Mattson LA, Sandin K, von Schoultz B 1993 Is sexual life influenced by transdermal estrogen therapy? A double blind placebo controlled study in postmenopausal women. Acta Obstetrica & Gynecologica Scandinavica 72: 656–660.

NFO Research Inc. 1999 AARP/Modern Maturity Sexuality Study.

O'Carroll R, Bancroft J 1984 Testosterone therapy for low sexual interest and erectile dysfunction in men: a controlled study. British Journal of Psychiatry 145: 146–151.

Orentreich N, Brind JL, Rizer RL, Vogelman JH 1984 Age changes and sex differences in serum dehydroepiandrosterone sulfate concentrations throughout adulthood. Journal of Clinical Endocrinology & Metabolism 59: 551–555.

Osborn M, Hawton K, Gath D 1988 Sexual dysfunction among middle-aged women in the community. British Medical Journal 296: 959–962.

Penev PD 2007 Association between sleep and morning testosterone levels in older men. Sleep, 30: 427–432.

Pfeiffer E, Davis GC 1972 Determinants of sexual behavior in middle and old age. Journal of the American Geriatric Society 20: 151–158.

Pfeiffer E, Verwoerdt GC 1972 Sexual behavior in middle life. American Journal of Psychiatry 128: 1262–1267.

Roger M, Nahoul K, Scholler R & Bagrel D 1980 Evolution with ageing of four plasma androgens in postmenopausal women. Maturitas 2: 171–177.

Rowland DL, Greenleaf W, Mas M, Myers L, Davidson JM 1989 Penile and finger sensory thresholds in young, aging and diabetic males. Archives of Sexual Behavior 18: 1–12.

Sarrel PM, Whitehead MI 1985 Sex and the menopause: defining the issues. Maturitas 7: 217–224.

Schiavi RC 1999 Aging and Male Sexuality. Cambridge University Press: Cambridge, UK.

Schiavi RC, Schreiner-Engel P, Mandeli J, Schanzer H, Cohen E 1990 Healthy aging and male sexual function. American Journal of Psychiatry 147: 766–771.

Sherwin BB 1991 The impact of different doses of estrogen and progestin on mood and sexual behavior in postmenopausal women. Journal of Clinical Endocrinology & Metabolism 72: 336–343.

Suh DD, Yang CC, Cao Y, Garland PA, Maravilla KR 2003 Magnetic resonance imaging anatomy of the female genitalia in pre-menopausal and post-menopausal women. Journal of Urology 170: 138–144.

Sulcová J, Hill M, Hampl R, Stárka L 1997 Age and sex related differences in serum levels of unconjugated dehydroepiandrosterone and its sulphate in normal subjects. Journal of Endocrinology 154: 57–62.

Tenover JL 2003 Androgens in older men. In Bagatell CJ & Bremner WJ (eds), Androgens in Health and Disease. Humana Press: Totowa, NJ, pp. 347–364.

Travison TG, Morley JE, Araujo AB, O'Donnell AB, McKinlay JB 2006 The relationship between libido and testosterone levels in aging men. Journal of Clinical Endocrinology & Metabolism, 91: 2509–2513.

Tsitouras PD, Martin CE, Harman SM. 1982 Relationship of serum testosterone to sexual activity in healthy elderly men. Journal of Gerontology 37: 288–293.

US Census Bureau 2000 http://www.census.gov/main/www/cen2000.html

Van Lunsen RHW, Laan E 2004 Genital vascular responsiveness and sexual feelings in midlife women: psychophysiologic, brain, and genital imaging studies. Menopause 11: 741–748.

Veldhuis JD, Iranmanesh A, Mulligan TY, Pincus SM 1999 Disruption of the young-adult synchrony between luteinizing hormone release and oscillations in follicle-stimulating hormone, prolactin, and nocturnal penile tumescence (NPT) in healthy older men. Journal of Clinical Endocrinology & Metabolism 84: 3498–3505.

Vermeulen A 2001 Androgen replacement therapy in the aging male — a critical evaluation. Journal of Clinical Endocrinology & Metabolism 86: 2380–2390.

Vestergaard P, Hermann AP, Stilgren L. Tofteng CL, Sorensen OH, Eiken P, Nielsen SP, Mosekilde L 2003 Effects of 5 years of hormonal replacement therapy on menopausal symptoms and blood pressure: a randomized controlled study. Maturitas 46: 123–132.

Warner P, Bancroft J and members of the Edinburgh Human Sexuality Group 1987 A regional service for sexual problems: a 3-year study. Sexual & Marital Therapy 2: 115–126.

Wiklund I, Karlberg J, Mattson LA 1993 Quality of life of post-menopausal women on a regimen of transdermal oestradiol therapy: a double-blind placebo-controlled study. American Journal of Obstetrics & Gynecology 168: 824–830.

Winn RL, Newton N 1982 Sexuality in aging: a study of 106 cultures. Archives of Sexual Behavior 11: 283–298.

Zumoff B, Strain GW, Miller LK, Rosner W 1995 Twenty-four-hour mean plasma testosterone concentration declines with age in normal premenopausal women. Journal of Clinical Endocrinology & Metabolism 80: 1429–1430.

Homosexuality and bisexuality

The historical background................................. 253
The position of women in society 254
The 20th century 255
The legal status of homosexuals and their relationships 259

The concept of sexual identity........................ 259
Gender differences... 261
Bisexual identity 261
The stability of sexual identity............................. 264

Cross-cultural comparisons............................ 265
Pre-industrial societies.................................... 265
Modern industrial societies 267

The prevalence of homosexual and bisexual
behaviours and identities 268
Sexual practices in same-sex interactions................. 270

The characteristics of homosexual men and women:
gender identities, personalities and mental health........ 270
Gender identities and gender role behaviour........... 270
Personalities 272
Mental health... 273

The status of relationships in the gay male
and lesbian world 275

The factors that contribute to or influence the development of sexual preferences and sexual identity were considered closely in Chapter 5 (see p. 159). The conclusion was reached that this developmental process is multifactorial, involving genetic factors, early learning, the impact of gender identity and quite possibly some specific changes that result from the further period of brain development during adolescence and early adulthood. The importance of socio-cultural factors was also emphasized, and this aspect in relation to homosexuality will be considered more closely in this chapter.

Our understanding has not been helped by the more or less universal emotional reaction to homosexuality. Whether an individual rejects homosexuals or regards them as victims of unjust repression, that individual's appraisal of evidence is likely to be biased. The person who is truly dispassionate and impartial on the subject is hard to find, a state of affairs that also applies to sexuality and gender issues in a more general sense. But with homosexuality, many aetiological theories have apparently been motivated by a need to absolve the homosexual of responsibility for his (or her) disposition, hence early ideas that homosexuality was a congenital anomaly (e.g. put forward in the 19th century by men such as Westphal and Lombroso), and therefore not a sin.

The idea that the homosexual individual comes, in some sense, between the typical male and the typical female, has prevailed for some time. As new scientific concepts relevant to sexuality, or new technologies for studying them, have emerged, there has been a predictable tendency to use them to address both gender differences and sexual orientation. Thus, when sex hormones were first identified, they were regarded as basic determinants of maleness and femaleness, although it soon became apparent that this was a misleading oversimplification. Hirschfeld (1914) put forward the view that homosexuality was a form of hormonal intersex; male homosexuals did not have enough testosterone and lesbians had too much. It was not until the 1940s, when it became possible to measure such hormones in the blood, that this idea was laid to rest.

Fausto-Sterling (2000), who reviewed this history, saw the science involved as sexist and male dominated. Since the advent of technology to measure the size of structures in the living brain, attention has been paid to structural differences in the brains of men and women and, inevitably, to the possibility that homosexual individuals came somewhere in between. With the recent introduction of functional brain imaging, a number of studies comparing brain activation in men and women have been reported (see Chapter 4), and comparison of brain activity in response to visual sexual or olfactory stimuli in heterosexual and homosexual men and women is now underway (see Chapter 5, p. 162). It is too early to reach firm conclusions from these new sources of data, but there is already enough evidence to convince us that biological factors are involved.

The historical background

The literature on historical aspects of homosexuality and its acceptance or persecution is now extensive. The 20th century will be considered closely, but for the earlier literature, going back to ancient Greece, making sense of the considerable range of interpretations of the evidence is beyond the scope of this book. There are certain themes, however, that should at least be acknowledged, and which are of relevance today. There seems to be general agreement that ancient Greece was in sharp contrast to later Judaism and Christianity in the attitudes to homosexuality. According to Crompton (2003), 'Love between males was honoured as a guarantee of military efficiency and civic freedom. It became a source of inspiration in poetry and art, was applauded in theatres and assemblies, and was enthusiastically commended by philosophers who thought it advantageous for young males to have lover-mentors' (p. 546). Such homo-eroticism, it would seem, was in addition to the more mundane heterosexuality of marriage. For the majority of those involved, being 'homosexual' rather than 'heterosexual' was simply not an issue. It is also apparent that to a considerable extent this homo-eroticism was intergenerational.

Ancient Rome was apparently different. There was less idealization, but male homosexuality per se was not condemned. However, whereas patriarchy was a dominant influence in ancient Greece, in Rome slavery possibly had a greater impact. The sexual exploitation of male slaves made the passive sexual role unacceptable to freeborn Roman men. Crompton (2003) concluded that this form of homophobia, which condemned the passive but not the active partner, helped pave the way for the horrendous persecution and execution of homosexuals in the Christian era, in particular passive male homosexuals. Such 'faith-inspired' intolerance of homosexuality in both men and women was evident in early Judaism and perhaps more strongly in Christianity, with a terrible history of executions which prevailed until the 19th century. Thomas Aquinas, the medieval Christian who strove to be rational in his interpretation of Christian dogma, justified the rejection of homosexuality along with all other non-procreative sex, including masturbation, on the grounds that they were 'treasonous rebellion against God'. As Crompton (2003) points out, it is important to keep in mind that the history of persecution of homosexuals has to be put in context with the even more numerous persecutions of heretics and witches. It is noteworthy how Crompton concludes his book with a positive statement about how Christianity, which through most of its earlier history preached both love and hate, has come in recent times to leave hate behind. Not everyone would agree with him. What has perhaps become increasingly apparent in recent times is the contrast between Christians (and those of other faiths) who are predominantly caring and tolerant, and those who continue to reject and stigmatize those who do not comply with their beliefs. This is perhaps the contrast between religious fundamentalism, characterized by certainty of what is 'right', and the more humble uncertainty of the spiritual but caring person, a distinction which has more to do with the personalities of the individuals involved than with the particular religious creed. The history of mankind is pervaded by episodes of horrific persecution committed by those who are certain that they are right and their victims are wrong, usually in the name of religion.

In spite of this entrenched homophobia, the age-asymmetric pattern, evident in ancient Greece and Rome, has persisted in Europe, to varying degrees, until relatively recently. Trumbach (2007) described two major turning points around 1700 and 1900. Before 1700, in southern Europe there was a large sex difference in age at marriage, with, on average, men aged 30 years marrying young women aged 15 years who had just reached puberty (see Chapter 6, Table 6.2, for recent cross-cultural data on this variable). Unmarried males therefore lived in a society in which young females were not available, resulting in sexual interaction between unmarried adult and adolescent males. The cut-off between adult and adolescent was apparently indicated by full beard growth, usually evident around the age of 25 years. In northern Europe before 1700, the age difference at marriage was much less, with men aged 25–27 years and women 23–24 years. Intergenerational sex among males still occurred but less frequently. Such male–male sexual behaviour, whether in Southern or Northern Europe, was illegal and considered immoral because of the homosexual rather than the intergenerational component.

Trumbach (2007) goes on to describe how, between 1700 and 1900, the 'social construction' of a heterosexual majority and homosexual minority became increasingly evident. This was apparent by 1750 in England, France and the Dutch Republic, by 1800 in central Europe, but in southern and eastern Europe not until around 1900. The homosexual minority became differentiated into those whose sexual preference involved adult males and those who preferred adolescents. An important dimension in this history is the gradual reduction in the age at puberty. Most scientific evidence has focused on puberty in the female, and this has shown gradually earlier onset over the past 200 years. But, although less marked, there has also been a reduction in the age at puberty of males (see Chapter 3, p. 28). During the 20th century there was an increasing taboo related to sex with adolescent and pre-adolescent males, leading to the cycles of 'moral panic' about adult–child sex documented by Jenkins (1998) and considered more closely in Chapter 16. In Chapter 4, the important stage of brain development in early adolescence, and its impact on behaviour, was considered (p. 60). As yet, however, we do not know to what extent this stage of brain development is dependent on the hormonal changes associated with puberty. It is conceivable that 200 years ago a 16-year-old peri-pubertal male may have been more mature behaviourally and emotionally than a 12-year-old peri-pubertal male today, at least in terms of the prevailing criteria of maturity, even though they were at the same stage of pubertal development. This may have altered the 'sexual appeal' of a peri-pubertal boy over this time period, but this is speculation and probably will remain so.

The position of women in society

Confronted with this long history of intergenerational sex between men and boys, it is appropriate to consider the relevance of the position of women. Bullough (1976) suggested that the ancient Greeks tolerated or even encouraged homosexuality as long as it did not threaten the family. Women, while having low status in most respects, were regarded as having the supreme purpose of bearing children, especially sons. As a consequence, their place was in the home, and it was in the home that young females stayed until they married.

This is the description of a sexually segregated society. Alongside this reproductive family unit, the men seemed to indulge in their love affairs with young boys as though it were a separate and perhaps even narcissistic exercise. From the many descriptions of this boy love, one is struck by the erotic identification the older man makes with a beautiful youth, as though he were trying to perpetuate or idealize his own youth. According to Boswell (1980) many Greeks viewed homosexual love as the only form of eroticism that could be 'lasting, pure and truly spiritual', though the 'lasting' component is questionable given the age factor: beautiful boys soon become men. Plato believed that only love between people of the same gender could transcend sex. It may also be relevant that romantic love was not regarded as a suitable basis for heterosexual marriage until well into the 18th century (Stone 1977; see Chapter 6). On the other hand, in such cultures as ancient Greece, being exclusively homosexual would be regarded very differently, and from the available evidence it appeared to be relatively unusual, and may even have been regarded as pathological.

There is much less to say about homosexuality between women in this early history. Much less has been written about women in general, underlining their lowly position in society. It is therefore tempting to see the apparent increase of female homosexuality and bisexuality in the 20th century reflecting the impact of the women's movement. Having been repressed by men for so long, it would not be surprising if women asserted themselves by denying the sexual importance of men.

The 20th century

When we look more closely at the history of homosexuality during the 20th century, at least in Europe and North America, four particular themes emerge: (i) the continuing persecution and suppression of homosexuality, (ii) the medicalization of homosexuality (particularly in the male), (iii) the gradual emergence of a campaign by homosexual men and women to protect their human rights and by some professionals to de-pathologize homosexuality, and (iv) the legal status of homosexuality and homosexual relationships.

Continuing socio-cultural suppression

The long history of execution of individuals because of their homosexuality, while now unusual, has not disappeared. Homosexuals were sent, together with Jews and other heretics, into the gas chambers by the Nazi regime of the 1940s, and there are more recent examples in extreme fundamentalist societies. Persecution of other kinds has continued more generally, though tending to peak at certain times. The emergence of a more publicly visible homosexual culture in certain large cities of the USA during the 1930s, mainly seen by the non-homosexual majority as a culture of effeminate homosexual men, or 'fairies', was followed by an intensification of anti-homosexual action, particularly imprisonment. In the period following World War II, homophobia was conflated with fear of communism, and homosexuals were excluded from many occupations, particularly associated with government, on the grounds of being a security risk. This distrust was found among the American public in a 1970 survey by Levitt & Klassen (1974). Nearly 60% of the respondents believed that the majority of homosexuals would be security risks in government jobs. About 40% believed that the majority of homosexuals tend to corrupt their co-workers. Three-quarters would deny a homosexual the right to be a clergyman, a school teacher or a judge and two-thirds would debar him from medical practice or government service. Nearly half agreed that homosexuality, by corruption, could cause a civilization's downfall, a view that has been expressed by historians in relation to ancient Greece and other social declines (Bullough 1976).

The role of the medical profession

The medical profession, through the 19th as well as the 20th century, has predominantly displayed a pervasive 'sex negativism', not confined to homosexuality (Bancroft 2005). For example, in 1955, in their evidence to the Wolfenden Committee, which was considering decriminalization of homosexuality, the British Medical Association (1955) included the following:

'The attempt to suppress homosexual activity by law can only be one factor in diminishing this problem. The public opinion against homosexual practice is a greater safeguard, and this can be achieved by promoting in the minds, motives and wills of the people a desire for clean and unselfish living... people who are mainly concerned with themselves and their sensations associate together and obtain from each other the physical and emotional experiences they desire. Personal discipline and unselfishness have little place in their thoughts. If this behaviour is multiplied on a national scale the problem to society is apparent for widespread irresponsibility and selfishness can only demoralize and weaken the nation. What is needed is responsible citizenship where concern for the nation's welfare and the needs of others takes priority over selfish interests and self-indulgence.'

If it were not for the first two sentences the reader might assume that this astounding statement referred to a substantial proportion of the heterosexual community. However, a series of individuals in the medical profession have risen above this sex negativism in one way or another. During the late 19th and early 20th century this mainly involved an attempt to compensate for the social stigmatization of homosexuality by identifying it as pathology, the conversion of sin into sickness. However much this might have been construed as more tolerant, it carried its own price: having to live with an identity which is pathological. At the end of the 19th century, Kraft-Ebbing (1886) gave homosexual men the chance to describe themselves, and in the process identify with each other, through his publication of their life histories, an early example of the 'Internet factor'. But he persisted in the view that homosexuality was psychopathology. Hirschfeld (1914), saw homosexuality as a congenital behavioural 'intersex' condition, which did not require treatment but rather help and support for those involved to enable them to accept this part of themselves. In various respects, Hirschfeld can be seen as an early campaigner for homosexual rights and an unprejudiced researcher of human sexuality, whose research movement in Germany was obliterated by the Nazis. Havelock Ellis (1915) used the term 'inborn sexual inversion' which did not, in his view, require treatment. He was, however, more negative about women expressing homosexual interests.

Most other explicit medical opinions emphasized pathology and the need for treatment. Freud (1942) acknowledged a bisexual potential in early sexual development, with 'arrested' development resulting in homosexuality. Psychoanalytic treatment, he suggested, was a possible solution, and some psychoanalysts have persisted with this view ever since. Henry (1941), though sympathetic to homosexuals and concerned about the many ways in which their human rights were violated, nevertheless regarded them as 'socially mal-adjusted'. To him the issue was not 'cure' but medical help to enable them to have better control over their impulses. In his documentation of sexual autobio-graphies, Henry, who subtitled his book *A study of homosexual patterns*, divided his male and female infor-mants into three groups: bisexuals, homosexuals and narcissists. He did not explain how he assigned indivi-duals to the 'narcissist' category, but this was presum-ably the psychoanalytic concept, described by Chesser (1949) as 'an autoerotic form of expression ... (which) denotes self love, the victim in the more extreme cases being totally unable to love another on anything approaching an adult level, if, indeed, at all, but remaining self-centred and self-absorbed ... In brief, narcissists are *in love with themselves*' (p. 130; italics in original). Obviously, narcissism, so defined, is not restricted to homosexuals.

Apart from psychoanalysis, no clear rationale for treating the 'psychopathology' that was homosexuality had emerged. Attempts to normalize the male homosex-ual's sexuality by the administration of testosterone had produced some suggestion of increased sexual desire but no evidence of its re-direction (Glass & Johnson 1944). Then, in the 1960s we entered the era of modern learning theory and the development of behaviour therapy or behaviour modification. Here the objective was not so much curing illness but modifying behaviour that was in some way unwanted. One of the more successful applications of this approach was the management of phobic anxiety, by means of graduated exposure, com-bined with some form of relaxation (e.g. systematic desensitization). Attention was also paid to the possibil-ity of modifying sexual preferences, reducing, for exam-ple, fetishism, transvestism or homosexuality, a chapter in this history which is of particular significance to me as, for a few years, I was involved in it. Soon after com-pleting my training in psychiatry, I collaborated with Isaac Marks and Michael Gelder in the treatment of fetishism and transvestism using electrical aversion ther-apy (Marks et al 1970). Around that time, MacCulloch & Feldman (1967) and McConaghy (1970) reported success, at least in some cases, in reducing homosexual and increasing heterosexual responsiveness by means of aversion therapy. I was interested to see if I could repli-cate their findings, using what I believed to be a better aversive procedure. I reviewed this literature, including my own research (Bancroft 1974; see Haldeman 1994 for a more recent review), coming to the conclusion that aversive procedures were ineffective, but more positive techniques to gradually increase the capacity for hetero-sexual response and behaviour without trying to sup-press homosexual interest, may have some value in those individuals who wanted to change. This, however, was around the peak of the gay rights movement, which will be considered more closely below, and I was

attacked for my contribution to 'brain-washing' homo-sexuals. This was a formative experience, causing me to reflect (Bancroft 1975). At no time had I considered homosexuality to be pathological, but stigmatization of homosexuality was still strong, gay rights had not yet achieved the breakthroughs that were to follow, and there were still many homosexual men (not women) who wanted to escape this stigma and sought help to do so. However, I also came to realize that, by pursuing this behaviour modification, I was unintentionally rein-forcing the medical pathologization of homosexuality. I also became aware of a further problem. Since the start of the 20th century, when clinicians like Schrenck-Notzing (1895), using hypnosis, and Moll (1911), using what he called 'association therapy', an early version of behaviour therapy, claimed some success in increasing heterosexual interest in homosexual men, there was con-cern that any evidence of the 'treatability' of homosexu-ality was evidence that it was acquired and hence sinful. Havelock Ellis (1915) concluded that any one who had changed as a result of such therapy could not have been a true homosexual in the first place. Masters & Johnson (1979), in their book on homosexuality, reported two series of cases: homosexual couples who were having sexual problems and who were given the same treat-ment as used for heterosexual couples, with good effect, and homosexual individuals who presented with 'homo-sexual dissatisfaction' and an opposite sex partner (mostly a wife or husband), the majority of whom, as a result of going through the treatment programme, were able to enjoy their heterosexual relationship more than previously. They called their treatment 'conversion' or 'reversion' therapy, depending on whether there had been any previous heterosexual interest. Clearly, as Masters & Johnson (1979) emphasized, their sample was 'highly selected' (p. 392) and certainly not represen-tative of homosexual men or women. Nevertheless, soon after this was published, following a prosecution of a British politician with a homosexual history, one com-mentator cited Masters & Johnson's results as evidence that homosexuality was always 'learnt', and it was there-fore justified to take steps to prevent it by fostering anti-homosexual values.

A challenge to the pathology model of homosexuality started to emerge in the 1950s with the work of Evelyn Hooker (1965), who used various psychometric tests to compare homosexual and heterosexual men, contrasting with much of the work by psychoanalysts (e.g. Bieber et al 1962) by recruiting homosexuals who were func-tioning well in their lives, rather than those seeking clinical help for psychological problems. She found that such 'normal' homosexual men showed a variability that was indistinguishable from heterosexual men in terms of personality characteristics. Her findings were repli-cated in a series of studies by Siegelman (1972, 1974, 1978), and we will return to this literature in the later section on the personalities of homosexual men and women. It is noteworthy that this research was carried out by psychologists, not psychiatrists, and, according to Minton (2002), gave considerable encouragement to the emerging homophile movement.

Those clinicians who continued to regard homosexuality as not only pathological but also immoral were not deterred by such evidence, and in the early 1990s there was a re-emergence of what is currently known as 'reparative therapy', which will be considered at the end of this historical section.

The rise of the homophile movement

The emergence of the voice of the homosexual community is an interesting story (Minton 2002), revealing a long-running attempt by the medical profession to keep control; the prevailing view was that information for the general public on such matters should first be sanctioned by the medical or legal profession (Bancroft 2005). In the 1920s Helen Reitman, a lesbian woman, inspired by Hirschfeld, started a project interviewing other lesbian women, with the intention of informing the world about homosexuality in women. In 1927 she changed her name to Jan Gay, reflecting the fact that 'gay' had become a popular code word among lesbians and homosexual men. Having completed a 70 000-word manuscript reporting her findings and an exhaustive search of the literature, she was confronted by the need to have medical authorization before anyone would publish it. She approached Robert Latou Dickinson, a gynaecologist who was also a pioneer sex researcher, and who co-authored, with Lura Beam, *A Thousand Marriages* (1931) and *The Single Woman* (1934) (see Chapter 6). He was keen to make use of Gay's work. Dickinson had played a key role in establishing in 1935 the Committee for the Study of Sex Variants, Inc. that sponsored the book authored by Henry (1941) mentioned earlier. Jan Gay's contribution was incorporated into this volume with a brief acknowledgement of her help in the foreword: 'much of the success has been due to the tact and resourcefulness which she has shown in bringing subjects and doctors together'. The fact that she did many or possibly a majority of the interviews did not qualify her for joint authorship; she was not medically qualified.

A comparable story is told by Minton (2002) of Thomas Painter, an educated homosexual man who wanted to contribute to our knowledge of homosexuality by detailing accounts of his own experiences and his observation of others. He was also taken on by Dickinson and contributed to the *Sex Variant* volume, but with no acknowledgement. Dickinson, however, introduced him to Kinsey, who expressed an interest in him. Here he encountered obstacles of a slightly different kind. He was keen to work on the Kinsey team and be trained to carry out the research interviews, but he eventually learnt that his homosexual status made this unacceptable. Kinsey required 'married heterosexuals' to collect his data, to minimize allegations of bias in the data collection. It is ironic that Kinsey encouraged his heterosexual interviewers to experiment with extramarital sex to reduce stereotypical attitudes and increase comfort with sexual variability. Painter was, however, welcomed by Kinsey as a volunteer and Kinsey encouraged him to archive his gradually growing collection of diaries and accounts, together with other relevant materials, at the Kinsey Institute. Kinsey and Painter were in conflict on one important issue. Painter supported a pathologized view of homosexuality. Kinsey considered this to be a matter of moral judgement and not objective science, commenting, 'If you know what the world should be told and persuaded to do about the homosexual before the scientific data are collected and objectively analysed, you cannot have much use for our project' (Minton 2002, p. 179). But Painter and Kinsey came to terms with this difference and continued a positive and co-operative relationship until Kinsey's death. It has, however, remained for Minton (2002) to bring Thomas Painter's efforts to understand male homosexuality into the literature.

The emergence of homosexual activist groups, initially called 'homophile groups' to emphasize a positive valence, confronts us with another interesting conflict: between those in the homophile movement who wanted gently to bring the medical profession and general public to see the positive features of the homosexual community, and those who lost patience and pursued a more confrontational approach. To some extent this reflected a more general emergence of confrontational political activism during the 1960s by feminists and other politically motivated groups. At this stage the homophile movement drew closer to the emerging civil rights movement, and the pressure of demonstrations, legal challenges and other forms of political activism steadily increased. By the 1970s efforts were focused on the American Psychiatric Association (APA), initially with demonstrations at APA meetings. Sensibly, the APA gave a voice to the gay rights movement at a subsequent APA conference in 1972. In a clever move, a gay psychiatrist, disguised and calling himself Dr Henry Anonymous, pointed out the number of gay psychiatrists in the profession who were forced to conceal their sexual identities. This 1972 panel proved to be a turning point. Robert Spitzer, a member of the APA's Committee on Nomenclature, agreed to pursue the issue, and by the end of 1973 this committee proposed the removal of homosexuality from the DSM, and its replacement with 'sexual orientation disturbance', a condition in which an individual was disturbed or sought help because of his sexual orientation. The APA Board approved the proposal. There was an inevitable reaction among APA members, and a demand for a referendum of the membership. Of the 10 000 psychiatrists who participated in the referendum, 58% voted in favour of the Board's decision, and 37% opposed (Minton 2002). The compromise in the 1974 APA proposal to retain the 'sexual orientation disturbance' or 'ego-dystonic homosexuality' category continued to provoke criticism from the homophile movement, and in 1986 this was also removed.

Needless to say, the 37% who opposed the original declassification did not disappear, and in various ways attempts to re-pathologize homosexuality have continued since. In some respects we have seen a reversal of 'sin to sickness', with a re-emphasis of the fundamental immorality of homosexuality and a collusion between religious groups and certain clinicians to pursue conversion of homosexual to heterosexual with what has become known as 'reparative therapy'. The psychiatrist Socarides and psychologist Nicolosi have led this reaction, forming the National Association for Research and Therapy in Homosexuality (NARTH), committed to defending the rights of therapists to treat dissatisfied homosexuals.

A recent episode in this history has focused renewed attention on reparative therapy. Spitzer, the psychiatrist who organized the removal of psychiatry from the DSM in 1974 had some form of conversion in terms of his attitudes and started to wonder to what extent it was possible to change homosexuals to homosexuals with reparative therapy. He therefore studied the outcome in 200 individuals (143 males and 57 females) and reported that many of them had changed. He published these results in the Archives of Sexual Behavior (Spitzer 2003) and the rest of that issue of the journal was filled with 26 commentaries on Spitzer's paper, all but three of which were critical, some very strongly. I wrote one of these commentaries, which contained the following:

'What can we learn from Spitzer's study? Its principal strength is the substantial size of his sample, much larger than most comparable studies. I also have no reason to doubt Spitzer's sincerity in carrying out this study. But there are some major limitations.'

First and foremost, the sample consists of men and women who principally sought treatment because of their religious beliefs, and who were presenting themselves as evidence that such change was both possible and desirable for others (for 93% religion was extremely or very important, and 78% had spoken in public about their 'conversion', in many cases in their churches). Assessment of change was entirely based on their recall of how things were before treatment. Given their powerful agenda of promoting such treatment, it would be surprising if they did not overestimate the amount of change. A similar problem exists with the evaluation of any treatment for which the patient has a vested interest in proving its worth. Spitzer addresses this issue by pointing out that simple bias of this kind would have produced a more clear-cut picture of reorientation and no gender difference. He is partially right, but he cannot justifiably conclude that, because there was not maximum distortion, distortion did not occur.

Secondly, it is very difficult to discern from this study just what the reparative therapy had involved. At best, it had been a long process, with a substantial minority still continuing in ongoing therapy after many years. There were a few hints at specific interventions, mainly of the self-control variety (e.g. 'thought stopping', 'avoiding tempting situations'), and an intriguing passing reference, at least for male homosexuals, to 'the demystification of the male and maleness', resulting in a decrease of romanticization and eroticization of men. But for the most part, there seemed to be a more general process involving group pressure and therapist reinforcement of the determination to be different, and as a result less immoral.

It was not clear how these subjects were recruited, although unquestionably they constituted a highly unrepresentative sample of those who had come under the influence of religion-driven reparative therapy. I could also take issue with Spitzer's criteria of change, and his title, which states that 200 subjects reported a change from homosexual to heterosexual orientation, when the paper reports a less substantial change for many, if not most, of them.

So where does this leave us? Let me put aside, for one moment, the politics and ethics of reparative therapy. There are good grounds, apart from this study, for concluding that sexual orientation is not always fixed early and immutable. Whereas the large majority of us identify as homosexual or heterosexual at a relatively early age, never change and have no inclination to attempt to change, there is a minority of unknown size whose sexual behaviour is less bound by an orientation or who are less certain about their sexual identity and who may go through processes of change without any involvement in reparative therapy or the like. It is noteworthy that Alfred Kinsey (Kinsey et al 1948) proposed his scales to capture the variability of sexual preference, not only across individuals, but also within the same individual over time. As the gay rights movement gathered momentum, Kinsey's view was rejected in favour of a clear dichotomy of 'straight or gay', with those who identified as bisexual regarded as deceiving themselves (e.g. Robinson 1976). In the past 15 years, the flexibility of sexual identity has again been acknowledged. In the AIDS era, the concept of 'men who have sex with men' is used as a more general descriptor than 'homosexual'.

The concept of reparative therapy, as described, raises some key ethical issues, the most fundamental being the distinction between medical treatment for a pathological condition and the imposition of moral values under the guise of medical treatment. If there were any grounds for regarding homosexual orientation as a pathology rather than a variant of human sexual expression, then treating the pathology might be justified. I would assert that there are no such grounds, and hence providing treatment on that basis is professionally unethical and, according to my value system, immoral. There is a long and disturbing history of medical practitioners imposing their moral values through their professional practice. The imposition of moral values, explicitly or implicitly, i.e. urging someone to undergo change because their current sexual orientation is immoral, should not be regarded as therapy, and in any case raises other ethical and moral issues. I would strongly advocate Surgeon General David Satcher's *The Surgeon General's Call to Action to Promote Sexual Health and Responsible Sexual Behavior* (US Department of Health and Human Services 2001). This calls for responsibility in our sexual lives (responsibility towards ourselves and our sexual partners), coupled with a respect for diversity. Thus, someone who believes that homosexuality is wrong is entitled to that opinion, but is not entitled to impose it on others, particularly if those others exercise responsibility in their sexual lives. Thus, the principle of responsibility facilitates the acceptance of diversity.

Robert Spitzer's findings are consistent with the idea that some people do change their sexual orientation in some respects during the course of their lives, but his findings do not justify the existence of reparative therapy. As defined, this constitutes vigorous reinforcement of homophobia and the social stigma experienced by those with homosexual identities in our society. Together, this results in widespread suffering for homosexual minorities and, no doubt, for many who are pressured into attempting such change, considerable conflict and unhappiness (Bancroft 2003).

My current policy as a counsellor in advising those who are uncertain about their sexual identity is outlined in Chapter 12 (see p. 377).

The legal status of homosexuals and their relationships

There has been some progress in the past 50 years, but there is still some way to go. At the start of the 21st century there are around 70 countries in which homosexuality is still illegal, but in most there have been changes in a positive direction. The story in the UK is a long and painful one. After a series of much publicized prosecutions of well-known people in the early 1950s, the Wolfenden Committee was set up to report on homosexual offences. Its report was published in 1957 (Wolfenden 1957) recommending that homosexual behaviour between consenting adults should no longer be a criminal offence. It also concluded that 'homosexuality cannot legitimately be regarded as a disease, because it is the only "symptom" and is compatible with full mental health in other respects'. However, it took another 10 years of intensive campaigning before the Sexual Offences Bill was passed in 1967. This decriminalized certain homosexual activities between consenting adults in private, a condition that was strictly enforced. The age of consent was 21 years. This Act did not apply to Scotland or Northern Ireland. In 1981, the legalization extended to Scotland and, in 1982, Northern Ireland. In the 1990s further attempts were made to equalize the age of consent at 16 years. In 1994, the age of consent was reduced to 18 years. In 1997, it became apparent that this discriminatory age of consent was violating Articles 8 and 14 of the European Convention of Human Rights. The British government then set about equalizing the age of consent, though in the process it had to override opposition from the House of Lords. It succeeded finally in 2000. The next important milestone was in 2004, with the Civil Partnership Act, which allowed same-sex couples to enter a civil union with many of the rights of full marriage. Around this time, various legal steps to outlaw discrimination on the basis of sexual orientation were taken.

The situation in the USA is more difficult to summarize because of the variability across states. The state of Massachusetts established marriage for same-sex couples in 2004, among much controversy. Several states have legalized registered partnerships, comparable to the civil unions in the UK (e.g. Hawaii in 1997, Vermont in 2000, Washington DC in 2002, New Jersey in 2004 and California in 2005). Other states have resisted, but their discriminatory policies, applied in specific cases, have been overruled by the Supreme Court. 'Gay marriage' remains an extremely divisive issue in the USA. The assumption is that marriage belongs to Christianity, and is being usurped. The reality is that marriage is a universal institution of human societies, and has evolved in varying forms across cultures. A close analysis of the legal story in the USA has been written by Pinello (2003).

Cross-cultural variations in the legal status of homosexuality will be considered in the section on cross-cultural factors, as it provides an informative view of socio-cultural attitudes to homosexuality cross-culturally.

The concept of sexual identity

In Chapter 5, I explained why I preferred the term 'sexual identity' to either 'sexual orientation' or 'sexual preference'. But the concept of 'identity' adds a substantial dimension to our thinking on sexuality. As Weeks (1995) puts it: 'Identities are troubling because they embody so many paradoxes: about what we have in common, and what separates us, about our sense of self and our recognition of others, about conflicting belongings in a changing history and a complex modern world, and about the possibility of social action in and through our identities' (p. 36). In many respects identity is a very subjective, personal experience. We should not expect to know much about other people's identities for that reason. This applies particularly to sexual identities and even more so to sexual identities in previous generations. We can consider how people tend to connect with others as examples of 'having identities in common,' and, as far as we can tell, there have been major changes in this respect during the second-half of the 20th century. Looking into the past, there were, for the large majority of people, limits to their knowing how similar they were to others, in general, not just in relation to sexuality. Identities were most obviously related to local community, social class and religion. Gender clearly played a major role in determining the individual's place in society, but sex was assigned, implicitly, to marriage, and we know little about how even married people experienced their 'sexual identities' in earlier generations.

In the historical section above, the emergence of a homosexual minority, at least in Europe, during the 18th century was described. However, this categorization was based on how people were seen by others rather than how they saw themselves. 'Sodomite' was a term used to stigmatize the homosexual male. There was probably more stigmatization of the passive than the active homosexual male, though there is no clear evidence on that point. Foucault (1978) made the following comment: 'The extreme discretion of the texts dealing with sodomy — that utterly confused category — and the nearly universal reticence in talking about it made possible a two-fold operation: on the one hand, there was extreme severity (of punishment) ... and on the other hand, a tolerance that must have been widespread, which one can deduce indirectly from the infrequency of judicial sentences...' (p. 101). This suggests some form of collective denial. In the mid-19th century, the emergence of concepts like 'third sex' or 'urnings', coined by Ulrichs (Kennedy 1980/81), and the various other concepts discussed earlier, that were introduced in the late 19th and early 20th century, must have challenged this collective denial, with a gradually more pervasive process of stigmatization. How homosexuals used this to describe themselves remains uncertain, but the eventual emergence of the homophile movement and a gay culture clearly had an impact.

In Chapter 6, we considered the emergence of individualism from the more traditional collectivism (see p. 204), with this process, probably first most evident in the USA, becoming one manifestation of Westernisation through much of the world. Modern technology has probably been fundamental to this process. People started to find out about those outside their local communities and churches by listening to the radio, and even more by watching television. Modern media in general have made us much more aware of other people outside our own communities, and of other cultures. The impact of the Internet has been and continues to be huge, promoting, among other things, sexual identities of an increasingly varied nature, both by connecting individuals to sexual stimuli, and to other individuals who are interested in them.

Kinsey and his colleagues did not use the concept of sexual identity (Kinsey et al 1948, 1953). At that time the extent to which a homosexual identity was adopted by individuals was unclear. Kinsey used the terms 'homosexual' and 'heterosexual' to describe behaviour, not individuals. This was consistent with his prevailing emphasis on individual variability. 'Males do not represent two discrete populations, heterosexual and homosexual. The world is not divided into sheep and goats ... It is a fundamental of taxonomy that nature rarely deals with discrete categories. Only the human mind invents categories and tries to force facts into separated pigeon-holes' (Kinsey et al 1948, p. 639). Consistent with that view, Kinsey developed his 'scales' that were designed to indicate the proportion of behaviour that was homosexual or heterosexual during a specific period in an individual's life. On this basis, Kinsey concluded that 4% of white males are 'exclusively homosexual throughout their lives, after the onset of adolescence'. A further conclusion was that '10% of males are more or less exclusively homosexual (i.e. rate 5 or 6 on the Kinsey scale) *for at least three years between the ages of 16 and 55* (p. 651, italics added). Kinsey was, in part, reacting negatively to the prevailing pathological typologies.

The 10% figure, which has subsequently been shown to predominantly reflect homosexual behaviour during adolescence (see p. 268), became a motivating and validating statistic for the gay rights movement that started to emerge a few years after Kinsey's death (Voeller 1990). But then we see the conversion of behaviour into identity and the empowering belief that 10% of men in the USA had homosexual identities, i.e. were gay. Here we see social action by groups connected through their sexual identities to counter the many ways in which they were being stigmatized. The story for lesbian women is somewhat different. According to some accounts, lesbian women were effectively discounted by gay men in this political campaign. This suggests that a male homosexual identity did not prevent you from being a traditional patriarchal 'sexist'. Instead we see the female perspective featuring in more general feminist politics, in which heterosexual, homosexual and bisexual women joined forces to counter the pervasive effects of patriarchy. The male gay rights movement also rejected bisexuality as an identity; this was regarded as a cover for men who were having difficulty accepting their gay identity.

In one important respect Kinsey was right in saying, 'Only the human mind invents categories and tries to force facts into separated pigeon-holes'. In this respect, 'the human mind' has acted collectively, resulting in what is now called 'social constructionism'. The emerging homosexual identities, apart from their impact on the individual's sense of self, were instrumental in bringing the homosexual community together so that they could take action. However, the essential validity of the data from the Kinsey scales suggests that the newly constructed sexual identities obscured variability in terms of sexual experience. Whatever precise label one uses, the implications of assigning oneself to a particular category of sexual orientation are substantial and go far beyond simple sexual partner choice. Apart from the negative consequences of being stigmatized, membership of such a 'club' can organize many aspects of life — where you live and socialize, who you meet and perhaps even what job you get (Hoffman 1968). Identifying as heterosexual has no such consequences. But, as Hooker (1967) pointed out, there is a range of homosexual 'clubs' that one can join, which vary in the extent to which members are 'out' with their homosexual identity, and also in the patterns of sexual activity that may result. This variability has obviously increased substantially since Hooker's report. The 1970s were a time of particularly rapid change (Altman 1985). During that decade gay men became far more visible, and there was the emergence of a gay economy, so that advertisers talked of the gay market (and politicians of the gay vote). Lesbians went through their own changes in a rather different way. There has been less of a lesbian economy, but whereas gay men became relatively apolitical, similar to other relatively affluent consumer groups, lesbians retained much more of a revolutionary fervour and remained closely linked to the women's movement.

The attention to sexual identity by the academic community did not really get underway until the 1970s (Cass 1990). Green (1974), in his book *Sexual Identity Conflict in Children and Adults*, described sexual identity as a fundamental personality feature with three components: (i) an individual's basic conviction of being male or female, (ii) an individual's behaviour, which is culturally associated with males or females (masculinity and femininity), and (iii) an individual's preference for male or female sexual partners. More recently, the first two components have usually been separated as 'gender identity', and the uncertain relationship between gender identity and sexual identity has been emphasized at various points in this book, and will be considered further below. Cass (1990) described six stages of sexual identity development, particularly relating to homosexual identity: (i) identity confusion, (ii) identity comparison, (iii) identity tolerance, (iv) identity acceptance, (v) identitiy pride and (v) identity synthesis (a blending of the sexual identity with other aspects of self-identity). Cass (1990) presents a useful description of this developmental schema that is compatible with the three-strand/six-stage model of sexual development described in Chapter 5. DeCecco (1990) presents a social constructionist view of gay identity, in which he rejects essentialist explanations of homosexuality. Since then 'queer theory' has been challenging the social construct of 'gay identity' (Gamson & Moon 2004), and we have also seen a seemingly endless emergence of new gender identities (see Chapter 9) that, while challenging our gender stereotypes, are of uncertain effect in terms of social action. More clear social action is evident in the role of the Intersex Societies in Britain and North America, which have been campaigning to change premature, and what they consider to be inappropriate, surgical interventions for infants born with intersex conditions (see Chapter 3, p. 52). A bisexual movement has emerged, involving both men and women, which will be considered further below. There has been a major impact of AIDS that will be considered further in Chapter 13. Clearly, the advent of AIDS reinforced much anti-homosexual prejudice when, in the early stages of the epidemic, it was seen as a 'gay disease'. But in addition it has challenged the gay community and caused many gay men to reflect, in particular on their relationships and the need for more commitment, a trend which may have already started before the epidemic hit (McWhirter & Mattison 1984). A further consequence of the epidemic has been closer attention to homosexual behaviour and its relation to disease transmission (see Chapter 14). The evidence that many men are having sex with other men without regarding themselves as being gay or having a homosexual identity led to a new label: MSM or 'men who have sex with men'. However, this label may be of more relevance to researchers than the men themselves (Weeks 1995).

There is little doubt that sexual identity is shaped by socio-cultural factors which themselves change over time, increasingly in this unstable modern world. Nevertheless, the socio-cultural factors act on a sexual developmental process that, as the evidence increasingly shows, is also influenced by biological factors. Given the seemingly accelerating mutability of the process of social construction at a socio-cultural level, is it relevant to question the stability of sexual identity at an individual level? The limited evidence of direct relevance will be considered later in the section on bisexuality.

Gender differences

As considered in Chapter 5, there are some striking gender differences in sexual identity. Firstly, in a man, sexual identity is determined principally by the gender of people he finds sexually attractive. In a woman it is determined less by gender and sexual attractiveness, at least in terms of physical appearance, and more by relational factors. A woman's sexual identity, therefore, is determined by the type of person with whom she establishes or wants to establish a close sexual relationship. The primary process is the establishment of an intense affectionate relationship. These two patterns, not surprisingly, have different stabilities over time. If we compare men and women who are not exclusively heterosexual, it is more common for women to move from heterosexual to homosexual identity and vice versa. Even more striking is a greater tendency for such women to identify as bisexual. Diamond (2007) has explored this potential for change over time in a longitudinal study of 89 non-heterosexual women aged 16–23 years, whom she has assessed on five occasions over a 10-year period. Obviously the majority of women show a stable sexual identity. But a key question is why some women eroticize intense same-sex relationships and others do not. Diamond (2007) postulates that in the absence of a typical and relatively stable male-type attraction to a particular gender, a variety of control parameters determine whether such emotional relationships, which can be with either women or men, become eroticized. She includes biological predisposition, early sexual experiences, cultural norms and, more simply, opportunities. She also postulates sex drive as being potentially relevant. Let us return to the three-strand model of sexual development, described in Chapter 5, and consider the integration of sexual arousability, gender identity and capacity for dyadic relationships that is postulated to occur around puberty, leading gradually to the sexual adult. In men, this appears to be organized relatively early, perhaps because of more specifically organized or established sexual attraction for one gender (usually female). In women, this early organizational effect is less evident, and a variety of factors, Diamond's control parameters, intervene to a variable extent across women to produce a less predictable and less stable outcome.

Bisexual identity

The concept of bisexual identity has been a challenging one both for the gay rights movement and for sex researchers. Kinsey disapproved of the term 'bisexual', partly because it described an individual rather than a behaviour and was in conflict with his determination to avoid categorization of individuals in terms of their sexual behaviour, and partly because it overlapped with the concept of hermaphroditism (Kinsey et al 1948). The gay rights movement dismissed bisexuality as a cover for homosexuality. There were understandable political reasons why, when in the process of struggling for their human rights they needed to distinguish between the homosexual and the heterosexual, and to assert that people are either one thing or the other. As mentioned earlier, the history of medicalization and attempts to 'treat' homosexuality have revealed that any evidence of 'treatability' is taken by some to justify defining homosexuality as acquired and hence sinful. The concept of an innate and immutable homosexual orientation therefore had political advantages. In fact, the limited evidence that homosexual orientation can be changed by medical intervention (e.g. Masters & Johnson 1979) probably applied to those who had already demonstrated bisexual potential, hence Ellis's (1915) comment that they could not have been proper 'inverts' in the first place.

Yet, the history covered briefly in this book, and the limited anthropological evidence, indicate a bisexual potential that has been, and probably continues to be, realized by many, at least at certain stages of their life. Thus, the concurrent bisexuality of the man in ancient Greece who enjoyed his sexual affairs with boys while maintaining a sexual relationship with his wife and fathering offspring, the sequential bisexuality of the Sambian youth who passed from his phase of ritualized homosexuality to a heterosexual marriage (p. 266) or the young teenage boy in European or North American society of 50 years ago, who was attracted to girls but enjoyed sexual interaction with other boys of his age because they were more available and possibly less daunting than girls, and because he had not yet learnt that this might be taken to mean he was a homosexual. Such bisexual potential has probably had much more scope for expression when clear socially constructed sexual identities have not been established, or at least have not become apparent to every one.

A pioneering approach to bisexuality was taken by Fritz Klein (1985). Having developed an interest in the concept, he established a Bisexual Forum in New York, a support group for bisexual men and women, which met weekly. Most of the people attending this group did so because they were confused about their sexual identity, assuming they had to choose between 'straight' or 'gay'. Only a few of them considered 'bisexual' as a third option when they first joined the group (Klein 1990). They discussed the use of the Kinsey Scale, which gave seven options rather than three, but this helped little. Klein (1990) illustrated this point with an example of a man who 'dearly loves his wife, has sex with her on the average of once a week, (but) also goes to the baths for sex with men on average once a month' (p. 278). Could this man's sexual orientation be determined by the number of female versus male partners, currently 1 vs 12, or by frequency of sexual activity (52 with his wife, 12 with males). In terms of love, he only loves his wife and has never had loving feelings for men. His sexual fantasies, on the other hand, were exclusively limited to men (in the past year). For social preference he enjoys the company of men and women equally. In terms of lifestyle, his life is almost exclusively in the heterosexual world. Klein did not comment on the extent to which he enjoyed sexual activity with his wife compared to men.

Klein's (1990) way of dealing with this complexity was to develop a multi-dimensional scale, based on the Kinsey scale, which he called the Klein Sexual Orientation Grid. Ratings from 0–6 (as with the Kinsey scale) were made for seven variables each for three conditions (past, present and ideal). The seven variables were sexual attraction, sexual behaviour, sexual fantasies, emotional preference, social preference, self-identification

and hetero/homo lifestyle. He acknowledges that this grid does not cover age of partner, difference between love and friendship or lust and limerence or whether sexual behaviours involve relationships that are monogamous or 'open' or 'casual'. Little attention has been paid in mainstream sex research to Klein's approach, although the *Journal of Bisexuality*, started by Klein in 2000, continues to be published. Weinrich et al (1993) explored the factor structure of the Klein Sexual Orientation Grid in two convenience samples, one including similar numbers of heterosexual, homosexual and bisexual men (total $n = 90$) and the other predominantly gay men, most of whom were HIV+ (total $n = 78$). They found one main factor on which all items of the grid loaded positively, and accounted for most of the variance. They also found weaker factors, one of which suggested that love (limerence), as opposed to lust, was an independent dimension of sexual orientation. It is perhaps not surprising that little attention has been paid to Klein's grid, given that it did not appear to add much to the conventional sexual identities. However, more attention needs to be paid to the love component, and we will return to that below.

In 1994, Weinberg et al published the results of their study of bisexuality. This was in two stages: in 1983 they interviewed 49 men and 44 women who identified as bisexual, who they recruited from the Bisexual Center in San Francisco. In 1984–1985 they carried out a questionnaire study, recruiting 84 men and 104 women who identified as heterosexual, 186 men and 94 women who identified as homosexual, and 116 men and 96 women who identified as bisexual. They recruited with the help of 'four San Francisco Bay Area organizations whose primary mission was to promote sexual freedom as well as provide support, education and information' (p. 136). These were the Bisexual Center, the Pacific Center for Gays and Lesbians, the Institute for the Advanced Study of Human Sexuality, and the San Francisco Sex Information Service, a telephone hotline. The following summarizes some of their conclusions.

The majority of the bisexual group established heterosexuality first in their lives and added homosexuality later. The establishment of a bisexual identity tended to occur late (in their 20s or later) when compared to the heterosexual- and homosexual-identified groups. For persons dealing with the confusion that results from dual attraction, a bisexual identity can stabilize, and lead to social support from others who identify as bisexual. The availability of a bisexual identity, as a socially available alternative supported by a bisexual subculture, is relatively recent. In their heterosexual- and homosexual-identified groups, identity usually was based on their earliest sexual experiences, even though many of them subsequently had sexual experiences that were discordant with this identity.

Weinberg et al (1994) assessed sexual preferences using Kinsey scales for three dimensions: sexual feelings, sexual behaviour and romantic feelings. They looked at how these three ratings combined in their three 'identity' groups (e.g. 000 for exclusive heterosexual, 666 for exclusive homosexual). They found five types of bisexual.

The most common was the 'heterosexual-leaning type', about 40% of the bisexual men and 50% of the women. These overlapped in many ways with those in the heterosexual group in being predominantly heterosexual but with some homosexual experience, differing most clearly in terms of their adopted bisexual identity. The least frequent type was the 'pure' bisexual, scoring 3 on each dimension; only 7% of the men and less than 4% of the women. The 'mid-bisexual' type, scoring from 2 to 4 with at least one 3, included about 20% of both men and women. The 'homosexual-leaning' type, who ranked themselves from 4 to 6, included 18% of the men and 13% of the women. The 'varied bisexual' type, who showed varied ratings with at least one 3-point difference between the variables (e.g. 103, 463, 414), included 15% of the men and 13% of the women. The distributions of ratings for each of the three variables are shown in Table 8.1. It is noteworthy that, for romantic feelings, almost 60% of the bisexual men and women rated themselves 0 or 1 (i.e. almost exclusively heterosexual).

Weinberg et al (1994) also reported some interesting gender differences. They found the role of pure sexual pleasure to be much clearer for men, and men experienced sexual pleasure earlier than women, whichever identity group they were in. For women it was not the pursuit of sex that was the central issue but rather the pursuit of intimacy. Men did not always satisfy women's emotional needs for intimacy and closeness, and bisexuality in a woman may centre around a close relationship with another woman in which there is little or no sex. 'For men it was easier to have sex with other men than fall in love with them. For women it was easier to fall in love with other women than to have sex with them' (p. 7).

Weinberg et al (1994) concluded that bisexual potential is universal among humans, and that those who develop a bisexual identity somehow disconnect sexual preference from gender; what they called an 'open gender schema'. Given the mounting evidence of a genetic or in some other way, biological contribution to the development of sexual identity, whether all males (or

TABLE 8.1 Kinsey ratings for sexual feelings, sexual behaviour and romantic feelings by men and women identified as heterosexual, homosexual or bisexual, given as percentages (Weinberg et al 1994)

A. SEXUAL FEELINGS

Kinsey rating	n =	Heterosexual Men	Heterosexual Women	Homosexual Men	Homosexual Women	Bisexual Men	Bisexual Women
		84	100	182	93	116	95
0		67.8	52.0	—	—	1.7	1.1
1		29.8	17.2	—	—	17.2	16.8
2		2.4	3.0	—	1.0	23.3	30.5
3		—	—	—	—	19.8	29.5
4		—	1.0	2.4	3.0	27.6	12.6
5		—	—	29.6	44.0	8.6	9.5
6		—	—	67.9	52.2	1.7	—

B. SEXUAL BEHAVIOUR

Kinsey rating	n =	Heterosexual Men	Heterosexual Women	Homosexual Men	Homosexual Women	Bisexual Men	Bisexual Women
		80	94	168	84	109	83
0		91.3	88.3	—	—	11.0	19.3
1		8.8	11.7	—	—	24.8	37.3
2		—	—	—	—	20.2	18.1
3		—	—	—	—	12.8	10.8
4		—	—	—	—	9.2	4.8
5		—	—	8.8	11.9	13.8	4.8
6		—	—	91.3	88.1	8.3	4.8

C. ROMANTIC FEELINGS

Kinsey rating	n =	Heterosexual Men	Heterosexual Women	Homosexual Men	Homosexual Women	Bisexual Men	Bisexual Women
		81	96	181	92	111	94
0		84.0	76.0	—	—	23.4	14.9
1		13.6	17.1	—	—	17.1	21.3
2		2.5	2.1	—	—	16.2	23.4
3		—	1.0	—	1.0	19.8	19.1
4		—	—	2.5	2.1	9.9	11.7
5		—	—	13.6	20.8	9.0	5.3
6		—	—	84.0	76.0	4.5	4.3

females) have a bisexual potential that eventually becomes directed in one direction or the other, or whether only some do, is as yet an unanswerable but important question.

Another interesting gender difference reported by Weinberg et al (1994) was that bisexual women reported a greater total number of partners than heterosexual or lesbian women, whereas bisexual men did not have more partners than gay men. A recent study of women is relevant to this finding (Sanders et al 2007). A convenience sample of 545 women, 82.6% heterosexually identified, 9% ($n = 49$) lesbian identified and 8.4% ($n = 46$) bisexual, completed a number of trait measures, including the SESII-W (see p. 16), the erotophilia/erotophobia scale (SOS; Fisher et al 1988) and the propensity for casual sex (Sociosexual Orientation Index; Simpson & Gangestad 1991) and also reported their lifetime number of sexual partners. Compared to the heterosexual women, the bisexual women scored significantly higher on scores of sexual excitation (SE from SESI-W), erotophilia and lifetime number of sexual partners, and significantly lower on sexual inhibition (SI from SESI-W). They also differed from the lesbian women on those same measures, except for SI, where there was no significant difference. In a huge BBC Internet survey of heterosexual, homosexual and bisexual women and men, Lippa (2007) found that bisexual women reported higher sexual desire than heterosexual and lesbian women. Heterosexual men, on the other hand, reported higher sexual drive than gay and bisexual men. These findings, which were consistent across cultures, together with those of Sanders et al (2007), support the idea that women who are most easily sexually aroused and less inhibited about sex are more likely to eroticize close affectional relationships, and given the apparently greater importance of emotional intimacy than specific sexual attraction in women (see p. 159) will do so with either women or men. From this perspective, bisexual women should not be seen as coming midway between heterosexual and lesbian women.

The case example given by Klein (see above) illustrates how an individual may establish a loving emotional relationship with a woman, which includes sexuality, but may continue to experience a 'non-relational' interest in sex with men. We can speculate about this pattern. If we start with a bisexual potential, evident in at least some men and possibly more women, and then focus on the integrative phase of the developmental process, postulated in Chapter 5 as a three-strand model (see p. 145), it is possible that such a man may establish a clear sexual attraction to males, which, as was proposed earlier, occurs during a critical period of male sexual development, but fails, for some reason, to integrate this sexual attractiveness component with capacity for establishing a close, dyadic relationship with another male. A residual bisexual potential allows some degree of sexualization of a close dyadic relationship with a female, and he is left with a lust for men and limerence for women (or at least one woman). With female sexual development, there is less evidence of a critical period for establishment of sexual attraction (see p. 159) and hence the expression of a

woman's sexuality is more dependent on her ability to incorporate it into a close dyadic relationship with another, either man or woman. Hence, we are less likely to see the lust separated from relationships, and it is more likely that women who proceed through more than one close relationship will show more variability in their sexuality. This explanation is compatible with a recent study of sexual arousal patterns in men (Rieger et al 2005). Sexual arousal was assessed by subjective ratings and measurement of erection in response to erotic films, showing either two men having sex or two women. One hundred and one men were categorized into heterosexual ($n = 30$), homosexual ($n = 38$) or bisexual ($n = 33$) on the basis of their Kinsey ratings of sexual attraction to men and women (those with ratings of 2–4 were categorized as bisexual). Whereas the bisexual group reported increased sexual arousal to both the male and the female stimuli, most of the bisexual group showed significantly more erectile response to the male stimuli than female (in a minority it was in the other direction). This led the authors to question whether male bisexuality exists rather than being a pretence to obscure homosexuality. It is possible that if different methods of stimulation had been used (e.g. narratives depicting sexual interaction between a man and woman who were in love), a different picture might have emerged. Maybe a proportion of men who identify as bisexual, lust after men, but are more able to sexualize a close emotional relationship with a woman.

The stability of sexual identity

We have seen in the above sections that individuals are distributed on the Kinsey scales, albeit with largest proportions at each end of the scale. What evidence is there that sexual identity, once established, remains stable over time? Diamond (2007) in her longitudinal study of women, has reported variability, but her sample did not include heterosexual women, and non-heterosexual women may be less stable in this respect for a variety of reasons. Kinnish et al (2005) explored this issue in men and women, including those with heterosexual, homosexual and bisexual identities at the time. Their convenience sample consisted of 420 men (39% heterosexual, 43% gay and 18% bisexual) and 342 women (35% heterosexual, 46% lesbian and 19% bisexual). They were asked to report their sexual identity and provide a Kinsey rating for three dimensions, similar but not identical to those used by Weinberg et al (1994), sexual fantasy, sexual behaviour, and romantic attraction, and to provide such ratings for 5-year periods in their lives, beginning with 16–20. A representative change score was computed for each dimension for each individual. One or more changes in sexual identity over the lifespan was reported by 3% of heterosexual men and women, 39% of gay men and 64% of lesbian women, and 66% of bisexual men and 77% of bisexual women. There were no gender differences for heterosexuals or bisexuals in this respect, but lesbian women reported significantly more change than gay men. Change scores for the three dimensions, fantasy, behaviour and romantic attraction,

TABLE 8.2 Lifetime changeability (Means ± SD) of sexual identity and orientation based on derived change scores in kinsey ratings for 5-year periods from age 16 (Kinnish et al 2005)

	Sexual fantasy	Romantic attraction	Sexual behaviour
HETEROSEXUAL			
Men	0.48 (1.09)*	0.26 (0.82)*	0.39 (0.88)
Women	0.97 (1.66)	0.58 (1.25)	0.45 (1.01)
HOMOSEXUAL			
Men	1.09 (1.82)*	1.89 (2.68)*	2.37 (2.84)*
Women	3.05 (2.91)	2.91 (3.29)	4.10 (3.01)
BISEXUAL			
Men	3.42 (2.46)	3.35 (2.78)	3.89 (2.87)
Women	2.94 (2.06)	3.34 (2.36)	3.83 (2.68)

*Male female comparison significant ($p < 0.05$)

are shown in Table 8.2. Although heterosexual men and women showed substantially lower mean change scores than the other two identity groups, statistical comparison of the three identity groups was not reported. Within sexual identity groups, heterosexual women reported significantly more change than heterosexual men in sexual fantasy and romantic attraction. Lesbian women reported significantly more change than gay men in all three dimensions. Bisexual men and women did not differ on any dimension. One-third of the total sample (66% of heterosexual men, 51% of heterosexual women, 33% of gay men, 9% of lesbian women, 5% of bisexual men and 1.5% of bisexual women) reported *no change ever* for any dimension of orientation. These findings challenge common assumptions about the immutability of heterosexual orientation, but leave us uncertain whether bisexual potential is universal.

Cross-cultural comparisons

The form of social labelling varies across cultures, and in some cultures the 'exclusive homosexual' label does not seem to exist or is at least rare. In many societies the label for such an individual does not occur in the language, i.e. it is not an emic concept.

Pre-industrial societies

Ford & Beach (1952), in their classic text, *Patterns of Sexual Behaviour*, reported that homosexuality was approved or tolerated in some form in 49 of the 78 pre-industrial societies studied. Female homosexuality was evident in 17. Blackwood (1985) reported on 95 cultures in which female homosexuality or female-to-male transsexualism occurred. Broude & Green (1980) found that, of the 70 societies for which there was sufficient data, homosexuality was present or common in 41%. The proportion of societies accepting homosexuality was about the same as that disapproving or rejecting it. When accepted, it almost always coexisted with heterosexuality in the same individual; in such a society, the person who was exclusively homosexual throughout his life

was unusual. This evidence was mainly gleaned from the Human Relations Area File, a collection of reports from anthropologists, travellers, writers, missionaries, etc. Many of the societies described no longer exist in the same form (Hotvedt 1983), and the impact of Westernization since these observations were archived could be considerable, at least in some societies (see below). The number of detailed anthropological studies of homosexual behaviour remains relatively small.

Carrier (1980), in reviewing the literature available at the time, emphasized that the main socio-cultural factors influencing attitudes to homosexuality were the attitudes to cross-gender behaviour and the availability of sexual partners. On the first issue, he divided societies into those that accommodated cross-gender behaviour and those that actively disapproved of it. In the accommodating societies there was usually an expectation that a few individuals will be 'born that way', and such a male showing feminine behaviour would be expected to relate sexually to a man and neither the behaviour nor the individuals would be labelled as homosexual. In disapproving societies, the negative reaction mainly came from men towards other males showing cross-gender behaviour. In such societies gender roles were sharply dichotomized, often with laws against cross-dressing, and cross-gender behaviour being equated with homosexuality. Carrier (1980) cited Mexico as an example of such a machismo culture. In such societies it was relatively acceptable for a man to act as the 'insertor' in sexual contact with a cross-gender male, providing that was not the exclusive pattern of his behaviour. Such behaviour could still be seen as an expression of male dominance. It is the 'insertee' who is stigmatized, who is seen to be anomalous in terms of gender and who is 'letting the side down' for the male gender.

As considered earlier in the changing history of homosexuality in Europe (see p. 255) availability of partners becomes a key issue when there are strong expectations that young women will remain virgins until marriage. Homosexual behaviour is then more likely amongst the unmarried. Polygamy may result in lesbian relationships between the wives, as in the Azande of Africa (Blackwood 1985).

In general, the prevailing patterns of sexual interaction in a society will reflect both the degree of of sexual segregation (in some societies males and females lead separate existences for most of their lives) and the degree of sexual stratification (i.e. the extent to which men hold more power). Hotvedt (1983) discussed some of the factors influencing the organization of such sexually dimorphic characteristics in early human societies. She noted that both sexual segregation and stratification were less evident in hunter–gatherer societies (of which the !Kung of the Kalahari desert remain one of the few existing examples), becoming more in evidence as societies became more horticultural (i.e. agriculture without the plough or irrigation) or pastoral (i.e. the herding of domesticated animals). Sexual stratification increased the likelihood of a link between masculinity and heterosexuality in the machismo culture. Segregation of the sexes increases the likelihood of homosexual behaviour being ritualized or institutionalized in some way.

One widely discussed example of institutionalized homosexuality of this kind is the sexual culture of Sambia, written about extensively by Herdt (1981; 2000 for a recent version). When studied, the Sambia were a mountain people in Papua New Guinea, one part of Melanesia. They were hunters who were also horticultural. They totalled around 2000 individuals, divided into six major groups composed of patrilineal clans, living with a number of other clans in hamlets. Their culture was unknown to the Western world until 1957. When first studied by Western anthropologists, it was a male-oriented culture of warlike competition between clans, or at least between hamlets, with an aggressive personality the main indicator of successful masculinity. There was considerable subjugation of women, who were moved from one clan or hamlet to be married into another. The society was strongly gender segregated. Children spent the first few years of their lives looked after by their mothers in the female component of the culture. At around the age of 10, boys were taken from their mothers by the male system and introduced into an all male 'dormitory' environment, apparently kept secret from the women. This was heavily sexualized. These young pre-pubertal boys were required to fellate the older boys and to ingest their semen. As the boy passed through puberty and became himself capable of ejaculating, he 'advanced' to the stage where he was fellated by younger boys. As an adult he entered an arranged marriage, and his first experience of heterosexual activity was after marriage. Apparently, some men continued to enjoy occasional fellation by young boys, but otherwise the majority remained heterosexual in their sexual activity thereafter. The justification of this sexual exploitation of the young boy was that insemination of semen was necessary for him to become effectively masculinized. Here, therefore, was a culture showing, at least among men, a clear institutionalized form of discontinuous sexual development, as discussed in Chapter 5 (p. 164), starting with a transient phase of sexual service to older boys, followed by a phase of sexual enjoyment of younger boys and leading onto a heterosexual marriage. This provides an example of age-structured (i.e. between men and boys) as well as ritualized homosexuality. However, orientation or sexual identity was not clearly evident, and instead one saw a bisexual potential, which was culturally compatible with heterosexual and reproductive marriage. To what extent men remained with a preference for sex with other males is unclear. One could argue that the sexual objects in this system were female-like; pre-pubertal boys previously restricted to a women's environment, and wives. Women and young boys might have shared features of sexual attractiveness, and certainly shared the absence of more obvious characteristics of the aggressive, war-like male.

While the Sambia appeared to give us a culturally determined, discontinuous but stable pattern, there have apparently been striking changes since Western influences impacted Melanesia. Knauft (2003) studied another, smaller Melanesian lowland society, the Gebusi. When he first visited them in 1980–1982 he found a pattern of ritualized homosexuality, differing somewhat from the Sambia in involving older post-pubertal boys as the sexual objects. When Knauft revisited the Gebusi in 1998 there were dramatic changes, with much evidence of Westernization. His impression was that ritualized homosexuality had disappeared, or at least was buried, and there was a much more open heterosexual interest among young men. It is difficult to know exactly what happens in circumstances such as these, but it provides an illustration of relative instability or at least mutability of what seemed like long entrenched customs. Knauft appeared to be witnessing a change from a culture that did not promote dichotomous sexual identities as we know them, to a modified culture incorporating concepts of heterosexual and homosexual identities from the West.

A relevant female example is the Lesotho of South Africa. A common pattern was for pairs of teenage girls, one slightly older, to establish an emotionally close relationship in which the older girl taught the younger one about being a woman. Sexual interaction between them often but not always occurred, from which the younger girl was able to learn about her emerging sexuality without fear of pregnancy (Gay 1985). A more recent report of the Lesotho by Kendall (1999) indicated that such special relationships had declined since the onset of Western influence and values.

When we look at our own culture, we find suggestions of a more covert discontinuous pattern involving male–male sexual interactions in early adolescence. Gagnon & Simon (1973) clarified the original Kinsey data to show that the 37% of men who had experienced orgasm in a sexual encounter with another male were mainly referring to early adolescent experience. This was not age-structured, as with the Sambia, but a pattern largely restricted to within early adolescent peer groups, concealed from the adult world. Although we lack good evidence of how this pattern may have changed over time in the USA, Schmidt et al (1994) showed, in Germany, that early adolescent same-sex interaction among boys declined substantially between 1970 and 1990 with, in contrast, little change in the initially much lower prevalence among girls. Although, in the case of the boys, this may in part reflect increased opportunities for sexual interaction with girls at this age, it is also possible that early adolescents are now much more aware of the identity implications of such behaviour and hence avoid it.

When we consider these contrasts between cultures, and at the same time recognize the potential for change, exemplified in the impact of Westernization on Melanesian cultures, which had presumably experienced long periods of stability before they were affected by Western ideas, the recent past of our own Western-type culture, as described in the previous paragraph, suggests one potentially important factor. The social construction of a male homosexual identity, as distinct from heterosexual, once it is adopted by society at large and helped in its dissemination by modern technology, leads to a directed stigmatization of 'the homosexual male'. Before the widespread establishment of this social construct, same-sex behaviour, not obviously replacing heterosexuality, is largely ignored, a form of the collective denial referred to earlier (p. 260), or institutionalized (or ritualized), as in the pre-Westernized Melanesian societies.

Overall, there is much less evidence of socio-cultural reinforcement of female homosexual or lesbian identities. This has been reflected in the paucity of legal sanctions against female homosexuality compared to male homosexuality. To a considerable extent, homosexuality among women has been less stigmatized, less recognized and less addressed by social processes. This may have contributed to the fact that sexual identities of women are less dichotomized and more flexible as discussed earlier. However, as with many contentious gender differences, there is probably an interaction between nurture and nature.

Modern industrial societies

Weinberg & Williams (1974) compared three different societies: the USA (represented by New York City and San Francisco), Denmark and The Netherlands. They found that attitudes to homosexuality were more negative amongst the general population in the USA than in the other two countries. There was other evidence of greater tolerance of, and less discrimination against, homosexuals in the two European countries, especially in The Netherlands, where government-backed agencies supported the needs of the homosexual community. It is likely that there have been substantial changes in all these societies since then, but there is a shortage of more up-to-date cross-cultural comparisons.

Changes in the law

At least in England, when changes in the law have occurred they have usually been associated with some recorded changes in public opinion. Thus, in England, shortly after the Wolfenden Committee recommended a change in the law in 1957, a Gallup poll showed nearly 25% in favour of such reform. By 1965, with the struggle to implement the recommendation still ongoing, 63% were in favour of reform, although 93% still saw homosexuality as a form of medical illness (Homosexual Law Reform Society Report 1966). By 2007, following change in the law banning discrimination against homosexual individuals in goods or services, a YouGov survey found that 85% supported the change (Muir 2007).

We can perhaps take the legal status of homosexuals, and how it varies cross-culturally, as one indicator of cross-cultural attitudes to homosexuality. In Europe there is reasonable consistency, with a diminution of anti-homosexual values manifested in laws against discrimination on the basis of sexual orientation, and an increasing number of European countries giving legal recognition to same-sex relationships. In the USA, as mentioned earlier, there is evidence of a divided nation in this respect, with 'gay marriage' having the most divisive effect. Let us consider how this compares with other parts of the world.

The following summary is based on an Internet survey by Ottosson (2006). Not all countries are listed but examples are given in each category to indicate the range of countries involved.

In 114 countries round the world, sexual relations between persons of the same sex are allowed (i.e. are not illegal). In at least 10 countries this has been the case since the 19th century or earlier (e.g. Argentina, Belgium, Brazil, France, Guatemala, Italy, Japan, Luxembourg, The Netherlands and Turkey). In 14 countries, the law has changed since 1990 (e.g. Bosnia-Herzegovina, Chile, China, Ecuador, Estonia, Ireland, Lithuania, Puerto Rico, Romania, Russia, South Africa, Ukraine, the UK and the USA). The remainder changed the law (or established the legal rights) at some stage between 1900 and 1990 (e.g. Austria 1971, Bulgaria 1968, Canada 1969, Denmark 1933, Finland 1971, Germany 1968/69, Jordan 1960, Israel 1988, New Zealand 1986, Norway 1972, Portugal 1983, Spain 1979 and Thailand 1957).

In 40 countries sexual relations between men and between women are illegal (e.g. Algeria, Barbados, Lebanon, Ethiopia, Libya, Morocco, Nepal, Pakistan, Saudi Arabia, Sudan and Tunisia). In a further 46 countries only sexual relations between men are illegal (e.g. Bangladesh, India, Jamaica, Kenya, Kuwait, Malaysia, Nigeria, Papua New Guinea, Singapore, Sri Lanka, Tanzania, Uganda and Zimbabwe).

In nine countries, not only is same-sex sexual activity illegal, it may also be subject to the death penalty (Iran, Mauritania, Pakistan, Saudi Arabia, Sudan, United Arab Emirates, Yemen, some parts of Nigeria and Somalia and Chechen Republic of Russia).

We should be cautious in extrapolating from the legal status to public attitudes, and this relationship may be more apparent in some cultures than others. In particular, we should not assume that those countries that have legalized same-sex sexual behaviour for the longest time will show the more accepting public attitudes. Italy is an interesting example: homosexuality has not been legally proscribed in Italy since 1890. Lingiardi et al (2005) described the coexistence of a strong Catholic culture and lack of legal discrimination as resulting in a 'don't ask, don't tell' attitude, which is perhaps a modern version of the collective denial that prevailed in much of

Europe pre-1900, and was considered earlier (see p. 260). Lingiardi et al (2005) went on to explore homophobic attitudes in Italians, finding them stronger among the Italian military than among university students, related to lack of personal knowledge of gay and lesbian people, conservatism and, interestingly, low self-esteem. Among their student sample, they found more homophobic attitudes among males than females.

In India, Bangladesh and other parts of South Asia, there is more focus on gender in determining social reactions. Thus sex between two men is illegal and clearly generates negative public reactions. Khan (2007) described a trinary system, which is based on how masculinity is defined. A man should desire not another man but someone who is not a man, and this includes a woman, a feminised male or a boy. This appears to be associated with further collective denial of the relevance of man–boy sex.

Herek (2004), who has researched anti-homosexual attitudes extensively, concludes that it is time that we stopped using the term 'homophobia'. Introduced in 1972 by George Weinberg, it was quickly adopted by the gay and homophile movements, obviously attracted to the term's pathologization of anti-homosexual attitudes. However, as Herek points out, the term tends to obscure the real and varied reasons why anti-homosexual attitudes exist.

It is clear that cross-cultural aspects of homosexuality, as well as the historical aspects discussed earlier, are of considerable importance to our understanding of homosexuality. It is to be hoped that our knowledge of cross-cultural aspects increases in the near future.

The prevalence of homosexual and bisexual behaviours and identities

Because of sampling problems, and lack of clear categorization by age, we cannot obtain a clear picture of the prevalence of male homosexual behaviour from Kinsey's data. In their sample of white males they made the following generalizations, based on the Kinsey ratings reported for different age periods (Kinsey et al 1948):

(i) 37% of males had at least some overt homosexual experience to the point of orgasm between adolescence and old age.
(ii) 50% of males who remain single until the age of 35 had such overt experience.
(iii) 10% of males are more or less exclusively homosexual (i.e. rate 5 or 6) for at least 3 years between the ages of 16 and 55.
(iv) 4% are exclusively homosexual throughout their lives.

The re-analysis carried out by Gagnon & Simon (1973) was mentioned earlier. By focusing on the college educated, the most representative part of the original sample, with most of them under 30 years of age when interviewed, the authors showed a substantial proportion

of the reported male homosexual behaviour had occurred during adolescence.

In 1969, Gebhard, in his report to the NIMH Task Force on Homosexuality, reviewed the literature on the prevalence of homosexuality in the USA and Western Europe, concluding that 4% of college educated males and 1–2% of the total adult female population were predominantly homosexual.

For the same reason that the gay community welcomed Kinsey's findings on homosexuality, the moral majority were disturbed by them. Their labelling of homosexuality as an immoral distortion was more easily maintained if it applied to a small proportion of the population. This same concern has remained as a strong reason for continuing opposition to sex surveys, for fear that they will show even larger proportions of the population as homosexual (Bancroft 2004). In fact, surveys since Kinsey have reported smaller percentages (reviewed below). Binson et al (1995), in reviewing a range of surveys, including the General Social Survey, found that homosexual behaviour was reported more frequently in urban than rural areas, and concluded that 'the oft-cited 10% estimate of homosexuality in the population may more closely correspond to the social world of white, educated homosexual and bisexual men residing in large urban areas, rather than the national population estimate' (p. 253).

Since the last edition of this book a number of large representative surveys have been reported, allowing a more confident assessment of prevalence, but, as the surveys were not focused specifically on homosexuality, only a limited amount of evidence related to homosexual behaviour.

Also, most of them have not asked about self-identified sexual identity, but only whether same-sex sexual behaviour had occurred.

Rogers & Turner (1991) combined three national US surveys of men (a 1970 Kinsey Institute survey, and 1989 and 1990 General Social Surveys), resulting in a combined total of 2449 men. 'Same gender sexual contact' was reported by 5–7% of men at some stage of their adult life. However, only 0.9% of the total reported same-sex contact during the previous year. Only 0.6% of the total indicated exclusively same-sex sexual contacts throughout their lives. In general, same-sex sexual contacts were more prevalent in urban than rural areas, and in never-married men, particularly those 35 years or older.

In the National Health and Social Life Survey (NHSLS) of 3432 men and women aged 18–59 (Laumann et al 1994), 4.9% of men and 4.1% of women reported any same-gender sex partners since the age of 18, and 2.7% of men and 1.3% of women reported such partners in the preceding year. In this survey participants were asked if they thought of themselves as heterosexual, homosexual or bisexual. Only 2.0% of men and 0.9% of women chose homosexual, and only 0.8% and 0.5% bisexual, respectively.

Johnson et al (1994) reported the findings from the large British National Survey of Sexual Attitudes and Lifestyles (Natsal I), a representative sample of around

TABLE 8.3 Percentages with same-sex experience in men and women aged 16 to 44 in the Natsal I (1990) and Natsal II (2000) surveys (Erens et al 2003)

	Men		Women	
	1990*	2000	1990*	2000
Ever had sexual experience with same-sex partner	5.3	8.4	2.8	9.7
With same-sex partner involving genital contact	3.7	6.3	1.9	5.7
Same-sex partner in last year	1.1	2.1	0.5	1.5

*Natsal I respondents 16–44 data, weighted to be comparable to Natsal II

12 300 men and 14 600 women aged 16–59. This survey was repeated 10 years later (Natsal II) with a more modest sized sample, around 11 000 men and women, and aged 16–44 (Erens et al 2003). A comparison of the two samples for the percentage of men and women who reported ever having had a same-sex experience, an experience involving genital contact, and a same-sex partner in the last year, is shown in Table 8.3. This shows significant increases in the later survey, particularly for women.

So far, the more detailed analyses reported from these two British surveys have come from Natsal I (Johnson et al 1994). For men, the likelihood of having a first homosexual experience increases steeply during the early teens and then, after 20, shows a gradual increase. For women, this likelihood increases steadily over the age range until the fifth decade. This gender difference is consistent with Kinsey's data. Intriguing age cohort patterns emerged, and differed for men and women. The percentage of men who reported any same-sex experience peaked in the 35–44 age group (7.1%) and declined in the 45–59 age group (4.2%). Furthermore, the 35–44 age group were twice as likely to report homosexual experience before the age of 16, accounting for much of their higher overall rate. In the Natsal II, the highest percentage was also in the 35–44 age group (8.1%), which was the oldest age group in that study. This pattern was not apparent in women. This consistent finding in men requires explanation. In Natsal I, the 35–44 age group would have been 15 in the mid-to-late 60s. If this age effect had moved to the 45–54 age group in Natsal II, it would have suggested a cohort effect. But as that age group was not included in Natsal II, we cannot reach that conclusion. Earlier, we had considered the findings of Schmidt et al (1994) that, in Germany, early adolescent same-sex interaction among boys declined substantially between 1970 and 1990, a change that was not apparent in females. It remains possible that, in the UK, an increasing awareness of homosexual identity, and the stigma associated with it, resulted in this decrease in teenage boys from 1970 onwards.

Johnson et al (1994) reported an interesting association between early same-sex experience and being at boarding school (a peculiarly British custom nearly always involving same-sex schools). Both men and women who had gone to boarding schools reported significantly more same-sex experience 'ever' but did not differ in terms of more recent experience.

Possibly the most informative survey so far in relation to homosexuality is the large Sex in Australia study (Grulich et al 2003; Smith et al 2003). Around 9700 men and 9600 women, aged 16–59 years, were assessed by computer-assisted telephone interviews. Prevalences of heterosexual, homosexual and bisexual identities, and of different degrees of sexual attraction and sexual experience, are shown in Table 8.4. Women were significantly less likely than men to report homosexual identity and significantly more likely to report bisexual identity. Women were significantly more likely than men to report homosexual experience, although when experiences not involving genital contact were excluded, the proportions for women and men were very similar (5.7% and 5.0%, respectively). Same-sex experiences during the past year were reported by 1.9% of men and 1.5% of women. Men with homosexual experience, however, reported many more lifetime same-sex partners than women with homosexual experience (means of 31.6 and 3.2). For both men and women, however, the 'homosexually identified' reported more same-sex partners than the number of opposite sex partners reported by the 'heterosexually identified'.

Men reporting homosexual identity were more likely to have had higher education and to have white collar, managerial or professional occupations than heterosexual men. The explanations for these associations are not yet clear, but it is possible that men experiencing some degree of same-sex attraction may find it easier to identify as gay when they have careers which strengthen their self-esteem and give them some protection against social stigma.

Bisexually identified women were significantly younger than lesbian-identified women. On the other hand, lesbian women were more likely to have had higher education and to be in managerial or professional

TABLE 8.4 Prevalences of sexual identities, sexual attraction and sexual experience in men and women in Australia (Smith et al 2003)

	Men (%)	Women (%)
SEXUAL IDENTITY		
Heterosexual	97.4	97.7
Homosexual	1.6	0.8*
Bisexual	0.9	1.4*
SEXUAL ATTRACTION		
Exclusively to opposite sex	92.9	86.5
Predominantly to opposite sex	4.5	11.0*
Equally often to both sexes	0.6	1.0*
Predominantly to same sex	1.1	0.6*
Exclusively to same sex	0.6	0.2*
SEXUAL EXPERIENCE		
Exclusively with opposite sex	92.9	88.3
Predominantly with opposite sex	4.0	7.5*
Equally often with both sexes	0.4	0.5
Predominantly with same sex	1.0	0.4*
Exclusively with same sex	0.6	0.1*

*Significant difference between men and women based on odds ratios

occupations than bisexual women. This raises the question of cause or effect: are women who are better educated and career orientated more likely to become lesbian, as a result of their personalities conforming less to the heterosexual stereotype (Sanders & Bancroft 1982) or do women who have developed lesbian identities seek out less heterosexist lifestyles as a consequence?

Younger women were more likely to report homosexual experience than older women. The authors comment on what appears to be a greater prevalence of female homosexual experience than in previous studies. They raised the possibility that, because of more open attitudes about homosexuality, younger women were more likely to be open about their experiences, while older women remain more likely to conceal them. They also suggest that there may be a difference across cultures, with some showing clearly more male than female homosexuality, and others showing little difference. This paper, however, preceded publication of the findings from Natsal II in the UK (Erens et al 2003), which found an increase in reporting of male same-sex behaviour in the 10 years since Natsal I, with an even greater increase in female same-sex behaviour. The possibility of an 'artefactual' increase due to greater readiness to report homosexual experience was considered. However, particularly for women, we should also consider the possibility that women are increasingly exploring same-sex relationships. If this is the case, it would be consistent with a more generalized reduction of the socio-cultural suppression of women's sexuality in the latter part of the 20th century, considered in Chapter 6.

Sexual practices in same-sex interactions

Men who have sex with men

Laumann et al (1994) found that of men who identified as homosexual, the large majority had engaged in oral sex (89.5% active, 89.5% receptive) and a somewhat smaller majority in anal sex (75.7% active, 81.6% receptive) with their male partners. For those who had same-sex experience in the previous year, the respective figures were 88.6% active and 94.3% receptive for oral sex, and 79.4% active and 77.1% receptive for anal sex. Of those who reported some sexual activity with a same-sex partner since the age of 18 years, 58.9% reported active and 69.9% receptive to oral sex, and 50% reported active and 53.4% receptive to anal sex.

Mercer et al (2004) reported on the sexual practices of the men who had sex with men (MSM) in the two Natsal surveys: 105 men in Natsal I and 155 in Natsal II. For the past year, 47.5% of Natsal I, and 62.6% of Natsal II MSM reported anal sex ('insertive' or active, 42.8% and 56.9%, respectively; receptive, 35.5% and 53.5%, respectively). The increase in the proportion reporting receptive anal sex was significant ($p = 0.028$). For the past year, 63.3% of Natsal I and 73% of Natsal II reported oral sex ('insertive' or active 62.2% and 71.0%, respectively; receptive, 57.4% and 71.4%, respectively). None of these differences between the two surveys for oral sex was significant.

Grulich et al (2003) from the Sex in Australia study reported on what happened during the most recent same-sex sexual encounter in their 187 MSM. Approximately three-quarters of encounters involved oral sex (75.9% active, 75.1% receptive). Approximately one-third involved anal sex (37.5% 'insertive', 29.8% receptive). On 88.7% occasions the man experienced orgasm.

Women who have sex with women

Overall, there are less data on sexual practices for lesbian women. In the NHSLS (Laumann et al 1994), of those who reported some sexual activity with a same-sex partner since the age of 18 years, 61.8% of the women reported active and 72.2% receptive oral sex. The numbers were too small to report for the 'sexual identity' or 'activity during the past year' group.

Johnson et al (1994), from the Natsal I study, reported an interesting difference in the prevalence of oral sex across the age groups, raising the possibility that this practice had increased among women who have sex with women. Of those who had had sexual experiences with other women, being the passive recipient of oral sex at some stage was reported by 80.1% of the 16–24 age group, 60% of the 25–34 age group, 57.8% of 35–44 age group, and 37.3% of the 45–59 age group. The percentages for these age groups reporting 'passive' oral sex in the past year were 42.3%, 20.3%, 9.0% and 3.0%, respectively. Being the active partner in oral sex, at some stage, was reported for these age groups by 67.8%, 57.7%, 53.7% and 34.7%, respectively, and in the past year by 30.0%, 23.4%, 9.0% and 3.0%, respectively.

Grulich et al (2003), in their 123 women who had sex with women, found that nearly all women reported manual stimulation by their partner (95.1%) or of their partner (90.8%) on their most recent sexual encounter, and nearly two-thirds reported oral sex (65.8% receptive and 62.1% active).

Bailey et al (2003) reported on 1218 women who identified as lesbian or bisexual; 803 of them were recruited from women attending two lesbian sexual health clinics in London, while the remaining 415 were recruited via groups for lesbians in England and Scotland. The most common sexual practices with other women reported were oral sex (72% often, 25% occasionally), vaginal penetration with fingers (84% often, 13% occasionally), mutual masturbation (71% often, 24% occasionally) and genital–genital contact (50% often, 42% occasionally).

The characteristics of homosexual men and women: gender identities, personalities and mental health

Gender identities and gender role behaviour

At various points in this chapter and in Chapter 5, when sexual development was closely considered, an interaction between gender identity and the development of sexual identity has been emphasized. The evidence of a link between gender non-conformity in childhood and subsequent homosexual identity has been well documented. What gender-related personality characteristics do we therefore find among adult gay men and lesbian women? This is a challenging question. As Sandfort (2005) put it, 'In the works of some scholars, the relation between gender and sexual orientation, primarily understood as a biologically determined phenomenon, almost comes across as a dogma. In traditional "gay and lesbian" work, the relation is almost completely ignored ... In these circles, it has been taboo for quite some time to even suggest that there might be a relation between effeminacy and male homosexuality' (p. 595). In the lesbian literature, on the other hand, the concepts of 'butch' and 'femme' remain very apparent, and seemingly less 'incorrect'.

We need to put this in historical context. As already reviewed, the heterosexual or non-homosexual world had developed stereotypes of homosexuality, and through history anti-homosexual feelings had been directed in particular at the 'passive' participant in male homosexual activity. The stereotype extended to viewing the active 'insertor' during anal sex as the masculine one, and the passive recipient of anal insertion, the feminine one. There is also a long history indicating that the active homosexual, in that sense, was regarded as more or less normal (albeit immoral), provided he did not restrict his sexual activities to penetrating passive men, but the passive recipient was not only seen as effeminate, but also more stigmatized and less acceptable, and, in more recent history, pathological. So the negative stereotypes were based on this dichotomy of the active masculine male and the passive feminine male. This pattern of stereotyping has still been evident in modern Latino cultures, although according to Sandfort (2005) this is changing: the 'activos' and passives have been joined by the 'modernos' or 'internacionales', who are more versatile (Carillo 1999). It is striking, however, how little recent attention has been paid to preferences among gay men for taking the active or passive role in sexual interaction. Bell & Weinberg (1978) found that nearly all their male homosexual subjects expressed a definite preference for one type of sexual activity. Being the recipient of oral sex was the most popular, with taking the active role in anal sex the second favourite. However, there appeared to be flexibility and adaptation and one could not easily divide them into the 'tops' or 'bottoms', in any predictable way, and in so far as one could judge, there was no clear association with gender identity.

In the recent large-scale community-based surveys reported in the previous section, extensive evidence was obtained about engagement in different patterns of sexual activity, with substantial proportions reporting the active insertor role in anal sex, and substantial proportions the passive insertee role, but with no indication of how many of them, if any, had clear preferences for one role or the other. The emerging picture is of adaptive flexibility that does not convey rigidly structured gender-related sex roles. However, it is probably politically incorrect to consider this issue, although with the current concerns about HIV and AIDS, which will be considered in a later chapter, better information about preferences for specific roles during sexual activity may be helpful. At this stage, there is little reason to believe that such specific aspects of sexual interaction (i.e. the insertor vs insertee) are determined by gender identity in gay men.

In the earlier literature, a number of studies reported on the proportion of homosexual men who showed effeminacy and these ranged from 14% to 27%, although usually based on unsystematic observation (Bancroft 1972). However, this evidence pointed to, at most, a relatively small minority. The use of more established methods of assessing masculinity and femininity was reported by Siegelman (1972), Freund et al (1974) and Schatzberg et al (1975), demonstrating significant differences between homosexual and heterosexual males in psychological measures of femininity, although no distinguishing characteristics in terms of body shape were demonstrated. Although gender non-conformity during childhood has been shown to have a strong association with later homosexual identity formation (see Chapter 5), its relation to adult gender identity is less clear. In Chapter 10 we consider a subgroup of gender non-conforming boys who grow up wanting to change into women and have heterosexual relationships with men. The proportion of gender atypical boys who would follow this sequence, while not yet established, is likely to be small. Harry (1983) presented evidence that such childhood gender non-conformity disappears during the adulthood of gay men — what he called 'defeminisation', a pattern also observed by others (reviewed in Skidmore et al 2006). Gagnon & Simon (1973), on the other hand, described how the young male homosexual, soon after acknowledging his homosexuality, often went through a crisis of masculine identity during which he may have adopted an effeminate identity or behaviour. They implied that in the majority, as the identity crisis was resolved, the need to be effeminate receded. It is as though the homosexuality conflicts with the prevailing criteria of masculinity until new criteria are adopted. Westfall et al (1975) described how effeminate behaviour may be exaggerated in social situations which provoke anxiety. As I wrote a long time ago (Bancroft 1972), 'The homosexual, if he is to achieve stability, usually needs to produce a special type of gender identity — "I am a homosexual". This then permits a reappraisal of what is consistent or inconsistent. It is in this respect that the influences of the homosexual subculture are so important, as it is difficult for an individual to establish an identity and role which does not receive some form of social recognition' (p. 70). Alternative ways of reacting to the demasculinizing challenge of homosexuality are to emphasize other ultra-masculine characteristics. Sandfort (2005) considered what he called a 'subculture coming out of the closet'; the emergence of the gay macho man and the leather man, and he raises questions about the extent to which these new 'gay masculinities' are reflections of 'straight masculinities' or something specifically gay. He comments on how these new expressions of masculinity are more self-conscious, and that 'traditionally, it is not men but women who have to worry about their appearance and this is exactly what these men are doing' (p. 608).

In the 1970s, masculinity and femininity started to be conceptualized and measured as two separate and independent dimensions (e.g. Bem 1974), rather than the bi-polar unidimensional concept of earlier years. Masculinity was defined in terms of instrumentality (e.g. dominance, independence and assertiveness) and femininity in terms of expressiveness (e.g. nurturance, compassion and interpersonal sensitivity) and early evidence indicated that homosexual men were similar to heterosexual men in terms of instrumentality, but scored higher than them in terms of expressiveness, whereas lesbian women were similar to heterosexual women in terms of expressiveness, but higher in instrumentality (Pillard 1991). Lippa (2005) presented the results from a series of his studies, mainly involving university students. He developed the concept of 'gender diagnosticity' (GD), a prediction of whether an individual was male or female based on expressed preferences for specific occupations (e.g. mechanical engineer, building contractor or stockbroker as predominantly male and florist, social worker or nurse as predominantly female; Lippa 2002). He had shown a clear differentiation of men and women using this method, and went on to use the measures to compare heterosexual and homosexual men and women. In addition to his GD ratings, he used a self-definition of masculinity and femininity (self-M-F) based on Storm's (1979) six item scale, which asks the respondent 'How masculine (feminine) is your personality?', 'How masculine (feminine) do you act, appear and come across to others?' and 'In general, how masculine (feminine) do you feel you are?'. Measures of 'instrumentality' and 'expressiveness' and some other 'big five' personality measures were also included. The biggest difference between heterosexual and homosexual men was in the GD: heterosexual men showed much clearer preferences for male-type occupations. They also rated themselves more masculine on the self-M-F. Homosexual men scored higher than heterosexual men for expressiveness, agreeableness, conscientiousness and neuroticism, all typically higher in women, and for openness to experience, which is typically higher in men than women. Lesbian women rated themselves more masculine on both the GD and the self-M-F, and, less strongly, rated higher for instrumentality and openness to experience. They were similar for expressiveness and, interestingly, the lesbian women scored lower on neuroticism than the heterosexual women. Bisexual men were noticeably more similar to homosexual than heterosexual men, whereas bisexual women were intermediate between heterosexual and lesbian women. In several respects, the homosexual and lesbian respondents showed more variability in their ratings than the heterosexuals, particularly for GD and self-M-F, and, in the case of lesbian women, for expressiveness.

The evidence therefore points to a blending of masculine and feminine traits in both gay men and lesbian women, which shows considerable variability across individuals. The extent to which this blend is determined by early, more biological, factors or by socio-cultural influences remains uncertain, but as with most aspects of homosexual development, a combination of nature and nurture seems likely, with the impact of gay cultures in their various forms being evident. This leads to the conclusion that alongside the emergence of a man's or woman's sexual identity, gender identity can also evolve and adapt, and that the cultural context is of crucial importance in that adaptive process. As with much else about sexual development, we should keep our minds open to the possibility of differences in these developmental processes between gay men and lesbian women.

Personalities

In Chapter 6 we considered the evidence relating personality variables to sexuality. The basic dimensions of personality have so far shown little predictable relationship to patterns of heterosexuality. The more sex-related measures derived from the Dual Control model (see p. 229) are of potential interest in understanding homosexual expression, though so far relevant data are limited. A sample of self-identified gay men ($n = 1379$) and an age-matched sample of heterosexual men ($n = 1558$), all recruited from various sources (67% from the Internet) to participate in studies of sexual risk-taking, were compared using SIS/SES (Janssen et al 2002; see p. 15). The gay men scored significantly higher on SES, our measure of propensity for SE (mean $\pm$ SD: gay 58.4 $\pm$ 8.2, heterosexual 55.9 $\pm$ 8.6, $p < 0.001$) and SIS1, propensity for SI due to fear of performance failure (gay 29.7 $\pm$ 6.0, heterosexual 28.0 $\pm$ 6.0, $p < 0.001$), but did not differ on SIS2, propensity for SI due to fear of sexual consequences (gay 27.4 $\pm$ 5.0, heterosexual 27.5 $\pm$ 4.6, not significant) (Bancroft et al 2005).

A comparison of lesbian, bisexual and heterosexual women, using the female measure of SI and SE propensity (SESII-W) was reported earlier in this chapter (Sanders et al 2007; see p. 264). Lesbian women scored lower than heterosexual women on SI and higher on erotophilia.

A further form of individual variability of potential relevance to the well-being of gay men and lesbian women is the relationship between negative mood and sexuality. This was considered in Chapter 4 (see p. 108). Whereas the majority of individuals experience no change or a decline in sexual interest or motivation in negative mood states, such as depression and anxiety, a proportion of gay and heterosexual men report an increase. This pattern can be problematic, resulting in some cases in 'out of control' sexual behaviour (see Chapter 11, p. 330), is relevant to certain types of sexual risk taking (see Chapter 14) and, as we have found it less frequently in men with stable relationships, may be a further barrier to integrating one's emerging sexuality into close emotional relationships.

Although we have found a comparable pattern in a minority of heterosexual women (Lykins et al 2006), we do not as yet have comparative data from lesbian or bisexual women.

Mental health

Although it can be confidently concluded that homosexuality is not a manifestation of psychopathology, there is increasing evidence that homosexual men and women are more likely to experience depression and other negative mood states. Given the level of stigma associated with homosexuality, it would be surprising if this was not the case. Let us look at the relevant evidence more closely.

Earlier studies did not use representative community-based samples and the potential for participation bias needs to be kept in mind. Siegelman (1972) found that although a non-patient group of male homosexuals showed more neuroticism than their heterosexual controls, this difference disappeared when the homosexuals with evidence of feminine identity were excluded. He replicated this finding in a British sample (Siegelman 1978). In other words, the neuroticism may be associated with feminine gender identity (or, as suggested earlier, the femininity may be part of a reaction of anxiety or insecurity). Saghir & Robins (1973) found no difference between their homosexual and heterosexual male subjects in terms of depression, anxiety or psychosomatic symptoms. However, their heterosexual group consisted of only single, unmarried males. Weinberg & Williams (1974) found their male homosexuals to be less happy than their heterosexual controls but to have no more psychosomatic symptoms. Bell & Weinberg (1978) found not only more psychosomatic symptoms, but also more loneliness, lower self-acceptance and more depression and suicidal ideas; 20% of their homosexual men had previously made a suicide attempt compared with 4% of their controls.

For lesbian women, early studies showed some similarities and some differences compared with gay men. Saghir & Robins (1973) found their lesbian women to show more depression than their heterosexual women but to be relatively unaffected by it. Kenyon (1974) found lesbians to be more neurotic than their heterosexual counterparts. Two studies (reviewed by Riess et al 1974) suggested that lesbians may have stronger or more adaptive personalities than heterosexual women, at least in terms of independence. In Bell & Weinberg's (1978) study, the lesbian women reported less current happiness, lower self-esteem and more suicidal ideas. For both their male homosexual and their lesbian subjects they found a higher incidence of seeking professional help in the past. This somewhat variable picture suggests that at least some homosexual men and women are vulnerable to mental health problems, but the evidence does not indicate how they differ from those that are more resilient or less affected, except for that suggestion in Siegelman's data (1978) that effeminacy may be a factor in male homosexuals.

The more recent literature is mainly based on representative samples, avoiding the potential confounding factors of recruiting from specific gay or lesbian groups. However, these newer studies have other kinds of limitations, most notably the varied ways in which homosexuals are defined, and given that most were surveys not specifically focused on homosexuality, or even heterosexuality, relevant questions were limited.

Several studies have reported an increased prevalence of mood and anxiety disorders and substance abuse. Cochran & Mays (2000), using the sample from the 1996 National Household Survey of Drug Abuse ($n = 9714$), found 194 who reported 'any same-gender partner' in the previous year. Of these nearly 75% did not meet the diagnostic criteria for any of six mental health-related syndromes assessed. However, 'homosexual' men showed significantly more major depression and panic attacks than heterosexual men, whereas 'homosexual' women reported significantly more alcohol or drug dependency. The authors concluded that there was a 'small increased risk in one year psychiatric morbidity'. They also appropriately pointed out that 'sexual behaviour is not a perfect correlate of sexual orientation'. It is not possible to say how many of their men or women with same-sex experience identified as homosexual, lesbian or bisexual.

Gilman et al (2001) used the National Comorbidity Survey, a nationally representative survey of 15- to 54-year-olds carried out in 1990–1992 ($n = 8098$). They used experience of sex with a same-sex partner in the previous 5 years as their criterion of homosexuality; 2.1% of men and 1.5% of women came into this category. Their conclusions were based on combining the men and women with same-sex experience, who they found to be at increased risk for anxiety, mood and substance use disorders, and for suicidal thoughts and ideas. The authors pointed out the limitation of not having assessed sexual identity, as 'sexual identity might be as important, or more important, for mental health than sexual behavior' (p. 937).

Sandfort et al (2001) studied a representative sample of Dutch men and women aged 18–64 years ($n = 7076$). They also used sexual activity with a same-sex partner in the previous year as their criterion for homosexuality; 2.8% of men and 1.4% of women came into this category. In their homosexual men they found an increased 1-year prevalence of mood and anxiety disorders, whereas in the homosexually active women there was increased prevalence of substance use disorders, a gender difference similar to that reported by Cochran & Mays (2000). Lifetime prevalence showed a similar picture, except that homosexual women reported more lifetime episodes of mood disorder than the heterosexual women.

Fergusson et al (1999) reported relevant findings from their New Zealand birth cohort of 1265 men and women assessed at intervals since birth until the age of 21. At the final assessment 1007 participants were asked about sexual orientation; 20 indicated gay, lesbian or bisexual (9 male and 11 male). However, because of the small numbers involved, they added on a further 8 subjects who identified as heterosexual but disclosed that they had had some same-sex sexual interactions since they were 16. With this combined group they found increased risk for major depression, generalized anxiety disorder, conduct disorder, nicotine dependence, other substance use or dependency, suicidal ideas or suicide attempts.

Jorm et al (2002) reported findings from a community survey of 4824 men and women in Canberra, Australia, the PATH Through Life Project. This had taken place in two stages: 20- to 24-year olds were interviewed in 1999–2000 and 40- to 44-year olds in 2000–2001. They asked specifically about sexual identity: 'Would you currently consider yourself to be predominantly: heterosexual, homosexual, bisexual, or don't know?' They presented this information according to their two age groups. For the 20- to 24-year olds ($n = 2331$), 1.0% of men and 1.8% of women chose homosexual, and 1.8% of men and 2.7% of women chose bisexual. For the 40- to 44-year olds ($n = 2493$), 1.6% of men and 2.0% of women chose homosexual, and 0.89% of men and 0.8% of women chose bisexual. After controlling for age and gender, bisexual orientation was associated with worse mental health than heterosexual orientation, with the homosexual group coming midway. The authors commented on the apparent decrease of bisexuality in the older age group, though they could not distinguish between an age effect, with bisexual identity becoming less likely as people gain more experience, and a cohort effect, with bisexuality being more accepted in the younger generation.

Three studies have focused specifically on suicidal ideation and behaviour. Remafedi et al (1998) used data from a Minnesota Adolescent Health Survey carried out in 1987, involving junior and senior public high school students. They were asked to describe themselves as 'mostly/100% heterosexual', 'mostly/100% homosexual' or 'bisexual' ($n = 34\,804$). The homosexual option was chosen by 119 (0.34%; 81 males and 38 females), the bisexual option by 275 (0.79%; 131 males and 144 females). Suicide attempts were reported by 28.1% of the homosexual and bisexual males, 20.5% of homosexual and bisexual females, 14.5% of heterosexual females and 4.2% of heterosexual males. Suicidal intent and attempts were significantly more frequent among the homosexual/bisexual males but not the females. Herrell et al (1999) reported on 103 pairs of middle-aged male twins from the Vietnam Era Twin Registry, where one of each pair reported a male sex partner after the age of 18 years. The homosexual twins were significantly more likely than the non-homosexual twins to report (i) thoughts about death, (ii) wanting to die, (iii) thoughts about suicide and (iv) a suicide attempt. After controlling for substance use and depression, these differences were still significant for (i), (iii) and (iv). No information was given, however, about the age at which these suicidal thoughts and experiences had occurred. In earlier studies (Bell & Weinberg 1978; Saghir & Robins 1973) suicide attempts in homosexual males were mainly during adolescence. A further report (deGraaf et al 2006), from the Dutch study considered earlier (Sandfort et al 2001), examined lifetime indicators of suicidal thinking in relation to same-sex partner experience, using similar markers of suicidality to Herrell et al (1999). Homosexual men differed from heterosexual men in reporting more of the four suicidal indices, whereas homosexual women differed only in showing more suicidal contemplation. After controlling for psychiatric morbidity, the increased likelihood of suicidality was reduced to some extent, but still significant in the homosexual men; the effect for homosexual women became insignificant. Among the homosexual men, perceived discrimination was a predictor of suicidality.

Two studies have explored quality of life in relation to homosexuality. Horowitz et al (2001) combined data from seven national surveys carried out by the National Opinion Research Center in the USA between 1988 and 1996 (combined $n = 11\,543$). Subjects were categorized according to the gender of their sexual partners (a) since age of 18 years and (b) in the last 12 months. Those who indicated that all of their sexual partners had been same sex for the time period were considered 'homosexual', and those with all opposite sex were considered 'heterosexual'. Those who indicated partners of both genders were classified as 'bisexual'. A variety of quality-of-life and mental health variables were assessed. Although there were some demographic and social background differences among the three orientation groups, they found little evidence of an association with quality-of-life or health indicators. It should be noted that their male and female groups were not assessed separately. A subsequent report from the Dutch survey considered earlier (Sandfort et al, 2001) found that quality of life was significantly less among their homosexual men, but did not distinguish their homosexual and heterosexual women (Sandfort et al 2003). The authors questioned whether the apparent difference to the Horowitz et al (2001) study was because they had analysed the males and females separately.

A further study of relevance to mental health and sexual orientation is the Sex in Australia survey, referred to earlier (Smith et al 2003). This incorporated a measure of psychosocial distress. For men, increased distress was associated with same-sex sexual attraction, rather than same-sex experience. In fact, the highest psychosocial distress scores were in those men who reported same-sex attraction but had not acted on that attraction. For women, increased distress was associated with both same-sex attraction and experience.

In a study comparing a convenience sample of gay men ($n = 1379$) to an age-matched sample of heterosexual men ($n = 1558$), gay men scored significantly higher on two trait measures, the Spielberger Trait Anxiety Inventory (Spielberger et al 1970) and the Zemore Depression Proneness Ratings (Zemore et al 1990), a trait measure for propensity for depression (Bancroft et al 2005).

There is now a substantial body of evidence that homosexual men and women are at increased risk for mental health problems, though there remains a lack of conclusive explanations of why. In attempting to answer this we should consider not just adulthood experience, but, perhaps in particular, the impact of uncertainty or perceived stigma related to sexual identity as the individual struggles with this phase of development during adolescence. The three-strand model of sexual development, employed in Chapter 5 to conceptualize heterosexual sexual development (see p. 145), is useful here also. The ability to form close emotional attachments may have been impaired as a consequence of alienation by parents, particularly fathers, during childhood. Landolt et al (2004) explored how, in gay men, childhood rejection by parents, which they construed as being probably a result of childhood gender non-conformity rather than the cause of it, was associated with attachment problems in adult relationships. The relative isolation from the peer group for those who are gender atypical creates further barriers to integration of the three strands. This integrative process is difficult enough for the average heterosexual, associated with a phase of emotional lability and propensity for depression in many of them. It will be even more problematic for those who are recognizing an emerging identity, which is stigmatized and likely to alienate them, at least for a while, from their families and peer group. The early establishment of a paradoxical relationship between negative mood and sexual response, considered earlier (see p. 111), may be a further complicating factor.

One of the limitations of the now extensive literature on homosexual orientation and mental health problems is the lack of information about whether the homosexual participants have established a homosexual identity or are still struggling with uncertainty; the latter group may well be more vulnerable. There was some indication of this in the Sex in Australia study (Smith et al 2003) where psychosocial stress was most marked in those experiencing same-sex attraction but were not acting on it; perhaps they represent the group with substantial internalized homophobia and who suffer as a consequence. The possibility that gender non-conformity will lead to more stigmatization, both from the heterosexual and from the homosexual communities, also has to be taken seriously, and this has been reviewed by Skidmore et al (2006). The need to conceal one's gender non-conformity adds an extra stress for such individuals. Several of these challenges may make it difficult for homosexually oriented individuals to establish a close, rewarding and stable sexual relationship, resulting in the additional burden of loneliness. Such relationships will be considered in the next section.

The status of relationships in the gay male and lesbian world

The evidence suggests that gay men have more sexual partners than lesbian women. This may be more a gender difference than one related to sexual orientation. If men, as is often assumed to be the case, tend to be more promiscuous than women, then the heterosexual version of the male has to contend with the restraining influence of his female partner. The homosexual male has no such constraint. On top of this has been a long-standing lack of encouragement or reinforcement for gay men to establish stable sexual relationships, an aspect of antigay attitudes which has been very evident in the recent opposition to gay marriage.

But homosexual men and women have the same needs for loving relationships and companionship as anyone else. How difficult has it been for them to achieve such relationships without the social reinforcement of marriage experienced by heterosexuals? Two early studies tell us something about this in the pre-AIDS era. Bell & Weinberg (1978), using factor analysis of many of the variables from their interview study, produced a typology of homosexuality; the same types emerged for their male and female subjects.

1. *Close-coupled.* These seemed to be comparable to the happily married faithful heterosexuals, living contentedly in a stable relationship with little sexual activity outside the relationship. They presented themselves as a particularly happy and well-adjusted group by any standards.
2. *Open-coupled.* Here the stable relationship was associated with a fair amount of 'extramarital' sexuality. Although not as well adjusted as the close-coupled, the males in this category seemed better able to cope with this lifestyle than the lesbians.
3. *Functionals.* These individuals were not in stable relationships and enjoyed a wide variety of sexual partners. They tended to be the most highly sexed group and were also somewhat younger. Presumably a proportion of them moved into other groups as they got older. Once again, the males in this category seemed to have fewer problems than the females.
4. *Dysfunctionals.* Individuals in this category conformed very much to the stereotype of the unhappy homosexual. They tended to have recurring problems in their relationships, often with sexual dysfunction and frequently feeling unhappy with their homosexual identities.
5. *Asexuals.* Comparable to the dysfunctionals, these individuals were characterized by a low level of sexual interest and hence were more inclined to live solitary existences.

The proportions of males and females found in these categories are shown in Table 8.5; more than a quarter of each gender were unclassifiable by this method. In addition, the lesbians included a much higher proportion of 'close-coupled'. The data for this study were collected in 1970, a time of major change in the gay world, and it is uncertain what proportions would be found today.

In Blumstein & Schwartz's (1983) study of American couples, gay male and lesbian couples were included. The reported frequency of love-making in these couples according to the duration of the relationship is shown in Figure 8.1. They found that initiation of love-making

TABLE 8.5	Typology of homosexuality (from Bell & Weinberg 1978)	
	Males (%) **($n = 686$)**	**Females (%)** **($n = 293$)**
Close-coupled	10	28
Open coupled	18	17
Functional	15	10
Dysfunctional	12	5
Asexual	16	11
Unclassifiable	29	28
Total	100	100

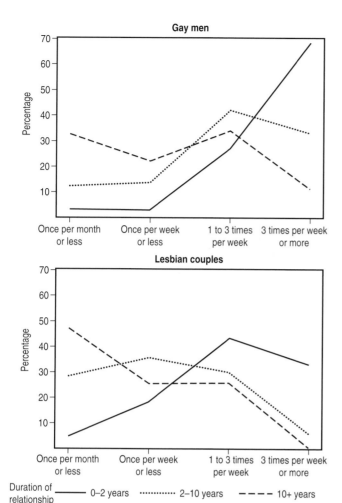

Fig. 8.1 Frequency of sexual activity in gay and lesbian couples by duration of relationship. (From Blumstein & Schwartz 1983.)

4. year 6–10, *building* (collaborating, increasing productivity, establishing independence, dependability of partner)
5. years 11–20, *releasing* (trusting, merging of money and possessions, constructing, taking each other for granted)
6. 20 years on, achieving security, restoring the partnership, remembering.

The end of the first year was a common time for male couples to split up. Expectations of fidelity were high but this was defined in terms of emotional commitment. Sexual exclusivity was expected by the majority at the start of the relationship, but this soon changed. In most of the couples there was an assumption of equality. This was an interesting if impressionistic study.

Since these early studies and the start of the AIDS epidemic, little research attention has been paid to established gay or lesbian relationships.

Deenen et al (1994) studied 320 men in gay relationships. They found emotional intimacy was the best predictor of satisfaction with the relationship, and that young gay men valued the emotional aspects more than older gay men. Schreurs (1993) reviewed the literature on lesbian couples and basically presented more questions than answers, as the majority of research has focused on the lesbian individual rather than the couple. She concluded that at that stage of research, lesbians and lesbian couples have more in common with heterosexual women than with gay men. She emphasized that emotional involvement was more important for most lesbian couples than sexuality per se, and, consistent with the findings for heterosexual women, lesbians are more likely to feel emotional closeness before they engage in sex. The variability in the literature could probably be explained by different lesbian subcultures having been sampled in the few studies that focused on couples.

Landolt et al (2004) considered the impact of childhood gender non-conformity on later attachment problems, but as yet it is not clear what the relationship is between gender non-conformity and established gay or lesbian relationships, though there is more likely to be a negative impact in gay male than in lesbian relationships.

With the recent increase in the possibilities of gay marriage or civil unions, there should be more opportunities to study the characteristics of those who succeed with long-term relationships. Frisch & Hviid (2006) reported on family correlates of both heterosexual and homosexual marriages in Denmark, where gay marriage has been possible since 1989. In a cohort of around 2 million Danish men and women, 1890 men and 1573 women married someone of their own gender between 1989 and 2001. Rates of such marriage were highest, not surprisingly, when they first became legalized. Since then rates of male same-sex marriage have stabilized, whereas female same-sex marriages have increased in recent years. However, this study was principally looking at the relationship between family characteristics and those who entered into heterosexual and homosexual marriages, and it is not possible to distinguish homosexuals who marry from those who do not on such a basis.

could be a problem, particularly for lesbian couples. They suggested that the woman's tendency to feel uncomfortable with the sexual initiator role contributed to a relatively low frequency of sex in lesbian relationships. They also found that lesbian couples were more likely to separate if one partner became sexually involved outside the relationship.

A further early study was published by McWhirter & Mattison (1984), who interviewed 156 established gay male couples whose relationships had lasted from 1 to 37 years. A friendship network was used to locate the couples, and many of them were interviewed on several occasions. They showed various joint lifestyles: some living together, some apart in the same town, while others lived in different parts of the country. McWhirter & Mattison described six stages in the evolution of these male relationships:

1. year 1, *blending* (merging, limerence, equalizing of partnership, frequent sexual activity)
2. year 2–3, *nesting* (home-making, finding compatibility, decline of limerence, ambivalence)
3. years 4–5, *maintaining* (reappearance of the individual, risk taking, dealing with conflict, establishing tradition)

Given the importance of stable relationships to the well-being of homosexual men and women, together with a likely positive impact of such relationships on public attitudes to homosexuality, we look forward to more research in this area.

REFERENCES

Altman D 1985 What changed in the 1970s? In Gay Left Collective (eds) Homosexuality: Power and Politics. Allison & Busby, London, pp. 52–63.

Bailey JV, Farquhar C, Oen C, Whittaker D 2003 Sexual behaviour of lesbians and bisexual women. Sexually Transmitted Infections 79: 147–150.

Bancroft J 1972 The relationship between gender identity and sexual behaviour: some clinical aspects. In Ounsted C, Taylor DC (eds) Gender Differences: Their Ontogeny and Significance. Churchill Livingstone, Edinburgh, pp. 57–72.

Bancroft J 1974 Deviant Sexual Behaviour: Modification & Assessment. Oxford University Press, Oxford.

Bancroft J 1975 Homosexuality and the medical profession. Journal of Medical Ethics 1: 176–80.

Bancroft J 2003 Can sexual orientation change? A long-running saga. Archives of Sexual Behavior 32: 419–421.

Bancroft J 2004 Kinsey and the politics of sex research. Annual Review of Sex Research 15: 1–39.

Bancroft J 2005 The history of sexual medicine in the United Kingdom. Journal of Sexual Medicine 2: 569–574.

Bancroft J, Carnes L, Janssen E, Goodrich D, Long JS 2005 Erectile and ejaculatory problems in gay and heterosexual men. Archives of Sexual Behavior 34: 285–298.

Bell AP, Weinberg MS 1978 Homosexualities. A Study of Diversity among Men and Women. Mitchell Beazley, London.

Bem SL 1974 The measurement of psychological androgyny. Journal of Consulting and Clinical Psychology 42: 165–172.

Bieber I, Dain HJ, Dince PR, Drellich MG, Grand HG, Gundlach RH, Kremer MW, Rifkin AH, Wilbur CB, Bieber TB 1962 Homosexuality: a Psychoanalytic Study. Basic Books, New York.

Binson D, Michaels S, Stall R, Coates TJ, Gagnon JH, Catania JA 1995 Prevalence and social distribution of men who have sex with men: United States and the Urban Center. The Journal of Sex Research 32: 245–254.

Blackwood E 1985 Breaking the mirror: the construction of lesbianism and the anthropological discourse on homosexuality. Journal of Homosexuality 11: 1–18.

Blumstein PW, Schwartz P 1983 American Couples. Morrow, New York.

Boswell J 1980 Christianity, Social Tolerance and Homosexuality. University of Chicago Press, Chicago.

British Medical Association 1955 Memorandum on Homosexuality drawn up by a Special Committee of the British Medical Association. BMA, London.

Broude GJ, Green SJ 1980 Cross-cultural codes on 20 sexual attitudes and practices. In Berry H III, Schlegel A (eds) Cross-cultural Samples and Codes. University of Pittsburg Press, Pittsburg, pp. 313–334.

Bullough VL 1976 Sexual Variance in Society and History. Wiley, New York.

Carillo H 1999 Cultural change, hybridity and male homosexuality in Mexico. Culture, Health and Sexuality 1: 223–238.

Carrier JM 1980 Homosexual behavior in cross-cultural perspective. In Marmor J (ed) Homosexual Behavior; a Modern Reappraisal. Basic Books, New York, pp. 100–122.

Cass VC 1990 The implications of homosexuality identity formation for the Kinsey model and scale of sexual preference. In McWhirter DP, Sanders SA, Reinisch JM (eds) Homosexuality/Heterosexuality: Concepts of Sexual Orientation. Oxford University Press, New York, pp. 239–266.

Chesser E 1949 Sexual behaviour. Normal and Abnormal. Medical Publications, London.

Cochran SD, Mays VM 2000 Relation between psychiatric syndromes and behaviorally defined sexual orientation in a sample of the US population. American Journal of Epidemiology 151: 516–523.

Crompton L 2003 Homosexuality & Civilization. Belknap Press, Harvard University, Cambridge, MA.

DeCecco JP 1990 Sex and more sex: a critique of the Kinsey conception of human sexuality. In McWhirter DP, Sanders SA, Reinisch JM (eds) Homosexuality/Heterosexuality: Concepts of Sexual Orientation. Oxford University Press, New York, pp 367–386.

Deenen AA, Gijs L, van Naersen AX 1994 Intimacy and sexuality in gay male couples. Archives of Sexual Behavior 23: 421–432.

De Graff R, Sandfort TGM, ten Have M 2006 Suicidality and sexual orientation: differences between men and women in a general population-based sample from the Netherlands. Archives of Sexual Behavior 35: 253–262.

Diamond LM 2007 A dynamical systems approach to the development of female same-sex sexuality. Perspective on Psychological Science 2: 142–161.

Dickinson RL, Beam L 1931 A Thousand Marriages. Williams & Wilkins, Baltimore.

Dickinson RL, Beam L 1934 The Single Woman: a Medical Study in Sex Education. Baltimore, Williams & Wilkins.

Ellis H 1915 Studies in the psychology of sex. Vol. 2, Sexual Inversion. Davis, Philadelphia.

Erens B, McManus S, Prescott A, Field J, Johnson AM, Wellings K, Fenton KA, Mercer C, Macdowell W, Copas AJ, Nanchahal K 2003 National Survey of Sexual Attitudes and Lifestyles II. Reference tables and summary report. National Centre for Social Research, London.

Fausto-Sterling A 2000 Sexing the Body: Gender Politics and the Construction of Sexuality. Basic Books, New York.

Fergusson DM, Horwood JL, Beautrais AL 1999 Is sexual orientation related to mental health problems and suicidality in young people? Archives of General Psychiatry 56:876–880.

Fisher WA, Byrne D, White LA, Kelley K 1988 Erotophobia–erotophilia as a dimension of personality. Journal of Sex Research 25: 123–155.

Ford CS, Beach FA 1952 Patterns of Sexual Behaviour. Eyre & Spottiswoode, London.

Foucault M 1978 The History of Sexuality. Volume 1: an Introduction. Translated by Hurley R. Random House, New York.

Freud S 1942 Three Essays on the Theory of SexualityTranslated by Strachey J 1949. Alcuin Press, Welwyn Garden City.

Freund K, Nagler E, Langevin R, Zajac A, Steiner B 1974 Measuring feminine gender identity in homosexual males. Archives of Sexual Behavior 3: 249–260.

Frisch M, Hviid A 2006 Childhood family correlates of heterosexual and homosexual marriages: a national cohort study of two million Danes. Archives of Sexual Behavior 35: 533–547.

Gagnon JH, Simon W 1973 Sexual Conduct: the Sources of Human Sexuality. Aldine, Chicago.

Gamson J, Moon D 2004 The sociology of sexualities: queer and beyond. Annual Review of Sociology 30: 47–64.

Gay J 1985 'Mummies and babies' and friends and lovers in Lesotho. Journal of Homosexuality 11: 97–116.

Gilman SE, Cochran SD, Mays VM, Hughes M, Ostrow D, Kessler RC 2001 Risk of psychiatric disorders among individuals reporting same-sex sexual partners in the National Comorbidity Survey. American Journal of Public Health 91: 933–939.

Glass SJ, Johnson R 1944 Limitations and complications or organotherapy in male homosexuality. Journal of Clinical Endocrinology 4: 540–544.

Green R 1974 Sexual Identity Conflict in Children and Adults. Duckworth, London.

Grulich AE, de Visser RO, Smith AMA, Rissel CE, Richters J 2003 Sex in Australia: homosexual experience and recent homosexual encounters. Australian and New Zealand Journal of Public Health 27: 155–163.

Haldeman DC 1994 The practice and ethics of sexual orientation conversion therapy. Journal of Consulting and Clinical Psychology 62: 221–227.

Harry J 1983 Defeminisation and adult psychological well-being among male homosexuals. Archives of Sexual Behavior 12: 1–20.

Henry GW 1941 Sex Variants: a Study of Homosexual Patterns. Hoeber, New York.

Herek G 2004 Beyond 'homophobia': thinking about sexual prejudice and stigma in the Twenty-First Century. Sexuality Research and Social Policy 1: 6–24.

Herdt GH 1981 Guardians of the Flutes. McGraw-Hill, New York.

Herdt G 2000 Why the Sambia initiate boys before age 10. In Bancroft J (ed), The Role of Theory in Sex Research. Indiana University Press, Bloomington, pp. 82–104.

Herrell R, Goldberg J, True W, Ramakrishnan V, Lyons M, Elsen SD, Tsuang MT 1999 Sexual orientation and suicidality: a co-twin control study in adult men. Archives of General Psychiatry 56: 867–874.

Hirschfeld M 1914 — Die Homosexualität des Mannes und des Weibes. Marcus, Berlin.

Hoffman M 1968 The Gay World. Basic Books, Southport.

Homosexual Law Reform Society Report 1966.

Hooker E 1965 Male homosexuals and their 'Worlds'. In Marmor J (ed) Sexual Inversion: the Multiple Roots of Homosexuality Basic Books, New York, pp. 83–107.

Hooker E 1967 The homosexual community. In Gagnon JH, Simon W (eds) Sexual Deviance. Harper & Row, London.

Horowitz SM, Weis DL, Laflin MT 2001 Differences between sexual orientation groups and social background, quality of life, and health behaviors. Journal of Sex Research 38: 205–218.

Hotvedt M 1983 Gender identity and sexual orientation: the anthropological perspective. In Schwartz MF, Moraczewski AS, Monteleone JA (eds) Sex and Gender. A Theological and Scientific inquiry. Pope John Center, St Louis, MI, pp. 144–176.

Janssen E, Vorst H, Finn P, Bancroft J 2002 The Sexual Inhibition (SIS) and Sexual Excitation (SES) Scales. I. Measuring sexual inhibition and excitation proneness in men. Journal of Sex Research 39: 127–132.

Jenkins P 1998 Moral Panic: Changing Concepts of the Child Molester in Modern America. Yale University Press, New Haven.

Johnson AM, Wadsworth J, Wellings K, Field J 1994 Sexual Attitudes and Lifestyles. Blackwell, Oxford.

Jorm AF, Korten AE, Rodgers B, Jacomb PA, Christensen H 2002 Sexual orientation and mental health: results from a community survey of young and middle-aged adults. British Journal of Psychiatry 180: 423–427.

Kendall K 1999 Women in Lesotho and the (Western) construction of homophobia. In Blackwood E, Wieringa S (eds) Female Desires: Same-sex Relations and Transgender Practices across Cultures. Columbia University Press, New York, pp. 157–178.

Kennedy HC 1980/81 The 'Third Sex' theory of Karl Heinrich Ulrichs. Journal of Homosexuality 6: 103–111.

Kenyon FE 1974 Female homosexuality—a review. In Loraine JA (ed) Understanding Homosexuality: its Biological and Psychological Bases. MTP, Lancaster, pp. 83–120.

Khan S 2007 Male intergenerational sexual relations in contemporary South Asia: India, Bangladesh, and Afghanistan (and Pakistan).Paper presented at International Academy of Sex Research, Vancouver, August 2007.

Kinnish KK, Strassberg DS, Turner CW 2005 Sex differences in the flexibility of sexual orientation: a multidimensional retrospective assessment. Archives of Sexual Behavior 34: 173–183.

Kinsey AC, Pomeroy WB, Martin CE 1948 Sexual Behavior in the Human Male. Saunders, Philadelphia.

Kinsey AC, Pomeroy WB, Martin CE, Gebhard PH 1953 Sexual Behavior in the Human Female. Saunders, Philadelphia.

Klein F 1985 Bisexualities: Theory and Research. Haworth, New York.

Klein F 1990 The need to view sexual orientation as a multivariable dynamic process: a theoretical perspective. In McWhirter DP, Sanders SA, Reinisch JM (eds) Homosexuality/Heterosexuality: Concepts of Sexual Orientation. Oxford University Press, New York, pp. 277–282.

Knauft BM 2003 What ever happened to ritualized homosexuality? Modern sexual subjects in Melanesia and elsewhere. Annual Review of Sex Research, 14: 137–159.

Kraft-Ebbing R von 1886 Psychopathia Sexualis. 12th edition translated by Klaf FS, 1965. Stein & Day, New York.

Landolt MA, Bartholomew K, Saffrey C, Oram D 2004 Gender nonconformity, childhood rejection, and adult attachment: a study of gay men. Archives of Sexual Behavior 33: 117–128.

Laumann EO, Gagnon JH, Michael RT, Michaels S 1994 The Social Organization of Sexuality: Sexual Practices in the United States. University of Chicago Press, Chicago.

Levitt EE, Klassen AD 1974 Public attitudes towards homosexuality: part of the 1970 National Survey by the Institute for Sex Research. Journal of Homosexuality 1: 29–43.

Lingiardi V, Falanga S, D'Augelli AR 2005 The evaluation of homophobia in an Italian sample. Archives of Sexual Behavior 34: 81–94.

Lippa RA 2002 Gender-related traits of heterosexual and homosexual men and women. Archives of Sexual Behavior 31: 77–92.

Lippa RA 2005 Sexual orientation and personality. Annual Review of Sex Research 16: 119–153.

Lippa RA 2007 The relation between sex drive and sexual attraction to men and women: a cross-national study of heterosexual, bisexual and homosexual men and women. Archives of Sexual Behavior 36: 209–222.

Lykins A, Janssen E, Graham CA 2006 The relationship between negative mood and sexuality in heterosexual college women. Journal of Sex Research 43: 136–143.

MacCulloch MJ, Feldman MP 1967 Aversion therapy in the management of 43 homosexuals. British Medical Journal 2: 594–597.

Marks IM, Gelder MG, Bancroft J 1970 Sexual deviants two years after electric aversion therapy. British Journal of Psychiatry 117: 173–185.

Masters WH, Johnson VE 1979 Homosexuality in Perspective. Little, Brown & Co, Boston.

McConaghy N 1970 Subjective and penile plethysmograph responses to aversion therapy for homosexuality: a follow-up study. British Journal of Psychiatry 117: 555–560.

McWhirter DP, Mattison AM 1984 The Male Couple: how Relationships Develop. Prentice Hall, New Jersey.

Mercer CH, Fenton KA, Copas AJ, Wellings K, Erens B, McManus S, Nanchahal K, Macdowall W, Johnson AM 2004 Increasing prevalence of male homosexual partnerships and practices in Britain 1990–2000: evidence from national probability surveys. AIDS 18: 1453–1458.

Minton HL 2002 Departing from Deviance: a History of Homosexual Rights and Emancipatory Science in America. University of Chicago Press, Chicago.

Moll A 1911 Die Behandlung sexueller Perversionen mit Vesonderer Beruchsichtigung der Assoziationstherapie. Zeitschrift fur Psychotherapie, Heft 1.

Muir H 2007 Majority support gay equality rights, poll finds. Guardian, 23 May 2007.

Ottosson D 2006 LGBT World legal wrap up survey. International Lesbian and Gay Association. www.stonewall.org.uk/documents/world_legal_wrap_up_survey__november2006.pdf.

Pillard RC 1991 Masculinity and femininity in homosexuality: 'inversion' revisited. In Gonsiorek JC, Weinrich JD (Eds) Homosexuality: Research Implications for Public Policy Sage, CA, Newbury Park, CA, pp. 32–43.

Pinello DR 2003 Gay Rights and American Law. Cambridge University Press, New York.

Remafedi G, French S, Story M, Resnicj MD, Blum R 1998 The relationship between suicide risk and sexual orientation: results of a population-based study. American Journal of Public Health 88: 57–60.

Rieger G, Chivers ML, Bailey JM 2005 Sexual arousal patterns of bisexual men. Psychological Science 16: 579–584.

Riess BF, Safer J, Yotive W 1974 Psychological test data on female homosexuality: a review of the literature. Journal of Homosexuality 1: 71–85.

Robinson P 1976 The Modernization of Sex: Havelock Ellis, Alfred Kinsey, William Masters and Virginia Johnson. Harper & Row, New York.

Rogers SM, Turner CF 1991 Male–male sexual contact in the USA: findings from 5 sample surveys, 1970–1990. Journal of Sex Research 28: 491–521.

Saghir MT, Robins E 1973 Male and Female Homosexuality: a Comprehensive Investigation. Williams & Wilkins, Baltimore.

Sanders D, Bancroft J 1982 Hormones and the sexuality of women — the menstrual cycle. Clinics in Endocrinology and Metabolism 11: 639–659.

Sanders SA, Graham CA, Milhausen RR 2007 Differences in sexual characteristics related to women's sexual orientation. Poster presented at International Academy of Sex Research, Vancouver, 2007.

Sandfort TGM 2005 Sexual orientation and gender: stereotypes and beyond. Archives of Sexual Behavior 34: 595–612.

Sandfort TGM, de Graaf R, Bijl RV, Schnabel P 2001 Same-sex sexual behavior and psychiatric disorders. Archives of General Psychiatry 58: 85–91.

Sandfort TGM, de Graaf R, Bijl RV, 2003 Same-sex sexuality and quality of life: findings from The Netherlands Mental Health Survey and Incidence Study. Archives of Sexual Behavior 32: 15–22.

Schatzberg AF, Westfall MP, Lumetti AB, Birk LC 1975 Effeminacy I. A quantitative rating scale. Archives of Sexual Behavior 4: 31–42.

Schmidt G, Klusmann D, Zeitzschel U, Lange C 1994 Changes in adolescents' sexuality between 1970 and 1990 in West Germany. Archives of Sexual Behavior 23: 489–513.

Schrenck-Notzing A von 1895 The Use of Hypnosis in Psychopathia Sexualis with Special Reference to Contrary Sexual Instinct. Translated by Chaddock CG, 1956.The Institute of Research in Hypnosis Publication Society and the Julian Press, New York.

Schreurs KMG 1993 Sexuality in lesbian couples: the importance of gender. Annual Review of Sex Research 4: 49–66.

Siegelman M 1972 Adjustment of male homosexuals and heterosexuals. Archives of Sexual Behavior 2: 9–25.

Siegelman M 1974 Parental background of male homosexuals and heterosexuals. Archives of Sexual Behavior 3: 3–18.

Siegelman M 1978 Psychological adjustment of homosexual and heterosexual men: a cross-national replication. Archives of Sexual Behavior 7: 1–12.

Simpson JA, Gangestad SW 1991 Individual differences in socio-sexuality: evidence of convergent and discriminatory validity. Journal of Personality and Social Psychology 60: 870–883.

Skidmore WC, Linsenmeier JAW, Bailey JM 2006 Gender nonconformity and psychological distress in lesbians and gay men. Archives of Sexual Behavior 35: 685–698.

Smith AMA, Riseel CE, Richters J, Grulich AE, de Visser RO 2003 Sex in Australia: sexual identity, sexual attraction and sexual experience among a representative sample of adults. Australian and New Zealand Journal of Public Health 27: 138–145.

Spielberger CD, Gorsuch RL, Lushene RE 1970 STAI Manual for the State Trait Anxiety Inventory. Consulting Psychologists Press, Palo Alto, CA.

Spitzer RL 2003 Can some gay men and lesbians change their sexual orientation? 200 participants reporting a change from homosexual to heterosexual orientation. Archives of Sexual Behavior 32: 403–417.

Stone L 1977 The Family, Sex and Marriage in England 1500–1800. Weidenfeld and Nicholas: London.

Storm MD 1979 Sex role identity and its relationship to sex role attributions and sex role stereotypes. Journal of Personality and Social Psychology 37: 1779–1789.

Trumbach R 2007 Male and female intergenerational sexual relations in Western Europe before and after 1900: marriage, prostitution, rape and same-sex relations. Paper presented at International Academy of Sex Research, Vancouver, August 2007.

Voeller B 1990 Some uses and abuses of the Kinsey Scale. In McWhirter DP, Sanders SA, Reinisch JM (eds) Homosexuality/Heterosexuality: Concepts of Sexual Orientation. Oxford University Press, New York, pp. 32–40.

Weeks J 1995 History, desire and identities. In Parker RG, Gagnon JH (eds) Conceiving Sexuality: Approaches to Sex Research in a Postmodern World. Routledge, New York, pp. 33–50.

Weinberg MS, Williams CJ 1974 Male Homosexuals: their Problems and Adaptations. Oxford University Press, New York.

Weinberg MS, Williams CJ, Pryor DW 1994 Dual Attraction: Understanding Bisexuality. Oxford University Press, New York.

Weinrich JD, Snyder PJ, Pillard RC, Grant I, Jacobson DL, Robinson SR, McCutchan JA 1993 A factor analysis of the Klein Sexual Orientation Grid in two disparate samples. Archives of Sexual Behavior 22: 157–168.

Westfall MP, Schatzberg AF, Blumetti AB, Birk CL 1975 Effeminacy II. Variation with social context. Archives of Sexual Behavior 4: 43–52.

Wolfenden 1957 Report of the committee on homosexual offences and prostitution. Cmnd. 247. : London. www.worldpolicy.orgglobalrights/sexorient/maps-gay.html.

Zemore R, Fischer DG, Garratt LS, Miller C 1990 The depression proneness rating scale: reliability, validity, and factor structure. Current Psychology: Research & Reviews 9: 255–263.

9

Sexual variations

Terminology: sexual minorities, variations, deviance, perversions or paraphilias?... 280
Sexual minorities 280
Sexual deviance 280
Sexual perversion 281
Paraphilias.. 281
Variations.. 281

Asexuality 281

Fetishism 283
The concept of fetishism.. 283

Parts of the body or partialism.................................... 283
Inanimate extensions of the body 284
Specific textures.. 284
The determinants of fetishism..................................... 284
Failure of incorporation of sexual learning into dyadic relationships 285
Abnormal learning 285

Sadomasochism 286
Determinants of sadomasochism............................... 286

'Multivariant sexuality' and conclusions 287

The history of human sexuality reveals a preoccupation with the immorality of sex. In much Christian thinking, there has been a struggle to accept sex as a normal aspect of life, with a pervasive 'sex-negativism' and a reluctant recognition that it is a 'necessary evil' to make reproduction possible. Thus it should be contained within marriage. The medical profession has, through much of this history, colluded with this position (Bancroft 2005). There have been substantial changes in the second half of the 20th century, with the emergence of more liberal, sex-positive attitudes, but counter-balanced by an ongoing sex-negativism from some sections of society. Gradually, however, the positive role of sex in establishing intimacy and binding relationships is being acknowledged, not only in the heterosexual married, together with awareness of how easily this positive component can be derailed. We are now seeing a shift in the involvement of the medical profession, particularly in their dealings with women, towards helping the maintenance of this positive component. In the process is a gradual acceptance of the extraordinary variability of human sexual expression illustrated 60 years ago by Kinsey's research. But this still leaves us with the challenge of defining what is acceptable, on either moral or socio-cultural grounds. The prevailing concept has been normal with an associated tendency to stigmatize anything regarded as abnormal. This chapter considers some of the better known examples of sex that are not regarded as normal, including the lack of sex, or asexuality. Apart from the aim of understanding these behavioural patterns better, so that those who experience them as problematic can be better helped, there is also scope in the process for increasing our understanding of the development of 'normal' sexual behaviour, which remains ill-understood. But let us first grapple with terminology.

Terminology: sexual minorities, variations, deviance, perversions or paraphilias?

Sexual minorities

In the last edition of this book this section was included in 'Sexual minorities', a neutral term, which acknowledges that there are many minority groups in society defined by their sexuality. The homosexual community, considered in the last chapter, is the largest and most important. In the next chapter we consider those with transgender identities. In this chapter we deal with a range of other sexual patterns that may be linked to minority groups for some, but be very individualized for others.

Sexual deviance

I used this concept in my earlier writing (e.g. Bancroft 1974). In conventional terms, deviance is behaviour that contravenes the norms of society. These norms combine the institutionalized norms or laws and the internalized and shared norms or mores. Gagnon & Simon (1967) distinguished between three types of sexual deviance. Firstly, *normal deviance,* which encompasses behaviour such as masturbation, premarital intercourse and oral sex, which, whilst frowned upon and even in some parts of the world still legally proscribed, is nevertheless carried out by large numbers of people. It is in this area that we are seeing the most obvious de-stigmatization. Secondly, *subcultural deviance,* which covers the more obvious sexual minorities, such as the homosexual and transgender subcultures. Thirdly, *individual deviance,* which includes sexual behaviours that are not clearly organized into subcultures or minority groups, exhibitionism being an example. The existence of a subculture with which the deviant individual can identify may be crucial to his or her well-being and adaptation. Having a social group within which one feels normal and accepted contrasts with feeling at all times abnormal and stigmatized. Such subcultures are far from static, however, and are constantly evolving and changing, reflecting the social attitudes of their time (see Chapter 10). In the mid-19th century, homosexuals had little opportunity for finding a homosexual subculture; now there is an international network of such organizations. Other types of deviant sexuality have generated their own organizations or subcultures and are continuing to do so. There are now well-established transgender organizations. An interesting example is the Paedophilia Information Exchange (PIE) formed in the 1970s. However, the social antagonism to paedophilia was such that any public meeting of this group generated considerable public hostility. Plummer (1979) likened this to the public reaction to homosexuality in the past, although it is less likely that attitudes to this form of behaviour will become more tolerant as time goes on. O'Carroll (1980), a member of PIE, made a serious but, in my view, unsuccessful attempt to defend the paedophiliac's sexual preference.

A further major change is the Internet. Internet 'communities' are not the same as 'real time' social groups, but they are providing increasing opportunities for individuals with unusual sexual interests to connect with others who are similar. Unfortunately, the term 'deviant' has grown to have pejorative connotations, so I am no longer using it.

Sexual perversion

This term, which has been widely used in the past, unequivocally means 'wrong', is hence stigmatizing, and for that reason should be avoided.

Paraphilias

This is the currently conventional medical term, used first by Stekel (1924) instead of 'perversion', and introduced into the DSM-III in 1980. Its Greek roots are *para* meaning 'besides' and *philia* meaning 'love' or 'friendship'. It covers a family of 'philias' and 'isms' mostly attributable to Money, who specialized in neology. Wikipedia (en.wikipedia.org) lists 106 terms in this category, most of them implying sexual behaviours that are rare and, beyond having a name to describe them, little understood. The better known 'philias' are necrophilia (sexual interest in dead bodies) and zoophilia (sexual interest in animals); examples of the more obscure are formicophilia (a subtype of zoophilia involving ants or other insects) and klismaphilia (love of enemas). This approach focuses attention on 'types' and not on explanatory mechanisms, and in addition imparts a somewhat confused medicalization (Moser 2001) that I prefer to avoid.

Variations

Henry (1948) used the term 'sex variants' in his study of homosexual patterns, which interestingly was sponsored by a Committee for the Study of Sex Variants, Inc. founded in 1935. The goals of this committee were 'to undertake, support and promote investigations and scientific research touching upon and embracing the clinical, psychological and sociological aspects of variations from normal sexual behaviour and of subjects related thereto...' (Henry 1948, p. *v*); a notably non-judgmental objective. More recently, Gosselin & Wilson (1980) published their book *Sexual variations; fetishism, sado-masochism and transvestism*. In this way, they minimized the emphasis on abnormality and pathology, and emphasized that such patterns of sexuality were not necessarily problematic for the individuals involved. I decided to use the term 'sexual variations' in this book.

This chapter focuses on three types of 'sexual variation': asexuality, fetishism and sado-masochism. These represent three aspects of sexuality: the presence (or absence) of a 'sexual drive'; the sexual stimulus, or type of person, that attracts you; how you interact with your sexual partner and what type of direct sexual stimulation is involved in that interaction. Our limited understanding of these three types will first be reviewed. An attempt will then be made to compare and contrast the possible explanatory mechanisms for each of them, and to consider in what way they inform us about human sexuality more generally. Variations which are illegal and likely to be harmful or disturbing to others (e.g. sadistic assault, exhibitionism and paedophilia) are considered in Chapter 16.

Asexuality

Given the extent of individual variability in human sexual expression, as documented so convincingly by Kinsey et al (1948, 1953), we can consider the extreme ends of the distributions of such factors as frequency of sexual activity and intensity of sexual desire. Those with 'hypersexuality' in these terms may have problems such as difficulty controlling their sexuality with various negative consequences. Similarly those with 'hyposexuality', or lack or absence of sexual desire, may experience this as a problem and be clinically diagnosed as having 'hypoactive sexual desire disorder'. Both types of problematic sex are considered further in Chapters 11 and 12. However, at both extremes there are likely to be individuals who are comfortable with either the high or low levels of their sexuality. Furthermore, this may determine their sexual identity in some respects. On the one hand, the highly sexed individual is likely to have a heterosexual, homosexual or bisexual identity, and to consider themselves highly sexed examples of such identities. But what of the 'asexual' individual with low or absent sexual interest?

This issue needs to be placed in historical context. As mentioned earlier, we have emerged relatively recently from a long phase of history when sexual expression was suppressed or contained by socio-cultural and religious influences. In those circumstances the asexual individual sat comfortably within many aspects of society, even marriage, as expressing the socio-culturally preferred 'default' position. Abbot (1999) has documented the long history of celibacy, institutionalized in various ways (e.g. Catholic priests) or adopted for a variety of reasons. The extent to which the celibate person is asexual is another matter; as we have recently been learning, not all Catholic priests remain celibate and some obviously have difficulty doing so. But now, in the modern era of relative 'sex positivism', celibacy requires more justification. Why would anyone, other than a Catholic priest, choose to be celibate in today's world?

Abbott (1999), having researched the history of celibacy, made an interesting personal revelation in her book. Most of her life she had been sexually active, but 'after clawing myself out from underneath the debris of a collapsed marriage, and assuming a new life in an unfamiliar city, I was not involved in a sexual relationship ... after *celebrating* the sense of liberation so many other women had derived from voluntary celibacy, I embraced it as a conscious choice' (p. 22). In this case we are seeing the adoption of celibacy, or interpersonal sexual inactivity, as an alternative to problematic sexual relationships. Some individuals obviously choose this alternative early in their developmental histories, and some of those may subsequently change their minds. This raises the vexed question of whether we choose our sexual identities or whether they evolve, which was considered in relation to homosexual and heterosexual identities in Chapter 5. Is 'asexuality' an identity that some people choose or does it evolve?

In recent years there has been increased attention to asexuality and debate about its nature. Jay (2003) is a self-identified 'asexual' who started a website for asexuals (www.asexuality.org), called AVEN (Asexual Visibility and Education Network). In his overview Jay writes 'An asexual is someone who does not experience sexual attraction. Unlike celibacy, which people choose, asexuality is an intrinsic part of who we are.' He goes on to describe the variability among self-identified asexuals with some wanting to be in close relationships, but without any sex, others preferring to lead more individual lives. He also comments that 'asexual' individuals can experience attraction to others, but the attraction is not sexual. However, on the basis of such non-sexual attraction, he suggests, asexuals can identify as gay, straight or bisexual; this is somewhat confusing.

Research into asexuality has only just started. Johnson et al (1994), in the first British NATSAL survey, asked their male respondents if they have felt sexually attracted to others, giving them six response options: (i) only to females, never to males, (ii) more often to females, and at least once to a male, (iii) about equally often to females and males, (iv) more often to males, and at least once to a female, (v) only ever to males or (vi) I have never felt sexually attracted to anyone at all. For female respondents, the first five options were in reverse order, and 0.8% of men and 1.2% of women selected option (vi). They asked similar questions about sexual experience rather than sexual attraction: 2% of men and 1.6% of women chose option (vi). Those who selected option (vi) for both sexual attraction and experience were 0.4% of men and 0.5% of women. Johnson et al (1994) did not comment further on these findings. Smith et al (2003) reported results from the Sex in Australia survey (9729 men and 9578 women aged 16–59), in which exactly the same questions had been asked about sexual attraction and experience. Those who selected option (vi) for sexual attraction were 0.2% of men and 0.6% of women, and for sexual experience were 3.3% of men and 3.1% of women. Bogaert (2004) carried out a secondary analysis of the British NATSAL 1994 data, focusing on the 'sexual attraction' question. He interpreted a positive answer to option (vi) as indicating lifelong asexuality, and explored possible predictors. Those selecting this option ($n = 195$; approximately 1%) were more likely to be female, to report religiosity, to have short stature, low education, low socio-economic status, and poor health. The 'asexual' women were more likely to report a late onset of menarche. He concluded that these findings suggest both biological and psychosocial determinants of 'asexuality'. Whilst these findings are of interest, the data has limitations. The choice of six options, listed above, does not allow the respondent to indicate a current absence of sexual attraction but experience of sexual attraction earlier in one's life. It is therefore questionable whether option (vi) should be interpreted as 'lifelong asexuality'. In addition there was no information about masturbation. It remains unclear, therefore, whether his 'asexual' subjects lacked sexual attraction to other people but were motivated to obtain sexual pleasure individually, and it is not possible to say whether any of them had fetishistic preferences.

Prause & Graham (2007) recruited 41 self-identified 'asexuals' from the AVEN website, mentioned earlier, and also the Kinsey Institute website and, with the addition of 732 undergraduates from psychology classes, had a 'non-asexual' comparison group of 1105 men and women. Both groups completed a range of questionnaires online, including the Sexual Desire Inventory (SDI; Spector et al 1996), which provides measures of both 'dyadic' and 'solitary' sexual desire, the Sexual Inhibition/Sexual Excitation Scale (SIS/SES; Janssen et al 2002), and the Sexual Arousability Inventory (SAI; Hoon et al 1976). Respondents were also asked open-ended questions about their perception of 'asexuality', its advantages and disadvantages. The 'asexuals' reported significantly lower 'dyadic' sexual desire (i.e. desire for sex with a partner), lower sexual arousability (SAI) and lower propensity for sexual excitation (SES), but did not differ significantly from the non-asexuals in their propensity for sexual inhibition (SIS) or their desire to masturbate. This study provides more detailed information about the characteristics of self-defined asexuals, and the authors concluded that low sexual desire is a primary feature of asexuality. There are various possible sampling biases, however. Many of the 'asexual' volunteers expressed a wish to understand the 'cause' of their asexuality, suggesting that this sample may have over-represented those who were concerned about their asexuality. In addition the 'non-asexual' comparison group was significantly younger than the asexual group, and the comparisons of these two groups on the questionnaire measures should be treated cautiously.

It is early days in the research of asexuality, and further research is certainly warranted. It would not be surprising, however, if this were to show that behind a shared identity of 'asexual' lies a heterogeneity of sexual characteristics, with some individuals being generally disinterested in sex of any kind and others having a range of reasons for currently avoiding sexual relationships.

Fetishism

An important component of sexual development is the emergence of sexual arousability in response to sexual stimuli. As considered in Chapter 5, there appears to be a critical period in the young male's sexual development when a connection between specific stimuli and sexual response is established. The precise mechanisms underlying this process are not understood, and as discussed in Chapter 5 the prevailing assumption that conditioning is involved is probably an oversimplification. These specific sexual signals, typically involving physical attributes of another person, usually serve to attract males to a suitable partner as well as to initiate sexual interaction. If we are successful in our sexual development, we are eventually able to sustain a relationship with a suitable partner in spite of the distractions of other sexual signals all around us. There are some important types of variability associated with this process. The most fundamental is whether the 'selected sexual signal' involves individuals of the same or opposite sex. This largely determines sexual identity (see p. 159). But on another dimension is the specificity of the signal. To what extent do we establish sexual preferences during this stage of development that remain specific and unchanged through most of our lives? Alternatively, to what extent do our specific preferences change as a result of later experiences and the influence of socio-cultural factors? It is striking that this issue has been almost totally ignored in the sexological literature on male sexuality. 'Male' or 'female' is specific and unchanging for the majority of men. But beyond that, there is considerable variability across individuals in the characteristics of the 'sexually attractive' other person, and also in how specific and constant those characteristics are. We will return to this issue when summarizing possible aetiological mechanisms.

So far this description characterizes male development, but is not so evident in female development, where attraction to a relationship is of more primary importance than attraction to a particular type of person. Sexual responsiveness to certain characteristics of the desired partner, or certain patterns of sexual interaction, may become established as a secondary stage.

Males often show preference for particular parts of the female (or male) body, e.g. for breasts, buttocks or legs, and for waist-to-hip ratios (see Chapter 6). To some extent preferences for the parts of the body may be culturally determined. In the west, the size of the breast considered most attractive has varied over time, as has the general body size (whether relatively thin or well built). In China, until recently, the 'lotus' or bound foot had a special sexual appeal (Money 1977). In a recent cross-cultural study, small feet in women and average size feet in men were generally preferred (Fessler et al 2005). When are such specific attributes to be regarded as fetishes?

The concept of fetishism

The word 'fetish', which from its Portuguese origins implies an artistically created artefact, also conveys a special symbolism or magical meaning — the love token or erotic icon. But we should consider such detachable tokens of the loved one alongside the physical attributes or body parts already mentioned. The fetishistic quality is a graduated one. The concept becomes more relevant as the subject becomes more preoccupied with the signal itself and less concerned with the associated partner. The fetish becomes more problematic as it serves to weaken rather than strengthen the sexual bond with the sexual partner and, in its most extreme form, makes the sexual partner, as a person, virtually redundant in sexual terms. Fetishism is rarely found in women, pointing to the link between fetishistic development and the more characteristically male pattern of development described above.

There are three principal categories of sexual signal or stimulus to consider: (i) a part of the body (partialism), (ii) an inanimate extension of the body, e.g. article of clothing, (iii) a source of specific tactile stimulation (e.g. the texture of a particular form of material).

Parts of the body or partialism

This category overlaps most obviously with the normal, but interest in specific body parts may over-ride any interest in the rest of the person or the body as a whole. Von Kraft-Ebbing (1965) gave a rich account of fetishes in the 19th century and there are some interesting differences with modern fetishism which presumably stem from changing attitudes to sexuality. He described hand fetishes as common at that time. He related this to a preoccupation with masturbation and a transfer from one's own masturbating hand to that of a girl. Hand fetishism is rarely seen nowadays (this author has never seen a case) whereas foot fetishism is possibly the most common form of partialism. It is, however, more difficult to provide as relevant an explanation for foot fetishism as Kraft Ebbing provided for hand fetishism. Sexual attraction to lame women or female amputees featured in Kraft-Ebbing's account and is still seen nowadays, though it is relatively rare (Marks et al 1970). Lawrence (2006) has postulated that the desire for amputation of a healthy limb, known as apotemnophilia, occurs in men who start with a fetish for amputees and who show a comparable transition of identity as seen in autogynephilic males who become transgendered (see Chapter 10).

Inanimate extensions of the body

Articles of clothing, boots and shoes are perhaps the commonest type of fetish. The use of women's clothes as fetishes overlaps with transvestism and will be considered further in Chapter 10. Some fetishes involve a link with babies rather than women, e.g. nappies (diapers).

Specific textures

One of the most common fetishes at the present time is rubber, particularly clothing made out of rubber. Other materials are leather and shiny black plastic. In Kraft-Ebbing's time, furs, velvets and silks were the popular textures.

Chalkley & Powell (1983) found 48 cases of fetishism referred to the Maudsley Hospital over a 20-year period (0.8% of all referrals). Only one was female (a lesbian with a fetish for breasts). Of the men, 15% showed partialism (mainly for legs). The remainder involved articles of clothing: 15% footwear, 23% rubber items. Seventeen men had one fetish, nine had two and the remaining 22 had three or more (to a maximum of nine different fetishes). In all, 25% of this group stole their fetish articles.

Gosselin & Wilson (1980) reported on 87 members of the Mackintosh Society for rubber fetishists and 38 members of the Atomage correspondence club for leatherites. They also contacted 133 members of a sadomasochistic club and 285 members of the Beaumont society for transvestites and transsexuals. Using the Eysenck personality questionnaire they found all four groups tended towards introversion and neuroticism though none of the groups had mean scores within the clinical range. Their social backgrounds were fairly unremarkable and they came from a normal socioeconomic cross-section.

Weinberg et al (1995) studied 262 members of a homosexual foot fetish organization, The Foot Fraternity, which promoted communication between its members by means of a newsletter. They reported a series of graphic accounts. 'Foot lovemaking' typically involved 'one man "worshipping" another man's feet by kissing, caressing, sucking and/or licking them' (p. 20). This interesting study not only describes clear fetishism among homosexual men, but also indicates considerable variability in the extent to which the fetish dominated the individual's sex life, or was associated with other psychological or interpersonal problems. In spite of their detailed report, however, one is left with no clear idea why a fetish for feet develops.

As with many other aspects of sexuality, the Internet has had an impact on the world of fetishism, providing not only a wide range of fetish stimuli but also the opportunity to identify with other fetishists and as a consequence to feel less abnormal. Junginger (1997) reviewed 'alternative sex forums' he found on the Internet in 1995, many of which were dealing almost exclusively with fetishes. From a selection of such sites, he counted different fetishes that were mentioned or depicted. Among articles of clothing, underwear was the most common, panties being the most frequent and, interestingly, diapers or nappies the second most frequent. Rubber and leather objects were both frequent, particularly rubber underwear and leather shoes or boots. Of the body parts mentioned, feet or toes were the most frequent. How the fetish object was used was also reported, with wearing, looking at or fondling being the most frequent.

Fetishism appears to be rare in women (Kinsey et al 1953). Apart from the case cited above, Stoller (1982) described three cases of fetishistic transvestism in women. The idea of female fetishism has been promoted, however. Gamman & Makinen (1995) published a book called Female Fetishism, which Ehrenberg (2000), in her review of this book, saw as a claim that 'the historical denial of fetishism among women is a phallocentric refusal to credit active female desire and libido' (p. 193). Devor (1996) reported that several feminist theorists considered the sexual use of dildos as fitting the definition of fetishism.

The determinants of fetishism

It is often assumed that fetishism results from the specific conditioning of sexual response to particular stimuli. In the male, the capacity for classical conditioning of erections to unusual stimuli has been demonstrated experimentally (Rachman & Hodgson 1968; Bancroft 1974) and it may be that erection is a peculiarly conditionable response. This may depend in part on the obviousness of penile erection so that cognitive processes may mediate in linking a sexual response to specific stimuli (e.g. 'that object produced an erection, it must have sexual significance'). The fact that women are much less aware of any genital response (see p. 131) may then help to explain the apparent lack of such fetishistic learning. A simple conditioning model is not sufficient, however. Other factors must operate to maintain the response. It has been suggested that, as with other sexual preferences, masturbation and orgasm in response to the fetish object will serve to reinforce and maintain the association (McGuire et al 1965). But it remains a puzzle to the learning theorist why in some individuals certain specific stimuli become discriminately reinforced, whilst in most individuals there is a generalization of learning which allows sexual preferences to evolve and to mature with experience, involving the whole person. This is a question of fundamental importance. Two possibilities warrant consideration: first, some interference with the incorporation of specific sexual learning into dyadic sexual relationships and, second, an abnormality in the learning process. As yet we can only speculate about the likely importance of either mechanism, and indeed, both may be involved.

Failure of incorporation of sexual learning into dyadic relationships

In Chapter 5, the process of normal sexual development was conceptualized as involving three developmental strands, gender identity, sexual responsiveness and the capacity for dyadic relationships, which, during childhood, are relatively independent of each other until around puberty when their integration starts, leading eventually to the sexual adult who is capable of maintaining a sexual relationship with one person. The integration of gender identity and sexuality is considered more closely in Chapter 10. Here we should consider the integration of sexual responsiveness and dyadic relationships. This, it has been postulated, is more crucial in male development because of the development of sexual attraction and the identification of sexually stimulating signals, in a relatively immutable fashion, at a critical stage in male development. If this sexual learning phase occurs too early, this might reduce the likelihood of appropriate incorporation into dyadic sexual relationships. Alternatively, or in addition, there may be other barriers to the development of dyadic relationships that effectively prevent the appropriate integration, resulting in a relatively impersonal establishment of sexual preferences. Gebhard et al (1965) expressed this view as follows:

'Many boys see their mothers' lingerie, many glimpse their sisters or other female relatives undressing, others have peeped — yet they do not develop fetishism. There must be the coincidence of early awareness of sexual arousal in connection with the fetish item so that the two are associated; following this there must be some imperfection in the development of sociosexual life which encourages the fetishism to grow in a compensatory way. There are probably many males who experienced the above mentioned coincidence, but whose incipient fetishism remained underdeveloped because of their subsequent adequate sex lives.'

(p. 419)

Weinberg et al (1995), in their study of homosexual foot fetishists, concluded that their findings did not support the 'compensation' hypothesis of Gebhard et al (1965), on the grounds that the majority of their sample reported their early fetish experiences as positive.

LaTorre (1980) reported an interesting experiment with male students, which warrants further study. These men, none of whom was in any established sexual relationship at the time, were randomly assigned to one of two groups. They were all shown pictures of young women together with an autobiographical account by each woman, and were asked to select those women they would most like to date. One group was told that the women they chose had not, when given the same task, chosen them; the other group were told that their chosen women had in fact chosen them. This experience of rejection or acceptance was repeated on two occasions, 2 weeks apart. In a further procedure, assumed to be unassociated with the first two, each man was asked to rate pictures of women's underclothes, feet, legs and women fully dressed, on scales of pleasantness, sexual arousability and acceptance. The rejected men evaluated the pictures of women more negatively than the accepted men and a further control group. In addition, the rejected men rated the pictures of women's underclothes and legs more positively than the pictures of women, which was not the case for the accepted men and controls. LaTorre (1980) suggested a possible relevance of these findings to the establishment of fetishism. While this experimental procedure is obviously of limited relevance to earlier sexual development, it is consistent with the idea that factors that discourage establishment of dyadic relationships may also discourage the establishment of 'whole person' sexual stimuli, and promote more fetish-like sexual interests.

Abnormal learning

Given the variety of fetishes, we can also consider the distinction between those that are part or extensions of the 'whole person', which may best be understood using the above 'failed integration' or compensatory model, and those that appear to be unrelated to a person. It may be that sexual learning at an early age, before any mature concept of sexuality has developed, permits more unusual associations to develop.

In some instances, fetishes are exceedingly bizarre and cannot be understood as extensions of the body and are more likely to be associated with some neurological abnormality such as temporal lobe epilepsy. In such cases, the stimulus can be seen as more random, the abnormality being in the disturbance of learning. Gosselin & Wilson (1980), in their study of 'rubberites', found that the interest in rubber originated between the ages of 4 and 10. From the ages of their subjects they concluded that many of them would have developed this interest around the early stages of World War II. They therefore speculated that such anxiety-provoking circumstances, combined with an often absent father and overprotective mother plus a lot of rubber articles in use at that time, provided the ingredients for this particular fetish to flourish. McConaghy (1993) noted that many of the fetishists seen in his clinical practice reported a strong interest in the fetish object earlier in childhood before it became sexually arousing. Weinberg et al (1995), in their study of homosexual foot fetishists, found that being sexually aroused by feet or footwear typically started around puberty. However, a number of their accounts indicated an earlier onset of interest and pleasure in feet, though not obviously sexual at that stage. However, it is not clear to what proportion of their group this applied.

Attention has been paid to the possibility that fetishism can result from brain abnormalities. A much quoted example is of a man with temporal lobe epilepsy (Mitchell et al 1954). Thinking of 'safety pins' gradually replaced sexual intercourse as his preferred sexual activity, and such thoughts could trigger epileptic seizures. Temporal lobectomy not only cured his epilepsy, it also removed the fetish for safety pins, with a return to more normal sexual interests. However, most people with temporal lobe disorders do not have such symptoms. The range of neurophysiological speculations to account for fetishism, and some interesting case histories, have been usefully reviewed by Mason (1997), who also provided a review of the relevant psychoanalytic literature. As yet, we can at best speculate about the origins of fetishism.

Sadomasochism

Sadism needs to be considered at two very different levels: as a factor in some forms of sexual violence and abuse, and as a component of ritualized sadomasochism, which is a consensual pattern of sexual interaction.

Sadistic sexual violence ranges from sexual assault or rape, in which the rapist is motivated by the desire to dominate his victim, to sadistic sexual murder. In its least serious forms this can be seen as a distorted manifestation of male dominance in sexual interactions. The most serious forms include some of the most ghastly crimes inflicted by one person on another; some graphic examples are provided by Hucker (1997). These aspects of sadistic violence are considered further in Chapter 16.

Although there is a clear difference between sadism as expressed in criminal behaviour and the ritualized versions of sadomasochochism enjoyed by both participants (often referred to as BDSM, for bondage, discipline, sadism and masochism), there remains considerable stigma associated with sado-masochism (Moser & Kleinplatz 2006). Mutually consenting BDSM, particularly between gay males, may be regarded as illegal, shown clearly by the Spanner case in the UK in the late 1980s when police discovered video recordings of the activities of a gay sadomasochistic sex club. Several of those involved, including some who had been the masochistic recipients, were sentenced to imprisonment for up to 4 years (Green 2001). It is therefore not surprising that those in the BDSM world are often very reluctant to reveal information about their behaviours or to allow researchers to observe them.

A number of studies of the ritualized forms of sado-masochism have nevertheless been published and were reviewed by Weinberg (2006). Most of this research has involved members of BDSM organizations. Although there is evidence of private clubs of this kind in London in the 18th and 19th centuries (Falk & Weinberg 1983), the earliest of the modern organizations, the Eulenspiegel Society, was founded in New York in 1971. These organizations tend to vary in what type of rituals they emphasize, but they typically involve patterns of dominance and submission, often with bondage, when the submissive partner is tied up or constrained and is, in a ritualized manner, at the mercy of the dominant partner, and the infliction of controlled amounts of pain (e.g. by 'spanking' or whipping). In gay male BDSM groups there is an additional component of 'hypermasculinity', with the wearing of clothes, most typically black leather, which have symbolic hypermasculine significance. In this respect there is some overlap with fetishism. In contrast, straight BDSM males tend to be more interested in humiliation. BDSM women, whether heterosexual or lesbian, tend to prefer bondage, spanking, or 'master–slave' scenarios (Levitt et al 1994).

An important aspect of the BDSM culture is the strict setting of rules and limits, which allow the participants to enjoy the BDSM experience without fear that it might go too far, and which include, for example, a prohibition of inebriation. Interestingly, in many BDSM groups, coitus or genital stimulation to induce orgasm is unusual (Moser 1998).

Although there are individuals, both males and females, who are primarily interested in playing the dominant, 'sadistic' role in such rituals, those who are primarily masochistic are the majority, and there is often an exchange of roles, so that the primarily masochistic individual comes to enjoy the sadistic role and vice versa. This overlap was recognized by Freud (1949) who wrote '... the most remarkable feature of this perversion is that its active and passive forms are habitually found in the same individual. A person who feels pleasure in producing pain in someone else during a sexual connection, is also capable of enjoying as pleasure any pain which he may himself derive from sexual relations' (p. 38).

Although evidence of the prevalence and developmental histories of sado-masochists is limited, they are somewhat more likely to be males. The age at which they became aware of their BDSM interests has been reported as between 18 and 20 by Sandnabba et al (1999), whereas in Breslow et al's (1985) study, half had become aware by age 14. This is a crucial developmental issue, which requires more research. The evidence for females shows a more consistently later awareness, often introduced by a partner (Hucker 1997). In general, BDSM rituals tend to be unacceptable to the sadomasochist's partner or spouse, resulting in the importance of clubs where the like-minded have opportunities to enjoy their sadomasochistic preferences with each other, and an increased likelihood of BDSM men and women being single or divorced.

Determinants of sadomasochism

As yet we understand little about the factors that lead to the development of sado-masochistic preferences. Kinsey et al (1953) reported that 12% of women and 22% of men had responded erotically to sadomasochistic stories. There is an important distinction between fantasy and reality. The use of fantasies of being raped or being forced into sexual activity by women during masturbation or intercourse is far from unusual (Wilson 1978), although few if any such women would enjoy such experiences in reality. However, some of them might learn to enjoy a ritualized version in which they know they are not going to be seriously hurt or be unable to stop when they want to. Fantasies of being sexually dominated may be used by young males early in their sexual development. For both females and males, particularly those who have grown up associating sexual pleasure with guilt, the arousing effect of being dominated may derive from a sense that one cannot be blamed for the experience. However, this is largely speculation.

Weinberg (2006), in his review, concluded that BDSM is predominantly about dominance and submission and not necessarily about pain. However, pain is commonly involved to some degree. Whether or not masochistic individuals seek pain, it is obvious that they can experience sexual arousal in the presence of pain. Moser gave a vivid account of his first experience of visiting a BDSM club as an observer. A woman was being subjected to 'a savage beating' to the extent that Moser was just about to object, when the woman experienced an intensely pleasurable orgasm (Moser & Kleinplatz 2006). In Chapter 4, we considered the paradoxical association between negative mood and sexual arousal that is evident in a minority of men and women. Perhaps moderate pain during sexual arousal may augment the arousal in some individuals. The commonest form of this is the love bite. This phenomenon is widespread amongst mammals. Kinsey et al (1953) found that 55% of women and 50% of men interviewed had responded erotically to such bites during love-making.

Much of the research reviewed by Weinberg has had a sociological or social psychological perspective, and has emphasized the impact of the BDSM culture in shaping the various rituals. However, we are left with fundamental but unanswered questions about why a minority of men and women develop sado-masochistic interests in the first place, leading them to identify with the BDSM culture. Although these questions include the importance of dominance and submission, and the impact of pain on sexual response, there is the further complication of the extent to which the sadistic and masochistic patterns of response can occur in the same individual. A closer examination of the sexual development of BDSM individuals is required.

Dominance and submission is a variant example of the 'interaction with partner' aspect of sexuality, and the infliction of pain, a variant of the 'direct sexual stimulation' aspect. Humiliation and embarrassment fit less easily into the 'four aspect' approach, and hypermasculinity among men is an interesting gender-related aspect.

'Multivariant sexuality'[1] and conclusions

This chapter has considered variations of three aspects of sexuality: the presence (or absence) of a 'sexual drive', the sexual signal, or type of person, that attracts you, how you interact with your sexual partner and what type of direct sexual stimulation is most effective.

Although the various kinds of sexual variations discussed in this chapter are scattered fairly widely through the population, with the exception of asexuality, they have a striking tendency to occur together. Even with 'asexuality', when defined as never having been attracted to either men or women, we cannot exclude the possibility that there is sexual drive which is directed at fetish objects rather than people. But fetishism and sado-masochism are commonly found in the same person, and may also be associated with one or more of the more obscure variations (Gosselin & Wilson 1980; Milne & Dopke 1997). Interest in bondage is not unusual amongst fetishistic transvestites (Buhrich & Beaumont 1981).

The frequency of these associations is of theoretical importance. It suggests that the conditions necessary for the development of one type of preference may facilitate the development of others. This potential may stem from some characteristic of the individual's nervous system that underlies sexual learning, e.g. the capacity for 'imprinting' sexual responses to a variety of stimuli, at least in the male. Alternatively, it may reflect difficulties in the interpersonal domain that make it difficult for the individual to incorporate his sexuality into a dyadic relationship. Lacking the framework for sexual expression that such a relationship normally provides, other varieties of sexual expression are given free rein. We remain uncertain about the relevance of either explanation, and careful study of such explanatory models is still needed. Freund & Blanchard (1993) suggested that with most variations there is a basic proneness to developmental error in locating erotic targets, but it is not clear that it is adding anything explanatory to what we already know.

We have the gender differences to take into account. As described in Chapter 5, there appears to be a critical period of male sexual development, around puberty, when sexual arousal to certain types of stimuli becomes an established pattern (see p. 189) and normally leads to the organization of sexual identity ('I am straight or gay'). There are substantial changes in brain structure and function around that stage, which may well account for this 'critical period'. This process is not apparent in females for whom sexual identity is more secondary to relational experiences, and less fixed as a consequence. Thus fetishism, a more or less exclusively male phenomenon, fits with this model. Sado-masochism on the other hand, is more about the nature of the relationship with a sexual partner (e.g. dominant or submissive, or humiliating) and here we see women showing sado-masochistic preferences, if somewhat later than men. The response to pain is in the category of 'specific types of sexual stimulation' and is probably equally relevant to males and females. The appeal of certain types of material, such as rubber, suggests a 'specific type of sexual stimulation'. Maybe this features in the sexual interests of some women (who enjoy wearing certain textures next to their skin) without it developing the characteristics of a fetish found in men.

But why only some men and women develop these specific variants remains obscure.

REFERENCES

Abbott E 1999 A History of Celibacy. DeCapo Press, Cambridge MA.

Bancroft J 1974 Deviant Sexual Behaviour: Modification and Assessment. Clarendon Press, Oxford.

Bancroft J 2005 A history of sexual medicine in the United Kingdom. Journal of Sexual Medicine 2: 569–574.

---

[1]In the last edition of this book I used the established phrase 'polymorphous perverse' at this point. I now prefer to avoid this term, and 'multivariant sexuality' is my attempt at a morally neutral alternative.

Bogaert A 2004 Asexuality: prevalence and associated factors in a national probability sample. Journal of Sex Research 41: 279–287.

Breslow N, Evans L, Langley J 1985 On the prevalence and roles of females in the sadomasochistic subculture: report of an empirical study. Archives of Sexual Behavior 14: 303–318.

Buhrich N, Beaumont T 1981 Comparison of transvestism in Australia and America. Archives of Sexual Behavior 10: 269–282.

Chalkley AJ, Powell GE 1983 The clinical description of 48 cases of sexual fetishism. British Journal of Psychiatry 142: 292–295.

Devor H 1996 Female gender dysphoria in context: social problem or personal problem. Annual Review of Sex Research 7: 44–89.

Ehrenberg M 2000 Review of female fetishism by L Gamman and M Makinen. Archives of Sexual Behavior 29: 193–194.

Falk G, Weinberg TS 1983 Sadomasochism and popular Western culture. In Weinberg T, Kamel GWL (eds) S and M: Studies in Sadomasochism. Prometheus Books, Buffalo, NY, pp. 137–144.

Fessler DMT, Nettle D, Afshar Y, de Andrade Pinheiro I, et al 2005 A cross-cultural investigation of the role of foot size in physical attractiveness. Archives of Sexual Behavior 34: 267–276.

Freud S 1949 Three Essays on the Theory of Sexuality. Translated by J Strachey. Imago, London.

Freund K, Blanchard R 1993 Erotic target location errors in male gender dysphorics, paedophiles and fetishists. British Journal of Psychiatry 162: 558–563.

Gagnon JH, Simon W 1967 Sexual Deviance. Harper & Row, New York.

Gamman L, Makinen M 1995 Female Fetishism. New York University Press, New York.

Gebhard P, Gagnon J, Pomeroy N, Christenson C 1965 Sex Offenders. Harper & Row, New York.

Gosselin C, Wilson G 1980 Sexual Variations: Fetishism, Transvestism and Sadomasochism. Faber & Faber, London.

Green R 2001 (Serious) sadomasochism: a protected right of privacy? Archives of Sexual Behavior 30: 543–550.

Henry GW 1948 Sex Variants: a Study of Homosexual Patterns. Hoeber, New York.

Hoon EF, Hoon PW, Wincze JP 1976 An inventory for the measurement of female sexual arousability: the SAI. Archives of Sexual Behavior 5: 291–300.

Hucker SJ 1997 Sexual sadism: psychopathology and theory. In Laws DR, O'Donohue W (eds) Sexual Deviance: Theory, Assessment and Treatment. Guilford, New York, pp. 194–209.

Janssen E, Vorst H, Finn P, Bancroft J 2002 The sexual inhibition (SIS) and sexual excitation (SES) scales: I. Measuring sexual inhibition and excitation proneness in men. Journal of Sex Research 39: 114–126.

Jay D 2003 Asexual visibility and education network. http://www.asexuality.org/home

Johnson AM, Wadsworth J, Wellings K, Field J 1994 Sexual Attitudes and Lifestyles. Blackwell, Oxford.

Junginger J 1997 Fetishism: assessment and treatment. In Laws DR, O'Donohue W (eds) Sexual Deviance: Theory, Assessment and Treatment. Guilford, New York, pp. 92–110.

Kinsey AC, Pomeroy WB, Martin CF 1948 Sexual Behavior in the Human Male. Saunders, Philadelphia.

Kinsey AC, Pomeroy WB, Martin CF, Gebhard PH 1953 Sexual Behavior in the Human Female. Saunders, Philadelphia.

Kraft-Ebbing R von 1965 Psychopathia Sexualis. Translation by Klaf FS. Stern & Day, New York.

La Torre R 1980 Devaluation of the human love object: heterosexual rejection as a possible antecedent of fetishism. Journal of Abnormal Psychology 89: 295–298.

Lawrence AA 2006 Clinical and theoretical parallels between desire for limb amputation and gender identity disorder. Archives of Sexual Behavior 35: 253–262.

Levitt EE, Moser C, Jamison KV 1994 The prevalence and some attributes of females in the sadomasochistic subculture: a second report. Archives of Sexual Behavior 23: 465–473.

Marks I, Gelder M, Bancroft J 1970 Sexual deviants 2 years after electric aversion. British Journal of Psychiatry 117: 173–186.

Mason FL 1997 Fetishism: psychopathology and theory. In Laws DR, O'Donohue W (eds) Sexual Deviance: Theory, Assessment and Treatment. Guilford, New York, pp. 75–91.

McConaghy N 1993 Sexual Behaviour: Problems and Management. Plenum, New York.

McGuire RJ, Carlisle JM, Young BG 1965 Sexual deviations and conditioned behaviour: a simple technique. Behaviour Research and Therapy 3: 185–190.

Milne JS, Dopke CA 1997 Paraphilia not otherwise specified. In Laws DR, O'Donohue W (eds) Sexual Deviance: Theory, Assessment and Treatment. Guilford, New York, pp. 394–423.

Mitchell W, Falconer M, Hill D 1954 Epilepsy with fetishism relieved by temporal lobectomy. Lancet ii: 626–630.

Money J 1977 Peking: the sexual revolution. In Money J, Musaph H (eds) Handbook of Sexology. Excerpta Medica, Amsterdam.

Moser C 1998 S/M (sadomasochistic) interactions in semi-public settings. Journal of Homosexuality 36: 19–29.

Moser C 2001 Paraphilia: a critique of a confused concept. In Kleinplatz PJ (ed) New Directions in Sex Therapy. Brunner-Routledge, Philadelphia, pp. 91–108.

Moser C, Kleinplatz PJ 2006 Introduction: state of our knowledge on SM. Journal of Homosexuality 50: 1–15.

O'Carroll T 1980 Paedophilia: the Radical Case. Peter Owen, London.

Plummer K 1979 Images of paedophilia. In Cook M, Wilson G (eds) Love and Attraction Pergamon Press, Oxford.

Prause N, Graham CA 2007 Asexuality: classification and characterization. Archives of Sexual Behavior 36: 341–356.

Rachman S, Hodgson R 1968 Experimentally induced 'sexual fetishism': replication and development. Psychological Record 18: 25–27.

Sandnabba NK, Santtila P, Nordling N 1999 Sexual behavior and social adaptation among sadomasochistically-oriented males. Journal of Sex Research 36: 273–282.

Smith AMA, Riseel CE, Richters J, Grulich AE, de Visser RO 2003 Sex in Australia: sexual identity, sexual attraction and sexual experience among a representative sample of adults. Australian & New Zealand Journal of Public Health 27: 138–145.

Spector L, Carey M, Steinberg L 1996 The Sexual Desire Inventory: development, factor structure and evidence of reliability. Journal of Sex & Marital Therapy 22: 175–190.

Stekel W 1924 Peculiarities of Behavior: Wandering Mania, Dipsomania, Cleptomania, Pyromania, and Allied Impulsive Acts (2 vols). English translation by J Van Teslar of Impulshandlungen (1922). Liveright, New York.

Stoller R 1982 Transvestism in women. Archives of Sexual Behavior 11: 99–116.

Weinberg TS 2006 Sadomasochism and the social sciences: a review of the sociological and social psychological literature. Journal of Homosexuality 50: 17–40.

Weinberg MS, Williams CJ, Calhan C 1995 If the shoe fits . . . : exploring male homosexual foot fetishism. Journal of Sex Research 32: 17–28.

Wilson GD 1978 The Secrets of Sexual Fantasy. Dent, London.

Transgender, gender non-conformity and transvestism

10

Introduction 289

Socio-cultural factors 289
Involvement of the medical profession 290

The incidence of transgender identity 291
The incidence of fetishistic transvestism 291

An interactive explanatory approach 292
Childhood gender identity discordance 293

Sexual identity 295
Biological factors 295
Sexual learning 296

The medical management of gender reassignment 296
Outcome of surgical gender reassignment 297
The assessment and selection process 297

Standards of care 300

Introduction

In this chapter we consider variations of gender identity and the complex and varied inter-relationships between gender identity and sexuality. Of primary importance is gender reassignment, when a person changes his or her gender identity and lives in the opposite gender role. Fetishistic patterns of sexuality can interact with gender identity in complex ways, the prime example being fetishistic transvestism. Sexual identity, whether one considers oneself heterosexual or homosexual, is a further important component of this interactive pattern.

The normal development of gender identity was considered in Chapter 3. A key distinction is between core gender identity, which is the sense 'I am a male' or 'I am a female', and gender role behaviour, patterns of behaviour or attitudes which are 'masculine' or 'feminine'. Core gender identity typically becomes established between the ages of 2 and 3, reflecting the appropriate stage of cognitive development, and basically does not vary thereafter. For the large majority of men and women, the fact that they are male or female is taken for granted throughout their lives. How masculine or feminine they feel or behave is another matter. While the young child has fairly simple gender constructs, less rigid gender stereotyping emerges as the child gets older, probably more so in females than males (see Chapter 3). In this respect the influence of socio-cultural factors is of paramount importance.

Socio-cultural factors

Variations in gender identity, with individuals not fitting clearly into socially prescribed male or female roles, are evident in most cultures, though with considerable differences across cultures in how such individuals are received. In some cultures a 'third gender' has been recognized and to a large extent accepted, e.g. the Hijras of India, a male sect who regarded themselves as a separate gender, neither male or female (Nanda 1993). In rural areas of the Balkans, since the early 1800s, some women have been living as a particular class of men (Gremaux 1993). Bullough (1991) provided a brief historical overview of how socio-cultural influences on gender role behaviour and its interaction with core gender identity have changed through history. The acceptance of the Hijras was, according to Bullough, a reflection of the androgyny of Hinduism. Christian societies, in contrast, have not only enforced a clear male–female dichotomy, but in the process have assumed a superiority of the male gender. It is of particular interest that at least until the 20th century, individuals who lived their lives as one gender and were discovered on their death to be of the other gender were nearly all women living as men. When their true gender was discovered this typically resulted in admiration rather than stigma. For a woman to have passed as a man was obviously regarded as an achievement. Bullough (1991) collected accounts of nearly 1000 such individuals. Within the Christian Church there were 30 women saints who were thought to be men when alive. Bullough was able to give only three historical examples of men living their lives as women.

This gender stereotyping and male 'superiority' in Christian societies became challenged during the 20th century. There was a new phase of scientific interest in the biology of sexual differentiation. In the 1910s, Steinach, in Austria, experimented with the use of hormones to change the sex of animals, and Hirschfeld's Institute for Sexual Science in Germany started to explore sex change surgery for patients they described as 'transvestites'. As a counter-challenge there were various institutions that strove to reinforce 'normal masculinity' and reduce the likelihood of 'effeminacy' in young males, e.g. the YMCA and the Scout Movement.

How many individuals in these earlier periods experienced gender dysphoria, i.e. discomfort with one's assigned gender and a wish to live one's life as the opposite gender, is not known. However, they clearly existed and for most of them there was little they could do about it, and the stigma associated with it, particularly in males, presumably resulted in most such individuals struggling but keeping it to themselves.

289

The interesting history of gender reassignment and transsexuality in the USA during the 20th century has been well documented by Meyerowitz (2002). A turning point was in 1952, when an American soldier, George Jorgensen, went to Denmark and received hormonal treatment followed by sex change surgery to become Christine Jorgensen. This was followed by massive media attention, and the seeking of gender change or reassignment surgery by numerous individuals in the USA and elsewhere. There is an interesting parallel here with the contrast between the media impact of Kinsey's publications around this time, and the relative lack of media and public attention to earlier sex surveys (see Chapter 6; p. 176). Much less attention had been paid to earlier attempts at sex change surgery. Presumably times had changed, both in terms of media technology and dissemination of information to the public, and in the public's response to such information. But post-Jorgensen the dream of changing gender became a real possibility for many gender dysphoric individuals. The organization of transsexuals into groups occurred, providing support and acknowledgement. An early example was the Beaumont Society in the UK, which has existed since the early 1960s (www.beaumontsociety.org.uk). This has provided opportunities for its members to cross-dress in company and from the start has welcomed not only those who have or who hope to undergo gender reassignment, but also those who simply cross-dress and do not seek other changes.

These subcultures also reflect a more general change in the second half of the 20th century, with gender stereotypes becoming less rigid, and the boundaries between male and female behaviour and manners of dress less enforced. The term 'transsexual' was first introduced in 1949 by Cauldwell, a psychiatrist, to describe people who wanted to change sex. However, in the subculture of sexual minorities that emerged in the latter part of the 20th century, transsexuals are seen as a subgroup of the 'transgendered', which includes lesbians with 'butch' or masculine gender identities and gay men with feminine gender identities, but also heterosexual transvestites. As the various sexual minorities have organized themselves into groups, the concept of gay lesbian bisexual transgender (GLBT) has emerged, covering the range. However, as Meyerowitz (2002) has documented, these groups have not sat comfortably together. In particular, feminists among them have rejected the concept of transgender mainly because it conflicts with their views about gender. Particularly in the 1970s there was a shift towards a more androgynous perspective, or as Bolin (1993) describes it, a shift from gender dichotomy to continuity. From a scientific feminist perspective, Fausto-Sterling (2000) has argued for continuity: 'complete maleness and complete femaleness represent the extreme ends of a spectrum of body types. That these extreme ends are the most frequent has lent credence to the idea that they are not only natural (that is produced by nature) but normal (that is they represent both a statistical and a social ideal).' She uses the varieties of intersex conditions (see Chapter 3) to support

her case (see Bancroft 2003 for a critique of this), but interestingly does not use the term 'transgender'. Given this shift towards a more androgynous or 'continuous' concept of gender within the sexual minority world, many transgendered individuals are not seeking surgical change, but some do, posing a challenge to the medical profession and resulting in allegations of 'medicalization' (Bolin 1993).

Involvement of the medical profession

The increase in requests for medical help with gender reassignment has resulted in a struggle within the profession. The use of such medical interventions, both hormonal and surgical, has been strongly opposed by some, as exemplified by the gradual closure of all gender identity clinics affiliated with university medical schools in the USA (Bolin 1993), resulting in a 'privatization' of this speciality. The persuasive evidence that gender reassignment has a positive outcome in the large majority of cases has, to some extent, countered this opposition. The current medical approach to gender reassignment will be considered later in this chapter. There has also been a struggle to explain these variations in gender identity in medically relevant terms. As is so often the case, the literature has been preoccupied with issues of diagnostic categorization, rather than understanding the determinants involved.

The DSM IV has a category of 'gender identity disorder' (GID), and this has two diagnostic criteria: the first, a strong and persistent cross-gender identification, i.e. the desire to be or the insistence that one is, of the other sex; the second, persistent discomfort or a sense of inappropriateness about one's assigned sex. GID may be associated with sexual attraction to males, to females, to both or to neither. Males are found in all four subgroups. Females with GID are almost all sexually attracted to females. It is noteworthy that beyond these specifiers of sexual attraction, 'sexual orientation' is not specified, and we will return to this issue. 'Transvestic fetishism' is included as a paraphilia; when a heterosexual male has recurrent, intense sexually arousing fantasies, sexual urges or behaviours involving crossdressing, which cause significant distress or impaired social functioning. This paraphilia may be associated with gender dysphoria.

One recurring theme in the clinical literature is that there are basically two male types, homosexual transsexualism and heterosexual fetishistic transvestism. The latter type has been described as 'autogynephilia' by Blanchard (1989), defined as a male's propensity to be erotically aroused by the thought or image of himself as a woman. This concept shifts the emphasis from a fetishistic reaction to women's clothes and the wearing of them, to a sexual responsiveness to the man's own body seen, in one way or another, as a woman's body. This is not fundamentally different from the concept of a fetish as described in Chapter 9, but is in some respects closer to a 'normal' pattern of sexual attraction, though dependent on various devices to create the illusion of a woman's body. In some cases this leads to a wish for gender reassignment — the 'autogynephilic transsexual'.

Controversy over this division into two types peaked with Bailey's publication of his book *The Man who would be Queen: the Science of Gender Bending and Transsexualism* (2003), which caused anger and outrage in the transgender community and disapproval among some clinicians working in this field. Apart from the simple binary distinction, Bailey presented each type as being basically driven by sexual needs. Hence the homosexual transsexual seeks gender reassignment so that he can attract men sexually, and preferably heterosexual men. The autogynephilic transsexual seeks gender reassignment because he desires the body of the woman that would result. In slightly less stark terms, Bailey (2003) explains 'those who love men become women to attract them. Those who love women become the women they love.' And for those who cross the gender boundary, 'one primary motive is lust' (p. xi–xii). No acknowledgement is given in this book to the fundamental role of gender identity in the lives of these individuals. Reducing their usually prolonged and disturbed journey through gender uncertainty to a matter of lust seriously demeans the new-found identities of these people, many of whom have finally found well-being and a comfortable sense of identity following gender reassignment.

Following the Bailey controversy, Blanchard (2005) revisited his concept of autogynephilia. Drawing the distinction between the term as descriptive of a particular pattern of behaviour and one which has explanatory value, he acknowledged that at one time or another he had advanced several explanations of autogynephilia, 'all or none (of which) may be true, false or something in between. Their accuracy is an empirical question that can be resolved only by further research' (p. 445). This is a welcome contrast to Bailey's unscientific 'certainty'.

For the remainder of this chapter I will use GID as an abbreviation of gender identity *discordance* rather than disorder, as it is less pathologizing. And, except when reporting the results of other researchers who used the term 'transsexual', I will use 'transgender' in place of 'transsexual', as I believe that the primary issue is more to do with gender than sexuality.

The incidence of transgender identity

In the last edition of this book I wrote the following: 'Much of the conceptual confusion in this field stems from the fact that surgical sex reassignment has become in some sense a reality. Prior to this being so, the person with gender identity confusion would have been less likely to see change of sex as a real alternative . . . . it is understandable that such a tangible and dramatic process as sex reassignment surgery should be seen as an escape route from a chronically disturbed or unrewarding existence. As a result, people who seek sex reassignment are a very heterogeneous group. A tendency to call them transsexuals because of their wish for surgery

TABLE 10.1	Estimated prevalence of transgender identity from various sources	
	Male	**Female**
1974 USA (Pauly 1974)	1/100 000	1/400 000
1981 Australia	1/24 000	1/150 000
1981 Sweden (Ross et al 1981)	1/37 000	1/103 000
1993 Netherlands (Bakker et al 1993)	1/11 000	1/30 000
1999 Scotland (Wilson et al 1999)	1/7 500	1/31 000

has created a spurious homogeneity. Sex reassignment with or without surgery is an end-point or at least a choice for people with very different developmental histories. They simply have in common the belief that escaping from one sex into the other will improve their lot.' (p. 356)

There have been no further developments that would lead me to revise that earlier statement. Estimates of incidence are based on those who seek help for gender reassignment or gender dysphoria. A number of attempts to estimate such incidence have appeared over the years, and are listed in Table 10.1. What is striking is a substantial increase, around 13-fold for both males and females, between 1974 and 1999. This is more likely to reflect an increased awareness and availability of gender reassignment surgery than an increase in transgender identity. The sex ratio was around 4:1 male to female in both 1974 and 1999, with some variation in between.

As shown in Table 10.1, Ross et al (1981) found higher prevalence of male to female transgender in Australia than Sweden, with the reverse for female-to-male. They suggested that cultural differences between the two countries lead to greater numbers of transsexuals seeking help in Australia than Sweden. Ross (1983) also reported that gay men in Australia identified themselves more strongly as feminine than their counterparts in Sweden. Australian culture probably reinforces clearly distinct gender stereotypes more so than Swedish culture. More rigid expectations about being male or female may generate greater anxiety and insecurity about gender identity in those who do not conform, for which gender reassignment offers one method of coping.

The incidence of fetishistic transvestism

The best estimate of the incidence of fetishistic cross-dressing comes from Langstrom & Zucker (2005). A representative sample of 2450 Swedish men and women, as part of a broader study of sexual attitudes and lifestyles, were asked 'Have you ever dressed in clothes pertaining to the opposite sex and become sexually aroused by this?' Positive answers were given by 2.8% of men and 0.4% of women. However, we do not know how many of these individuals repeated this behaviour and, if so, over what period of time.

An interactive explanatory approach

Let us return to the drawing board and consider how various factors might interact to lead along different routes to this end point of wishing to escape from one sex into the other.

What is clear is that both gender identity and sexuality are involved, with the latter needing to be considered at two levels: sexual identity (see Chapter 5) and patterns of sexual arousability (e.g. fetishistic), but how they interact is complex and varied. Some time ago I attempted to conceptualize this interactive process, based mainly on the principles of cognitive consistency that were in fashion at that time (Bancroft 1972). The idea proposed was a basic tendency to strive for consistency between our gender identity, our sexual identity and our pattern of sexual responsiveness. In Chapter 5 the three-strand model was proposed to help us conceptualize normal sexual development. In this, the strand of gender identity, which is in most respects the first to become established in the developmental process, and the strand of 'sexual responsiveness', together with the strand of 'capacity for dyadic relationship' are viewed as relatively independent during childhood until puberty approaches, when they start to integrate. Normally this integration results in patterns of sexual response consistent with the gender identity and subsequently sexual identity, e.g. 'I am a male, I am sexually attracted to females and I am heterosexual'. How this integration leads to a homosexual identity is less obvious. However, there is consistent evidence that boys who show gender non-conformity during childhood have an increased likelihood of ending up with a homosexual identity (see below). The principal uncertainty is the extent and the manner to which these two components are causally related. Are childhood gender identity and the direction of sexual attraction (i.e. to males or females) the result of some common early biological factor, or are they in fact independent of each other? Does the male develop sexual attraction to males to achieve consistency with a female gender identity? Or does the gender identity change to be consistent with the direction of sexual attraction and assumed sexual orientation? Either way, the importance of culturally available sexual identities is clear; in a culture or a period of history where 'homosexual identity' is less clearly established and available to the emerging adolescent, this integrative process may be more difficult to resolve, leaving the individual with uncertainties, confusion and associated dysthymia. In today's world, an individual with discrepant gender identity (the boy with gender non-conformity) may experience the emergence of same-sex sexual attraction, and the resolution of inconsistency by the recognition that 'I am a homosexual', which carries different gender identity implications ('a homosexual male doesn't have to be masculine'). Another developmental sequence is that a heterosexual identity emerges, made possible by a clear change in gender identity. 'I am sexually attracted to males, I am a woman (trapped in a man's body), hence I am a heterosexual woman.' All possible combinations of gender identity and sexuality can occur in male-to-female transsexuals. A genetic male may change into a female and be attracted to males (i.e. heterosexual post-reassignment). Another may change into a woman and be attracted to another woman (i.e. lesbian post-reassignment). Two of my male-to-female patients, having both gone through reassignment within a year of each other, started a relationship and have been living happily as a lesbian couple for the past 20 years. In some, sexuality is unimportant post reassignment, and if sexual interactions with a man occur they are more to reinforce the female gender identity than to provide sexual pleasure. Sexual interest post reassignment can be further lowered by the effects of hormones used in the male-to-female reassignment process (i.e. oestrogens and sometimes progestagens, or antiandrogens). In female-to-male transsexuals, a heterosexual relationship with a woman is usually pursued, seldom if ever a homosexual relationship with a man. Not infrequently, the heterosexual relationship with a woman emerges from a lesbian relationship with the same women prior to reassignment. In such cases the attitudes and needs of the partner can be important (e.g. a preference for a man without a penis rather than another woman). The impact of hormonal reassignment in the female-to-male (i.e. the administration of testosterone) is more likely to have a sexually enhancing than inhibiting effect.

The distinction between these alternative developmental trajectories raises the question of the relative importance of sexual orientation and gender identity. Is there a greater need in some individuals for a heterosexual identity that would be sufficient to promote gender identity change to achieve consistency? Alternatively, is the need for a particular gender identity sufficient to determine the sexual identity, which then reinforces the gender identity? And in what way do these two types of individuals differ? These are questions we cannot as yet answer.

A further source of variability in the developmental sequence is the establishment of sexual arousability. In most individuals, the emerging pattern of sexual responsiveness becomes focused on sexually attractive others, is consistent with gender identity and leads to a sexual identity, whether heterosexual or homosexual. But alternative patterns of sexual responsiveness can arise, and the concept of fetishism, more or less an exclusively male phenomenon, was considered in the previous chapter. Being sexually aroused by a 'thing' rather than a person may make the establishment of consistency more difficult in the developmental process. However, most fetishists end up with a clear heterosexual or homosexual identity. Fetishistic transvestism, however, has the potential for disrupting the developmental process. A fetish for particular articles of women's clothing may be relatively uncomplicated in this respect. However, transvestism involves the wearing of women's clothing and the associated perception of the cross-dressed self as, in some sense, a woman. Here there is a curious and unexplained variation from the more normal appeal of a woman's body. Most heterosexual males fantasize, use images of or respond to the body of an attractive woman, dressed to a variable extent. The fetishistic transvestite generates the 'attractive woman' by translating his own body. It is not clear what related mechanism(s) distinguish such an individual from a 'normal' heterosexual male, or from other fetishists. It may not be unusual or in any sense abnormal for a man to imagine part of his body as belonging to a woman and to enjoy caressing it. This could be seen as an ingenious process of 'adaptive perception'. But when this process becomes established as a fetishistic pattern, then the potential consequences are very different.

It is well established in the literature that many fetishistic transvestites not only continue their fetishistic practices over long periods of time, but may also establish otherwise normal heterosexual relationships and marriage. In my clinical experience, it is not unusual for the fetishistic transvestism to recede in importance once a rewarding sexual relationship becomes established, only to re-emerge when the sexual relationship runs into difficulties. How many men have an early fetishistic pattern that disappears in this way not to return, we do not know. In some instances the partner is agreeable to incorporating the fetish (cross-dressing) component into the couple's sexual interactions. It is also established that in a proportion of cases the fetishistic pattern changes. In particular, the sexually arousing aspect of wearing women's clothes becomes accompanied, and eventually replaced, by a non-sexually arousing experience of being dressed as a woman. There are two outcomes of this process. The man may establish what can be called a 'dual-role' pattern of transvestism, in which he spends most of his time in his usual male role, but also some of his time in the female role. A married individual in this category typically enacts his female role outside his marriage, family and work setting. Although we are restricted to clinical impressions because of the lack of good longitudinal data of such life histories, my impression has been that such individuals may maintain this dual role for many years. The other outcome, however, involves an increasing wish to change into a woman permanently, with associated bodily change. This usually has major adverse effects on any current relationship. Occasionally a female partner or wife of such a man may be willing to adapt to having a 'female' sexual partner. But this is the exception. Such an individual is likely, sooner or later, to present at a gender problem clinic seeking medical help with gender reassignment. We do not know what determines which of these outcomes prevails. Reliance on retrospectively recalled information about earlier stages of development is potentially confounded by an understandable tendency for the gender-change cross-dresser to recall his earlier experiences in ways which are consistent with his current gender identity preference, strengthening his claim for gender reassignment in the process. But it is clear that many of the fetishistic transvestites who change in this way do so after many years. The oldest person I have seen in this category was 70 when he asked me for help with gender reassignment. He had spent most of his life as a double-role transvestite, and was now hoping that

he could achieve some consistency of gender identity before it was too late.

Having considered the variety of developmental trajectories towards the wish for gender reassignment, let us now look at some of the various contributory factors more closely.

Childhood gender identity discordance

To what extent can GID in adolescents and adults be linked to GID in childhood? Goldman & Goldman (1982), in their cross-cultural study of the sexual thoughts of children, asked 'If you could have chosen, would you have chosen to be a boy or a girl?' Among 7-year-olds, 10% of Australian and 13% of North American boys would have chosen to be a girl. For 13-year-old boys, it was 20% for Australian and 7% for North American. Among 9-year-old girls, 10% of Australian and 27% of North American would have chosen to be a boy. Among 15-year-old girls it was 10% and 20% respectively. It is difficult to know how to interpret children's answers to this question, and they did vary substantially across age and country. The reports of mothers, presumably based on more manifest tendencies, are probably more valid for our purpose. Using the Child Behaviour Checklist in a normal control group of children, 1–2% of mothers of boys and 3–4% of mothers of girls reported their child's 'wish to be of the opposite sex' (Zucker & Bradley 1995). It therefore seems likely that GID is more common in children and that most children grow out of it. The possibility therefore remains that there is a link to later GID in those who, for one reason or another, do not grow out of it. At all ages, but particularly in adolescence and more so in males than females, GID is associated with other behavioural problems (Zucker & Bradley 1995). Let us consider GID in children more closely.

Boys

Green (1976) pioneered the study of boys with GID, comparing them to normal children. Typically they showed a marked interest in cross-dressing (three-quarters of them starting before their fourth birthday, all by their sixth), chose female roles in make-believe games, preferred playing with girls' toys, especially dolls, avoided rough and tumble sports and tended to be loners, relating better to girls than to other boys. They were often particularly adept at play-acting. Green described a number of factors that were sometimes found in the upbringing of these boys and which may have had aetiological significance, although it is not possible to say whether any of them were necessary or sufficient or even causative and they occurred with considerable variability. These factors included the following:

1. Parental indifference to feminine behaviour in a boy during his first year. In about 50% of Green's cases, help was sought by parents because of pressure from outside the family (e.g. school). Paradoxically when parents are concerned about the behaviour, it is more likely to be the mother than the father.

2. Parental encouragement of feminine behaviour during the first years. In about 10% of cases, the mother wanted a daughter so badly she tended to see her baby son as a girl.
3. Repeated cross-dressing of a young boy by a female. About 15% of these mothers cross-dressed their sons; less frequently sisters or grandmothers were responsible.
4. Maternal over-protection of a son and inhibition of boyish or rough and tumble play. Presumably this parental attitude is likely to operate by undermining masculine identity.
5. Excessive maternal attention and physical contact, resulting in lack of separation and 'individuation' of a boy from his mother. This was regarded by Stoller (1979) as of fundamental importance in childhood GID, though Green only found evidence of it in about 20% of cases.
6. Absence of or rejection by father. A third of the feminine boys were separated from their father before the age of 4. In general, when fathers were present, the boys were more likely to be closer to their mothers than were the control boys.
7. Physical beauty of a boy, influencing adults to treat him in a feminine manner. About a third of the feminine boys were pretty children.
8. Lack of male playmates during early years of socialization. About one-third of boys were deprived of the opportunity for contact with male peers. In other cases, avoidance of male peers reflected existing gender identity problems.

Green failed to find any difference in the pattern of parental role division (e.g. who was dominant, and in which sphere) between the families of his feminine and his normal boys. This is not surprising as in many cases the feminine boys have normally masculine brothers. The one factor which Green (1976) regarded as close to a necessary variable was the lack of discouragement of the feminine behaviour for an appreciable period of time and presumably during critical periods of gender identity development. This was true in nearly every family he studied.

Girls

Young girls with typically boyish interests are considerably more common than their male counterparts. Such behaviour is also regarded as more acceptable and hence parents seldom seek help for this as a problem. Paradoxically we therefore have less systematic information about 'tomboy' girls than we have about the much less common 'sissy' boy. Green et al (1982) compared tomboys and non-tomboys aged 4–12 years. These two groups of girls differed considerably in various aspects of behaviour, such as sex-typed preferred toys, gender of peer group, participation in sports, roles taken in playing house and the stated wish to be a boy. However, there were few discernible differences in their families. As yet we lack follow-up studies of tomboy girls into adulthood. But, in contrast to the effeminate boy who usually carries into adulthood considerable problems relating to his gender identity, the tomboy girl seldom

has any difficulty in adapting to an adult female role (Devor 1996). This also usually applies to those girls who are masculinized due to endocrine abnormalities (see Chapter 3) even though they may continue to show some typically male characteristics, e.g., putting careers before marriage or preferring male-type clothes.

Asking adult transgender individuals about their childhood and family is another source of information, though subject to recall bias of various kinds. Early studies of adult female-to-male transsexuals found a marked degree of tomboyism reported during childhood (Green 1974; Pauly 1974). A disturbed parental relationship was also commonly reported, the majority with a weak or depressive mother or an aggressive, excessively masculine and often alcoholic father. Encouragement by both parents of masculinity in the daughter appeared to be common (Pauly 1974). However, in contrast, Benjamin (1966) stated that in 56% of his 122 cases of adult male to female transsexualism, there was no evidence of parental encouragement of feminine behaviour during childhood. Nearly half of Green's (1974) group of 30 adult male-to-female transsexuals reported a normal male self-concept during childhood. This difference between female and male transgendered is consistent with feminine behaviour in boys being more stigmatized than masculine behaviour in girls.

In a more recent review, Cohen-Kettenis & Gooren (1999) found evidence of differences in recalled child-rearing patterns between transsexuals and controls. Male-to-female transsexuals characterized their fathers as less warm, more rejecting, and more controlling. Female-to-male transsexuals, in comparison to controls, rated both parents as more rejecting and less warm, but only their mothers as more overprotective. It may be that the family constellations typically found in these cases serve to reinforce masculine traits, which are in any case common amongst girls, but in these particular cases this may lead to more marked gender identity discordance. Such family influences are not always found however and should not be considered necessary for transsexual development. It is also difficult, with retrospective evidence of this kind, to distinguish between family patterns which might increase the likelihood of, and those which are a reaction to, gender non-conformity in the child.

While childhood GID may therefore be relevant to transgender identity in adulthood, the commonest outcome is homosexual orientation. Green (1985) found that 30 of 44 GID boys became homosexual or bisexual in orientation. Bailey & Zucker (1995) reviewed the relevant literature for males and found this outcome consistent across prospective studies. They estimated that around 51% of boys but only 6% of girls with the requisite degree of cross-gender behaviour will become homosexual. Furthermore, men with homosexual identity were much more likely to recall cross-gender behaviour during childhood than heterosexual men. Adult transgender identity has occurred infrequently in the prospective studies of GID boys; there was only one case in Green's series. Possibly more would have come into this category later in adulthood; transgender identity tends to become evident at a much later age than homosexual identity.

But this also reflects the relative rarity of adult transgender compared with homosexual orientation. Bailey & Zucker (1995) did not comment on transgender outcomes. There is a lack of comparable studies in women.

Childhood GID may therefore contribute to transgender identity in adults, but given the relative frequency of GID in children, that outcome is rare.

Sexual identity

What impact does sexual identity have on the emergence of transgender identity? Based on over 500 new transsexual patients a year seen at the Charing Cross Gender Identity Clinic, Green (2002) reported that, whereas in the past the large majority of male-to-female transsexuals indicated an exclusive sexual interest in men, with gender reassignment resulting in their achieving heterosexual status, more recently, approximately one-third are sexually attracted to females only and aspire to be lesbians after gender reassignment. In an earlier study, Bentler (1976) reported on 42 male-to-female transsexuals following sex reassignment surgery. Before surgery, approximately a third considered themselves homosexual, a third heterosexual and a third were categorized as asexual (they had not experienced enjoyable sex with a woman but were not homosexual, although half of them regarded themselves as heterosexual in spite of lack of experience). Almost all of these individuals considered themselves heterosexual following sex reassignment. More recently, Lawrence (2005) reported on 232 male-to-female patients of one surgeon. Before surgery, 54% had been predominantly attracted to women and 9% to men. After surgery, the figures were 25% and 34% respectively. In various respects, the sexual activity of these male to female transgendered was substantially less post surgery. This was particularly striking in those who had reported fetishistic transvestism or autogynophilia prior to surgery, underlining the primarily gender rather than sexual objectives of the reassignment.

A number of writers have suggested that avoidance of homosexuality is an important determinant of transsexualism. This is probably most often observed in the female transsexual who typically is aware of a normal or strong sexual attraction to females from late childhood or early adolescence (Pauly 1974). Commonly there is a rejection of these homosexual feelings and a flight into heterosexuality. Sexual relationships with boys are tried out but invariably found unsatisfactory. The resistance to accepting a homosexual identity continues, however, and they are likely to choose as sexual partners girls who have had no previous homosexual experience. By regarding themselves as boys they can then maintain a heterosexual identity, the previous existence of masculine interest and mannerisms making this a more feasible solution. The transsexual role is thus serving the primary purpose of permitting the desired sexual relationship. During love-making, direct stimulation of the transsexual's breasts or genitalia by the partner is usually avoided, to minimize this tangible evidence of anatomic femaleness (Pauly 1974).

A large majority of fetishistic transvestites regard themselves as heterosexual; they may enjoy fantasies in which they relate sexually to men, but only if they are seeing themselves as women at the time. Usually they are sexually attracted to women and, as already indicated, many of them have enjoyed heterosexual relationships.

Biological factors

Genetic factors

Evidence from twin studies of the heritability of gender atypical behaviour in 3- to 4-year-olds and in 7- and 10-year-olds, was considered in Chapter 3 (see p. 31). However, four monozygotic pairs of female twins *discordant* (Segal 2006) and two monozygotic pairs *concordant* (Knoblauch et al 2007) for female-to-male transsexualism have been reported. Green (2000) has reported gender dysphoria in 10 sibling or parent–child pairs, suggesting a familial pattern. As yet, therefore, we have no understanding of whether or how genetic factors influence gender identity development.

Brain function

There is limited evidence of differences in brain structure in the transgendered. This was considered in Chapter 4 (see p. 60). The central region of the bed nucleus of the solitary tract (BNST) has been shown to be smaller in six male-to-female transsexuals than in heterosexual or homosexual men, and more similar to the size in women, raising the possibility that it is related in some way to core gender identity (Zhou et al 1995). Further research showed that the difference in size was related to the number of neurons (Kruijver et al 2000). The gender difference in the size of the BNST may not become established until adolescence (Chung et al 2002), raising the question, as with other gender and sexual identity-related differences in brain structure, of how much is cause and how much is effect, i.e. to what extent does this structural difference in the brain of adolescence result from behavioural differences during childhood?

Several early studies reported a high incidence of epilepsy or abnormal electroencephalograms in transsexuals, interestingly more so in female-to-male transsexuals (Hoenig & Kenna 1979).

Hormones

Abnormalities resulting from exposure to hormones prenatally were considered in Chapter 5. Whereas masculinization of behaviour and occasionally homosexual orientation occurs in women with congenital adrenal hyperplasia, no case of transgender in such individuals has been reported. Dessens et al (1999), however, found three transgender individuals (one male to female, two female to male) in a follow-up study of 243 individuals who had been exposed to anticonvulsants (mainly barbiturates) in utero. Such drugs have been shown in animal studies to interfere with sexually dimorphic, non-mating linked behaviour as well as having other adverse behavioural effects (Reinisch & Sanders 1982). This could result either from direct effects on the brain or indirectly by altering hepatic metabolism of steroids.

So far, in male-to-female transsexuals, no relevant differences in their adult reproductive hormone levels or responsiveness of the brain to positive or negative feedback mechanisms have been clearly identified (Gooren 1986; Cohen-Kettenis & Gooren 1999). However, Henningson et al (2005) examined polymorphisms in the genes for the androgen receptor, aromatase and the oestrogen β receptor in 29 male-to-female transsexuals and 229 male controls, and found some association between all three polymorphisms and transsexuality. This opens up some important possibilities that warrant further research.

With female transsexuals, the story is somewhat different. Although the majority show no evidence of physical or endocrine abnormalities, a number of studies have reported raised testosterone levels (Sipova & Starka 1977), menstrual irregularities or evidence of polycystic ovarian disease (Futterweit et al 1986). Seyler et al (1978) reported some evidence of impaired positive feedback in female-to-male transsexuals, but this was not found by Gooren (1986). Clearly such abnormalities are not *necessary* for female-to-male transsexual development. A particular caution is required in investigating such cases to ensure that any endocrine abnormalities are not due to the surreptitious use of exogenous hormones.

Sexual learning

The role of learning and conditioning in the development of fetishes was discussed in the previous chapter. The fetish component of male cross-dressing is common, particularly during adolescence when the pattern of erotic responsiveness is being established. Typically the pubertal boy discovers that women's clothes have an erotic effect. They are an obvious extension of a woman's body and in the case of underclothes have been in contact with her genitalia. Frequently the clothes used belong to the boy's mother or sister and may reflect guilt-ridden, incestuous feelings. The fetish effect of the clothing may be enhanced by the texture of the material, particularly when worn next to the boy's own body. Starting off as an erotic aid to masturbation, the simple fetish object, by being worn, initiates the process of female role identification. Though this is difficult to understand, it may be that given certain types of imagination, one's own body can be used to create 'another person' with more effect than by using fantasy alone. Certainly the descriptions of fetishistic cross-dressers suggest the 'creation of a woman' and it is unusual for them to imagine involvement of that woman with another man. This emphasizes the heterosexual orientation of the majority of fetishistic cross-dressers, but also increases the likelihood that the sexually arousing effect is dependent on producing this doppelganger sexual partner (Bancroft 1972).

It may also be that such a boy is already sensitized to female identification. The fetish object is chosen not only because of its sexual significance but also because it appeals to an already established cross-gender tendency.

Thus, Buhrich & Beaumont (1981) and Buhrich & McConaghy (1985) found that 50% of fetishistic transvestites had been cross-dressing before the behaviour had obvious sexual connotations. They divided their fetishistic transvestites into two groups according to whether they reported early transsexual ideas. Interestingly, these two groups did not differ in the frequency of early prefetishistic cross-dressing.

Whatever the factors that initiate this behaviour, the sexually arousing effect of cross-dressing serves to perpetuate the pattern. Typically it leads to masturbation and orgasm, following which the spell is broken and the clothes removed immediately, often with a degree of disgust or other negative feelings.

The male fetishistic cross-dresser may continue to show a very simple fetish pattern just using or wearing one article of female clothing (usually underwear) or he may use more and more as time goes on until he becomes intent on creating as convincing an illusion of a woman as possible. As described earlier, he may eventually move out of the fetish pattern and become primarily concerned with cross-gender identification.

It is striking that fetishistic transvestism is generally regarded as a heterosexual phenomenon. Fetishism may, however, play a role in homosexual development, though this has received much less attention. Probably the best known 'fetish' in the gay world is leather (Jay & Young 1979). To what extent this is worn because it reinforces both a homosexual and masculine identity is not clear. But it is conceivable that in a proportion of gay men wearing leather has a fetish quality, and may even make their own bodies sexually arousing to them. This possibility warrants research.

At the present time, biological mechanisms sufficient to account for either transgender or fetishistic transvestism are yet to be found, though a range of biological factors may be influencing the picture in ways not yet understood. The more or less universal occurrence of cross-gender behaviour across a wide variety of cultures points to some early or even biological determination. However, cultural factors may have considerable impact on how such propensities are expressed.

The medical management of gender reassignment

In this book, most forms of clinical help relating to sexuality are described in Chapter 11. With transgender the situation is sufficiently different to justify including medical management in this chapter. This is because for many transgendered individuals the medical component is a fundamental part of their gender transition. The clinician is faced with a request for help with this transition, and the challenge for the clinician is to assess whether such help is appropriate. Before considering the clinician's approach more closely, let us first put this in context by reviewing the evidence of the outcome of gender reassignment.

Outcome of surgical gender reassignment

There have now been several reviews of the outcome of gender reassignment surgery (Abramowitz 1986; Green & Fleming 1990; Pfafflin & Junge 1998; Carroll 1999) and their conclusions were summarized by Carroll (2007). Lawrence (2003) reported on 232 male-to-female surgical reassignments all carried out by one surgeon between 1994 and 2000. Using a 0–10 scale to rate happiness with result, 86% scored 8 or higher. None reported consistent regret about having the surgery, and any regret that was reported was about disappointment with the functional outcome of the genital reconstruction, rather than with the gender reassignment per se.

In spite of methodological limitations, there is overall consistency in the findings of improvement or a satisfactory outcome in 66% to 90% of cases, for both male-to-female and female-to-male reassignments. The greatest improvements were in self-satisfaction, interpersonal interaction and psychological well-being. The cosmetic results of the surgery were more variable, reflecting variability of skill among surgeons as well as improvements in relevant surgical techniques over the years. Sexual functioning is often impaired. Given the extent of overall satisfaction, this underlines the primary importance of gender ·identity over sexuality. Abramowitz (1986) found a poor outcome in around 8% of cases. Pfafflin & Junge (1998) reported that less than 2% regretted the surgery. In spite of the fact that the surgical possibilities for converting female genitalia to male are less than in the reverse direction, female to males showed a more positive psychosocial outcome than male to females (Pfafflin & Junge 1998). Apart from it being generally easier for female-to-males to pass effectively in their chosen gender, they also tended to have less mental health problems pre-surgery.

Those whose transgender emerged from a previous phase of fetishistic transvestism or autogynephilia were more likely to regret reassignment or have more negative outcomes than those whose gender identity discordance was primary. The reasons for this are not established. Predictors of a poor outcome are personality problems of various kinds and a history of depression.

In general, these more recent reviews convey a more positive picture than those cited in the previous edition of this book, which was based on much more limited evidence. This may reflect more effective selection of suitable cases by referring clinicians as well as improvements in surgical techniques.

Overall, there is strong support for gender reassignment improving the mental health and quality of life for both male-to-female and female-to-male transgendered individuals. However, surgical reassignment is only part of the reassignment process, and careful selection of those who are recommended for surgical reassignment is important and will be considered more closely in the following section.

The assessment and selection process

The majority of individuals referred to a gender identity clinic or a sexual health clinic with issues relating to transgender will be seeking clinical help in order to obtain surgical gender reassignment. A small proportion may be unsure about their gender identity and seek guidance and advice. The clinician should keep in mind the point made earlier, that seeking gender reassignment is an endpoint of a variety of developmental sequences, and there is consequently no simple diagnostic procedure for selecting those suitable for surgery.

The issue of surgery is indeed central to the whole topic. As discussed earlier, the existence of sex reassignment surgery, in spite of its considerable limitations, has provided a goal or a would-be solution for a wide variety of gender identity problems, sometimes referred to collectively as gender dysphoria. However, the well-being of the transgendered after sex reassignment depends only partly on the surgery. Yet this aspect looms large; many transgendered patients want nothing else and will go to great lengths to obtain surgery. This determination, often combined with more than adequate intelligence, and a wealth of information of mixed quality on the Internet and obtained through transgender support groups, means that they probably know the literature on transgender and surgical reassignment as well as most clinicians and better than many. This may lead to them presenting their histories in ways that are most likely to convince the clinician. This sets apart transgender issues from most other issues that confront clinicians. Rather than seeking medical help for a health problem, this is a matter of recruiting the clinician's help in achieving a particular goal defined by the patient.

The consequent difficulty in placing any reliance on past history has been one important reason why responsible clinicians have relied on the real-life test — the ability of the transgendered individual to live fully in the chosen gender role for a reasonable period of time before anything irreversible like surgery is undertaken. It is of particular importance to confront the patient with the fact that most of the problems of sex reassignment, being accepted as a member of that sex, working in that role, living from day to day as a woman rather than a man or vice versa, will not be solved by surgery, particularly genital surgery. Self-confidence may be increased, which undoubtedly helps. Intimate relationships may become possible and provide one of the most important consequences of the change. But the many day-to-day problems that must be overcome first require patience and relearning, not surgery. Thus it is important to demonstrate that these primary adjustments can be made before embarking on major irreversible steps. The transgendered person who sees the surgery as a solution for most of his or her problems has an increased likelihood of regret post surgery. Such a person, faced with disillusionment after surgery, may seek more and more surgical change in search of well-being.

The main assessment of the transsexual patient is therefore a continuous one, in which the clinician gets to know the patient over a period of months, developing a sense of mutual trust. This does not have to be viewed as 'therapy' but as counselling in the process of the real-life test, and 'reality-confrontation' — making sure that the individual interprets his or her experiences during the test realistically. During that time the patient is trying out new behaviours, gradually working through a programme that will make it clearer to both the patient and the clinician whether a more permanent sex change is likely to be beneficial. My policy has been to make it clear from the outset that I am prepared to help with the non-surgical aspects of reassignment but that this takes time. Decisions about surgical help come much later and involve other people. This makes it easier for patients to express ambivalence, which would be less likely if they felt they had to present a consistent story before anyone was prepared to take them seriously. Having known some patients over many years, it became clear to me that the transsexual urge varies in intensity and may depend on situational factors, such as the views of the current sexual partner. This variable natural history warns us on the one hand to avoid rapid irreversible decisions and on the other to be cautious in interpreting reports of treatment claiming to remove transsexual feelings. But given a cautious and conservative approach I believe there are individuals who will benefit from permanent sex reassignment, including surgery. In the UK at the present time it is possible to obtain surgical reassignment within the National Health Service (NHS) in a few specialized centres.

The guidelines of the Harry Benjamin International Gender Dysphoria Association are given at the end of this chapter (HBIGDA 2001). What follows now is based on my clinical approach.

The initial contract

The extent to which the therapist is prepared to help should be made clear at the outset. Along the lines described above, it is emphasized that time will be needed, a trusting relationship between therapist and patient should be allowed to develop and nothing irreversible will be done for some time. The reasons for this cautious approach are given — principally that only some patients end up happier in the newly assigned role and that others change their mind before they get to that stage. Decisions to be taken in the process will eventually be irreversible and considerable care is required to ensure that the correct choice is made, not only by the patient but also by the clinician.

At this stage the difficulties in obtaining surgery are stressed and the practical limitations of surgery discussed. Factual information about legal status (e.g. the inability to be legally married in some countries, but with an increasing option of 'civil unions') and the biological limitations (e.g. it will not be possible to have children in the new role) are pointed out. Usually the patient will accept such a contract, though the clinician may well find pressure for more rapid progress being brought to bear at an early stage. It is important to make the contract a two-way affair. It is unreasonable to expect the patient to wait months simply to provide the clinician with information to help him make up his mind. Something should be given in return.

Practical steps

From an early stage the patient who feels certain that he or she wants to change should be encouraged to spend more time 'passing' in the desired role, becoming increasingly ambitious and adventurous as time goes on. Initially this may mean going out at night cross-dressed and walking in the street. Later, people in shops should be approached and so on. The clinician can give useful advice about what to do and where to go, plus more tangible benefits, such as providing a letter for the patient to carry around, authorizing the cross-dressing behaviour as part of a medically supervised treatment programme. This will often remove the fear of being harassed by the police.

When the patient feels ready, he or she can be invited to come to the clinic cross-dressed. The therapist can then provide more direct feedback about how effective the person is in that role.

Usually transsexuals are cut off from their own families, but occasionally it is helpful for the therapist to explain the nature of the problem to relatives, who sometimes provide extremely valuable support in the patient's future endeavours. It is particularly important to meet and get to know any sexual partners. These are much more likely to exist with female-to-male transsexual partners. They are important because often their attitude may play a major part in the patient's motivation for surgery. I have had experience with several female-to-male transsexuals whose strong desire to have surgery receded dramatically when they changed partners. Usually the issue is whether either the patient or the partner is prepared to accept the relationship as a homosexual rather than a heterosexual one.

Alongside more practical, positive advice, the therapist should be carrying out the continuous process of reality confrontation with both the patient and any partner who is involved. As trust in the counselling relationship develops, the therapist should be making sure the patient is aware of the enormous difficulties ahead. There is no place for false optimism, since the patient's (and the clinician's) ultimate decision depends on the patient's ability to overcome these problems. Physical appearance is a key factor. Some patients have no difficulty looking the part. For others it will remain a formidable problem, usually because of their facial structure. The older the person, the less of a problem this is likely to be.

In the male-to-female transsexual, beard growth is usually a problem, making effective facial make-up difficult. Facial electrolysis is the only real solution. This is a very time-consuming and expensive business. At a relatively early stage the patient can be advised to seek this treatment. It is difficult to obtain electrolysis within the NHS. In any case, it may be desirable to give the responsibility for this to the patient in the first instance. The treatment goes on for months, with one or two sessions per week. One advantage of electrolysis is that, though it is irreversible, it takes long enough for many uncertainties to be resolved and if sexual reassignment is eventually abandoned, loss of facial hair is not a major problem.

Alternatives to sex reassignment should periodically be reconsidered. The most important are the transvestite 'dual role' (see p. 293) and the homosexual role. For many transsexuals, particularly female-to-male, life would be so much easier for them if they could accept and feel comfortable with a homosexual identity. Sometimes the extreme and rigid rejection of homosexuality reveals a personality that may not fare well after surgery (Morgan 1978).

In general, one is looking for evidence that, apart from the gender dysphoria, the patient has a realistic view of the problems to be faced and of his or her abilities to overcome them.

More specific forms of training may be introduced stage by stage. Voice training is often helpful. Oates & Dacakis (1986) provided a useful review of the evidence of sex differences in speech and indicated that modification of speech involves not only pitch and intonation patterns, but also vocal loudness, voice quality, vocabulary usage, articulatory precision and conversational style. Social skills training with video feedback may be useful in increasing the authenticity of gender role behaviour (Yardley 1976). Sometimes transsexuals caricature the role they seek and need to tone down mannerisms. Help with make-up and hairstyles is often needed.

At some stage the patient, if still intent on pursuing the programme, is encouraged to start living and working full-time in the new role. This usually means moving to a new place to live and changing jobs. This is often the most difficult stage. Absence of any previous employment in the new role makes applying for jobs difficult as references may not be available. The therapist can provide some help, e.g. by contacting the Disablement Resettlement Officer or arranging for a period of time on a government training scheme to learn some new skill. Medical reassurance can be given to the would-be employer. But the patient will have to take the main responsibility for finding employment.

For some female-to-male transsexuals, large breasts can make this stage particularly difficult, and mastectomy may have to be considered at this relatively early stage in the programme if further progress is to be made.

Hormone treatment

The use of hormones also requires careful thought (Gooren 1999). Although many of their effects are reversible, this step should be seen as a definite move towards permanent reassignment that should not be started too early. In the male-to-female transsexual, oestrogens with or without progestagens are used. Their effects are difficult to predict with certainty but are likely to include some breast enlargement (usually not enough, so that mammoplasty will eventually be required), redistribution of fat in a more feminine pattern, softening of the skin and usually a reduction in sexual interest. No effect on the voice is to be expected. Some authorities believe that the addition of progestagen to the oestrogen leads to more breast enlargement, but there is no evidence to support this view. Patients should be screened for contra-indications to taking steroids (e.g. hypertension, liver disease, history of thrombotic disorders) and should be warned of the risks of taking hormones. It is sensible to carry out some endocrine investigations initially to establish a baseline. It is then advisable to start with a low dose and increase gradually in case unpleasant side effects, such as nausea, occur. Ethinyloestradiol is the most widely used oestrogen and can be given in doses up to 0.05 mg daily. This can be increased to 0.1 mg daily if there has been no satisfactory response after 3 or 4 months. If progestagen is to be given, a combined oral contraceptive provides a convenient method, though before surgery it should be taken continuously. Antiandrogens may also be combined with oestrogens. They may further slow down hair growth and enhance breast growth, though a reduction in sexual interest is even more likely. Cyproterone acetate 50 or 100 mg daily is appropriate. It is a requirement of most surgeons to stop steroids temporarily when surgery is carried out to reduce the risk of post-operative thrombosis.

For the female-to-male transsexual the appropriate hormone is testosterone. This can be expected to increase body and facial hair, though to what extent is difficult to predict, to cause some enlargement of the clitoris and probably increase clitoral sensitivity, increase muscle bulk and body weight and deepen the voice. Menstruation may be less heavy or stop and a slight reduction in breast size may occur but neither of these effects should be assumed. Again it is advisable to build up the dose gradually. Genetic females vary considerably in their sensitivity to testosterone (see Chapter 4) and the minimum dose to obtain the desired effect should be the goal. Transdermal administration, using testosterone gel, is the favoured method at present. This allows gradual increase of the dose.

The adolescent

Increasingly individuals with transgender issues are being seen at younger ages. This presents the clinician with a difficult challenge. The HBIGDA standards of care (HBIGDA 2001) clearly set 18 years as the minimum before recommending surgical reassignment. This is probably sensible. However, the prevalence of psychological and personality problems, particularly in the male-to-female transgendered, may in part result from the gender dysphoria and associated peer group stigmatization that they experience during adolescence, a phase crucial for development of personality and emotional reactivity. If one were to know that a 12-year-old with transgender identity was going to persist as transgendered, there would be advantages to early gender reassignment, and the prospect of a more stable personality and emotional state in adulthood. But one cannot be sure, and adolescence is a time of many changes. Gooren (1999) now considers postponement of puberty in such cases to allow a longer period for grappling with gender identity issues before the often powerful impact of pubertal development hits. Hence the transgendered girl, wanting to be male, can be traumatized by the onset of menstruation. Similarly, the transgendered boy when he experiences voice change and facial hair growth with puberty. Caution is required with such cases, but the postponement of puberty approach warrants evaluation, and such cases should be carefully followed up.

Suitable for surgery or not?

The objective of the clinical assessment of a transgendered patient seeking gender-reassignment surgery is to establish, with a reasonable level of clinical confidence, whether the patient is likely to benefit from surgical reassignment. The purpose of the 'real life test' that is required as part of this assessment, is to establish that, without surgery, the patient can nevertheless make a good adjustment in the desired gender role, be accepted by others and, if possible, obtain employment in the new role. The addition of the surgical component is not going to make much difference to those adjustments, apart from the increased self-confidence that might result. It is part of the clinician's role to inform and persuade the patient that surgery will not solve most of the problems of acceptance and adjustment, and will be most relevant to the establishment of a new sexual relationship. Hence the need for the patient to show that considerable pre-surgical adaptation can be achieved.

In addition to basic adaptation to the new role, an important criterion of suitability for surgery is the individual's level of psychological stability and resilience. The psychiatric history is obviously of importance, though it is appropriate to acknowledge that the gender dysphoric individual, particularly during the emotional upheavals of adolescence, may have had mental health problems as a result of his or her dysphoria. The question is whether he or she has matured enough to be able to cope better with the challenges and new 'emotional upheavals' of gender role change. The 'real life test' is a practical and reasonably effective way of addressing that question, which is why a sufficient period of time (at least 18 months in my clinical practice) is required before the decision about surgery is taken. The introduction of hormones can be made earlier because, although they do have some relatively irreversible effects, they are less substantial than those following surgery. An informative case history of a male-to-female transgendered person who eventually went through surgery and subsequently regretted it is given by Olsson & Möller (2006); this is a good example of how personality problems can make the transition difficult.

Surgery

For the male-to-female transsexual, this usually involves orchidectomy and penectomy, with preservation of scrotal and penile skin. The fashioning of a vaginal tube uses the penile skin and usually an additional split-skin graft. The labia are fashioned out of the scrotal skin. The operation may be done in one or two stages. Post-operative complications are common and may be troublesome. Urethral stricture or urethrovaginal fistulae may occur. Most common is a fibrosis of the artificial vaginal barrel,

leading to shortening or even closure. This can be corrected with further surgery (McEwan et al 1986). If successful, the vagina can eventually be used for sexual intercourse and pleasurable erotic sensations, including orgasm may be experienced.

For the female-to-male transsexual the surgical options are less satisfactory. Mastectomy has already been mentioned. Hysterectomy and oophorectomy are relatively straightforward, but the creation of a penis (phalloplasty) or scrotum presents formidable difficulties. Although attempts have been made (e.g. see Hoopes 1968; Noe et al 1978 for early accounts) results have been far from satisfactory with particular difficulty in avoiding urinary fistulae. It should also be kept in mind that even when a penis is surgically constructed and allows relatively normal urination, it will not have the capacity to become erect, limiting its use in subsequent sexual interaction. It is questionable whether phalloplasty justifies the time, expense and substantial risk of post-operative complications, until there is a breakthrough with new surgical techniques.

Post-operative care

The counselling relationship should obviously continue post-operatively and may well be needed for some considerable time. Hormones should also be continued, particularly if testes or ovaries are removed.

Those considered unsuitable for surgery

The transgendered are often impatient in their pursuit of surgical treatment and if they believe that such help is not going to be forthcoming, they may well move on to seek help elsewhere. This may preclude a sufficient 'real life test'. Those who have been adequately assessed and are judged to be unsuitable for surgery may not accept the decision and may go elsewhere in search of surgery. In some cases a positive decision about surgery should not be made until there has been some other long-term change (e.g. effective treatment of depression). Ongoing support will then be needed until it is appropriate to reconsider surgery. Those who have established a good relationship with a therapist may well accept this state of affairs. In those for whom surgery is considered to be unsuitable, alternative approaches to their dealing with their gender identity issues should be explored (for a useful overview see Carroll 2007).

Transgendered males and females need a great deal of help and the clinician is advised not to get involved with their management unless prepared to offer long-term help and support.

Standards of care

The Harry Benjamin International Gender Dysphoria Association periodically publishes standards of care for hormonal and surgical reassignment (HBIGDA 2001). Their main points include the following:

1. Clinical decisions about both hormonal and surgical reassignment should be made by clinical behavioural

scientists with appropriate experience of the diagnosis and treatment of psychological and sexual problems, as well as experience of working with patients with gender dysphoria.

2. The wish for sex reassignment should have existed for at least 2 years.
3. The clinician should have known the patient for at least 3 months before recommending hormonal and 6 months before recommending surgical reassignment.
4. This recommendation should be supported by a second appropriately qualified clinical behavioural scientist.
5. The patient should have lived full-time in the preferred role for *at least* 1 year before surgery is recommended.

REFERENCES

Abramowitz SI 1986 Psychosocial outcomes of sex reassignment surgery. Journal of Clinical and Consulting Psychology 54: 183–189.

Bailey JM 2003 The Man who would be Queen: the Science of Gender-Bending and Transsexualism. Joseph Henry Press, Washington DC.

Bailey JM, Zucker KJ 1995 Childhood sex-typed behavior and sexual orientation. Developmental Psychology 31: 43–55.

Bakker A, van Kesteren PJ, Gooren LJG, Bezemer PD 1993 The prevalence of transsexualism in the Netherlands. Acta Psychiatrica Scandinavica 87: 237–238.

Bancroft J 1972 The relationship between gender identity and sexual behaviour: some clinical aspects. In Ounsted C, Taylor DC (eds) Gender Differences: their Ontogeny and Significance. Churchill Livingstone, Edinburgh, pp. 57–72.

Bancroft J 2003 Review of A. Fausto-Sterling's 'Sexing the Body'. Archives of Sexual Behavior 32: 289–291.

Benjamin H 1966 The Transsexual Phenomenon. Julian Press, New York.

Bentler PM 1976 A typology of transsexualism: gender identity, theory and data. Archives of Sexual Behavior 5: 567–584.

Blanchard R 1989 The concept of autogynephilia and the typology of male gender dysphoria. Journal of Nervous and Mental Disease 177: 616–623.

Blanchard R 2005 Early history of the concept of autogynephilia. Archives of Sexual Behavior 34: 439–446.

Bolin A 1993 Transcending and transgendering: male-to-female transsexuals, dichotomy and diversity. In Herdt G (ed) Third Sex, Third Gender: Beyond Sexual Dimorphism in Culture and History. Zone Books, New York, pp. 447–486.

Bullough V 1991 Transvestism: a re-examination. Journal of Psychology and Human Sexuality 4: 653–657.

Buhrich N, Beaumont T 1981 Comparison of transvestism in Australia and America. Archives of Sexual Behavior 10: 269–282.

Buhrich N, McConaghy N 1985 Pre-adult feminine behavior of male transvestites. Archives of Sexual Behavior 14: 413–420.

Carroll RA 1999 Outcomes of treatment of gender dysphoria. Journal of Sex Education and Therapy 24: 128–136.

Carroll RA 2007 Gender dysphoria and transgender experiences. In Leiblum SR (ed) Principles and Practice of Sex Therapy. 4th edn. Guilford, New York, pp. 477–508.

Chung WC, DeVries GJ, Swaab DF 2002 Sexual differentiation of the bed nucleus of the stria terminalis in humans may extend into adulthood. Journal of Neuroscience 22: 1027–1033.

Cohen-Kettenis P, Gooren LJG 1999 Transsexualism: a review of etiology, diagnosis and treatment. Journal of Psychosomatic Research 46: 315–333.

Dessens A, Cohen-Kettenis P, Mellenbergh G, Poll N, Koppe J, Boer K 1999 Prenatal exposure to anticonvulsants and psychosexual development. Archives of Sexual Behavior 28: 31–44.

Devor H 1996 Female gender dysphoria in context: social problem or personal problem. Annual Review of Sex Research 7:44–89.

Fausto-Sterling A 2000 Sexing the Body: Gender Politics and the Construction of Sexuality. Basic Books, New York.

Futterweit W, Weiss RA, Fagerstrom RM 1986 Endocrine evaluation of 40 female to male transsexuals: increased frequency of polycystic ovarian disease in female transsexualism. Archives of Sexual Behavior 15: 69–78.

Goldman R, Goldman J 1982 Children's Sexual Thinking. Routledge & Kegan Paul, London.

Gooren LJG 1986 The neuroendocrine response of luteinising hormone to estrogen administration in the human is not sex specific but dependent on the hormonal environment. Journal of Clinical Endocrinology and Metabolism 63: 589–593.

Gooren, LJG 1999 Hormonal Sex Reassignment. IJT 3, 3, http://www.symposion.com/ijt/ijt990301.htp

Green R 1974 Sexual Identity Conflict in Children and Adults. Duckworth, London

Green R 1976 One hundred and ten feminine and masculine boys: behavioural contrasts and demographic similarities. Archives of Sexual Behavior 5: 425–446.

Green R 1985 Gender identity in childhood and later sexual orientation: follow-up of 78 males. American Journal of Psychiatry 142: 339–341.

Green R 2000 Family co-occurrence of 'gender dysphoria': ten sibling or parent–child pairs. Archives of Sexual Behaviour 29: 499–508.

Green R 2002 Sexual identity and sexual orientation. In Pfaff D, Arnold A, Etgen A, Fahrbach S, Rubin R (eds) Hormones, Brain and Behavior. Vol. 4, Academic Press, Elsevier, Amsterdam. pp. 463–485.

Green R, Fleming DT 1990 Transsexual surgery follow-up: status in the 1990's. Annual Review of Sex Research 1: 163–174.

Green R, Williams K, Goodman M 1982 Ninety-nine 'tomboys' and 'non-tomboys': behavioural contrasts and demographic similarities. Archives of Sexual Behavior 11: 247–266.

Gremaux R 1993 Woman becomes man in the Balkans. In Herdt G (ed) Third Sex, Third Gender: Beyond Sexual Dimorphism in Culture and History. Zone Books, New York, pp. 241–284.

HBIGDA 2001 Harry Benjamin International Gender Dysphoria Association. The standards of care for gender identity disorders (6th version). International Journal of Transgenderism 5(1). Retrieved 21 May 2007 from www.symposion.com/ijt/soc_2001/index.htm.

Henningson S, Westberg L, Nilsson S, Lundstrom B, Ekselius L, Bodlund P, et al 2005 Sex steroid-related genes and male-to-female transsexualism. Psychoneuroendocrinology 30: 657–664.

Hoenig J, Kenna JC 1979 EEG abnormalities and transsexualism. British Journal of Psychiatry 134: 293–300.

Hoopes JE 1968 Operative treatment of the female transsexual. In Green R, Money J (eds) Transsexualism and Sex Reassignment. Johns Hopkins, Baltimore, pp. 335–352.

Jay K, Young A 1979 The Gay Report. Summit, New York.

Knoblauch H, Busjahn A, Wegener B 2007 Monozygotic twins concordant for female-to-male transsexualism: a case report. Archives of Sexual Behavior 36: 135–137.

Kruijver FPM, Zhou J-N, Pool CW, Hofman MA, Gooren LJG, Swaab DF 2000 Male-to-female transsexuals have female neuron numbers in a limbic nucleus. Journal of Endocrinology & Metabolism 85: 2034–2041.

Langstrom N, Zucker KJ 2005 Transvestic fetishism in the general population. Journal of Sexual and Marital Therapy 31: 87–95.

Lawrence AA 2003 Factors associated with regret following male-to-female sex reassignment surgery. Archives of Sexual Behavior 32: 299–315.

Lawrence AA 2005 Sexuality before and after male-to-female sex reassignment surgery. Archives of Sexual Behavior 34: 147–166.

McEwan L, Ceber S, Daws J 1986 Male to female surgical genital reassignment. In Walters WAW, Ross MW (eds) Transsexualism and Sex Reassignment. Oxford University Press, Oxford, pp. 103–112.

Meyerowitz J 2002 How Sex Changed: A History of Transsexuality in the United States. Harvard University Press, Cambridge.

Morgan AJ 1978 Psychotherapy for transsexual candidates screened out of surgery. Archives of Sexual Behavior 7: 273–284.

Nanda S 1993 Hijras: an alternative sex and gender role. In Herdt G (ed) Third Sex, Third Gender: Beyond Sexual Dimorphism in Culture and History. Zone Books, New York, pp. 373–418.

Noe J, Sato R, Coleman C, Laub DR 1978 Construction of male genitalia: the Stanford experience. Archives of Sexual Behavior 7: 297–304.

Oates JM, Dacakis G 1986 Voice, speech and language considerations in the management of male to female transsexuals. In Walters WAW, Ross MW (eds) Transsexualism and Sex Reassignment. Oxford University Press, Oxford.

Olsson S-E, Möller A 2006 Regret after sex reassignment surgery in a male-to-female transsexual: a long-term follow up. Archives of Sexual Behavior 35: 501–506.

Pauly IB 1974 Female transsexualism. Archives of Sexual Behavior 3: 487–526.

Pfafflin F, Junge A 1998 Sex reassignment: thirty years of international follow-up studies after sex reassignment surgery: a comprehensive review 1961–1991. Retrieved May 21 2007 from www.symposion.com/ijt/books/index.htm.

Reinisch JM, Sanders SA 1982 Early barbiturate exposure: the brain, sexually dimorphic behavior and learning. Neuroscience and Biobehavioral Reviews 6: 311–319.

Ross MW 1983 Femininity, masculinity and sexual orientation: some cross-cultural comparisons. Journal of Homosexuality 9: 27–36.

Ross MW, Walinder J, Lundstrom B Thuwe I 1981 Cross-cultural approaches to transsexualism. Acta Psychiatrica Scandinavica 63: 75–82.

Segal NL 2006 Two monozygotic twin pairs discordant for female-to-male transsexualism. Archives of Sexual Behavior 35: 347–358.

Seyler L E, Canalis E, Spare S, Reichlin S 1978 Abnormal gonadotrophin secretory responses to LHRH in transsexual women after diethyl-stilboestrol priming. Journal of Clinical Endocrinology and Metabolism 47: 176–183.

Sipova I, Starka L 1977 Plasma testosterone values in transsexual women. Archives of Sexual Behavior 6: 477–481.

Stoller R 1979 Gender disorders. In Rosen I (ed) Sexual Deviation. 2nd edn. Oxford University Press, Oxford, pp. 109–138.

Wilson P, Sharp C, Carr S 1999 The prevalence of gender dysphoria in Scotland: a primary care study. British Journal of General Practice 49: 991–992.

Yardley KM 1976 Training in feminine skills in a male transsexual: a preoperative procedure. British Journal of Medical Psychology 49: 329–339.

Zhou J, Hofman M, Gooren L, Swaab D 1995 A sex difference in the human brain and its relation to transsexuality. Nature (London) 378: 68–70.

Zucker KJ, Bradley SJ 1995 Gender Identity Disorder and Psychosexual Problems in Children and Adolescents. Guilford Press, New York.

The nature of problematic sexuality

11

Sexuality in the context of a relationship 303

The medicalization of sexual problems 304
In the male.. 304
In the female.. 305

Conceptualizing sexual problems — the fundamental
role of inhibition... 305
The impact of socio-cultural factors 306
When is a sexual problem a 'dysfunction'? 306
The three windows approach... 306
The three categories of sexual problem 307

Problems of reduced sexual interest
or responsiveness 307
Sexual problems in men.. 307
Sexual problems in women.. 308

Prevalence of problems in the community 310

People who attend sexual problem clinics
and their problems 313

Understanding problems of reduced interest
or responsiveness 316
Through the first window — the current situation..................... 316

Through the second window — vulnerability to
sexual problems 319
Through the third window — factors that alter
sexual function 327
Problems of altered sexual response or interest in men
and women with homosexual or bisexual identities 328

Problematic sexual behaviour.. 329
High-risk sexual behaviour 329
'Out-of-control' sexual behaviour.................................... 330
Other types of problematic sexual behaviour 334

Problems with sexual or gender identity 335
Sexual identity 335
Gender identity 336

The classification of sexual problems............................ 336
The historical context 336
Towards a better classification of sexual problems.................. 338

The benefits of being sexual 338
Sexual barriers to parenthood....................................... 338
Barriers to establishing a rewarding sexual relationship........... 338
Barriers to experiencing sexual pleasure 339
Explaining a barrier.. 339
Conclusion.. 339

In this final section of the book we will be considering the various ways that sexuality can be problematic, how to assess such problems and how best to help with or treat them.

Since the last edition of this book, there have been major relevant changes requiring a new approach and method of conceptualization. In various ways, the theoretical models used in this edition, particularly the Dual Control model, will be influential in this process, and many of the themes in the last edition will still be evident.

Of the various factors that have had impacts in the last 15 years, one of the most important has been the new involvement of the pharmaceutical industry in the treatment of sexual problems. Whereas in the last edition there was a limited amount to consider as far as pharmacological treatments were concerned, that has all changed, at least for men. The most notable change has resulted from the serendipitous discovery of the effect of sildenafil on erectile function — the Viagra story detailed in Chapter 4 (see p. 76). This demonstrated that there was a large market for drugs that enhanced or improved sexual response. It has led, not surprisingly, to the search for a Viagra for women, confronting us with how little we really understand about sexual problems in women. So we are in the midst of vigorous debate, controversy and active research, and hopefully much will come of it, not necessarily pharmacological. In this introduction, we will consider some of the key issues that have emerged during this phase, before moving on to present a revised approach to the 'psychosomatic circle' and its relevance to sexual problems.

Another new factor of major significance is the Internet. Problematic use of the Internet will be considered later in this chapter.

Sexuality in the context of a relationship

As presented in Chapter 4, sexual arousal is a physiological response. It involves physiological mechanisms that do not always work as we expect them to. However, it differs in an important way from most other physiological response systems that are fundamental to our existence; it is in many respects a response system that involves interaction with another person. Obviously, we can get sexually aroused when alone, but problems with our arousal responses are most often experienced in the context of a relationship. This underlines the importance of keeping the interactive relationship component in mind when striving to explain and help with sexual problems. The history of involvement of the medical profession in helping people with sexual problems shows a preoccupation with the responsiveness of the individual. In some cases this is appropriate; there are various ways that pathological mechanisms, such as vascular disease or neuropathy, can directly interfere with an individual's sexual arousal. But the relevance of the sexual relationship is usually ignored, mainly because few in the medical profession know how to assess or deal with it.

As we have seen at various places in this book, the relationship is of fundamental importance to the sexuality of most women, in terms of their sexual identity (see Chapter 5), their sexual well-being (see Chapter 6), and in older women, many of whom do not have a sexual partner, to whether they feel any sexual need or interest (see Chapter 7). The woman's physiological responses contribute less than the relationship aspects to her sexual well-being (Bancroft et al 2003a).

In the case of the male there are two types of relationship to consider: the sexual relationship with his partner and the relationship between the man and his penis. I elaborated on the second type in an earlier paper: 'Relationship is an apt term because so often the penis seems to have a life, if not a mind, of its own. It's not just that it can't be taken for granted; often out of apparent perversity of spirit, it fails to provide its owner support when he most needs it' (Bancroft 1989, p. 7). In contrast to the relevance of genitalia to women, the penis plays a fundamental role in a man's identity as a male. As Zilbergeld (1992) puts it: '... male socialization and cultural expectations place a very heavy burden on a very small part of the man's anatomy'(p. 28). As a consequence, the psychosomatic process is central to a man's experience of sex. In contrast to a woman, a man judges both his level of sexual arousal and his effectiveness as a lover on the basis of what is happening in his penis. The equation of male sexuality with 'power' is inherent in the term 'potency'. The term 'impotent' captures the sense of 'loss of power' with significance well beyond the man's capacity for sexual pleasure. 'Impotent' is a pejorative term, originally used to describe ejaculatory as well as erectile dysfunction (ED). The female equivalent is 'frigid', which interestingly focuses on the woman's lack of response to the man, not on her own pleasure. The term 'frigidity' has largely disappeared from the medical literature; the term 'impotent', while used less than previously, is still very much in evidence, at least for describing erectile problems (Bancroft 1992).

The medicalization of sexual problems

In the male

Male sexual dysfunction, mainly erectile, attracted the interest of surgeons in the 1930s (Johnson 1968). That was a passing phase. For some years after that, the prevailing wisdom was that ED was 90% psychological in its origins, though apart from psychoanalysis, which was of limited relevance, psychological treatments were not available. Things changed in the 1970s. On the one hand, Masters & Johnson (1970) started a new era of psychologically-based therapy for sexual problems. On the other hand, urological and vascular surgeons re-entered the field. We will be considering Masters and Johnson's treatment approach in the next chapter. The surgical approaches initially focused on the penis (and not the man attached to it), with various types of penile implant to provide a relatively permanent erection, or vacuum devices to induce an erection followed by tight bands at the base of the penis to prevent loss of an erection once established. With technological development, implants became more sophisticated, involving a small pump implanted into the scrotum that allowed the man to inflate the implant when needed. Alongside these surgical treatments a veritable diagnostic industry emerged. Men are sufficiently troubled by impotence that they will pay to get it sorted out. Given that the surgical methods of treatment were mostly irreversible, reducing if not eliminating the possibility of a return of normal erectile function, the approach was to demonstrate the 'organic' (hence irreversible) nature of the erectile problem. Two types of diagnostic procedure were used. The first was used to distinguish between 'organic' and 'psychogenic' problems; initially the principal method used was measurement of nocturnal penile tumescence (NPT; see Chapter 4, p. 69) with the occurrence of relatively normal NPT taken as evidence of psychogenicity and the lack of normal NPT as indicating an 'organic' problem. The second type of procedure focused on specific aetiologies of 'organic' impotence, in particular vascular and neurological abnormalities. In the 1980s a new and important dimension was added. It was discovered that injection of smooth muscle relaxants into the corpora cavernosa would typically induce erection. This initially was used for diagnostic purposes, the assumption being that such injections were assessing the peripheral mechanisms of erection and not their control by the brain. Soon intracavernosal injections became widely used as a form of treatment. These methods used as treatment will be revisited in Chapter 12.

This phase of intensive diagnostic investigation did result in a substantial amount of new knowledge about erectile function and dysfunction. In terms of diagnosis relevant to treatment, however, it was flawed because of the assumption that the penis could be investigated independently of the man attached to it. It soon became apparent, for example, that psychogenic factors could suppress the erectile response to intracavernosal injections (Granata et al 1995). NPT is suppressed in states of depression, which do not involve malfunctioning of the genital response system but rather a depression-related reduction in central excitatory tone (see p. 388). Men with vascular impairment could have a substantial worsening of any ED as a result of psychological reactions to the basic impairment. In other words, the relationship between the man and his penis had been largely ignored in this phase of medicalization.

The next phase followed the introduction of Viagra in the late 1990s. This is effective in inducing erection in around two-thirds of men with ED, but it is noteworthy that the long-term use of this medication is uncertain, and side effects are not trivial. This will be considered further in Chapter 12, but the relevance to this discussion is that, until recently, very little attempt has been made to assess the impact of drugs like Viagra on the sexual relationship, or on the partner (Rosen et al 2006 report a pilot study). The impact of an expensive drug (not usually covered by health insurance), that enhances erectile response for several hours, may impose a 'sexuality' on the relationship which is not necessarily welcomed by the partner, and this may be particularly relevant to older age groups (Potts et al 2003). In the last five years, attention has turned to the treatment of premature ejaculation (PE), using relatively short-acting serotonin re-uptake inhibitors. This will also be considered in Chapter 12.

Overall, the medicalization of male sexual problems has resulted in an increase in our knowledge of peripheral physiological mechanisms, the availability of new and often effective pharmacological treatments, but in the process, a reinforcement of the socio-cultural focus on male 'potency', and little or no progress in furthering our understanding of the impact of the relationship on male sexual response and vice versa.

In the female

When we turn to the medicalization of women's sexuality we find a very different and well documented history (e.g. Veith 1965; Maines 1999; Thompson 1999), which reminds us that the need to suppress or limit women's sexuality has been more evident during some historical periods than others. During the Victorian era, for example, 'respectable' women were seen as not particularly sexual. Women who clearly enjoyed sex were at risk of being hospitalized for insanity, or subjected to surgical procedures such as clitoridectomy (Bancroft 2005). This was followed by a long period when the medical profession paid little or no attention to women's sexuality. The introduction of oral contraceptives in the 1960s produced an interesting response from the medical profession (Watkins 1998; Marks 2001). The pill was acceptable if used by married women to control fertility, but not for women in general to enjoy sex free from the fears of unwanted pregnancy. The exceptional and continuing lack of research on possible adverse effects of steroidal contraceptives on women's sexuality will be addressed in Chapter 15. Then there was a phase of further neglect, which came to an end around the turn of the century for two principal reasons. Firstly, an increasing awareness that widely used drugs, such as serotonin re-uptake inhibitors for depression and anxiety, had sexual side effects in women as well as men. The introduction of a few drugs without such side effects (see Chapter 13 for more detailed discussion), marketed with that message, motivated the pharmaceutical industry to take women's sexuality seriously. Secondly, the major commercial impact of Viagra led to interest in the possibility of a 'Viagra for women'.

One of the most striking examples of this phase was a paper published in the *Journal of the American Medical Association* (Laumann et al 1999). Using data from the NHSLS, the national survey of men and women in the USA reviewed in Chapter 6, it was reported that 43% of women suffered from sexual dysfunction. This led them to conclude that 'sexual dysfunction is a largely uninvestigated yet significant public health problem... With the affected population rarely receiving medical therapy for sexual dysfunction, service delivery efforts should be augmented to target high-risk populations.' (p. 544) Their reports of 'sexual dysfunction' were based on very limited information, and will be considered more closely below. Nevertheless, these findings have been widely disseminated in the media and the medical literature. The approach to conceptualizing sexual problems that follows can be understood to some extent as a reaction to this era of medicalization of sexual problems in both men and women.

Conceptualizing sexual problems — the fundamental role of inhibition

As we strive to comprehend the nature of sexual problems, the Dual Control model, which runs through this book (starting with Chapter 2), confronts us with a fundamental issue. It postulates a basic inhibitory mechanism that is adaptive; inhibition of sexual arousal and response is appropriate and necessary to avoid sexual activity occurring in unsuitable or potentially disadvantageous circumstances. The assumption is that two types of inhibition are involved: an inhibitory tone, normally present, which has to be reduced (or counteracted by increased sexual excitation) for sexual response to occur; and inhibitory responses that are reactive to the circumstances. These mechanisms were closely considered in Chapter 4. Information processing is clearly involved, but it is likely that reactive inhibition results from automatic rather than conscious processing. Our findings using measures of inhibition and excitation proneness, reviewed in Chapter 6, are consistent with inhibition as an adaptive mechanism. In both men and women we find close to normal distributions for inhibition scores, not compatible with the idea that inhibition is a dysfunctional response restricted to a minority of individuals. Our evidence also shows that men and women who score at the high end of the distribution are more likely to report problems of impaired sexual response; those at the low end are more likely to engage in high-risk or otherwise problematic sexual behaviour. The evidence for these two associations will be revisited in this chapter. Although there is considerable overlap between inhibition scores for men and women, the distribution for women is shifted towards the high inhibition end to a significant extent; i.e. women tend to have higher propensity for inhibition than men (see p. 229). Once the concept of adaptive inhibition is accepted, then a crucial distinction needs to be made between inhibition that is adaptive, given the circumstances, and that which is maladaptive or dysfunctional. Given the distributions we have found, we should not expect a clear distinction. A key and as yet unanswered question is whether propensity for inhibition constitutes a personality trait that is determined by genetic or early learning mechanisms, or whether it can be altered by circumstances or by pathological processes during adulthood. One relevant finding considered in Chapter 7 is an apparent increase in sensitivity of the smooth muscle in erectile tissues to inhibitory signals from the brain with increasing age, and also in men with diabetes (see p. 243). It is possible that alteration of brain function, e.g. temporal lobe disorders, can have a comparable effect, though mediated centrally rather than peripherally. This remains a crucial issue for future research.

Propensity for sexual excitation, as measured by our scales, also shows normal distributions in men and women. The low and high ends of the distributions are also associated with problematic sexuality, whereas the mid range can be considered adaptive. Here it is much more likely that both central and peripheral mechanisms resulting from ageing, pathological or pharmacological processes will reduce the propensity for excitation; reduced sexual arousability with ageing and in states of depression are good examples, and many more involving metabolic or endocrine abnormalities can be given (see Chapter 13).

In relation to both excitation and inhibition proneness, this therefore confronts us with the question of whether we are measuring a trait or a state. That requires further research. The Dual Control model, however, helps us make a clear distinction between two types of problem: *reduced sexual responsiveness*, associated with increased inhibition, reduced excitation or both, and *problematic behaviour*, which results in part from lack of adaptive inhibition and is amplified by high excitation proneness.

The impact of socio-cultural factors

As yet, there is no evidence of ethnic or racial differences in propensities for either excitation or inhibition proneness. What are likely to vary across cultures are the contexts, meanings or scripts that invoke reactive inhibition. As discussed in Chapter 6, the substantial changes in women's sexuality documented through the 20th century, at least in North America and Europe, reflect a lessening of socio-cultural suppression of women's sexuality (see p. 232). The evidence from cross-cultural comparisons reviewed in that chapter also suggests that these changes have been world-wide to some extent, but with ethnic differences still apparent. To what extent this reflects differing degrees of socio-cultural suppression across cultures or ethnic differences in the susceptibility to socio-cultural suppression (e.g. ethnic differences in propensity for inhibition) is at present unanswerable. However, socio-cultural factors are crucial to understanding how sexual problems are experienced in different cultures. In multi-racial societies, such as the USA and much of Europe, this is of considerable clinical relevance, not only in assessing and diagnosing sexual problems, but also in treating them with psychological methods. This will be considered further in Chapter 12. Some evidence of ethnic differences in how sexual problems are experienced in older men and women was considered in Chapter 7 (Dennerstein & Lehert 2004; Avis et al 2005; Laumann et al 2005).

When is a sexual problem a 'dysfunction'?

It was probably Masters & Johnson in 1970 who initiated the current use of the term 'sexual dysfunction'. Prior to 1970 its use was restricted to sexual side effects caused by medication or surgery. The dictionary definition of 'dysfunction' is of a medical term meaning 'malfunctioning, as of a structure of the body' (Random House 1983). The concept of 'sexual dysfunction' strongly implies that the sexual response system is malfunctioning. The early use of this term was principally intended to convey psychological malfunctioning; at that time most 'sexual dysfunctions' were considered to be psychogenic. Over the past 20 years the emphasis, at least for men, has shifted to 'organic' dysfunction and, as indicated earlier, to a prevailing mind–body dualism that makes the clear distinction between 'psychogenic' and 'organic' causes. In this book, the emphasis is on psychosomatic interaction, and hence the mind–body dualism is considered obsolete and unhelpful. Keeping in mind that sexual arousal and response involve psycho-neurophysiological mechanisms, it becomes appropriate to identify components of the psychosomatic circle that may be contributing to its malfunction, but not appropriate to separate them out as distinct aetiologies. According to the Dual Control model, the high and low levels of inhibition and excitation proneness, observed at the ends of the distribution, can be considered potentially malfunctional. Hence, keeping in mind that the boundary between malfunction and function is not clear-cut, the concept of 'dysfunction' has heuristic value. It then becomes necessary to distinguish between sexual problems that are adaptive, or at least understandable reactions to present circumstances, and those that are the result of malfunction.

The three windows approach

This is a way of conceptualizing the approach to careful clinical assessment of anyone complaining of or reporting a sexual problem. Through the first window, to what extent is the current situation or relationship likely to result in 'adaptive' inhibition of sexual interest and response? Through the second window we look for evidence that the individual with a problem has experienced that type of problem periodically through his or her sexual life, or whether indeed the problem is of long duration; this requires a careful sexual history, including coverage of early experiences of relevance (e.g. child sexual abuse (CSA)). Given that there is no clear demarcation between malfunction and adaptive reactive inhibition, a judgment is made as to whether this individual is or has become more vulnerable to inhibitory reactions to circumstances, i.e. more than one would expect most people to be. Through the third window, one looks for any evidence of physical or pathological factors of relevance. If there is positive evidence through the first window, but not the second or third, then the current problem can appropriately be regarded as 'adaptive', and help focused on dealing with the situations that have provoked the adaptive reaction (e.g. stress or relationship difficulties). If there is explanatory evidence obtained through either the second or third window, the concept of 'sexual dysfunction' is appropriate. Through the second window, the dysfunction is of the 'psychosomatic trait' variety, i.e. where the characteristic responsiveness to circumstances makes that individual vulnerable. Through the third window, one is likely to be seeing factors of relatively recent onset, which may involve altered or disturbed brain mechanisms (e.g. depressive illness) or impaired physiological response systems (e.g. peripheral vascular disease), or pathological conditions which can have both peripheral and central effects (e.g. hypogonadism). Sexual side effects of drugs come into this category. It is questionable whether the effects of ageing should be seen as viewed through the second or third window. However, in this chapter, we will consider it through the third window.

The more detailed application of this approach in taking a clinical history will be considered in the next chapter, but we will use it below to organize our consideration of aetiological factors.

So far we have used the three windows to seek explanation for reduced sexual responsiveness. To what extent do they help us to identify problematic sexual behaviour, the second of our two categories of sexual problem? We can use the first two windows in a similar way, and the third window in a more limited sense. Through the first window, to what extent is someone engaging in inappropriate behaviour, such as extramarital sexuality, in ways which are both atypical for that person and understandable given current circumstances (e.g. provoked by the behaviour of one's spouse)? Through the second window, has a pattern of 'out-of-control' sexual behaviour, such as excessive use of the Internet for sexual purposes, been evident at other times in that individual's life, suggesting vulnerability? Could this be explained by a low propensity for sexual inhibition and high propensity for sexual excitation? Through the third window, is there evidence of an abnormal mental state, such as clinical depression, hypomania, obsessive–compulsive disorder or schizophrenia, which might account for a relatively recent onset of problematic sexual behaviour?

The three categories of sexual problem

The remainder of this chapter will be in three parts, focusing on three categories of sexual problem: (i) problems of reduced sexual interest or response, (ii) problematic sexual behaviour and (iii) problems with gender or sexual identity.

Problems of reduced sexual interest or responsiveness

In the next section our understanding of the psychosomatic mechanisms that lead to reduced sexual interest or responsiveness, or pain associated with sexual activity, will be summarized for men and women. The literature on the prevalence of the more common problems, as assessed in surveys, will be reviewed, followed by a brief review of the problems presented by men and women attending sexual problem clinics.

The three windows approach will then be used to look more closely at the factors that can adversely affect sexual interest and response, which need to be addressed in any comprehensive clinical assessment.

Sexual problems in men

Erectile problems

As considered in Chapter 4, there is a clear distinction between sexual arousal and orgasm/ejaculation in male sexual response. Penile erection is a tangible and crucial component of a man's experience of sexual arousal. The awareness of an erection not only signifies the sexual nature of central processes, but also acts as a powerful stimulant in the psychosomatic circle, further enhancing the arousal process. The lack of erection therefore has a significant negative effect in a situation where sexual arousal is wanted. This underlines the psychosomatic nature of ED. Whether or not there are peripheral explanations for impaired erection (e.g. vascular disease), the man's reaction will play a large part in how problematic the erectile impairment becomes. Hence we see an interaction between personality related psychological processes and peripheral physiological mechanisms. This has commonly been conceptualized as 'performance anxiety', though there is a striking lack of research on this component of male sexual dysfunction. In Chapter 4 we considered three central response patterns, each of which may be clinically relevant, although probably varying in importance across individuals: first, distraction from the sexual stimuli due to concerns about performance failure, second, insufficient reduction of inhibitory tone and, third, reactive inhibition in response to a negative appraisal of the situation. Further research may tell us whether these three patterns can be distinguished clinically. At this juncture, however, we can consider erectile difficulty as one type of male sexual problem, leaving the clinician with the need to weigh the relative importance of physical and psychological factors in each case. Erectile problems vary in severity; in some men the problem only occurs on a proportion of occasions of sexual activity. The problem may be a failure to sustain the erection after vaginal entry, some degree of erection but insufficient rigidity of erection to allow vaginal entry, or minimal or no erectile response. Variable degrees of erection with a tendency to lose erection when vaginal entry is being attempted is suggestive of inhibition being involved, with concern about performance having an adverse effect. A more or less complete absence of erectile response is suggestive of a basic failure of the erectile mechanism (e.g. from vascular or neurological impairment).

Lack of sexual desire

Sexual desire in the male is linked with erectile responsiveness for most men. 'Incentive motivation' for sex can be experienced in the absence of erection. Conversely, a man can experience lack of sexual desire without necessarily losing the capacity for erection. However, he may well need direct tactile stimulation to demonstrate that capacity. If we keep in mind the conceptual overlap between sexual desire and sexual arousal (see p. 64) then we will not be surprised to find that many men with low sexual desire also report a reduction in 'spontaneous' erections. The relationship, however, can work in the opposite direction. A man who is unable to experience erection, for whatever reason, may well find that his level of sexual interest goes down. This is an interesting form of individual variability, not as yet adequately explained. Some men persist with significant levels of sexual desire while confronted by impairment of erectile response. In other men, both decline to become consistent, although this may take some time to happen. This issue of change towards consistency between different aspects of the sexual arousal complex will be considered further in relation to women.

Premature ejaculation

The link between orgasm, seminal emission and ejaculation was considered in Chapter 4 (p. 89) where it was proposed that ejaculation results from a combination of orgasm and seminal emission, with muscular contractions as part of the orgasmic response resulting in the expulsion of the seminal emission, otherwise known as ejaculation. Clearly, in normal circumstances, arousal precedes orgasm and, in some way as yet not understood, triggers orgasm. The seminal emission is also triggered, although again the mechanism is not understood, and it is uncertain whether the 'trigger' is the same for orgasm and seminal emission. Premature ejaculation (PE) is a problem when the man is unable to delay orgasm and ejaculation as he would wish. In severe cases, not only may seminal emission precede vaginal entry, the orgasmic component may be so reduced that the usual orgasm-associated muscle spasms do not occur and the semen oozes out of the urethra rather than being 'ejaculated' (see p. 88). One possible explanation for this phenomenon is that the seminal emission is triggered at a stage when sexual arousal is minimal or absent, so that the associated orgasm, presumably linked to the seminal emission, is minimal. As yet we do not know exactly what is happening with PE, although this appears to be a specifically male phenomenon, which to some extent is common, though varying considerably in degree. What is notable is that the post-ejaculatory refractory period is in no way reduced in such cases.

Learning control of ejaculation is a normal requirement for many men; initially, when first involved in vaginal intercourse, they may ejaculate quickly as a result of their intense sexual arousal. With time, most men learn to control this, often without awareness of the learning process. For some men, however, this process of gaining control is particularly difficult, and is probably aggravated by their worrying about it.

Delayed or absent ejaculation

This is much less common than premature or rapid ejaculation. Here, the evidence from the effects of SSRIs (see p. 403), which often block orgasm in women as well as ejaculation in men, suggests that the primary problem is with the triggering of orgasm. Other variations of ejaculation sometimes occur. 'Dry-run' orgasm is when a man experiences an orgasm but no semen is ejaculated. This can be caused by drugs (see p. 87), which suggests that a specific block of seminal emission is occurring, without orgasm being affected.

Pain during sexual response

Pain associated with sexual response sometimes occurs in men. This may be associated with sexual arousal, if arousal is prolonged and not terminated by ejaculation/orgasm. In such cases the pain is usually experienced in the testes. In other cases the pain accompanies ejaculation, and a range of factors may account for this, which will be considered later. More common is 'chronic pelvic pain syndrome' which may adversely affect the man's capacity for sexual response and enjoyment, but which is not confined in its effects to sexual activity (Luzzi 2003). These varieties of male sexual pain will be considered more closely in Chapter 13 (see p. 383).

Sexual problems in women

Vaginal dryness

Conceptualizing sexual problems in women is more difficult. This is partly because of the more complex and less well-understood relationship between vaginal vasocongestion and other components of sexual arousal, which were considered closely in Chapter 4. Thus vaginal dryness may be a problem, because of the likelihood of discomfort or pain with penile entry when the vagina is not adequately lubricated. But the dryness is not necessarily accompanied by lack of sexual arousal in other respects. Conversely, a woman may experience lack of sexual arousal and yet have some degree of vaginal lubrication. Thus, in contrast to the role of penile erection in men, vaginal response is not central to the experience of sexual arousal in women. Whether clitoral engorgement would be more closely related than vaginal response remains uncertain but, in any case, it is unlikely to have the same significance as penile erection in men; women are much less aware of what is happening in their clitoris, and an erect clitoris is less crucial for their sexual interaction. The experience of lack of sexual arousal in women is not only manifested by a lack of 'excitement' in a general sense, but also a lack of enhanced pleasurable sensitivity to touch in the genital and other erotic regions of the body (e.g. breasts).

Lack of arousal and/or desire

The relationship between sexual arousal and sexual desire in women is particularly challenging. For many women, there is a clear overlap between 'desire' and arousal, i.e. awareness of 'incentive motivation' is usually accompanied by some degree of central arousal, whether or not any genital response is perceived. We also need to keep in mind that sexual desire is less well understood in women. The 'object of desire' has been little studied and may well vary considerably across women. As discussed in Chapter 6, there may be different kinds of sexual desire in women, and, if so, this has a bearing on what women experience when they complain of loss of desire, and how it should best be treated clinically. The idea was proposed that for many women the desire is 'to be desired', a manifestation of the female basic pattern (see p. 222). The incentive is the emotional engagement with a partner who desires you. In other women, the desire may be for sexual pleasure, as it is typically for men. For many women, both types of incentive may be involved. On another dimension, women may have experienced desire spontaneously and notice a reduction of such spontaneous incentive motivation, whether it is of the basic pattern type or the pleasure seeking type. For other women, desire is 'receptive' or 'reactive', i.e. the desire is stimulated by the sexual approach of one's partner. Some women may experience both spontaneous and receptive desire at different times. Low sexual desire is therefore a heterogeneous problem category for women, requiring considerable clinical assessment before relevant determinants, and hence the most likely form of effective treatment, can be identified. In some cases, there is considerable overlap with problems of sexual arousal. In other cases, the capacity for sexual arousal may be relatively unaffected, whereas the desire to experience it is reduced.

Problems with orgasm

As in men, relationship between sexual arousal and orgasm, and in particular the trigger mechanism that leads from arousal to orgasm, are not understood. As discussed in Chapter 4, the capacity to have orgasm triggered probably varies considerably across women; some progress readily to orgasm if sufficient arousal occurs, others may require more specific or intense stimulation to make the transition and yet other women experience the transition rarely or never. So in identifying a problem, one needs first to assess to what extent sexual arousal occurs. It is only appropriate to see the problem as orgasmic if it is clear that sexual arousal that would normally precede the orgasm is not itself a problem.

Pain during sexual activity

Also known as dyspareunia, this is a much more common and important problem for women than for men. Pain may be experienced following any tactile stimulation of the vulva (e.g. vulvo-vestibulitis) or associated with vaginal penetration by an erect penis or finger (e.g. vaginismus) or with deep thrusting during vaginal intercourse (e.g. endometriosis). Careful diagnostic assessment is required to determine the cause of such pain and is described in detail in Chapter 12. The various gynaecological or medical causes of pain are further considered in Chapter 13.

Vaginismus is a term used to describe an apparent obstruction which makes vaginal penetration by a penis, and usually a finger or tampon, difficult or impossible, and which, according to conventional clinical wisdom, results from contraction of the pelvic floor muscles surrounding the outer third of the vagina (see p. 34). Attempts to penetrate may cause pain, and hence this needs to be distinguished from other causes of dyspareunia.

Vigorous debate is in progress about how best to conceptualize dyspareunia and vaginismus, and this will be considered more closely in the later section on understanding sexual problems.

Persistent genital arousal disorder (PGAD)

This is a recently recognized but fairly uncommon problem, also referred to as persistent sexual arousal disorder. It was first reported by Leiblum & Nathan (2001), who identified five descriptive features: (i) genital and breast vasocongestion and sensitivity, persisting for hours or days, (ii) which resolve only temporarily following orgasm and may require multiple orgasms to obtain relief; (iii) the feelings of genital response are unassociated with any sense of sexual desire or excitement, (iv) are intrusive and disturbing and (v) can be triggered by a variety of non-sexual stimuli. With further evidence, obtained in an Internet-based survey, cases have also been reported where orgasms occur spontaneously and maybe frequently. No consistent cause for this syndrome has been identified, though some cases are apparently related to medication use (Leiblum 2007). There is also an interesting distinction to be made between women who experience this disturbing problem and those who get spontaneous vaginal response that is relatively pleasant and not so intrusive and persistent (Leiblum et al 2007a). One possible reason for the distinction is a paradoxical relationship between negative mood and sexual response in the first group (Leiblum et al 2007b). We will return to this possibility later. At present there is no evidence of the prevalence of PGAD but it appears to be relatively rare.

The move towards consistency

In terms of categorizing sexual problems in women, there is also the issue of consistency between the various components of the sexual response cycle over time, referred to briefly in the above section on male problems. In an early study (Bancroft et al 1982), we compared the patterns of sexual response in women with and without sexual problems. We concluded that for most women sexuality presents a consistent pattern of 'goodness' or 'badness'. Lack of sexual desire, arousal and orgasm tend to go together. However, this consistent pattern may take time to become established, and how the woman presents her problem may depend on when in this developmental sequence she is assessed. This point can be illustrated with a fairly common scenario. In the early stages of a relationship in which the man has a tendency to ejaculate rapidly, the woman becomes sexually aroused, lubricates, experiences pleasure, but is left unsatisfied as the sequence is terminated prematurely by the rapid ejaculation. Over a period of time, which may take years, the absence of a satisfying orgasm may change into a lack of sexual arousal, and subsequently into a loss of sexual desire. The 'consistency' may, however, vary across women; for some women, experiencing orgasm is unimportant, and other, more relational factors determine whether she is left unsatisfied, and whether this develops into a more consistent pattern of low desire and low arousal. This change towards consistency may therefore occur in a variety of contexts, and needs to be carefully evaluated during clinical assessment. But its developmental nature is of crucial clinical importance, as the factor that needs to be changed may have been more evident at an earlier stage of the relationship.

Prevalence of problems in the community

Simons & Carey (2001) reviewed 52 studies, published in the previous 10 years, reporting the prevalence of sexual dysfunctions. There was considerable variability in prevalence rates across studies. It was pointed out that more than a third of the studies provided no definition of the dysfunctions they reported, and of those claiming to be using DSM-IV criteria, most failed to do so for one reason or another. Similar difficulty in comparing prevalence rates across studies, particular studies of women, was reported by Fugl-Meyer & Fugl-Meyer (2006), reviewing European studies, and Paik & Laumann (2006) reviewing studies from the USA. Graham & Bancroft (2006) concluded that using normal community-based surveys to identify sexual dysfunction, whether according to DSM-IV criteria or not, was not feasible; there is insufficient detailed evidence to allow a clinical diagnosis to be made. Surveys can be useful, however, in assessing the association between the reporting of sexual problems and factors of potential causal relevance. In the next section we consider relevant findings from a number of representative community samples.

Data from the NHSLS survey (Laumann et al 1999) were mentioned earlier, and its unsuitability for identifying sexual dysfunction was emphasized. However, it is a valuable data set in its own right. It also warrants comparison with results from the British NATSAL 2000 (Mercer et al 2003) and the Australian Study of Health and Relationships (ASHR; Richters et al 2003). These used exactly the same questions, except for differences in how the

duration of the problem was assessed, which are of considerable relevance, and there were some differences in inclusion criteria. In the NHSLS, for each of the items, the respondent was asked 'During the last 12 months has there been a period *of several months or more* when you...,' with a yes or no answer. NATSAL, using the same questions, offered two response options: (i) *lasting at least one month* in the past year and (ii) *lasting at least six months* in the past year, which they termed a 'persistent' problem. In the ASHR, the question was 'During the last year has there been a period of one month or more when...'. In the NHSLS and NATSAL studies, analysis was restricted to those who had at least one sexual partner in the previous year; in the NATSAL this was at least one heterosexual partner. The ASHR reported on those who were sexually active (including masturbation), and in the case of questions about sex with a partner, only those 'who had a partner'. The findings from these three surveys, and others cited in this chapter, are shown in Table 11.1.

Laumann et al (1999) considered anyone who answered 'Yes' to any of their questions to be experiencing sexual dysfunction. Mercer et al (2003) more prudently interpreted the positive responses from the NATSAL as 'self-reported problems related to sexual function' rather than sexual dysfunction. Richters et al (2003) used the term 'sexual difficulties' to refer to 'a range of conditions relevant to sexual satisfaction' and opened their paper with a strong critique of the concept of sexual dysfunction.

The comparison of the two durations from the NATSAL is striking. For each item, the percentage reporting a problem for at least 1 month during the past year is substantially higher than those reporting persistent problems (at least 6 months). This is not surprising, but it emphasizes the extent to which alteration of sexual interest or function can be short term, consistent with the problem being reactive to current circumstances, and hence less likely to reflect a 'dysfunction' as defined above. When comparing the NATSAL to the NHSLS data, 'lacked interest in sex', the most commonly

TABLE 11.1	Percentage reporting sexual problems in the past year from the NHSLS (Laumann et al 1999), NATSAL 2000 (Mercer et al 2003) and Richters et al (2003)							
	NHSLS		**NATSAL**				**ASHR**	
	≥**Several months**		≥**1 month**		≥**6 months**		≥**1 month**	
	Men	**Women**	**Men**	**Women**	**Men**	**Women**	**Men**	**Women**
n =	1410	1749	4888*	4826*	4877*	4818*	8517*	8280*
Lacked interest in having sex	3.0	33.4	17.1	40.6	1.8	10.2	24.9	54.8
Were unable to come to a climax[†]	8.3	24.1	5.3	14.4	0.7	3.7	6.3	28.6
Came to a climax too quickly[†]	28.5	10.3	11.7	1.3	2.9	0.2	23.8	11.7
Experienced pain during intercourse	3.0	14.4	1.7	11.8	0.3	3.4	2.4	20.3
Did not find sex pleasurable	8.1	21.2	–	–	–	–	5.6	27.3
Felt anxious about performance	17.0	11.5	9.0	6.7	1.8	1.5	16.0	17.0
Had trouble achieving or maintaining an erection (men)	10.4	–	5.8	–	0.8	–	9.5	–
Had trouble lubricating (women)	–	18.8	–	9.2	–	2.6	–	23.9
At least one of the above problems	31.0	43.0	34.8	53.8	6.2	15.6	46.5	70.9

*Weighted
[†]'Experience an orgasm' was added to this item

reported problem, was consistent across the two studies; it was much higher in women than men, with the NHSLS percentages for 'at least several months' coming between the 'at least 1 month' and 'at least 6 months' figures from NATSAL. For the other items, however, the percentages were higher in the NHSLS than for the 'at least 1 month' figure for NATSAL. The reasons for this are not clear. The higher rates in the Australian survey for lack of sexual interest and the composite variable (at least one problem in past year) may reflect differences in the inclusion criteria (e.g. including individuals who masturbated but did not have a sexual partner).

One important difference between the three samples is the age range; the NHSLS range was 18 to 55 years; NATSAL, 16 to 44 years; ASHR, 16 to 59 years. This could help to explain the higher rates in the NHSLS, although it is not clear why this should be so for 'came to a climax too quickly' in men, which does not show an increase with age. There was also a curious difference for women on this variable. It is unusual for women to complain of 'coming too quickly', yet 10.3% in NHSLS (Laumann et al 1994) and 11.7% of the Australian sample reported this, compared to 1.3% in NATSAL. This item was not included in the later NHSLS paper (Laumann et al 1999). This raises methodological questions about what appear to be almost identical items in these three surveys.

The composite variable of 'at least one of the above problems' (the origin of '43% of women having a sexual dysfunction') shows much higher rates for women than for men in all three studies and duration categories. Laumann et al (1999) reported on the association between these various sexual problems and other factors of possible causal relevance. Age had a clear effect in men, with older men reporting more lack of sexual interest, erectile problems and difficulty ejaculating. For women, in contrast, problems were more likely in the younger age groups, particularly pain during sex and anxiety about sex. Being married, and also having more education, was associated with fewer sexual problems in both men and women. Black women were more likely than white women to report lack of sexual desire, but less likely to report pain or lubrication problems. Hispanic women were generally less likely to report problems, and Hispanic men were less likely to report anxiety about sex. Laumann et al (1999) also carried out latent class analyses to group their sexual problems into categories. This resulted in three categories for each gender: low desire, arousal disorder and sexual pain for women, and PE, ED and low sexual desire for men. Men with poor health were more likely to report each of the three male categories, whereas this association was only evident for 'sexual pain' in women. Economic problems (e.g. decrease in family income) increased likelihood for all three categories in women but only ED in men. Men with liberal attitudes about sex were more likely to report PE. Overall, emotional and stress-related problems were associated with increased likelihood of sexual difficulties in all phases of the sexual response cycle, although these associations were stronger in women. Associations between childhood experiences of sexual abuse or exploitation and arousal disorder in women and ED and PE in men were found, and are considered further in Chapter 16.

Richters et al (2003) reported on the associations between 'sexual difficulties' in their subjects and age, and the following are significant. In men, lack of sexual interest was least frequent in the 20–29 year and most frequent in the 50–59 year age group. Men over 40 were more likely to report problems with erections and difficulty in ejaculating. PE was not associated with age. For women, lack of sexual interest was least likely in the 16–19 year group, but did not differ significantly between the other age groups. Women aged 50–59 were more likely than younger women to report orgasm difficulty. Older women were more likely to report vaginal dryness but, interestingly, pain during sex was reported more by younger women. Older women worried less about their body looking unattractive during sex (not shown in Table 11.1). Among other variables assessed, men with poorer physical health, or taking medication for cardiovascular disease or hypertension, were more likely to report sexual difficulties, although, somewhat surprisingly, no association was found with diabetes. Women with poorer physical health or a physical disability were more likely to report a sexual difficulty. No significant association was found for the use of medication for cardiovascular disease or hypertension, or the diagnosis of diabetes.

Mercer et al (2005) also examined possible predictors of reported sexual problems in the NATSAL 2000 survey. These problems will be referred to in the following summary as 'brief' (for at least 1 month in the past year) and 'persistent' (at least 6 months in the past year). They found no clear association between age and reporting of 'brief' problems for either men or women. The more persistent problems, however, increased with age for both men and women. Married and co-habiting men were less likely than single men to report 'brief' sexual problems; for women it was the other way round. After controlling for age, marital status was not associated with persistent problems in either men or women. Women with young children were more likely to report both brief and persistent sexual problems. Neither racial group nor level of education was predictive. Both men and women who found it difficult to talk about sex with their partner were more likely to report both brief and persistent problems. Men with poor health were more likely to report both brief and persistent problems; in women this was apparent only for brief problems and this was only marginally significant. A strong negative association was found between being 'sexually competent at first sexual experience' and reporting problems, both brief and persistent. 'Sexually competent' was a composite variable, covering absence of duress or regret, autonomy of decision and use of a reliable method of contraception at first sexual intercourse. Both this and the variable referring to difficulties in talking about sex point to the importance of personality factors and early learning of some kind. Overall, these findings also have to be interpreted cautiously because of uncertainty about the direction of causality. But the distinction between brief and persistent enhances their relevance.

While these findings are of value and interest, it is important to keep in mind that they are based on very limited information about sexual problems, raising the possibility that some of the predictors (e.g. education) may have influenced how the questions were answered more than indicating what the individuals had actually experienced. It is also difficult, as the authors acknowledge, to be sure of the direction of causality in several of the significant associations.

The French ACSF (Spira et al 1994) included limited questions about sexual dysfunctions, although more detailed for men than women. They distinguished between a problem being experienced 'often' and 'sometimes'. The results are presented in Table 11.2. In view of the way the likelihood of a problem was assessed (e.g. how does one decide between often and sometimes; how similar are people's decisions in this respect) it is difficult to compare these findings with the NHSLS or NATSAL. It is perhaps reasonable to conclude that the choice of 'often' indicates that it is problematic. Unfortunately, no assessment of the associations between these variables and others of possible causal relevance has yet been published.

It will be increasingly apparent, as we move through this chapter, that the identification of sexual dysfunction, as defined earlier, and the distinction from reactive problems, is more challenging for women than for men. Osborn et al (1988), in an interview study of 436 English women aged 35 to 59 and in a sexual relationship, derived operationally defined problems of impaired sexual interest, infrequent orgasm, dyspareunia and vaginal dryness. Thirty-three per cent met the criteria for one or more of these problems. In addition, they asked each woman whether she regarded herself as having a sexual problem; only 10% of women answered 'yes', and nearly a third of those did not meet any of the authors' operational criteria for the 'problem'. Fugl-Meyer & Fugl-Meyer (1999), in a 1996 survey of 1335 Swedish women, aged 18–74, identified 'sexual disabilities' in terms of sexual interest, vaginal lubrication, orgasm and dyspareunia. Each of these questions was followed by the question 'Has this been a problem in your sexual life during the past year?'. Forty-seven per cent met the criteria for one or more of the disabilities, but the proportion of each disability group where the woman regarded the disability as a problem varied from 69% for dyspareunia to 43% for decreased interest. Dunn et al (1998) studied a sample of 979 English women aged 18 to 75, 75% of whom were married. They were asked 'On what proportion of occasions that you made love in the past 3 months did you have a problem being aroused?'. There were four response categories: 'never', 'rarely', 'often' and 'always'. A further question asked about how often climax was experienced. Questions about experiencing pain or vaginal dryness were answered yes or no, with no indication of frequency. Forty-one per cent of women were identified as having a problem in at least one of these four respects. Apart from the question on sexual arousal, which referred to 'having a problem', there was no indication whether the women themselves regarded these operationally defined problems as problems. Women were asked, however, if they would like to receive help for sexual problems if it was available; 39% said yes, but only 46% of those women were in the operationally defined problem groups.

Because of this recurring lack of concordance between what researchers consider a sexual problem or dysfunction and what the woman herself thinks, a deliberate attempt was made in the recent Kinsey Institute survey (Bancroft et al 2003a) to assess these two issues separately, so that associations between them could be more closely assessed. In this survey all women were in a heterosexual relationship of at least 6 months' duration. The intention was to avoid using questions which implied problems (e.g. 'Do you have a problem with . . . ?'). Instead we asked women to indicate whether they were distressed or worried about (a) their sexual relationship and (b) their own sexuality, without asking why. In addition, we asked detailed questions about their sexual experiences during the last 4 weeks. Having established how often sexual interaction with the partner had occurred, a series of questions asked on how many of those occasions specific responses occurred (e.g. pleasant genital sensations, feeling aroused or excited, feeling pleasure or enjoyment, having vaginal lubrication, experiencing an orgasm, or pain or discomfort). Also, on how many of the occasions did her partner have erectile difficulties or rapid ejaculation? Sexual interest was assessed separately; 'During the past 4 weeks, about how often did you think about sex with interest or desire?'. Response options were 'not at all', 'once or twice, 'once a week', 'several times a week', 'at least once a day'. Care was taken to avoid response options with problematic implications (like 'often' versus 'sometimes' or 'rarely'). Marked distress about the sexual relationship was reported by 19.8% and about their own sexuality by 14.7% of women; 24.4% reported marked distress about either their sexual relationship, their own sexuality or both.

We then defined 'problems' as the relative absence of specific responses (or lack of sexual interest) during the past 4 weeks. The detailed results are reported in Bancroft et al (2003a); the following are some examples. Seventy-one women (7.2% of the sample) reported no sexual thoughts during the past month. Of these women,

TABLE 11.2	Sexual problems as reported by sexually active men and women in the ACSF (Spira et al 1994)		
		Often (%)	Sometimes (%)
MEN			
You do not have an erection (impotence)		7	12
You ejaculate too early, even before entering your partner		5	16
You ejaculate too soon, on or shortly after entering your partner		10	27
It takes you too long to ejaculate once you have entered your partner		4	16
You fail to ejaculate at all		2	5
You don't have an orgasm		7	7
You feel no or insufficient sexual desire		3	16
WOMEN			
You have painful intercourse		5	10
You don't have an orgasm		11	21
You feel no or insufficient sexual desire		8	33

32% reported marked distress about their relationship, and 24% about their own sexuality. Impaired sexual response was indicated by feeling aroused, feeling pleasant tingling in the genitals and enjoying the genitals being touched on less than 50% of occasions. Ninety-eight of the sexually active women (12.2%) were in this category; of these 41% reported marked distress about their sexual relationship, and 29% about their own sexuality. 69 women (9.3%) had no orgasm during sexual activity with their partner; of these, 41% reported marked distress about their sexual relationship, and 35% about their own sexuality. In each type of problem, as defined by the researchers, a substantial proportion of women reported no marked distress about either their sexual relationship or their own sexuality.

Using multinomial logit, we explored predictors of the two types of sexual distress. The strongest predictor of both types of distress was the measure of mental health (MCS12). Physical health, as measured by the PCS12, was also predictive, but more strongly for 'own sexuality' than 'sexual relationship'. Of the five indicators of the woman's response during sexual activity, subjective response during sexual activity was a strong predictor of distress about the sexual relationship ($p < 0.001$), and less strongly of distress about own sexuality ($p < 0.05$). This composite variable was derived from (i) feeling emotionally close to partner 80% or more of the time, (ii) feeling indifferent less than 20% of the time and (iii) having unpleasant feelings less than 20% of the time. Impaired physical response (defined above) was just significant in predicting distress about the relationship ($p = 0.04$), but not for distress about their own sexuality. Frequency of orgasm, difficulties with vaginal lubrication and pain during sex were not predictive of either. As discussed earlier (p. 211) 'frequency of sexual thoughts' was modestly significant in predicting distress, but paradoxically, it was more frequent thoughts (thinking about sex every day) that were predictive, and only of distress about the relationship.

In a British study, King et al (2007) assessed 401 women attending their general practitioner, asking questions about their sexual experiences in the last 4 weeks, and any associated difficulties. They applied ICD-criteria of sexual dysfunction and also asked the women whether they considered themselves to have a sexual problem. According to the ICD-10 criteria, 38% of women had a diagnosis of sexual dysfunction. However, only 18% of women qualified for the diagnosis *and* considered themselves to have a sexual problem, and only 6% regarded the problem as moderate or severe. Twenty per cent of women were diagnosed as having a sexual dysfunction but did not consider themselves to have a problem, 19% had a problem but did not meet the criteria for sexual dysfunction and 42% had neither a problem nor a diagnosis. Although a clinician would not make a diagnosis of sexual dysfunction on the basis of 1 month's sexual activity, this study is further evidence of the limited overlap between definitions of female sexual dysfunction and how women conceptualize sexual problems

Overall, where these associations have been explored in women, we find the reporting of sexual problems is more clearly associated with the level of general wellbeing and quality of the relationship than with aspects of the woman's sexual interest or physiological sexual response. Obviously, we have to be cautious in drawing conclusions about the direction of causality in these associations. It is also important to understand the relevance of distress to the diagnosis of a sexual dysfunction. Distress indicates the woman's concern about her sexual relationship or her own sexuality; it does not help in understanding the reasons for that concern and is of limited relevance in distinguishing between a problem and a dysfunction. The absence of distress, in a woman who has no sexual desire or sexual responsiveness, does not exclude the existence of a dysfunction, though it is of obvious relevance in terms of clinical needs and management. We will return to this issue at the end of the chapter when we consider current views of the diagnostic classification of sexual dysfunctions.

People who attend sexual problem clinics and their problems

Given the variable associations between sexual function and the individual's perception of a sexual problem, it is of some interest and relevance to look at the problems for which men and women seek help when they attend a sexual problem clinic. Such people have not only recognized a problem in their sexual lives, they have taken the step of seeking help for it. For most such clinics, the patient has usually gone through one or more steps before getting there, e.g. consulted with their general practitioner or a specialist, such as a gynaecologist, who has made the referral. In a proportion of cases it is the patient who makes initial contact with the specialist clinic.

In the last edition of this book, I referred to a report on referrals to a co-ordinated group of sexual problem clinics in Edinburgh between 1981 and 1983 (Warner et al 1987). Since then a number of reports of sexual problem clinic attenders within the UK have been published. As the Edinburgh sample remains the largest, the results from this will be presented in some detail, followed by a comparison with the more recent studies.

The various Edinburgh clinics were situated in gynaecological and psychiatric outpatient departments, a family planning clinic and a local marriage guidance centre. They were all specifically for sexual problems. There were 1194 referrals during that time. The percentage of males presenting was 45% and of females 48%. In 7%, both partners had problems and presented as a couple. In 56% of cases, the referral was by general practitioners, 10% were self-referred, while the remainder came from a variety of agencies, including hospital consultants. The types of problems presented are shown in Table 11.3.

For men, ED was clearly the most commonly presented problem, whilst low sexual desire was relatively infrequent, and it was rare for men to complain principally of lack of sexual enjoyment. In women low sexual interest was the most common.

Table 11.4 lists the problems regarded as most important in each case, but also the extent to which they co-occurred with other problems. In the Edinburgh

TABLE 11.3 Principal problems of men and women presenting at a sexual problem service in Edinburgh (problems of those presenting as couples, both with problems of equal importance, are not included)

Male problems	%	Female problems	%
Low sexual interest	7	Low sexual interest	35
Lack of enjoyment	1	Lack of enjoyment	12
Other orgasmic problems	5	Orgasmic dysfunction	7
Dyspareunia	1	Dyspareunia	11
Erectile failure	50	Vaginismus	13
Premature ejaculation	13	Sexual aversion	3
			3
Problems relating to homosexuality	3	Problems relating to homosexuality	0.2
Transsexualism	4	Transsexualism	2
Sexual deviance	2		
Sexual offences	3		
Miscellaneous	12	Miscellaneous	15
Total	100		100
	(n = 533)		(n = 577)

TABLE 11.4 The most common types of sexual problems in men and women attending a sexual problem clinic, showing the main problem, associated problems (ranked second or third) and the percentage for whom a problem was listed amongst the first five (from Warner et al 1987)

			Male presenters				
Problem	**Main complaint**	**Problem listed (max. 5)**	**Associated problem ranked second or third (% of row)**				
	(n = 535) (% of total)	(n = 615*) (% of total)	**Low interest**	**Low enjoyment**	**Erectile failure**	**Premature ejaculation**	**Other orgasmic problem**
Low interest	6	16		13	32	12	
Erectile failure	50	54	11			15	
Premature ejaculation	13	24			18		

			Female presenters				
Problem	**Main complaint**	**Problem listed (max. 5)**	**Associated problem ranked second or third (% of row)**				
	(n = 577) (% of total)	(n = 657*) (% of total)	**Low interest**	**Low enjoyment**	**Orgasmic dysfunction**	**Dyspareunia**	**Vaginismus**
Low interest	36	49		50	16	13	
Low enjoyment	12	38	46		24	18	
Orgasmic dysfunction	7	20	20	24			
Dyspareunia	11	20	20	27			
Vaginismus	14	15		10		17	

*In this column, men and women presenting as couples are also included, producing a larger n.

survey it was possible to specify up to five problems, ranked in order of importance, for each individual. The first ranked problem is shown as the main complaint. The second column in Table 11.4 shows the percentage of presenters for whom the complaint was indicated amongst the five choices, and second and third rank problems are also shown. In men we see that PE was an additional problem in 15% of men with erectile failure, whereas erectile problems were present in 18% of men with PE as their main problem. A third of men with low sexual interest also had erectile failure. Amongst the women we see a strong association between low interest and low enjoyment, though in part this reflected a common difficulty in women in making a clear distinction between the two. We see that more women have orgasmic dysfunction as a secondary problem than as the main complaint, so that in all, 20% of women had this difficulty to some extent.

The most striking impression from these tables is the extent to which men complain principally of problems with their genital responses (i.e. erection or ejaculation) whereas women predominantly complain of lack of interest or enjoyment, i.e. the subjective quality of the sexual experience. This is entirely consistent with the more recent evidence reviewed earlier. There were important relationships between sexual problems and age. In general male presenters were older than female (Fig. 11.1); of the men, those presenting with PE were younger than those with ED (Fig. 11.2). The age distributions for the main types of female problem are shown in Figure 11.3. The bimodal distribution for orgasmic dysfunction may reflect the different age of presentation of primary and secondary

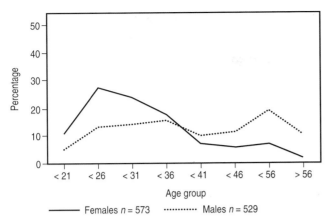

Fig. 11.1 Age distribution of men and women presenting at sexual problem clinics in Edinburgh. The two distributions differ; $p < 0.001$. (From Warner et al 1987.)

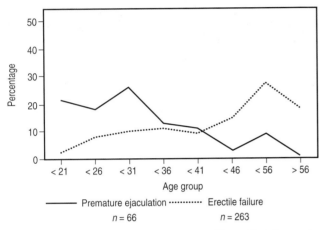

Fig. 11.2 Age distribution of men presenting with erectile failure and premature ejaculation. The two distributions differ; $p < 0.001$. (From Warner et al 1987.)

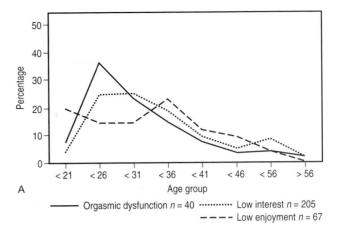

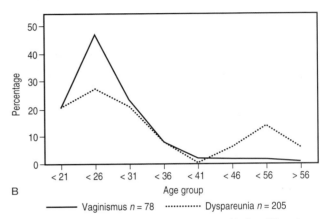

Fig. 11.3 Age distribution of women presenting with five different complaints at sexual dysfunction clinics. (From Warner et al 1987.)

problems; unfortunately this survey did not make that distinction. The bimodal distribution for dyspareunia, with a second peak in the older age group, reflects the post-menopausal causes of this problem (see p. 246).

There were some differences in the pattern of referrals to the differently situated clinics. Thus 70% of cases of dyspareunia and 44% of vaginismus were referred to the clinic in the gynaecology department, whereas the majority of problems relating to deviant sexuality or sexual offences were referred to the psychiatrically-based clinic.

Catalan et al (1990) reported a consecutive series of 200 couples referred to the Oxford Sexual Problems clinic, based in the psychiatric outpatients department. Bancroft & Coles (1976) published an earlier report from this same clinic. The gender ratio for those with the presenting sexual problems was almost identical, and the problems were very similar in their proportions to those from the Edinburgh study. The age difference between male and female presenters was also similar. An important finding was that around a third of the couples were having significant marital or relationship problems, though it was often not easy to establish the causal relations between these and the sexual problem. This information was not provided by Warner et al (1987) for the Edinburgh sample.

Hirst et al (1996) reported a series of 458 referrals to the Guy's Hospital Sexual Problem Clinic in London, for the period from 1989 to 1993. This clinic is run by the Department of Psychiatry, but deals with sexual problems with both physical and psychological causal factors. There were some similarities and differences when compared with the Edinburgh sample. The gender ratio was different; 66.2% men and 32.8% women. The frequencies of presenting problems were similar. Of the 303 men, 40.2% presented with ED, 11.2% with PE, 8.9% with low sexual desire, 3.3% with delayed/absent ejaculation (DE) and 1% with dyspareunia. Of the 155 women, 35.5% presented with low sexual desire, 15.5% with vaginismus, 14.2% with dyspareunia, 4.5% with anorgasmia and 1.9% with arousal difficulties. However, 17.4% of the women (and 2.3% of the men) were categorized as 'childhood sexual abuse', with no further details of how their sexual lives were currently affected. The age distributions were similar, although the distribution for men presenting with ED showed a clear peak in the 25–30-year group and a further larger peak between 55 and 65 years. This may reflect an increase in help-seeking by younger men as a result of new developments in treatment for ED.

Hems & Crowe (1999) reported a consecutive series of 135 patients referred during 1996 to the Maudsley Hospital Psychosexual Dysfunction Clinic in London. Their findings were similar to those of Hirst et al (1996).

In the UK, another source of counseling for sexual problems is from marriage guidance centres, most of which, since the 1970s, have included counselors trained in sex therapy. Roy (2004) reported a survey of 131 of the sex therapists in Relate, the English, Welsh and Northern Irish marriage guidance service, who gave information about 592 cases, 86% of which involved couples. An important difference from the earlier studies was that close to 50% of cases were self-referrals to Relate. In the NHS-based clinics in the previous studies, the large majority would be referred by a health professional. In 51% the woman was considered to have the main sexual problem, 28% the man, 21% both partners. Of the male presenters, 23% had low sexual desire, 30% erectile problems and 19% PE. However, a further 24% had more than one problem, and details of these were not reported. For the female presenters, 53% had low sexual desire, 24% vaginismus, 7% anorgasmia, 4% dyspareunia and 12.5% more than one problem (not otherwise specified). It is difficult from this paper to establish the ages of those who had the presenting problem, and somewhat surprisingly, the proportion with marital or relationship problems other than sexual was not reported.

Overall, there is some consistency across these studies. Erectile problems continue to be most commonly presented by men, and PE next most frequent. There may have been a change to more younger men seeking help for erectile problems, and possibly fewer men seeking help for PE. The Relate study also raises the possibility that men are now more likely to seek help for low sexual interest. This needs to be replicated. With women, low sexual interest remains the most commonly presented problem, and with a continuing tendency for younger women to be seeking help. Lack of enjoyment, as a complaint, has not been reported in the more recent studies.

Understanding problems of reduced interest or responsiveness

The focus of this section of the book, and indeed much of the book, is to further our understanding of sexual problems so that we can better explain why they occur and how to treat them. The conventional process of diagnostic classification, while ostensibly intended to have the same outcomes, is not used to structure this chapter. The reasons for this, together with a tentative proposal for an alternative approach to diagnostic classification, will be considered later (p. 336). The scheme that follows makes use of the three windows approach described earlier.

Through the first window — the current situation

In this section we focus on the various circumstantial factors, particularly those relevant to the sexual relationship, which can impact on an individual's sexual responsiveness and hence the couple's sexual interaction.

Feeling secure and 'letting go'

In order for sexual arousal to occur and to allow it to continue to orgasm, the individual needs to 'let go' and to some extent lose control. In a sexual relationship there is the additional need to feel safe enough to allow these things to happen in front of another person. Even when there are no physiological problems with our sexual response systems, the sexually aroused state makes us vulnerable and requires a lowering of our defenses. We are vulnerable because we let go but also because we may be seen to fail. For the woman, orgasm is a particular challenge in this respect requiring her to let go and momentarily lose control; for the man, his sense of vulnerability is more about not responding sufficiently or ejaculating too quickly. Any factors that reduce this sense of security and trust are likely to have negative sexual consequences.

Expectations of sex

Men tend to assume that they will ejaculate during love-making and to regard this as the end of active proceedings. Women are less likely to assume that their orgasm, if they experience one, brings love-making to a halt; this in part reflects the differences in the post-orgasmic refractory period in the two sexes (see p. 90) but is not simply a physiological difference. The importance of orgasm, particularly to women, varies considerably. Many women are content not to experience orgasm, at least not every time. Others are put under pressure from their partners to 'come' as if it were a test of the male's potency.

Communicating about sex

A fundamental requirement for a good sexual relationship to be sustained over time is the ability for both partners to communicate what they like and what they do not like. It is commonplace for one partner to assume that he or she knows what the other partner likes or enjoys, and because their partner enjoyed something on a previous occasion, they would always enjoy it. This issue commonly contributes to the establishment and continuation of problems. Both partners should be able to indicate, on any occasion, what they would like to do, and what they would prefer not to do. This two-way communication needs to be in place, and is often one of the goals of treatment; it is one application of the 'self-assert and self-protect' principal that is fundamental to any intimate relationship (see p. 347).

Misunderstandings and lack of information

Particularly important are misinformed beliefs about what is 'normal' and hence desirable. Norms about frequency of sexual intercourse may impose pressure on a couple who lag behind the national average. It is commonly believed that it is normal for both partners to reach orgasm at the same time; anything else is failure. The woman who requires clitoral stimulation for orgasm may believe herself to be abnormal or immature. Certain positions during intercourse may be seen as normal, anything else as 'kinky' and hence unacceptable. A couple may not realize that their enjoyment of oral sex is widely shared and fear that they are in some way peculiar for engaging in it.

As a couple gets older, the woman may misinterpret her male partner's normal decline in erectile responsiveness as evidence of loss of love or sexual attraction to her, still assuming that a normal man should get a full erection without his partner touching his penis. In some cultures, the man believes that each time he ejaculates he is losing some of his irreplaceable life-energy. Many other examples could be given.

Simple lack of knowledge about the elementary anatomy and physiology of sex can lead to problems. As described in Chapter 12, most sex therapists spend 20 to 30 minutes in an early treatment session going through the basics of sexual anatomy and response. It is nevertheless important to be cautious about attributing too much to simple ignorance. Whereas learning of sexual technique is normally necessary, even amongst animals, failure to learn may stem from more than lack of appropriate education. Acknowledging ignorance may be easier for some people than acknowledging fear or guilt. Sometimes the change that follows a simple provision of information is as much a consequence of the 'permission' that implicitly (or explicitly) accompanies that information.

Unsuitable circumstances and lack of time

The middle-class, reasonably affluent sex therapist usually has an image of good sex that, if it does not involve making love under a warm sun on a tropical beach, at least requires privacy and comfort. All too often, less affluent sexual partners have neither privacy nor comfort for their lovemaking. Living in over-crowded conditions, they may have children sleeping in the same room or able to hear much of what happens through the walls. What private space they can find may be cold and uncomfortable. It is important to recognize that such situational factors can be of primary importance.

For both the affluent and the less affluent, pressure of work may seriously interfere with one's sex life, which becomes squeezed into those few minutes remaining between a full and exhausting day and a fitful sleep. The rejuvenation of sexual feelings that so often happens on holiday is testimony to the negative effects of our day-to-day pressures. Our sexual relationships, if they are to flourish, have to be nourished with adequate time in the right circumstances.

Concerns about pregnancy

Fear of pregnancy, of an understandable and rational kind, has probably succeeded in spoiling more sexual relationships than any other single factor. In the days before effective birth control was available, and when there was a comparatively high maternal and infant mortality, it was perhaps surprising that women were able to develop relaxed, enjoyable sexual relationships at all. Much of the emergence of female sexuality in the second half of the 20th century must be attributed to the liberating effect of modern contraception. There are nevertheless some women for whom sex cannot be comfortably separated from reproduction. Only when there is some risk of conception are they able to enjoy sex. If such a woman is also fearful of the practical consequences of having more children then she is certainly likely to have difficulty in her sexual relationship. Sometimes the male partner may be keen to have a child, or another child, and hence is opposed to the use of contraception. This is a major issue in some cultures. Women may go along with this, but as a consequence may be less able to enjoy their sexual interactions.

Couples who are striving to get pregnant, organizing their sexual activity around the fertile phase of the woman's cycle, may find that their normal capacity for letting go and enjoying their love-making is impaired.

Concerns about sexually transmitted infections

There is good evidence that the use of a condom, as a barrier to sexually transmitted infection, is less likely in those who regard their relationship as established (see Chapter 15). The non-use is a form of declaration of commitment. However, fears of infection, or of the infidelity of one's partner increasing the risk of infection, may arise and undermine the sense of security needed for sexual response and enjoyment.

Low self-esteem and negative mood

Our ability to feel safe and comfortable when relating to a sexual partner is lessened if we are feeling bad about ourselves — if something has happened to lower our self-esteem. This may be specifically related to body image — we may feel uncomfortable with our specific bodies, dislike their shape, thinking they are too fat or too thin or just not attractive. This is probably more often an issue for women, who rely more on their physical appearance for their self-esteem than men do. If a man is experiencing failure in his job, he feels less effective, less potent as a man and this can adversely affect his sexual relationship. Sometimes the problem is compounded by a need to reassert himself sexually when he is failing to do so in other ways — a return to the adolescent use of sex as a self-esteem booster. Sometimes low self-esteem is best understood as a symptom of a depressive illness, which will be considered later.

As reviewed earlier, there is consistent evidence of a relationship between negative mood, particularly depression, and sexual problems in women. There is also such evidence for men but less frequent, reflecting the fact that, particularly for those in mid-life, episodes of depression are more common in women than in men. The direction of causality is by no means clear in such associations, but it is a reasonable assumption that in the majority of cases the sexual problem is either caused or aggravated by the negative mood. The extent to which the negative mood can be explained as a reaction to other current circumstances, is also variable, and a crucial aspect of psychiatric assessment in such cases. The complex and variable relationships between different types of negative mood and sexual response and interest were considered in Chapter 4 (p. 106) and as a source of individual variability will be considered further below, as viewed through the second window.

Relationship problems

There are two emotions which cause havoc with sexual relationships: resentment and insecurity. Often the two are closely related, with insecurity resulting in behaviour that makes you or your partner feel resentful and vice versa.

Anger is a normal emotion which is bound to arise from time to time in any close relationship. For most people, anger interferes with their sexual feelings. Some couples may use sex as a way of making up after a row, which usually means that they have already started to resolve their angry feelings when their love-making starts. Others seem able to dissociate sex from other aspects of their relationship with surprising effect, though one wonders what sex means to them in interpersonal terms. For most people, anger and good sex are incompatible though there are some important exceptions, which are considered through the second window. What is particularly relevant to sexual problems is chronic unresolved resentment. It is often striking how much couples are reluctant to recognize the link between some long-standing feeling of hurt or resentment and a decline in their sexual relationship. This stems from the link between anger and insecurity. For many people, full acknowledgement of the extent of their resentment is too threatening, as it may lead to the loss of their partner or rejection.

The ability of a couple to cope with the inevitable vicissitudes of an ongoing relationship depends to a great extent on their methods of communication. This involves the communication of both information and feelings, which together allow us to assert ourselves and to protect ourselves as two individuals in a relationship. We shall consider such processes more closely when dealing with sex therapy in Chapter 12, as these principles provide much of the basis of effective counselling. Ineffective communication not only sustains but also often aggravates problems. How common it is to find couples conforming to a stereotype of the nagging wife who is only too ready to communicate (i.e. complain) and the silent husband who withdraws into his long-suffering shell. An imbalance of this kind has powerfully destructive effects — the husband feels increasingly resentful about being nagged while the wife, in addition to her burning resentment, feels herself increasingly trapped in this unattractive role of the nagging woman, lowering her self-esteem even further. Dealing inappropriately with anger is often the crux of the problem. Some of us grow up learning to avoid outward expression of anger if at all possible. Others fear that if they get angry they might lose control and some irreversible physical or psychological harm would result. Others are reluctant to acknowledge the intensity of their anger towards the person they believe they do or should love. Often, such individuals have seldom if ever experienced full-blown anger in a key relationship and so have not learnt that relationships can indeed survive such storms.

One of the fundamental reactions to being hurt is to be able to express that hurt at the time. The cause of the hurt is then clear. This is what we mean by self-protection. Both individuals in a pair need to do this, and to expect the other to do the same.

Adapting to marriage or a committed relationship — the first 5 years

During this initial period there are important tasks of separation from both family and premarital friends, organization of household arrangements, the management of money, commitment to work and to leisure. Any of these aspects may reveal that one or other of the partners is not ready or willing to make the commitment to the relationship that marriage, in its conventional form, or committed co-habiting demands. In the last few decades, many of the traditional views about marriage have been challenged, mainly by women because they have least to gain from the old view of marriage and most to gain from appropriate change. Nevertheless, expectations still abound and often those of husband and wife do not coincide.

The bartering approach to marriage is a common cause of problems. The assumption is made that in return for material security and companionship the wife will provide sex. If she feels she is missing out on her side of the bargain she will be less inclined to provide sex, or at least her enjoyment of it. Her sexual pleasure becomes a form of currency and both partners suffer the consequence of its withdrawal.

The traditional expectation of wife as home-keeper and child-rearer, often held firmly by both partners, may place the modern wife at a disadvantage compared with her husband. She becomes cut off from her peer group (in particular her previous workmates); she may be relatively isolated in a semi-rural housing estate, reliant on inadequate public transport. More often than not she is separated from her own mother and extended family, and if she has more than one child of preschool age there are demands on her patience and resources that are seriously underestimated in our society. This is a stressful time and yet both she and her husband are inclined to the view that she has everything she has always wanted — a home of her own, little children and a loving husband. Her reaction to this situation may make her feel a failure and hence even more depressed than the circumstances already warrant. She then finds herself unduly dependent on her husband, who will seem to be much more self-sufficient. Unless he is perceptive and responsive, he will not meet her needs and the seeds of resentment and low self-esteem are sown.

If both partners recognize the size of the wife's task during this early parenting phase of marriage, then mutual support may see them through and sex, if it is working well, can continue to provide a powerful binding force in their relationship. However, many couples have much to learn before their sexual relationship works well. The majority of young couples, particularly those with a minimum amount of previous sexual experience, have a lot of finding out to do, not just about each other but also about themselves, before their sexual relationship settles down to be comfortable and predictably enjoyable.

For some couples, this period of sexual adjustment goes badly, either because of other interpersonal problems or because of specific difficulties in coping with their sexual responses. Perhaps the commonest example is when the man has a tendency to ejaculate too quickly, and the woman is a little slow to respond. Each may worry about this discrepancy, further aggravating the problem. PE becomes established and the woman gradually loses interest in sex as her way of coping with repeated frustration and disappointment. All too often the problem is tolerated for many years but eventually becomes inextricably tangled with other causes of resentment in the relationship. Once again, poor or inhibited communication (which may be specifically related to sexual matters) has served to turn what should be a normal developmental stage into a chronic difficulty. Sometimes the couple will seek help at an early stage and often benefit from simple counselling with surprising ease.

For those who have established a satisfactory sexual relationship prior to marriage, it is not unusual to experience a sexual decline in the first year or two of marriage. The traditionalist might say that they are paying the price for foregoing premarital chastity but their premarital experience has shown them how good sex can be; it provides a discomforting contrast. Usually in such cases, sex was better before marriage because it was not taken for granted, and for many women was a means of expressing their love. After marriage they are 'contracted to provide it'. In a comparable way the man may, after marriage, feel under pressure to perform sexually.

The first 5 years are the commonest time for marital breakdown to occur.

Phase 2 — the next 20 years

When two young people get married, they still have a great deal of development and growth as individuals ahead of them. After the first phase of adjusting to one another, they may have substantial social changes to cope with, either upwards with career improvement, or downwards with unemployment, problems with alcohol or even chronic illness. The parental role creates its own demands and can lead to tension in the marriage in a variety of ways. Parenting adolescent children, when anxieties about one's children's sexuality are often paramount, may have repercussions on the sexuality of the marital relationship.

As considered in Chapter 5, sex is used to bolster our self-esteem during adolescence — to feel sexually admired is to feel good. The need for this type of reassurance may not only continue into early marriage but will recur at times when, for other reasons, our self-esteem is low. The woman may feel that her physical attractiveness, previously so important to her, is now waning as she gets older. The man in a similar way may feel less virile or less attractive as he sees younger men moving into the ascendancy. Either may then look for reassurance either in overt extramarital affairs, or more commonly by flirtations that, whilst not involving overt sex, may nevertheless be threatening and hurtful to the partner.

Often crises, either for the individual or the relationship, are followed by important stages of personal growth and maturity. Sometimes progress for one partner can be threatening for the other, who may try to resist such change. Of particular importance is the move from traditional dependence of the wife to a state of independence as she establishes a role for herself in her own right, which does not depend on being a mother or someone's wife.

Causal mechanisms

A wide range of factors and circumstances in the current situation has been considered through this first window. A number of mechanisms may be involved in translating these circumstances into an impairment of sexual interest or response. The most important is probably reactive inhibition. This conclusion is based on the assumption that ongoing appraisal of the circumstances leads to inhibition as a basically adaptive mechanism, i.e. switching off sexually because of the need to focus on other issues. Also, the impact of negative emotions, such as unresolved resentment, may increase inhibition or make it less likely that inhibitory tone is reduced. The impact of chronic stress and fatigue or tiredness is less well understood, and may involve other mechanisms either resulting in increased inhibition or reduced capacity for excitation (Bancroft 1999).

The most likely consequences sexually are reduced sexual desire and arousability, which in the male may be manifested as reduced erectile responsiveness. This may then be amplified by a negative feedback effect (see Fig. 4.1). When arousal is reduced then other consequences may follow; in women this can involve pain during sexual intercourse, subsequent anticipation of which then serves to keep the problem going. Women may also be less likely to experience orgasm either because of reduced arousability, or possibly direct inhibition of orgasm. As yet we have little direct evidence of the effects of these circumstantial factors, but it is reasonable, in treatment, for the therapist to work with the couple at resolving or correcting the circumstantial factors in the expectation that normal sexual interest and responsiveness will then return.

Through the second window — vulnerability to sexual problems

Although a wide range of factors that can impact on our sexuality were identified through the first window, it is also clear that individuals and couples vary substantially in the extent they are affected by such factors, particularly in terms of an associated inhibition of sexual response. In this section we consider explanations for this variability, focusing on the relevant characteristics or earlier relevant experiences that individuals bring into a relationship that indicate their particular vulnerability.

Such vulnerability may have been apparent in earlier episodes in the current relationship or in earlier relationships. It is also important to identify those cases where the problem has been long-standing, and hence not sufficiently explained by current circumstances.

We can consider different aspects of vulnerability under the following headings: negative attitudes, belief and values about sex, earlier negative or traumatic sexual experiences, and constitutional variations in sexual responsiveness and propensity for inhibition.

Negative attitudes, beliefs and values

Sex is bad

When we consider the adult silence and implied taboo that surrounded the subject of sex during the childhood of so many of us, it is not surprising that many children develop and harbour peculiar or primitive fears or beliefs about sex that remain in adult life because they are not challenged. Most commonly we learn to view sex as wrong, naughty, dirty, or even evil. Such strong negative values may be incompletely resolved when we start our sexual relationships and serve to temper or even inhibit what should be spontaneous pleasures. We may feel that sexual pleasure is always wrong or we may feel sufficiently unsure about it that we must conceal its occurrence from everyone (except possibly our partner). We certainly must not be seen, or even heard, indulging in any form of sexually pleasurable activity. On no account must we give our children any reason for thinking that we enjoy sex and so on.

Identifying sex as bad may have other results. Some people learn to enjoy sex in spite of the 'bad' image by confining sexual pleasure to 'bad' or at least illicit relationships. Illicit sex is exciting; respectable sex, as part of a good, loving relationship is unacceptable. Sometimes in such cases, part of the excitement stems from the risk involved of getting caught or being found out. The variable ways in which human beings learn to associate emotional states with sexual response have been considered at various places in this book (see Chapter 4) and will be considered further below. However, while we are becoming more aware of these variable mood–sexuality associations, we still understand little about how they arise.

One possible explanation for the need to exclude sexual pleasure from a loving relationship is when the relationship is too closely identified with the child–parent relationship, particularly when Oedipal anxieties have not been resolved. Although I do not accept the almost ubiquitous role that most psychoanalysts assign to Oedipal feelings, they may well be important in some cases. It may be that when an especially close father–daughter or mother–son relationship leads to active denial of the sexuality involved, trouble is to be expected in a subsequent marriage. The sexuality in such parent–child relationships is not likely to be overt, but rather implicit. This results in sexual feelings being recognized to some extent but regarded as taboo.

Sex is disgusting

Disgust is an intriguing and under-researched emotion (Ekman 2003). Lazarus (1966) suggested that it is a combination of approach and avoidance. If we simply want to avoid something, we feel frightened of it, but if we have strong mixed feelings about it we may feel disgust. Disgust may be elicited by 'moral repugnance' or 'oral incorporation' (i.e. taking offensive objects or material into one's mouth). Miller (1997) commented on the suspension of disgust that characterizes intimacy; this is evident, for example, in a mother changing her baby's nappy. This is also relevant to sexual intimacy; 'someone else's tongue in your mouth can be a sign of intimacy because it can also be a disgusting assault … Consensual sex means the mutual transgression of disgust-defended boundaries' (p. 137). A 9-year-old boy, at an age when disgust in many forms holds a fascination, is likely to react to any explicit evidence of sexual interaction with disgust. An aspect of sexual development that has received little attention is how and when we learn to replace disgust with intimacy. But the connection between the two underlines the importance of the need to feel secure, mentioned earlier. The sense of vulnerability in a sexual interaction in part stems from fear that one's sexuality, or one's 'sexual parts' will be regarded as disgusting.

Sometimes, the disgusted patient shows a dramatic breakthrough of sexual pleasure during treatment, which would support Lazarus's idea. Disgust may be directed specifically at the penis or the vagina, the vaginal smell or the ejaculate or vaginal fluid. It may occur in those who learned to associate sex and excretion, particularly those who are generally fastidious about their body cleanliness. This type of disgust, reflecting a more general personality characteristic, may be more difficult to resolve.

It is important to remember that in a state of sexual arousal we may tolerate or even enjoy sensations or smells that in a non-aroused state we might find somewhat offensive. Sexual disgust may therefore arise or become established when there are other factors blocking normal sexual arousal. In those instances, it is obviously of secondary importance.

The need for self-control

Sexual arousal may threaten our need for *self-control*. Some people who have not experienced orgasm may be threatened by the image of it. Others have experienced orgasm during masturbation and feel unable to allow such abandonment to happen in front of another person. This may reflect a general need to keep control, particularly in the sort of person who never likes getting ruffled or showing too much emotion. In others, the fear may stem from the intensity of sensation involved and the extent of loss of control experienced. They may dislike their physical appearance during orgasm; they may fear losing control of bowel or bladder function. They may be aware of becoming vulnerable, not only because momentarily they are unable to protect themselves, but also because they may lay themselves open to ridicule or rejection by their lover.

Sexual pleasure may be feared as a road to promiscuity. This is particularly likely to be a problem for a woman who may feel that if she lets herself go and really enjoys sex, she will have difficulty in controlling herself and become promiscuous. In some cases, she may have passed through a relatively promiscuous phase earlier in her development. After a stage of sexual restraint she enters a reasonably stable and respectable marriage but at the expense of loss of sexual abandonment. Any attempt to recapture earlier sexual enjoyment may bring fears of returning promiscuity.

The need to maintain contact

In Fisher's (1973) study of female orgasm, he found one particular feature that distinguished between women with high and low orgasmic attainment. 'The low orgasmic woman . . . feels that people she values and loves are not dependable, that they may unpredictably leave her. She seems to be chronically preoccupied with the possibility of being separated from those with whom she has intimate relationships'. These women tended to have detached or absent fathers during their childhood and adolescence. Fisher suggested that their difficulties in letting go for orgasm resulted from their fear of losing contact with the loved one. This interesting finding needs to be replicated. Certainly, for many people, men and women, orgasm means 'taking off' for a few moments on a solitary 'trip'. Those who are only comfortable with sex as an expression of love may enjoy the shared experience of the earlier stages of love-making but feel uncomfortable when they find themselves moving into this 'solitary' phase. Such a reaction may not completely prevent orgasm, but may temper its intensity.

Earlier traumatic or negative sexual experiences

The type of negative experience that has received the most attention is sexual abuse or exploitation during childhood or adolescence. The literature on the effects of such abuse is reviewed in Chapter 16 and will only be briefly considered here. To the extent that such earlier experiences were traumatic or unpleasant at the time, the occurrence of long-term negative consequences is not surprising, although clearly individuals vary in their ability to cope with and adjust to such traumas. What is somewhat paradoxical about the findings in this literature is that probably the commonest outcome in community surveys is what has been called 'sexualization', meaning an earlier onset of voluntary sexual activity, more sexual partners when young, more sexual risk taking. The explanations for such an outcome are not well understood, and there is a lack of relevant research designed to explore possible determinants. It should not be assumed, however, that this 'sexualized' pattern is predictive of good, enjoyable sex once a relationship is established. There appear to be a number of possible barriers to the establishment of sexual intimacy in such individuals. One hypothesized pattern, considered more closely in Chapter 16, is that when the sexual trauma or exploitation occurs at a relatively early stage of sexual and emotional development, a connection between negative emotion and sexual arousal is established. As considered later in this chapter, this paradoxical pattern, which is far from rare, may result in sex being used as a mood regulator, and as such may become a barrier to intimacy. Another pattern that is a more understandable outcome of CSA is an avoidance of sexuality in adolescence and adulthood. This may not appear in community surveys because such individuals are reluctant to talk about it. A third pattern, which I have encountered in my clinical practice but not in the related literature, is a sense of guilt stemming from the memory of enjoying the 'sexual abuse' experience as a child, yet being confronted by a consistent message that children are 'asexual'. Such individuals therefore see themselves as in some way responsible for the abuse, and this is a barrier to their feeling comfortable about their sexuality in adulthood.

Another mechanism, which is by no means restricted to experiences of sexual abuse, may depend on an earlier experience of sex, or even a non-sexual experience, such as a gynaecological examination, which was painful. A woman who has previously experienced such pain (it is less likely to be a man) may have a tendency to anticipate further pain, which can interfere with her ability to respond, and enjoy the experience.

Constitutional variations in sexual responsiveness and propensity for inhibition

Men and women clearly vary in their capacity for sexual response and orgasm. This can be reflected in their propensities for sexual excitation or inhibition, measures of which, as we considered in Chapter 6, show close to normal distributions. Assuming that these are measures of an established trait, they are of relevance to how an individual engages in a sexual relationship or reacts to the range of challenges reviewed through the first window.

Let us first look at the evidence available so far that links measures of excitation and inhibition proneness to sexual problems.

Vulnerability to sexual problems in men

Erectile problems

In a non-clinical convenience sample of 1558 heterosexual men (mean age 34.5 years $\pm$ 11.3) who completed the SIS/SES questionnaire (Bancroft et al 2005a), we asked about problems with erection and rapid ejaculation, with the following three questions:

1. In your sexual activities with a sexual partner, have you had difficulties in obtaining or keeping an erection in the past 3 months?
2. The same as (1) except the time period was 'ever'.
3. In your sexual activities with your partner have you ever had a problem in ejaculating (i.e. 'coming') too quickly?

Possible answers for each were 'never', 'occasionally', 'less than half the time' and 'most of the time'. In answering question 1 (ED past 3 months), 3.5% said most of the time, 4.1%, less than half the time, and 38.6% occasionally. For question 2 (ED ever), there were 3.9%, 3.6% and 43.3%, respectively. Answers to question 3 (Rapid ejaculation ever) were 7.1%, 5.8% and 43.1%, respectively. As these were not representative samples we cannot use them to assess the prevalence of such problems, but we can use them to examine the relationship of such problems to our SIS/SES measures. Using ordinal logit to predict the reporting of erectile problems in the past 3 months, with SES, SIS1, SIS2, age, and trait measures of depression proneness (Zemore Depression Proneness Ratings; ZDPR) and anxiety proneness (Spielberger Trait Anxiety Inventory; STAI) as independent variables, SIS1 and age were significant positive predictors of erectile problems.

SES, SIS2, ZDPR and STAI were not predictive. We found no association between SIS/SES scores and reporting of rapid ejaculation, though we did find that STAI was a significant predictor.

We then collected data, including SIS/SES scores (ZDPR and STAI were not included), from a series of 172 men attending sexual problem clinics. Of these, 116 presented with ED only, 15 with PE, 2 with low sexual desire and 30 with various combinations of the first three problems. In all, 146 men had ED and these were compared with an age-matched sample of 446 men from our non-clinical studies. The mean scores for SES and SIS1 for the clinic group with ED, and the four subgroups of the non-clinic sample for ED 'ever', are shown in Figures 11.4 and 11.5. These show that both SES and SIS1 scores from the clinic

group were very similar to those from men in the non-clinic sample who reported ED 'most of the time'. Once again we found no association between SIS/SES scores and PE (Bancroft et al 2005b).

We thus have strong evidence of an association between SIS1 (positive), SES (negative) and erectile problems. At this stage, it is not clear, particularly in the clinic attenders, whether SIS/SES scores indicate vulnerability (i.e. are 'trait' measures) or reflect the impact of the dysfunction (i.e. are 'state' measures). Both SES (negatively) and SIS1 (positively) are correlated with age in our non-clinic samples. The lack of this correlation in our clinic sample is not surprising; the two samples were matched for age, and most of the younger men in the clinic sample had ED. Interestingly, SES was more clearly

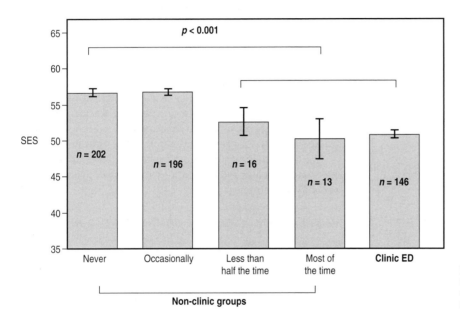

Fig. 11.4 SES scores in the ED 'ever' groups from a non-clinical sample compared to clinic attenders with erectile problems. (From Bancroft et al 2005a.)

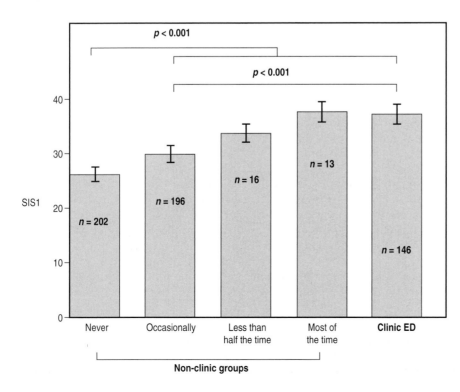

Fig. 11.5 SIS1 scores in the ED 'ever' groups from a non-clinical sample compared to clinic attenders with erectile problems. (From Bancroft et al 2005a.)

reduced in cases of ED with evidence of organic aetiology (e.g. impaired waking erections). This may indicate that SES is more of a 'state' measure, which can be influenced by both ageing and physical factors. What can we conclude about SIS1 in this respect? As considered in Chapter 6, there is now evidence from a twin study of heritability of SIS1 and 2, but not of SES (Varjonen et al 2007). If valid, this finding suggests that propensity for inhibition is more of a trait aspect of vulnerability, although, as discussed earlier, a trait which can be amplified by the effects of ageing (see p. 243).

Premature ejaculation

The lack of any association between SIS/SES scores and PE is noteworthy. This may be because the questions in the SIS/SES focus on sexual arousal rather than the ease or speed of reaching orgasm. It may also indicate that the inhibitory systems affecting arousal and orgasm/seminal emission are different. As yet we cannot make that distinction.

The developmental aspects of ejaculatory control are of interest. There is a natural tendency for most young males to ejaculate quickly and the longer the period since last ejaculating, the quicker it is likely to be, reflecting greater arousability. Kinsey, in his volume on men (Kinsey et al 1948), regarded rapid ejaculation as an indication of potency. He also suggested a social class difference in this respect: 'At lower educational levels, it is usual for the male to try to achieve an orgasm as soon as possible after effecting genital union. Upper level males more often attempt to delay orgasm' (p. 580). However, with increasing sexual experience, greater control over ejaculation usually develops. This is partly because of the dampening effects of the ageing process and also because of the lessening of novelty, and hence arousability, that comes with a long-term sexual relationship. But some process of learnt control is probably also involved. This represents a source of individual variability; some men are unable to learn this control and they remain with what is generally known as PE. It is becoming increasingly apparent that we do not understand the reasons for this. Conventional wisdom has assumed that to improve his control a man learns to recognize when he is getting close to the point of ejaculatory inevitability so that he can temporarily reduce the level of stimulation and allow his arousal to subside a little. This is the rationale for treatment methods such as the 'stop–start' technique introduced by Semans (1956) or the 'squeeze' technique introduced by Masters & Johnson (1970), both of which will be described in Chapter 13. However, such treatments are not always successful, or produce improvement that is not sustained. Conventional wisdom has also considered anxiety to aggravate PE if not actually cause it, with performance anxiety resulting from PE making the problem worse (Cooper 1969; Masters & Johnson 1970). In our recent study reported above (Bancroft et al 2005a) we found STAI, a trait anxiety measure, to be predictive of rapid ejaculation. However, one needs to distinguish between variability in the speed of ejaculation, which may be more difficult to control in states of anxiety, and the chronic condition of PE, which

may become a cause of anxiety and low self-esteem. Increasing attention is now being paid to the possible mechanisms underlying this problem.

The effectiveness of serotonin reuptake inhibitors (SSRIs) in delaying ejaculation has recently fostered a new phase of interest in PE in the pharmaceutical industry. On the basis of such pharmacological effects, Waldinger (2002) concluded that PE is a neurobiological problem-based on lack of sensitivity of serotonin inhibitory mechanisms. He also reports limited evidence that it may be heritable (Waldinger et al 1998). However, much of the mystery still remains. As discussed in Chapter 4, there is some form of interaction between orgasm induction, seminal emission and the triggering of muscle contraction that expels the semen, turning seminal emission into ejaculation. But the precise sequence of physiological events is not as yet understood (Levin 2005). We should not conclude that, because SSRIs delay ejaculation, abnormal serotonergic mechanisms are the cause of PE. SSRIs also delay orgasm in women, and to some extent reduce genital arousal in men and women. The ejaculation process does, however, lend itself to psychophysiological assessment, and some progress has been made in that area (Rowland et al 1997). In a recent review, Rowland et al (2007) reached a number of conclusions from this research, including the following. Men with PE do not report higher subjective arousal than normal controls. Their erectile responses to visual sexual stimuli (VSS) alone are less than those of normal controls. But when vibrotactile stimulation is combined with VSS, their erectile responses are similar to controls. Men with PE do not differ from controls in their preferred intensity of vibrotactile stimulation. Heart rate changes when responding to sexual stimulation, however, are different in men with PE who show an acceleration of heart rate as they become more aroused. Normal controls show a deceleration at least until orgasm and ejaculation occurs. This suggests a difference in the balance of sympathetic and parasympathetic system activation during sexual arousal. Given that sympathetic activation is involved in seminal emission and orgasm, this could well indicate some basic autonomic difference that accounts for the PE. Men with PE are more likely to experience negative affect (supported by our reported association with STAI; see above), but the relevance of this to the aetiology of PE remains uncertain.

There is a strong association between PE and erectile failure. Typically, a man with lifelong problems of ejaculatory control develops erectile problems in middle age. The nature of this association is also not understood. It remains a possibility that men with PE who develop ED may differ in some neurophysiological way from men with PE who do not develop ED.

The origins of these psychoneurophysiological patterns underlying PE therefore remain unknown. However, because in most cases, the problem has been evident from the start of a man's sexual career, it is reasonable to regard this as a constitutional characteristic appropriately considered through our second window. The question of whether this is a pattern that results from early learning or is genetically determined remains unanswered. It is difficult to see how such a pattern could be learnt before the onset of ejaculation, unless it is a pattern which does not only have relevance to ejaculation. Waldinger et al (1998) reported limited evidence of a familial pattern. Presumably PE, unless so severe that intravaginal emission is not possible, is compatible with fertility (though I have seen no directly relevant evidence on that point). If so there would be no particular tendency for any underlying genetic pattern to be 'bred out'.

Delayed or absent ejaculation (DE) is a much less common problem and has consequently received little research attention. Obviously there are some medical conditions, as well as medication side effects, that interfere with normal orgasm and ejaculation, and they will be looked at through the third window. But in the majority of cases without such explanations, this difficulty is reported from the start of their sexual careers, and hence it is likely to reflect some constitutional characteristic. Rowland et al (2007) have recently started to investigate this problem. Over an 8-year period, 5% of men referred for psycho-physiological assessment (i.e. 74 out of 1400) were diagnosed as having inhibited or retarded ejaculation. Excluding those cases with clear somatic aetiology or ejaculatory problems secondary to ED, only 2% ($n = 29$) remained; 27 of these were assessed in the laboratory and compared with three other dysfunctional groups; men with PE alone ($n = 47$), with ED and PE ($n = 14$), and ED alone ($n = 39$). In response to sexual stimulation in the laboratory, men with DE were similar to the PE group and better than the two ED groups in erectile response but reported less subjective sexual arousal than the PE group, and were similar to the two ED groups in that respect. This suggested a lowered central arousal component, which could well explain the delayed orgasm and associated ejaculation. This could be regarded as comparable to orgasmic difficulty in women. The question then arises whether this is a result of lowered excitation proneness or increased inhibition proneness. In our recent study of men attending sexual problem clinics, the small number with the complaint of DE ($n = 9$) had normal SES scores and a hint of increased SIS 1 for their age (Bancroft et al 2005b). Most were students attending the Kinsey Institute Sexual Health Clinic, and several of them overcame their difficulty with counseling. Their mean SIS/SES scores, with the mean and SD from a non-clinical age-similar student sample given in parentheses, were as follows: SES, 58.9 (57.2 ± 7.9); SIS1, 31.5 (27.1 ± 4.1) and SIS2, 28.7 (27.7 ± 4.8). There was therefore a suggestion of higher SIS1 in the DE group, which might have been significant with a larger n. The idea of increased inhibitory tone, which we postulate is measured by SIS1, is probably of likely relevance to this problem, and requires further study. The evidence, reported earlier, that SIS1 and SIS2 are to some extent heritable, raises the question of why such traits, if expressed as inability to ejaculate, are not 'bred out' of the male population. Our small sample, however, was predominantly young and such men may often overcome the difficulty sufficiently to allow them to become fathers.

Low sexual desire

What constitutional characteristics might we expect to relate to the experience of 'low sexual desire' in men? In Chapter 6, the concept of 'asexuality' was briefly considered. Individuals self-identifying as asexual scored lower on the SES scale of the SIS/SES. A low propensity for sexual excitation is likely to be associated with low sexual desire, at least in men. In our earlier non-clinical studies we did not ask about sexual interest or desire. More recently, Janssen (unpublished data) used our standard question about frequency of sexual thoughts, which we use as a measure of sexual interest (see p. 221), with 774 men completing his questionnaire on the Kinsey Institute website. SES was the strongest positive predictor of the frequency of sexual thoughts ($p < 0.001$). SIS1 was also a significant negative predictor, but only just ($p = 0.03$). This is consistent with propensity for sexual excitation being a key component of one's level of sexual desire, but with inhibitory tone also likely to be relevant. In our clinical sample (Bancroft et al 2005b) we had only two men whose problem was restricted to low sexual desire, and they had markedly high SIS1 (mean 45.0), and fairly low SES (mean 47.0) scores.

Vulnerability to sexual problems in women

Dyspareunia and vaginismus

As mentioned earlier, sexual intercourse requires a woman to be physiologically prepared for vaginal penetration. Any of the problems identified through the first or second windows, particularly those associated with negative attitudes or beliefs about sex, may interfere with this, resulting in attempts at vaginal penetration being uncomfortable or painful. Also, earlier negative, particularly painful experiences, including painful vaginal examinations, may result in anticipation of pain and a negative feedback which make the prophesy self-fulfilling. But in addition, there are a variety of local disorders that lead to pain during sexual activity, such as vaginal or vulvar infection, post-episiotomy scarring and pelvic pathology such as endometriosis. Pain and tenderness of the vulva and vestibular area are often referred to as vulvo-vestibulitis, and if a burning pain persists without tactile stimulation or pressure, the term 'vulvodynia' may be used. If the primary problem is difficulty in allowing vaginal penetration, due to tightness of the pelvic floor muscles that surround the vagina, the term 'vaginismus' is used. As we shall see, there is often an overlap of symptoms in conditions with different aetiologies. A crucial clinical requirement is an effective differential diagnosis of the cause of the pain, and this process is considered closely in Chapter 12.

There is an ongoing and vigorous debate around this issue, largely thanks to the pioneering research of Binik and his colleagues in Montreal. Binik (2005), in an article in *Archives of Sexual Behavior*, criticized the DSM-IV classification of dyspareunia as a sexual dysfunction (i.e. 'sexual pain disorder'). He proposed that instead, dyspareunia should be classified as a pain disorder, best dealt with by pain specialists. Twenty commentaries on the Binik paper followed in the same issue, most of which disagreed, in one way or another, with Binik's proposal. Leaving aside the implications of DSM criteria (which will be considered more closely at the end of this chapter), there is an aspect of dyspareunia that has been strikingly absent from this literature. Given the fact that vaginal intercourse involves invasion of the woman's body space by a man's erect, and sometimes large, penis, there is a need to understand why this is not uncomfortable or painful for most women most of the time. We have some understanding of this, which will be considered below, and we can therefore see specialized mechanisms that enable painless vaginal penetration as representing a response pattern as specifically sexual as penile erection in the male. Just as the male has to develop a rigid erection for vaginal intercourse to take place, so also does the woman require a 'sexual preparation' of her vulva and vagina. Binik (2005) likens vaginal pain to other types of pain that disrupt our behaviours (e.g. headache or shoulder pain) hence his proposal to view pain during sexual intercourse as a pain disorder rather than a sexual problem. There are causes of erectile failure in the male such as vascular impairment or peripheral nerve damage that are similar to those found in other disorders. And in some cases of erectile failure we turn to the vascular specialist or neurologist for help or guidance. But the majority of cases of erectile failure involve a complex psychosomatic process that the clinical sexologist is best able to manage. In my view, therefore, a woman's genital pain during sexual activity should be carefully assessed to distinguish between problems in this specific sexual response system and less sexually relevant mechanisms such as altered pain sensitivity, or local inflammation or pathology that causes pain. The first step in this diagnostic process is best carried out by a clinical sexologist rather than a pain specialist. I would, however, make the following proviso: the appropriate clinical sexologist for this purpose is one who has experience in vaginal examinations. This does not mean full gynaecological training, though that would obviously be an advantage, but the ability to carry out a vaginal and vulval examination sensitively and cautiously, to locate areas of inflammation or tenderness, and resistance to finger insertion into the vagina (a speculum would not normally be used in such assessments), to help the woman to become more at ease and better informed about her genitalia (see Chapter 12, p. 369 for a more detailed description), and all of this combined with the necessary skills and sensitivity to carry out sex therapy. In a proportion of cases, such assessment would result in referral to a gynaecologist or pain specialist. This therefore means that any sexual problems clinic that takes referral of women with sexual pain should have at least one member of the team with the above training and skills. Binik (2005) recommends a team approach to the individual, i.e. the woman with sexual pain is assessed by more than one person, including a psychologically trained therapist and a physical therapy (pelvic floor) specialist. For this particular type of patient I would advocate someone who combines these necessary skills.

Let us now revisit some of the basic physiological mechanisms, described in Chapter 4, which are involved in the preparation of the vulva and vagina for pleasurable rather than painful vaginal intercourse. Three such mechanisms are of obvious relevance: (i) an 'automatic' increase in vaginal blood flow and associated vaginal lubrication in any potentially sexual situation, whether or not the woman feels sexually aroused or even interested (see p. 79), (ii) a specialized and complex neurological network which results in vaginal or cervical stimulation raising the pain threshold (see p. 83) and (iii) appropriate levels of muscle tone in the pelvic floor muscles, particularly those that surround the lower third of the vagina (p. 34), which if too tense can make vaginal entry difficult and possibly painful. Given these specialized mechanisms that normally determine whether coitus can occur in a non-noxious manner, we should not be surprised if such mechanisms might not always work sufficiently or appropriately. What constitutional factors might impact on each of these mechanisms?

Vaginal lubrication, while of fundamental importance to a woman's genital response, is not well understood. It is dependent on increase in vaginal blood flow, but its relation to sexual arousal is unclear (see Chapter 4, p. 80). Psycho-physiological studies of women with dyspareunia and their VPA response to different types of erotic stimuli have shown somewhat inconsistent results (Wouda et al 1998 Brauer et al 2006; see p. 80). But it remains a relevant possibility that women who anticipate pain in a sexual encounter may not only become less sexual aroused but also may have less vaginal lubrication, increasing the likelihood of vaginal discomfort or pain. As yet, however, we have no way of characterizing those women who are particularly vulnerable to such an effect. Oestrogen deficiency, as found in post-menopausal women, is related to vaginal dryness (see p. 246), although the relationship is probably more complex than conventional wisdom has assumed and the association between oestrogen levels and vaginal discomfort or pain is also unclear; vaginal dryness is not infrequent in pre-menopausal women (see Chapter 7, p. 246). In psycho-physiological studies comparing pre- and post-menopausal women, Laan & van Lunsen (1997) and Laan et al (2003) found significantly lower baseline levels of VPA in post-menopausal women, but the VPA responses to erotic stimuli did not differ between the two groups (see p. 248). It has been recognized for some time that post-menopausal women who are sexually active are less likely to experience vaginal dryness than those who are inactive, interpreted by some as indicating that sexual activity is good for the vagina. But in both pre- and post-menopausal women we are not in a position to distinguish cause from effect; does pain or discomfort result from vaginal dryness, or does vaginal dryness result from anticipation of pain or discomfort or do both causal mechanisms interact?

The existence of special mechanisms to increase pain threshold following vaginal and cervical stimulation has only recently been recognized (see p. 83) and has not so far been taken into consideration when striving to explain dyspareunia. However, the complexity of the relevant nerve supply to the vulva and vagina has been acknowledged (Binik et al 1999), and the possibility of some alteration of neuronal sensitivity has been suggested. Studies of women with vulvo-vestibulitis have shown enhanced sensitivity to pain not only in the vulvo-vestibular region, but in other parts of the body as well (Pukall et al 2002; Granot et al 2004). Increased intraepithelial innervation in the vulvar tissues has been demonstrated in women with vulvo-vestibulitis (Bohm-Starke et al 1998; Westrom & Willen 1998). Genetically determined mechanisms that prevent organisms normally present in the vagina (in particular the yeast, *candida albicans*) from infecting the tissues are deficient in some women with vulvo-vestibulitis (Babula et al 2005).

Factors which influence tension in the pelvic floor muscles are likely to vary among women. Some women appear to be particularly apprehensive about anything entering their vagina, not only an erect penis, but also a finger or a tampon. This is relevant to the condition known as vaginismus. In most cases, this appears to be a relatively restricted fear of vaginal penetration; sometimes this is associated with negative feelings or embarrassment about the genitalia combined with a lack of understanding about their structure and function; in a minority the phobia about vaginal penetration is part of a more generalized apprehension about sex.

A crucial point is that there are a variety of developmental sequences that lead to the establishment of pain during sexual activity. For example, a woman starting with simple vaginismus may, because of recurrent pain when sexual intercourse is attempted, develop increased pain sensitivity of the vulva and vestibule. A woman who develops vulvo-vestibulitis associated with recurrent *Candida* infections, may show pelvic floor contractions when vaginal entry is attempted. Varying developmental patterns, such as these, result in overlap of specific manifestations of sexual and genital pain. It is therefore important to understand the developmental sequence in each woman — what came first and how it evolved.

There are mechanisms involved in many cases of dyspareunia, particularly in the vulvo-vestibulitis category, which are comparable to those in other kinds of pain disorder, and vulvo-vestibulitis has proved particularly difficult to treat (see Chapter 13). Vaginismus, on the other hand, has long been regarded as one of the more treatable sex dysfunctions. I agree with Binik that this condition has not been adequately researched, and the overlaps with other types of genital pain problems are important and need to be better understood. But I have

not as yet been persuaded to change my mind about the management of vaginismus and its generally good prognosis. Although I have not systematically reported on the cases I have treated in my career, and there have been many, I very much concur with the report by Hawton & Catalan (1990) on a consecutive series of 30 couples in which the woman was diagnosed as having vaginismus. The characteristics of these couples were compared with those of 76 couples presenting with other kinds of female sexual dysfunction. The vaginismus couples were younger and had shorter relationships than the comparison group, their general relationships were rated more positively, they reported better communication about sex, the women with vaginismus reported less sexual aversion, and more interest in sex, and more sexual arousal and pleasure from sexual activities providing that vaginal intercourse was not on the agenda, and they were more highly motivated for treatment. At the end of treatment, 43% reported their problem resolved, and a further 37% largely resolved. A minority showed little or no improvement and such resistant cases often present with sexual problems more comprehensive than the vaginismus. The method of treatment is important, and is not simply a matter of graded dilatation, and this will be considered closely in Chapter 12. In addition, specific medical conditions relevant to genital pain will be considered in Chapter 13.

Propensity for sexual inhibition

As yet we have less evidence of the associations between measures of sexual excitation and inhibition proneness and reporting of sexual problems in women. Sanders et al (2007) have recently used their SESII-W, developed to measure sexual excitation and inhibition proneness in women (see p. 229), in a non-clinical sample of 540 heterosexual women (mean age 33.7 ± 13.9 years). The women were also asked four questions about sexual problems: one general question, 'to what degree, if any, would you say you experience sexual problems?' (with six response categories from 'not at all' to 'very strongly'); and three questions about lifetime experience of specific sexual problems: 'Have there been any times in your life when you had (i) difficulty becoming or staying sexually aroused, (ii) difficulty in reaching orgasm/climax or (iii) low sexual interest?'. The response options were 'never', 'less than half the time', 'about half the time', 'more than half the time', 'all of the time'. For the first general question about current problems, 5.4% answered 'strongly/very strongly' and 10.4% 'moderately'. For the three specific questions the results are shown in Table 11.5. The extent to which these problems

TABLE 11.5   Women's responses to 'Have there been times in your life when you had...? (from Sanders et al 2007)

	Never (%)	Less than half the time (%)	About half the time (%)	More than half the time (%)	All the time (%)
Difficulty becoming or staying sexually aroused	37.5	45.2	8.9	6.9	1.5
Difficulty in reaching orgasm/climax	21.4	39.4	15.8	15.8	7.6
Low sexual interest	45.0	34.9	10.2	7.4	2.4

n = 540; percentages shown

could be predicted by the SESII-W was explored with multiple regression, using all eight of the SESII-W subscales, together with a number of demographic and background factors as independent variables. Five of the subscales make up the 'sexual excitation' factor ('arousability', 'sexual power dynamics', 'smell', 'partner characteristics' and 'setting') and three make up the 'sexual inhibition' factor ('arousal contingency', 'concerns about sexual performance' and 'relationship importance'). Two of the inhibition subscales were of particular interest: 'arousal contingency' was predictive of all of the sexual problems and 'concerns about sexual performance' was predictive of arousal and orgasm difficulty. 'Arousal contingency' is an intriguing subscale. It consists of three items: 'When I am sexually aroused, the slightest thing can turn me off', 'It is difficult for me to stay sexually aroused' and 'Unless things are "just right" it is difficult for me to become sexually aroused'. Together these three items suggest a fragility of sexual arousal and response, the precise nature of which is not yet clear. Distractibility is obviously involved, but probably not 'general distractibility', rather a sensitivity to certain types of distraction. This suggests a predominantly inhibitory pattern of response, but closer examination of how women experience these items is required. 'Concerns about sexual function' are more suggestive of performance anxiety (e.g. 'If I am worried about taking too long to become aroused, this can interfere with my arousal') and it then becomes difficult to sort out which is cause and effect.

The only other study to report the use of the SESII-W in women involved sexually active pre-menopausal women, none of whom complained of sexual problems (Bradford unpublished findings). Significant negative correlations were found between the Arousal Contingency sub-scale and scores from the Female Sexual Function Index (Rosen et al 2000) for desire ($r = -0.5$), arousal ($r = -0.6$), lubrication ($r = -0.34$) and sexual satisfaction ($r = -0.36$). A significant positive correlation was also found with trait anxiety (STAI). These findings increase the likelihood of a causal relationship between arousal contingency and the sexual problems in the Sanders et al (2007) study.

It may be informative to explore how these excitation and inhibition measures relate to different types of sexual desire or different objects of desire. In particular, the distinctions between desire for sex, characteristic of male sexual desire and important for some women, and desire for emotional closeness and desire to be desired, both aspects of the female basic pattern, warrant attention. Would the predictive power of the various subscales of the SESII-W differ across these different types of desire?

Orgasmic function also needs to be considered from the perspective of the basic pattern model. It has been argued earlier (see Chapter 4) that female orgasm is a by-product of the male basic pattern and has no reproductive function in women. Consistent with this is some preliminary evidence of heritability of orgasmic capacity in women (Dunn et al 2005). This is not surprising; if female orgasm was necessary for reproduction, the lack of orgasmic capacity in females would have been 'bred out' during evolution. Thus, in considering the very variable reporting of orgasmic experiences among women, we need to consider that women are variable in their orgasmic capacity for genetic reasons, and that absence of or diminished capacity for orgasm is a difference which does not need to be regarded as a dysfunction. Loss of the ability to experience orgasm in a woman who has typically been orgasmic previously is another matter. One can argue along similar lines for the relevance of various patterns of female sexual response and desire. This point will be revisited when we grapple with a proposal for a new classification of sexual problems.

Through the third window — factors that alter sexual function

A key component of a comprehensive clinical assessment is to look for factors that alter or impair an individual's capacity for sexual response and sexual interest. These will be considered under three headings: (i) the effects of ageing, (ii) factors related to ill-health and (iii) sexual side effects of medication.

The effects of ageing

As ageing is a normal and inevitable process, there is a case for considering its effects through the second window. The impact of ageing on sexuality is very variable, however, and parallels the effects of age-related disease processes, particularly in men. For that reason, it will be considered here. It is important not to interpret the consequences of normal ageing as dysfunctional, but to encourage older couples to accept and adapt to these changes, even though some will want to explore treatment to restore their sexual responsiveness.

The effects of ageing on sexual interest and response were considered closely in Chapter 7. A more predictable, linear age effect is observed in men, although the extent of the effect varies considerably across individuals. A key component of this change appears to be a reduction in the NA-mediated central arousal system, and this may be related to a reduction in responsiveness of T receptors, both in the brain and peripherally, as well as a reduction in circulating levels of T. Other age-related changes directly affect the responsiveness of peripheral mechanisms such as penile erection, on the one hand reducing the effectiveness of vascular mechanisms, and on the other hand increasing the sensitivity of erectile smooth muscle to inhibitory signals from the brain (see p. 243). The effects of ageing on the sexuality of women is much more complex, involving a variety of factors which are secondarily related to age, e.g. the lack of a sexual relationship, which is more common in older women than in older men because of women's greater life expectancy, and which has more of an impact on the sexuality of women than of men. Changes in women's sexuality show a less linear decline, with more substantial reduction around mid-life. Yet the extent to which these changes can be attributed to the menopause per se is uncertain. The psychological impact of the end of fertility may be more important in some women than the hormonal or other physiological changes related to the menopause, and depressive episodes, which have an important effect on a woman's sexuality, are more common at that stage of life.

Health problems

There is a wide range of health problems that adversely affect sexuality, which will be considered more closely in Chapter 13. Here we will consider them briefly. A pathological process may directly interfere with sexual function (e.g. neuropathy impairing erectile response), or illness may have less direct physical effects due to metabolic disturbance or general lack of well-being and energy, or may have indirect psychological effects (e.g. body image concerns after mastectomy or ileostomy).

Affective disorder

It is important to keep in mind the distinction between negative mood, which is reactive to circumstances, and a more endogenous mood disorder, although clinically a clear distinction is often not possible. In the first case, the reactive inhibition of sexual interest or response is more appropriately identified through the first window, requiring change or resolution of the problem evoking the negative reaction. In the second case, we are dealing with a more physiological change in brain function, which may be associated with a reduction of the capacity for sexual arousal and response. In such cases treatment is primarily aimed at improving the affective disorder.

The mechanisms by which negative mood may influence sexuality and individual variability in the relation between negative mood and sexuality were considered in Chapter 4. Paradoxical associations between negative mood and sexuality and how they relate to problematic sexual behaviours are considered further in the last part of this chapter.

Psychotic illnesses, such as schizophrenia, can have sexual manifestations that are likely to be complex (see p. 388) and will be discussed in Chapter 13.

Neurological disorders

Brain abnormalities, including brain tumours, injury or the effects of vascular impairment and dementia, may affect sexuality depending on the part of the brain affected. Abnormalities or injuries to the spinal cord can affect the crucial connections between the brain and peripheral responses. Various types of neuropathy can impair function of peripheral nerves necessary either for the sensory or the motor components of sexual response.

Peripheral vascular disease

Small vessel disease, and less often large vessel abnormalities, can impair the vascular responsiveness of the genitalia in both men and women, though the impact on sexual function is likely to be greater in the male.

Endocrine disorders

Testosterone deficiency and hyperprolactinaemia are associated with reduced sexual interest and responsiveness in men. The effects of such hormonal changes in women are less predictable (see Chapter 4).

Diabetes mellitus

Diabetes mellitus is a condition commonly affecting sexual responsiveness, particularly in men, but to some extent in women. These effects may result from a range of pathological changes that occur in diabetes, including peripheral vascular disease, peripheral neuropathy and changes in brain function.

Gynaecological conditions

Problems such as endometriosis and retroverted uterus may result in pain during sexual activity.

Genital infections

Genital infections, which are often sexually transmitted, can cause pain or soreness during sexual activity. In some sexually transmitted infections (e.g. syphilis) there are systemic effects that can indirectly affect sexual function. These are considered more closely in Chapter 14.

Sexual side effects of medications

A variety of medications can adversely affect sexuality, most commonly by impairing orgasm in women or ejaculation in men (e.g. SSRIs) or by interfering with genital response (e.g. anti-hypertensives) or by altering sex hormone levels (e.g. steroidal contraceptives). These are considered more closely in Chapter 13 (and in the case of steroidal contraceptives in Chapter 15).

Problems of altered sexual response or interest in men and women with homosexual or bisexual identities

In most respects, the sexual problems encountered by gay men and lesbian women are similar to those of heterosexuals, but with some interesting differences.

Sandfort & de Keizer (2001) reviewed the limited literature on sexual problems in gay men, reporting on 19 studies, four involving HIV positive gay men. The impact of HIV infection on sexual function will be considered further in Chapter 14. They stressed the importance of not seeing these problems in heterosexual terms; in particular, they pointed out the absence of any equivalent of vaginal intercourse; in gay male sex each sex role is completely reversible. They found only one study, however, which directly compared sexual problems in gay and heterosexual men, and this was based on only seven and eight men in the two groups. They concluded that little could be learnt from this literature, perhaps because the majority of research attention had focused on safe and unsafe sex, rather than on functional and dysfunctional sex. Sandfort & de Keizer (2001) speculated that gay men find sexual failure more embarrassing and suffer more performance anxiety as a consequence.

The following three studies were included in Sandfort & de Keizer's (2001) review. Masters & Johnson (1979), during a 10-year period, treated 56 gay male couples seeking help for sexual dysfunction. There were only two cases of PE and none of ejaculatory failure. The remainder all complained of ED, though four were also sexually aversive. In a further study, Paff (1985) reported on the types of sexual dysfunction in gay men seeking treatment from therapists identified with the gay movement. Broadly speaking, their problems were similar to those of heterosexual men, with some interesting differences. Aversion towards anal sex was one charactistically gay male problem, whereas PE seemed to be less common than amongst heterosexual men. Rosser et al (1998) assessed the frequency and duration of pain during anal intercourse. In a sample of 277 men with experience of anal intercourse, only 25% reported 'no to extremely mild pain'; 63% reported occasional to fairly frequent pain of mild to moderate severity. Twelve per cent reported pain that was too severe to allow the anal intercourse to continue. It is relevant to compare this with vaginal intercourse in women. As considered in Chapter 4 (see p. 83), not only does a woman usually have vaginal lubrication before penile insertion, there are other specialized mechanisms to reduce pain sensitivity from vaginal penetration. It is unlikely that such mechanisms are relevant to anal penetration.

In a Kinsey Institute study, a large, non-clinical sample of homosexual men ($n = 1379$) were compared with an age matched sample of heterosexual men ($n = 1558$) and all were asked limited questions about problems with erections and rapid ejaculation (Bancroft et al 2005a). Erectile problems were reported more frequently by gay men, though in most cases this was 'occasional' ED (during the past 3 months, 33% gay and 23.1% heterosexual). The percentages reporting ED most of the time were similar in the two groups (for the past 3 months; 3.6% for gay and 3.3% for heterosexual men). We looked for evidence that gay men were more prone to performance anxiety, as Sandfort & de Keizer (2001) had speculated. The gay men scored significantly higher on SIS1, our measure of propensity for inhibition due to fear of performance failure, than our heterosexual sample. SIS1 may be influenced by actual erectile problems, so we excluded those men reporting ED in the past 3 months, and homosexual men still scored significantly higher on SIS1. We then selected the one item that most clearly described performance anxiety, 'If I feel I have to respond sexually, I have difficulty getting aroused'. The gay men scored significantly higher on this item. Rapid or premature ejaculation (PE) was assessed by one question, 'In your sexual activities with a sexual partner have you ever had a problem in ejaculating (i.e. "coming") too quickly?'. PE was reported more frequently by heterosexual men ('most of the time'; 4.5% gay, 7.1% heterosexual). Interestingly, in contrast to the heterosexual men, gay men were more likely to report PE in the older age groups. Cove & Boyle (2002) pointed out that PE in heterosexual men was often a consequence of a pressure not to ejaculate before their female partner had reached orgasm, whereas this was not an issue in gay sex, whether anal or oral insertion was involved.

These findings suggesting greater concern about erectile function in gay men and about ejaculatory control in heterosexual men need to be replicated and examined more closely. They may reflect some interesting and clinically important differences in how gay and straight men experience sex.

When we consider the sexual problems of lesbian women we once again have less published evidence to guide us. Masters & Johnson (1979) treated 25 lesbian couples, and in every case the problem was categorized as anorgasmia. Because of Masters & Johnson's way of conceptualizing sexual dysfunction, this did not distinguish between specific orgasmic problems and a more general lack of sexual arousal. They commented, however, that amongst the lesbians who were usually in committed relationships, sexual fakery was less common than amongst heterosexual women, and attributed this in part to the lesbian's ability to admit orgasmic difficulty to her partner with less loss of face than her heterosexual counterpart. Nichols & Shernoff (2007) comment that lack of sexual interest or a discrepancy of sexual interest between lesbian partners are the most common sexual problems presented for treatment. Vaginismus and pain are rare complaints because of the lesser emphasis on and need for vaginal penetration.

Clearly, there are differences in the dynamics of same-sex relationships that, in some respects, may be less problematic and, in other respects, may be more so than those of opposite sex relationships, and these may need to be addressed in same-sex couples seeking help to improve their sexual relationships. There are also consequences of homosexual stigmatization with which heterosexuals do not have to contend.

Problematic sexual behaviour

In this section sexual behaviours are examined that either interfere with an individual's relationship, work or well-being, or incur risk of unwanted pregnancy, sexually transmitted infections or other negative consequences. Here it is the behaviour, either because of its high frequency, or because of the potential negative consequences, that is the issue. Problems with sexual responsiveness may be relevant to some extent, but more because of a persistent sexual response than an impaired one. A key conceptual distinction is between sexual behaviour at the high end of the 'normal' continuum, and behaviour which is qualitatively different from 'normal' sexual behaviour. The issue of when 'hypersexuality' is a statistical variation or an inherent problem was considered by Orford (1978) some time ago. With high levels of sexual interest, problems may arise in a sexual relationship because of the resulting discrepancy of need between the two sexual partners. This may not only lead to dissatisfaction with the sexual relationship in either or both partners, but also increase the likelihood of 'extra-marital' relationships with the associated potential for negative consequences, particularly for the primary relationship. In this section we focus on sexual behaviour that involves poor risk management, with a range of possible negative consequences, and sexual behaviour which is 'out of control'.

High-risk sexual behaviour

Sexual behaviour can involve risk in a number of ways. The most common examples include unwanted pregnancy, sexually transmitted infection, negative consequences for one's primary sexual relationship (e.g. extra-marital sex) or legal consequences (e.g. sex with an under-aged partner). Most individuals avoid such risks, but some do not. To what extent can we understand such propensity for sexual risk taking? This is of considerable potential importance in designing interventions to reduce high-risk sexual behaviour (HRSB). Obviously, the processes determining high- and low-risk sequences of sexual behaviour are complex, involving a range of interacting factors (Bancroft 2000).

HRSB, and our attempts to explain why some individuals are more likely to engage in it than others, is looked at closely in Chapter 14, with particular reference to the risk of sexually transmitted infections. The risk of legal consequences from inappropriate sexual behaviour is considered in Chapter 16.

'Out-of-control' sexual behaviour

Most of the relevant literature has employed two currently fashionable concepts: 'compulsive sexual behaviour' or 'sexual addiction'. As we will see, both concepts have potential explanatory value, but probably only for a proportion of cases. Barth & Kinder (1987) argued for the use of 'impulse control disorder' as a description, which, in contrast with the compulsivity and addiction labels, is consistent with DSM criteria, but which, beyond inferring a problem of self-control, has little explanatory value. In the past, other labels, such as nymphomania, satyriasis and hypersexuality, have been used (Rinehart & McCabe 1997). Two types of behaviour may be involved: masturbation, probably the most common, and behavioural interactions with others, of various kinds. Such patterns which break the law (e.g. exhibitionism and paedophilia) are considered in Chapter 16. However, in many such cases, the issue is not one of being out of control but rather of being illegal and hence likely to get the individual into serious trouble. A new and exceedingly important development is the use of the Internet. This was considered in Chapter 6 (p. 226) and while a large number of men and women use the Internet for sexual purposes, the majority do not find it a problem, nor does it get out of control. But in some it does, and out-of-control Internet sex is the fastest growing aspect of this problem area. With the Internet we see, in many cases, a blending of the masturbatory and interactive patterns referred to above. Individuals vary in this respect, and some, particularly men, use the Internet as an almost limitless extension of their out-of-control masturbatory behaviour. For others, interaction with others, via chat rooms and other devices, is of importance, even though masturbation is likely to be the principal pattern of sexual release. The extent to which Internet interactions allow modifications and variations in how one presents oneself and how one interacts is considerable, and as yet we do not know how much this characteristic contributes to the undermining of self-control. A collection of essays on the topic has been edited by Cooper (2002).

The literature on sexual compulsivity and sexual addiction has been preoccupied with issues of definition, particularly pertaining to DSM-IV, and very little with

possible causal explanations for why, in such cases, sexual behaviour becomes problematic. While statements are often made about likely mechanisms, e.g. anxiety reduction or mood regulation, these are seldom based on reported data, but apparently on clinical impression, leading Gold & Heffner (1998) to title their review paper *Sexual addictions; many conceptions, minimal data*. Explaining such behaviour is of fundamental importance.

A few data-based studies have examined potentially relevant co-morbidity. Raviv (1993) found that 32 self-identified sex addicts had higher mean scores on SCL-90-R scales for anxiety, depression, obsessive–compulsiveness and interpersonal sensitivity, than 38 controls. In an uncontrolled study of 36 subjects with self-defined out-of-control sexual behaviour, Black et al (1997) found a high prevalence of co-morbidity with psychiatric conditions, most notably lifetime histories of substance use disorders (64%), anxiety disorders (50%) and mood disorders (39%) (see also Quadland 1985).

There is increasing evidence that out-of-control sexual behaviour can be reduced by mood elevating drugs such as the SSRIs (Stein et al 1992; Fedoroff 1993; Kafka 2000) which has been taken as support for the idea that the problem relates to affective disorder, at least in a proportion of cases. However, we do not yet know the extent to which such pharmacological benefits, when they occur, result from improvement in mood or specific inhibition of sexual response or both. Given the high prevalence of sexual side effects with such drugs (see Chapter 13, p. 403), inhibition of sexual response is likely to be relevant.

Following a small study of self-defined sex addicts (Bancroft & Vukadinovic 2004), in which 29 men and 2 women were interviewed and completed questionnaires, and compared with a large age-matched control group, an attempt was made to postulate a range of possible causal mechanisms which are testable with further research. These will be briefly reviewed, with illustrations from that study.

Negative mood and 'out-of-control' sexual behaviour

The impact of negative mood on sexuality was considered closely in Chapter 4 (p. 106). While for most people negative mood, both depression and anxiety, is associated with a reduction of sexual interest and/or response, there are a minority of individuals who report a paradoxical tendency for sexuality to be increased during negative mood states. This is of obvious relevance to out-of-control sexual behaviour.

According to the Dual Control model (Chapter 2, p. 15), in situations that induce negative mood, sexual interest and arousal is normally inhibited to allow maximum focus on the coping process. One postulate, therefore, is that paradoxical increase in sexual interest in negative mood states requires unusually low levels of inhibition of sexual response (as measured by SIS2), and relatively high levels of sexual arousability (as measured by SES). As presented in Chapter 4, we found support for this in heterosexual men, but more limited support in gay men, while in women, there was support for the association with high arousability, but not low inhibition proneness (see p. 108). We have also postulated (Bancroft et al 2003b) that the paradoxical effect of anxiety on sexuality is an example of 'excitation transfer' (Zillman 1983), when arousal induced in association with anxiety becomes incorporated into response to sexual stimuli in those with low inhibition of sexual response.

In our study of sex addicts, 27 subjects (87%) stated that their sexual 'acting out' was predictably affected by their mood. Seventeen subjects reported being more likely to sexually act out when depressed, and 19 when anxious or stressed. Eleven subjects (9 men and both women) reported an increase in acting out in states of both depression and anxiety. Two men said that they were *less* likely to act out when depressed; no one said this in relation to anxiety. As a group their scores on the mood and sexuality questionnaire (MSQ; see p. 108) were significantly higher than those of the controls ($p < 0.001$), indicating their greater likelihood of being sexually responsive in negative mood states. The sex addicts also scored significantly higher on a trait measure of proneness to depression, and propensity for sexual excitation (SES), but did not differ from controls in the two scales for propensity for inhibition (SIS1 and 2).

An association between negative mood and out-of-control sexual behaviour therefore appears to be highly relevant. However, the mediating mechanisms may vary and are not just a matter of 'using sex as a mood regulator'. Three patterns can be considered:

1. Those individuals who retain sexual interest or responsiveness in states of depression may pursue sexual contact with another person to meet depression-related emotional needs, e.g. establishing personal contact through sex, feeling validated by another person, enhancing one's self-esteem by feeling desired by another person. These are direct examples of 'mood regulation'.
2. Sexual stimulation may be used to distract one's attention from the issues, which when thought about induce negative mood. This assumes that negative affect is being kept at bay by the distraction. As Baumeister & Heatherton (1996) put it, 'the source of emotional distress is not present in the immediate situation, but is highly available in memory (e.g. just after a major rejection or failure experience). Under such circumstances, people will seek to distract themselves to prevent themselves from thinking about the upsetting event' (p. 5). This pattern seems more relevant to episodic use of sexual behaviour than typical patterns of out-of-control sexuality.
3. The tendency for sexual interest and arousability to be increased in negative mood states characterized by increased arousal, i.e. states of anxiety or stress, as a result of 'excitation transfer' (Zillman 1983). For most individuals this does not happen because the circumstances that induce the negative affect also lead to an inhibition of sexual responsiveness. But in those who do not show this inhibitory pattern, excitation may occur and lead to establishment of learnt or even conditioned associations between negative mood and

sexual arousal. This pattern is most likely to be manifested in solitary or masturbatory patterns of behaviour. Once the arousal has been transferred into sexual arousal, there is a strong intrinsic need to pursue sexual release through orgasm, which, once this is recognized as a recurring and out-of-control pattern, induces further negative mood.

In some individuals, depression can be associated with anxiety, allowing for a blending of patterns 1 and 3.

A key question is why some individuals have the capacity for these atypical and potentially problematic interactions between mood and sexuality. As reported in Chapter 4 (p. 110), we found a negative correlation between MSQ score and age in heterosexual men, indicating that such paradoxical patterns are more likely in younger men, and presumably lessening for most as they get older. This begs the question of when such an association becomes established. Is it possible that this paradoxical mood–sexuality relationship is developed during childhood or early adolescence as a consequence of early experiences that combine sexual response with negative mood, such as CSA or induced guilt about masturbation? This is a researchable question. Coleman (1986) has postulated that the predisposition to use substances or behaviours to alleviate emotional pain may reflect an 'intimacy dysfunction' that could result from CSA or neglect. It would not be surprising if an early established pattern of increased sexual arousal and interest, in association with negative mood, could become a barrier to the normal incorporation of one's sexuality into close, intimate sexual relationships. In our study of sexual risk taking in heterosexual men (Bancroft et al 2004) we found that men in exclusive, monogamous relationships had lower MSQ scores (i.e. were less likely to report this paradoxical pattern).

'Out-of-control' sexual behaviour as a result of impaired inhibition

Goodman (1997), in his useful review of the theoretical basis of sexual addiction, proposed impaired behavioural inhibition as one causal factor. Inhibition of sexual response is, according to the Dual Control model, an adaptive mechanism across species. The concept of 'low propensity for sexual inhibition' has already proved useful in explaining some aspects of high-risk sexual behaviour (see next section).

The neurobiology and psychopharmacology of sexual inhibition is complex, and is considered closely in Chapter 4. However, serotonin does appear to play a crucial role. Kafka (1997) has proposed that a dysregulation of central monoamine function underlies out-of-control sexual behaviour. Goodman (1997) reminds us, however, of the difficulties in localizing complex effects within the central nervous system, or relating them to specific neurotransmitters, and the case has been made for formulating 'conceptual systems' in the brain, based on function rather than specific neurotransmitter mediation or anatomic localization (Bancroft 1999). There is, however, a clear need for well-designed, controlled studies of SSRI treatment for men and women with out-of-control sexual behaviour, in which groups are carefully selected and matched for indicators of impaired inhibition as well as other behavioural characteristics.

While direct investigation of serotonergic mechanisms in the central nervous system are difficult in humans, developments in the genetics of neurotransmitters offer a new and potentially informative approach to explaining individual differences. Do individuals who develop out-of-control patterns of sexual behaviour have lower levels of serotonin transporter gene markers (Lesch et al 1996)? Another new approach to the study of central inhibitory mechanisms is the use of brain imaging (e.g. Rédoute et al 2000; Stoléru et al 1999), which shows that certain areas of the brain are deactivated during response to sexual stimuli, which has been interpreted as a reduction or 'switching off' of inhibitory tone. Brain imaging studies of sexual arousal were reviewed in Chapter 4. The techniques are still at an early stage of development, particularly for exploring complex processes such as sexual arousal. But it could be informative to compare the patterns of brain activity in response to sexual stimuli in individuals with out-of-control sexual behaviour and normal controls.

One fundamental issue, in considering the role of inhibition, is whether the problem lies in conscious mechanisms of self-regulation, or in the neurophysiological mechanisms of inhibition of sexual response and their apparent variability across individuals as postulated by the Dual Control model. In other words, to what extent is out-of-control or unregulated sexual behaviour similar to other out-of-control behaviours like binge eating or overspending? Or to what extent is it a problem peculiar to control of sexual response? Let us consider both possibilities.

Self-regulation

Baumeister & Heatherton (1996) provided a useful theoretical approach to failure of self-regulation, which they described as a multi-faceted process, which can break down in several different ways. They paid little attention to sexual behaviour in this article, but their theoretical analysis is relevant in several respects. They described three ingredients of self-regulation: (i) standards, (ii) monitoring and (iii) the operative phase of regulation. Standards are of interest, in particular the dilemma of conflicting or incompatible standards, which can undermine regulation. For five of the male sex addicts in our study, religion was very important. It is not difficult to see how, in such cases, the unquestionable moral unacceptability of most types of sexual behaviour conflicts with one's sexual impulses, undermining any sensible pattern of regulated sexual behaviour. Thus, an individual who believes masturbation is evil, and who has strong impulses to masturbate on the Internet, is unable to see that a regulated pattern of masturbation can be a responsible way of dealing with one's sexual needs. Coleman (1986) proposed that highly restrictive attitudes to sexuality can result in inability to conform, starting off a cycle of guilt, pain and compulsivity.

Monitoring is clearly important to effective self-regulation, and Baumeister & Heatherton (1996) suggest that alcohol, as well as fatigue and stress, can impair normal monitoring. Sexual arousal may also have this effect, and this is considered further in the section on HRSB in Chapter 14 (p. 430). An important aspect of monitoring, discussed by Baumeister & Heatherton (1996), is 'transcendence' or focusing one's awareness beyond the immediate situation, so that more distal concerns or consequences are kept in mind. In our study of sex addicts (Bancroft & Vukadinovic 2004) we found some indications of a dissociative tendency that could contribute to 'out-of-control' behaviour by undermining, if not eliminating, this transcendence. When asked to describe a typical state of mind while acting out, 14 (45%) gave descriptions suggestive of some degree of dissociation. The following are illustrative examples, each from a different subject: '. . . an overpowering drive. . .nothing else is under consideration'; '. . . numb, completely zoning out, not present, not conscious of reality'; '. . . trancelike state . . . kills time and pain. . .numb like a dream'; 'when I'm sexually aroused, I click out'; '. . . feel detached from what is happening'; '. . . like a drug to numb out.' It is possible that such explanations are used as post hoc justifications. But dissociation has not been explored in the relevant literature, and warrants closer study.

These general aspects of self-regulation, about which there is a substantial literature (Baumeister et al 1994), are clearly relevant to out-of-control sexual behaviour.

'Automatic' inhibition

In considering the role of 'automatic' or subconscious inhibition, the problem of persistent genital arousal disorder is of interest and relevance. This was described on p. 309, and has only recently received attention in the literature. It appears to be a uniquely female problem and this in itself requires explanation. One of the two women in our sex addicts study fits this diagnosis, describing herself masturbating as 'like a gerbil on a wheel'.

Leiblum et al (2007a) identified at least two subtypes of persistent genital arousal, which they referred to as PGAD and non-PGAD. The main difference was that the PGAD group was more likely to report their genital response and arousal as continuous and overwhelming and distressing, whereas women in the non-PGAD group would at least some of the time report pleasurable feelings associated with the genital response, and overall be less distressed by it. In a further web-based survey, 76 women with PGAD were significantly more likely to be depressed and to report panic attacks than 48 women in the non-PGAD category, and to monitor their physical sensations in a somewhat obsessive–compulsive manner. The association between genital response and negative mood is clearly relevant to this phenomenon, but this aspect is not necessarily different to that experienced by men. Two gender differences in sexual response may be relevant. First, women have much less refractory inhibition after orgasm than men (see p. 90); thus orgasms are less likely to have a limiting effect. It would however be interesting to compare the post-ejaculatory refractory period in men with out-of-control sexual behaviour and normal controls. Another uniquely female aspect of genital response is the automatic increase in vaginal blood flow which occurs in the presence of any sexually relevant stimulus, whether or not the woman finds the stimulus appealing (see p. 80). This response may initiate a process of monitoring in certain women, leading to the augmentation and persistence of the response because of the impact of negative emotions (Leiblum & Chivers 2007). As yet, however, we can only speculate about the explanation of PGAD, which could certainly lead to out-of-control sexual behaviour, particularly masturbation, in women.

Clearly, regulation of sexual behaviour does not depend on physiological mechanisms of inhibition alone, and it is likely that a combination of deliberate self-regulation and neurophysiological inhibition of sexual response are involved (Bancroft 2000). In out-of-control sexuality, impairment of both aspects, in various combinations, may be responsible.

'Out-of-control' sexual behaviour as an addiction

Another explanatory mechanism proposed by Goodman (1997) is 'aberrant function of the motivational reward system'. As yet we can say little about the relevance of reward and incentive mechanisms to out-of-control sexual behaviour. But the possibility exists that some change in sensitivity of the incentive reward system may occur as part of the establishment of an out-of-control pattern, sharing in common changes associated with chronic use of 'drugs of addiction' (Robinson & Berridge 2000) and possibly behavioural addictions of various kinds (Holden 2001). Brain imaging offers possibilities for future research on this issue, as exemplified by a study of gambling by Breiter et al (2001). Without further evidence, however, the concept of sexual addiction is best seen as an analogy, which may be useful, at least for some individuals, when used in therapeutic programmes.

'Out-of-control' sexual behaviour as an obsessive–compulsive disorder

A few studies have looked for evidence of obsessive–compulsive personality among sex addicts, usually finding a small minority in this category (e.g. Black et al 1997, 15%; Shapira et al 2000, 15%). According to the DSM-IV, out-of-control sexual behaviour is excluded from the obsessive–compulsive category on the grounds that 'the person usually derives pleasure from the activity and may wish to resist it only because of its deleterious consequences' (American Psychiatric Association 2000, p. 422). Compulsive thoughts of obsessive–compulsive type often do have sexual content, but typically they are accompanied by negative mood and no sexual arousal. We would anticipate that most people with obsessive–compulsive personalities and a propensity for mood disorders would experience a decline in sexual arousability during negative mood states, as is the case for most other people. But there are likely to be exceptions. Warwick & Salkovskis (1990) described two men whose obsessive–compulsive symptoms included intrusive sexual thoughts accompanied by penile erection. The awareness of the erection intensified the anxiety and

hence reinforced the process. Is it possible that occasionally there is a combination of obsessive–compulsive tendencies and a low propensity for inhibition and/or high propensity for excitation of sexual response, with an atypical, sexualized type of compulsive behavioural pattern resulting? If so, one would expect to find evidence of other obsessive–compulsive phenomena in such individuals.

A key component of obsessive–compulsive phenomena is their ego-dystonic nature, usually manifested by some attempt to resist compulsive urges. In our study of sex addicts, subjects were asked whether they found themselves trying to resist the urge to act out or whether, at the time, it was something they genuinely wanted to do. Eleven men and one of the women indicated that they tried to resist, but most of them did not give a convincing description of resistance (e.g. 'I tell myself not to do it, but I do it anyway'). The two most convincing accounts of resistance were from men with obsessive–compulsive personalities. In both cases the sexual acting-out was masturbation. One man had intrusive thoughts about teenage boys, or a compulsion to look at pictures of them. This would lead to considerable guilt and resistance, and he would obtain a very transient calming effect by masturbating, followed quickly by renewed guilt and depression. It should be noted here that the resistance was to the intrusive thoughts about boys rather than the masturbation. The other man described ruminative preoccupation with sexual thoughts, which would lead to masturbation followed by a need to take a shower because of the 'dirtiness' of the act.

Thus some forms of out-of-control sexual behaviour can be appropriately regarded as atypical obsessive–compulsive phenomena, but this clearly applies to a small minority.

Conclusions

In striving to understand out-of-control sexual behaviour, we should be expecting a range of aetiological mechanisms, associated with different behavioural patterns, which share in common the two key features of addictive behaviour as described by Goodman (1997), i.e. (i) a recurrent failure to control the sexual behaviour and (ii) continuation of the behaviour in spite of harmful consequences. At this stage, it is therefore premature to attempt some over-riding definition relevant to clinical management until we have a better understanding of the various patterns and their likely determinants. The concepts of 'compulsivity' and 'addiction' may prove to have explanatory value in some cases, but are not helpful when used as general terms for this class of behaviour problem. Stein et al (2001) proposed that, until we have a better understanding of the subtypes, 'hypersexuality' should be used. In my opinion, 'out-of-control' sexual behaviour is a more appropriate non-specific term, as it focuses on the issue of control rather than high levels of sexuality. However, there are now a number of clinically relevant hypotheses, and research is clearly needed to put them to the test.

Other types of problematic sexual behaviour

Autoerotic asphyxia

After sexual violence, probably the most disturbing sex practice is autoerotic asphyxia (AEA or hypoxyphilia). This involves either self-strangulation (by hanging or ligature) or suffocation by breathing inside a bag, inhaling fumes. In some way, it has a sexually enhancing effect, but usually those who engage in this do so secretly and it is only discovered when the person fails to stop in time and dies accidentally. Such cases may be misinterpreted as suicide (e.g. by hanging), but there is usually other evidence of sexual activity to be found (e.g. nudity, pornographic material) and commonly evidence of other sexual variations (e.g. bondage, transvestism, anal stimulation, mirrors for self-observation).

This phenomenon has a long history. The occurrence of penile erections in men who had been publicly executed by hanging has been observed on many occasions, sometimes associated with ejaculation. Ellis (1905) wrote of 'the impulse to strangle the object of desire, and the corresponding craving to be strangled' (p. 151). According to Hirschfeld (1938), 'The *motif* of strangulation recurs again and again in extreme cases of masochism'. He goes on to tell the story of a very talented musician, Kotzwarra, who lived in London. 'He became a voluptuary of the first magnitude and was always thinking of ways of intensifying erotic pleasure by artificial means. He had been told that a hanged person experienced for several minutes a very pleasant sensation, owing to the accelerated circulation of blood and the distension of certain vessels' (p. 446). He paid a number of prostitutes to hang him transiently. In 1791 after he had persuaded a prostitute to 'hang' him for 5 minutes, she found, when she released him, that he was dead.

Deaths of this kind are now being reported with increasing frequency. In the USA in 1979, 250 cases were reported, in 1983 the number had more than doubled (Uva 1995). To what extent this is an actual increase or an increase in its recognition is not yet clear — probably both. It is most common in adolescence. Sheehan & Garfinkel (1988) re-evaluated adolescent hanging deaths in two counties in Minnesota, over a 20-year period (1965–1985), and concluded that 31% were probably accidental due to AEA and not suicidal as originally assumed. Suicide rates for 15–19 year old Americans increased fourfold from 2.7 per 100 000 in 1950 to 11.3 per 100 000 in 1988, and between 1980 and 1992, 67 369 persons aged less than 25 committed suicide. Hanging is the second most common method of suicide among males (Jenkins 2000). It is therefore possible that many cases of accidental death associated with AEA are assumed to be suicide, and in such cases, the families may conceal the relevant evidence because they have even greater difficulty coming to terms with the AEA explanation than with suicide.

Blanchard & Hucker (1991) studied the coroners' records of such deaths in two Canadian provinces between 1974 and 1987, involving 117 males, aged 10 to 56 years (median 24 years) and with a third being younger than 19, 73% unmarried and four men (3.4%) homosexual. The methods of asphyxiation used were hanging (80%), strangulation (5%), suffocation (4%), inhaling gas or solvent (6%), chest compression (0.8%) and the remainder with various combinations of the first four methods. In 35.9% of cases there was no evidence at the death scene of any other sexual variation. In the remaining 64% there was evidence of bondage (e.g. ankles tied), or transvestism, anal stimulation and 'fantasy props'. Noteworthy was the association between these other indicators of sexual variation and age. In the younger individuals, bondage and transvestism were less likely. This was interpreted to suggest that AEA practitioners elaborate their masturbatory rituals as they get older. However, Blanchard & Hucker (1991) conceded that their findings were also consistent with there being at least two types of AEA practitioners with different developmental histories.

AEA deaths do occur in females (Hazelwood et al 1983; Byard et al 1993), though the majority are in males. However, there may be even greater non-recognition of AEA in females because they are less likely to display other evidence of sexual activity or sexual variations.

The evidence obtained from individuals who practice AEA and have so far survived is very limited. Friedrich & Gerber (1994) assessed five adolescent AEA practitioners, aged 14 to 17. They all had very disturbed backgrounds with physical and/or sexual abuse in most of them. One boy (aged 14), who was a serious risk taker, described how he and his two step-brothers engaged in a 'choking game'; one of his step-brothers had choked him at least 100 times. He also described choking himself to the point of passing out, and combined this with masturbating. Another boy, aged 16, masturbated 8 to 10 times a day using a practice he called 'choking'. According to his description, he would wedge his neck between the wall and a bedpost that he had positioned on an incline so that after releasing the bedpost it would slide away. This use of a safety mechanism of this kind is quite common with AEA practitioners, but obviously does not always work. Friedrich & Gerber (1994) pointed to the more general pattern of risk taking in these five boys and suggested that this might be a requirement for the establishment of AEA.

Money et al (1991) published the personal account of an AEA practitioner who they had successfully treated. 'Nelson', the individual's assumed name, grew up in a morally strict household, had hearing impairment, and symptoms suggestive of childhood autism, though this was not diagnosed as such, and clearly had difficulties interacting and relating to his peer group. He also suffered from asthma, and according to Money and his colleagues, many boys who die as a result of AEA have a history of asthma.[1] Because of a tendency to wander at night he was tied down in his crib. Thus, bondage and breathlessness became associated. As a child he was gender atypical, preferring to play with girls and having an interest in girls' underwear. When he was 11, a girl

---

[1] I have not found any other reference to this potentially important association.

neighbour drowned, and this remained a highly traumatic emotional experience for Nelson, who felt guilty that he had not saved her. Sometime after this he started masturbating, and for several years his predominant fantasy was of having sex with each of his nieces 'and then strangling them all in a row'. All the imagined strangling ended in orgasm. 'I spent most of eighth grade staring at girls from school and masturbating while having fantasies about them being strangled or drowned' (p. 77). His AEA started when he was 16. 'I strangled myself in front of an angled mirror, using nylon pantyhose . . . and pretended the whole time that a homosexual killer was throttling me . . . After I choked to the point where my dizziness got too much for me, I broke off the panty hose, fell to the floor as if I were dead, and immediately masturbated until I climaxed in a super, great orgasm . . . I always promised to myself that I would never do it again. But when it struck, there was no stopping it' (p. 22). In their closing commentary, Money et al (1991) marveled at the fact that in spite of Nelson's gruesome fantasies, no one ever got hurt. In someone with a different personality, it may have been a different story.

The determinants of autoerotic asphyxia

These accounts of 'survivors' of AEA involve individuals with substantial sexual and psychological problems of various kinds. However, the evidence obtained about people who have killed themselves with AEA presents a very different picture. Adolescent victims are usually well-adjusted, non-depressed high achievers (Uva 1995). In 1994, considerable media attention resulted from the death of a British Member of Parliament, who had clearly died as a result of AEA, associated with transvestism.

What is the mechanism that links asphyxia to sexual arousal, orgasm or pleasure? Ellis (1905) commented 'respiratory excitement has always been a conspicuous part of the whole process of tumescence and detumescence, of the struggles of courtship and of its climax, and . . . restraint upon respiration, or, indeed, any restraint upon muscular and emotional activity generally, tends to heighten the state of sexual excitement associated with such activity' (p. 154). It has been widely assumed in the more recent literature that asphyxiation results in a euphoric 'high', but it is not clear whether this is experienced during the hypoxia or immediately following it, or whether it is due to acute hypoxia or acute hypercapnia (increased CO_2). Increasing the arterial CO_2 has a powerful effect in increasing cerebral blood flow; inhaling 5% CO_2 increases it by 50%; 7% CO_2 doubles it. Reducing arterial O_2 has a similar but less pronounced effect (Brust 2000). Conventional medical descriptions of the effects of acute hypoxia or hypercapnia do not acknowledge any positive effects. According to Moxham (2000), acute severe hypoxia causes anxiety, restlessness, sweating and, if sufficiently severe, confusion. Acute hypercapnia causes restlessness, confusion and flapping tremor. The immediate effects of correcting these states are not usually described in detail. The precise mechanism therefore remains unexplained.

How do individuals discover AEA? Of relevance is an apparently widespread practice among teenagers, called the 'choking game', in which young boys choke each other, apparently because it induces a pleasant 'high' that is not dependent on sexual arousal. This 'choking game' is also known in the adolescent community as Space Monkey, Blackout, Rising Sun, or Knockout (Pearlstein 2003) or Suffocation Roulette (Shlamovitz et al 2003). In spite of the fact that this can result in accidental death, there has been scant attention in the medical literature. Shlamovitz et al (2003) published a case report on a 12-year-old Israeli boy who had been referred because of recurrent syncope. On questioning, the boy described a game in which the player takes a deep breath and holds it while another participant hugs him strongly from behind until he feels dizzy and passes out. He had experienced this on several occasions, the last time resulting in him falling and hitting his head, leading to the referral. According to his description the game involved a group of boys, did not have any sexual context and seemed to be driven by peer pressure and risk seeking rather than erotic impulses. Ming Chow (2003) welcomed this publication and drew attention to the risk of death involved. Such games, he indicated, produce a dizzy sensation, which the children regard as 'cool'. In July 2005 CBS News reported on three recent deaths, one involving a 13-year-old girl. It is striking and somewhat disturbing that we remain in so much ignorance about this dangerous practice, and that it receives so little attention from the medical profession. However, if this 'game' is part of adolescent culture, it would not be surprising if some adolescents try it on their own and discover a sexually enhancing effect leading to the establishment of AEA.

Whether it is the 'choking game' or AEA, we are left with a difficult challenge in knowing how best to prevent it. In 2001, together with my colleague Carol McCord, I was asked for advice by a local school where, in the previous two years, two 13-year-old boys had died, assumed to be the result of AEA. We were very conscious of the possibility that by giving children warnings we might be leading them to experiment. One of the principal researchers on this topic, Dietz (1989), has been unwilling to discuss the problem on television for that reason.

Problems with sexual or gender identity

Sexual identity

Earlier in my career, and before the era of 'gay liberation', it was not unusual for a homosexual man to seek treatment to become heterosexual, though exceedingly unusual for a lesbian woman to do so. Today, with greater acceptance of gay and lesbian identities and much more opportunities to be part of gay or lesbian groups or subcultures, requests for such help are rare for both men and women. Sometimes an individual is uncertain about their sexual identity and seeks help to resolve the uncertainty. Sometimes the issue is whether bisexuality actually exists or whether it is a defense against acknowledging a gay or lesbian identity. One example of uncertainty, presented by a man attending my clinic at the Kinsey Institute, involved strong sexual attraction to other males but a difficulty in having a loving, emotional relationship with another man, whereas he could envisage such a relationship with a woman. These are issues more to do with the incorporation of ones sexuality into dyadic relationships (see p. 146) than with sexual identity per se, and equally important in individuals with heterosexual identity. Helping to resolve such issues is discussed in Chapter 12.

The era of attempting to convert homosexuals into heterosexuals, mainly evident in the 1960s (see Chapter 8) passed, partly because of the failure of such attempts (Bancroft 1974) but also because of the lessening of stigma associated with the emergence of the gay rights movement, reinforced by the 'depathologization' of homosexuality in the DSM in 1974. However, religious condemnation has once again taken over from medical pathologization, leading to a resurgence of 'reparative' therapy for homosexuals, motivated by the moral unacceptability of homosexual behaviour. Paradoxically, one of the leading figures in the process of excluding homosexuality from the DSM, Robert Spitzer, involved himself in evaluating and reporting the effectiveness of 'reparative therapy'. Details of this study, together with my reactions to it, are given in Chapter 8 (see p. 258). There, I strongly advocated Surgeon General David Satcher's *Call to Action to Promote Sexual Health and Responsible Sexual Behavior* (US Department of Health and Human Services 2001). This calls for responsibility in our sexual lives (i.e. responsibility towards ourselves and our sexual partners), coupled with a respect for diversity. Thus, someone who believes that homosexuality is wrong is entitled to that opinion, but is not entitled to impose it on others, particularly if those others exercise responsibility in their sexual lives. Thus, the principle of responsibility facilitates the acceptance of diversity.

Within that principle, there are grounds for therapists and counselors to help individuals who are uncertain about their sexual identity, and an ethically acceptable approach to such help is considered in Chapter 12.

Gender identity

In most cases of individuals seeking clinical help for problems related to gender, they are doing so to obtain medical authorization of their gender reassignment and the use of hormonal and surgical procedures for that purpose. Such clinical involvement, as it represents crucial steps in the development of gender identity in these individuals, are considered in Chapter 9. There are, however, some individuals who are struggling with uncertainty about their gender identity, and seek guidance. This type of help will be considered in Chapter 12.

The classification of sexual problems

The historical context

What are the purposes of a classification system for sexual problems? Such a system is generally assumed to be a diagnostic system. The role of diagnosis in general medicine is relatively straightforward; the heuristic value of most medical diagnostic categories is that they convey information about aetiology, the most appropriate form of treatment and prognosis. Clearly, as our understanding of pathology increases our diagnostic criteria become more sophisticated. Diagnostic categories in psychiatry are less straightforward (Kendall 1975). Early in the 20th century, Adolph Meyer's priority was in understanding the sick person in terms of life's experiences, rather than fitting the symptoms into some diagnostic category. Menninger was in favor of abandoning diagnosis. Today there is general agreement that a diagnostic system should exist within psychiatry, but less attention is paid to its therapeutic or prognostic significance. Carson (1991) in his critical evaluation of DSM-IV, saw it as a method of increasing reliability of diagnosis, so that clinicians would be more likely to agree, while sacrificing validity, resulting in diagnostic categories that were consistently applied but were of limited clinical use.

In my view, we face the same dilemma with current diagnostic classifications of sexual problems, which are essentially psychosomatic in nature. The DSM-IV system in particular is of very uncertain value in identifying aetiology and planning treatment. Given this uncertainty, its value in organizing our thinking and research about sexual problems remains in doubt. This has been particularly noteworthy in relation to women's sexual problems (Bancroft et al 2001).

In revising this section, I carefully considered what impact the DSM-IV or its predecessors had had on the development of my thinking as a sex researcher and of my clinical practice as a sex therapist. I came to the conclusion that the impact was more or less confined to categorizing cases for the clinic records, and during my 10 years in the Kinsey Institute Sexual Health Clinic this mainly related to a patient's ability to get treatment covered by health insurance. In the previous two editions of this book neither the DSM nor the ICD systems featured. Yet in reading the recent literature for this third edition, I have been repeatedly struck by the extent to which researchers and clinicians in the field of sexual problems are preoccupied with DSM categorizations. A good example was the article by Binik (2005), where the focus was on whether dyspareunia should go into the 'sexual pain' or 'pain disorder' sections of the DSM-IV (see p. 324). On the other hand, I believe that a classificatory system, or at least an explanatory model which covers the range of sexual problems, and with implications for treatment as well as research, would be of value. What are the prospects for this?

As we approach the development of DSM-V, the next 'official' psychiatric classification system that will cover sexual problems, there is active controversy and debate about how sexual problems should be classified, particularly sexual problems in women. *The Journal of Sex and Marital Therapy* dedicated an issue (2001; Volume 27, Number 2) to a report on The International Consensus Development Conference on Female Sexual Dysfunction: Definitions and Classifications, and 36 commentaries on this report from researchers and clinicians in the field. There were those who believed the conventional DSM approach should be maintained to provide continuity, and there were others, this author included, who believed that a fundamental change was required if the classification system is to have any heuristic value in clinical or research terms. Before too long, we will see what the DSM-V brings us, and in the meantime it is appropriate to put the current DSM-IV into historical context.

Although in their first book Masters & Johnson (1966) put forward their idea of a sexual response cycle, basically the same in men and women, in their second book (1970) they categorized sexual dysfunction for men and for women quite differently. With the male they focused on impotence (primary and secondary), with PE and ejaculatory incompetence as additional categories. With the female they focused on orgasmic dysfunction, with vaginismus as an additional, specifically female dysfunction. Dyspareunia was considered relevant to both men and women. Kaplan (1974) used the concept of 'general female sexual dysfunction', noting that this was 'usually called frigidity' (p. 361). In addition, she described 'orgastic dysfunction', drawing the distinction between inhibition of the vasocongestive and orgasm components of sexual response. Both Kaplan and Masters and Johnson therefore continued to use the conventional but pejorative terms for the principal types of male and female dysfunction, i.e. impotence and frigidity.

The first two editions of the *Diagnostic and Statistical Manual of Mental Disorders* (DSM) did not use the concept sexual dysfunction. DSM-I, under the general heading of 'psychophysiological autonomic and visceral disorders', included the terms frigidity and impotence, PE of semen, and vaginismus in a list of supplementary terms for the urogenital system. In DSM-II only dyspareunia and impotence were listed as examples of psychophysiologic genito-urinary disorders.

In 1980, the concept of psychosexual dysfunction appeared in the third edition of the DSM (American Psychiatric Association 1980). The DSM approach to sexual dysfunction was clearly based on Masters and Johnson's ideas; although interestingly, not their ideas about sexual dysfunction but rather their concept of the sexual response cycle (Masters & Johnson 1966), modified by Kaplan's (1974) addition of sexual desire as a separate component. This resulted in male and female diagnostic categories that were conceptually similar: 'inhibited sexual desire' (neither 'inhibited' nor 'sexual desire' were defined), 'inhibited sexual excitement', 'inhibited orgasm' and 'functional dyspareunia', each with a male and female version. 'Functional vaginismus' was included as a specifically female dysfunction and PE as a male dysfunction.

The current DSM classification (DSM-IV; American Psychiatric Association 2000) defines sexual dysfunction as characterized by disturbance in sexual desire and in the psycho-physiological changes that characterize the sexual response cycle, causing marked distress and interpersonal difficulty. The concept of inhibition no longer features. Thus there is hypoactive sexual desire

disorder and sexual aversion disorder, defined in the same way for men and women. Female sexual arousal disorder is defined as 'a persistent or recurrent inability to attain, or to maintain until completion of the sexual activity, an adequate lubrication-swelling response of sexual excitement' (p. 504), and for the male version, erection is the relevant response. Orgasmic disorder (i.e. delayed or absent orgasm) and dyspareunia are defined in basically the same way for men and women. Vaginismus is a specifically female disorder. PE is a specifically male disorder.

'Distress' as an essential diagnostic criterion was new in the DSM-IV, and it is questionable that it should be used in that way. Distress, it could be argued, is a reaction to the dysfunction and thus has no explanatory value. It is of clinical relevance, but mainly because it determines whether the individual is motivated to change or wants help; the person who is not distressed by the dysfunction, or whose sexual relationship is not affected by it, is unlikely to seek treatment. It does not help in deciding which treatment is most likely to be effective. On the other hand, if our goal is to conceptualize sexual dysfunction in women's terms, capturing the problems and difficulties which are the principal concern for women, then we need to understand what worries or distresses them. The relation between distress and sexual desire is also likely to be complex and as yet not well understood.

The ongoing use by the DSM of the sexual response cycle as a predictable sequence of basically physiological events, essentially the same in women and men, can be seen as an attempt to redress the societal view, which has prevailed in the past, that women's sexuality was something fundamentally different to that of men. Given that such a distinction was central to the long-standing societal repression of female sexuality, challenging this distinction had obvious socio-political significance, and may have been regarded by some as 'politically correct' for that reason. However, although Masters and Johnson proposed a 'sexual response cycle' that in physiological terms was basically the same for women and men, they also emphasized the impact of socio-cultural factors on women's sexuality: 'negation of female sexuality, which discourages the development of an effectively useful sexual value system, has been an exercise of the so-called double standard and its socio-cultural precursors' (1970, p. 216). They go on to say 'socio-cultural influence more often than not places woman in a position in which she must adapt, sublimate, inhibit or even distort her natural capacity to function sexually in order to fulfill her genetically assigned role. *Herein lies a major source of woman's sexual dysfunction*' (p. 218; italics in original). Masters and Johnson did not appear to equate the sexual dysfunctions of men and women, either in their diagnostic categories, or in the above, telling statement. But if their earlier ideas on the sexual response cycle were used by clinicians to achieve 'political correctness' through the DSM process, 'political correctness' can be regarded as no longer the same on this issue. There is now growing recognition of, and emphasis on, gender differences in sexuality, a recurring theme in this book. Alternative models of sexual response (Basson 2000) and new, women-centered definitions of sexual problems in women (Tiefer 2001) have been proposed. And, as early studies evaluating the effects of Viagra in women have proven disappointing (Basson et al 2002), even the pharmaceutical industry is moving toward a 'politically correct' view that there are fundamental differences between men and women's sexuality. Pfizer recently publicly announced that, after 8 years of work, they are terminating their research programme evaluating the effects of Viagra on women, citing greater complexity of women's sexual response and a 'disconnect between genital changes and mental changes' in women as reasons (Harris 2004).

The following section is aimed at progress towards improved clinical diagnosis, and, after empirical evaluation, towards a clinically relevant diagnostic classification.

Towards a better classification of sexual problems

Based on the conceptual approach to understanding sexual problems that has prevailed in this book, the following represents a move towards a classificatory system with heuristic value, both clinically and scientifically. The three windows approach provides a structure for considering aetiological mechanisms (see p. 306): (i) understandable inhibitory reactions to the current life situation (e.g. relationship problems), (ii) vulnerability to inhibitory response as shown in the individual's past history and (iii) effects of psychiatric or medical disorders, or side effects of medication.

The starting point is to acknowledge that sexual activity is not essential for health, and that some individuals live long and rewarding lives without sex. Sex on the other hand, is necessary for reproduction ('assisted fertilization' is changing this to some extent). It is also a central feature in the primary relationships of most of us. But even within sexual relationships, there is considerable variability of sexual responsivity and interest in men and even more so in women. This raises the question of when a 'diagnosis' is needed or appropriate. The following approach differs from conventional systems in placing primary emphasis on the purpose or function of sexual activity, rather than specific physiological components of the individual's sexual response.

The example of asexuality

Some people are relatively 'asexual'; they have little desire for sexual contact with another person and consequently have no particular wish to establish a sexual relationship (see p. 281). We do not know how many people come into this category, nor how stable their asexual identity is, but do we need to regard such asexuality as a dysfunction? The proposed answer is that if an individual has been asexual in this way since adolescence, then this should be regarded as a difference rather than a dysfunction. If an individual becomes asexual after a period of relatively 'normal' sexual function, then a dysfunction may have arisen, and a thorough assessment would be required to establish the cause for this change and hence the best method of treatment. However, the individual may not be concerned about it and hence does not seek treatment. If an asexual individual decides that he or she would like to change, and become sexual, then clinical assessment is appropriate to see if there are factors which, with help, might change to allow that individual to become more sexual (e.g. the long-term presence of beliefs or attitudes which suppress sexual expression in an individual whose sexuality is relatively easily suppressed).

Thus, as exemplified by the asexuality model, we need to distinguish between *differences* which are not considered problematic by those experiencing them, *changes*, for those who have previously benefited from sexuality and for some reason have become less able to do so, and *a desire to be different* in those for whom sex was previously unimportant but who have now become interested in the benefits of being sexual and are experiencing some barriers to obtaining them, or those who throughout their lives have been unable to benefit from sexuality and who wish to do so.

The benefits of being sexual

Sexual activity can lead to three types of benefit: (i) reproduction, rewarding for those who want to have children and raise a family, (ii) a rewarding sexual relationship, and (iii) sexual pleasure.

We can now consider the various barriers to obtaining these three types of benefits.

Sexual barriers to parenthood

Apart from issues of fertility (ovulation in the female, and fertile sperm in the male; see Chapter 15), conception is unlikely when a male is unable to develop an erectile response sufficient for vaginal entry and/or ejaculate intravaginally, or a female is unable to accept vaginal penetration by an erect penis without significant pain. There is as yet no evidence that lack of orgasm in the woman reduces her fertility. If fertility is an issue, the need to time sexual intercourse to occur around ovulation can result in psychological pressure, which in the vulnerable individual or couple may result in or aggravate failure of genital response.

Barriers to establishing a rewarding sexual relationship

There are sexual requirements for two people to succeed in a sexual relationship, whether or not they wish to have children. In the male, problems with erection and ejaculation, and a significant lack of interest in sexual interaction are all barriers. In the female, lack of interest in or reward from engaging in sexual interaction, including vaginal intercourse, or the occurrence of pain or discomfort when vaginal intercourse is attempted, are all barriers to establishing a sexual relationship. The nature of the 'necessary' reward for the woman may vary, however. For some women the reward is the emotional closeness, the experience of being desired that results from sexual interaction, and giving her partner sexual pleasure (the basic pattern; see p. 131). Such a woman who is willing to interact sexually, who enjoys the emotional closeness, but does not become obviously sexually aroused or does not experience an orgasm, does not have a barrier to establishing a sexual relationship and is not necessarily dysfunctional. For other women, sexual pleasure and orgasm for themselves may be equally or more important (the superadded component; see p. 133). For such a woman, difficulty in becoming sexually aroused or experiencing orgasm during sexual interactions with her partner may be a barrier to establishing and maintaining a rewarding sexual relationship.

Although couples vary in their expectation of who initiates sexual interaction, the tendency is to see the male as being mainly responsible. Women may feel more comfortable initiating once they are in an established relationship, but many women still expect their male partner to initiate at least as often if not more so than them. This is relevant to how problematic low sexual interest becomes. Lack of sexual interest in the woman, as shown by lack of initiation of sexual activity, may not be a problem providing she is responsive to her partner's initiations. Lack of interest in the man is likely to be problematic for both partners.

PE may be a problem mainly because it results in premature termination of sexual interaction, leaving the partner frustrated. It may also be a problem because it becomes associated with performance anxiety in the man, with resulting impairment of his genital response and his sexual pleasure.

Barriers to experiencing sexual pleasure

Two people may have a rewarding and intimate sexual relationship but either or both partners may not be experiencing the sexual pleasure they have come to expect. For the man, establishment of a firm erection, and the associated increase in erotic sensitivity of the penis, are important for his sexual pleasure, whether or not he participates in vaginal intercourse. Orgasm and ejaculation are part of his expected pleasure, unless circumstances restrict the possibilities for this (e.g. during early 'dating'). Erotic sensitivity in other parts of his body and response to tactile stimulation by the partner contribute to his sexual pleasure, but are typically less important than the pleasure from genital stimulation and orgasm.

Women, by comparison, are more variable in the sources of their pleasure, as conceptualized by the distinction between the basic pattern and superadded components of sexual reward referred to earlier. A woman's normal pattern of sexual response and pleasure will determine what is for her the development of a barrier to sexual pleasure.

For both men and women, loss of sexual interest or desire may be regretted because of the associated lack of pleasurable sexual activity, even when there is no negative impact on the sexual relationship.

Explaining a barrier

Whereas all three barriers may co-exist, it is helpful to establish which barrier is the main reason for seeking help. The next step is to decide how best to explain this barrier, i.e. if it is an understandable reaction to current circumstances (i.e. the first window), if there is evidence of vulnerability to maladaptive inhibition (i.e. the second window) and if there is evidence of an age-related, psychiatric, medical or medication-induced impairment of sexual responsiveness or interest. By identifying the relevant barrier, and which of the three types of explanation are relevant (and there may be more than one), the appropriate treatment programme will be more easily selected.

Conclusion

This proposal for a classificatory system has emerged from my clinical experience and thoughts about a heuristically valuable approach, but has not yet been evaluated in any systematic manner, and such an evaluation is required before putting it forward as an alternative to the DSM-IV. Its application in treatment will be considered in the next chapter, together with some clinical examples.

REFERENCES

American Psychiatric Association 1980 Diagnostic and Statistical Manual of Mental Disorders. 3rd edn (DSM-III). Psychiatric Association, Washington DC.

American Psychiatric Association 2000 Diagnostic and Statistical Manual of Mental Disorders. 4th edn (DSM-IV). Psychiatric Association, Washington DC.

Avis NER, Zhao X, Johannes CB, Ory M, Brockwell S, Greendale GA 2005 Correlates of sexual function among multi-ethnic middle-aged women: results from the Study of Women's Health Across the Nation (SWAN). Menopause 12: 385–398.

Babula O, Lazdane G, Kroica J, Linhares IM, Ledger WJ, Witkin SS 2005 Frequency of Interleukin-4 (IL-4) − 589 gene polymorphism and vaginal concentrations of IL-4, nitric oxide and mannose-binding lectin in women with recurrent vulvovaginal candidiasis. Clinical Infectious Diseases 40: 1258–1262.

Bancroft J 1974 Deviant Sexual Behavior: Modification and Assessment. Oxford: Oxford University Press.

Bancroft J 1989 Man and his penis — a relationship under threat? Journal of Psychology and Human Sexuality 2: 7–32.

Bancroft J 1992 Leading comments. The vocabulary of sex therapy: labels. Sexual and Marital Therapy 7: 5–9.

Bancroft J 1999 Central inhibition of sexual response in the male: a theoretical perspective. Neuroscience & Biobehavioral Review 23: 763–784.

Bancroft J 2000 Individual differences in sexual risk taking by men: A psycho-socio-biological approach. In Bancroft J (ed) The Role of Theory in Sex Research. Indiana University Press, Bloomington, pp. 177–212.

Bancroft J 2005 The history of sexual medicine in the United Kingdom. Journal of Sexual Medicine 2: 569–574.

Bancroft J, Coles L 1976 Three years experience in a sexual problems clinic. British Medical Journal 1: 1575–1577.

Bancroft J, Vukadinovic Z 2004 Sexual addiction, sexual compulsivity, sexual impulsivity or what? Towards a theoretical model. Journal of Sex Research 41: 225–234.

Bancroft J, Tyrer G, Warner P 1982 The classification of sexual problems in women. British Journal of Sexual Medicine 9: 30–37.

Bancroft J, Graham CA, McCord C 2001 Conceptualizing women's sexual problems. Journal of Sexual & Marital Therapy 27: 95–104.

Bancroft J, Loftus J, Long JS 2003a Distress about sex: A national survey of women in heterosexual relationships. Archives of Sexual Behavior 32: 193–208.

Bancroft J, Janssen E, Strong D, Carnes L, Vukadinovic Z, Long JS 2003b The relation between mood and sexuality in heterosexual men. Archives of Sexual Behavior 32: 217–230.

Bancroft J, Janssen E, Carnes L, Goodrich D, Strong D 2004 Sexual activity and risk taking in young heterosexual men: the relevance of sexual arousability, mood, and sensation seeking. Journal of Sex Research 41: 181–192.

Bancroft J, Carnes J, Janssen E, Long JS 2005a Erectile and ejaculatory problems in gay and heterosexual men. Archives of Sexual Behavior 34: 285–297.

Bancroft J, Herbenick D, Barnes T, Hallam-Jones R, Wylie K, Janssen E, and members of BASRT 2005b The relevance of the dual control model to male sexual dysfunction: the Kinsey Institute/BASRT Collaborative Project. Sexual and Relationship Therapy 20: 13–30.

Barth RJ, Kinder BN 1987 The mislabeling of sexual impulsivity. Journal of Sex and Marital Therapy 13: 15–23.

Baumeister RF, Heatherton TF 1996 Self-regulation failure: an overview. Psychological Inquiry 7: 1–15.

Basson R 2000 The female sexual response: a different model. Journal of Sex & Marital Therapy 26: 51–64.

Basson R, McInnes R, Smith MD, Hodgson G, Koppiker N 2002 Efficacy and safety of sildenafil citrate in women with sexual dysfunction associated with female sexual arousal disorder. Journal of Women's Health 11: 367–377.

Baumeister RF, Heatherton TF, Tice DM 1994 Losing Control: How and Why People Fail at Self-Regulation. Academic Press, San Diego.

Binik YM 2005 Should dyspareunia be retained as a sexual dysfunction in DSM-V? A painful classification decision. Archives of Sexual Behavior 34: 11–21.

Binik YM, Meana M, Berkley K, Khalife S 1999 The sexual pain disorders: is the pain sexual or is the sex painful? Annual Review of Sex Research 10: 210–235.

Black DW, Kehrberg LLD, Flumerfelt DL, Schlosser SS 1997 Characteristics of 36 subjects reporting compulsive sexual behavior. American Journal of Psychiatry 154: 243–249.

Blanchard R, Hucker SJ 1991 Age, transvestism, bondage, and concurrent paraphiliac activities in 117 fatal cases of autoerotic asphyxia. British Journal of Psychiatry 159: 371–377.

Bohm-Starke N, Hilliges M, Falconer C, Rylander E 1998 Increased intra-epithelial innervation in women with vulvar vestibulitis syndrome. Gynecologic & Obstetric Investigation 46: 256–260.

Brauer M, Laan E, ter Kuile MM 2006 Sexual arousal in women with superficial dyspareunia. Archives of Sexual Behavior 35: 191–200.

Breiter HC, Aharon I, Kahneman D, Dale A, Shizgal P 2001 Functional imaging of neural responses to expectancy and experience of monetary gains and losses. Neuron 20: 619–639.

Brust JCM 2000 Circulation of the brain. Appendix C. In Kandel ER, Schwartz JH, Jessell TM (eds) Principles of Neural Science. 4th edn. McGraw-Hill, New York, pp. 1302–1316.

Byard RW, Hucker SJ, Hazelwood RR 1993 Fatal and near-fatal autoerotic asphyxial episodes in women; characteristic features based on a review of nine cases. American Journal of Forensic Medicine and Pathology 14: 70–73.

Carson RC 1991 Dilemmas in the pathway of the DSM-IV. Journal of Abnormal Psychology 100: 302–307.

Catalan J, Hawton K, Day A 1990 Couples referred to a sexual dysfunction clinic. Psychological and physical morbidity. British Journal of Psychiatry 156: 61–67.

CBS News 2005 'Choking game' s deadly trend. July 28th 2005

Coleman E 1986 Sexual compulsion vs. sexual addiction: The debate continues. SIECUS Report July: 7–11.

Cooper A 1969 A clinical study of 'coital anxiety' in male potency disorders. Journal of Psychosomatic Research 13: 143–147.

Cooper A (ed) 2002 Sex and the Internet: a Guidebook for Clinicians. Brunner-Routledge, New York.

Cove J, Boyle M 2002 Gay men's self-defined sexual problems, perceived causes and factors in remission. Sexual and Relationship Therapy 17: 137–148.

Dennerstein J, Lehert P 2004 Women's sexual functioning, lifestyle, mid-age, and menopause in 12 European countries. Menopause 11: 778–785.

Dietz PE 1989 Television inspired autoerotic asphyxiation. Journal of Forensic Sciences 34: 58.

Dunn KM, Croft PR, Kackett GI 1998 Sexual problems: a study of the prevalence and need for health care in the general population. Family Practice 15: 519–524.

Dunn KM, Cherkas LF, Spector TD 2005 Genetic influences on variation in female orgasmic function: a twin study. Biology Letters 1: 260–263.

Ekman P 2003 Emotions Revealed. Times Books, New York.

Ellis H 1905 Studies in the Psychology of Sex. Volume 1, Part 2. Random House, New York (published 1941).

Fedoroff JP 1993 Serotonergic drug treatment of deviant sexual interests. Annals of Sex Research 6: 105–121.

Fisher S 1973 The Female Orgasm. Basic Books, New York.

Friedrich WN, Gerber PN 1994 Autoerotic asphyxia: the development of a paraphilia. Journal of the American Academy of Child and Adolescent Psychiatry 33: 970–974.

Fugl-Meyer AR, Fugl-Meyer KS 1999 Sexual disabilities, problems and satisfaction in 18–74 year old Swedes. Scandinavian Journal of Sexology 2: 79–105.

Fugl-Meyer AR, Fugl-Meyer KS 2006 Prevalence data in Europe. In Goldstein I, Meston C, Davis S, Traish A (eds) Textbook of Female Sexual Dysfunction. Taylor & Francis, London, pp. 34–41.

Gold SN, Heffner CL 1998 Sexual addiction: many conceptions, minimal data. Clinical Psychology Review 18: 367–381.

Goodman A 1997 Sexual addiction. In Lowinson JH, Ruiz P, Millman RB, Langrod JG (eds) Substance Abuse: a Comprehensive Textbook. Williams & Wilkins, Philadelphia, pp. 340–354.

Graham CA, Bancroft J 2006 Assessing the prevalence of female sexual dysfunction with surveys: what is feasible? In Goldstein I, Meston C, Davis S, Traish A (eds) Textbook of Female Sexual Dysfunction. Taylor & Francis, London, pp. 52–62.

Granata A, Bancroft J, Del Rio G 1995 Stress and the erectile response to intracavernosal prostaglandin E1 in men with erectile dysfunction. Psychosomatic Medicine 57: 336–344.

Granot M, Friedman M, Yarnitsky D, Tamir A, Zimmer EZ 2004 Primary and secondary vulvar vestibulitis syndrome: systemic pain perception and psychophysical characteristics. American Journal of Obstetrics and Gynecology 191: 138–142.

Harris G 2004 Pfizer gives up testing Viagra on women. New York Times Feb 28th.

Hawton K, Catalan JP 1990 Sex therapy for vaginismus: characteristics of couples and treatment outcome. Sex and Marital Therapy 5: 39–48.

Hazelwood RR, Dietz PE, Burgess AW 1983 Autoerotic Fatalities. Heath (Lexington Books), Lexington MA.

Hems SA, Crowe M 1999 The psychosexual dysfunction clinic at the Maudsley Hospital: a survey of referrals between January and December 1996. Sexual and Marital Therapy 14: 15–25.

Hirschfeld M 1938 Sexual Anomalies and Perversions. Encyclopaedic Press, London.

Hirst JF, Baggaley MR, Watson JP 1996 A four-year survey of an inner-city psychosexual clinic. Sexual and Marital Therapy, 11: 19–36.

Holden C 2001 'Behavioral addictions': do they exist? Science 294: 980–982.

Jenkins AR 2000 When self-pleasuring becomes self-destruction: autoerotic asphyxiation paraphilia. The International Electronic Journal of Health Education 3: 208–216. http://www.iejhe.siu.edu

Johnson J 1968 Disorders of Sexual Potency in the Male. Pergamon: Oxford.

Kafka MP 1997 A monoamine hypothesis for the pathophysiology of paraphilic disorders. Archives of Sexual Behavior 26: 343–357.

Kafka MP 2000 Psychopharmacologic treatments for nonparaphilic compulsive sexual behaviors. CNS Spectrums 5: 49–59.

Kaplan HS 1974 The New Sex Therapy. Brunner/Mazel: New York.

Kendall R 1975 The Role of Diagnosis in Psychiatry. Blackwell: Oxford.

King M, Holt V, Nazareth I 2007 Women's views of their sexual difficulties: agreement and disagreement with clinical diagnosis. Archives of Sexual Behavior 36: 281–288.

Kinsey AC, Pomeroy WB, Martin CE 1948 Sexual Behavior in the Human Male. Saunders, Philadelphia.

Laan E, van Lunsen R 1997 Hormones and sexuality in postmenopausal women: a psychophysiological study. Journal of Psychosomatic Obstetrics & Gynecology 18: 126–133.

Laan E, van Driel E, van Lunsen RHW 2003 Sexual responses of women with sexual arousal disorder to visual sexual stimuli [in Dutch]. Tijdschrift Seksuologie 27: 1–13.

Laumann EO, Gagnon JH, Michael RT, Michaels S 1994 The Social Organization of Sexuality. Sexual Practices in the United States. University of Chicago Press, Chicago.

Laumann EO, Paik A, Rosen RC 1999 Sexual dysfunction in the United States: prevalence and predictors. Journal of the American Medical Association 281: 537–544.

Laumann EO, Nicolosi A, Glasser DB, Paik A, Gingell C, Moreira E, Wang T for the GSSAB Investigators Group 2005 Sexual problems among women and men aged 40–80y: prevalence and correlates identified in the global study of sexual attitudes and behaviors. International Journal of Impotence Research 17: 39–57.

Lazarus RS 1966 Psychological Stress and the Coping Process. McGraw Hill, New York.

Leiblum SR 2007 Persistent genital arousal disorder. In Leiblum SR (ed) Principles and Practice of Sex Therapy, 4th edn. Guildford, New York, pp. 54–83.

Leiblum SR, Nathan SG 2001 Persistent sexual arousal syndrome: a newly discovered pattern of female sexuality. Journal of Sexual and Marital Therapy 27: 191–198.

Leiblum SR, Chivers M (2007) Normal and persistent genital arousal in women: new perspectives. Journal of Sex and Marital Therapy 33: 357–376.

Leiblum S, Seehuus M, Brown C 2007a Persistent genital arousal: disordered or normative aspect of female sexual response. Journal of Sexual Medicine 4: 680–689.

Leiblum S, Seehuus M, Goldmeier D, Brown C 2007b Psychological, medical and pharmacological correlates or persistent genital arousal disorder. Journal of Sexual Medicine 4: 1358–1366.

Lesch KP, Bengel D, Heils A, Sabol SZ, Greenberg BD, Petri S, et al 1996 Association of anxiety-related traits with a polymorphism in the serotonin transporter gene regulatory region. Science 274: 1527–1531.

Levin R 2005 The mechanisms of human ejaculation — a critical analysis. Sexual and Relationship Therapy 20: 123–131.

Luzzi G 2003 Male genital pain disorders. Sexual and Relationship Therapy 18: 225–235.

Maines RP 1999 The Technology of Orgasm. Johns Hopkins Press, Baltimore.

Marks LV 2001 Sexual Chemistry: a History of the Contraceptive Pill. Yale University Press, New Haven.

Masters WH, Johnson VE 1966 Human Sexual Response. Churchill, London.

Masters WH, Johnson VE 1970 Human Sexual Inadequacy. Churchill, London.

Masters WH, Johnson VE 1979 Homosexuality in Perspective. Little, Brown, Boston.

Mercer CH, Fenton KA, Johnson AM, Wellings K, Macdowall W, McManus S, Nanchalal K, Erens B 2003 Sexual function problems and help seeking behaviour in Britain: national probability sample survey. British Medical Journal 327: 426–427.

Mercer CH, Fenton KA, Johnson AM, Copas AJ, Macdowall W, Erens B, Wellings K 2005 Who reports sexual function problems? Empirical evidence from Britain's 2000 National Survey of Sexual Atitudes and Lifestyles. Sexually Transmitted Infections 81: 394–399.

Miller WI 1997 The Anatomy of Disgust. Harvard University Press, Cambridge.

Ming Chow K 2003 Deadly game among children and adolescents. Annals of Emergency Medicine 42: 310.

Money J, Wainwright G, Hingsburger D 1991 The Breathless Orgasm: a Lovemap Biography of Asphyxiophilia. Prometheus, Buffalo, NY.

Moxham J 2000 Respiratory failure: definition and causes. In Ledingham JGG, Warrell DA (eds) Concise Textbook of Medicine. Oxford University Press, Oxford, pp. 491–492.

Nichols M, Shernoff M 2007 Therapy with sexual minorities: queering practice. In Leiblum SR (ed) Principles and Practice of Sex Therapy. Guilford, New York, pp. 379–415.

Orford J 1978 Hypersexuality: implications for a theory of dependence. British Journal of Addiction 73: 299–310.

Osborn M, Hawton K, Gath D 1988 Sexual dysfunction among middle-aged women in the community. British Medical Journal 296: 959–962.

Paff BA 1985 Sexual dysfunction in gay men requesting treatment. Journal of Sex & Marital Therapy 11: 3–18.

Paik A, Laumann EO 2006. Prevalence of women's sexual problems in the USA. In Goldstein I, Meston C, Davis S, Traish A (eds) Textbook of Female Sexual Dysfunction. Taylor & Francis, London, pp. 23–33.

Pearlstein S 2003 Teens see asphyxial game as a drug-free high. (Explain dangers to our young patients.) Family Practice News 33: 38.

Potts A, Gavey N, Grace VM, Vares T 2003 The downside of Viagra: women's experiences and concerns. Sociology of Health & Illness 25: 697–719.

Pukall CF, Binik YM, Khalife S, Amsel R, Abbott FV 2002 Vestibular tactile and pain thresholds in women with vulvar vestibulitis syndrome. Pain 96: 163–175.

Quadland MC 1985 Compulsive sexual behavior: definition of a problem and an approach to treatment. Journal of Sex and Marital Therapy 11: 121–132.

Random House Dictionary of the English Language (Unabridged edition) 1983 Random House, New York.

Raviv M 1993 Personality characteristics of sexual addicts and pathological gamblers. Journal of Gambling Studies 9: 17–30.

Rédoute J, Stoleru S, Grégoire MC, Costes N, Cinotti L, Lavenne F, Le Bars D, Forest MG, Pujol J-F 2000 Brain processing of visual sexual stimuli in human males. Human Brain Mapping 11: 162–177.

Richters J, Grulich AE, de Visser RO, Smith AMA, Rissel CE 2003 Sexual difficulties in a representative sample of adults. Australian and New Zealand Journal of Public Health 27: 164–170.

Rinehart NJ, McCabe MP 1997 Hypersexuality: psychopathology or normal variant of sexuality? Sexual and Marital Therapy 12: 45–60.

Robinson TE, Berridge KC 2000 The psychology and neurobiology of addiction: an incentive-sensitization view. Addiction 95: 91–117.

Rosen R, Brown C, Heiman J, Leiblum SR, Meston CM, Shabsigh R, Ferguson D, D'Agostino R 2000 The Female Sexual Function Index (FSFI): a multidimensional self-report instrument for the assessment of female sexual function. Journal of Sex & Marital Therapy 26: 191–208.

Rosen R, Janssen E, Wiegel M, Bancroft J, Althof S, Wincze J, Segraves RT, Barlow DH 2006 Psychological and interpersonal correlates in men with erectile dysfunction and their partners: a pilot study of treatment outcome with sildenafil. Journal of Sexual & Marital Therapy 32: 215–234.

Rosser BRS, Short BJ, Thurmes PJ, Coleman E 1998 Anodyspareunia, the unacknowledged sexual dysfunction: a validation study of painful receptive anal intercourse and its psychosexual concomitants in homosexual men. Journal of Sex & Marital Therapy 24: 281–292.

Rowland DL, Hotsmuller EJ, Slob AK, Cooper SE 1997 The study of ejaculatory response in the psychophysiological laboratory. Journal of Sex Research 34: 161–166.

Rowland DL, Tai W, Brummett K 2007 Interactive processes in ejaculatory disorders: psychophysiological considerations. In Janssen E (ed) The Psychophysiology of Sex. Indiana University Press, Bloomington, pp. 227–243.

Roy J 2004 A survey of relate psychosexual therapy clients, January to March 2002. Sexual and Relationship Therapy 19: 155–166.

Sanders SA, Graham CA, Milhausen RR 2007 Predicting sexual problems in women: the relevance of sexual excitation and sexual inhibition. Archives of Sexual Behavior, 37: 241–251.

Sandfort TGM, de Keizer M 2001 Sexual problems in gay men: an overview of the empirical research. Annual Review of Sex Research 12: 93–120.

Semans J 1956 Premature ejaculation: a new approach. Southern Medical Journal 49: 353–358.

Shapira NA, Goldsmith TD, Keck PE, Khosia UM, McElroy SL 2000 Psychiatric features of individuals with problematic Internet use. Journal of Affective Disorders 57: 267–272.

Sheehan W, Garfinkel BD 1988 Adolescent autoerotic deaths: a case study. Journal of the American Academy of Child and Adolescent Psychiatry 27: 367–370.

Shlamovitz GZ, Assia A, Ben-Sira L, et al 2003 'Suffocation roulette': a case of recurrent syncope in an adolescent boy. Annals of Emergency Medicine 41: 223–226.

Simons JS, Carey MP 2001 Prevalence of sexual dysfunctions: results from a decade of research. Archives of Sexual Behavior 30: 177–219.

Spira A, Bajos N, the ACSF Group 1994 Sexual Behaviour and AIDS. Avebury, Aldershot.

Stein DJ, Hollander E, Anthony DT, Schneier FR, Fallon BA, Liebowitz MR et al 1992 Sertonergic medications for sexual obsessions, sexual addictions, and paraphilias. Journal of Clinical Psychiatry 53: 267–271.

Stein DJ, Black DW, Shapira NA, Spitzer RL 2001 Hypersexual disorder and preoccupation with internet pornography. American Journal of Psychiatry 158: 1590–1594.

Stoléru S, Grégoire MC, Gérard D, Decety J, Lafarge E, Cinotti L et al 1999 Neuroanatomical correlates of visually evoked sexual arousal in human males. Archives of Sexual Behavior 28: 1–21.

Tiefer L 2001 Arriving at a 'new view' of women's sexual problems: background, theory, and activism. In Kaschak E, Tiefer E (eds) A New View of Women's Sexual Problems. Haworth Press, Binghamton, NY, pp. 63–98.

Thompson L 1999 The Wandering Womb: A Cultural History of Outrageous Beliefs about Women. Prometheus, Amherst.

US Department of Health and Human Services 2001 The surgeon general's call to action to promote sexual health and responsible sexual behavior. US Government Printing Office, Washington, DC. http://www.surgeongeneral. gov/library/sexualhealth

Uva JL 1995 Autoerotic asphyxia in the United States. Journal of Forensic Sciences 40: 574–581.

Varjonen M, Santilla P, Hoglund M, Jern P, Johansson, A, Wager I, Witting K, Algara M, Sandnabba NK 2007 Genetic and environmental effects on sexual excitation and sexual inhibition in men. Journal of Sex Research 44: 359–369.

Veith I 1965 Hysteria: the history of a disease. University of Chicago Press, Chicago.

Waldinger MD 2002 The neurobiological approach to premature ejaculation. Journal of Urology 168: 2359–2367.

Waldinger MD, Rietschel M, Nothen MM, Hengeveld MW, Olivier B 1998 Familial occurrence of primary premature ejaculation. Psychiatric Genetics 8: 37.

Warner P, Bancroft J, members of the Edinburgh Human Sexuality Group 1987 A regional clinical service for sexual problems: a three year survey. Sexual and Marital Therapy 2: 115–126.

Warwick HMC, Salkovskis PM 1990 Unwanted erections in obsessive–compulsive disorder. British Journal of Psychiatry 157: 919–921.

Watkins ES 1998 On the Pill: a Social History of Oral Contraceptives, 1950–1970. Johns Hopkins University Press, Baltimore.

Westrom LV, Willen R 1998 Vestibular nerve fiber proliferation in vulvar vestibulitis syndrome. Obstetrics & Gynecology 91: 572–576.

Wouda J, Hartman PM, Bakker RM, Bakker JO, van de Wiel HBM, Weeijmar Schultz WCM 1998 Vaginal photoplethysmography in women with dyspareunia. Journal of Sex Research 35: 141–147.

Zilbergeld B 1992 The man behind the broken penis: social and psychological determinants of erectile failure. In Rosen RC, Leiblum SR (eds) Erectile Disorders: Assessment and Treatment. Guilford Press, New York, pp. 27–54.

Zillman D 1983 Transfer of excitation in emotional behavior. In Cacioppo JT, Petty RE (eds) Social Psychophysiology: a Sourcebook. Guilford Press, New York, pp. 215–240.

Helping people with sexual problems: assessment and treatment options

Treatment of sexual problems — the historical
background 344

PART 1
Problems of reduced sexual interest
or response 346

Sex therapy for the couple 346

Sex therapy for the individual 353

The outcome of sex therapy for couples 355

Pharmacological and hormonal treatments 360

Other non-pharmacological methods of treatment 366

Outcome of integrated psychological and
medical treatment 366

The current status of treatment for problems of
impaired sexual response or interest 367

Assessment for treatment — when to treat and which
treatments to use 367

Clinical illustrations 374
Case study 1 374
Case study 2 374
Case study 3 375

Treatment of same sex couples 375

PART 2
Problematic sexual behaviour 376
'Out of control' sexual behaviour 376

PART 3
Sexual or gender identity problems 377
Sexual identity problems 377
Gender identity problems 377

In the previous editions of this book there were two separate chapters for assessment and treatment of sexual problems. Since then there have been a number of substantial changes in the field. As mentioned in the last chapter, in the section on medicalization, new pharmacological treatments have become available, the most notable being the PDE-5 inhibitors such as sildenafil, for the treatment of erectile dysfunction (ED). This has resulted in a shift in the medical world from the specialist, in particular the urologist, to the primary care physician as the source of prescribed treatment, accompanied by a dramatic reduction in the use of specialized methods of assessment, particularly of erectile function. There is increasing evidence, however, that treating ED with a prescription and a minimum of assessment is associated with benefits that are often transient or unacceptable in the longer term. Simply focusing on the erectile response by means of a drug, with no attention to other factors in the man's current life or relationship which might be contributing to the problem, and no attention to how his partner feels about the problem or the solution, while solving the problem for some, will be insufficient for many (e.g. Althof 2002; Leiblum 2002). Exactly the same principles apply to other sexual problems. At the same time there is a shortage of good evidence of the effectiveness of psychological treatments, and this issue will be addressed later in this chapter. This is in large part because of the complexity of evaluating treatments that focus on the couple and involve changing interpersonal dynamics. A specific dysfunction, such as erectile failure, then becomes one of several facets of the situation requiring change. As will be concluded later, that is no justification for the absence of adequately powered treatment outcome studies, but it is to some extent an explanation.

In these circumstances, there has been an understandable shift towards integrating pharmacological and psychological methods of treatment, well reviewed by Rosen (2007) in relation to ED. Whereas such integration was proposed in the last edition of this book, it will now become more of an organizing principle in this section.

There are two further important aspects. In the last chapter, by using the three windows approach the need for considering a wide range of causative factors was emphasized. Whereas much can be done in the course of clinical assessment, I have been increasingly impressed in my own career as a sex therapist by the powerful way that the early stages of sex therapy provide assessment through the first window (e.g. relationship problems) and through the second window (e.g. negative attitudes to sex). This is partly because the carefully graduated behavioural programme helps to identify the key problems or causes of inhibition, and also because, in the process, a positive patient–therapist relationship becomes established, making it easier to uncover and discuss sensitive issues. I now see the early stages of a behavioural programme for the couple as a key component of the assessment process; hence, the combination of both assessment and treatment in this one chapter, and a description of available treatment methods given before considering how assessment helps to decide on which to use. Secondly, as has been known for some time, a wide range of medical conditions can impact on an individual's sexuality and hence the sexual relationship of that individual. In the earlier 'medicalized' phase of intensive vascular and neurological investigation, the focus was on the medical condition, without sufficient consideration of the individual and the relationship. Important consequences of that approach were that insufficient attention was paid to (i) the psychological component of the psychosomatic process, which can be of crucial importance even when relevant somatic pathology has been identified, and (ii) the part that sexuality was playing in the relationship and the various ways in which a couple can adapt to medically induced changes in sexual function.

Given the complexity of sexual relationships and the variety of patterns that can lead to sexual problems, and given the importance of a sexually satisfying relationship for the well-being and health of men and women in long-term relationships, it is clearly desirable for there to be specialist clinical services available that allow the full range of assessment and treatment. The Kinsey Institute Sexual Health Clinic and the integrated group of Edinburgh clinics I was involved in earlier in my career (Warner et al 1987), I consider to be in this category. But the reality is that such services are the exception, and, if anything, are becoming less in evidence than previously. This chapter, however, is written with such a clinic in mind. In this era of evidence-based medicine, there will be a need to demonstrate clearly the advantages of such a service if they are to increase in the future. The challenges involved in that process are considerable and will be considered more closely later in this chapter. As I retire I must fervently hope that those remaining in and joining this field will grapple and succeed with that task.

The types of sexual problem presented at sexual problems clinics were reviewed in the previous chapter, based on studies of patients or clients attending such clinics in the UK. In this chapter we will consider three categories of problem: (i) problems of reduced sexual interest or response, (ii) problematic sexual behaviour, and (iii) problems with gender or sexual identity. In each category we will describe the treatment options currently available and then consider the assessment required before making an appropriate treatment plan. In the first category the principal focus for both treatment and assessment is on the couple. Treatment and assessment when only an individual is involved is also covered.

In each of the first two problem categories most of those seeking help will be heterosexual, but some will be gay men or lesbian women or bisexual. The extent to which their problems differ was considered in Chapter 11. The principles of treatment and methods of assessment, however, are basically the same for same sex and opposite sex couples. The third category involves individuals who have a problem with identity. Most often it is gender identity that is at issue; men who feel themselves to be women, or vice versa, and who seek help in living their lives in the preferred gender. Occasionally, there is concern about sexual identity; e.g. am I gay or bisexual? Can I become straight?

Treatment of sexual problems — the historical background

Given how fashions in treatment tend to come and go, it is of some importance to place current approaches to treatment in a historical context. The dominant influence in the first half of the 20th century was psychoanalysis. Sexual problems, whether experienced as dysfunction or deviance, were regarded as symptoms of disorders of personality development; hence their effective treatment was seen to require psychoanalytic therapy, usually of a fairly prolonged kind. The essence of this approach was described by Rosen (1977): 'Full analysis is usually four or five times weekly, and extends for many years because of the time necessary to effect structural changes in the personality concerning events in earliest childhood which are totally unconscious'. Much reliance is placed on analysing the 'transference', which is a process 'whereby the patient, following the basic rule of free association, relives within the therapeutic situation past psychic events in their fullest recall ... The therapist is regarded as being the other person or persons in that past relationship or experience... The process of verbalizing such reliving, which partakes of abreaction in its emotional expression ... is known as working through'. In this way the defences against these early stresses are gradually relinquished and conflicts resolved. However, 'because one is dealing in the sexual disorders with pleasurable aspects which the patient does not wish to give up, and painful guilts, anxieties, and losses the patient does not wish to encounter, progress is slow and proceeds against constant resistance' (Rosen 1977; pp 1260–1261). Not surprisingly, given the cost and time involved, such treatment was available to only a few of those with sexual problems, and the benefits that those few obtained have not been clearly documented.

The psychoanalytic approach has always been countered to some extent by a more pragmatic and directive view of psychological treatment, in which learning or relearning or the acquisition of healthy habits has been the basic theme. In an early crude form this was shown in the various attempts to discourage masturbation, believed to lead to all types of problems, sexual and otherwise. Towards the end of the 19th and in the early parts of the 20th century hypnosis enjoyed a vogue, and is still in evidence to a limited extent today. Von Schrenck-Notzing (1895) wrote a monograph on the use of hypnotherapy in the treatment of various sexual problems. He derived the principles of treatment from the more general principles of education, the aim of which was 'to create a series of habits by means of direct persuasion, acts, imitation and admiration'. Using 'suggestion' in its widest sense, he regarded all education as a combination of coordinated and well-considered suggestions. He believed sexual problems stemmed from 'faulty habits'. Whilst such approaches seem crude today, they contain much of the essence of more modern behavioural methods.

Over the years a number of practical approaches have been advocated such as progressive relaxation (Schultz 1951), a 'stop–start' method for controlling premature ejaculation (PE) (Semans 1956), the use of graded dilators for vaginismus and self-stimulation techniques for unresponsive women (Hastings 1967). These were essentially empirical, atheoretical approaches.

Modern behaviour therapy became established in the 1950s and 1960s. Practical behavioural approaches were based on the theoretical principles of learning derived from laboratory experiments. This basis claimed to endow such treatment with a scientific respectability, in contrast to the more mundane 'commonsense' of earlier practical approaches. This scientific respectability has proved to be an illusion, as the early theoretical assumptions have failed to be justified, but it did motivate many scientifically minded clinicians to explore these treatment approaches. Much of the 'scientism' of early behaviour therapy, shown in careful methods of measuring change, was a reaction against the unscientific nature of psychoanalysis. As a consequence of these early theoretical constraints, treatment of sexual problems was mainly confined to those conditions which fitted an appropriate experimental learning model, hence the early emphasis on aversive conditioning and the modification of 'undesirable' sexual behaviours, such as homosexuality. These aversive procedures, which evoked considerable ingenuity amongst their innovators, seem of very limited relevance nowadays, not simply because of their doubtful efficacy. They gave way to more positive approaches — learning new behaviours rather than actively discouraging old ones (Bancroft 1974). Behaviour therapy for the much more widespread problems of sexual dysfunction received very little attention. Occasional case reports of the use of systematic desensitization for sexual dysfunction (e.g. Lazarus 1963; Wolpe 1969) appeared, but were few compared to the literature on the treatment of deviant sexuality.

Alongside the psychoanalytically and behaviourally oriented therapists were those advocating surgical, pharmacological or mechanical methods of treatment. In the 1930s there was a brief interest in a variety of surgical procedures for impotence, such as cautery and the passage of cold sounds, tightening of the perineal musculature, the application of testicular diathermy or galvanic stimulation of the perineal musculature (Johnson 1968). Not surprisingly, in view of the lack of any sensible rationale, such methods had a short history. The main surgical procedure used for treating female dysfunction was Fenton's operation for vaginismus, and posterior wall vaginal repairs were sometimes carried out to increase vaginal tightness.

Surgical treatment of erectile failure then entered a new and important phase. The 1940s saw the first attempts at inserting penile splints, implants or prostheses. In the 1970s and 1980s there was a dramatic increase in these methods, accompanied by considerable technical ingenuity. Vascular surgery for erectile problems attributed to vascular pathology was also being explored. This growth in surgical interventions was accompanied by increased interest in methods of investigation and diagnosis, ostensibly to identify those cases where organic aetiology justified surgical treatment. The tendency to see sexual dysfunction as *either* organic *or* psychogenic prevailed, in spite of unremitting evidence that both types of factor were, more often than not, involved. There were some benefits to the field, if not to the individual patients; substantial progress was made in understanding the peripheral physiological mechanisms of sexual response, particularly erection, although much less progress in understanding what was happening in the brain.

Non-surgical mechanical devices have been on the scene for some time. The coital training apparatus of Loewenstein (1947) was an early example. More recently we have seen penile rings and vacuum devices for inducing erection mechanically. These will be considered later.

Pharmacological agents to help sexual difficulties remained elusive. The search for the effective aphrodisiac is, needless to say, older than alchemy (Taberner 1985). The story in relation to penile erection was recounted in Chapter 4, first with the discovery of the effects of drugs injected into the penis, and then the big breakthrough with Viagra. The impact of this serendipitous discovery on the pharmaceutical industry, and the recognition of a huge market waiting out there, inevitably led to attention to the sexuality of women. As yet, the industry has failed to find the 'Viagra for women', but there has been no lessening of the search for other drugs that might enhance women's sexual arousal or increase their sexual desire. Currently available pharmacological or hormonal treatments will be reviewed in this chapter.

The history of psychological methods is also of interest. In the UK a new approach to sexual counselling emerged within the Family Planning Association. This was mainly under the influence of Michael Balint, who had applied his psychoanalytic training to devise ways for general practitioners to achieve more limited aims in a short time with a wide range of problems (Balint 1957). In 1958, Balint, together with a group of family planning doctors, started to apply these principles to the sexual problems that presented in family planning clinics. A central feature was the vaginal examination, not only used for diagnostic and educational purposes, but also as a powerful method of eliciting emotional reactions relating to the genitalia and their functioning (Tunnadine 1980). Over the next few years, a treatment approach and programme of training was devised and established as the Institute of Psychosexual Medicine. The closest to a documentation of this approach was the published proceedings of the *First International Conference on Psychosexual Medicine* (Draper 1983). Little has been written on this approach since. Mathers et al (1994) reported a study of the effects of training, but precisely what was being trained remained obscure. One obtains a somewhat clearer idea of how underlying problems are identified than the method of resolving them. Consistent with its psycho-analytic origins, this approach focuses on the individual, not the couple (Duddle 1994). Nevertheless, it is of interest and, from a historical perspective, presents one of the first attempts to bridge the psycho-somatic gap in treatment.

In the development of modern sex therapy, 1970 proved to be a crucial year. Masters & Johnson (1970) published *Human Sexual Inadequacy*, claiming impressive results in a large number of couples with sexual dysfunction, using an intensive but very brief treatment method lasting only 2 weeks. They also presented follow-up data for at least 5 years.

The impact of this book was enormous and the repercussions are still continuing. Their method of appraising outcome and their presentation of results were open to criticism. Their approach was atheoretical. But it has remained the most influential text in the psychological treatment of sexual problems ever since. The method of couple therapy described in this chapter is largely based on Masters & Johnson's approach. More recent attempts to evaluate the efficacy of this approach have been less positive than Masters & Johnson's original claims of success. A more realistic and less simplistic view has emerged which recognizes the considerable heterogeneity of problems that present for sex therapy, with their widely differing therapeutic needs and prognoses, and the substantial complexity that results from working with two people rather than one.

Possibly helped by Masters & Johnson's atheoretical approach, the eclecticism that followed has been refreshing, particularly compared with the polemic that prevailed between psychodynamic and behaviourally oriented therapists working in other fields. Kaplan (1974) set an example in her attempts to combine behavioural and psychoanalytic principles. Whereas the traditional behavioural approach has value when modifying specific aspects of behaviour (e.g. phobic anxiety, obsessional rituals, smoking), sex therapy more often than not has to deal with the complexities of the relationship. Although specific behavioural techniques may be helpful, and, as we shall see, play a part in couple therapy, their effects are usually mediated by highly complex inter- and intrapersonal processes. It is thus not surprising that sex therapists developed their eclecticism at a relatively early stage. As we shall see in the next section, this treatment approach involves a behavioural programme that serves to identify the key problems underlying the sexual difficulty and invites a variety of psychotherapeutic techniques to resolve them.

We are also seeing less polarization between psychological and physical methods. In the past the amount of dialogue between the exponents of these contrasting approaches was minimal. In the past 20 years, there has been growing collaboration between surgical, physiological and psychological researchers, which has been reflected in a more eclectic approach to treatment (e.g. Hatzichristou et al 2004).

PART 1 Problems of reduced sexual interest or response

In the first part of this chapter we will consider the various forms of treatment available, including evidence of their efficacy, followed by a section on assessment and the development of a treatment plan. This is based on the assumption that many cases will benefit from an integration of psychological and pharmacological methods, but also on the basic premise that in the majority of cases, the sexual problem is enacted within a relationship and the treatment programme should be designed for the couple rather than the individual. Close attention is paid to the principal method of sex therapy for couples, partly because the early stages of this method are particularly effective in identifying the key problems and hence the most appropriate final treatment plan, whether or not an integrated approach is followed.

Sex therapy for the couple

Although, consistent with Masters & Johnson, my earlier accounts of this treatment method have been largely atheoretical, I have now become much more theoretical in my approach, as is evident throughout this book. In particular, the Dual Control model now guides how I conceptualize the treatment process. This model is developed more fully in Chapters 2 and 4.

From this theoretical perspective, the main objective of psychological treatment is to identify and reduce inhibition of sexual response. Using the three windows approach, described in Chapter 11, issues identified through the first window are likely to be relevant because of the ongoing reactive inhibition that they evoke. Through the second window, the individual's propensity for inhibition becomes more relevant, which may not in itself be easy to change, although the individual and the couple may be helped to develop different ways of dealing with it. Through the third window we considered the impact of physical factors, most of which adversely affect sexual response by lowering the capacity for sexual excitation. The above theoretical framework is relevant to sex therapy in a number of ways. Sex therapy, as we define it here, may reduce 'reactive inhibition' by identifying factors relevant to the individual or the couple, which invoke inhibition, and finding ways to make them less inhibiting. Problems stemming from relationship difficulties are in this category, as are problems resulting from poor communication between the couple and misinformation about normal sexual response. In people with longstanding negative attitudes about sex, involvement in sexual activity may also provoke inhibition. Therapy aims at modifying negative attitudes. Problems resulting from high inhibitory tone and associated fear of failure (reflected in high SIS1 scores) or from low excitation proneness (low SES scores) may be more difficult to resolve. However, the impact of both effects may be lessened by changing expectations, seeking modified behavioural and sexual response goals, and considering the possibility of integrating pharmacological treatment into sex therapy.

The following account, as described, is designed for heterosexual couples, but the same principles and approach can be used for same-sex couples.

Goals of treatment
These include:

- helping each person to accept and feel comfortable with his or her sexuality
- helping the couple to establish trust and emotional security during sexual interaction
- helping the couple to enhance the enjoyment and intimacy of their love-making.

A fundamental point is that these goals do not include reversal of specific sexual dysfunctions. There are exceptions (e.g. for the treatment of PE or vaginismus) which will be described later, but the overriding principle is that, on the assumption there is no abnormality of the basic physiological mechanisms involved in sexual response, normal sexual function (in terms of sexual desire, arousal and genital response) will return once reactive inhibition is lessened and the above goals are achieved. In cases where impairment of physiological mechanisms does exist, the above goals of sex therapy may still be appropriate, even though the expected amount of change in sexual response is lessened as a result. Alternatively, sex therapy in such cases may be combined with medication. The decision to do this is not necessarily made at the outset, but becomes more obviously indicated as a result of each partner's reaction to the early stages of sex therapy.

Stages of treatment

The key elements of the therapeutic process are:

a. Clearly defined tasks are given and the couple asked to attempt them before the next therapy session.
b. Those attempts, and any difficulties encountered, are examined in detail.
c. Attitudes, feelings and conflicts that make the tasks difficult to carry out are identified.
d. These are modified or resolved so that subsequent achievement of the tasks becomes possible.
e. The next tasks are set, and so on.

The key is the nature of the tasks set. These have two purposes: (i) to move the behavioural interaction in the right direction and (ii) identify obstacles to behavioural change. Sometimes the behavioural assignments result in change without any additional treatment needed. In most cases, however, obstacles to change are identified and need to be resolved by treatment.

We will now consider the requisite behavioural assignments, for which Masters & Johnson's (1970) term 'sensate focus' is often used, the 'obstacles' likely to emerge, and the psychotherapeutic interventions to deal with them.

The non-genital phase — stages 1 and 2

Self assert and self protect. Each partner is instructed to practise 'self-asserting' and 'self-protecting', that is making clear what 'I' like, prefer or find unpleasant or threatening. It is often difficult to state 'I would like...' or 'I would prefer not...' instead of the more usual 'Shall we...?' or 'Why don't you...?' It is often regarded as unselfish and hence preferable to think or guess what your partner would like rather than making clear your own wishes. Given a reluctance to hurt the partner, misunderstandings remain concealed and persist as a result. However, providing each partner states his or her own wishes and expects that the other will do the same, there is no cause for resentment and differences are resolvable through open negotiation. The therapist advises the couple to try this style of communication in relatively trivial, non-sexual situations before applying it to sexual tasks (e.g. 'I would like a cup of tea, would you?'). The emphasis on 'I' is maintained throughout the course of treatment.

A 'contract' is also negotiated for the early treatment sessions that no attempt will be made by either partner to touch genital or breast areas or to attempt intercourse. The importance of this, at this early stage, for reducing performance anxiety and allowing both partners to feel safe, is explained. Moreover, it is emphasized that the non-genital stages of interaction are valuable in their own right. The couple is advised to have no more than three sessions of love-making before their next appointment; only a limited agenda can be properly covered at each meeting with the therapist. The couple decides when those sessions occur, and the more spontaneous they are the better. But they are specifically asked to alternate who suggests and initiates a session. Until the next therapy session, they should restrict their interactions to stage 1, as follows:

Stage 1. The objective is to 'touch your partner without genital contact and *for your own pleasure*'. The person who has 'invited' or initiated the session, touches the partner's body, other than the out-of-bounds areas, in whatever way is pleasurable; the objective is for the *person touching* to enjoy the experience. The partner being touched has only to 'self-protect' (i.e. to say 'stop' if anything unpleasant is felt). Roles are then reversed. They should not expect to get strongly aroused, but may do so. The goal is to relax and enjoy the process.

The therapist ensures that these steps have been carried out with both partners feeling secure before proceeding to stage 2.

Stage 2. '*Touching your partner without genital contact, for your own, AND your partner's pleasure*' is now the goal. Sessions continue as before, the couple alternating who initiates, with active touching carried out by one person at a time. Now, however, the person being touched gives feedback as to what is enjoyable as well as what is unpleasant. The toucher can use this information to give as well as to receive pleasure. The ban on genital contact continues.

A partner may express concern that the ban on intercourse will lead to unresolved sexual arousal and frustration. Reassurance is given that such frustration only arises if one is not clear what to expect. Explicit acceptance of limits obviates this. However, if after a session either partner is left aroused and in need of orgasm, it is acceptable to masturbate on one's own.

Issues often identified during stages 1 and 2

Misunderstandings about the treatment and motivation for change

Precise 'homework' assignments quickly demonstrate the couple's motivation. Difficulty in understanding and accepting the assignments may stem from the therapist's failure to clarify the process adequately or from having failed to establish a positive therapeutic relationship. In some cases, the treatment style conflicts with personal values about sex. A couple may complain that they dislike the lack of spontaneity — the feeling that the therapist not only instructs them but 'looks over their shoulder' at what should be an intimate affair. Although these feelings are perfectly understandable, it is gently pointed out that treatment is a temporary bridge between the problematic situation and a rewarding sexual relationship. The therapist also explains that these two stages are of sufficient relevance to a normal sexual relationship that it would be worthwhile for any couple to go through them periodically. Finally, it is pointed out that the therapist's initially very directive role will change as treatment proceeds and control is progressively handed back to the couple.

Difficulty in accepting the approach may reflect reluctance in one or both partners for treatment to succeed. At an unconscious or at least unacknowledged level, they may seek failure to justify ending the relationship, accepting a non-sexual one or engaging in an extramarital affair.

Accepting limits, especially on genital touching and intercourse, is often difficult and discussion of why this is the case is often fruitful. Although failure to understand the rationale behind the limits may be responsible for this difficulty, more often other factors are involved. The limits may be rejected on the grounds, for example, that it is unreasonable to expect a 'normal' man to become sexually aroused and not follow through to orgasm.

Issues of trust and interpersonal security

The above steps are an effective way to test trust between the couple. Breaking the ban or reluctance to maintain it, when examined closely, provides valuable information to the therapist (and subsequently to the couple). It may emerge that one partner believes the other is unlikely to keep to the ban once sexually aroused. This is an opportunity to inform the couple that feeling secure is key to the realization of sexual pleasure in any relationship. An essential feature of sexual pleasure is being able to let oneself go and become 'sexually abandoned'. At the same time, this involves letting down one's defences, making one vulnerable to hurt or rejection in the process. By the same token, exposing oneself in this way, in the presence of another person, and surviving the experience emotionally unscathed, has a binding effect. Thus, insecurity is likely to impair sexual enjoyment, and the insecurity may reflect a fear of rejection or sexual betrayal.

Other problems in the relationship and current situation

In Chapter 11, we considered relevant factors in the couple's current situation that might be resulting in inhibition of sexual response or interest. These were observed 'through the first window' (p. 316). Most of these factors, if they are relevant, are likely to surface during these first two stages, particularly the following: 'not feeling secure and being unable to let go', 'inappropriate expectations of sex', 'poor communication about sex', 'misunderstandings and lack of information', 'unsuitable circumstances and lack of time', 'low self-esteem and negative mood', and 'relationship problems'. Common unresolved problems stem from the couple's difficulty in adapting to each other. The most crucial form is veiled resentment, often related to the bartering aspect of a sexual relationship, when one partner is participating in sex at least partly to gain non-sexual benefits from the other in return. When such factors are relevant, therapy may be sabotaged because one partner feels that the sexual difficulty is being resolved before the other conflicts have been addressed.

Relevant sexual attitudes

The goal of 'touching your partner for your own pleasure' is often difficult to understand and accept, particularly for men. It is, however, often a fruitful first step in treatment. It may uncover deeply held attitudes such as 'you should only enjoy sex if you are giving pleasure to your partner', which may be central to the overall problem. These are part of the 'vulnerability' of the individual considered through the second window (p. 319).

The requirement for clear alternation of who invites and initiates sessions is an effective way to elicit problematic attitudes such as the widely held belief that 'nice' women don't initiate sex, they wait for their partners to do so. Providing structured, therapist-sanctioned alternation helps the reluctant initiator to overcome this difficulty.

The emphasis on 'self-assertion' and 'self-protection' often elicits relevant problems in the non-genital phase. The idea that it is all right to assert one's wish to do something specific sexually, confident that one's partner will indicate clearly if it is unacceptable, is revolutionary for many couples. Implementing this principle, which is of general relevance to close relationships, avoids second guessing what one's partner wants. The common assumption that 'you should know what your partner enjoys' is challenged, and the importance of ongoing effective communication is highlighted. One should not assume that because your partner enjoyed some specific activity on one occasion, it will be equally enjoyable on another.

Adding the genital component

Before moving on to stage 3, the therapist provides basic information about the anatomy and physiology of sexual response in both sexes, emphasizing those aspects that are often misunderstood and underlie dysfunction. This account is given no matter how well informed the couple may be. Providing the therapist does this well, the process of being explicit and detailed, with appropriate illustrations, adds a positive and comfortable feel to the information, which for many has previously been lacking. This is also an opportunity to introduce the vocabulary to be used for discussion and reporting back once genital contact begins.

Before giving the next set of assignments, the therapist stresses how important it is for the couple to maintain the changes achieved in the non-genital phase. It is all too easy, when genital contact becomes involved, for either or both partners to lose sight of open communication, the principles of 'self-assert and self-protect' and the value of 'touching for one's own pleasure'.

Stage 3. Touching with genital contact included. Alternating who initiates and who touches still applies, with genital areas and breasts now included. It is emphasized that the enjoyable types of non-genital touching identified in stages 1 and 2 should continue. In addition, the couple is encouraged to explore positions that allow genital touching (see, for example, Figs. 12.1 and 12.2). Questions about their reactions to different positions may reveal important feelings and attitudes.

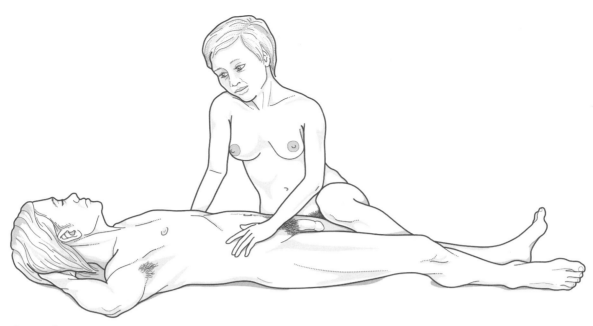

Fig. 12.1 Sensate focus.

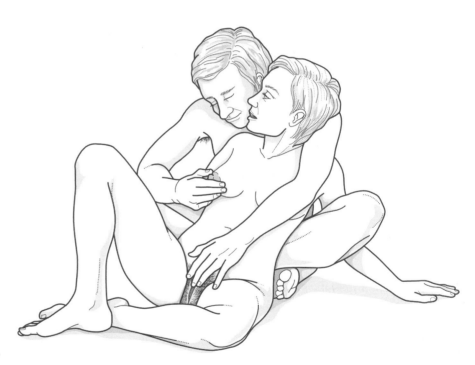

Fig. 12.2 Armchair position. This allows the man to touch the breasts and vulva of the woman in a non-threatening position. The woman can clearly guide her partner's hand.

Communicating what one finds pleasurable about being touched often presents difficulties at this stage. The therapist emphasizes that pleasure will vary, making open communication important. Their goal is to relax and enjoy the experience. The partner being caressed may or may not become sexually aroused; if ejaculation or orgasm happens it does not matter and need not signify an end to the session.

The couple have been warned from the outset about the 'spectator role', that is being a detached observer of oneself or one's partner rather than an active participant. This detachment generates performance anxiety and interferes with normal sexual response. A useful method is to concentrate on the local sensations experienced while touching or being touched (i.e. 'lend oneself to the sensations'). If this fails, a simple relaxation procedure can be used. If that doesn't work, the partner is informed that a problem has arisen and a temporary halt is requested. The session is resumed after a short period of conversation or other activity.

If PE is a problem, the couple are introduced at this stage to the 'stop–start' (Kaplan 1974) or 'squeeze' (Masters & Johnson 1970; see Fig. 12.3) techniques and asked to incorporate either of them into the touching sessions (see references for details of these techniques). In the case of vaginismus, gradual vaginal dilatation with finger or graded dilators is used. The timing of these techniques and whether they should be carried out

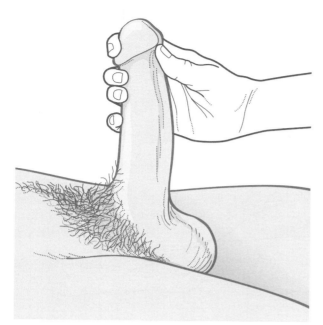

Fig. 12.3 Squeeze technique in the management of premature ejaculation. If the 'stop–start' technique fails to control ejaculation, squeezing the penis in the manner shown can be used by the partner to delay ejaculation when the man indicates that ejaculation is imminent.

individually or conjointly will be discussed further in relation to individual therapy.

Stage 4. Simultaneous touching with genital contact. Once the couple are comfortable with the preceding stages they can now move on to this stage, when touching is done by both partners simultaneously. Difficulty in taking the initiative and asserting oneself is often identified at this point.

Issues often revealed during stages 3 and 4

Other aspects of the sexual vulnerability of the individual, as considered through the second window, may be revealed once genital contact becomes involved. These were considered in Chapter 11 (p. 320). They include negative attitudes about sex ('sex is bad', 'sex is disgusting'), issues of self-control and fear of losing control, and the impact of earlier traumatic experiences, including sexual abuse as a child.

Appraising progress so far

These first four stages, before any attempt at vaginal intercourse is attempted, usually provide a substantial amount of information, which may enable the therapist to discuss with the couple whether sex therapy should continue on its own, whether individual sessions should be used to deal with PE or vaginismus, whether medication should be incorporated, or whether some other form of intervention should be considered. Stages 1 and 2 are likely to elicit problems relevant to the first window, i.e. relevant current circumstances, including relationship problems. In stages 3 and 4, when genital touching is added, the vulnerability of each individual is likely to be revealed or at least hinted at. It is an objective of treatment to recognize and discuss such vulnerabilities, and in the process enable the partner to have more empathy and understanding.

With the introduction of genital touching, to what extent is genital response occurring in each partner? If

it is lacking, can this be explained by continuing negative feelings or concerns about performance failure? If so, more time at this stage may be needed, looking closely at the relevant factors before passing on to stage 5. If, however, there are no indications of continuing psychological factors operating, yet genital response or arousal is lacking, the introduction of medication should be considered. This will be considered more closely later.

The gradual inclusion of vaginal intercourse

Stages 5 and 6. Vaginal containment. Once genital and body touching is progressing well and the man is achieving a reasonably firm erection (or has started to gain control over ejaculation during manual stimulation), and the woman is aware of some genital response, including vaginal lubrication, some vaginal containment is added to the session. The use of these structured assignments has helped discourage the couple from regarding lovemaking as divided into foreplay and intercourse. During a touching session, the woman may adopt the female superior position and, at some stage, introduces the penis into her vagina (Fig. 12.4). This not only makes it easier for her to guide the penis but also allows her partner to remain in a 'non-demand position', with the woman in control and able to stop or withdraw whenever she wants. The couple are instructed to try vaginal containment for short periods at first, without other movement or pelvic thrusting, concentrating on the sensations of the 'penis being contained' or the 'vagina being filled'. Duration is gradually extended. Stage 5 merges into stage 6 when movement and pelvic thrusting are allowed, although initially for brief periods only. Again, one is breaking down the 'big divide' between foreplay and intercourse that, if present, provokes anxiety whenever the step from one to the other is anticipated. Instead, subtle behavioural steps merge into intercourse.

The couple are encouraged to practise stopping at any point, at the request of either partner, to counter the common notion that love play once begun must continue until its physiological conclusion, with no escape en route. The confidence that either partner can say 'stop' at any stage, without incurring anger or hurt in the other, is a basic feature of a secure sexual relationship. The couple are also advised to experiment with different positions and methods of touching to discover what they find enjoyable.

Issues often identified during stages 5 and 6

Performance anxiety

Concern that one will not respond sexually or will lose one's response is a common feature of sexual problems. As indicated earlier, this is one way in which inhibition of sexual response can be invoked. The use of graded behavioural steps helps to identify when performance anxiety arises. It may become clear that the partner's expectations aggravate this problem. The therapist counsels that there is no need for any particular response to occur at any particular time, that for many couples responses occur on some occasions but not others, that pleasure and intimacy can occur without genital response, as experienced during the first part of the programme, and

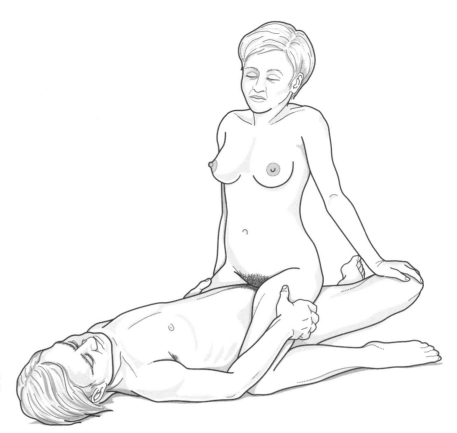

Fig. 12.4 The female superior position, in which the woman is above to control entry of the penis into her vagina. It also allows her to feel safe and not trapped under her partner's body, whilst at the same time permitting the man to relax without the responsibility for vaginal entry.

that each partner should feel free to call a halt at any stage without worry that the other will become upset or critical.

Ignorance or incorrect notions about sex

Misunderstandings are numerous. A widely held notion is that an erection indicates advanced sexual arousal and the need for intercourse, at a time when the woman may only be starting to respond. Erection is obvious to both partners whereas genital response in the female, involving vaginal lubrication and clitoral tumescence, may pass unnoticed. Genital responses occur, however, with similar speed in men and women, and often as the initial response to sexual stimulation (see Chapter 4, p. 74). The belief that if an erection subsides it cannot return needs correction. Another common belief is that 'normal sex' means simultaneous orgasm. The notion that a woman should experience orgasm from vaginal intercourse alone and that failure to do so or that reliance on clitoral stimulation indicates an abnormality, needs to be dispelled. The therapist stresses that only a small proportion of women on a minority of occasions achieve orgasm without clitoral stimulation, either by themselves or their partners.

The psychotherapeutic component

So far we have considered the appropriate behavioural steps and possible obstacles to their being carried out. Let us now consider what else the therapist can do to help resolve those obstacles.

Facilitating understanding

Understanding why one has difficulty in carrying out a particular task is crucial since this leads to reappraisal of the problem and related beliefs and values. For example, a woman may be reluctant to initiate love-making, since she feels this reflects improper enthusiasm. She then feels vulnerable to her partner's refusal should she try to initiate, and this is yet further evidence of its unacceptability. Men are conditioned differently. Rejection of their advances is much less threatening to self-esteem. By re-examining such assumptions, acknowledging, for example, that it is appropriate for the woman in an established relationship to take initiatives, and that both partners may decline at any time, cognitive re-structuring follows. This may occur implicitly and between therapy sessions. What can the therapist do to facilitate it?

1. Setting further tasks may help to focus on the specific problem. Identifying differences in the reaction to two subtly different tasks may be particularly useful. Why, for example, is it easier to show a partner what is unpleasant than to convey what is pleasurable?
2. Encourage examination and correct labelling of feelings experienced at the time of difficulty (e.g. fear, guilt, disgust or anger).
3. Encourage the couple to work out an explanation for their difficulty in carrying out a task. Therapists may offer likely hypotheses and evidence for and against, but the couple should be encouraged to provide the explanation. This underlines the educational aspect of the therapy process, and the importance of the couple understanding why they overcome a problem so that they can take a similar approach should problems recur in the future. But this is not likely to happen unless the couple recognize that they need to understand a

particular difficulty. The therapist can facilitate this by asking the couple to repeat the homework assignments. 'Socratic questioning' may help; the therapist, with an explanation in mind, poses questions encouraging the couple to view the situation in a particular way. The therapist may offer more than one explanation, inviting the couple to consider the options.

Making explicit the couple's commitment to specific changes

As obstacles are encountered, the therapist establishes explicitly whether both partners want to surmount them (e.g. does the woman want to be able to initiate? Does the man who finds his partner's genitalia repellant want to overcome that feeling?) In other words, is the obstacle a 'resistance' regarded by the patient as unwelcome (i.e. ego-alien), or is it consistent with his or her value system and therefore not in need of change?

Setting further behavioural steps designed to tackle the difficult problems stemming from fears of a 'phobic' kind require a graded approach. A woman who fears vaginal entry is asked briefly to insert her own finger a short distance. Such a small step does not overwhelm the patient with anxiety, and she can then be encouraged to 'stay with' the anxious feelings until they start to subside. The steps are then gradually extended.

Reality confrontation

The causes of anxiety can be challenged on a rational basis. When anxiety is ego-syntonic and the patient does not wish to overcome a resistance, the therapist should consider whether this is compatible with the aims of treatment. Thus, a suggestion that masturbation may help to achieve orgasm or overcome inhibition may be rejected on the grounds that masturbation is unacceptable. An alternative approach should be offered, which may be possible if he or she is in a sexual relationship. If, on the other hand, a patient objects to touching his or her partner's genitals, the therapist points out the incompatibility of this objection with the goals of treatment.

Patients may need to be confronted with other inconsistencies between belief and action or between their understanding and the facts. For instance, the view that 'normal' women experience orgasm from vaginal intercourse has to be challenged. Giving permission is often a crucial role for the therapist, who may be required to make explicit the differences between the values of patient and therapist.

Facilitating the expression of emotion

Negative emotions are often crucial in establishing or maintaining a sexual problem. The first step in coping with these is to label them correctly. Resentment within the relationship is common. More often than not, its appropriate expression is required before it resolves. The therapist assists in three ways: (i) educates the couple about ways that unexpressed emotions adversely affect them and the benefits of appropriate expression, (ii) helps the couple to identify instances when unexpressed emotions are likely to have caused problems and (iii) encourages the couple to work out effective ways to communicate feelings.

General tactics

The rationale of therapy may need to be clarified more than once. It is often better understood after the first attempts at the behavioural assignments. The couple are told that treatment recommendations are based on common sense, not magic. The therapist carefully explains why an assignment is necessary and the patient is encouraged to seek clarification of any matter that seems ambiguous or uncertain. This not only allows the patient to voice doubts about therapy, but also highlights its educational function.

Other relevant non-specific features include reassurance, promoting hope, showing warmth and empathy, reinforcing specific behaviour by responding to it with pleasure or praise, and 'inoculating against failure' by preparing the couple for possible setbacks so that when they do arise, they will not feel discouraged but rather make constructive use of them.

Although sex therapy varies in duration, 12 sessions over 4–5 months is typical, and is determined by the particular needs of the case. Treatment begins weekly with the interval between sessions extended once major issues like unexpressed resentment, communication problems or undue passivity have been dealt with. The last two or three sessions are spaced out over a few months so that the couple have an opportunity to consolidate their progress and cope with any setback before ending treatment.

Open-ended arrangements about length of treatment are best avoided. A specified number of sessions are agreed on at the outset with the proviso that progress will be assessed and a decision made on that basis whether to continue for longer. In cases where sex therapy seems the obvious choice at the assessment stage, a contract of 10 sessions with scope for a further two to four is sensible. Where there is uncertainty about whether other treatment modalities, such as medication, may need to be combined with sex therapy or replace it, a contract of three or four sessions is appropriate, with the understanding that reassessment will occur at the end of the fourth session. In general, a couple's ability to benefit from sex therapy is usually evident by the fourth session. Hawton & Catalan (1986) found that early response to treatment predicted a good outcome, whereas couples who drop out usually do so around the third or fourth session.

Masters & Johnson 1970 advocated a dual-therapist (male and female) team, but this requires justification on economic grounds. There are obvious advantages: both male and female points of view are represented and collusion between therapist and one partner is more easily avoided. Moreover, one therapist can remain more objective while the other is interacting with the couple. Against this, in addition to the doubling of therapist time, the co-therapist relationship is not necessarily easy, making the choice of co-therapist crucial. Co-therapy requires time outside treatment sessions for adequate discussion between therapists. Co-therapy, however, is an excellent model for training, provided that the experienced therapist takes care not to monopolize.

Whereas management of sexual problems, as presented in this chapter, requires access to medical skills, the characteristics of an effective sex therapist, using the approach described here, are determined more by personality, experience and training than by a particular professional background. In my experience in training sex therapists, doctors, psychologists, social workers, nurses and marriage guidance counsellors have all proved to be effective.

Sex therapy for couples is indicated for problems of wide-ranging complexity. At one extreme, a behavioural programme with little therapist intervention will suffice; at the other, considerable psychotherapeutic skills are required. Most cases fall between these extremes. The basic framework is, however, similar across the range.

Sex therapy for the individual

A proportion of patients presenting with problems of impaired sexual response or desire have no current sexual partner. Not infrequently, the sexual problem is a reason why they are not currently in a relationship. Obviously, couple therapy is not a possibility for them. Others do have partners but either they will not participate in treatment or the patients do not want to involve them. Individual or group therapy may be the only available option. However, if individual therapy is to be used then it is crucial that there are treatment goals that are not dependent on interaction with a partner. Thus a man who has erectile problems only evident in sexual interaction with a partner, is not likely to be helped by individual sex therapy. On the other hand, a man with PE who has difficulty controlling ejaculation, even when masturbating on his own, may benefit from individual therapy. Similarly, a woman with vaginismus may benefit from individual treatment even if she is in a relationship, though it is usually a good idea to involve the partner at a later stage, if possible. Someone with low sexual desire or inhibitory beliefs and atitudes, may be helped on an individual basis.

The patient–therapist relationship

In individual sex therapy the nature of the patient–therapist relationship requires special attention. A dependent 'doctor–patient' relationship between the patient and the therapist is more likely to develop in individual than in couple therapy. It is therefore particularly important to spell out the limits of the therapeutic relationship. The onus for change lies with the patient, not with the therapist. The relationship is primarily an educational one between two adults, one providing expertise, the other making use of that expertise in an active way. In these circumstances, the sex of the therapist has an added importance. The vicarious sexuality of a psychotherapeutic relationship should never be denied. When the focus of therapy is the patient's sexual life, this is even more important. In some cases this may be a therapeutic advantage. A shy inhibited male, lacking self-confidence and fearing rejection by all women, may find the vicarious

sexuality of the relationship with a female therapist reassuring. However, such advantages of the sexuality of the therapeutic relationship rely on the taboo against therapist–patient sex being firmly upheld (Bancroft 1981). For others a good relationship with a therapist of the same sex may be more important not only in reinforcing the patient's gender-related self-esteem but also providing a model of certain behaviours.

The basic principles of treatment

The principles of behavioural psychotherapy, already described for couple therapy, are also applicable to the individual, with a combination of behavioural, educational and psychotherapeutic components. The main difference is that as a relationship is not directly involved in treatment, a more idiosyncratic, tailor-made set of assignments is necessary from the start. When working with a couple, stage 1 can be appropriately started without delay; the behavioural steps, at least for the first part of treatment, are pre-determined as they are of relevance and value to any couple, with or without a sexual problem. For the individual, more time is usually needed in the initial assessment and behavioural analysis before appropriate assignments are identified.

Let us consider some particular types of treatment objective when working with the individual.

Marked sexual inhibition or absence of sexual desire

A person with such a problem may complain that his or her rather negative approach to sex is a barrier to establishing a rewarding sexual relationship, but a normal relationship is desired or children wanted.

Many such people have difficulty in accepting with comfort their sexual feelings and bodily responses. This may be an aspect of their general personality that avoids any form of undue hedonism or loss of control, or it may be more specifically linked to avoidance of, or discomfort with, sexual pleasures. The 'sensate focus' approach, described above for the couple, may be relevant to such a person, but carried out on an individual basis; sessions involve 'sensate focus' on one's own. The patient is asked to agree to limits — no genital touching initially — but to spend time exploring the feel of the body, the effects of different types of touch or stimulation, perhaps experimenting with a variety of stimuli such as creams, lotions, water baths, vibrators, etc. Patients are encouraged to make time and space just for themselves, to pamper themselves, to listen to good music, read interesting erotic literature, look at pictures, enjoy nice smells and so on.

Advocating such an approach may quickly uncover negative attitudes about body pleasure and sexuality. It may also reveal discomfort with body image. As described in Chapter 11, feeling bad about one's body does not enhance sexuality. There may be rational grounds for such negative feelings, e.g. being overweight, too thin or unfit. If so, there may be good reasons for suggesting specific goals to improve self-image, e.g. dieting, exercise, and yoga.

Step by step, individuals are encouraged to explore their genitalia in privacy, and with the use of a good mirror. This should eventually lead to gentle genital caressing whilst continuing the earlier body caressing. Negative attitudes about masturbation may be crucial at this stage. The beginnings of sexual excitement in response to such self-caressing may lead the patient to stop suddenly, fearing where the arousal may lead. Fears of loss of control may have to be resolved before further progress can be made.

Relaxation exercises may be usefully incorporated into this sort of programme, mainly to allow the individual to reduce tension before embarking on the pleasuring exercises and also to enhance body awareness. Much of the loss of erotic sensitivity that people experience is because they dissociate themselves from their bodily and tactile sensations by focusing their minds on other matters. An important objective is to 'tune in' to the sensations they are experiencing, either in the part of the body that is being touched or the part that is doing the touching. Avoidance of the spectator role is particularly important at this stage. Kegel's exercises for increasing tone and control over the pelvic floor muscles may be useful for some women, giving them an increased sense of awareness and control over their own bodies.

As in couple therapy, each new behavioural step may encounter some emotional block that then has to be identified and worked through. The principle of desensitization may be useful. Pictures of certain types of sexual activity may arouse anxiety and gradual repeated exposure to such pictures, accompanied by the reassurance and 'permission' of the therapist, who looks at the pictures with the patient, may serve to desensitize this anxiety. Taboo words or ideas may lose their threat by their repeated use or discussion during therapy. The therapist is therefore employing a combination of education, giving permission, desensitization and the psychotherapeutic resolution of emotional blocks and conflicts when appropriate.

Lack of sexual interest that results from active psychophysiological inhibition may respond to this approach. Initial assessment (see below) should have given some indication of this aetiology before choosing this treatment approach. It is important to point out, however, that although an individual may lack any spontaneous sexual interest or desire, this does not preclude him or her from responding to appropriate stimulation with sexual arousal and pleasure. As we discussed in Chapter 6, there are many women who seldom if ever experience spontaneous sexual desire and yet are able to respond with pleasure to their partner's advances. Lack of desire of this kind may be more problematic in a man, particularly if both he and his partner expect him to take the initiative.

Those individuals with lack of sexual desire may find it helpful to use erotic films or literature as well as novel forms of tactile stimulation, such as vibrators.

Sexual problems in women

Vaginismus

This problem, as considered on p. 324, has become a focus of controversy in the past few years. The main issue involves the nature of the 'obstacle' to vaginal entry, and the extent to which it is a problem of muscle contraction or spasm, or a problem of behavioural avoidance. The woman presents with a difficulty or impossibility in allowing entry of an erect penis or even her own finger into her vagina. Attempts to do so result in pain and encounter resistance, suggestive of muscle tightening or spasm around the lower third of the vagina.

Treatment involves a carefully graduated approach to vaginal insertion. The first step is for a careful and sensitive examination by the therapist, and the partial insertion of the tip of the examining and well-lubricated finger. If the woman can tolerate this, the finger is left in this position for a minute or so before withdrawal. Either at the same session or a later session, this is done again, aiming for slightly more insertion. Once acceptance of the therapist's finger in the vagina is established, the woman is encouraged to insert her own finger in the same way, during the therapy session. Once she is able to do this, she is instructed to do so on her own at home, keeping the finger inserted for increasing periods so that she can adjust to the sensation. The next step is the involvement of graded vaginal dilators. These vary in width with the smallest being similar to a finger, and the largest, bigger than most erect penises. The therapist first inserts the smallest dilator, and then asks the woman to insert it herself. This is followed by regular sessions on her own (e.g. once a day) during which she gradually replaces smaller with larger dilators, leaving each one in the vagina for several minutes at a time. For women in a relationship, it can be helpful to involve the partner in this process in its later stages. As the woman continues with this vaginal dilatation exercise she can, at an appropriate stage, explore limited penile insertion with her partner, emphasizing that the same graduated approach should be maintained. It is a good idea for the woman, once penile entry is acceptable, to periodically use her larger dilators to reinforce the learning process.

Vaginismus is often one of the easiest sexual problems to treat, hence the frequent success with individual as well as with couple therapy. However, in some women the vaginismus is one manifestation of a more substantial reluctance to participate in 'adult' sexual interaction, reflecting a more general developmental personality problem. Such cases may be very difficult to treat, requiring either skilful couple therapy or long-term individual therapy.

Anorgasmia

It is important to emphasize to women seeking such treatment that orgasmic function is very variable in women, that absence of orgasm does not preclude a woman having a satisfactory and enjoyable sexual relationship and that experiencing an orgasm is much more important for some women than others. In this way one can counter what has become a socio-cultural pressure on women to be orgasmic. Consistent with the concept of a basic pattern and superadded components of women's sexuality, considered at various points in this book, an anorgasmic woman who is capable of enjoying sexual activity with a partner is not 'dysfunctional' (see Chapter 11, p. 339). Nevertheless, a woman may want to explore the possibility of experiencing orgasm.

Women who are unable to experience orgasm, even on their own during masturbation, may be helped with an individual 'sensate focus' approach progressing gradually to genital stimulation, with the use of a vibrator as a possibility. Starting with the non-genital stages, as described above for individuals with sexual inhibition, and progressing on to graduated genital stimulation, the key is to avoid 'performance demand' but to emphasize the pleasure that occurs without orgasm. By prolonging such pleasurable stimulation orgasm may eventually occur, but it is not seen as a goal in any particular session. Once orgasm does occur, it will often recur more easily on subsequent sessions, as if the inhibition barrier had been lowered.

The capacity for orgasm acquired during such an individual approach does not necessarily generalize to sexual involvement with a partner. It will do in a proportion of cases, but may need additional couple therapy for that reason. Heiman (2007) provides an overview of the treatment of anorgasmia in women.

Sexual problems in men

Delayed or absent ejaculation

Males who have never been able to ejaculate, even during masturbation on their own, may be helped to overcome this by following an individual sensate focus programme, similar to that described above for anorgasmia in women. The important guiding principle is an assumption of inhibition blocking the orgasm, which can be reinforced during attempts to ejaculate. Hence, during the sessions of graded self-stimulation, attention should be diverted from reaching orgasm to the extent that if the man feels he might be getting close he stops the stimulation. In this way the arousal is allowed to build up without the interfering inhibition. Then what typically happens is that orgasm and ejaculation occurs when he is not expecting it. This appears to substantially reduce subsequent inhibition, perhaps because ejaculation has now occurred and no disaster ensued! However, the graduated approach should continue after this first ejaculation until he gradually builds up his confidence and his ability to feel positive during sexual arousal. Men with this problem vary considerably in how readily they are able to overcome this. Younger men presenting with this problem are often the easiest to help, probably because they have a better prognosis to start with but have sought treatment earlier than most men do. We drew this conclusion at the Kinsey Institute Sexual Health Clinic, which, being based on a university campus, attracted young students who would have been less likely to seek help if they needed to go through the usual referral process. We had a number of young men, unable to ejaculate, who responded well to this individual approach.

Premature ejaculation

Whether this problem can be helped by individual therapy depends on the extent to which ejaculation is poorly controlled during masturbation. If there is scope for improving control during masturbation, rather than with a partner, then an individual programme may be beneficial. A sensate focus approach is used, encouraging the male to explore his body and enjoy various types of tactile stimulation before reaching the phase of penile stimulation. Then he is taught the principles of the 'stop–start' technique, as originally advocated by Semans (1956). The objective here is to learn to recognize when he is getting close to the point of 'ejaculatory inevitability' (see p. 323). Initially he should err on the side of recognizing this early; at which point he stops penile stimulation and allows his arousal to subside. After a break he resumes stimulation, following the same sequence. With practice he becomes able to continue for longer before stopping. Two things appear to be happening here; he is getting better at anticipating ejaculatory inevitability and he is probably learning to delay and control it. With this advantage he is then able to monitor his sexual stimulation during sexual interaction with a partner stopping or withdrawing in time to avoid ejaculation, and gradually finding that his control is improving. As discussed earlier (p. 349), this same approach can be incorporated into couple therapy.

Erectile problems

Problems with erection are more difficult to treat on an individual basis, particularly when performance anxiety is a major factor. It is often assumed in such cases that erections during masturbation will be unaffected and that if they are, some organic factor is involved. This is not the case, however, as masturbation may become an important test of erection and also suffer the effects of performance anxiety. If that is so, individual sensate focus may help the individual regain his erections during masturbation and increase his self-confidence to some extent. How best to tackle sexual encounters with a partner can be usefully discussed. Usually performance anxiety is much more troublesome if the man has to conceal it from his partner. Being able to share one's concern and obtaining a sympathetic and caring response is half the battle. He should therefore avoid sexual encounters where the reaction of his partner to sexual failure will be unpredictable. He should be encouraged to see himself as someone needing a relatively stable and secure relationship for his sexuality to be properly expressed, rather than as a potential sexual athlete. When he does find a partner he can trust he should prepare himself with some convincing reason for not engaging in sexual intercourse too quickly. If he has chosen his partner sensibly this will not be a problem, as she may also be happier to take things slowly. Engaging in mutual caressing with a clear commitment not to attempt intercourse (as in the early stages of couple therapy) may well allow him to experience full erection and increase his self-confidence. During the counselling sessions, his experiences during such encounters can be discussed and the appropriate lessons learnt from them.

In some men with erectile problems, their histories suggest a more basic difficulty in incorporating sex into a loving relationship, or of tolerating sexual intimacy. In such cases more long-term individual psychotherapy should be considered.

The outcome of sex therapy for couples

Uncontrolled outcome studies

The largest series of treated cases for which outcome and long-term follow-up has been reported from any one clinical service remains that of Masters & Johnson 1970. They used an unusual method for reporting outcome, giving the failure rate rather than the success rate. This led to considerable confusion, as many interpreted a 20% failure rate to mean an 80% success rate, and provoked much criticism (e.g. Zilbergeld & Evans 1980). Masters & Johnson defended their position at the World Congress of Sexology in Washington in 1983 (Masters et al 1983). They first admitted that their method was less than satisfactory, but that it reflected the state of the art at the time. They quoted Bergin, an authority on psychotherapy outcome studies, as saying in 1971: 'It is impossible to conclude very much from gross studies of therapeutic effects'. They justified their use of failure rates as follows: 'When symptoms were not reversed, it was quite obvious; whereas when symptoms were reversed little was known about whether that actually constituted sexual health'. After comments that they were reluctant to ask questions about the frequency and effectiveness of specific sexual responses, as it would encourage the goal-oriented attitude that they aimed to avoid, they went on to describe the criteria that were in fact used for each type of dysfunction. For erectile impotence, failure was adjudged if erection sufficient for coitus was not maintained on at least 75% of opportunities. They pointed out, however, that at their end of treatment assessment, this would probably be based on only three or four such opportunities. With PE, failure was the inability to maintain coital thrusting long enough for the partner to be orgasmic in the majority of opportunities, or if the partner had difficulty with orgasm herself, the inability to delay ejaculation 'for the length of time he wished'. Women with orgasmic dysfunction were failures if they 'did not reach orgasm in a consistent fashion during sexual opportunities... 50% being a general guide'. Masters & Johnson's defence contains some special pleading, but they do make an important point — the difficulties of defining success when evaluating sex therapy. As I intend to argue, no one has yet satisfactorily resolved that problem. This is an important issue because more often than not the specific dysfunction is only one aspect of the sexual relationship and therapy can achieve substantial improvement in the quality of the relationship whilst leaving the dysfunction largely unaltered, as, for example, in some cases of erectile failure of organic origin.

There has been a striking lack of treatment outcome studies over the past 15 years. Heiman & Meston (1997), in their review of this literature, cited 90 studies of psychological or behavioural treatment, yet only 2 of them had been published since 1990, and 60 of them before 1980. For that reason I will present much of the account that appeared in the last edition of this book as there is little new to add, and I will consider later why this extraordinary decline in controlled outcome research occurred after an initial phase of enthusiasm.

The results reported by Masters & Johnson 1970 in more than 500 couples are shown in Table 12.1. They also reported a 5-year follow-up of 313 couples who were 'non-failures' at the end of treatment and found a relapse rate of only 5.1%, most commonly with

TABLE 12.1 Failure rates reported by Masters & Johnson (1970)	
Sexual problem	**Percentage failure**
Orgasmic dysfunction	
Primary	16.6
Secondary	22.8
Vaginismus	0
Erectile dysfunction	
Primary	40.6
Secondary	26.3
Premature ejaculation	2.2
Ejaculatory incompetence	17.6

secondary ED (11.1%). It is difficult to escape the conclusion that Masters & Johnson were unusually successful with their treatment, particularly when taking their 5-year follow-up data into consideration. Why they were so successful remains uncertain. It is likely that they were highly effective therapists. The couples they treated travelled from all over the USA to obtain their help, and were required to stay in a hotel close to the Masters & Johnson's clinic for 2 weeks while having daily therapy sessions. This may well have proved effective in selecting only the highly motivated. Subsequent studies have demonstrated the importance to outcome of lack of motivation in at least one of the partners. It is also possible that at that time, in what can be considered a new era of sex therapy, accompanied by much public attention and acclaim to Masters & Johnson's earlier physiological research, couples with less severe problems were seeking help. After this initial phase of enthusiasm, and possibly because of the increased availability of self-help manuals and informative literature for the general public, we may have seen a shift towards more difficult and intractable problems being presented. But this is all speculation.

A number of reports have given a crude global assessment of outcome at the end of therapy. Thus, Bancroft & Coles (1976) reported on 78 couples entering therapy in their Oxford clinic: 32% showed a successful outcome, 31% worthwhile improvement and 32% no change or dropped out. These were similar to results reported elsewhere in the UK at that time (Duddle 1975; Milne 1976). Hawton (1982) later reported a further 100 couples treated at Oxford. At the end of treatment the problem was rated as resolved or largely resolved in 66%, slightly improved in 12% and unchanged in 21%. The best outcomes were for vaginismus and ED.

Heisler (1983) reported outcome in 998 couples assessed for sexual problems by marriage guidance counsellors with special training in sex therapy. Twenty-five per cent were deemed not suitable for such treatment and 28% failed to complete treatment once started. This left 47% who completed treatment. Of those, 70% showed a marked improvement. Warner et al (1987) reported on 1194 referrals to sexual problem clinics in Edinburgh during a 3-year period. Of these, 478 (51% of those with a current partner) were offered couple therapy. At the time of the report 40% of these couples had completed treatment and 35% had dropped out of treatment. For those who completed or dropped out, the outcome was reported to be good in 35%, and moderate in 25%. The best outcome was for vaginismus.

None of the reported attempts at long-term follow-up following therapy have been anywhere near as successful, in terms of making contact, as Masters & Johnson had been with their 5-year follow-up. The reasons for this difficulty remain unclear, and may not simply reflect relapse. Treatment of this kind, focusing closely on a relationship, may be followed several years later by a reluctance to revisit what was often a painful and taxing experience. In any case we must be cautious in generalizing from follow-up data with high non-response rates. Arentewicz & Schmidt (1983), reporting on 262 treated couples, attempted a follow-up by questionnaire at 1 year and from 2.5 to 4.5 years after the end of treatment. However, they obtained information from only 50% at 1 year and 42% at the later follow-up (Table 12.2).

Dekker & Everaerd (1983) attempted to follow up 140 couples from 5 to 8 years after treatment, using postal questionnaires. Only 46% responded appropriately. Of those for whom information was available, 21% had separated or divorced. The authors concluded that improvement obtained during treatment was fairly stable during the follow-up period in those couples staying together. DeAmicis et al (1985) attempted to follow up 104 couples 3 years after sex therapy. Of these 37 couples (36%) could not be contacted, 18 couples (17%) refused to respond, leaving 49 who were located, but only 38 (36%) returned complete data. They found some evidence of treatment gains being maintained, but there was a fair amount of relapse, particularly with problems of low sexual desire. Watson & Brockman (1982) followed up 116 couples but were only able to obtain information from 53% of them, with follow-up periods averaging 13 months. Of 29 couples who had improved

at the end of treatment and who were followed up, 16 (55%) had maintained their improvement. A total of 35% of couples had separated, though these were significantly more likely to be amongst those who had not responded to treatment or had not been treated. Heisler (1983) attempted to follow up couples who had been treated by marriage guidance counsellors but succeeded in only 36% of cases. Within that subgroup, 59% had maintained or increased their improvement whereas 41% had shown some return of problems. Hawton et al (1986) proved somewhat more successful in contacting their ex-patients. Of 140 couples who had entered therapy 1–6 years earlier, at least one partner was contacted and usually interviewed in 75% of cases. Recurrence of or continuation of the presenting problem was experienced at some stage during the follow-up period by 75% of couples, though in a third of them this did not cause concern. Almost a half of those who had experienced these recurrences were able to deal with them effectively, often by adopting strategies learnt during therapy. In all, 17% of the relapsing couples had sought further help; 13% of the original group had separated.

The outcome for different types of sexual dysfunction also presented a confused picture. The most consistent findings for good results were with vaginismus (Masters & Johnson 1970; Arentewicz & Schmidt 1983; Bramley et al 1983; Hawton et al 1986) and poor results for low sexual desire (DeAmicis et al 1985; Hawton et al 1986). The evidence of prognosis for orgasmic dysfunction and erectile failure was much more variable, and in the latter case may reflect varying degrees of selection of cases without organic impairment. PE, whilst often helped initially, appears to relapse much more often than Masters & Johnson's figures would indicate. Arentewicz & Schmidt (1983) made this interesting comment: 'Maybe therapists too readily considered PE a purely

TABLE 12.2	Changes in sexual functioning classified by type of sexual problem at end of treatment and at follow-up (Arentewicz & Schmidt 1983)				
	Orgasmic dysfunction	Vaginismus	Erectile dysfunction	Premature ejaculation	Total
At end of treatment					
n	108	27	57	31	223
Dropped out	24%	11%	13%	13%	17%
No change	2%	0%	4%	0%	2%
Slightly improved	4%	11%	4%	3%	5%
Improved	50%	11%	30%	43%	40%
'Cured'	19%	67%	49%	40%	35%
After 1 year (compared with end of treatment)					
n	51	16	29	15	111
The same	39%	56%	48%	33%	43%
Better	25%	19%	14%	13%	29%
Worse	24%	12.5%	24%	47%	25%
Separated	12%	12.5%	14%	7%	12%
After 2–4 years (compared with 1 year follow-up)					
n	44	14	23	13	94
The same	50%	64%	48%	15%	47%
Better	18%	7%	9%	46%	18%
Worse	18%	14%	26%	31%	21%
Separated	14%	14%	17%	8%	14%

technical problem and so were distracted from dealing with deeper rooted problems between the partners or in the patient'.

More recently, a report was issued on psychosexual therapy by counsellors at Relate (previously the National Marriage Guidance Council) in the UK (McCarthy & Thorburn 1996). Relate's sex therapy service was established in 1974, with counsellors trained in Masters & Johnson's 'sensate focus' approach, very different to standard marriage guidance counselling. However, normal marriage guidance counselling skills are very relevant to the psychotherapeutic component of sex therapy, as described earlier in this chapter. At the time of this report there were 230 counsellors trained as sex therapists working within 115 Relate centres around the country. Between 1992 and 1994, 3693 couples were assessed for sexual problems. In 71% of the couples, the woman had a sexual problem: lack of sexual interest 38.7%; orgasmic problems 16.5%; vaginismus 8.1%; dyspareunia 7.2%; other 0.5%. In 57.2% of the couples, the man had a sexual problem: erectile problem 26.3%; PE 18.8%; lack of sexual interest 7.1%; retarded ejaculation 4.9%; other 0.9%. Thus in 28.2% of couples both partners presented with a problem; the commonest combination was PE in the man and lack of interest in the woman. Forty seven per cent of the couples proceeded into treatment after the assessment process, and of these 1076 (29.1% of the total) completed treatment. According to therapists' ratings, improvement occurred in 70% of women with lack of sexual interest, 48% with orgasm difficulties and 80% with 'vaginal entry problems' (e.g. vaginismus), and in 74% of men with erectile problems, 74% with PE and 55% with delayed ejaculation.

Controlled treatment outcome studies

Modern sex therapy, particularly that derived from Masters & Johnson's approach, has been popular amongst behaviour therapists. The early days of behaviour therapy were characterized by a striving for scientific respectability, mainly by carrying out controlled evaluation of treatment using group designs. For much of my earlier career I was involved in such treatment outcome research. At that stage I never doubted that it was the right thing to do. However, subsequent and somewhat painful salutary experiences led me to attach over-riding importance to the marked prognostic variability in couples presenting for help with sexual problems, and the need to control for such variability in any attempt at a methodologically sound outcome study.

When in Oxford I was involved in two attempts at controlled outcome studies. In the first (Mathews et al 1976), two components of Masters & Johnson's method were defined: the behavioural component (stages 1 through 6 as described earlier, which was called 'directed practice') and the counselling component. In a randomized treatment study of 36 couples with sexual problems, three treatment methods were compared: (i) the combination of 'directed practice' and counselling, (ii) 'directed practice' with minimal therapist contact (by postal contact) and (iii) counselling with an alternative behavioural component, 'systematic desensitization' of anxieties about sex. At the end of treatment, there was a trend towards better results with 'directed practice' plus counselling ($p < 0.1$), but this was not significant at 4 months follow-up; a rather modest outcome! The second attempt was possibly the first study to assess the combination of pharmacological and psychological treatment, comparing two pharmacological treatments in the process, testosterone (T) and diazepam (Carney et al 1978). Women with 'sexual unresponsiveness' were randomly assigned to either weekly or monthly sex therapy sessions (i.e. 'directed practice' plus counselling) and, within each sex therapy group, assigned to receive either sublingual T or diazepam. No differences in outcome were found between the weekly and monthly sex therapy groups. However, women receiving T showed significantly more improvement than those in the diazepam group. This left us with the impression that oral T was an effective treatment at least in combination with sex therapy. However, two attempts to replicate this finding failed. In each case T was compared not with diazepam but with placebo. Placebo was as effective if not more so than T (Dow & Gallagher 1989; Mathews et al 1983; see p. 119). One possible explanation for this failure to replicate was that in the original study diazepam was having an adverse effect, possibly by reducing the effectiveness of counselling, whereas T was having no effect.

In Edinburgh we carried out a comparable study with male sexual dysfunction (Bancroft et al 1986), comparing T with placebo, both in combination with sex therapy. We found trends in favour of placebo; but there is no reason why T should be *less* beneficial than placebo in men. We also found that in spite of randomization there were differences in the two treatment groups (i.e. T and placebo) *before* treatment in variables that were found to have prognostic significance. In some cases these pre-treatment differences reached statistical significance. It was apparent that they could have accounted for the post-treatment differences, making the results *uninterpretable*. We had been unlucky in our randomization. But this experience emphasized the importance of balancing for pre-treatment variables of prognostic significance. In our case we had an imbalance of statistically significant proportions. But such significance levels are arbitrary and their biasing effect on the results depend on the *degree* of the difference, not on whether it is statistically significant.

If prognostic variability is not controlled, there are two important negative consequences. If one treatment group has a better prognosis than the other, bias will be introduced, inflating or cancelling out real treatment effects or producing spurious effects where none exist (as probably happened in our ill-fated study). Secondly, if prognostic variability is not taken into account in the analysis it will add to the experimental error. Since the statistical significance of a treatment effect is measured in relation to this residual error, moderate treatment effects will remain undetected, unless the sample size is increased substantially. Anyone who has clinical experience of sex therapy will know how variable couples are in their response to treatment. Some improve with apparent ease and little therapeutic effort; others are notably resistant to change. This variability in outcome is likely to be at least as great if not greater than the differences between a 'good' and a 'bad' treatment method. Thus, it is not difficult for genuine and worthwhile treatment effects to be obscured by the prognostic variability. We reported our ill-fated study as a cautionary tale (Bancroft et al 1986) and in the second part of the paper examined in detail the methodological issues involved (Warner & Bancroft 1986). This experience confronted us with the need to first identify and then control for the key prognostic variables.

There have been a few, more recent controlled trials of cognitive behaviour therapy (CBT) for sexual problems. Van Lankveld et al (2006) randomly assigned 117 women with primary vaginismus to cognitive-behavioural group therapy, cognitive-behavioural bibliotherapy or a waiting list. Twenty-one per cent dropped out before completing treatment. At the end of treatment 9% of those with group therapy and 14% with bibliotherapy reported successful intercourse whereas none did so at the end of the waiting period. At 12 months follow-up, 21% of those who had received group therapy and 15% of those with bibliotherapy reported successful sexual intercourse. The authors concluded that there was a modest treatment effect, and commented that it was much lower than that reported in uncontrolled studies. They suggested that the 3-month duration of the treatment programmes may have been too short, and that their cases may have been more severe than other case series. Before entering this programme 69% of the women had sought professional help, but the nature of the help, and the extent to which it focused on the vaginismus, was not made clear in this paper. Apart from no consideration of potential prognostic factors, I have two principal concerns with this study. A waiting list control seems inappropriate when assessing the impact of treatment on a life-long condition of this kind, in contrast to medical or psychological conditions of more recent onset that have a greater likelihood of spontaneous remission. More important are the limitations of the treatment methods involved. Clearly, they were informative for the couples, and this is an important component. In addition, they involved a hierarchical approach to vaginal penetration, with the woman's finger, subsequently her partner's finger and a plastic dilator preceding attempts at penile insertion. However, a potentially important difference when compared with the treatment described on p. 354, which is typical of most of the reported treatment studies of vaginismus, is absence of initial finger and dilator insertion by the *therapist*. This, if done sensitively, could make a crucial difference to reassuring the woman and facilitating her homework assignments of this kind, though it does restrict this component of treatment to a therapist experienced at vaginal examinations. Further controlled studies of vaginismus should control for this potentially crucial component.

Trudel et al (2001) reported on the treatment of hypoactive sexual desire (HSD) in women, claiming their study was a rare example of a 'study of HSD using a standardized treatment program, a control group and a scientific methodology'. Couples were recruited through newspapers and 74 couples participated. A reasonably precise set of criteria for the diagnosis of HSD was used, which allows comparison with subsequent studies. Thirteen established questionnaires were used to assess mood, marital, psychological and sexual functioning. The treatment involved 12 weekly group couple sessions (4–6 couples per group) and a pair of male and female therapists. The treatment followed a 'cognitive-behavioural, multimodal therapeutic program' involving nine therapeutic techniques: analysis of immediate and long-term causal factors related to HSD, sexual information, couple intimacy exercises, sensate focus, communication skills training, emotional communication skills training, mutual reinforcement training, cognitive restructuring and sexual fantasy training. The control group was a waiting list; half of the couples were assigned to wait 3 months and were assessed at the beginning and end of the wait period before proceeding with the same treatment. At 1 year follow-up, 36% of women were symptom free. However, it is not clear how many of the 74 women were assessed at that stage; only 45 of them completed all the questionnaires. This is a useful study, with a number of strengths, including detailed (possibly too detailed) assessment and reporting of couples' reactions to the various components of the treatment. The method of recruitment may be important, and one wonders how such a group would compare with those referred to a clinic for treatment. The value of delaying treatment for 3 months as a form of control is limited, and only the one treatment programme was used. Once again, no information is given about the characteristics of those who did and did not respond, which could be of prognostic relevance.

A controlled comparison of three methods of treating vulvo-vestibulitis (Bergeron et al 2001), is considered in Chapter 13 (see p. 385), as this condition is more appropriately regarded as a pain disorder rather than a sexual dysfunction.

Prognostic indicators of response to sex therapy

Most available evidence of variables which predict outcome in couple therapy have been derived as by-products of controlled treatment outcome studies which were not designed primarily for this purpose (e.g. Mathews et al 1976, 1983; Whitehead & Mathews 1986), or from retrospective case note studies (e.g. Glover 1983). One systematic prospective study aimed primarily at prognosis has been reported by Hawton & Catalan (1986). A series of 154 couples, receiving Masters & Johnson-type therapy, were assessed before treatment for levels of sexual knowledge, motivation for treatment, how much the therapist liked the couple, global ratings of the quality of both general and sexual relationship, and psychiatric status. The initial response to treatment was assessed after the third treatment session. Outcome was assessed by the therapist after the last treatment session, whether or not treatment had been completed. Failure to complete treatment was significantly associated with lower social class and lower motivation on the part of the male partner, poorer general relationship and poorer progress by the third treatment session. Outcome of the whole group was related to the quality of the general relationship as rated by the therapist and female partner (though not by the male), and to motivation of the male partner. The extent to which couples were carrying out their homework assignments by the third session was also highly predictive of outcome. The prognostic importance of the general relationship was found in a number of early studies (e.g. Cooper 1969; Lansky & Davenport 1975; Leiblum et al 1976; Mathews et al 1976; Snyder & Berg 1983; Whitehead & Mathews 1986).

In 1992, Hawton reviewed the research literature on sex therapy. He was able to report some further progress in identifying prognostic factors. Further findings from the Oxford clinic had been reported by Catalan et al (1990). Of 200 consecutive cases assessed, 110 (55%) were offered sex therapy. However, only 77 started treatment and of those 42 completed it. Completion of treatment was associated with higher motivation for treatment, the quality of the general relationship and lower initial ratings of anxiety in the presenting partner.

Attention to prognostic factors in relation to specific types of sexual problem has also been limited. In a study of couples where the woman had low sexual desire, completion of treatment was associated with the motivation of the male partner (Hawton et al 1991). In couples where the man had ED (Hawton et al 1992), completion of treatment was less likely when the female partner had a history of psychiatric disorder, or had experienced less sexual pleasure previously, or when there was poor communication in the general relationship. It was also less likely in couples from lower socio-economic groups. This confronts us with the fact that sex therapy, as usually administered, advocates a pattern of male–female sexual interaction appropriate in the American and British middle classes, but which might fit uncomfortably in other socio-cultural contexts.

Empirical validation

In Heiman and Meston's (1997) review of the literature on treatment outcome studies, the American Psychiatric Association's (APA, 1995) two categories of 'empirical validation' were assessed. They concluded that 'well-established' treatments had been reported for primary anorgasmia in women and ED in men, and 'probably efficacious' treatments for secondary anorgasmia, vaginismus and PE. Only two of the cited studies involving behavioural treatment had been published since Hawton's (1992) review. Prognostic factors, however, were not addressed.

In various ways, the available prognostic evidence points to the importance of partner characteristics as well as those of the person with the presenting problem, and hence underlines the relevance of a couple approach. In his conclusions, Hawton (1992) emphasized the need for more controlled outcome research, but with the proviso that key prognostic factors would be controlled in the design.

There is also a need to identify prognostic factors that relate to the specific method of treatment in use. When we compare two forms of treatment, we are assuming crucial differences in the treatment process (e.g. one method may focus on communication skills, the other on anxiety management). In such circumstances, we need measures of the relevant pre-treatment status (i.e. communication skill or anxiety) that will indicate prognosis. We then require our two treatment groups to be adequately matched on both these variables.

The accumulation of evidence about prognostic factors is not going to make the task easier. The greater the number of such factors identified, the more complex (and impracticable) a balanced design becomes. Warner & Bancroft (1986) considered the possibility of using a single composite prognostic variable derived from appropriate multivariate analysis (e.g. discriminant function).

More research is certainly required in this respect if we are to expect worthwhile benefits from treatment outcome studies in the future. The immediate research needs are of three types: the study of commonsense prognostic indicators, such as general relationship and motivation, along the lines of Hawton & Catalan's (1986) study, the development of appropriate methods of measuring these variables and producing composite prognostic scores (e.g. discriminant function scores), and the analysis of treatment processes that will allow the identification and measurement of patient characteristics relevant to that process.

Pharmacological and hormonal treatments

For male problems

Erectile dysfunction

Phosphodiesterase-5 inhibitors

The most important development in this field was the serendipitous discovery that sildenafil, a phosphodiesterase-5 (PDE-5) inhibitor, enhances erectile response. The Viagra story that followed was briefly described in Chapter 4, together with the implications for our understanding of normal erectile response. There is now an extensive literature demonstrating the efficacy of sildenafil in the treatment of ED, which has been well reviewed by Rosen & McKenna (2002). They reviewed 12 placebo-controlled studies involving, together, more than 2500 men from around the world, and all using the International Index of Erectile Function (IIEF; Rosen et al 1997) as the principal outcome measure. In one study, a comparison was made with a sexually functional age-matched control group (Dinsmore et al 1999). This showed that the men with ED increased their percentage of maximum response, as measured by the IIEF, from 34.2% at baseline to 72.6% with sildenafil, compared to 86.1% for the controls. It is difficult with most of these studies to establish what proportion of men failed to get a clinically useful response to treatment. Meuleman et al (2001), however, reported that after 26 weeks of treatment 79% reported improved erections with sildenafil, and 27% with placebo. In most studies, there is evidence of a dose–response effect, with available tablets of sildenafil containing 25, 50 or 100 mg. The most common side effects are headache, flushing and dyspepsia, and they are also dose related.

Two further PDE-5 inhibitors have been developed and are now in use: tadalafil (Cialis) and vardenafil (Levitra). Evidence of their effectiveness has been demonstrated (e.g. Padma-Nathan et al 2001 (tadalafil); Porst et al 2001; Fisher et al 2005 (vardenafil)) and they are both comparable to sildenafil in this respect. The main differences between the three drugs are in their speed and duration of action. Sildenafil should be taken about 1 h before sexual activity and has a half-life of around 3.5 h. Tadalafil should be taken at least 30 min before sexual activity, and has a half-life of 17.5 h; treatment effect can persist for 24–36 h. Vardenafil is pharmacokinetically similar to sildenafil, but is more potent, with a dose range of 5–20 mg. These three compounds are similar in their side effects, though the duration of these relate to the half-life of the drug. One advantage of tadalafil is that its absorption is not delayed by food intake, which can be a problem with the other two. For all three drugs, the most important and dangerous drug interaction is with nitrates used for ischaemic heart disease, and this is a strong contraindication for the use of PDE-5 inhibitors.

Most of the controlled outcome studies have used groups with mixed aetiologies for the ED, with the majority having an 'organic' component. Some studies have looked at groups with specific aetiologies. In men with diabetes, 60–65% show improvement of erectile function with PDE-5 inhibitors, which is lower than the outcome in typical mixed aetiology groups, but still substantially better than placebo (Rendell et al 1999; Boulton et al 2001). As yet no clear associations between treatment response and specific diabetic complications or glycaemic control have been reported. In men with ischaemic heart disease, around 70% have shown improvement in erectile function, although side effects have been more frequent in these patients (Conti et al 1999). In men with spinal cord injury, who typically have ED because of loss of neural activation of erection, results have been particularly good, with 80–88% reporting improvement (Giuliano et al 1999; Sanchez et al 2001). Several studies have assessed treatment in men with ED following prostatectomy, and overall the results have been disappointing, particularly in those men who have not received nerve-sparing surgery (reviewed by Rosen & McKenna 2002). Seidman et al (2001) found significant improvement in erectile function in men with ED who in addition reported untreated mild to moderate depression. They also found some associated improvement in mood and well-being that followed the improvement in erectile function.

In spite of these impressive results from numerous placebo-controlled trials, the longer-term use of PDE-5 inhibitors appears to be limited. In a recent large study, in eight countries, of more than 25 000 men, aged 20–75 years, 16% were found to have ED. In a second phase, 2912 of the men identified with ED were followed up; 58% of them had sought medical help for the ED, but only 16% were currently using PDE-5 inhibitors (Rosen et al 2004b). Various reasons were given for discontinuation, including lack of appropriate information from the physicians, fear of side effects, partner concerns and distrust of medications (Rosen 2007). Leiblum (2002) has pointed out that the advantages of PDE-5 inhibitors may be less for men in relationships with chronic conflict or lack of desire in either partner. Such men are typically excluded from controlled treatment trials. Men with ED often have high expectations of success with PDE-5 inhibitors, having been influenced by the media 'hype' around these drugs. When the drug fails to work or loses its effect after initial success, it can be particularly devastating for the man (Tomlinson & Wright 2004). Also, the reactions of the partner to a drug-induced erection aren't always favourable (Potts et al 2003; see p. 304).

Anti-adrenergic drugs

The complex role of noradrenaline (NA) in sexual response was elaborated in Chapter 4. NA transmission is largely responsible for the 'central arousal' component of sexual arousal, manifested by feelings of excitement and peripheral activation with increased blood pressure and heart rate. In the periphery, in contrast, NA is largely responsible for the inhibitory tone in erectile smooth muscle. Thus, increase in NA activity centrally is associated with arousal and decrease in NA activity peripherally with genital response (see p. 67). A number of drugs influence NA transmission, though the receptors involved are complex. Drugs which antagonize pre-synaptic α2 receptors increase the amount of NA at the synapse, and hence enhance NA transmission. Drugs which antagonize post-synaptic α1 receptors block NA-mediated smooth muscle contraction.

Yohimbine, originally derived from plants, is predominantly an α2 antagonist that has a long history as a putative aphrodisiac. A number of placebo-controlled trials of its use in the treatment of ED have been reported, but with various design deficiencies. Riley (1994), in reviewing this literature, concluded that yohimbine has a modest therapeutic benefit over placebo, and is generally well tolerated.

In the early 1990s, a more specific α2 antagonist was developed by Syntex in the hope of maximizing the possible benefits of yohimbine. This compound, delequamine, was investigated in a series of laboratory studies, assessing both nocturnal penile tumescence (NPT) and erectile and cardiovascular responses to erotic stimuli, in men with and without ED (see Chapter 4; for review see Bancroft 1995). The results were consistent with a central arousal enhancing effect, but this was only apparent in younger men with ED, raising the possibility that central NA arousal may be diminished with ageing (see p. 70). The results were also consistent with the idea that men with ED have increased α2 tone centrally, which reduces their capacity for central arousal in response to sexual stimuli. This compound did not make it through phase 3 studies, showing only modest effects.

Phentolamine is an α1 and α2 antagonist used medically to treat hypertensive crises. It has been used, in combination with papaverine, to induce erection by intra-cavernosal injection (see p. 78). In this case, the effect is presumably mediated by its α1 antagonist effect. In the penis, α2 receptors are found both pre- and post-synaptically. The post-synaptic α2 receptor probably has similar effects to the α1 receptor. In an earlier study, idazoxan, an α2 antagonist, had no effect when injected intracavernosally (Brindley 1984) probably because the pre- and post-synaptic effects cancelled each other out. The effects of phentolamine administered systemically are therefore of interest. Is it possible that it could improve sexual arousal by both blocking the peripheral α1 receptors and enhancing central arousal by blocking the α2 receptors in the brain? Goldstein et al (2001) reported two studies: one parallel group and the other crossover in design. In the parallel group study, significantly greater improvement in erectile response occurred with phentolamine than with placebo and was dose related. In the crossover study the differences were in the same direction but not significant. Long-term follow-up resulted in high attrition, but of those staying in the study, phentolamine continued to have beneficial effects. In a Mexican study (Ugarte et al 2002), sildenafil was found to be significantly more effective than phentolamine.

Dopamine agonists

Given the central role of dopamine (DA) in both incentive motivation and central control of genital response (see Chapter 4), and the negative sexual effects of most DA antagonists (see Chapter 13), the effects of DA agonists are of obvious interest. However, the pharmacology of dopaminergic agents illustrates the complexity of the role of DA in the brain. DA antagonists may show their main sexual effect in reducing sexual interest (see Chapter 13). The main effects of dopamine agonists, like apomorphine, are to induce genital (i.e. erectile) response, probably via the oxytocinergic system (Heaton 2000). Cocaine and amphetamine, both drugs of addiction, increase DA activity either by inhibiting re-uptake (cocaine) or increasing release (amphetamine) of DA. These effects are presumably mediated via the incentive motivation system (see p. 67).

The pharmacological pursuit of DA-induced enhancement of sexual interest or response provides an interesting episode in the history of sexual pharmacology. In the 1980s Eli Lilly became the first pharmaceutical company to develop a drug specifically for this purpose, quinelorane, a D2 dopamine agonist. Extensive animal studies had shown its pro-sexual effects, including studies of primates (e.g. Pomerantz 1991). Phase 2 treatment studies in humans encountered substantial problems with side effects, mainly nausea and dizziness, leading to its abandonment clinically (Crenshaw & Goldberg 1996). I was involved in one of these controlled studies, and can recall one subject who developed a convincing erection but was unable to get off the bed because as soon as he lifted his head he would go round in circles.

The DA agonist that has received the most attention is apomorphine. Early studies, while showing positive effects on erection, also demonstrated substantial side effects (reviewed by Rosen 1991; Segraves 1995). The development of a sublingual route of administration (Apomorphine SL) was intended to lessen side effects by avoiding absorption via the liver. A number of studies have evaluated the effects of apomorphine SL in the treatment of ED.

In a placebo-controlled study of 296 men with ED, of mixed aetiology and severity, 3 mg of apomorphine SL was significantly better than placebo in improving erections; 4 mg was not more effective than the 3 mg dose, but produced more side effects, nausea being the most frequent (Dula et al 2001). Similar results were reported in two European studies (Stief et al 2002; von Keitz et al 2002). Apomorphine SL is taken around 30 min before sexual activity. Although all of these studies, each funded by a pharmaceutical company, concluded that apomorphine was effective in the treatment of ED, it is evident that nausea severely limits 'on-demand' use, and only a minority of men have been willing to continue with the drug after completing the studies (Uckert et al 2006). Two further crossover studies have directly compared apomorphine SL with sildenafil: Eardley et al (2004) included men with ED who had not previously received pharmacological treatment for the problem, but who had mixed aetiologies, and Perimenis et al (2004) included men diagnosed as having arteriogenic ED. Both studies showed a clear superiority of sildenafil over apomorphine. Perimenis et al (2004), whose study is unusual in focusing on a specific aetiology, pointed out that 20% were not satisfied with either treatment.

Melanocortin agonists

The new phase of interest in melanocortins was considered in Chapter 4 (p. 130). The first human study relevant to treatment involved the use of melanotan-II, a non-selective melanocyte receptor agonist, administered subcutaneously (Wessells et al 2000). Subjects were monitored by Rigiscan for several hours following administration in their own home, and instructed to avoid deliberate sexual stimulation. This resulted in erections occurring in 17 out of 20 men with ED, and also an increase in sexual desire. But severe nausea in some men and a relatively long time before onset of action, around 2 h, limited the clinical value of this preparation.

Interest then shifted to bremelanotide (PT-141) a metabolite of melanotan-II, and a menalocortin analogue. In one placebo-controlled laboratory study (Diamond et al 2004), intranasal administration of PT-141 was found to enhance erections in response to visual sexual stimuli (VSS) in men with ED who had already found sildenafil to be effective. In a second study, using the same design but administering PT-141 subcutaneously and involving men with ED who had not responded to sildenafil, a similar positive effect on response to VSS was observed (Rosen et al 2004a). Side effects similar to those with apomorphine did occur, and were more marked in the second study, partly because of the higher plasma levels with subcutaneous than with intra-nasal administration, and also because the blood levels were sustained for longer. Vomiting, when it occurred, was 6–15 h after administration. The subcutaneous route had been used in the second study because it was anticipated that the ED subjects resistant to sildenafil would require higher plasma levels of PT-141. That proved not to be the case. Large-scale phase 3 studies with this compound are underway at the time of writing.

The effects of both apomorphine and bremelanotide are of theoretical interest as, in contrast to the PDE-5 inhibitors, they appear to be influencing sexual response centrally. This raises some fundamental questions about treatment effects and the nature of the ED. When ED is considered to be dependent on altered responsiveness in the penis, it is questionable whether such centrally acting treatments would be effective. As yet such issues have not been addressed. It remains to be seen whether the propensity for side effects limits the clinical value of these new treatments. They illustrate the crucial point that it is difficult to manipulate central mechanisms in the brain pharmacologically without inducing a range of other unwanted effects.

A theme throughout this literature is an absence of attention to the characteristics of those who respond and how they differ from those who do not. Only in this way are we likely to identify prognostic markers. We have postulated, for example, that men with psychogenic ED showing high inhibition (SIS1) scores on the SIS/SES will do better with a drug that reduces peripheral inhibitory tone, such as phentolamine, than a drug which acts through the excitatory pathways, such as sildenafil (Bancroft & Janssen 2001). That remains to be tested. Apart from the studies, mentioned earlier, which have focused on men with different medical conditions (e.g. diabetes), the rest of the controlled outcome literature involves mixed aetiology groups. I have so far found no study of medication that focuses on psychogenic ED. It is time for the field to be developing and testing hypotheses that would increase our understanding of the mechanisms involved as well as improving the selection of the most appropriate treatment for a particular patient. The initial excitement and enthusiasm for PDE-5 inhibitors as an overall solution discouraged such research.

Intracavernosal injections

As indicated in Chapters 4 and 11, the discovery that certain drugs injected into the corpus cavernosum induced erection was an important phase in the history of sexual medicine, and contributed to our understanding of erectile physiology. Whereas initially intracavernosal injection (ICI) was used as a method of investigation, it soon became a form of treatment by self-injection. The best-established compound for ICI, and the only one approved for this purpose, is prostaglandin E1 (alprostadil or Caverject), a potent smooth relaxant and vasodilator. Erections occur within 5–20 min of the injection. The main side effect is penile pain, and the most serious is priapism. Any erection following ICI that lasts more than 4 h should be reported and dealt with medically.

Other compounds that have been used 'off label' for ICI are papaverine and phentolamine, an α1 and 2 adrenergic antagonist (see above) either separately or combined.

A preparation of alprostadil that is applied intra-urethrally (MUSE) is available. In a direct comparison with ICI administration, the ICI was more effective and preferred (Shabsigh et al 2000).

Gene therapy

A new approach to the treatment of ED which is at a very early stage of development is gene therapy. The principles are complex (for a detailed overview see Gonzalez-Cadavid et al 2001). Much of the relevant work has been done by Melman and his colleagues, and in 2006 they reported their first, preliminary clinical results (Melman et al 2006). As explained in Chapter 4 (see p. 78), the key process in penile erection is relaxation of the smooth muscle of the corpora cavernosa and also penile arterial walls. At the cellular level this complex process involves the balance of potassium (K^+) outflow and calcium (Ca^{2+}) influx, with maintenance of smooth muscle contractile tone depending on a sufficient concentration of Ca^{2+}. In response to signals intended to produce erection, the K^+ channels open, resulting in an outflow of K^+ and hyperpolarization that limits Ca^{2+} entry. The focus of Melman's approach is to produce an increased expression of K^+ channel genes, which are believed to be reduced by ageing or disease processes like diabetes. They have developed a 'naked' DNA plasmid that they call hMaxi-K, which is administered by single-dose intracavernosal injection. The hope is not only to enhance erectile response but to do so for a relatively long period (several months). So far such injections have not resulted in any adverse effects. In their first clinical report, in which varying doses of the gene were administered to 11 men, 2 out of the 11 reported improved erectile function, which was maintained through the 24 weeks of the study. The two responders were among the five receiving the higher doses of the gene plasmid. Interestingly, one of the two responders was not only the youngest in the group (aged 42) but also the only one to be diagnosed as having psychogenic ED. Obviously, further studies are required before the therapeutic potential of this approach can be evaluated.

Premature ejaculation

The high prevalence of delayed or absent orgasm or ejaculation as a sexual side effect of antidepressants, particularly selective serotonin re-uptake inhibitors (SSRIs; Rosen et al 1999a; and see p. 403), in men and women, has drawn attention to the use of such drugs for treating PE. This was first reported with clomipramine, a tricyclic antidepressant atypical in having serotonin reuptake inhibition in common with SSRIs. Subsequent controlled studies have also shown treatment effects with SSRIs, including paroxetine, sertraline and fluoxetine (reviewed by McCullough 2001). A new SSRI with rapid onset and short duration of action specifically designed for use to delay ejaculation in men with PE has been developed, but so far has not been approved by the US FDA for this purpose.

More recently PDE-5 inhibitors have been explored as treatment for PE. The most persuasive explanation for their delaying ejaculation has been given by Abdel-Hamid (2004). Whereas it may seem paradoxical that a class of drug shown to be effective in enhancing erectile response should also delay ejaculation, it becomes less so when one considers that the effects on erection result from nitrergically mediated relaxation of smooth muscle in the erectile tissues, and also that seminal emission involves smooth muscle contraction. Abdel-Hamid (2004) reviewed the evidence that nitrergic transmission was involved in relaxing smooth muscle in the prostate, vas deferens and seminal vesicles. However, McMahon et al (2006) reviewed 14 studies reporting a positive effect of PDE-5 inhibitors on PE, and concluded that only one study met the criteria for appropriate methodology and assessment. Interestingly, that study was their own (McMahon et al 2005)! They also concluded that the evidence for the usefulness of PDE-5 inhibitors is probably limited to secondary PE, where there is typically some degree of associated ED. At this stage we should reserve judgment on the use of PDE-5 inhibitors for PE.

Delayed or absent orgasm/ejaculation

At the present time there is no accepted pharmacological treatment for delayed or absent ejaculation or orgasm that is not secondary to some other disorder or is a side effect of medication. Difficulty in ejaculating occurs in hypogonadism, and this will be considered in the next section.

Low sexual desire

As indicated earlier, erectile response and sexual desire are closely related in men, and in many cases (though not all) men with ED experience loss of sexual desire (see Chapter 11). Less often, it is the desire that goes first, with ED following, and sometimes it is not easy to be sure which came first, even with a careful history. The mechanisms that lead to consistency between sexual desire and erectile function are not well understood (see p. 307). If sexual desire was dependent on the same central neuroendocrine mechanisms as erectile response, one might expect sexual desire to increase when using pharmacological treatments that act centrally (e.g. apomorphine) to enhance erection. If, on the other hand, loss of sexual desire is a psychological reaction to the ED, then one might expect increase in desire when treating ED with peripherally acting agents such as PDE-5 inhibitors. Unfortunately, the now extensive literature on pharmacological treatment of ED, reviewed briefly above, has paid scant attention to these issues, and it remains uncertain when and to what extent we can expect improvement in sexual desire when effectively treating ED.

The most treatable cause of loss of sexual desire in men is hypogonadism. This is considered closely in Chapter 4 and, in older men, in Chapter 7. In those cases where androgen deficiency is demonstrated, T replacement is indicated. Currently the most favoured route of administration is trans-dermal, either using cream, or preferably skin patches that provide a more controlled release into the skin. One advantage of the trans-dermal route is that the hormone is absorbed into the skin and then released more gradually into the circulation, maintaining relatively physiological levels. In comparison, intramuscular injections of T (e.g. T enanthate) produce supraphysiological levels in the circulation, which then steadily decline. Oral routes (e.g. methyltestosterone)

are complicated by considerable metabolism during the first pass through the liver, hence the need for higher doses, and some risk of hepatic toxicity. One oral preparation, T undecanoate, is absorbed via the lymphatic system and hence avoids the liver initially. While the absorption is variable, depending on fat content of the diet, it has been used in Europe for androgen replacement for many years (Gooren 1994).

If loss of sexual desire is associated with hyperprolactinaemia (see p. 129), treatment with a dopamine agonist is indicated. Most experience has been with bromocriptine, but pergolide, quinagolide and cabergoline have all been used for this purpose (Molitch 2004).

For female problems

Given the considerable uncertainty about the nature of sexual problems in women that prevails at the present time, it is not surprising that the effectiveness of pharmacological methods in the treatment of women's sexual dysfunction is unclear and probably limited. In a recent review of this literature Nijland et al (2006) identified 25 randomized placebo-controlled studies, but they excluded 14 because they did not use a 'validated' method for identifying female sexual dysfunction. All of the excluded studies involved hormonal manipulation of some kind and included some of the seminal studies in the literature (e.g. Sherwin et al 1985). Of the 11 studies included, four involved administration of sildenafil, the first PDE-5 inhibitor, which has proved to be effective in enhancing erectile response in men. The remaining seven studies all involved T administration, either trans-dermal or oral (as methyltestosterone). Nijland et al (2006) paid little attention to the results, but concentrated on the lack of consistency in the outcome measures, with several of them based on what they call 'the traditional linear sexual response model' moving from sexual desire to arousal to orgasm. They question what such changes might mean to the women involved, commenting 'first of all, a woman's motivation for sexual activity is frequently for reasons other than sexual desire and/or sexual thoughts and fantasies, and its absence does not equate to dysfunction. Second, emotional well-being and positive emotional responses during sexual activity are reported to contribute more to sexual satisfaction than physical or genital aspects of sexual response' (p. 773). In several respects I agree with them. However, they conclude, 'a universally accepted method for defining the FSD population is needed and as a result a consensus should be reached for appropriate inclusion and exclusion criteria for FSD trials' (p. 774). The issue of classification is considered more closely in Chapter 11 (p. 338). Unfortunately, Nijland et al (2006) make no proposals for such definitions, and indeed it can be argued that more basic research is needed before attempting such a definition. Controlled treatment studies, whether involving 'satisfactorily diagnosed FSD' or not, may be helpful in this respect, as were several of the earlier and more recent studies on hormone administration to women. In the course of this book I have proposed certain concepts that, if they prove to have any validity or heuristic value, will be relevant to this task (see discussion of the basic pattern etc., in Chapters 4 and 6). It is reasonable to suppose that if women vary in their pattern of sexuality, they may vary in their response to pharmacological or hormonal manipulations, and their treatment needs will differ when they encounter sexual 'dysfunctions'. What is particularly striking is the contrast between this literature, with all of its complexities and inconsistencies, and the comparable literature for men. For example, almost all the controlled outcome studies of PDE-5 inhibitors and ED have used the IIEF (Rosen et al 1997) as the outcome measure. Furthermore, the results reported have typically been restricted to the 'domain' of erectile function, composed of six questions. And in many of these papers they simplify the findings by referring to two of these questions: Q3: When you attempted sexual intercourse, how often were you able to penetrate (enter) your partner? and Q4: During sexual intercourse how often were you able to maintain your erection after you had penetrated your partner? Apart from the fact that much of this literature has tended to ignore the other domains, such as sexual desire, this demonstrates how simple (one could say 'simplistic'), by comparison, are our concepts of sexual function in the male compared to the female.

So far, as the review by Nijland et al (2006) makes clear, most relevant evidence involves administration of hormones, mainly androgens, to women, with most studies restricted to surgically or naturally menopausal women. These studies have been examined closely in Chapter 4. Another hypothesis promoted in this book is that women vary in their behavioural sensitivity to androgens. This would explain why a substantial proportion of women (at least 50%) can experience major reduction in circulating androgens, as a result of steroidal contraception (see p. 446) or ovariectomy, without obvious adverse effects on their sexuality. I have also hypothesized (p. 133) that such women are more likely to be in the basic pattern category; they may not need the effects of T but will need adequate oestrogenization for satisfactory vaginal response. The women who do need T may be those who enjoy sexual arousal and orgasm. Obviously, there is going to be no clear cut off between these groups in these respects. But a fundamental need that arises from this perspective is to identify markers of the T sensitive woman. It is striking that absolutely no attention has been paid in the rest of the literature to this general idea that there may be different types of women who would respond differently to pharmacological or hormonal treatments, with one exception, considered below. From this perspective what is important is a universally accepted method for defining the different patterns of women's sexuality, which require a different treatment when they go wrong, rather than defining the FSD population. With male as well as female sexual problems, the pharmaceutical industry and the clinical researchers working with them have paid virtually no attention to distinguishing between those who do and those who do not respond to a treatment. The emphasis has been on getting a large enough sample to achieve statistical

significance for what, as an average for the total group, is a modest improvement. Let us now look more closely at the limited evidence.

Problems with sexual arousal and orgasm

Although it has been suggested that nitrergic neurotransmission is as important to genital response in women as in men, the evidence was considered in Chapter 4 (p. 80) and it was concluded that whereas nitric oxide is involved, other mechanisms of neurotransmission are probably more important in women (e.g. vasoactive intestinal polypeptide). Nevertheless, the impact of PDE-5 inhibitors on women's sexual response is of interest, and it remains a possibility that nitrergic neurotransmission is more important in the clitoris than the vagina. The effects of sildenafil in women with sexual problems have been explored in four studies. The most substantial evidence comes from two placebo-controlled multi-centre international studies of women with sexual problems funded by Pfizer Ltd (Basson et al 2002). One study involved 577 women who were either pre-menopausal or post-menopausal and receiving hormone replacement (HRT). They were regarded as 'oestrogenized'. They were randomly assigned to one of four groups, receiving one of three doses of sildenafil (10, 50 or 100 mg) or placebo. The other study involved 204 post-menopausal women not receiving HRT, regarded as 'oestrogen deficient', who were randomized to 50 mg sildenafil or placebo, but with the option of increasing the dose to 100 mg or reducing it to 25 mg, or placebo equivalents. In terms of sexual response and ability to participate in sexual activity, no differences were found between sildenafil and placebo in either study, and there were no differences between different doses of sildenafil, apart from side effects being more marked with the higher dose. This study, however, used a relatively heterogeneous group of women in terms of their sexual problems. Only 40–50% had a primary diagnosis of female sexual arousal disorder (see p. 308), the remainder being diagnosed with hypoactive sexual desire disorder or female orgasmic dysfunction. Is it possible that the women who reported improvement in this study differed from those who did not in their type of sexual problem, or in their normal pattern of sexual response? This was not reported. Basson & Brotto (2003), in a placebo-controlled laboratory study of 30 oestrogenized post-menopausal women with impaired sexual arousal and orgasm, found that those women who showed less increase in vaginal pulse amplitude (VPA see p. 79) in response to erotic films, showed more increase in subjective arousal and reduction in latency to orgasm when taking sildenafil compared to placebo. Caruso et al (2001) compared two doses of sildenafil and placebo in 53 pre-menopausal women who complained of reduced arousal and capacity for orgasm, but did not report low sexual desire. They found a significant improvement in sexual arousal and orgasm with sildenafil compared to placebo, though no difference between the two doses of sildenafil. It therefore remains possible that a subgroup of women who experience normal sexual interest and subjective arousal but lack vulval and vaginal response, might benefit from such treatment. Further research is required on this issue.

Low sexual desire

Most of the relevant evidence involves the administration of T. This was reviewed in Chapter 4. There is evidence that administration of T to women with low sexual desire, whether pre- or post-menopausal, can result in increased desire. But the results are variable and a number of uncertainties remain. First is the possibility that only some women are sensitive to T, as considered above. Secondly, much of the positive evidence comes from studies producing supraphysiological levels of T. Are positive effects due to a 'pharmacological' rather than a 'hormone replacement' effect and could this be mediated by effects on mood and well-being? Thirdly, is it possible that the effects of T, at least in some cases, depend on its aromatization oestradiol (E)? As pointed out in Chapter 4, there has been surprisingly little attention to comparing the effects of different dosages of E administration on sexuality and well-being in women. In addition, we have to contend with the fact that the safety of long-term use of T (or other androgens) in women has not been established. At the present time, therefore, T is an option for treating low sexual desire in women, but in each individual case clear benefits should first be demonstrated and the cost–benefit analysis carefully evaluated before long-term use.

Other pharmacological agents

Uckert et al (2006) reviewed a number of studies of drug effects on women's sexuality that should be considered preliminary and warranting further research. In each case these drugs have first been shown to be effective in studies of dysfunctional men (see above). These include prostaglandin E1 applied to the vulvar area prior to vaginal intercourse (Padma-Nathan et al 2003), phentolamine, an α1 and α2 antagonist (Rosen et al 1999b), apomorphine, a dopamine agonist (Bechara et al 2004), bupropion, an antidepressant (Segraves et al 2004) and bremelanotide (PT-141), a melatonin receptor agonist (Diamond et al 2006).

Other non-pharmacological methods of treatment

For the male

Vacuum constriction devices

Inducing erection by creating a vacuum around the penis and then retaining the erection by applying a constriction ring around the base of the penis has been an option for ED for many years. Vacuum constriction devices (VCDs) are commercially available, and have become more technologically sophisticated over the years. A VCD-induced erection should be maintained for no more than 30 min to avoid ischaemic damage. Complications are relatively minor, but include penile pain, difficulty ejaculating while wearing the device and minor bruising. Peyronie's disease (see Chapter 13) has been raised as a complication, but there is no clear evidence of this. A number of studies have assessed VCD use and are reviewed by Donatucci

(2001). In one study, Rigiscan monitoring showed an average rigidity of the induced erection of more than 80%. In most studies the VCD was only used on a long-term basis by a minority of patients, ranging from 69% to 19%. Some studies have reported beneficial effects of combining VCD with ICI, when neither works well on its own.

As with ICI, there is limited acceptability of this method for long-term use even when it is effective at inducing erection. But it remains an option that suits some men and their partners.

Penile implants

Surgical implantation of penile prostheses or 'splints' was introduced in the 1970s. The earlier prostheses, known as 'malleable', consisted of an inner twisted metal wire with an outer silicone cover. After insertion this provides a permanent semi-rigid erection, sufficient for vaginal intercourse, but not easily 'put away' after use! This type of prosthesis has largely given way to more modern inflatable devices, which incorporate a small pump, implanted in the scrotum, and two inflatable cylinders in the penis. An erection is produced by squeezing the scrotal pump, and can be deflated. The most modern and technically sophisticated are the three-piece prostheses, which have a third component, a reservoir, placed intra-abdominally, containing the fluid that is pumped into the cylinders. These more complex devices, needless to say, are much more expensive than the earlier malleable variety, and the surgery involved is more demanding. This form of treatment should also be regarded as a last resort, as following such surgical implantation normal erection is no longer possible. The various types of implant are described by Wang & Lewis (2001) and their complications by Mulcahy (2001).

For the female

There are few if any non-pharmacological treatment methods for women that have been evaluated. Vibrators are widely used and often recommended as a component of treatment (e.g. for primary anorgasmia). Kegel's exercises, to strengthen the pelvic floor muscles and increase the woman's awareness of her pelvis, have often been advocated but their value has been disputed by some. Surgical treatment for vulvo-vaginitis will be considered in Chapter 13, as this is regarded more as a pain condition than a sexual problem.

Outcome of integrated psychological and medical treatment

A recent international consensus concluded that if one accepts a 'biopsychosocial' model of sexual dysfunction, there are compelling reasons for doubting that any single intervention, such as drug treatment, will be sufficient in most cases (Althof et al 2005). This has led Rosen (2007), one of the pioneers in the drug treatment of sexual dysfunction, to recommend an integrated medical and psychological approach to the problem of ED.

However, after the discouragement from earlier studies of combined psychological and pharmacological treatment, considered earlier, no further research attention was paid to integrated treatments until recently. Althof (2006) reviewed a number of recent studies of that kind. In one study (Melnick & Abdo 2005), men with psychogenic ED were assigned to (i) a 6-month course of 'theme-based psychotherapy', (ii) sildenafil treatment or (iii) a combination of the two. Using the criterion of 'normalization of IIEF scores' (i.e. erectile function domain scores of 26 or higher), only the combined treatment group showed significant improvement. In contrast to 6 months of psychotherapy, Phelps et al (2004) evaluated a one-session (60–90 min) psycho-educational intervention combined with sildenafil, and compared this with sildenafil used alone. The combination resulted in higher treatment satisfaction scores. Two studies compared ICI treatment with and without counselling, and found advantages to the combination over ICI alone (Lottman et al 1998; Titta et al 2006). For men with psychogenic ED, Wylie et al (2003) compared couple therapy alone and in combination with instructions in the use of a vacuum device. Those with the combined regime did better. So far these more recent evaluations point to the benefit of an integrated approach.

The current status of treatment for problems of impaired sexual response or interest

The evidence favours the integration of psychological and pharmacological or other non-psychological treatments. But whatever approach is indicated, the therapist should aim to work with the couple whenever possible.

The potential for response to treatment, particularly in the longer term, varies considerably, reflecting a wide range of aetiological factors of a psychological kind, and a range, in severity and type, of physiological factors.

There are no grounds for concluding that either psychological or medical interventions are ineffective, but with a better understanding of prognostic indicators, treatment could be more effectively planned.

Whereas there is a crucial need for good controlled treatment outcome studies, research is needed to optimize the value of such studies. In particular, comprehensive methods for assessing prognosis are needed, which would allow different types of prognostic factors to be integrated into a limited number of 'prognostic' scales. These should be designed for particular types of sexual problem and particular types of therapeutic intervention, for example a good overall prognostic scale to assess likelihood of response in women treated for low sexual desire, or in men treated for ED. Although more research on prognostic factors is warranted, particularly for some specific sexual problems, enough prognostic factors have been identified to allow a start to this process. Relatively large numbers of couples entering therapy of different kinds need to be assessed and their results incorporated into a meta-analysis. This will obviously require substantial cross-centre and cross-researcher collaboration, which would be made more possible by government funding for that purpose.

In the meantime, I have no doubts about recommending the integrated treatment approach described in this chapter. We have much to learn to improve treatment, but in the meantime many people need help.

Assessment for treatment – when to treat and which treatments to use

Usually, those with problems relating to impaired sexual response are referred (or refer themselves) to the clinic as a couple with one partner having the problem. Not infrequently, only the partner with the problem is referred. In such cases, a strong recommendation is made that the other partner should attend for the assessment process. If, however, this does not happen, then the assessment and treatment process for individual therapy is used (see p. 353). However, the fact that the partner will not attend, or the referred individual does not want the partner to attend, warrants close scrutiny and is likely to be highly informative (i.e. why is the partner not attending?).

The initial assessment interview

One hour is normally allowed. The following objectives should be clear: an initial description of the nature of the problem; identification of other assessments required (e.g. physical examination; blood tests); evidence of the commitment and motivation of each partner to improve the relationship; assessment of the mental state of each partner.

The first few minutes are intended primarily to establish rapport and to set the patient or couple at ease. At this stage both partners are seen together. The contents of the referral letter are discussed, when appropriate, to check that it presents a correct picture and to give patients an idea of what the clinician already knows about them. Their feelings about coming to the clinic are then explored, providing an opportunity to express anxiety, embarrassment or ambivalence.

The next stage of the interview is carried out on an individual basis. One of the partners, usually the one without the presenting problem, is asked to wait outside. After about 20 min they change round and the last 10 min or so of the interview are used to see the couple jointly again.

During the course of each individual interview the following points are addressed, at least to some extent:

1. The precise nature of the sexual problem and the current level of sexual desire or spontaneous interest.
2. The history of the sexual problem. The early stages in the development of a problem are often of crucial significance to understanding aetiology and selecting treatment. Were there particular times of change in the sexual relationship and if so what was going on in their lives at those times?
3. The nature of the general relationship and other details of the immediate family and children. It is of particular importance to assess the extent of marital disharmony.

4. Psychiatric history: the recognition of depression is important. Its relevance to sexual desire has already been emphasized (p. 106). If too severe, it may interfere with counselling and more specific treatment of depression may be indicated first. However, it is important to recognize that depressed mood is commonly a reaction to marital or sexual difficulties, and by acknowledging the importance of those difficulties and tackling them directly, considerable improvement in mood may result.

5. Medical history. Evidence of recent health (e.g. exercise) or illness is important. Particularly careful enquiry should be made about any drugs being used and for how long. Earlier medical history may be important in understanding the early stages of a sexual problem, e.g. did if first become noticeable after a transient physical illness or accident? The extent to which a medical condition has been diagnosed and appropriately treated should be established. Details of relevant investigations and specific treatment for such conditions are given in Chapter 13. Sexually transmitted infections and their treatment are covered in Chapter 14.

6. Contraceptive history. Contraceptives may interfere with sexual enjoyment in a variety of ways (see Chapter 15) and may occasionally be the principal cause of the problem. A reappraisal of suitable contraception is therefore appropriate at this stage. Sometimes, when the couple are keen to start a pregnancy, and are partly seeking treatment for that reason, they may be reluctant to use any contraception. They should nevertheless be encouraged to do so, after explaining that it is more sensible to concentrate on improving the sexual relationship first. There are various ways in which striving to conceive can interfere with the treatment process.

7. Use of alcohol or recreational drugs Establish the typical number of units taken by each partner in a week. Alcohol may impact on a sexual relationship in several ways. The immediate effects of some degree of intoxication can alter the dynamics of the relationship and how emotions are felt and communicated. In the long term, there may be adverse effects on sexual function. Similar problems may be associated with use of recreational drugs, though they have been less well studied (see Chapter 13, p. 407).

8. Attitudes to the sexual problem and possible treatment. By the end of the initial interview the couple's attitudes and expectations about the nature of the problem and suitable treatment should be apparent. One or both of them may prefer to see their problem in physical terms and deny the importance of psychological factors. This will determine the acceptability of different treatment methods; counselling, particularly involving the partner, may be rejected on those grounds. The attitude of the partner is also crucial. Is he or she prepared to accept any responsibility for tackling the problem? Sometimes strong rejection by partners of any involvement in treatment may indicate some fear that they also have problems they would rather not acknowledge. Special efforts by the therapist may then be required gradually to win the trust and confidence of the partner. In such cases, decisions about treatment may need to be delayed until further interviews have been completed.

In the final part of the interview, with the couple together, the clinician describes his or her initial impression of the nature of the problem and a recommended programme of assessment and treatment.

Let us now closely consider some of the more important points that need to be covered during assessment of each partner, whether or not presenting with the problem; first with women and then with men. Only part of this information is likely to be obtained at the initial assessment session.

Assessing the woman

How has she been reacting recently during sexual activity? Does she find herself becoming excited or aroused? How does she experience this? Does she find that being touched by her partner is pleasurable, and if so which parts of the body does she particularly enjoy being touched? Does sexual activity make her feel emotionally close to her partner?

Does her vagina lubricate during love-making? Has there been any pain or soreness during sexual activity? When is the pain experienced? Does it occur from simply touching her vulva? Does she experience this pain at other times as well? Is it on initial entry of the penis, easing once the penis is inserted? Is it felt at the entrance of the vagina or deeper in the vaginal barrel? Is it brought on by deep thrusting, or simply by movement of the penis inside the vagina? Does the vagina feel sore after intercourse and for how long? Is the pain related to posture during love-making? Does she have a tendency to back pain and if so does she get backache after sexual intercourse?

Does she usually experience orgasm during love-making? If she does not, has this always been the case? If so, has she been able to experience orgasm during masturbation on her own? Has the absence of orgasm during sexual activity with her partner been a cause of concern for her? If she used to experience orgasm, but no longer does, when did that change and what were the circumstances? If she does usually experience orgasm, how enjoyable is this for her? Questions about orgasm often lead to hints that direct clitoral stimulation is required. This should be made explicit and appropriate reassurance given. How does she feel if she doesn't experience an orgasm? Is there any indication of performance anxiety about orgasm?

Does she masturbate on her own? (Attitudes to masturbation are often informative.) If she does, and this usually results in orgasm, how does this compare with orgasm during sexual activity with her partner?

Does she feel spontaneous sexual desire? It is often necessary to make the clear distinction between spontaneous desire and desire which is part of a response to a sexual approach by her partner. When she feels sexual desire, what in particular is she desiring? How often does she feel spontaneous sexual desire?

Does she find her partner sexually attractive? Has this changed? Does she feel sexually attracted to others, apart from her regular partner?

What sort of lover is her partner? Does he have problems with erection or does he ejaculate too soon? How sensitive is he to her needs? Can she communicate with him about what she enjoys or does not enjoy? How does she feel about his body; does she mind touching or caressing his genitalia?

What attitude does the woman have to her own body? Is she comfortable with nakedness? Does she have a particular concern about weight and is there evidence of abnormal eating patterns?

How does she experience menstruation? Does her sexual desire vary predictably with her menstrual cycle? Does she have substantial perimenstrual mood change? If so, what effect does this have on her relationship? How does she cope with her periods? Are they heavy or painful? Has she been having other gynaecological problems, in particular vaginal infections, soreness or discharges?

If this is not her first long-term sexual relationship, how does it compare with previous relationship(s)? Were her early sexual experiences positive? This is an opportunity to invite information about sexual abuse during childhood or adolescence, though some women only feel safe enough to reveal such experiences once they have established a secure therapeutic relationship.

Indications for physical examination of the female

1. A complaint of pain or discomfort during sexual activity.
2. Recent history of ill-health or physical symptoms apart from the sexual problem, and where no adequate clinical assessment has already been carried out.
3. Recent onset of loss of sexual desire with no apparent cause.
4. Any woman in the peri- or post-menopausal age group with a sexual problem.
5. History of marked menstrual irregularities or infertility.
6. History of abnormal puberty or other endocrine disorder.
7. When the patient believes that a physical cause is most likely, or suspects there is something abnormal about her genitalia.

The timing of the physical examination is important. For women who are particularly apprehensive about being examined it may be appropriate to delay until a more secure therapeutic relationship has developed, though in such cases it should be made clear that an examination needs to be carried out at some stage. In pre-menopausal women, it is sensible to avoid the menstrual phase of the woman's cycle.

Physical examination of the female

Whilst a general physical examination, including cardiovascular system, central nervous system, respiratory system, etc. is often necessary, it is the genital examination which is of special relevance to the assessment of sexual problems and which requires our particular consideration and this should be preceded by a careful abdominal examination, in particular to look for areas of tenderness on palpation.

The psychological reaction of the patient to the genital examination may give important information in addition to the direct results of the examination itself. The impact that the whole procedure has on the relationship between the examining clinician and the patient is important, particularly if the clinician is also to be the therapist. The impact is also likely to be different when the clinician is of the opposite sex to the patient. If the examination is carried out in a sensitive manner it may have a constructive, positive effect on the therapeutic relationship. If carried out insensitively it may make treatment with that particular clinician difficult if not impossible.

How the examining clinician maintains his or her own comfort in this situation may be crucial. Some adopt an attitude of indifference to the patient's sexuality, deflect any reference to the topic with hearty jocularity, or deter it with an aloof aseptic clinical approach. Some tend to heavy-handedness during genital examination, to ensure that gentleness of touch is not mistaken for a caress. If the examination is to achieve its aims, however, it must be conducted in a gentle, relaxed, unhurried but thorough manner. An adequate sexological examination also calls for close and detailed visual inspection of the genitalia, to a greater extent than usual in routine examinations, when a cursory glance is usually regarded as more appropriate than a prolonged gaze. Opportunities should be taken to explain details of the patient's anatomy and physiology during the examination process. The use of a mirror can be valuable for that purpose.

There is therefore a need to combine the sensitivity and perceptive awareness of the trained therapist with the physical expertise of the gynaecologist or urologist.

Genital examination

Some women have described vaginal examinations as distasteful, embarrassing and physically uncomfortable experiences, from which they have emerged feeling demeaned or sullied — an experience which detracts from their sense of sexual self-respect. In contrast, the aim during the examination of a patient with sexual dysfunction should not be merely to avoid inflicting discomfort and embarrassment but also to contribute to the therapeutic process, endorsing the patient's sexuality and enhancing her sense of sexual self-assurance.

In Western cultures, the doctor should usually maintain eye contact and relevant conversation with the patient during the vaginal examination. But he should also be sensitive to the patient's cultural and personal background. For example, women from traditional Muslim or Hindu cultures may prefer to conceal their faces behind a sari or sheet during the examination or if their face is exposed, may adopt an expression of exaggerated distaste, as if to demonstrate their respectability. The style of the examination should therefore be adapted to the individual patient.

Good lighting from an adjustable source is important. If during examination the patient's abdomen and thighs are kept covered by a draping sheet, she will be more ready to abduct her thighs widely, which is essential if the examination is to be comfortable and informative.

The examination process should be very much guided by the woman's history, in particular pain history. The clinician should demonstrate sensitivity and caution in relation to pain. If vulvar pain or burning has been reported, a careful visual examination of the vulva should be carried out, with very gentle opening of the labia to facilitate this. Are there any areas of inflammation, apparent lesions or ulcers? Vivid illustrations of such lesions are provided by Margesson & Stewart (2006). In the absence of visible lesions, a careful exploration of sensitivity of the vulvar surfaces should be carried out using a moist Q-tip. This may elicit relatively discrete areas or a more generalized vulvar sensitivity. The diagnostic process then needs to discriminate between localized pathologies, including infections, such as herpes simplex, candida, trichomonas or herpes zoster, inflammatory conditions such as lichen planus and squamous cell carcinoma. In the absence of any such explanation the diagnosis of vulvo-dynia or vulvo-vestibulitis should be considered. This is an ill-understood condition, with uncertain treatment (Margesson & Stewart 2006; and see Chapter 13, p. 385).

The next step is the vaginal examination. Self-lubricated disposable plastic gloves should be worn, with a trace of lubricating jelly, and the labia minora are gently held apart by the fingers of the left hand, thus everting their moist medial surfaces while the examining finger is introduced. If the woman has reported pain on vaginal insertion of a penis or finger or tampon, she may well show evidence of tension when the vaginal examination is imminent, i.e. she will be less willing to abduct her legs widely, or tend to draw away when the vulva is touched and may grimace when even gentle vaginal examination is attempted, and the muscles surrounding the lower vagina will be found to be tight. In these circumstances, successive steps of the examination should be conducted gradually, with continuing verbal encouragement and reassurance.

In women with vaginismus and marked contraction of the perivaginal muscles (see p. 34) entry of the examining finger may be impossible, and any attempts to insert it painful. In severe cases marked tensing of body musculature with arching of the back and firm adduction of the thighs gives an early indication of the diagnosis as well as preventing access to the vaginal area. Patience and sensitivity are then essential. Vaginismus can only be properly diagnosed by vaginal examination and will not be apparent if examination is carried out under general anaesthesia. In cases when vaginismus seems likely from the history and considerable apprehension about an examination is expressed by the woman it may be advisable to delay examination until a more trusting relationship with the clinician has been established. Even so, it should be made clear at the start that an examination will eventually be necessary. In women with a marked aversive response to examination, it can be carried out in steps on a number of occasions. First, the patient is assured that only visual examination of the vulva will be involved, requiring abduction of her thighs. On the second occasion, the doctor's finger will simply be placed in the opening of the vagina but not inserted, and so on. This procedure, in addition to being gradual, demonstrates firmness combined with trustworthiness on the part of the doctor. The diagnosis of vaginismus, currently controversial, is discussed on p. 324.

For visual examination of the vaginal wall it is advisable to use a smaller than normal size of bivalve speculum. It should be near body temperature and the blades should be lubricated with a thin film of jelly. The handle of the speculum should be directed posteriorly to ensure minimal contact with the more sensitive areas of the clitoris and urethral meatus and to allow the speculum to remain at full depth within the vagina when opening the blades, minimizing the stretching of the introital ring, which is especially sensitive in nulliparous women.

To inspect adequately the vaginal aspects of a perineal scar the speculum should be gently rotated through 90° before withdrawal so that the blades are spread laterally and the length of the vaginal wall is exposed to view posteriorly. In this way small tags of tender granulation or ridges of scar tissue are not overlooked.

Further vaginal examination includes a combination of finger insertion and gentle abdominal palpation to look for evidence of deep sensitivity or pain. When considering possible causes of pain on deep penetration or thrusting, it is important to remember the elongation of the vagina and elevation of the uterus which normally occur during sexual arousal. Deep discomfort may be due to impairment of this normal functional response or to pelvic pathology or a combination of both. The presence of deep dyspareunia warrants a full gynaecological assessment that may include laparoscopy or ultrasound.

Relevant pelvic pathologies include:

1. *Pelvic inflammatory disease.* Infection may involve the adnexa (salpingitis) or the pelvic connective tissue (parametritis). There will be deep tenderness on palpation in the lateral fornices and on displacement of the cervix. It is worth noting here that cervical erosions, which are common, are not a manifestation of pelvic infection and are not a cause of dyspareunia.
2. *Endometriosis.* Even small deposits of endometriosis, if located (as they often are) in or near the pouch of Douglas (i.e. the peritoneal cavity between the rectum and uterus), will usually cause intolerable pain during coitus. The tender nodules can often be felt on vaginal examination.
3. *Uterine retroversion* (see Chapter 3, p. 35). The majority of patients with retroversion of the uterus do not experience pain during intercourse unless there is some additional complicating feature such as prolapsed ovary in the pouch of Douglas, retroversion fixed by adhesions or retroversion with impaired arousal and therefore no uterine elevation. Apart from the body of the retroverted uterus, other

swellings in the pouch of Douglas, such as a low-lying fibroid or a fixed ovarian tumour, can similarly cause discomfort.

4. *Vaginal vault scarring*. The normal ability of the vaginal vault to dilate during sexual arousal may be impaired in a parous woman by scarring resulting from a deep cervical laceration at the time of delivery or from hysterectomy. In the latter case, granulations may also be present at the site of the vault suture line.

In some women discomfort during coitus is not experienced at the introitus, nor on full penetration, but during coital movement, which causes pain in the vaginal walls at an intermediate depth. This may be due to vaginal infection (e.g. thrush or *Trichomonas*) in a milder form without associated vulvar infection and pain. Frictional contact with the vaginal walls during thrusting elicits the discomfort and the woman is often left with the sensation of post-coital rawness for several hours. The diagnosis is based on microscopic examination of the vaginal fluid. Women using oral contraceptives sometimes experience vaginal dryness and consequent discomfort, and may also be more vulnerable to active infection by *Candida albicans* present in the vaginal flora (see Chapter 14).

Vaginal obstetric scars also need to be considered in parous women. If an episiotomy has been sited too far laterally or a vaginal laceration has extended to the middle third of the lateral vaginal wall, the resulting scar may overlie the inner margin of the levator ani muscle. This area is particularly sensitive (and can also be an important source of erotic stimuli), so that severe dyspareunia is likely and will be localized to the affected side of the vagina.

Assessing the man

Erectile problems In assessing erectile problems, establish whether full erection can occur in any situation or at any stage during love-making. If so, at what stage does it start to fail? Loss of erection on attempting vaginal entry usually has a psychological explanation, although rarely it can result from a postural effect in someone with vascular disease and the 'pelvic steal' syndrome. Are erections painful or deformed in any way, suggesting Peyronie's disease?

When did the problems with erection start? Was it a relatively sudden onset, or was there a more gradual development of erectile difficulty? The latter is suggestive of organic factors or the effects of ageing. Do problems with erection only occur during sexual interaction with the partner, and do they occur usually during masturbation or on other occasions when vaginal intercourse is not imminent? Erections present on waking in the morning or during the night are evidence of normal sleep erections. Full erections occurring on waking or during masturbation or during non-coital interactions with the partner are suggestive of a psychogenic causation of an erectile problem. However, the absence of such erections does not exclude psychogenic causation. The diagnostic significance of sleep erections will be discussed more fully later in this chapter.

Premature ejaculation is a more difficult problem to specify, because it is a matter of how much control the man believes he has, and how much he believes he should have. Does ejaculation occur before vaginal entry and, if not, how soon after vaginal entry? Has this problem been present since the start of the man's sexual career or has it developed or got worse recently? How does his partner react to this difficulty? Does the man feel under pressure to delay his ejaculation for the sake of his partner? There is a particular need to distinguish between problems of ejaculation, erection and sexual desire. Late-onset PE may be secondary to erectile failure, perhaps as a result of the performance anxiety engendered by the erectile problem, although if that is the case then it is likely that there was some lack of control previously. As discussed in Chapter 11, the role of performance anxiety in the causation of PE is not clear, but may serve to aggravate an existing problem. Also, with erectile impairment, the time taken to elicit an erection may be prolonged, whereas that required to produce ejaculation is not. This can give the impression of PE. Careful questioning is necessary to distinguish between these various situations.

How soon after PE can the man become aroused again? When ejaculation occurs quickly as a result of high arousal and with a long interval since his last ejaculation, it is usually possible for arousal to return in a relatively short time, at least during that same love-making session. When PE is accompanied by performance anxiety, and low levels of sexual arousal, the post-ejaculatory refractory period tends to be complete and very prolonged.

Absent or delayed ejaculation also requires careful description. Does the problem occur only in the presence of the partner (e.g. is he able to ejaculate normally when masturbating on his own) or is it only a problem intravaginally (i.e. can he ejaculate outside the vagina during love play with his partner)? Does he get seminal emissions during sleep? Relatively frequent 'wet dreams' in a man who is unable to ejaculate when awake suggests an inhibitory mechanism. Are any medications being used which might interfere with orgasm or ejaculation? Does orgasm occur without ejaculation (a 'dry run' orgasm, without the seminal emission component, may be drug-induced or due to a neurological deficit), or is there evidence of retrograde ejaculation into the bladder (e.g. cloudiness of the first urine passed after orgasm)?

Low sexual desire. The assessment of sexual desire is somewhat easier in men than in women, as it is more readily manifested as a desire to initiate sexual activity. But the main difficulties are deciding whether a loss of sexual desire preceded or followed some other sexual dysfunction, such as erectile failure, and distinguishing between desire and concern about sexual performance, which can become a preoccupation. Loss of desire following erectile failure is of little help diagnostically; it is likely to be an understandable response to the genital failure, although it is noteworthy that some men experience no decrease in desire in spite of loss of erectile function. The explanation for this difference is not yet established. But loss of sexual desire that clearly preceded other dysfunctions may have important causes, such as hormonal deficiency, which need to be identified. In such cases the erectile failure can then be a psychological response to the loss of desire but may also be a later manifestation of the hormonal deficiency (see p. 111). As discussed in Chapter 11, the aetiology of loss of sexual desire is complex and heterogeneous and may require much more careful history-taking than is often necessary with other types of sexual problem.

The man's attitude to his general health may be important. Concern about sexual function is sometimes part of a general hypochondriacal pattern. Concerns about body image are sometimes important, but less often, it seems, than with women. The use of tobacco and excessive alcohol are potentially important factors (see Chapter 13, p. 405).

The occurrence of pain during sexual activity needs careful enquiry. Where is the pain experienced? Is it in the glans, shaft of the penis or elsewhere in the groin or scrotum? Is it a pain, a soreness to touch or an unpleasant hypersensitivity? At what point during the sexual response sequence does it occur? Is it associated with ejaculation, or does it occur with prolonged arousal and then is relieved by ejaculation? Is there ever blood in the ejaculation? Is it a skeletal pain associated with movement or posture during sexual intercourse?

Indications for physical examination of the male

These include the following:

1. Recent history of ill-health, or physical symptoms apart from the sexual problem, if clinical assessment has not already been carried out.
2. Complaint of pain or discomfort associated with sexual activity.
3. Recent onset of loss of sexual desire with no apparent cause.
4. Any man aged over 50 with sexual problems.
5. Past history of abnormal puberty or other endocrine or genital problem (e.g. mumps orchitis, torsion of the testicles).
6. When the patient believes a physical cause to be most likely or is in some way concerned about his body or genitalia (e.g. penis too small or bent, difficulty retracting the foreskin).

Genital examination of the male

In general, the comments about the need for sensitivity to the patient's feelings when examining women also apply to examination of men. Genital examination can be carried out with the man either lying or standing.

The size and consistency of the testes should be assessed. Normal adult size is 15–25 mL, approximately 4 cm in length. The presence of scrotal swellings, such as hydrocele or spermatocele, should be noted. Large swellings may be a cause of embarrassment or mechanical problems during sexual activity. They may also conceal testicular pathology. Varicoceles, nearly always on the left, are easy to identify but are of uncertain relevance to sexual function.

The shaft of the penis should be examined by palpation. Pulsation in the penile arteries can often be palpated between thumb and index finger. Indurated plaques in one or other corpora cavernosa may be felt, probably indicating Peyronie's disease (see Chapter 13, p. 382) or indurated scarring following penile trauma.

In uncircumcised men, the foreskin should be examined carefully. Can it be fully retracted? Are there any sites of tenderness, resulting from small tears? Torn or tight foreskin (phimosis) may cause pain during intercourse. Difficulty in replacing the retracted foreskin may indicate a tendency to paraphimosis when, following coitus, the tight collar of foreskin remains withdrawn, causing swelling and pain in the glans. Unfortunately, it is not always possible to assess these problems when the penis is not erect.

Pain during intercourse may also be caused by infection under the foreskin (balanitis) or genital thrush or herpes (see Chapter 14, p. 416).

Pain accompanying ejaculation is sometimes a symptom of chronic prostatitis, vesiculitis or epididymitis. In such cases, a rectal examination is indicated, though often no such cause for the pain can be found. It is important to remember that rectal examination can be an unpleasant and demeaning experience for both men and women and should be carried out with sensitivity and care. The opportunity can be used, however, to assess anal tone and innervation in response to light touch and pinpoint, as an assessment of sacral reflexes. Also the bulbocavernosus reflex is an indicator of intact pudendal nerve function. It is elicited by squeezing the glans penis whilst the examiner's finger is inserted into the patient's rectum. A positive response is shown by reflex contraction of the anal sphincter. It is observable in 70% of normal men (Bors & Blinn 1959) but false negatives are common.

When erectile or ejaculatory function is impaired, neurological assessment of the pelvis and lower limbs may be indicated. This is also an opportunity to check peripheral pulses in the lower limbs for evidence of peripheral vascular disease.

Laboratory investigations

Checking urine for sugar is a simple procedure that can be done in the clinic and should be carried out for every man presenting with secondary erectile problems, and probably also those with late-onset ejaculatory disturbance, to exclude the possibility of diabetes.

Other tests should be based on appropriate clinical indications, derived either from the history or the physical examination. Indications for hormone measurement in men present the main difficulty. Any clinical evidence of hypogonadism (i.e. small testes, deficient body hair, gynaecomastia, etc.) requires measurement of plasma T, gonadotrophins and prolactin, preferably in more than one sample. Sex hormone-binding globulin measurement enables estimation of free T (see p. 112). Loss of sexual interest in men under the age of 50, with no other obvious cause, justifies hormonal assay, whereas in men over 50 the onset of ED also warrants hormonal assessment (Buvat & Lemaire 1997).

Prolactin also presents a problem in this respect. Hyperprolactinaemia in men is rare (see p. 129). It is usually (though not always) accompanied by lowered T. In men with loss of sexual desire and low T, prolactin should also be checked. In men under 50 with unexplained loss of sexual desire, prolactin should be checked even if T levels are normal.

Assessment of erectile function

Nocturnal penile tumescence

The occurrence of erections during REM sleep (NPT) is a normal phenomenon described in Chapter 4 (p. 69). Assessment of NPT has been used as a diagnostic procedure in men with ED. Presence of normal ED reduces the likelihood of 'organic' aetiology, although impairment of NPT does not exclude psychogenic causation. Comprehensive monitoring of NPT requires three nights in a sleep laboratory and hence it is now seldom used. However, portable Rigiscan devices can be given to the patient to use at home, and can be helpful provided the patient is given clear instructions how to use them, and is capable of doing so (Levine & Elterman 2001). Their use can be helpful in those cases where aetiological uncertainty persists and when, according to the patient, there is no indication of full erections on waking.

Other physiological assessment

Neurological or vascular assessment is sometimes indicated, particularly if surgical treatment for ED is being considered. Such procedures are reviewed by Rosen et al (2004c) and will also be addressed in relation to specific medical causes of ED in Chapter 13.

Psychometric assessment for men and women

There are now a large number of pencil and paper tests to assess aspects of sexuality. In general these have been developed for research purposes, and in most cases their validation has been based on demonstrating differences between clinical and non-clinical samples (for recent reviews see Daker-White 2002; Meston & Derogatis 2002; Rosen et al 2004c) and have not been shown to have value in distinguishing between sexual dysfunctions with different aetiologies (e.g. Blander et al 1999). In most cases this is because the instrument identifies presence or absence of problems, with limited attention to the degree of severity. A few instruments show a more continuous distribution of scores allowing identification of a 'normal range'. An early example was the Sexual Arousal Inventory for women (Hoon et al 1976). In Chapter 6 the limited evidence of relations between personality measures and sexual behaviour was reviewed. The Sexual Orientation Inventory (Fisher et al 1988), which measures what its developers called 'erotophobia-erotophilia', is more a measure of attitudes, and although it does provide a relatively continuous measure of such attitudes, these have not been used to distinguish between different aetiologies in sexual dysfunction, or in predicting response to different types of treatment. A first attempt to explore the clinical usefulness of the SIS/SES, our measure of propensities for sexual inhibition and sexual excitation, was considered in Chapter 11 (see p. 321). We found some evidence that low sexual excitation scores (SES) in men with ED were suggestive of 'organic' aetiology. More work is needed in exploring such measures in both men and women with sexual problems. We have also postulated that with ED, men who score high on SIS2 (inhibition due to threat of performance consequences) are likely to benefit from psychological treatment, and men with low SES scores are more likely to benefit from pharmacological treatment with PDE-5 inhibitors (e.g. sildenafil). Men with high SIS1 scores (inhibition due to threat of performance failure) may benefit from a combination of psychological treatment and drugs capable of reducing inhibitory tone such as phentolamine (Bancroft & Janssen 2001). However, these hypotheses await adequate testing. Since we developed the SIS/SES questionnaire, however, I have found it helpful in a number of cases to have SIS and SES scores measured and discussed with the patient during the assessment.

Presenting a treatment plan

After the initial assessment, the clinician should start to present recommendations for a treatment plan. Sometimes, these are clear from the start; in other cases, the need for further assessments, sometimes involving referral to a specialist clinic, are required before recommendations can be confidently made. In the large majority of cases, the point is made from the outset that, whatever precise treatment plan is followed, both partners need to remain involved. In any case, it is the responsibility of the clinician to give adequate information about what any specific treatment plan will involve before asking the couple to make a decision about whether to accept it. In this process they should be encouraged to ask questions.

The clinician may use the three windows approach to organize the findings during assessment. To what extent are there indications through the first window of why the couple are experiencing problems sexually? These may be individually based (e.g. depression in one partner), circumstantial (current stress of one kind or another, affecting both partners) or relationship based (evidence of factors likely to induce inhibition of sexual interest or response). With the first two types of explanation, the feasibility of resolving those issues as a first step should be discussed. If relationship based, then couple sex therapy should be recommended, as described earlier in this chapter.

It should then be made clear that such therapy has the added advantage of clarifying the key causative factors as it proceeds. It may become clear, for example, that there are additional factors reducing sexual responsiveness that warrant use of pharmacological methods. These can then be integrated into the ongoing couple therapy.

If there are indications through the second window of vulnerability of one of the partners, these should be discussed, with proposals to consider these as sex therapy proceeds and, when appropriate, modifying the goals of treatment to take them into account. There may also be grounds for use of pharmacological methods (e.g. to reduce inhibitory response patterns; see p. 363).

PE and vaginismus are typical examples. In some cases, particularly with vaginismus, a more individual programme may be warranted (see p. 354), although in general one should strive to keep the partner involved in some way.

If there are explanations apparent through the third window, these should then be discussed with the couple. This may indicate the need for further assessment and specific treatment (e.g. undiagnosed hypogonadism in the male, vulvo-vestibulitis in the female) or accepting the limitations imposed by a medical condition and working with the couple to help them adapt to these. If sexual side effects of medication are considered likely, the possibilities for change of medication should be discussed, and this may involve communicating with the clinician responsible for prescribing the medication.

As discussed earlier in this chapter, some individuals present for treatment who either have no current partner or whose partner is clear that he or she will not become involved. As discussed on p. 353, this has clear implications for the goals of treatment. But otherwise a similar approach to presenting a treatment plan can be employed.

Clinical illustrations

Case study 1

Mary and Peter had lived together for 4 years. Mary complained that she only experienced orgasm during masturbation, not during intercourse. A crucial issue arose when the stage 1 assignment was presented. Peter doubted he could accept the ban on genital touching and intercourse. The rationale was carefully explained a second time. Notwithstanding, he feared that he would become sexually aroused during a session and felt he could not be held responsible for what might ensue. Once aroused, he expected to continue with intercourse. He attributed this to his 'normal maleness'. Would he be in danger of raping his partner if he became aroused, he was asked. Peter admitted this was unlikely. He conceded he had been able to accept limits during courting days, before they started to have intercourse.

Asked if she would lose control were she to become aroused, Mary replied negatively. Both were confronted with the stereotypes of the controlled woman and the uncontrolled man. Offered a reasoned argument that such stereotypes were imposed by societal not biological factors, Peter was asked if he preferred to see himself as a 'sexual animal' and did he feel more masculine as a result. What did control mean to Mary? She described how, given her insecurity during love-making, she was unable to let go. Could this be relevant to her orgasmic difficulty? Peter felt that it probably was. With the importance of feeling safe in a sexual relationship highlighted, Peter agreed to accept the limits of stage 1.

This couple revealed highly relevant attitudes in their reaction to the initial behavioural assignment, which helped to explain why Mary was probably, though unwittingly, inhibiting her arousal and orgasm.

How does this case fit the classification system proposed at the end of Chapter 11? Mary's presentation indicated barriers to (i) having a rewarding sexual relationship and (ii) sexual

pleasure. Although at initial assessment it was not clear whether these barriers were due to factors in the current situation (first window) or to a vulnerability in Mary (second window), this was quickly clarified once sex therapy started. This was a first window relationship issue, resolvable by modifying the dynamics of the sexual interaction. For this purpose Peter needed to recognize his contribution to the problem.

· ·

Case study 2

Jane and Bob, both 25 and married for 3 years, had stopped all sexual activity when Jane found herself unable to touch Bob's genitals. After participating without difficulty in stages 1 and 2, a key issue arose during stage 3, once genital touching was on the agenda. Jane felt a strong feeling of disgust but could not explain it. The therapist suggested that her disgust might be a mixture of attraction and repulsion (an interesting idea, with therapeutic value as it allows for a positive component of an otherwise negative emotion; see p. 320). Jane was then requested to define the difference between touching Bob's penis and other parts of his body she was prepared to touch. After an unconvincing attempt to do so in terms of texture and shape, she was asked what it meant to be disgusted by something Bob found pleasurable. She then expressed the fear he would lose control if she made him aroused. Bob was surprised at Jane's lack of trust.

Following this therapy session, Jane began to touch Bob's penis, although initially she felt mildly nauseous while doing so. Over the following 2 weeks she began to enjoy her own genitals being touched, a new experience, and described feeling aroused. She was, however, still reluctant to touch Bob's penis more than briefly. Why was she able to enjoy being touched but hesitant to give Bob his pleasure? She felt confident she herself would not lose control but expected Bob to do so when he approached orgasm. What did this loss of control mean to her and, what consequences did she fear? She described the break in communication that occurs when partners are approaching and experiencing orgasm. The break constituted a threat to her; she needed to remain in contact. She was invited to describe other situations where a similar break in communication might occur, such as Bob falling asleep. This was not a concern because she knew she could wake him if necessary. Asked how the time scale of Bob going to sleep compared with his reaching orgasm, she acknowledged with surprise that the latter 'time out' was, by comparison, brief.

This couple illustrates how a behavioural assignment can, with appropriate inquiry, expose relevant attitudes and beliefs which are difficult to sustain when they are clearly identified and challenged (a clear example of cognitive restructuring). Jane's 'reactive inhibition', invoked by the threat of losing contact with Bob when he was experiencing orgasm, may reflect a long established tendency for her to feel that sex was justified if it involved expressions of love and intimacy, which were threatened by the departure from intimacy that Bob's orgasm entailed.

This couple presented with a barrier to them establishing a rewarding sexual relationship. In the assessment of this case it was not clear to what extent this was a vulnerability issue in Jane, as seen through the second window or a reaction to the relationship, seen through the first window. As therapy progressed, the second window explanation became clearly more important, indicating vulnerabilities.

· ·

Case study 3

Jeff, 62, and Amanda, 32, had recently married after a relationship of 9 years. Jeff presented with erectile problems and difficulty ejaculating intra-vaginally. His history included a childhood marred by emotional and physical abuse. He described himself as having a 'tainted view of sex'. He first married when aged 20, attracted by his wife's 'normal' family. He regretted the marriage from an early stage. Having children was a major issue; she wanted several, he did not. He would pretend to ejaculate inside her. After they had two children, sexual activity declined markedly.

Jeff suffered from long-standing depression and had received a variety of antidepressants continuously for 15 years.

Amanda described the relationship as good but felt that sex presented a 'wall' between them. She wanted to feel closer sexually and was keen to have a child. She had stopped taking oral contraceptives 6 months previously, and had found herself more easily sexually aroused since. Jeff felt he was too old and not healthy enough to have another child.

Jeff's history revealed significant factors through all three windows. Through the first window was continuing difficulty in their current relationship, which was, in part, related to the child issue. A clear history of Jeff's negative attitude to sex going back to his childhood was obvious through the second window. He did not feel comfortable about enjoying sex. There was also the potentially relevant point about 'pretending to ejaculate' with his first wife. Was this a manifestation of a long-standing ejaculatory difficulty or did it reflect a long-standing conflict over having children? The use of antidepressants was seen through the third window. To what extent was his ejaculatory difficulty due to drugs like sertralin and fluoxetine, which Jeff had been taking?

Before starting sex therapy agreement was obtained from Jeff's psychiatrist for a trial withdrawal of sertraline; bupropion, an antidepressant which he had also been taking and which is not associated with sexual side effects, would be continued. With no consequent worsening of his depression, a limited contract (five sessions) course of sex therapy was started. An agreement was also negotiated to avoid pregnancy for the next 6 months.

During stages 1 and 2, Jeff experienced a distinct reduction in performance anxiety. He had difficulty initially touching for his own pleasure; giving Amanda pleasure was in the forefront of his mind. After a while, he enjoyed and valued the touching ('it was a lot of fun'), since he was able to dissociate this non-genital touching from the negative aspects of sex he associated with sexual intercourse. Amanda felt at first that the assignment was artificial and 'forced', but then found that touching 'made me feel close'. She had difficulty keeping to the limits, and was quite aroused by the end of these early sessions. Jeff, interestingly, found himself wondering 'what's coming next' when Amanda touched him, an indication of his concern about her 'breaking the ban' and putting pressure on him to respond.

As they continued with stage 2 sessions, both of them felt aroused. They broke the ban on one occasion, with Jeff touching Amanda's vulva. This resulted in her having a series of orgasms, whereas Jeff lost his erection. Following this, Jeff was reluctant to initiate further sessions. At the next meeting with the therapist, they were asked to move on to stage 3 and genital touching, with Jeff paying particular attention to when and why he started to feel any performance anxiety, given that there was still a clear ban on vaginal entry. He was also instructed not to attempt to ejaculate. They progressed well over the next few sessions. Jeff revealed, however, that he had difficulty communicating verbally during the sessions, and was instructed to practice talking. This was clearly related to his negative attitudes about sex. He was also prescribed sildenafil to enhance his erections, while still maintaining the ban on vaginal intercourse. He had tried sildenafil before but without benefit. This time, taking the sildenafil initially made him feel more performance anxiety, but this settled down. Amanda then started to express distress about her wish to have a child.

The couple continued to make good progress, with Jeff's sexuality much improved. The combination of medication (i.e. sildenafil) with sex therapy worked well. Longer term improvement, however, will probably depend on their resolving the issue about having a child.

How can this treatment be viewed from our theoretical perspective? Jeff completed our questionnaire during the early assessment. He had a high SIS1 score (a measure of propensity for inhibition due to the threat of performance failure), suggesting a high inhibitory tone and susceptibility to performance anxiety. His SIS2 score (inhibition due to the threat of performance consequences) was moderately raised, consistent with his 'reactive inhibition' associated with Amanda's wish to get pregnant. His SES (propensity for sexual excitation) was somewhat low, reflecting his age and possible effects of medication or other health issues. Sex therapy was effective in enabling them as a couple to deal with Jeff's performance anxiety, and this had the added benefit of enabling the sildenafil to be more effective at improving his low arousability. Therapy also achieved cognitive restructuring of negative sexual attitudes and beliefs that had been a barrier to sexual pleasure, with consequent reduction of reactive inhibition during sexual activity.

This complex case demonstrated all three barriers: to parenthood, to a rewarding sexual relationship and to sexual pleasure. In addition, there were relevant relationship issues through all three windows which needed to be addressed and which required an integrated treatment approach. In spite of substantial improvement, the 'barrier to parenthood' remained a significant issue.

· ·

These brief case summaries illustrate the extent to which relevant diagnostic information is elicited as a consequence of the early stages of sex therapy, leading in the third case to a clear rationale for an integrated approach.

Cases will vary in the extent to which such factors can be identified in the initial assessment. For that reason, where there is uncertainty, embarking on a sex therapy programme may be the most effective way to identify the treatment needs. In this respect, sex therapy differs from most other treatment approaches, particularly pharmacological, in not having any adverse consequences. The early stages of sex therapy (i.e. stages 1 to 3) can be usefully enacted by any couple in a sexual relationship, whether or not they are experiencing sexual problems.

Treatment of same-sex couples

As considered in Chapter 11, the sexual problems encountered by same-sex couples are to a large extent similar to those in opposite sex relationships, and the treatment approaches, as outlined above, are equally appropriate. Obviously, when exploring the likely determinants of such problems, there are likely to be some differences in the relevant factors, resulting from some degree of difference in the dynamics of same-sex relationships. Nichols & Shernoff (2007) provided a useful review of some of these differences. In gay male couples, problems of pain or anticipation of pain with anal intercourse may be presented, and can be dealt with in a comparable way to the management of vaginismus in heterosexual couples, with the need to exclude local causes for increased pain sensitivity. An interesting way to approach potential differences in the sexual problems of same-sex couples is to consider the problems which in opposite-sex couples result from the interaction of the male and female patterns. Thus, the evidence indicating more concern about erectile function in gay men and more concern about PE in heterosexual men, summarized in Chapter 11 (p. 329), reflects the fact that gay men are not troubled about 'coming' too quickly, before their partner does, but may be concerned, for a number of reasons which would be less relevant to a heterosexual interaction, about their ability to get an erection (Sandfort & de Keizer 2001). Lesbian couples will vary considerably in whether either or both partners fit the superadded category (see Chapter 6), or whether both are in the basic pattern. Two lesbian women who both seek intimacy rather than sexual pleasure may find that neither initiates sexual interaction, leading to what has been termed 'lesbian bed deaths'. Nichols & Shernoff (2007) consider the various ways that these more essentially same-sex dynamics may lead to problems and how they can be helped. It is reasonable to conclude, however, that the same basic principles of assessment and therapy as those described earlier for heterosexual couples apply. Problems relating to sexual identity are considered in the third part of this chapter.

PART 2   Problematic sexual behaviour

Problems of high-risk sexual behaviour are seldom presented as such for treatment in a sexual health clinic. Interventions to reduce high-risk behaviour are, nevertheless, important, and will be considered further in Chapter 14.

'Out of control' sexual behaviour

This is an important clinical issue, the treatment of which has not been well studied. On the basis of research guided by the Dual Control model, there are a number of principles that can be considered in such treatment and may prove to have clinical value.

One factor of particular relevance is the tendency to be more sexual during negative mood states (Bancroft & Vukadinovic 2004). In the case of anxiety, the behavioural pattern most often associated involves masturbation (see p. 108). This can be problematic in several ways, including an associated preoccupation, and a resulting barrier to sexual intimacy with one's partner. With depression, as discussed in Chapter 11, the effects are more variable, and may include a transient mood elevating effect of sexual activity, a need for contact with or validation by another person, and an undermining of concern about negative consequences (the 'what the heck' phenomenon). Although such effects may lead to sexual interaction with one's primary partner, which need not be problematic, they are often associated with pursuit of casual sex, with a range of potential negative consequences.

With both anxiety and depression, when clinical assessment shows them to have some causal role in the 'out of control' sexuality, the patient should be encouraged to examine and become familiar with the typical sequence of events. In what circumstances does negative mood lead to out of control behaviour? What are the stages that typically intervene between awareness of the negative mood and enactment of the sexual behaviour? The therapist can guide and monitor the patient's attempts to carry out such behavioural analysis, with the objective of identifying stages in the sequence which lend themselves to alternative and less problematic sequences. Once such strategy is identified and agreed, the therapist maintains contact as a way of motivating the patient to employ them, and of monitoring the patient's attempts to do so.

An alternative approach is pharmacological. In particular, selective serotonin re-uptake inhibitors (SSRIs) have been advocated (Kafka 2007). As considered in Chapter 4, serotonin plays a key role in the sexual inhibition system, and hence it would not be surprising if SSRIs, by increasing serotonergic activity at the synapse, increased inhibition and hence reduced the problematic sexual behaviour. In addition, SSRIs are antidepressants, and hence beneficial effects on mood may also be relevant. There is a need for well-controlled research on the use of SSRIs in the management of 'out of control' sexual behaviour. Until then, SSRIs can be regarded as an additional option. A different approach is hormonal; antiadrogenic drugs, such as cyproterone acetate or medroxyprogesterone acetate (MPA), have been widely used in the management of sexual offenders, and this is considered in Chapter 16. They are also an option for managing 'out of control' behaviour. They can, however, have negative effects on mood, which may be a confounding factor in such cases. Pharmacological or hormonal therapy, as with pharmacotherapy for sexual dysfunction, should be integrated into a psychological treatment approach. It is particularly important, when possible, to carry out the behavioural analysis, as described above, before starting on medication.

PART 3   Sexual or gender identity problems

Sexual identity problems

The history of 'treatment' for homosexuality and the pre-vailing interest in 'reparative therapy' for homosexuals, driven by moral and religious concerns, is reviewed in Chapter 8. An occasional problem presented nowadays at a sexual health clinic is uncertainty about one's sexual identity. Therapists' responses will depend on their attitudes and values concerning homosexuality. My relevant personal values involve issues of responsibility and the importance of using sex to foster intimacy in a close ongoing relationship. Neither is dependent on the gender of those involved. The clinical response I advocate involves a series of crucial sequential steps.

Step 1. Make it absolutely clear that, whatever the patient's values or beliefs might be, the therapist has no difficulty whatsoever in accepting and valuing either a homosexual or a heterosexual or a bisexual identity. The issue is which is right for that person. It is a responsibility of the therapist to be explicit about her or his moral values as they impact on the treatment process so that the patient can choose whether to work with that therapist or not.

Step 2. Make it clear that in order to find out what type of sexual relationship works best, it may be necessary to experience more than one type of relationship, involving partners of either gender. Furthermore, during a lifetime, more than one successful relationship may be experienced, involving same sex and opposite sex partners at different times.

Step 3. Emphasize the need to take time to work out what is right. The therapist, who is better designated as a counsellor in this context, facilitates this process of search and discovery as appropriate. This may involve helping the patient to identify the different 'compartments' of his or her sexuality, and how to incorporate them into a sexually rewarding, intimate and loving relationship. This is more education than therapy.

Gender identity problems

The involvement of the medical profession in gender reassignment is sufficiently central to the transgender experience, that it was covered in Chapter 10. Such medical management typically involves patients who have decided they want gender reassignment and are seeking the necessary medical help to implement it. Some individuals may be uncertain, however, and seek guidance for that reason. In my experience, I have encountered few in that situation. The appropriate therapist's help, however, follows the same principles as used for those who are clear about their wishes. As detailed in Chapter 10, this includes ensuring that the individual is fully informed about what is possible, and

encouraging experimentation with 'passing' as the other gender to see how it feels. Some individuals, and they are usually male, find that a long-term solution is a part-time female existence (Carroll 2007), and this option can be defined. It is also appropriate to point out that clear differentiation into male and female is less socially determined than it has been in the past, and that there is increasing 'gender bending' by individuals who prefer to avoid being seen as either male or female, but as a worthwhile human being. It is becoming increasingly possible to connect with other like-minded 'gender benders' via the Internet.

REFERENCES

Abdel-Hamid IA 2004 Phosphodiesterase 5 inhibitors in rapid ejaculation: potential use and possible mechanisms of action. Drug 64: 13–26.

Althof S 2002 When an erection alone is not enough: biopsychosocial obstacles to lovemaking. International Journal of Impotence Research 14(suppl 1): S99–104.

Althof S 2006 Sexual therapy in the age of pharmacotherapy. Annual Review of Sex Research 17: 116–131.

Althof SE, Leiblum SR, Chevret-Measson M, Hartman U, Levine SB, McCabe M, Plaut M, Rodrigues O, Wylie K 2005 Psychological and interpersonal dimensions of sexual function and dysfunction. Journal of Sexual Medicine 2: 793–818.

APA 1995 American Psychological Association: training in and dissemination of empirically-validated psychological treatments: report and recommendations. The Clinical Psychologist 48: 3–24.

Arentewicz G, Schmidt G 1983 The Treatment of Sexual Disorders. Basic Books, New York.

Balint M 1957 The Doctor, his Patient and the Illness. Pitman Medical, London.

Bancroft J 1974 Deviant Sexual Behaviour: Modification and Assessment. Clarendon Press, Oxford.

Bancroft J 1981 Ethical aspects of sexuality and sex therapy. In Bloch S, Chodoff P (eds) Psychiatric Ethics. Oxford University Press, Oxford, pp 160–184.

Bancroft J 1995 Are the effects of androgens on male sexuality noradrenergically mediated? Some consideration of the human. Neuroscience and Biobehavioral Reviews 19: 325–330.

Bancroft J, Coles L 1976 Three years' experience in a sexual problem clinic. British Medical Journal 1: 1575–1577.

Bancroft J, Janssen E 2001 Psychogenic erectile dysfunction in the era of pharmacotherapy: a theoretical approach. In Mulcahy J (ed) Male Sexual Function: A Guide to Clinical Management. Humana Press, Totowa, NJ, pp 79–90.

Bancroft J, Vukadinovic Z 2004 Sexual addiction, sexual compulsivity, sexual impulse disorder or what? Towards a theoretical model. Journal of Sex Research 41: 225–234.

Bancroft J, Dickerson M, Fairburn CG, Gray J, Greenwood, J, Stevenson N, Warner P 1986 Sex therapy outcome research: a reappraisal of methodology. 1. A treatment study of male sexual dysfunction. Psychological Medicine 16: 851–863.

Basson R, Brotto LA 2003 Sexual psychophysiology and effects of sildenafil citrate in oestrogenised women with acquired genital arousal disorder and impaired orgasm: a randomized controlled trial. British Journal of Obstetrics & Gynaecology, 110: 1014–1024.

Basson R, McInnes R, Smith MD, Hodgson G, Koppiker N 2002 Efficacy and safety of sildenail citrate in women with sexual dysfunction associated with female sexual arousal disorder. Journal of Women's Health and Gender-Based Medicine 11: 367–377.

Bechara A, Bertolino MV, Casabe A, Fredotovich N 2004 A double-blind randomized placebo controlled study comparing the objective and subjective changes in female sexual response using sublingual apomorphine. Journal of Sexual Medicine 1: 209–214.

Bergeron S, Binik YM, Khalifé S, et al 2001 A randomized comparison of group cognitive-behavioral therapy, surface electromyographic biofeedback, and vestibulectomy in the treatment of dyspareunia resulting from vulvar vestibulitis. Pain 91: 297–306.

Blander DS, Sanchez-Ortiz RF, Broderick GA 1999 Sex inventories: can questionnaires replace erectile dysfunction testing? Urology 54: 719–723.

Bors E, Blinn K 1959 Bulbocavernosus reflex. Journal of Urology 82: 128.

Boulton AJ, Selam JL, Sweeney M, Ziegler D 2001 Sildenafil citrate for the treatment of erectile dysfunction in men with Type II diabetes mellitus. Diabetologia 44: 1296–1301.

Bramley H M, Brown J, Draper K C, Kilvington J 1983 Non-consummation of marriage treated by members of the Institute of Psychosexual Medicine: a prospective study. British Journal of Obstetrics and Gynaecology 90: 908–913.

Brindley GS 1984 Pharmacology of erection. Paper presented at 10th Annual meeting International Academy of Sex Research, Cambridge, England.

Buvat J, Lemaire A 1997 Endocrine screening in 1,022 men with erectile dysfunction: clinical significance and cost-effective strategy. Journal of Urology 158: 1764–1767.

Carney A, Bancroft J, Mathews A 1978 Combination of hormones and psychological treatment for female sexual unresponsiveness: a comparative study. British Journal of Psychiatry 132: 339–346.

Carroll RA 2007 Gender dysphoria and transgender experiences. In Leiblum SR (ed) Principles and Practice of Sex Therapy. 4th edn. Guilford, New York, pp. 442–476.

Caruso S, Intelisano G, Lupo L, Agnello C 2001 Premenopausal women affected by sexual arousal disorder treated with sildenafil: a double-blind, cross-over, placebo-controlled study. British Journal of Obstetrics and Gynaecology 108: 623–628.

Catalan J, Hawton K, Day A 1990 Couples referred to a sexual dysfunction clinic: psychological and physical morbidity. British Journal of Psychiatry, 156: 61–67.

Conti CR, Pepine CJ, Sweeney M 1999 Efficacy and safety of sildenafil citrate in the treatment of erectile dysfunction in patients with ischaemic heart disease. American Journal of Cardiology 83: 29C–34C.

Cooper AJ 1969 Disorders of sexual potency in the male: a clinical and statistical study of some factors related to short term prognosis. British Journal of Psychiatry 115: 709–719.

Crenshaw TL, Goldberg JP 1996 Sexual Pharmacology. Norton, New York.

Daker-White G 2002 Reliable and valid self-report outcome measures in sexual (dys)function: a systematic review. Archives of Sexual Behavior 31: 197–210.

DeAmicis LA, Goldberg DC, LoPiccolo J, Friedman J, Davies L 1985 Clinical follow up of couples after treatment for sexual dysfunction. Archives of Sexual Behavior 14: 467–489.

Dekker J, Everaerd W 1983 A long term follow up study of couples treated for sexual dysfunction. Journal of Sexual and Marital Therapy 9: 99–113.

Diamond LE, Earle DC, Rosen RC, Willett MS, Molinoff PB 2004 Double-blind, placebo-controlled evaluation of the safety, pharmacokinetic properties and pharmacodynamic effects of intranasal PT-141, a melanocortin receptor agonist, in healthy males and patients with mild-to-moderate erectile dysfunction. International Journal of Impotence Research 16: 51–59.

Diamond LE, Earle DC, Heiman JR, Rosen RC, Perelman MA, Harning R 2006 An effect on the subjective sexual response in premenopausal women with sexual arousal disorder by Bremelanotide (PT-141), a melanocortin receptor agonist. Journal of Sexual Medicine 3: 628–638.

Dinsmore WW, Hodges M, Hargreaves C, Osterloh IH, Smith MD, Rosen RC 1999 Sildenafil citrate (Viagra) in erectile dysfunction: near normalization in men with broad spectrum erectile dysfunction compared with age-matched healthy control subjects. Urology 53: 800–805.

Donatucci CF 2001 Vacuum erection devices. In Mulcahy J (ed) Male Sexual Function: A Guide to Clinical Management. Humana Press, Totowa, NJ, pp. 253–262.

Dow MGT, Gallagher J 1989 A controlled study of combined hormonal and psychological treatment for sexual unresponsiveness in women. British Journal of Clinical Psychology 28: 201–212.

Draper K 1983 Practice of psychosexual medicine. Libby, London.

Duddle CM 1975 The treatment of marital psychosexual problems. British Journal of Psychiatry 127: 169–170.

Duddle M 1994 Training in psychosexual medicine. British Medical Journal 308: 1440.

Dula E, Bukofzerb S, Perdok R, George M, and the Apomorphine SL study group 2001 Double-blind, crossover comparison of 3 mg apomorphine SL with placebo and with 4 mg apomorphine SL in male erectile dysfunction. European Urology 39: 558–564.

Eardley I, Wright P, Macdonagh R, Hole J, Edwards A 2004 An open-label, randomized, flexible-dose, crossover study to assess the comparative efficacy and safety of sildenafil citrate and apomorphine hydrochloride in men with erectile dysfunction. British Journal of Urology International 93: 1271–1275.

Fisher W, Byrne D, White LA, Kelley K 1988 Erotophobia-erotophilia as a dimension of personality. Journal of Sex Research 25: 123–151.

Fisher WA, Rosen RC, Mollen M, Brock G, Karlin G, Pommerville P, Goldstein I, Bangerter K, Bandel T-J, Derogatis LR, Sand M 2005 Improving the sexual quality of life of couples affected by erectile dysfunction: a double-blind, randomized, placebo-controlled trial of vardenafil. Journal of Sexual Medicine 2: 699–708.

Giuliano F, Hultling C, El Masry WS, Smith MD, Osterloh IH, Orr M, Maytom M 1999 Randomized trial for sildenafil for the treatment of erectile dysfunction in spinal cord injury. Annals of Neurology 46: 15–21.

Glover J 1983 Factors affecting the outcome of treatment of sexual problems. British Journal of Sexual Medicine 10: 28–31.

Goldstein I, Carson C, Rosen R, Islam A 2001 Vasomax for the treatment of male erectile dysfunction. World Journal of Urology 19: 51–56.

Gooren LJ 1994 A ten-year safety study of the oral androgen testosterone undecanoate. Journal of Andrology 15: 212–215.

Gonzalez-Cadavid NF, Ignarro LJ, Rajfer J 2001 Gene therapy for erectile dysfunction. In Mulcahy JJ (ed) Male Sexual Function: A Guide to Clinical Management. Humana, Totowa, NJ, pp. 371–386.

Hastings DW 1967 Can specific training procedures overcome sexual inadequacy? In Brecher R, Beecher E (eds) An Analysis of Human Sexual Response. Deutsch, London, pp. 221–235.

Hatzichristou D, Rosen RC, Broderick G, Clayton A, Cuzin B, Derogatis L, Litwin M, Meuleman W, O'Leary M, Quirk F, Sadofsky R, Seftel A 2004 Clinical evaluation and management strategy for sexual dysfunction in men and women. Journal of Sexual Medicine 1: 49–57.

Hawton K 1982 The behavioural treatment of sexual dysfunction. British Journal of Psychiatry 140: 94–101.

Hawton K 1992 Sex therapy research: has it withered on the vine? Annual Review of Sex Research 3: 49–72.

Hawton K, Catalan J 1986 Prognostic factors in sex therapy. Behaviour Research and Therapy 24: 377–385.

Hawton K, Catalan J, Martin P, Fagg J 1986 Long term outcome of sex therapy. Behaviour Research and Therapy 24: 665–675.

Hawton K, Catalan J, Fagg J 1991 Low sexual desire: sex therapy results and prognostic factors. Behaviour Research and Therapy 29: 217–224.

Hawton K, Catalan J, Fagg J 1992 Sex therapy for erectile dysfunction: characteristics of couples, treatment outcome, and prognostic factors. Archives of Sexual Behavior 21: 161–175.

Heaton JPW 2000 Central neuropharmacologic agents and mechanisms in erectile dysfunction: the role of dopamine. Neuroscience and Biobehavioral Reviews 24: 561–569.

Heiman JR 2007 Orgasmic disorders in women. In Leiblum SR (ed) Principles and Practice of Sex Therapy. 4th edn. Guilford, New York, pp. 84–123.

Heiman JR, Meston CM 1997 Empirically validated treatment for sexual dysfunction. Annual Review of Sex Research 7: 148– 194.

Heisler J 1983 Sexual therapy in the National Marriage Guidance Council. NMGC, Rugby.

Hoon EF, Hoon PW, Wincze JP 1976 An inventory for the measurement of female sexual arousability: the SAI. Archives of Sexual Behavior 5: 291–300.

Johnson J 1968 Disorders of Sexual Potency in the Male. Pergamon, Oxford.

Kafka MP 2007 Paraphilia-related disorders: the evaluation and treatment of nonparaphilic hypersexuality. In Leiblum SR (ed) Principles and Practice of Sex Therapy. 4th edn. Guilford, New York, pp. 442–476.

Kaplan HS 1974 The New Sex Therapy. Brunner/Mazel, New York.

Lansky MR, Davenport AE 1975 Difficulties in brief conjoint treatment of sexual dysfunction. American Journal of Psychiatry 182: 171–175.

Lazarus AA 1963 The treatment of chronic frigidity by systematic desensitisation. Journal of Nervous and Mental Disease 136: 272–278.

Leiblum SR 2002 After sildenafil: bridging the gap between pharmacological treatment and satisfying sexual relationships. Journal of Clinical Psychiatry 63(Suppl. 5): 17–22.

Leiblum SR, Rosen RC, Pierce D 1976 Group treatment format: mixed sexual dysfunctions. Archives of Sexual Behavior 5: 313–322.

Levine LA, Elterman L 2001 Nocturnal penile tumescence and rigidity testing. In Mulcahy JJ (ed) Male Sexual Function: A Guide to Clinical Management. Humana, Totowa, NJ, pp. 151–166.

Loewenstein J 1947 Treatment of Impotence. Hamish Hamilton, London.

Lottman PE, Hendriks JC, Vruggnik PAS, Meuleman EJ 1998 The impact of marital satisfaction and psychological counseling on the outcome of ICI-treatment in men with ED. International Journal of Impotence Research 10: 83–87.

Margesson LJ, Stewart EG 2006 Overview of vulvar pain: pain related to a specific disorder and lesion-free pain. In Goldstein I, Meston C, Davis S,

Traish A (eds) Textbook of Female Sexual Dysfunction. Taylor & Francis, London, pp. 480–495.

Masters WH, Johnson VE 1970 Human Sexual Inadequacy. Churchill, London.

Masters WH, Johnson VE, Kolodny RC, Meyners JR 1983 Outcome Studies at the Masters & Johnson Institute. Paper presented at 6th World Congress of Sexology, Washington, May 1983.

Mathers N, Bramley M, Draper K, Snead S, Tobert A 1994 Assessment of training in psychosexual medicine. British Medical Journal 308: 969–972.

Mathews A, Bancroft J, Whitehead A, Hackmann A, Julier D, Bancroft J, Gath D, Shaw P 1976 The behavioural treatment of sexual inadequacy: a comparative study. Behaviour Research and Therapy 14: 427–436.

Mathews A, Whitehead A, Kellet J 1983 Psychological and hormonal factors in the treatment of female sexual dysfunction. Psychological Medicine 13: 83–92.

McCarthy P, Thorburn M 1996 Psychosexual Therapy at Relate: a report on cases processed between 1992 and 1994. Relate, London.

McCullough AR 2001 Ejaculatory disorders. In Mulcahy JJ (ed) Male Sexual Function: A Guide to Clinical Management. Humana, Totowa, pp. 351–370.

McMahon CG, Stuckey B, Andersen ML, Purvis K, Koppiker N, Haughie S, Boolell M 2005 Efficacy of sildenafil citrate (Viagra) in men with premature ejaculation. Journal of Sexual Medicine 2: 368–375.

McMahon CG, McMahon CN, Leow LJ, Winestock CG 2006 Efficacy of type-5 phosphodiesterase inhibitors in the drug treatment of premature ejaculation: a systematic review. British Journal of Urology International 98: 259–272.

Melman A, Bar-Chama N, McCullough A, Davies K, Christ G 2006 hMaxi-K gene transfer in males with erectile dysfunction: results of the first human trial. Human Gene Therapy 18: 1165–1176.

Melnik T, Abdo C 2005 Psychogenic erectile dysfunction: a comparative study of three therapeutic approaches. Journal of Sex and Marital Therapy 31: 243–256.

Meston CM, Derogatis LR 2002 Validated instruments for assessing female sexual function. Journal of Sex and Marital Therapy 28(suppl.1): 155–164.

Meuleman E, Cuzin B, Opsomer RJ, Hartmann U, Bailey MJ, Maytom MC, Smith MD, Osterloh IH 2001 A dose-escalation study to assess the efficacy and safety of sildenafil citrate in men with erectile dysfunction. BJU International 87: 75–81.

Milne HB 1976 The role of the psychiatrist. In Milne HB, Hardy SJ (eds) Psychosexual Problems. Bradford University Press, Bradford.

Molitch ME 2004 Prolactin in human reproduction. In Strauss JF, Barbieri RL (eds) Yen & Jaffe's Reproductive Endocrinology, 5th edn. Elsevier Saunders, Philadelphia, pp. 93–124.

Mulcahy JJ 2001 Penile implant complications: prevention and management. In Mulcahy JJ (ed) Male Sexual Function: A Guide to Clinical Management. Humana Press, Totowa, NJ, pp. 279–292.

Nichols M, Shernoff M 2007 Therapy with sexual minorities: queering practice. In Leiblum SR (ed.) Principles and Practice of Sex Therapy. Guilford, New York, pp. 379–415.

Nijland E, Davis S, Laan E, Weijmar Schultz W 2006 Female sexual satisfaction and pharmaceutical intervention: a critical review of the drug intervention studies in female sexual dysfunction. Journal of Sexual Medicine 3: 763–777.

Padma-Nathan H, Brown C, Fendl J, Salem S, Yeager J, Harninger R 2003 Efficacy and safety of topical alprostadil cream for the treatment of female sexual arousal disorder (FSAD): a double-blind, multicenter, randomized, and placebo-controlled clinical trial. Journal of Sex and Marital Therapy 29: 329–344.

Padma-Nathan H, McMurray JG, Pullman WE, Whitaker JS, Saoud JB, Ferguson KM, Rosen RC 2001 On demand IC351 (Cialis) enhances erectile function in patients with erectile dysfunction. International Journal of Impotence Research 13: 2–9.

Perimenis P, Gyftopoulos K, Giannitsas K, Markou SA, Tsota I, Chrysanthopoulou A, Athanasopolous A, Barbalias G 2004 A comparative crossover study of the efficacy and safety of sildenafil and apomorphine in men with evidence of arteriogenic erectile dysfunction. International Journal of Impotence Research 16: 2–7.

Phelps JS, Jain A, Monga M 2004 The PsychoedPlusMed approach to erectile dysfunction treatment: the impact of combining a psychoeducational intervention. Journal of Sex and Marital Therapy 30: 305–314.

Pomerantz SM 1991 Quinelorane (LY 163502), a D2 dopamine receptor agonist, acts centrally to facilitate penile erections of male rhesus monkeys. Pharmacology, Biochemistry and Behaviour 39: 123–128.

Porst H, Rosen RC, Padma-Nathan H, Goldstein I, Giuliano F, Ulbrich E, Bandel T 2001 The efficacy and tolerability of vardenafil, a new, oral, selective phosphodiesterase type 5 inhibitor, in patients with erectile dysfunction. The first at-home clinical trial. International Journal of Impotence Research 13: 192–199.

Potts A, Gavey N, Grace VM, Vares T 2003 The downside of Viagra: women's experiences and concerns. Sociology of Health & Illness 25: 697–719.

Rendell MS, Rajfer J, Wicker P, Smith M 1999 Sildenafil for treatment of erectile dysfunction in men with diabetes; a randomized controlled trial. Journal of the American Medical Association 281: 421–426.

Riley AJ 1994 Yohimbine in the treatment of sexual disorder. British Journal of Clinical Practice 48: 133–136.

Rosen I 1977 The psychoanalytic approach to individual therapy. In Money J, Musaph H (eds) Handbook of Sexology. Elsevier/North Holland, Amsterdam, pp. 1245–1270.

Rosen RC 1991 Alcohol and drug effects on sexual response: human experimental and clinical studies. Annual Review of Sex Research 2: 119–179.

Rosen RC 2007 Erectile dysfunction: integration of medical and psychological approaches. In Leiblum SR (ed.) The Principles and Practice of Sex Therapy. 4th edn. Guilford, New York, pp. 277–312.

Rosen RC, McKenna KE 2002 PDE-5 inhibition and sexual responses: pharmacological mechanisms and clinical outcomes. Annual Review of Sex Research 13: 36–88.

Rosen RC, Riley A, Wagner G, Osterloh IH, Kirkpatrick J, Mishra A 1997 The International Index of Erectile Function (IIEF): a multidimensional scale for assessment of erectile dysfunction. Urology 49: 822–830.

Rosen RC, Lane RM, Menza M 1999a Effects of SSRIs on sexual function: a critical review. Journal of Clinical Psychopharmacology 19: 67–85.

Rosen RC, Phillips NA, Gendrano III NC, Ferguson DM1999b Oral phentolamine and female sexual arousal disorder: a pilot study. Journal of Sex and Marital Therapy 25: 137–144.

Rosen RC, Diamond LE, Earle DC, Shadiack AM, Molinoff PB 2004a Evaluation of the safety, pharmacokinetics and pharmacodynamic effects of subcutaneously administered PT-141, a melanocortin receptor agonist, in healthy males and patients with an inadequate response to Viagra. International Journal of Impotence Research 16: 135–142.

Rosen RC, Fisher WA, Eardley I, Niederberger, Nadel A, Sand M 2004b The Multinational Men's Attitudes to Life Events and Sexuality (MALES) study: prevalence of erectile dysfunction and related health concerns in the general population. Current Medical Research and Opinion, 20: 607–617.

Rosen RC, Hatzichristou D, Broderick G, Clayton A, Cuzin B, Derogatis L, Litwin M, Meuleman E, O'Leary M, Quirk F, Sadofsky R, Seftel A 2004c Clinical evaluation and symptom scales: sexual dysfunction assessment in men. In Lue TF, Basson R, Rosen R, Giuliano F, Khoury S, Montorsi F (eds) Sexual Medicine: Sexual Dysfunctions in Men and Women. Health Publications-2004. Editions 21, Paris, pp. 173–220.

Sanchez RA, Vidal J, Jauregui ML, Barrera M, Recio C, Giner M 2001 Efficacy, safety and predictive factors of therapeutic success with sildenafil for erectile dysfunction in patients with different spinal cord injuries. Spinal Cord 39: 637–643.

Sandfort TGM, de Keizer M 2001 Sexual problems in gay men: an overview of the empirical research. Annual Review of Sex Research 12: 93–120.

Schultz JH 1951 Autogenic Training. Grune & Stratton, New York.

Segraves RT 1995 Dopamine agonists and their effect on the human penile erectile response. In Bancroft J (ed.) The Pharmacology of Sexual Function and Dysfunction. Excerpta Medica: Amsterdam, pp. 225–234.

Segraves RT, Clayton A, Croft H, Wolf A, Warnock J 2004 Bupropion sustained release for the treatment of hypoactive sexual desire disorder in pre-menopausal women. Journal of Clinical Psychopharmacology 24: 339–342.

Seidman SN, Roose SP, Menza MA, Shabsigh R, Rosen RC 2001 Treatment of erectile dysfunction in men with depressive symptoms: results of a placebo-controlled trial with sildenafil citrate. American Journal of Psychiatry 158: 1623–1630.

Semans J 1956 Premature ejaculation: a new approach. Southern Medical Journal 49: 353–358.

Shabsigh R, Padma-Nathan H, Gittleman M, McMurray J, Kaufman J, Goldstein I 2000 Intracavernous alprostadil alfadex is more efficacious, better tolerated, and preferred over intraurethral alprostadil plus optional actis: a comparative, randomized, cross-over, multicenter study. Urology 55: 109–113.

Sherwin BB, Gelfand MM, Brender W 1985 Androgen enhances sexual motivation in females: A prospective, crossover study of sex steroid administration in the surgical menopause. Psychosomatic Medicine 47: 339–351.

Snyder DK, Berg P 1983 Predicting couples' response to brief directive sex therapy. Journal of Sexual and Marital Therapy 9: 114–120.

Stief C, Padley RJ, Perdok RJ, Sleep DJ 2002 Cross-study review of the clinical efficacy of apomorphine SL 2 and 3 mg: pooled data from three placebo-controlled, fixed dose cross-over studies. European Urology Supplements 1: 12–20.

Taberner PV 1985 Aphrodisiacs. The Science and the Myth. Croom Helm, London.

Titta M, Tavolini IM, Dal Moro F, Cisternino A, Pierfrancesco B 2006 Sexual counseling improved erectile rehabilitation after non-nerve-sparing radical retropubic prostatectomy or cystectomy; results of a randomized prospective study. Journal of Sexual Medicine 3: 267–273.

Tomlinson J, Wright D 2004 Impact of erectile dysfunction and its subsequent treatment with sildenafil: a qualitative study. British Medical Journal Online, 29 March 2004.

Tunnadine P 1980 The role of genital examination in psychosexual medicine. Clinics in Obstetrics & Gynaecology 7: 283–291.

Trudel G, Marchand A, Ravart M, Aubin S, Turgeon L, Fortier P 2001 The effect of a cognitive-behavioral group treatment program on hypoactive sexual desire in women. Sex & Relationship Therapy 16: 145–64.

Uckert S, Mayer ME, Jonas U, Stief CG 2006 Potential future options in the pharmacotherapy of female sexual dysfunction. World Journal of Urology 24: 630–638.

Ugarte F, Hurtado-Coll A 2002 Comparison of the efficacy and safety of sildenafil citrate (Viagra) and oral phentolamine for the treatment of erectile dysfunction. Journal of Sexual Medicine 14 (Suppl 2): S48–S53.

Van Lankveld JDM, ter Kuile MM, de Groot HE, Melles R, Nefs J, Zandbergen M 2006 Cognitive-behavioral therapy for women with lifelong vaginismus: a randomized waiting-list controlled trial of efficacy. Journal of Consulting & Clinical Psychology 74: 168–78.

Von Keitz AT, Stroberg P, Bukofzer S, Mallard N, Hibberd M 2002 A European multicentre study to evaluate the tolerability of apomorphine sublingual administered in a forced dose-escalation regimen in patients with erectile dysfunction. BJU International 89: 409–415.

Von Schrenck-Notzing A 1895 The Use of Hypnosis in Psychopathia Sexualis with Special Reference to Contrary Sexual Instinct. Translated by Chaddock C G, 1956. The Institute of Research in Hypnosis Publication Society and Julian Press, New York.

Wang R, Lewis RW 2001 Penile implants: types and current indications. In Mulcahy J (ed.) Male Sexual Function: A Guide to Clinical Management. Humana Press, Totowa, NJ, pp. 263–278.

Warner P, Bancroft J 1986 Sex therapy outcome research: a reappraisal of methodology. 2. Methodological considerations - the importance of prognostic variability. Psychological Medicine 16: 855–863.

Warner P, Bancroft J, members of the Edinburgh Human Sexuality Group 1987 A regional service for sexual problems: a 3-year study. Sexual and Marital Therapy 2: 115–126.

Watson JP, Brockman B 1982 A follow up of couples attending a psychosexual problem clinic. British Journal of Clinical Psychology 21: 143–144.

Wessells H, Gralneck D, Dorr R, Hruby VJ, Haldey ME, Levine N 2000 Effect of an alpha-melanocyte stimulating hormone analog on penile erection and sexual desire in men with organic erectile dysfunction. Urology 56: 641–646.

Whitehead A, Mathews A 1986 Factors related to successful outcome in the treatment of sexually unresponsive women. Psychological Medicine 16: 373–378.

Wolpe J 1969 The practice of behavior therapy. Pergamon, New York, pp. 72–90.

Wylie KR, Hallam-Jones R, Walters S 2003 The potential benefit of vacuum devices augmenting psychosexual therapy for erectile dysfunction: RCT. Journal of Sex and Marital Therapy 29: 277–242.

Zilbergeld B, Evans M 1980 The inadequacy of Masters & Johnson. Psychology Today August: 29–43.

Sexual aspects of medical practice

13

Some general principles 381

Andrology 382
Penile problems 382
Prostate disease 383
Chronic pelvic pain and other causes of pain during
sexual activity 383
Abnormalities of pelvic and penile blood flow 384
Hypogonadism 384

Gynaecology 385
Dyspareunia and genital pain disorders 385
Gynaecological surgery 385
Gynaecological malignancy 386
Breast cancer and mastectomy 387

Psychiatry 387
Depression and anxiety 387
Schizophrenia 388
Learning disability 389

General medicine 390
Diabetes mellitus 390
Cardiovascular disease 395

Neurology 397
Epilepsy 397
Multiple sclerosis 398
Parkinson's disease 398
Spinal cord injuries 399

Sexual side effects of medication 401
Pharmacological treatment of hypertension 402
Psychotropic drugs 403
Other drugs 405

Sexual aspects of alcohol and drug addiction 405
Alcohol and alcoholism 405
Drugs of addiction 407

Some general principles

The wide variety of pathological and psychological mechanisms capable of interfering with sexual function was described in Chapter 11. Whilst it is probably true that the majority of sexual problems are not caused by medical conditions (i.e. third window factors), there are few medical or surgical conditions that do not have sexual implications. In this chapter we aim to place these sexual aspects of clinical practice into perspective, and focus on those medical conditions that not only have an impact on sexuality, but are also of theoretical interest.

The physician or surgeon will be confronted with the sexual lives of his patients in a number of ways. A sexual problem may be the presenting symptom of an illness; erectile dysfunction (ED) as the first evidence of diabetes mellitus (DM) is one example. The medical problem may be linked to sexual activity, a sexually transmitted infection being the most obvious example (see Chapter 14). In most acute illnesses sexual interest or enjoyment is likely to be impaired, if not abolished, but usually this is of little consequence while the person is acutely ill. In the recovery phase, however, there may be concern or anxiety about when to resume sexual activity, whether it is safe to do so, and whether normal sexual function will be regained.

The possible effects of a clinical condition on a patient's sexuality can be summarized under the following headings:

1. The *direct physical* effects of the condition:
   a. specific interference with genital or other physiological components of sexual response, as with vascular impairment or neurological damage
   b. non-specific effects, such as pain, general malaise, fatigue and lack of sexual desire, immobility with arthritis or spasticity making postural changes normally expected during sexual activity difficult or impossible.
2. The *psychological* effects of the condition:
   a. on the *individual,* such as embarrassment, feeling sexually unattractive, or generally experiencing a loss of self-esteem as a result of the condition
   b. on the *relationship.* A man who is sexually disabled after an accident or stroke may become dependent on his wife in a number of ways, resulting in a relationship which is more like child–parent than the adult–adult relationship which existed before the accident. This may make it difficult for either or both partners to continue with an active sexual relationship. The existence of a life-threatening illness, such as cancer, can also disrupt the sexual relationship because the healthy partner feels guilty about seeking sexual pleasure in such circumstances
   c. concern about effects of sexual activity on the condition. The existence of ischaemic heart disease (IHD) or severe hypertension may result in fear in either partner that sexual activity, particularly the excitement associated with orgasm, will be harmful.
3. The effects of *treatment* on sexuality:
   a. drug effects
   b. effects of surgery, causing damage to genital structures or their neurological or vascular control
   c. psychological effects of treatment, particularly surgery resulting in disfigurement.

Of particular importance are those conditions that result in chronic physical handicap. The extent to which sexual function is impaired by the handicap will vary, but sexual repercussions, depending often as much on

psychological as physical factors, occur in a large proportion of the handicapped population. Stewart (1975)
investigated a sample of 215 physically disabled individuals drawn from a survey of the general population,
and representing a wide variety of physical problems
and degrees of disability. Of this sample, 23% were
unmarried compared with 16% of the same age group
in the normal population; 54% of the disabled subjects
were currently experiencing difficulties in their sexual
lives. A further 18% had done so since the onset of their
disability and had either overcome the problem or come
to terms with it. In about 45% the sexual problem was
attributed to physical factors; in 15% to predominantly
psychological factors and in 30% to a combination of
the two. Physical problems ranged from impairment of
genital responses to mechanical difficulties in adopting
suitable postures for love-making. Psychological reactions included unfounded fears about the consequences
of sexual activity, loss of self-esteem and changes in the
marriage, resulting from the handicap, which interfered
with a good sexual relationship.

Obviously the needs of these patients include basic
commonsense advice about overcoming practical problems, reassurance and encouragement to experiment.
Such simple counselling should be based on a proper
understanding of the sexual consequences of the condition in question, as well as awareness of the psychological
idiosyncrasies of the individual. One should not assume
that a handicapped person wants or needs sex. On the
other hand, the professional should create no barriers to
discussing sexual matters. Fundamental to much of this
simple counselling is 'giving permission' to approach
love-making in ways which may be regarded as unconventional. Also important is the communication between
the handicapped individual and the partner. Those without partners should not be ignored, however. They also
have their sexual needs and anxieties. They may need
'permission' to masturbate and in some instances practical help to do so, such as the woman who was unable to
reach her genitalia because of severe arthritis but was
able to use a vibrator with a special extension. One of
the commonest barriers between the professional and
the handicapped patient is the difficulty that non-
handicapped people have in acknowledging that disabled
people have sexual feelings. Obviously such attitudes
have to be resolved before the professional can hope to
help the patient in this area of his or her life.

In some cases, more substantial sexual counselling, as
described in Chapter 12, will be required. Any well-
organized clinical service for the handicapped should
have access to a specialized sexual health clinic for those
who need it.

Those working in sexual health clinics must also be
prepared to see many patients with physical disease
which may or may not be relevant to their sexual problem. This is particularly likely to be the case with men
presenting with ED. In the Edinburgh 3-year clinic survey (Warner et al 1987) 52% of those presenting with
erectile problems had such a condition. The types of clinical problems encountered are shown in Table 13.1.

TABLE 13.1	Evidence of organic disease in two series of men presenting with erectile dysfunction to (i) a regional service (Warner et al 1987) and (ii) a sexual problem clinic in a general hospital (Western General, Edinburgh)	
	Regional service 1981–84 $n = 262$	General hospital 1984–87 $n = 207$
Type of organic problem	Percentage with organic problem	
Arterial disease	32	26
Neurological disease	21	12
Urological disease	29	43
Skeletal problem	4	14
Diabetes mellitus	19	13
Other endocrine disease	6	3
Infertility	4	7
Miscellaneous conditions	14	28
Any organic problem	52	73

For the remainder of this chapter we will focus on a
number of specific conditions, organized according to
the medical specialty most likely to encounter them.
There are many more that could be considered but those
selected hopefully cover most of the basic issues.

Andrology

Penile problems

Peyronie's disease

This condition interferes with normal erection, causing a
deformity of the erect penis, which can be embarrassing
or painful, and sometimes interfering with ejaculation.
The condition is believed to start as an inflammation of
the connective tissue of the tunica albuginea (see p. 35),
leading to fibrosis and the formation of a palpable plaque.
The penis bends towards the side of the lesion during
erection, presumably because of unequal filling pressures
in the two corpora cavernosa. The cause is unknown,
although a wide variety of mechanisms, including trauma
and genetically determined abnormalities of the immune
system, have been implicated. The estimated incidence
has varied across studies, from 0.03% to 3.2%, but the
majority of cases apparently resolve spontaneously (Chun
et al 2001). Reflecting the uncertainty about aetiology and
prognosis, a wide variety of treatments have been tried,
including vitamin E, corticosteroids and verapamil, an
injectable calcium channel blocker. None has been shown
convincingly to be effective (Chun et al 2001). In cases
where there is a simple bend of the erect penis in one
direction, the deformity can often be corrected surgically.
However, this is only recommended when the lesion
has proved to be persistent. Nesbit's operation is the
most widely used procedure, with a good success rate
(Graziottin et al 2001).

Priapism

Priapism is a persistent erection that may be painful. Two types of priapism have been identified and are well reviewed by Wessells (2001).

Low-flow priapism results from occlusion of the venous drainage from the corpora cavernosa, and is typically painful. This represents an emergency as unless it is relieved within 24 h or so, there is a considerable likelihood of permanent erectile failure resulting. This is thought to result from the fibrin deposition and eventual fibrosis that follows a prolonged period of anoxic venous stasis. The blood is dark, acidotic and with high CO_2 content. There are many causes of this condition, the most important being sickle cell disease, and the use of intracavernosal injections of muscle relaxants for the investigation or treatment of ED. A variety of prescription drugs also occasionally have this effect, the best known being trazadone, which has α1 adrenergic-blocking effects (see Chapter 4, p. 70). The first line of management of this acute condition is to aspirate blood from the corpora and to inject phenylephrine, which is an α1 adrenergic agonist. If this fails then surgical intervention to produce a shunt is required.

High-flow priapism typically results from blunt trauma which damages the erectile tissues, leading to uncontrolled arterial flow into the cavernous tissue that overloads the venous outflow. The blood is bright red and well oxygenated; the priapism tends to be less rigid than the low-flow type and is usually not painful. This may require assessment by colour Doppler angiography to locate the site of the fistula, which is then usually treated either by arterial embolization or arterial ligation.

Prostate disease

In the majority of men beyond their mid-40s, there is an enlargement of the suburethral glands surrounding the prostatic part of the urethra. In approximately 10% of these men, this will cause some narrowing and obstruction of the urethra as well as compression of the normal prostatic tissue. In time, this may lead to incomplete emptying of the bladder with loss of bladder tone, back pressure effects on the kidney and the risk of infection. This is the commonest indication for prostatectomy. Less common and more serious is malignant change in the prostate. Chronic prostatitis is also sometimes treated by surgical removal of the gland. None of these conditions in themselves should interfere with sexual function, but it is often assumed that surgical treatment will.

There are four types of operation:

1. *Transurethral prostatectomy* is the most widely used method and carries the lowest morbidity when used by experienced surgeons. The adenomatous tissue is removed through a special endoscope inserted along the urethra (Notley 1979).
2. *Suprapubic prostatectomy*, the earliest form of operation to be used, involves an abdominal incision and access to the prostate through the bladder.
3. *Retropubic prostatectomy*, now more favoured than the suprapubic approach, also involves an abdominal incision but gains access to the prostate and bladder neck by passing between the pubic bone and the bladder.
4. *Perineal prostatectomy* involves access through a perineal incision.

The retropubic and perineal approaches are used for radical prostatectomy in cases of prostatic carcinoma as more extensive clearance is possible.

The incidence of erectile problems is lowest after transurethral resection (approximately 5%) and slightly higher (10–20%) for the suprapubic and retropubic methods. In all three, however, disturbance of ejaculation is usual, resulting in retrograde ejaculation in 30–90% of cases (Kolodny et al 1979; Pearlman 1980). Radical prostatectomy, because of the need to remove any possible malignant tissue, has a much higher incidence of ED post-operatively (90–100%). This is likely to be due to nerve damage, vascular damage or both (Novak et al 2000). This situation has been improved by the development of 'nerve sparing' procedures (Walsh & Donker 1982), but this does not eliminate the possibility of post-operative ED. This risk, together with the likelihood that ejaculation will be impaired, needs to be carefully considered when deciding on the best treatment approach, and when to pursue it. There is undoubtedly an important need for adequate counselling pre-operatively as well as the opportunity for discussing sexual function in the post-operative recovery period.

Chronic pelvic pain and other causes of pain during sexual activity

Chronic pelvic pain syndrome (CPPS), sometimes called chronic prostatitis (CP), is an extremely common problem, affecting around 30% of men at some stage of their life, and is little understood (Schneider et al 2005). It is manifested as chronic or recurring pain in the inguinal, testicular, retropubic or perineal regions, often worse during sexual activity, and dysuria. Only a small percentage of such men are shown to have either acute or chronic bacterial infection of the prostate, and it is not clear why the source of the problem is usually assumed to be the prostate. Painful ejaculation, delayed ejaculation, pain during vaginal intercourse and erectile impairment may all occur (Lobel & Rodriguez 2003). The psychosomatic aspects of the pain experience are likely to be complex, and require similar consideration to those related to chronic pelvic pain in women, which is considered further in the next section. Smith et al (2007) studied couples in which the male partner had been diagnosed as CPPS/CP, and compared them with a control group of couples. The female partners reported a tendency to experience pain themselves during attempts at vaginal intercourse. The shared sexual problem, however, was not associated with any substantial impairment of their relationship in other respects.

Other causes of pain

Painful retraction of a foreskin that is too tight may be experienced during the first attempt at intercourse or may become a problem with tightening or scarring following inflammation or local infection. Small tears in the frenulum of the foreskin may occur during vigorous intercourse or masturbation and become exquisitely painful. Any painful lesion or inflammation of the penis may be relevant, herpetic infections being one of the more common causes. Pain may be experienced during intercourse with deformities of the penis that cause bending or bowing during erection. Such deformity is commonly associated with hypospadias (a congenital anomaly in which there is incomplete development of the penis and the urethra opens at some point along the underside of the penis). This bending is sometimes called 'chordee'.

Hypersensitivity of the glans penis following orgasm and ejaculation is common. This may be so extreme that the man fears ejaculation occurring. This obviously can have a powerful inhibitory effect on his sexual performance and enjoyment.

The young male quite commonly experiences an aching sensation, usually in the testicular or inguinal region, following prolonged periods of sexual arousal not resolved by ejaculation. The discomfort presumably results from vasocongestion and is fairly quickly relieved following ejaculation.

Abnormalities of pelvic and penile blood flow

Since the 1970s considerable attention has been paid to possible abnormalities of penile blood flow. Identification of abnormalities in arterial supply to the penis in men with ED has been taken as evidence of a vascular cause for the ED. Vascular surgery to improve the arterial supply to the corpora cavernosa has been reported. As described in Chapter 4 (see p. 74) normal erection involves closure of the venous drainage and consequent cessation of blood flow out of the erectile tissues. Abnormalities in venous drainage have been identified as causes of ED. Surgical ablation of key venous pathways has been carried out to counter such problems.

Numerous techniques for assessing blood flow have been employed, including penile arteriography and colour duplex Doppler ultrasound. In recent years it has become increasingly clear that many variations of arterial supply occur without impairment of erectile function, methodological uncertainty about measuring blood flow and venous drainage has increased (Sanchez-Ortiz & Broderick 2001), and the efficacy of the various surgical procedures remains uncertain. A recent sexual medicine committee report recommended that adequate outcome research and follow-up is required demonstrating the efficacy of such surgical procedures before they can be justified for general clinical use (Mulcahy et al 2004).

Hypogonadism

The fundamental role of testosterone (T) in male sexual development and function was reviewed in Chapter 4. Much of the evidence of this role comes from studies of men with hypogonadism and T replacement. Hypogonadism and associated failure of T production (and usually of sperm production) may result from abnormalities of the testis or of the stimulation and control of the testis by the hypothalamus and pituitary.

Primary testicular failure is typically associated with high levels of gonadotrophins, as there is absence of negative feedback on pituitary control resulting from the low T levels. It is therefore called hypergonadotrophic hypogonadism. The commonest cause is Kleinfelter's syndrome (see Chapter 5) in which the presence of an extra X chromosome (XXY) results in failure of testicular development and hypogonadism in a proportion of cases. Other causes include trauma and infection (e.g. mumps orchitis).

Testicular failure secondary to lack of normal stimulation by gonadotrophins from the pituitary is called hypogonadotrophic hypogonadism. One condition associated with this is Kallman's syndrome. This is an abnormality of the hypothalamus resulting in a lack of gonadotrophin-releasing hormone (GnRH) required to stimulate the pituitary to release gonadotrophins. This syndrome, which occurs in 1 in 7500 males, is associated with impairment of smell (anosmia) and a number of other abnormalities sometimes occur (e.g. colour blindness).

A rare but treatable cause of male hypogonadism is hyperprolactinaemia. This most often results from a prolactin-secreting adenoma of the pituitary gland. As considered in Chapter 4 (see p. 129) the impact of prolactin in high concentrations on sexual function is not well understood. However, hyperprolactinaemia is typically associated with loss of sexual interest, and in a proportion of cases there is an associated hypogonadotrophic hypogonadism (Franks & Jacobs 1983). Testicular function usually improves once the hyperprolactinaemia is corrected (surgically or by use of dopamine agonists).

Hypogonadism may develop in men with diabetes (p. 392) or with the metabolic syndrome associated with obesity. Relative hypogonadism, associated with ageing in men, is considered in Chapter 7 (see p. 241).

T deficiency resulting from hypogonadism in men is typically associated with loss of sexual interest, erectile response may be impaired, ejaculation is impaired or absent, and there is likely to be loss of energy, muscle wasting and reduced body hair growth. As reported in Chapter 4, such manifestations are readily corrected by T replacement. This can be administered orally or intramuscularly, but there is an increasing preference for transdermal administration, which maintains more physiological levels and avoids complications of 'first pass' through the liver (Seftel 2007). In cases of hypogonadotrophic hypogonadism, when infertility is an issue, pulsatile GnRH or gonadotrophin administration can be considered; it is much more expensive than T replacement (Wu 2000).

Gynaecology

Dyspareunia and genital pain disorders

The ongoing debate and controversy about the nature of sexual pain disorders in women was considered closely in Chapter 11 and the prevalence of pain during sexual activity, which varies across studies, was shown in Table 11.1. The problem in distinguishing between different conditions that lead to pain during sexual activity, either involving vaginal penetration or more simply tactile stimulation of the vulva and vestibule, and the considerable overlap in how they are manifested during clinical examination, was acknowledged, and the importance of identifying the developmental sequence in making the correct diagnosis was emphasized. In this section, we focus on some of the underlying conditions.

Vulvar vestibulitis syndrome and vulvodynia

Vulvar vestibulitis syndrome (VVS) is characterized by severe pain when the vestibule is touched or vaginal entry is attempted and signs of erythema confined to the vulvar vestibule (Friedrich 1987). Vulvodynia is the term used to describe a more persistent or intermittent burning pain not only resulting from tactile stimulation or pressure. Pukall et al (2002) using a calibrated method of determining touch and pain sensitivity, showed that not only did women with VVS have extremely low pain threshold in the vulvar vestibular region, compared with controls, but they also showed lowered pain threshold in other parts of the body.

The aetiology of this condition is not understood. Binik (2005) listed a number of related factors which had been reported and which probably interact in various ways. Women with VVS are more likely to report early use of oral contraceptives, recurrent yeast infections, and indicators of an increased vulnerability to chronic inflammation, including a genetic disposition. The vulvar vestibular region is susceptible to a variety of infections, several of which can be sexually transmitted and which will be considered further in Chapter 14. The impact of early oral contraceptive use may be to increase susceptibility to such infections, though this has not been conclusively shown. Added to these factors related to infection and inflammation may be a non-specific tendency to sensitization of peripheral and central neurons involved in the processing of pain, resulting in a reduced pain threshold (Coderre et al 1993). Adding to the complexity is an ill-understood relationship between pain and depression. This has also arisen in another poorly understood pain condition, fibromyalgia, the most widely used treatment for which is the use of tricylic anti-depressants that in some way alter pain sensitivity (Mease 2005). Not surprisingly, women with VVS are often depressed, and it is difficult to understand the causal relationship between the depression and the pain. Anti-depressants have sometimes been used in the treatment of VVS (McKay 1993).

Not surprisingly, VVS is a difficult condition to treat, and a wide variety of methods have been tried. Bergeron et al (2001) reported a study of 78 women with VVS who were randomly assigned to one of three contrasting treatment methods; cognitive behavioural therapy (for 12 weeks), surface electromyographic biofeedback from the pelvic floor musculature (for 12 weeks), or vestibulectomy (surgical excision of the vestibular area to a depth of 2 mm and a width of 2 cm, up to the urethra). Each group showed significant reduction of pain compared to pre-treatment, but the vestibulectomy method was significantly more successful than the other two. A surgical procedure such as vestibulectomy is an extreme approach and it must be hoped that with better understanding of this condition less extreme but effective treatments will become established.

Chronic pelvic pain

A variety of gynaecological or intra-abdominal pathologies can be associated with chronic pelvic pain, which may be accentuated during vaginal intercourse. Endometriosis may result in areas of tenderness near the vagina, causing pain particularly with deep thrusting during penile–vaginal intercourse. Pelvic inflammatory disease or prolapsed ovaries may have a similar effect. As with VVS and other chronic pain disorders, depression is often an understandable but complicating factor, and problems in the sexual relationship are not surprisingly evident in many cases, again raising questions of 'cause or effect' (Schlesinger 1996; Randolph & Reddy 2006).

Gynaecological surgery

Hysterectomy

This is the most common major gynaecological operation. In the USA, in 1997, 5.6 per 1000 women underwent hysterectomy (Farquhar & Steiner 2002). In post-menopausal women, the usual indications are prolapse of the uterus or cervical or uterine malignancy, and for such conditions there are few alternative options. In pre-menopausal women, the most common indications are dysfunctional uterine bleeding and fibroids. In the UK, menorrhagia is the reason for more than 10% of outpatient referrals to gynaecologists, and about half of such women undergo hysterectomy within 5 years of referral (Coulter et al 1991). In such cases there are alternatives to hysterectomy and it is therefore important to have a clear idea about the likely post-operative effects. Here we consider such effects on the woman's sexuality.

There are various forms of hysterectomy, e.g. 'total', involving removal of the uterus and cervix, and 'subtotal', removing the uterus but retaining the cervix. Oophorectomy is done in a proportion of cases, most often because it is regarded as a safeguard against future ovarian cancer. As the hormonal contribution of the post-menopausal ovary is now better recognized (see p. 42) this is done less often than it used to be.

There are various ways in which hysterectomy could adversely affect a woman's sexuality. Damage to the autonomic nerve supply responsible for genital response could occur (see Chapter 3, p. 39). Damage to the pelvic floor muscles and suspensory ligaments could alter the experience of orgasm. Even if the ovaries are left intact, there is some evidence that alteration to ovarian blood flow following hysterectomy can lead to premature ovarian failure (Maas et al 2003). Some women may feel de-feminized by the surgery, and in some cases the reaction of the partner may be negative. However, hysterectomy is carried out in women who are suffering in some way, and who may well be experiencing adverse sexual consequences pre-surgery. An improvement in sexual well-being following effective treatment of their gynaecological problem would not be surprising. In addition, as discussed elsewhere in this book, women vary in what is important for their sexual well-being; an alteration in the precise pattern of genital response or orgasmic experience may be more relevant to some women than others. And whereas there may be a reduction in circulating testosterone, particularly following bilateral oophorectomy, T appears to be important for the sexuality of some women and not others (Chapter 4, p. 127). Given that these various factors have not been adequately taken into account, it is not surprising that the literature is inconclusive, leading Maas et al (2003) in their review to conclude: 'there is no scientific proof for either a worsened or an improved sexual function as a result of the surgical procedure' (p. 105). One of the most consistent predictors of sexual problems post-operatively, is evidence of sexual difficulties pre-operatively. However, pre-operative dyspareunia is often reduced or relieved following hysterectomy (Bradford & Meston 2006).

Given the number of women who undergo hysterectomy it is to be hoped that the predictors of good and poor sexual outcomes will be better identified so that women can be better informed before making the decision whether to accept surgery in those cases where alternative treatments are available. A substantial amount of outcome research has been reported but in many cases is methodologically flawed. Perhaps the next phase of research should focus on careful assessment of women's sexuality and mental state, carried out pre-operatively primarily to look for prognostic indicators that can be validated in subsequent controlled outcome studies. As Bradford & Meston (2006) point out, however, it is crucially important that such predictors should not be restricted to the woman's state in the immediate pre-operative period, which is likely to be confounded by the effects of the gynaecological condition.

Vaginal repair

Surgical repair of the vagina is indicated when there is a degree of prolapse. In the less severe forms, the bladder is prolapsed, producing a cystocele interfering with bladder emptying. The rectum is less often prolapsed as a rectocele. These conditions result from weakening of the pelvic supporting tissues, and occur in older women who have borne children. Further weakening of the supporting tissue which accompanies ageing often leads to a progression of the prolapse which in

its more extreme form results in complete eversion of the vagina and descent of the uterus, the so-called procidentia.

Surgical repair involves either the anterior wall of the vagina (anterior colporrhaphy), the posterior wall and perineum (posterior colpoperineorrhaphy) or a combination of the two procedures. Sometimes a vaginal hysterectomy is carried out in addition.

Interference with sexual functioning after these operations may result from undue narrowing of the vaginal introitus, shortening of the vagina or the presence of tender scar tissue. Francis & Jeffcoate (1961) followed up 243 women after vaginal repairs: 177 had had anterior and posterior repairs, the remainder anterior repair only. Subsequent problems with sexual intercourse were substantially more frequent when a posterior repair was involved, leading the authors to conclude that posterior repair should be avoided if possible. With either operation, if intercourse is to be resumed, it should begin reasonably soon (say after 6 weeks) and should be seen as an important part of the vaginal rehabilitation process.

Gynaecological malignancy

The four most common malignancies of the genital tract are carcinoma of the endometrium, ovary, cervix and vulva. Endometrial carcinoma is important sexually mainly because of its oestrogen dependency, with the need for oophorectomy and the consequent hormonal deficiency. The cause of ovarian carcinoma is ill-understood. It is difficult to diagnose and is often identified at an advanced stage of the disease. Hence the prognosis tends to be much worse than for the other three types. Its relevance to sexuality is mainly because of the hormonal implications of ovarian removal and the major threat to life that is involved.

The majority of cases of carcinoma of the cervix and vulva are caused by specific types of the human papilloma-virus (HPV) (Beral 2000). This sexually transmitted infection will be considered further in Chapter 14. Cervical carcinoma, which is much more prevalent in Third World countries than the West, is the end state of a sequence which starts with dysplasia, and develops through 'carcinoma in situ' to reach its invasive form. The risk of cervical cancer is increased in women who are poor, have little education, started sexual intercourse at a young age, and have had many sexual partners and sexually transmitted infections. Screening for cervical cancer is carried out using cervical smears (or 'Pap smears', named after Papanicolaou who started them, rather than papilloma virus).

The method of treating cervical carcinoma is a controversial issue. The cure rate for surgery and radiotherapy is similar, so that the implications of the two methods for quality of life have gained in importance. Several studies have suggested that radiotherapy causes ovarian decline, soreness of the vagina with a risk of stenosis and more sexual problems than occur with surgical treatment. Overall the evidence is conflicting (Andersen 1984).

Vulval carcinoma is much less common than cervical cancer. In younger women it is likely to be caused by HPV, but not in older women. It commonly affects the labia (70%) and less commonly the clitoris (13%). Its treatment is noteworthy because of its mutilating nature. Surgery may include removal of all labial tissue and the clitoris, depending on the extent of carcinoma. The impact of such a procedure on the woman's sexuality is likely to be considerable. Andersen (1984) studied 15 such women post-operatively and found evidence of a reduced capacity for sexual arousal, though, interestingly, orgasmic capacity was retained in some women, even those who had their clitoris removed. Similarly, Weijmar Schultz et al (1986) studied 10 women post-operatively and found that half of them made a satisfactory sexual recovery, including orgasm. Radiotherapy or chemotherapy is usually restricted to the more advanced cases.

With all types of gynaecological malignancy, therefore, many women will need post-operative counselling to enable them to return to a rewarding sexual life (Andersen 1984).

Breast cancer and mastectomy

Breast cancer is the most common form of malignancy in women. One in eight women (13%) are likely to develop breast cancer at some stage in their life (American Cancer Society 2006). Controversy continues about the best clinical management. Radical mastectomy has been the most common procedure in the past. Increasingly, breast-sparing 'lumpectomy' combined with radiotherapy or chemotherapy is being used as an alternative.

There is now an extensive literature of studies comparing these two approaches, but the results have been inconsistent, reflecting variations in methodology of various kinds (for review see Weijmar Schultz et al 1992). The evidence is consistent, however, in finding negative effects of mastectomy on body image, well-being and sexual function. A more recent, large and longitudinal study was reported by Engel et al (2004). More than 900 women, treated between 1996 and 1998, were followed up and assessed at intervals over 5 years; 57% received breast-conserving therapy (BCT) and 43% mastectomy. The BCT group showed significantly more improvement during the follow-up in their ratings of body image and sexual function, across the age groups, leading the authors to conclude that BCT should be encouraged for all age groups.

Psychiatry

To what extent do people suffering from psychiatric illness experience sexual difficulties? The relevance of personality, including neuroticism, to sexual difficulties was discussed in Chapter 6 and the relationship between mood and sexual response was looked at in some detail in Chapter 4. Depression remains an important issue. Watson (1979) estimated that 30% of women and 14% of men attending his sexual problem clinic had a present or past psychiatric illness, usually affective in type.

Depression and anxiety

Beck (1967) found that loss of sexual interest was reported by 61% of severe depressives compared with 27% non-depressed controls. Cassidy et al (1957) found that sexual activity had decreased in 63% of depressed patients compared with 39% of medically sick, non-depressed control subjects. Reduced libido affected 83% of the depressed males and 53% of the females. Woodruff et al (1967) found ED in 23% of men with a primary affective disorder. Mathew & Weinman (1982) found significantly more loss of sexual interest in a group of drug-free depressed men and women than in their control group. They did not find differences in genital dysfunctions. Schreiner-Engel & Schiavi (1986) studied men and women with low sexual desire as their primary problem. Although not depressed at the time of assessment, the low sexual desire group had a significantly higher incidence of depressive illness in the past. Typically, the initial episode of depressive disorder coincided with or preceded the onset of loss of sexual desire. Further suggestion of a relatively irreversible impact of depressive illness on sexuality was reported by Cyranowski et al (2004). In a study of women at mid-life, after controlling for any current depressive mood, women with a recurrent history of major depressive disorder reported less physical pleasure in their sexual relationships. It is not yet possible to say whether this pattern results from a basic biological alteration in their sexual response system, or is secondary to recurrent difficulties in their relationships resulting from or aggravated by the recurrent depression.

In the Massachusetts Male Aging Study, a community study, Araujo et al (1998) reported an association between ED and depressive symptoms, after controlling for other potentially confounding factors, such as age and physical health. Although they found an association between ED and loss of sexual interest, there was, somewhat surprisingly, no direct association between depression and loss of sexual interest. In the Zurich Cohort Study, a longitudinal study of men and women between the ages of 20 and 35 years, an association between depression and loss of sexual interest was found in both men and women, though more marked in the women (Angst 1998). In this study, 'depression' included major depressive illness, dysthymia and recurrent brief depression. An association between depression and sexual problems was also reported by Kennedy et al (1999).

Clinical evidence of the association between anxiety and sexual problems is much more limited. Ware et al (1996), using the Sexual Function Questionnaire, found higher rates of sexual dysfunction in men and women with anxiety disorders, compared with normal controls (13 males and 24 females). Angst (1998), in the Zurich Cohort Study, reported that loss of sexual interest was associated with generalized anxiety disorder, but was not associated with panic disorder, agoraphobia or social phobia. Van Minnen & Kampman (2000), on the other hand, found that women with panic attacks were more likely to have hypoactive sexual desire or sexual aversion than controls. Figueira et al (2001) found that panic disorder patients were more likely to report sexual problems, particularly sexual aversion, than social phobics, whereas premature ejaculation was the most common sexual problem in men with social phobias. Given the emphasis that has been placed on 'performance anxiety' as a factor aggravating sexual problems, it is striking how little attention has been paid to this form of anxiety in relation to sexual function (Norton & Jehu 1984).

As indicated in Chapter 4, the association between negative mood and sexuality is not always in the same direction. In a mixed gender group of 57 depressives, Mathew & Weinman (1982) reported that whereas 31% had loss of sexual interest, 22% reported increased sexual interest. In Angst's (1998) study, 26% of depressed men reported decreased and 23% increased sexual interest, compared with 11% and 7%, respectively, of their non-depressed male group. This paradoxical pattern was less prevalent in women. Only 9% of their females reported increased interest when depressed with 35% reporting decreased sexual interest (compared with 2% and 32%, respectively, of their non-depressed group). In a study of cognitive behaviour therapy as a treatment for depression in men (Nofzinger et al 1993), those who failed to respond to treatment had significantly higher levels of sexual interest than both those who responded and their non-depressed control group. Furthermore, this high sexual interest, non-responding group was more anxious as well as having more intermittent depression. This led Nofzinger et al (1993) to wonder whether sexuality variables might be useful in categorizing different types of affective disorder. It is apparent that asking about *increased* sexual interest in negative mood states has been very unusual and if more studies had covered this possibility there may have been more consistency in the literature.

An association between depressed mood and reduced sexual appetite is not surprising. Although the paradoxical association between depression and increased sexuality occurs in a minority of men and women (see Chapter 4, p. 108), for most people sexuality is most readily expressed at times when they are feeling generally well. For many, the presence of negative thoughts about self and low self-esteem lower their sense of sexual worth. This is presumably a non-specific effect and we should expect it to operate during more prolonged states of depressed mood. There may, however, be a more specific link. A common biochemical change in cerebral monoamine function may link mood with sexuality, but as yet we can only speculate on its nature. Nocturnal penile tumescence (NPT) is impaired in depressed men, improving as the depression is treated, whether by cognitive or pharmacological means (Roose et al 1982; Thase et al 1987). NPT is considered more closely in Chapter 4 (p. 112). This association suggests that in states of depression there is a lowering of central excitatory tone, but this is not necessarily specific to sexual excitation.

The paradoxical increase in sexual activity or interest during negative mood states that occurs in a minority of individuals requires a different explanation. Some possible explanations were considered in Chapter 4 (p. 110).

Sexual interest and activity are often increased in states of mania or hypomania. Disinhibited sexual behaviour leading to promiscuity or socially inappropriate actions is quite common in this condition (Clayton et al 1965; Segraves 1998) though diminished sexual interest can also occur. Once again, we have to consider at least two possibilities: that the increased sexuality reflects the general increase in well-being and energy, a non-specific effect, or that the biochemical basis may have a parallel effect on sexuality. Again, we can only speculate, though more detailed studies of these associations and their response to treatment in both depressive and manic states may throw further light on this very fundamental issue.

Schizophrenia

Given the frequency and importance of schizophrenia, consideration and research about the impact of this illness on sexuality is strikingly limited. There are various aspects that need to be considered. Given the typical age of onset of this illness, and the tendency for non-psychotic, pre-schizophrenic aspects of personality to precede its onset, to what extent is normal sexual development affected? In what ways is sexuality manifested during the psychotic illness? What are the effects of treatment on sexual function? How do schizophrenic men and women in treatment or remission deal with sexuality in their lives?

The lack of attention to these issues could be considered a form of 'denial' on the part of the psychiatric profession, but there have been some exceptions. One example is a review by Rowlands (1995). He revisited Bleuler's studies from Zurich in the 1940s, in which he categorized the 'erotic lives' of schizophrenic patients prior to their illness (Bleuler 1978). His first category is 'non-erotic': individuals who had no experience of romantic or sexual relationships prior to their illness. This included 24% of his male and 36% of his female patients. The second group he described as 'erotically discrete', with evidence of normal relationships: 43% of males and 14% of females. The third group was 'erotically active', with several relationships and many problems associated with them: 16% of males and 42% of females. The remainder included individuals with deviant sexuality of various kinds. Following up these patients through the course of their illness and treatment, he found that more than half remained unmarried, and of those who married a high proportion became divorced. Rowlands (1995) reviewed other evidence that is broadly consistent with Bleuler's findings.

In early studies, both males and females with schizophrenia showed less reduction of sexual interest than did patients with other types of psychiatric illness, though the females with schizophrenia showed more loss of interest than the males (Gittleson & Levine 1966; Gittleson & Dawson-Butterworth 1967). Friedman & Harrison (1984) in a small, controlled study of schizophrenic women found that sexual dysfunction was more common amongst the schizophrenic women, both before and after the onset of the psychosis. Of the schizophrenic women, 60% had never experienced orgasm.

The psychotic phenomena of schizophrenia in many cases have a sexual content. In one study of males, hallucinations involving the genitalia occurred in 30%, delusions of genital change in 20% and of sex change, or being no longer a man, in 27% (Gittleson & Levine 1966). The figures for female schizophrenics were very similar (36, 24 and 25%, respectively; Gittleson & Dawson-Butterworth 1967). According to Connolly & Gittleson (1971), these sexual hallucinations are significantly associated with gustatory and olfactory hallucinations.

The continuation of sexual interest in the presence of bizarre sexual ideas or highly abnormal patterns of personal interaction may account for the psychotic sexual behaviour or sexual attacks that occasionally occur in schizophrenics.

Although a substantial proportion of individuals with schizophrenia have few or no sexual relationships, there is a minority who are sexually active, and in some cases, in problematic ways. In a sample of 128 patients hospitalized for schizophrenia, 42 (33%; 32 males and 10 females) reported sexual activity in the preceding 6 months, 30 of them (71%) reported infrequent use of contraceptives, and 21 (51%) had been treated previously for STDs (Buckley et al 1997). Not only among those with schizophrenia but also with other acute psychiatric illnesses there is a troubling prevalence of undetected HIV infection (Sacks et al 1992). According to Rowlands (1995) occurrence of high-risk sexual behaviour is not apparently dependent on the current level of psychopathology, and may be more determined by pre-morbid levels of sexual behaviour.

Much more attention has been paid to the sexual impact of psychotropic medication (Lilleleht & Leiblum 1993; Kelly & Conley 2004). There are two particular reasons for this. Sexual side effects of such medication are common in this patient group. Also, the fact that the earlier psychotropic drugs were predominantly dopamine antagonists had been used as evidence of the importance of dopaminergic mechanisms in schizophrenia. Both of these issues will be considered more closely in the section on sexual side effects of medication later in this chapter (see p. 404). However, it can be pointed out that the newer psychotropics, or second-generation anti-psychotics such as clozapine, are much less dependent on dopamine antagonism, and yet are effective. This underlines the need for caution in extrapolating from the specific effects of medication to the mechanisms underlying the disease process.

Clearly the sexual side effects of psychotropic drugs are an important issue, underlining the need to have a better understanding of the role of sexuality in the lives of those with schizophrenia. Along with this is an obvious need to provide appropriate education and counselling about sexuality to patients in this category and their partners.

Learning disability

Approximately 3% of the population has a learning disability (LD). We know remarkably little about the sexuality of these individuals, though there has been no shortage of beliefs and assumptions. They are believed to show uncontrolled or inappropriate sexual behaviour, which in the case of males leads to sexual offences, and in females, promiscuity. Until recently, many parents of those with LD, and most professionals looking after them, were unable to acknowledge the acceptability of any form of sexual expression. To some extent these assumptions become self-fulfilling prophecies. By segregating them, separating the sexes and giving them no opportunity to learn appropriate sexual expression, they are more likely to manifest their sexuality inappropriately, with public displays of masturbation or unsolicited sexual approaches.

In the past these negative attitudes have been linked to a 'eugenic' concern that the 'mentally defective' would overbreed, resulting in 'national degeneracy' (Craft & Craft 1978). This has even led to policies of involuntary sterilization for the institutionalized. By the mid-1940s, this attitude was changing as people began to realize that only a small proportion of LD is genetically determined and that this group has in any case a low fertility (Hall 1975).

The limited available evidence suggests that those with LD are somewhat less sexually active than those with more normal intelligence and that the greater the degree of handicap, the less sexual they are likely to be (Hall 1975). Gebhard (1973) reported 84 men with LD and compared them with a control group of men who had never been convicted of crime or sent to a mental institution. Evidence of pre-pubertal sex play indicated somewhat less heterosexual experience but somewhat greater homosexual experience for the LD men than for the controls. The proportion (4%) who, as children, had sexual contacts with adults was very similar in the two groups. Almost half of the LD men had engaged in pre-pubertal masturbation, compared with a third of the control men, though after puberty, the incidence in the two groups was very similar. However, for each post-pubertal age group, the frequency of masturbation was less for those with LD than for the controls. Not surprisingly, the men with LD had less post-pubertal heterosexual experience. Their greater incidence of homosexual experience was only noticeable up to the age of 15 years. This tendency may well reflect the lack of any opportunity or encouragement to explore heterosexual relationships, plus a tendency for them to be sexually exploited by some homosexual males.

Those with LD may be more prone to get involved in sexual offences for a number of reasons. Their natural tendency to relate to people of similar mental age may result in their making sexual approaches to children. Gebhard et al (1965) found that the 'feeble-minded' (i.e. IQ less than 70) were somewhat over-represented in those committing non-violent offences against female children, incest with adults, peepers and exhibitionists. They were not over-represented amongst the sexual aggressors.

The learning disabled are usually naive and vulnerable hence easily exploited; they may also act impulsively. However, their difficulties with sex derive less from poor self-control than from lack of appropriate learning. For reasons already described, most institutions for those with LD have in the past been sexually repressive and over-protective. As a consequence, such individuals have had very few opportunities to explore and learn about close personal relationships, particularly with members of the opposite sex. Typically they have been given no sex education, on the basis that a little information would cause more problems than it would solve. Whereas the normal child can often compensate for lack of sex education by finding out for himself, from peers or by reading, the person with LD remains virtually cut off from useful information.

There is now increasing recognition that those with LD have special sex educational needs (Savarimuthu & Bunnell 2003). Because of their very limited intelligence, information must be given in extremely simple terms, and because of their very short attention span, in small amounts and repeatedly. They need to learn clear and simple rules that allow for sexuality in its proper place. The fact that sex should be in private is especially important, as is the need for proper consent for involving any would-be sexual partner. Girls with LD have a special need to learn about menstrual hygiene. Given such clear rules and limits, sexuality may provide one of the few pleasures in the extremely limited lives of these unfortunate people. It is a particularly cruel world that denies them even that.

The limitations of the learning disabled do not affect their capacity for love, though they may need opportunities to learn how to express that love. Marriage may be successful not only in enhancing the well-being of the couple but also in reducing the need for institutional care. Mattinson (1975) investigated 32 married couples living in the community, all of whom had been regarded as learning disabled before marriage. Nineteen couples felt their partnership to be supportive and affectionate. In six, there was no obvious resentment but there were signs of marital stress; in four, one partner was over-dependent and there was expressed resentment and the other three had obviously unsatisfactory marriages. Craft & Craft (1978) studied a further group of such married couples. Some were living in institutions, some in hostels, some in the community with fairly regular support and some were leading independent lives. They found no correlation between the degree of handicap and the success of the partnership.

The question of children in such marriages is a controversial one. It is widely assumed that children in these circumstances will be handicapped and their parents unable to care for them. Neither assumption is necessarily true. Reed & Reed (1965), in an extensive follow-up study, found that where both parents had IQs of less than 70, 40% of the children born to them had LD but the mean IQ of those children was 74. Where only one parent had an IQ of less than 70, then 15% had LD and 54% had IQs greater than 90. There was thus the expected tendency to 'regress towards the mean'. In Mattinson's (1975) 32 couples, the average number of children was 1.5, lower than the national average for the same age group. Only 7.5% of the children had LD.

Many learning disabled couples use contraception or choose to be sterilized. For the unmarried, contraception is more problematic. For those who are unreliable in their use of oral contraceptives, long-acting injectable progestagens can be considered. This raises ethical issues that have to be taken seriously.

A comprehensive review of many of these aspects of service provision for the learning disabled was edited by Craft (1994).

General medicine

Diabetes mellitus

DM is a state of chronic hyperglycaemia due to inadequate insulin activity. This may be the consequence of failure of insulin production by the pancreas, usually referred to as type I or insulin-dependent diabetes. This typically starts before the age of 30 years, and around 5–10% of diabetics come into this category. The more common form of diabetes involves increased insulin resistance, usually referred to as type II or non-insulin-dependent diabetes. This has a later onset and is often associated with overweight, and is treated with oral hypoglycaemic drugs or diet. A proportion of type II diabetics develop a need for insulin. Diabetes of either form affects more than 5% of the population in the USA (CDC 2005). This classification oversimplifies what is being increasingly realized as a complex metabolic abnormality, with varied causes. It produces or is associated with a wide variety of metabolic and degenerative effects, many of which are not understood. It has a particular tendency to damage peripheral and autonomic nerves and to cause degenerative changes in small blood vessels, but also has relevant effects within the brain. As we shall see, there are various ways in which such changes may interfere with sexual function.

Sexual problems in male diabetics

The tendency for diabetic men to suffer from ED has been recognized for nearly 200 years. Surveys of diabetic men have consistently shown a high prevalence of erectile problems. In a Scottish study (McCulloch et al 1980), 563 males attending a diabetic outpatient clinic were interviewed. They were shown to be representative of the clinic population. In this group the prevalence of erectile problems of at least 6 months' duration was 35%. There was a clear relationship with age, showing a considerable amplification of the age-related pattern reported in non-diabetic men by Kinsey et al (1948) (see Fig. 13.1). There was an increasing prevalence of erectile failure with increasing duration of the diabetes. Whilst diabetics treated with diet alone were less susceptible, there was no obvious difference between those needing insulin and those using oral hypoglycaemic agents. There was an association between erectile failure and the presence of retinopathy, peripheral neuropathy and autonomic neuropathy. ED was seen in all patients aged 50 years or more with proliferative retinopathy and in all those aged 35 years or more with autonomic neuropathy. It was not, however, unusual to find erectile

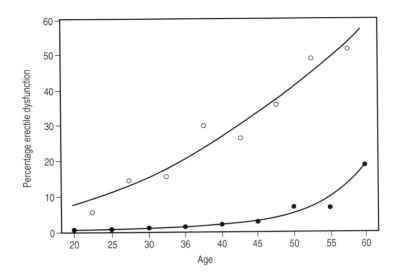

Fig. 13.1 The age incidence of erectile dysfunction in diabetic and non-diabetic men. Open circles, diabetic men (McCulloch et al 1980); solid circles, non-diabetic men (Kinsey et al 1948).

problems in men without any evidence of these diabetic complications. These authors concluded that diabetic ED has a multifactorial aetiology. They went on to follow up 466 of these patients over a 5-year period (McCulloch et al 1984). Of the 275 who were originally free from erectile problems, 28% became dysfunctional during the follow-up period. Factors which predicted this deterioration included age, alcohol intake, initial glycaemic control, intermittent claudication and retinopathy, the development of neuropathic symptoms, and poor glycaemic control during the 5 years.

Of the 128 who were initially dysfunctional, only 9% remitted and they were young, with diabetes of short duration, and often with features suggesting psychogenesis. Also of interest was the finding that, in the group without other diabetic complications to begin with, those with erectile problems were more likely to develop retinopathy or neuropathy than those with no erectile problems. This suggests that in some cases erectile failure is an early sign of other vascular or neurological damage. Jensen (1986) in a 6-year follow-up study of a smaller group of diabetic men, found some whose sexual dysfunction improved without treatment, in spite of evidence of peripheral or autonomic neuropathy.

Weinhardt & Carey (1996) reviewed the literature on the prevalence of ED among men with diabetes; estimates varied from 7% to 85% and they attributed this variability to methodological inconsistencies. They derived an average rate of 35% compared to 11% in healthy controls. This fits well with the study of McCulloch et al (1980), cited above.

A detailed investigation of the nature and development of diabetic sexual dysfunction was reported by Fairburn et al (1982). Twenty-seven patients with diabetic ED were interviewed at length. In all but three the first sign of the problem was a decline in either the strength or the duration of erection. Initially intermittent or variable, this became more consistent and severe as time went on. In three men, changes in ejaculation were the first symptoms to be noticed; one developed premature ejaculation for no good reason, the other two noticed a loss of the normal pumping sensation accompanying ejaculation; erectile problems developed later.

Changes in the pattern of ejaculation developed in half of the whole group; four described orgasm without emission, but in only one of these was there any evidence of retrograde ejaculation. This type of 'dry run orgasm' was found to be relatively common in diabetics by Klebanow & MacLeod (1960). Retrograde ejaculation into the bladder appears to account for only a small proportion of these cases. There was no association between the pattern of sexual dysfunction and the presence of either retinopathy or autonomic neuropathy. There was, however, a tendency for those men with obvious psychological problems to show a more classical psychogenic picture, i.e. loss of sexual interest but continuing morning erections. Certain distinct patterns of psychosomatic interaction emerged. In most, the initial erectile problem was followed by anxiety or distress. In some this anxiety gave way to a lessening of sexual interest and avoidance of sexual activity. In others, the couple worked through the anxious phase, came to accept that a physical factor was involved, and resumed sexual activity within the limits imposed by the erectile impairment. Some accepted the erectile failure with little apparent concern, as though it provided an escape from a sexual relationship that had not been particularly rewarding.

These findings raise the importance of the interaction between psychological and physical mechanisms, and we will return to this psychosomatic component. Let us first consider more closely the evidence of relevant pathological mechanisms in diabetes.

Relevant aetiological mechanisms associated with diabetes mellitus

Central autonomic dysregulation

Men with DM and ED typically show impaired sleep erections (NPT) during sleep monitoring (e.g. Schiavi & Fisher 1982). This has often been interpreted as showing the 'organic' nature of diabetic ED, with the assumption that this results from peripheral impairment. However, studies of men with DM who do not have impaired erectile function have also shown a reduction in REM sleep and associated NPT (Schiavi et al 1985; Nofzinger et al 1992; Schiavi et al 1993). It is therefore likely that deficient glycaemic control associated with DM can cause central autonomic dysregulation. This is not necessarily accompanied by erectile failure, but it probably increases the vulnerability to other factors associated with ED. It should also not be assumed that this central dysregulation is irreversible.

Peripheral autonomic and non-autonomic neuropathy

There is evidence of both autonomic and peripheral nerve damage in diabetic men with erectile failure (Ellenberg 1971; Faerman et al 1974). Lincoln et al (1987) found evidence of diminished VIPergic (see p. 78) and cholinergic as well as adrenergic transmission in the penises of diabetic men with ED.

Peripheral neuropathy is manifested as numbness, paraesthesiae, burning pain or weakness and there is clinical evidence of diminished tendon reflexes, vibration and tactile sensation together with muscle wasting in the lower limbs. Its functional significance in erectile failure is not clear except in causing diminished response to tactile stimulation. Ejaculatory disturbance is likely to result from neural dysfunction, which may be of a subtle kind. An association between ejaculatory and bladder dysfunction is to be expected because of their common neural control.

Peripheral vascular impairment

Based on animal studies, diabetes is believed to cause generalized endothelial cell dysfunction, involving, in part, reduced activity of NO synthetase (NOS). This results in increased prevalence of vascular disease in both type I and type II diabetics (Saenz de Tejada et al 2004).

Narrowing or obstruction of the arterial supply to the erectile tissues is commonly found in diabetic men with ED. In a study on 78 such men, with an average age of 56 years, and an average onset of the ED 10 years after diagnosis of DM, were assessed with a duplex ultrasound scan following intracavernosal injection of prostaglandin E1 (Wang et al 1993). Moderate or severe cavernous artery insufficiency was observed in 68 (87%) of the men. The severity of this pattern was related to age, longer duration of DM, hypertension, cigarette smoking and alcohol abuse. This demonstrates the complex interaction between DM, age and a range of other health-related factors.

Responsiveness of erectile smooth muscle

As described in Chapter 4 (p. 78) the development of erection depends in part on the relaxation of erectile smooth muscle, whereas flaccidity of the penis is determined in part by an 'inhibitory tone', mediated by noradrenaline (NA), a peripheral manifestation of central inhibitory mechanisms. Several in vitro studies of erectile smooth muscle, obtained during surgery from diabetic men with ED have shown impairment of nitrergically mediated relaxation, although this effect is probably not specific to diabetes (Saenz de Tejada et al 2004). Christ et al (1992) showed that in vitro, the sensitivity of erectile smooth muscle to NA-mediated contraction was increased in men with DM. As reported in Chapter 7 (p. 243), it was also increased with ageing. The precise mechanism involved is not yet certain, and

is probably not simply a matter of enhanced responsiveness of the NA receptors (see p. 79). So, if this effect proves to be relevant to in vivo function, it is a further example of how DM and ageing have similar effects, and the potential relevance of this mechanism to the impact of psychological factors is considered below.

Hypogonadism

Men with diabetes tend to have low levels of plasma T (Barrat-Connor et al 1990). This is more likely with type II DM, obesity and older age, and, given the interrelationship between these three factors, it remains unclear to what extent it is the diabetes per se that is responsible (Betancourt-Allbrecht & Cunningham 2003). The interaction between age and obesity is complicated, however, by the fact that age is associated with an increase and obesity with a decrease in SHBG (see Chapter 7, p. 241). One study of hypogonadism associated with DM found low LH levels, suggesting an impairment of the hypothalamic control of T production (Dhindsa et al 2004). However, as considered in Chapter 7, a comparable, if less marked change occurs with ageing. This is yet a further example of how diabetes and ageing produce similar results and may compound each other's effects.

Effects of psychological mechanisms

A number of studies have commented on the existence of psychological factors evident in many diabetic men with ED. The psychosomatic nature of sexual function, as considered in Chapter 11, would lead us to expect this. Given the complexity of potential aetiological factors already considered, it would be surprising if some individuals were not more vulnerable to the pathophysiological effects of diabetes than others.

Multifactorial evidence

In addition to the work of McCulloch et al (1980, 1984), a number of other studies have examined a range of relevant mechanisms in men with diabetes and ED.

In an early study by the author (Bancroft et al 1985), which measured erection, penile pulse amplitude and blood pressure response to erotic stimuli in diabetic men with ED and normal controls, it was found that diabetics with evidence of both sympathetic and parasympathetic neuropathy (based on cardiovascular reflex tests) showed significantly greater impairment of both erectile and penile pulse amplitude response when compared with diabetic men without evidence of autonomic neuropathy (see Fig. 13.2).

The presence of severe (i.e. exudative or proliferative) retinopathy was associated with a significant reduction in penile pulse amplitude response but not erectile response to erotic stimuli. It is noteworthy that in this study the presence of small vessel disease in the retina was associated with reduction of pulse amplitude in the penis. The relevance of penile pulse amplitude response to erection remains uncertain. This response was assessed in a study in a number of studies of functional and dysfunctional men, showing some interesting patterns that warrant further research (Bancroft & Bell 1985; Bancroft

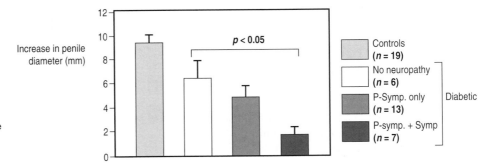

Fig. 13.2 Erectile response to visual erotic stimuli in diabetic men with erectile function, with and without autonomic neuropathy, and in normal non-diabetic controls (Bancroft et al 1985).

et al 1985; Bancroft & Smith 1987). Unfortunately, this response has been totally ignored in the literature since. In a recent discussion I revisited it, drawing parallels with vaginal pulse amplitude (VPA) response (Bancroft 2007).

The diabetic ED group was also divided into those with and those without evidence of psychogenic factors. The psychogenic group showed significantly lower blood pressure but a significantly greater erectile response to the erotic stimuli than the non-psychogenic group, pointing to an impairment of some aspects of central arousal in the psychogenic cases (see Fig. 13.3).

Buvat et al (1985) compared 26 dysfunctional diabetics with 26 diabetic controls. The two groups were almost identical in terms of Doppler wave-form analysis and blood pressure of the penile arteries, latency time for the bulbocavernosus reflex and cystometrogram. The authors did find that urine flow rates were substantially lower in the dysfunctional group, though they concluded that this may be a consequence of the sexual difficulty and the anxiety associated with it. The association between urinary flow control and erectile response remains an intriguing issue, largely unresearched. Buvat et al (1985) also found more consistent evidence of abnormalities on the Minnesota Multiphasic Personality Inventory which led them to conclude that neither neuropathic nor arteriopathic factors are a sufficient explanation, whereas psychogenic factors were at least contributory in about 50% of cases.

A comprehensive study of 500 men with erectile problems, 100 of whom were also diabetic, showed that both neurological (including NPT) and vascular mechanisms were more evident in the diabetic than the non-diabetic men, except for those aged 65 years or older, where the groups did not differ (Hirshkowitz et al 1990). This led the authors to suggest that 'diabetes may foreshadow some of the age-related pathophysiological processes associated with ED '(p. 53).

Conclusions

ED in diabetic men is clearly multifactorial in origin. Psychogenic factors are undoubtedly important, and in some cases may be the only significant cause. In others they may interact with physical factors along the lines described in Chapter 11. In some cases the physical damage is sufficient on its own. The relative importance of autonomic neuropathy, peripheral neuropathy and vascular damage remains a controversial issue, though neuropathic factors are likely to be more important in younger diabetics.

There may be subtle changes in autonomic control of erection that precede overt ED. In turn, erectile failure may precede other clinical manifestations of autonomic neuropathy.

Peripheral arterial disease is commonly associated with ED in non-diabetic men. The vulnerability of the diabetic to both large and small vessel atherosclerosis makes it likely that vascular impairment at least contributes to erectile problems in some cases, and when severe enough may be a sufficient explanation, particularly in older diabetics.

Treatment of erectile dysfunction in diabetic men

In a placebo-controlled study, sildenafil was shown to be superior to placebo in improving erections in men with ED and DM (Rendell et al 1999). After 12 weeks, 56% of the sildenafil group and 10% of the placebo group reported improved erections. These results are less successful than those reported in mixed-aetiology groups (see Chapter 12, p. 360). It is also important to note that exclusion criteria included retinopathy and neuropathy, as well as the usual exclusion criteria for PDE-5 inhibitors (i.e. stroke or myocardial infarction (MI) within the previous 6 months, hypo- or hypertension). Thus, PDE-5 inhibitors are likely to be helpful in a reasonable proportion of diabetic men with ED, but not all. Other methods such as intracavernosal injections or vacuum devices (see Chapter 12) are alternative options. It is nevertheless important to manage the ED, whether using a PDE-5 inhibitor or not, in the context of integrated couple therapy (see Chapter 12, p. 343).

Diabetes in women

Virtually no attention was paid to the sexual problems of diabetic women until Kolodny (1971) reported a higher incidence of orgasmic dysfunction in diabetic women than in a control group (35% and 6%, respectively). There is no obvious reason why orgasm per se should be affected by diabetes in either men or women. Orgasmic dysfunction in a woman, as described in Chapter 11, should only be diagnosed if it is clear that the woman becomes sufficiently aroused during sexual activity, but is unable to progress to orgasm. This criterion was not clearly met in the Kolodny study.

During the 1980s four further controlled studies were reported (Jensen 1981; Tyrer et al 1983; Whitley & Berke 1984; Schreiner-Engel et al 1985). No association between

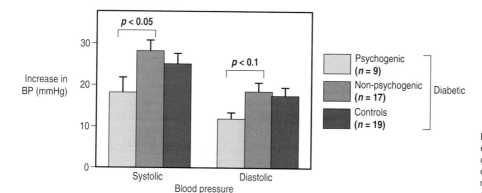

Fig. 13.3 Blood pressure response to visual erotic stimuli in two groups of diabetic dysfunctional men (with and without evidence of psychogenic causation) and a group of normal non-diabetic controls (from Bancroft et al 1985).

diabetes and orgasmic dysfunction was found in any of the four studies, but in each there was some evidence of impaired vaginal lubrication, though usually insufficient to cause problems. In a fifth uncontrolled study, Newman & Bertelson (1986) assessed 81 women with type I diabetes; 47% were diagnosed with sexual dysfunction, mainly 'inhibited sexual excitement', low sexual desire and dyspareunia. The women with sexual problems were more depressed and less satisfied with their sexual relationships.

Ellenberg (1977) had earlier found no difference in sexual response between diabetic women with and without autonomic neuropathy, and this was the case also in the Danish (Jensen 1981) and Scottish (Tyrer et al 1983) studies. Whitley & Berke (1984), on the other hand, did find that women with autonomic neuropathy were more likely to report problems with vaginal dryness.

Schreiner-Engel et al (1985) assessed sexual function with the Derogatis sexual function inventory. They found little evidence of impaired sexual response, but they did find that their diabetic women showed lower levels of sexual desire, scored lower on a global measure of sexual functioning and reported less satisfaction with their relationships. These authors wondered whether the existence of a chronic disease like diabetes would have adverse effects on the dynamics of a long-term relationship. Somewhat in contrast, diabetic women in the Scottish study (Tyrer et al 1983) were more likely to report a beneficial effect of their diabetes on their marriage (21%) than a detrimental effect (9%). Jensen (1985), on the other hand, found that both men and women with diabetes were more likely to have sexual problems if they had made a poor psychological adjustment to their illness.

One difference between the study of Schreiner-Engel et al and the Danish and Scottish studies was that in the former both type I and type II diabetics were involved, whereas in the other two studies only type I cases were included. Schreiner-Engel et al (1986) went on to investigate the relevance of the type of diabetes in a further study of diabetic women. Type I (or insulin dependent) and type II (or non-insulin dependent) diabetes are also distinguished by their age of onset. In this study, the type I group had an average age of onset of 17.6 years; for type II it was 35.9 years. Other potentially important differences were that the type II women were heavier and more likely to be post-menopausal than

their age-matched controls. Using a similar method of assessment as in their previous study, they found that the type I women were virtually indistinguishable from their age-matched controls, whereas the type II women differed in a number of ways. These women rated themselves as less sexually attractive, less happy and satisfied with their sexual partners and sex life in general, less interested in and more likely to avoid sexual activity, less likely to lubricate and more likely to experience dyspareunia, and less likely to experience orgasm with their partners.

The lack of orgasm was correlated with menopausal status, whereas none of the parameters correlated with weight. Although requiring replication, these interesting findings suggest that the stage of the life cycle and in particular of the relationship at the time the diabetes develops may be more important in relation to sexual function than the diabetic process itself, at least in women. The type I women would usually have been diagnosed before marriage and this would be reflected in their choice of partner, who would be likely to be caring and supportive. For the type II women there would be no such selection process to prepare the couple for a chronic illness.

In 1993, Wincze et al reported a comparison of 7 type I diabetic women, not complaining of sexual difficulty, with seven well-matched non-diabetic controls. Their VPA responses and subjective ratings of sexual arousal were measured while watching erotic films. The diabetic women showed significantly less VPA response than the controls but did not differ in their subjective ratings of sexual arousal.

In a more recent controlled study, 97 women with type I diabetes and 145 non-diabetic controls were assessed for sexual problems (Enzlin et al 2002). A limitation of this study is that only four questions were asked about sexual problems: (i) decreased libido, (ii) increased libido, (iii) vaginal dryness and (iv) orgasm difficulty. The only one of these problems reported significantly more frequently by the diabetic women was vaginal dryness, which was referred to as 'arousal' throughout the text. The only significant predictor of sexual problems in both groups was depression.

Drawing together the findings from these various studies two themes emerge. Diabetic women may experience sexual problems in the same way as non-diabetic women, and the importance of depression as a predictor of sexual difficulty emerged in several studies. In addition, a recurring theme across several of these studies was the issue of vaginal dryness, and both with interview and with psychophysiological assessment this was not necessarily associated with impaired sexual arousal. This is consistent with the idea that diabetes interferes with vaginal lubrication response, but does not interfere with other aspects of the woman's sexual experience. This reflects the separate role of vaginal lubrication, which was considered closely in Chapter 4 (see p. 79). This limitation can and often is dealt with in ways that avoid making the sexual experience negative.

Diabetic women are vulnerable to a number of other sex-related problems, apart from sexual dysfunction. They are prone to vaginal infections when their diabetes is not well controlled. Reproduction is also surrounded with hazards. Not only is fertility impaired, there is also a tendency to spontaneous abortion, premature births and intrauterine death. Large babies are more common in diabetic (and pre-diabetic) women, increasing the likelihood of complications at delivery, as well as perinatal morbidity. Contraception also has its problems, as steroidal contraceptives may disturb the diabetic control.

It is therefore gratifying how well sexually adjusted most diabetic women are, and the weight of evidence points more to the psychological impact of the diabetes on the relationship than the disease process itself as the cause of sexual problems when they occur. Although physical factors are more important in the male diabetic, it seems probable that these interpersonal factors are important for them also.

As yet no controlled treatment studies of sexual problems in diabetic women have been reported. The general counselling approach, described in Chapter 12, is appropriate, and the more specifically diabetic problem of vaginal dryness can be remedied in a variety of simple ways.

Cardiovascular disease

Most disease of the cardiovascular system results from a variable combination of atheromatous degeneration and narrowing of the arteries, and raised blood pressure. Sometimes the arterial disease is confined to the heart, producing IHD with angina of effort and a predisposition to MI. In other cases, the main effects are in more peripheral vessels, causing ischaemic pain during exercise (intermittent claudication) and other peripheral manifestations. The importance of hypertension varies, but there is a marked tendency for raised blood pressure of any duration to be associated with arterial disease. The patient may present with symptoms of high blood pressure, of chronic arterial insufficiency or acutely, following an MI.

The association between cardiovascular disease and sexual problems or concerns is complex. But it is now clear that erectile failure may be an early manifestation of arterial disease, and that the vessels supplying the penis may be especially vulnerable to atheromatous degeneration. It is worth bearing in mind that the penile arteries undergo frequent straightening and convoluting through the life cycle as erections come and go. Apart from the coronary arteries, there are probably no other medium-sized arteries that are submitted to so much mechanical distortion — a factor that could contribute to their vulnerability.

We can consider the sexual problems associated with cardiovascular disease in three ways: direct effect of the disease process on sexual function, the psychological reactions to the disease and the sexual consequences of treatment (this is covered later in this chapter).

Most of the limited evidence in the literature is confined to IHD and hypertension. The ability to attribute sexual dysfunction to the vascular disease is limited without adequate control for other aetiological factors.

Ischaemic heart disease

Men with IHD have up to a fourfold increase in likelihood of developing ED (Mickley 2002, cited in Sumanen et al 2005). The impact of IHD on the sexuality of women has been less studied, and given the complexity of factors that can influence women's sexual well-being, we should not expect any simple associations. Probably the most direct equivalent in the woman to the ED that results from vascular impairment in the man would be impaired vaginal lubrication. As considered in the previous section, there is increasing evidence of this effect of diabetes in women, but we do not yet have the evidence to assess this association in relation to cardiovascular disease.

Of particular importance to the clinician is the fact that ED may be the first symptom of IHD, and this possibility should be kept in mind during assessment in a sexual health clinic, with referral for cardiovascular investigations when there are other risk factors increasing the likelihood. Wabrek & Burchell (1980) interviewed 131 men after acute infarction; two-thirds reported a significant sexual problem before the heart attack and of these 64% involved erectile difficulty, 28% a substantial decrease of sexual interest and activity and 8% premature ejaculation.

A Finnish study assessed 105 men and 29 women who had experienced MI, and 102 men and 83 women who had experienced angina (A) (Sumanen et al 2005). When compared to matched control groups, the importance of sex was significantly lower in men and women in the MI groups, but not in the A groups. Both men and women in the MI groups reported a significantly greater recent decline in sexual interest than controls; in the A groups, only the men did so. A key question is the extent to which these differences between those who had experienced MI and those who had only experienced angina was due to different degrees of vascular pathology, or rather different psychological reactions, with experience of MI increasing fear of death from a further infarction.

The psychological reactions of the partner also need to be considered. The prospect of one's spouse dying during the process of making love is especially horrifying.

Hypertension

The effects of hypertension on sexual function are uncertain. In an early study of men (Bulpitt et al 1976), treated hypertensives were compared with untreated hypertensives and age-matched normotensive controls. The prevalence of ED in the three groups was 24.8%, 17.1% and 6.9%, and of ejaculatory failure, 25.6%, 7.8% and 0%, respectively. Hanon et al (2002, cited in Salonia et al 2006) studied 459 hypertensive men and women in France. Sexual problems were reported by 49% of men and 18% of women. But there were no control groups. The importance of control groups was illustrated in a study by Dhabuwala et al (1986). They compared 50 men following MI with 50 controls matched for age, hypertension, diabetes and smoking. They found little difference between the two groups in the incidence of sexual dysfunction. Burchardt et al (2002) sent detailed questionnaires to women attending a hypertension clinic in New York and concluded that sexual dysfunction was common and overlooked in women with hypertension. However, apart from having no control group, their response rate was only 16%. Given the detailed nature of the questionnaires sent out, it is highly possible that those women prepared to complete them were not representative of the total sample contacted.

At the moment there is no reason to believe that hypertension per se impairs erectile function or genital response in women, but the untreated hypertensive may well have some degree of peripheral arterial disease.

Sexual problems in men and women may be associated with problems in the relationship that can be stressful, and could aggravate the hypertension. The man or woman with hypertension may fear that sexual activity will raise their blood pressure to a dangerous level.

Several of the drugs used to treat hypertension have sexual side effects, which are considered later.

Counselling the patient with cardiovascular disease

In this, as in many other areas of medical care, the advice given to the male patient with cardiovascular disease about his future sex life may be of crucial importance to his health, and even his survival. For middle-aged men, there is some suggestion that regular sexual activity may reduce the likelihood of fatal MI (Ebrahim et al 2002). Little attention has been paid to advising women with cardiovascular disease about their sexual activity. It is reasonable, however, to assume that the following guidelines, explicitly for men, are of equal relevance to women.

It is also helpful to have some information about the 'exercise' effects of typical sexual activity on cardiac function. The best evidence comes from an early study by Hellerstein & Friedman (1970). They monitored cardiovascular function during a variety of activities in a number of men following MI. In 14 of their subjects, sexual activity occurred during the monitoring period (carried out in their own homes). The increase in heart rate and blood pressure, which was maximal around orgasm, was somewhat less than that occurring during modest physical activity of a non-sexual kind. It is nevertheless important to remember that the degree of excitement and hence cardiovascular arousal may vary according to the circumstances of the sexual act. Ueno (1963) studied the circumstances of sudden death in Japan and found that death during sexual activity, whilst fairly rare (0.6% of sudden deaths), was much more likely to occur during extramarital sexual encounters. One should obviously be cautious in interpreting these data; the married woman whose husband dies during lovemaking may well conceal this fact. For the partner involved in an extramarital liaison, perhaps in a hotel room, concealment is much more difficult. But if there is any validity in this finding, it points to the extra exciting effects of novel or risky sexual situations. Larson et al (1980) showed that sexual activity was comparable to exercise involving climbing 22 steps in normal men, and slightly less demanding than climbing steps in men following MI.

Whilst familiarity in these circumstances is beneficial for the heart patient or hypertensive, it is also sensible to avoid more athletic sexual performances. There is, however, likely to be reduced risk as the post-infarct patient becomes physically fitter. Stein (1977) found that men who underwent an exercise training programme after their myocardial infarct showed a decline in their peak heart rate during intercourse, compared with men who did not undergo such training.

The resumption of sexual activity should be seen as comparable to other forms of physical activity. Gradual rehabilitation is advisable and if a patient is apprehensive about his or her performance on resuming sexual activity, it may help for him or her to masturbate alone in the first instance. In general, if moderate exercise such as climbing two flights of stairs or a short brisk walk can be managed without undue difficulty, sexual activity of a calm, non-athletic kind should be equally manageable.

The occurrence of angina during sexual activity should be judged in the same way as angina occurring during exercise. Coronary dilators can be used before intercourse, although activity should not continue in the presence of persisting ischaemic symptoms. A short rest or even a slowing down may suffice in some instances. Sexual activity after substantial intake of food or alcohol should be avoided.

Although it is advisable to enquire about background factors with the patient alone, it is also important to discuss the same issues with the spouse and to go over the main points of sexual rehabilitation with the couple together.

In treating hypertension, the possibility of sexual side effects of drugs should be discussed in a way not to alarm the patient or generate performance anxiety, but to point out that adjustment of the dosage or change of drug can be used if necessary to reduce such effects. If the patient is not told of these possible sexual side effects, he may not only fail to mention them when they arise, but may cease to take the drug regularly because of them.

Neurology

Epilepsy

A link between epilepsy and sexuality featured in the medical writings of antiquity. Sexual behaviour, particularly masturbation, has in the past been seen as a cause of epilepsy (Money & Pruce 1977). The similarity between orgasm and an epileptic seizure has often received comment. Kinsey et al (1953) made a serious comparison between these two equally mysterious neurophysiological phenomena (see Chapter 4, p. 85).

In modern medicine, the sexual implications of epilepsy are threefold:

1. *The sexual manifestations of epileptic seizures.* A range of sexual sensations, erection, ejaculation or orgasm can occur as part of an epileptic seizure, and are most likely to be associated with temporal lobe lesions. Pelvic or sexual movements, occurring during or after a seizure are more likely to be associated with frontal lobe lesions. Such experiences, however, are rare (Lundberg 1992).
2. *The provocation of a seizure by sexual activity.* Although only a few such cases have been reported in the literature (e.g. Mitchell et al 1954; Hoenig & Hamilton 1960), it may be more common as epileptic patients are unlikely to report such associations unless specifically asked (Lundberg 1992).
3. *The sexuality of epileptic individuals in between their seizures.* Many epileptic men and women report sexual problems of one kind or another. In most studies the association has been with temporal lobe epilepsy. Gastaut & Collomb (1954) found that 26 of 36 patients with temporal lobe epilepsy had 'hyposexuality', not only a lack of interest in sexual intercourse but also lack of sexual curiosity, erotic fantasies or sensual dreams. Usually this became evident after the onset of the epilepsy. Blumer (1970) reported that 29 out of 50 patients with temporal lobe epilepsy showed 'global hyposexuality' and often an inability to achieve orgasm. Taylor (1969) studied 100 temporal lobe epileptics who underwent temporal lobectomy. Before the operation, 56% had sexual problems, usually reduced sexual activity and indifference with 'a bland denial of interest in sex'. Kolarsky et al (1967) used a register of a central epileptic clinic in Prague and intensively investigated a group of 86 males. Sixteen (19%) were hyposexual and this was usually associated with temporal lobe epilepsy. Herzog et al (1986 a,b) reported further evidence of hyposexuality in men and women with temporal lobe epilepsy, particularly involving the right temporal lobe. They also found considerable overlap with endocrine abnormalities. In contrast, Jensen et al (1990) compared 86 men and women with epilepsy with diabetics and normal controls, assessed in the same way. They found no more sexual dysfunction in the epileptic group than the controls. It is possible that this contrast reflects milder cases in this study than in earlier ones.

More recently, Morell & Guldner (1996) reported on 116 women with epilepsy (99 with a localized epileptic focus, and 17 with more generalized epilepsy). More than one-third of the women in both groups reported reduced sexual arousability. Those with localized epilepsy were more likely to report dyspareunia, whereas those with generalized epilepsy, orgasmic difficulty. In contrast with earlier studies, low sexual desire was not reported.

Occasionally hypersexuality is reported. It is usually episodic and most often is manifested as excessive masturbation (Taylor 1969; Blumer 1970). The occasional association between epileptic disorder and fetishism and transvestism was mentioned in Chapter 9, and other types of abnormal sexual preference may be more likely in epileptics, especially those with temporal lobe focus (Kolarsky et al 1967).

The reasons for these associations between epilepsy and sexual disturbance are likely to be complex. Epilepsy still carries considerable stigma, and children with epilepsy are more likely to be overprotected and to have personality problems for this reason alone. They may lack self-confidence, fear rejection or failure, and, particularly when with another person, fear the effects of sexual excitement because of its similarity to epileptic phenomena. Sexual disturbance is more likely to arise on this basis if the onset of the epilepsy is in childhood rather than if it occurs after normal adult sexual development is established (Taylor 1972). This may indicate a direct neurological interference with normal sexual development (see Chapter 5). The relevance of the temporal lobe is of considerable interest in this respect. It has been suggested that excessive neuronal activity of the limbic portions of the temporal lobe produce a suppression of sexual behaviour, whereas lack of such activity leads to increased sexuality. This is supported by the characteristics of the Kluver–Bucy syndrome, a state produced by surgical removal of both temporal lobes. This condition has been studied in primates, and something comparable has been observed in humans (Terzian & Orr 1955). Amongst a number of other bizarre features, there is a tendency to hypersexuality, usually in the form of masturbatory or aimless sexual mounting behaviour. These findings are consistent with recent evidence of brain activity associated with sexual response, considered closely in Chapter 4. In particular, inhibitory tone, which requires to be reduced for sexual arousal to occur, appears to be temporal lobe based (Stoléru & Mouras 2007).

Although lack of sexual appetite is the most commonly reported problem in epileptics, there is also evidence that women have difficulty in responding to sexual stimulation with increased arousal and men have problems establishing normal erections (Lundberg 1977). This could also reflect impairment of limbic function. In humans, there is some evidence of improvement in hyposexuality as fits are brought under control. The effects of unilateral temporal lobectomy on the characteristic hyposexuality are rather less predictable. Some patients improve, whereas others get worse (Taylor & Falconer 1968; Blumer 1970). The effects of anti-convulsants on endocrine status (considered later in this chapter) are consistent with a substantial amount of the hyposexuality in epileptics being iatrogenic. In the study by Jensen et al (1990), in which the prevalence of low sexual interest and erectile problems was no greater than in the control group, more than half were using carbamazepine. This anti-convulsant does not increase sex hormone-binding globulin, and consequently reduce free T, in the way that most anti-convulsants, such as phenytoin do. The subjects in this study were endocrinologically normal. Thus, the higher incidence of sexual problems in other series could be due to the endocrine effects of other anti-convulsants. Such effects may be relevant to women as well as men (Penovich 2000).

Multiple sclerosis

In multiple sclerosis (MS), the basic lesion is demyelination of nerve fibres. It can affect subjects at any age from 12 to 60 years, but most commonly has its onset in the 20s or 30s. It is about twice as common in women as in men. Its basic cause is not known, but may involve an abnormality of the immune response of the nervous system, with abnormal reactions to certain virus infections. Demyelination can occur anywhere in the nervous system, hence the manifestations of the disease are protean. MS may be quite localized; it has a tendency to come and go, leading to remissions and relapses. The prognosis is extremely uncertain, as there must be many people who have had mild or transient forms of this disease and have never seen a neurologist. In a proportion of cases, however, impairment becomes permanent and may be severe.

Sexual problems are common in MS patients. They may stem from the non-specific consequences of physical handicap and the strains that these impose on sexual relationships. Also, sufferers from MS may be particularly prone to anxiety and depression, which will take their own toll of sexual happiness (Burnfield 1979). Specific effects of the disease on sexual function are also to be expected. Impairment of peripheral autonomic nerves or their spinal pathways may lead to failure of genital responses such as erection, similar to the neural effects of diabetes. Ejaculation may be impaired in the presence of normal erections. Sensation may also be affected, resulting in diminished response to tactile stimulation or sometimes hypersensitivity which can make either genital touch or orgasm unpleasant (Lundberg 1980). Spasticity, particularly of the leg adductors in women, may interfere with normal love-making in a distressing fashion.

Sexual problems are associated with disturbances of bladder or bowel function or other peripheral autonomic symptoms more commonly than with more central lesions (Ghezzi 1999). However, an interesting association between brain damage from MS and orgasmic difficulty has been reported. Barak et al (1996) included brain magnetic resonance imaging (MRI) in a comprehensive assessment of MS patients. Anorgasmia correlated significantly with brain stem and pyramidal abnormalities, and with the total area of lesions or plaques observed on the MRI.

Lilius et al (1976) gave a questionnaire to 302 men and women with moderately severe MS: 64% of the men and 39% of the women reported sexual problems or cessation of sexual activity. Of the men with problems, 80% had erectile difficulties and 56% diminished libido. General weakness, spasticity of limb muscles and loss of genital sensation were given as reasons by some of the men. Of the women with problems, 48% reported low interest in intercourse, 49% diminished clitoral sensitivity and 57% difficulty in attaining orgasm. Spasticity and dryness of the vagina were also mentioned.

Vas (1969), investigating men with mild MS, found 47% with erectile problems. This was commonly associated with disturbance of body sweating. Lundberg (1980) compared 25 women with established MS but minimal disability with 25 migraine sufferers of similar age. Thirteen (52%) of the MS women had sexual problems compared with 3 (12%) of the control group. Reduced libido, orgasmic difficulty and altered genital sensitivity were the most common complaints. McCabe et al (1996) obtained questionnaire data from 37 men and 74 women registered with the MS society in Australia; the refusal rate was very low. Sexual problems were common and varied; 65% of the men and 80% of the women reported at least one sexual problem. In men, ED (19%) and low sexual interest (12%) were the most common; in women, it was low sexual interest (29%) and orgasmic difficulty (24%). No association was found between the presence of sexual problems and the duration of the MS or the level of disability. Overall, those who were in relationships were mostly positive about their relationships. However, the partner without MS was not assessed.

The reasons for reduced libido in MS are not clear. Impaired sensation may be relevant as sexual desire is often activated by awareness of one's genitals, particularly in men. Central neural pathological mechanisms may also be involved. It is probably most often a psychological reaction to the sexual problem or to other aspects of the condition, and the associated depression, which are mainly responsible.

Parkinson's disease

This is a progressive degenerative disease of the central nervous system, relatively common in those beyond middle age (prevalence of around 1 per 1000 rising to 1 per 200 in the elderly; Marsden 2000). Its manifestations are a characteristic tremor, rigidity, a poverty and slowness of movement (akinesia) and postural changes (flexion of the limbs, neck and trunk and postural instability). Although this specific pattern of degeneration can be associated with other more generalized degenerative conditions, Parkinson's disease (PD) specifically involves degeneration of the substantia nigra, in the mid brain, and its dopaminergic connection with the striatum of the basal ganglia (i.e. the caudate nucleus and putamen). This connection is the meso-striatal dopaminergic system, described in Chapter 4 (see p. 62), which is crucial to the control of motor activity. In addition to major neuronal loss in the substantial nigra there is a substantial loss of dopamine throughout the meso-striatal system (Marsden 2000).

Parkinson-like symptoms are common side effects of dopamine antagonists such as anti-psychotic drugs and calcium channel blockers used in the treatment of hypertension (see p. 404).

The central role of dopamine (DA) in this condition and also in many aspects of sexual response, makes PD of theoretical interest to sexology. However, although the motor coordination controlled by the meso-striatal system is relevant to normal sexual behaviour, it is not clear to what extent DA activity becomes impaired in the other DA systems of more direct relevance to sexual arousal and motivation (i.e. the meso-limbic and the incerto-hypothalamic (or A14) DA systems; see Chapter 4, p. 67).

Sexual problems are common in men and women with PD (Koller et al 1990; Welsh et al 1997). Bronner et al (2004) assessed 32 women and 43 men with PD. Of the women, 87% reported difficulty with sexual arousal, 75% with reaching orgasm and 47% with low sexual desire. Of the men, 68% reported ED, 41% premature ejaculation, 39% retarded ejaculation and 65% 'sexual dissatisfaction'.

Lundberg (1992, 2006) describes the various ways that PD may lead to sexual problems. Muscle rigidity and akinesia may impair performance of sexual activity; autonomic nervous system dysfunction (Koller et al 1990) may directly impair genital response, orgasm and ejaculation; psychological reactions to the disease and their impact on the relationship may adversely affect the sexual relationship. The specific role of DA presents us with an intriguing puzzle. Given the central role of DA in incentive motivation, as well as genital response, if the depletion in DA was not restricted to the meso-striatal system (which it may be) then loss of sexual desire and arousability might result. In some individuals with PD, treatment with L-dopa, now the most widely used medication for PD, but also dopamine agonists like bromocriptine, have produced an increase or normalization of sexual desire and erectile capacity not dependent on improvement in the specific PD symptoms. However, in other cases, such treatment is associated with negative sexual effects (Bronner et al 2004). This remains an unresolved paradox, which may reflect the extent to which pharmacological manipulation of the DA systems, in either direction, may disrupt their function. More research is required on this issue.

Spinal cord injuries

Spinal cord injuries (SCI), most commonly resulting from traffic accidents, are tragic and all too common. The majority affected are men. They tend to be young, and with modern methods of treatment have good life expectancy with no particular risk of progression of the disability. Their sexual capacity is therefore of considerable importance. Lesions low in the spinal cord result in paralysis and loss of sensation in the lower limbs (i.e. paraplegia). Higher lesions may cause paralysis and loss of sensation in all four limbs (i.e. quadriplegia).

The earlier literature mainly focused on men, but in recent years there has been increasing attention to the effects of spinal cord injury in women. Useful early reviews were provided by Cole (1975) and Higgins (1979). Evidence of the relationship between the type of sexual impairment and type of injury is not only of clinical importance, but also of relevance to our understanding of the neuroanatomy and neurophysiology of sexual response. The complexity of the neural control of sexual response, orgasm and ejaculation was considered in Chapter 4. A basic theme is the distinction between reflexive genital response, which depends on intact connections with the sacral cord (mainly S2–4) and 'psychogenic' genital response, which depends on outflow from the thoracic cord (see p. 74). A 'reflexive' response depends on appropriate tactile stimulation, even if the individual with SCI is unable to feel the stimulation. 'Psychogenic' stimulation involves central control of genital response in the brain, which may be elicited by fantasy or visual stimuli. Normal sexual response obviously involves an interaction between the two. A crucial component of such response mechanisms is inhibition; normally there is inhibitory tone from the brain, which requires to be reduced before genital response occurs (see p. 72). A complete transection above the sacral level may leave the reflexive component intact while cutting off the inhibitory signals from the brain. This explains why in some men with SCI, reflexive erections occur with minimal peripheral stimulation, even though the man is unable to feel the response. What is often uncertain with SCI is the extent to which the spinal cord pathways are completely or partially transected by the lesion. These different factors, together with the substantial psychological and relational consequences of such injury, account for the considerable variability in the sexual consequences of SCI.

Effects in the male

In men with complete cord lesions who have recovered from the initial phase of spinal shock, some reflexive erection is to be expected, providing that the sacral segments of the cord are not destroyed. In general, the higher the level of the lesion, the more likely there are to be reflexive erections (Higgins 1979). The completeness and duration of such erections do vary, however, and may be partly due to variable degrees of damage. Psychogenic erections, by contrast, are more likely to continue with lower lesions that are incomplete, though usually they are also associated with some reflexive responsiveness. There are, however, a number of men described in the literature with lesions below the level of T8 who had psychogenic erections in the absence of reflexive responses (Higgins 1979). This is understandable if we accept that psychogenic erections do not require the sacral nerve supply to be intact.

Ejaculatory capacity tends to be more impaired than erection. Ejaculation is unlikely in men with complete lesions (ranging from 0% to 7% in different series) but with incomplete lesions ejaculation, to some extent, is possible in about two-thirds of cases. It is more likely to occur with lower than with higher level lesions, though the evidence is far from conclusive (Higgins

1979). It is more difficult to be certain about the incidence of orgasm. Lack of awareness of any pelvic sensations must make recognition of orgasm difficult. However, as considered in Chapter 4 (see p. 84) orgasm is a complex process that involves extensive activity within the brain as well as peripheral changes. Thus, even if there is loss of sensation peripherally, the central changes are likely to be experienced, although probably altered in some way. In terms of experiencing the orgasm, therefore, it may be more a matter of the process by which it is triggered, and this process is not well understood (see p. 87). Many paraplegic men do describe orgasmic experiences without their necessarily being associated with ejaculation. These orgasmic experiences are often followed by a period of comfortable resolution, comparable to that of a normal orgasm (Cole 1975). Those few men with upper motor neuron lesions and spasticity of the lower limbs who do ejaculate may experience considerable reduction in the spasticity following ejaculation, which can be gratifying (Bors & Comarr 1960). A heightening of erotic sensitivity in areas above the lesion is not unusual, though the neurophysiological mechanism involved is not understood (Bors & Comarr 1960; Cole 1975). In some men with cord injuries above the fourth thoracic vertebra sexual stimulation and, in particular, ejaculation, may lead to excessive excitation of the autonomic nervous system — the so-called autonomic dysreflexia. This may result in a marked rise in blood pressure and headache or flushing, sweating and cardiac arrhythmia (Elliott & Krassioukov 2005).

Alexander et al (1993) assessed 38 men with SCI (median age 26 years). Twenty-three of them (61%) engaged in penile–vaginal intercourse to some extent post-injury, but the sexual activity that was enjoyed the most was oral sex, though the details of this (e.g. who was orally stimulated) were not given. They categorized this sample as 'quadriplegic complete' (QC; $n = 16$), 'quadriplegic incomplete' (QI; $n = 6$), 'paraplegic complete' (PC; $n = 12$) and 'paraplegic incomplete' (PI; $n = 4$). Only four men, all in the PC group, were unable to get any erection. Around a half of the two complete groups (QC and PC) obtained an erection from manual stimulation only. Those with incomplete lesions (QI and PI) were more likely to respond to mental stimulation. The duration of erection was shortest in the PC group. Twenty-two of the total sample (58%) were unable to ejaculate; 15 (39.5%) no longer experienced orgasm. The PI group, over all, was most likely to report impaired sexual response. The body areas most responsive to erotic touch were typically those with preserved sensation above the level of the injury. As with earlier studies, the association between level and completeness of the SCI and sexual function varied to a considerable extent.

Effects in the female

The limited evidence so far suggests that the sexuality of women with spinal injuries is somewhat less affected than it is in men. Fitting et al (1978) investigated 24 women; 20 (85%) had had sexual relationships since

the injury and 13 (54%) were involved in a relationship at the time of the interview. Thirteen women had complete spinal lesions and of these, seven found sexual relations to be 'very enjoyable'. Eight of the 11 women with incomplete lesions reported the same. The subjective feelings expressed by the women did not appear to correlate with the level of injury. Although it was not stated, one assumes that these women had little or no awareness of genital sensations. Six of them spontaneously mentioned experiencing orgasm, though differing from their pre-injury experiences. One woman described her orgasm as 'a fuse box gone haywire'. Two-thirds stated that concern about their bowel and bladder dysfunction had interfered with sexual expression. Spasticity may occasionally cause problems, particularly if the adductors are involved (Cole 1975).

More recently, Sipski and colleagues have reported a series of studies of women with SCI. These included psychophysiological assessment of sexual response during visual erotic stimulation, and combined with manual stimulation. In a separate condition, women were left alone to stimulate themselves to orgasm, if possible. Sixty-eight SCI women were assessed, plus an 'able-bodied' control group of 21 women (Sipski et al 2001). The measure of genital response was VPA. The relevance of this response to woman's sexual arousal is uncertain, as discussed in Chapter 4 (see p. 80). However, it is of importance for vaginal lubrication. VPA increased significantly in both the SCI women and the controls, although to a significantly greater extent in the controls. They went on to divide the SCI group according to the degree of preservation of light touch and pinprick sensation, at three different levels of the cord: T6–9, T11–L2 and S2–5. Most striking was the division based on T11–L2 sensation. Regardless of the level of the injury, VPA response was significantly reduced in those with marked sensory impairment below T11–L2. This pattern was not evident when the women were divided according to the sensory impairment at the other two levels. Notably, cardiovascular and subjective measures of arousal were not significantly different between the SCI and control groups. Orgasm was significantly less likely in the SCI group; however, 44% of the SCI women (compared with 100% of the controls) were orgasmic in the laboratory, although this took significantly longer than with the controls, and this ability was not related significantly to the level or degree of the lesion. Women were asked to describe how they had experienced the orgasm and, interestingly, blind raters were unable to discriminate between the descriptions of the SCI women and the controls.

Orgasmic experience in women with complete SCI has also been reported by Komisaruk et al (1997). Komisaruk and colleagues have used such evidence, together with studies showing perception of vaginal/cervical stimulation in such women, as evidence of the sensory pathways associated with the vagus nerve, which escape spinal lesions (Komisaruk et al 2006). Sipski et al (2001) concluded that their findings, summarized above, and including a study of the effects of inducing anxiety (Sipski et al 2004), did not support Komisaruk's interpretation, and instead advocated the role of sympathetic activation in sexual response. This way of interpreting 'sympathetic nervous system' effects was critically discussed in Chapter 4 (see p. 80). Although the effects of spinal cord lesions offers scope for furthering our understanding of the neurophysiology of sexual arousal and orgasm, it is fair to say that as yet such evidence has not produced conclusive results.

Fertility and spinal injuries

Fertility in women with spinal injuries is relatively unaffected. Menstruation usually resumes within 6 months of the injury, and it is not unusual for SCI women to experience menstrual pain. Pregnancy may occur and continue to normal delivery, although there is an increased risk of urinary infection, anaemia and premature labour (Griffith & Trieschmann 1975). Contraception is therefore an important issue in these women if they are sexually active. Steroidal contraceptives are probably contraindicated because of the increased risk of thrombosis. Diaphragms are impractical and intra-uterine devices have to be used with extra caution because of the absence of pelvic sensation and the small risk of uterine perforation or pelvic infection. The appropriateness of sterilization should not be assumed, however, as many women have coped with motherhood from a wheelchair when provided with additional support (Cole 1975).

For the male with spinal injuries, fertility is much less likely. As mentioned above, few ejaculate and among those who do, spermatogenesis is not always normal. This could be related to scrotal temperature, which is notably higher than in normal men (Brindley 1982). The endocrine status of cord-injured men is usually normal (Kolodny et al 1979). Artificially induced ejaculation (e.g. electro-ejaculation; Brindley 1982) may be possible and, if the ejaculate is fertile, may be used for artificial insemination. Ejaculation has occasionally been obtained by applying a vibrator to the penis.

Counselling men and women with spinal injuries

Sexual enjoyment, if still possible, may be an important option for someone with an otherwise severely restricted life. The married paraplegic or quadriplegic, largely dependent on the spouse for so many things, may both want and need to give sexual pleasure to his or her partner. Self-esteem may be severely affected by the physical incapacity, particularly in a man who relied on his physical prowess before the injury. The retention of erectile function may have extra importance for such a person. Male paraplegics capable of having erections were found by Berger (1951) to have higher self-esteem than those who had loss of erectile response. Lindner (1953) found that those who were unable to get erections had more physical complaints and bodily preoccupations. In some cases the need for sexual activity produces difficulties in the marital relationship; the partner may sometimes resent having to be available sexually as well as taking so many other responsibilities.

Most of the issues involved in counselling people with spinal injuries are common to the general field of physical handicap, discussed earlier in this chapter. The younger age of this population compared with some other disabled groups is associated with a relatively high level of sexual awareness and interest, the importance of sexuality for self-esteem and concern with fertility. More specific issues are often of a practical, commonsense nature, involving catheters, sphincter control, spasticity and physical positioning during love-making (Cole 1975). It is important in the early stages not to reach conclusions about sexual impairment before sufficient time has elapsed to judge the degree of recovery. Whilst it is important to accept the realities of an irreversible and static disability, there does seem to be scope for developing and enhancing new forms of sexual pleasure. An approach to love-making involving exploration and discovery is therefore required. Encouragement or even 'permission' to do this may be needed.

Sexual side effects of medication

The sexual side effects of drugs are receiving increasing attention, mainly for the reason that there is now much more public awareness of such side effects, and they have become a significant factor in the marketing success of one drug compared with another. They are, in any case, of fundamental clinical importance as they may determine whether patients continue to take their medication. In addition, such pharmacological effects, particularly when they differ between different drugs, are of considerable theoretical interest. However, as we shall see, the explanations for such differences are complex and often not well understood. A further challenge, in many cases, is the distinction between an effect of a drug and a symptom of the condition for which the drug is being used. This is particularly relevant when, as is often the case, no clinical assessment of pre-treatment sexual function is carried out. Sometimes the patient or doctor may prefer to blame a drug rather than be confronted with other possibly more threatening alternative explanations. In appraising the likelihood of a drug-induced sexual effect, the following questions should be asked:

1. What proportion of people taking the drug are affected in this way? Most often we have evidence of assumed side effects in a small proportion, say 5–10%. Obviously the higher the proportion, the more likely it is that the drug is responsible. But we have to allow for the possibility of relatively idiosyncratic reactions to a drug, as well as for variability in the functional importance of a particular pharmacologically sensitive mechanism.

2. How specific is the observed effect? If interference with a discrete mechanism is repeatedly observed, a drug effect is more likely. The best early example of this was the selective blocking of seminal emission by certain α-adrenergic blockers, leaving orgasm, erection and sexual interest unaffected (see below). Unfortunately, it has been unusual for investigators to ask sufficiently careful questions to distinguish between failure of emission and failure of orgasm. Inhibition of both could result from some central impairment of sexual arousability or even as a

non-specific effect of general sedation. Erectile failure could be due to a peripheral or a central pharmacological effect or alternatively result from a psychological reaction to some other effect, such as ejaculatory failure. It is particularly difficult to distinguish between pharmacological and psychological mechanisms when loss of sexual interest is the problem.

3. Is there a pharmacological basis for the suspected drug effect? This question is made more difficult by the relatively mixed pharmacological action of so many modern drugs, and the variable extent to which they cross the blood–brain barrier.

Pharmacological treatment of hypertension

The story of the recognition of sexual side effects of anti-hypertensive medication is an interesting one. Early in my career there were enough pharmacological grounds for such effects to make me interested in researching them. I approached the local hypertension clinic to see if I could study their patients. I was discouraged from doing so on the grounds that talking to patients about such side effects would put the idea into their heads, causing 'sexual side effects' as a result; denial was the preferred option. Soon after, however, the story started to gradually unfold (Crenshaw & Goldberg 1996).

The first major study (Bulpitt & Dollery 1973; Bulpitt et al 1976) compared three groups of men: hypertensives receiving hypotensive drug treatment, hypertensives before receiving any treatment and normotensive controls. The proportions reporting ED in each group were 24.6%, 17.1% and 6.9%, respectively. There were significantly more men with ED in the treated hypertensive group than amongst the controls; the untreated group came midway but was not significantly different from either. Ejaculatory failure was reported by 25.6%, 7.3% and 0%, respectively. The treated group showed significantly more ejaculatory problems than either of the other two. From this evidence it seemed likely that ejaculatory problems resulted from drug treatment, whereas erectile problems could have resulted either from the hypertension itself or from the treatment. Erectile failure is also more likely than ejaculatory failure to result from psychological factors. Only men were involved in this research.

In 1981, the Medical Research Council (MRC 1981) reported a single-blind placebo-controlled study of treatment of moderate-to-mild hypertension. In this study, hypertensive women were included, but only the men were asked questions about sex. Patients were randomly assigned to a thiazide diuretic (bendroflumethiazide), propanalol, a β-blocker, or placebo. The diuretic was associated with twice as much ED as propanalol, which was contrary to 'clinical wisdom' at that time.

In 1986, comparison of captopril, a new ACE inhibitor, with propanalol and methyldopa was reported (Croog et al 1986). Captopril was associated with no sexual side effects in contrast with the other two drugs. This study, sponsored by Squibb, the manufacturer of captopril, was widely advertised by the company, resulting in considerable media attention (Crenshaw & Goldberg 1996). Again only men were included.

In 1991, we saw perhaps the first attempt to assess sexual side effects in women. Wassertheil-Smoller et al (1991) compared men and women on a diuretic (chlorthalidone), a β-blocker (atenolol) or placebo, but varied the dietary conditions. Interestingly, both men and women on a weight-losing diet experienced minimal sexual side effects on the diuretic, as compared to the 'normal diet' or 'low salt diet' groups.

Let us briefly review the relevant pharmacological evidence, mainly restricted to men, and involving drugs many of which are no longer used for regular management of hypertension, before summarizing the current status of anti-hypertensive therapy and its effects on sexual function. A much more comprehensive review is provided by Crenshaw & Goldberg (1996).

Ganglion blockers such as hexamethonium or pentolinium, which block both sympathetic and parasympathetic post-ganglionic fibres, predictably produce complete erectile and ejaculatory failure. They are seldom used now except for the management of acute hypertensive crises. Adrenergic neurone-blocking drugs, such as guanethidine or bethanidine, depress the function of post-ganglionic adrenergic nerves, affecting both α and β mechanisms. Their use was associated with erectile problems in 40–67% and ejaculatory problems in 40–79% of patients (Pritchard et al 1968; Bulpitt & Dollery 1973). Unfortunately in these studies it was not established whether failure of ejaculation was also associated with failure of orgasm. Money & Yankowitz (1967), however, described clearly the occurrence of orgasm without ejaculation in men taking guanethidine. These drugs are seldom used nowadays.

Methyldopa is a different form of hypertensive agent which has marked central as well as peripheral anti-adrenergic effects. Erectile and ejaculatory problems occur significantly less often than with the adrenergic neurone blockers (Pritchard et al 1968; Bulpitt & Dollery 1973) but loss of libido has been reported in up to 25% of men and women using this drug, depending on the dosage involved (Kolodny et al 1979). This would be consistent with the central effect but also may be secondary to a general sedating effect; tiredness is the most common side effect with this drug. Methyldopa is now seldom used to treat hypertension, except, for some reason, in pregnant women (Swales 2000). Clonidine, an α2 agonist, has mainly central effects, including sedation, and hence is seldom used for routine anti-hypertensive treatment.

β adrenergic blockers (e.g. propanolol) have a relatively low incidence of sexual side effects, and it remains unclear why some individuals are susceptible and not others. Riley (1980a) described a man who experienced erectile failure within 2 days of starting propanolol that was reversed as quickly on stopping the drug. He reacted similarly to further propanolol, but not to acebutolol. Both drugs are β-blockers but only propanolol crosses the blood–brain barrier, suggesting that in this case erectile problems resulted from some central pharmacological effect. Labetolol is a hypotensive drug that acts by both α and β blockade. Riley & Riley (1983) in controlled studies with volunteers demonstrated that labetolol increases the time taken to reach orgasm in women and ejaculation in men, without affecting erection in the male subjects.

α1 antagonists, as one would expect from their pharmacological effect (see p. 67), have not been blamed for erectile problems, but may interfere with ejaculation. In one study (Pentland et al 1981), indoramin, an α1 antagonist used not only for hypertension, but also for asthma and migraine, interfered with ejaculation in two-thirds of men using it, whereas in the same study, no such effect was produced by clonidine or placebo. In this study, all men affected described normal erections and orgasms in spite of the ejaculatory failure, indicating that the effect was specifically on seminal emission (see Chapter 4, p. 87).

Angiotensin-converting enzyme (ACE) inhibitors, such as captopril, have not been implicated as causing sexual problems. Calcium-channel blockers (e.g. verapamil) also have a relatively good record in this respect. However, calcium channel blockers produce a wide range of pharmacological effects, including dopamine antagonism, and hence it would not be surprising if they had a negative effect on sexual interest, or erectile function. It should not therefore be assumed that they are free of such effects.

Management of essential hypertension tends to vary from country to country. In the UK, according to Swales (2000), β-blockers tend to be the first treatment method in men and women under 60 years and diuretics for those over 60 years of age. Because of non-sexual side effects, ACE inhibitors and calcium channel are reserved for those who do not respond to first treatment, as are α1 blockers, which are likely to interfere with ejaculation.

Psychotropic drugs

Drugs used to influence psychological states are particularly difficult to evaluate from the sexual point of view. The psychological states for which they are prescribed are likely to have sexual repercussions and most of the drugs used today have a rich mixture of pharmacological actions. Psychotropic drugs can be considered under three broad headings: (i) tranquillizers, sedatives and hypnotics; (ii) anti-depressants; and (iii) neuroleptic or anti-psychotic drugs.

Tranquillizers, sedatives and hypnotics

The benzodiazepines are the most commonly used drugs in this category, both as tranquillizers (e.g. chlordiazepoxide and diazepam) and hypnotics (e.g. nitrazepam). Their pharmacological action is complex and in addition to sedation there is also a reduction of serotonergic activity (Crenshaw & Goldberg 1996). This may explain the rather inconsistent effects on sexual function, as there could be both negative and positive effects. Riley & Riley (1986), in a placebo-controlled study of normal volunteers, found that a single dose of diazepam delayed orgasm in women. It is not known whether this effect would occur in anxious women. The use of benzodiazepines is widespread, and there is relatively little evidence of sexual side effects. Zolpidem is a more recent hypnotic, which has benzodiazepine-like sedative effects, but without the anti-convulsant and muscle relaxant effects. As yet there is no evidence of adverse sexual effects (Crenshaw & Goldberg 1996).

Anti-depressants

There are now two principal types of anti-depressant: tricyclics (e.g. imipramine and amitryptyline) and selective serotonin re-uptake inhibitors (SSRIs; e.g. fluoxetine, paroxetine and sertraline). Monoamine oxidase inhibitors (MAOIs, e.g. phenelzine and tranylcypromine) the earliest class of anti-depressant, are now seldom used because of the risk of dangerous drug interactions.

The extensive literature on sexual side effects of anti-depressants has been reviewed by Montgomery et al (2002). They concluded that the majority of the reported evidence was inconclusive because of methodological shortcomings, and in many cases an inadequate distinction between different types of adverse sexual effects. Effects on orgasm, for example, have not been asked about until relatively recently. Sexual side effects are commonly reported with most types of tricyclics and SSRIs. They are less often reported with pharmacologically atypical anti-depressants such as bupropion, meclobemide, reboxetine, mirtazapine and nefazadone. However, as yet such drugs have been much less widely used, and sexual side effects were not so well recognized with more conventional anti-depressants until they had been in use for many years. Bupropion, which pharmacologically is metabolized into a NA and DA re-uptake inhibitor, has been associated with less sexual side effects in direct comparison with sertraline (Croft et al 1999) and various other SSRIs (Modell et al 1997). This is consistent with bupropion having a dopaminergic and central norepinephric effect. Nefadazone, which is similar to trazadone, with a clear 5HT2 antagonist effect, but without the histaminergic sedative effect of trazadone, has been shown to have less sexual side effects than SSRIs (Gregorian et al 2002).

In the recent literature, which has more comprehensively assessed sexual function, one side effect stands out: delayed ejaculation or orgasm is the most commonly reported sexual side effect in men and in women. Across studies, 30–60% of patients on SSRIs report orgasmic or ejaculatory difficulty. In a number of studies this problem only came out with direct questioning, and was not otherwise mentioned (e.g. Monteiro et al 1987). This effect has been more evident with SSRIs than with tricyclic anti-depressants, and is sufficiently predictable that it is now being exploited as a pharmacological treatment of premature ejaculation. In all of the randomized-controlled comparisons of SSRIs with atypical anti-depressants, like bupropion and nefazadone, the side effect which most consistently showed a significant difference was orgasmic dysfunction in women and delayed ejaculation in men, being more frequent with SSRIs. Although a number of studies have directly compared one SSRI with another, they have generally found no significant difference (Rosen et al 1999).

Although this relatively predictable effect of SSRIs on orgasm and ejaculation is consistent with a serotonergic inhibitory effect, what is puzzling is why inhibition of orgasm/ejaculation is so much more predictable than inhibition of erection or other components of genital response. This reflects our relative lack of understanding of inhibitory systems as they affect sexuality, as well as uncertainty about specific receptor effects of different drugs. The recently demonstrated role of the nucleus paragigantocellularis in inhibiting erectile response, probably dependent on serotonergic mediation, leaves one wondering where 5-HT is acting to more specifically inhibit orgasm/ejaculation. Given the rise in 5-HT in the lateral hypothalamus following ejaculation in rats (Lorrain et al 1997), this may be one brain area where serotonergic inhibition of ejaculation takes place. Other brain areas, such as the postero-medial bed nucleus of the stria terminalis, and the medial parvicellular sub-parafascicular nucleus of the thalamus, have been shown to be active around the time of ejaculation (Veening & Coolen 1998).

Various attempts to counter sexual side effects of anti-depressants have been made by adding a further compound to block the mechanisms assumed to be causing the sexual side effect. In women, placebo-controlled studies, with the addition of buspirone (5HT1A agonist), and amantadine (thought to increase DA availability) (Michelson et al 2000), mirtazapine (5HT2 and α2 antagonist), yohimbine (α2 antagonist), and olanzapine (mixed dopaminergic and serotonergic action) (Michelson et al 2002), and ephedrine (Meston 2004) have all failed to show any significant benefit. In a study of both men and women, the addition of bupropion was no better than placebo in this respect (Masand et al 2001). The one apparently successful reduction of anti-depressant-induced sexual side effects was obtained with sildenafil in men (Nurnberg et al 2003). Improvement in erectile function with sildenafil, when attributable to anti-depressant use, is to be expected; because of its assumed peripheral effect, sildenafil enhances the excitatory arm of the erectile system, whatever factor may have reduced excitation previously. But as considered in Chapter 12, sildenafil has been used effectively in the treatment of premature ejaculation. Although Abdel-Hamid (2004) emphasizes the effect of sildenafil on the smooth muscle contraction in seminal emission, we also have to consider the possibility of central nitrergic effects, plus the recent finding that SSRIs have been demonstrated to reduce the production of NO by NOS (Finkel et al 1996). Limited evidence from three single case studies suggests that PDE-5 inhibitors, in this case tadalafil, may reduce SSRI-induced sexual side effects in women (Ashton & Weinstein 2006) and this warrants further research.

An earlier study evaluating the effects of tricyclics and MAOIs on sexual function was reported by Harrison et al (1985). They studied 36 men and 47 women who were clinically depressed. Each person received imipramine (tricyclic), phenelzine (MAOI) or placebo, in increasing dosage. Decrease in sexual function occurred in 8% of men and 16% of women on placebo, 80% of men and 57% of women on phenelzine and 50% of men and 27% of women on imipramine. For men the differences between active drug and placebo were significant for both anti-depressants; for women, only for phenelzine.

Clomipramine is an interesting anti-depressant that inhibits re-uptake of both serotonin and NA. Everitt (1979) found that the sexuality of female rhesus macaques was 'switched off and on' within 3 days of starting and stopping clomipramine. Once again, the best documented effect of clomipramine is inhibition of ejaculation or inhibition of female orgasm (Segraves 1985), and given the predictable effect of SSRIs on orgasm, it is probably the serotonergic action of clomipramine which is responsible for this.

Anti-psychotic drugs

Dopamine antagonism is generally regarded as the key factor in most anti-psychotics, particularly at the D2 receptor, and mainly in the meso-limbic DA system. However, the meso-limbic system is involved in a range of 'motivated' behaviours, including sexual behaviour. The disordered sexuality which features in the symptoms of acute schizophrenia was considered earlier (see p. 388), but it is of some interest, both clinical and theoretical, to consider the impact of anti-psychotics on the sexuality of men and women with schizophrenia.

The prevalence of sexual dysfunction in patients treated with anti-psychotic medication is reported to be around 60% in men and from 30–90% in women (Smith et al 2002). Recognizing the problems that schizophrenic patients, treated or not, had in engaging in sexual relationships, Smith et al (2002) assessed sexual function in a way that was not relationship dependent. In a comparison with normal controls, sexual interest in those with schizophrenia did not differ, whereas ED and ejaculatory dysfunction in men, and orgasmic dysfunction in women, were significantly more prevalent. However, in the men, ejaculatory problems were much more common than erectile problems. They interpreted the normal levels of sexual interest as possibly resulting from the normalizing effects of the treatment, although they did not speculate on whether this was due to an increase or a reduction of sexual interest to normal levels. They also found some relationship between prolactin levels and problems with sexual arousal (erection in men and vaginal response in women), and sexual interest in women. From this they concluded that the principal sexual side effects of the medication resulted from the drug-induced hyperprolactinaemia. The relevance of increased prolactin was considered closely in Chapter 4, where it was argued that the prolactin level in the blood is a marker of the dopaminergic–serotonergic balance in the tubero-infundibular system, and quite possibly in other dopaminergic systems as well (see p. 92), and is itself an epiphenomenon. However, in comparing different anti-psychotic drugs, it is a useful marker in determining the level of dopamine antagonism.

Knegtering et al (2004) compared the effects of two atypical anti-psychotics, risperidone which produces hyperprolactinaemia and is therefore relatively dopamine antagonistic and quetiapine, which does not raise prolactin. They found fewer sexual side effects with quetiapine. Similar results were reported by Nakonezny et al (2007). In a further study (Knegtering et al 2006), risperidone, an anti-psychotic which increases prolactin levels, was compared with olanzapine, which does not. Less sexual dysfunction was found in the olanzapine group. A reduction in DA activity, which would explain the increased prolactin, could well explain the 'normalization' of sexual interest and impairment of genital response in schizophrenic men and women (see Chapter 4). However, it is less clear why dopamine antagonism would result in suppression of orgasm or ejaculation, which are more frequent sexual side effects. But we should keep in mind the complex dopaminergic–serotoninergic balance, and a shift towards serotonergic dominance would be consistent with orgasmic inhibition.

Butyrophenones (e.g. haloperidol) are anti-psychotics with similar pharmacological effects to phenothiazines, though probably with less anti-adrenergic, anti-histaminic and anti-cholinergic, and more anti-dopaminergic effects. Benperidol is a butyrophenone which is marketed specifically for controlling unwanted sexual behaviour (see Chapter 16, p. 502). In an early controlled study, benperidol was found to reduce self-rated sexual interest more than either chlorpromazine or placebo, though it did not alter the psychophysiological responses to erotic stimuli (Tennent et al 1974).

Other drugs

Anti-convulsants

As described earlier in this chapter, sexual problems, particularly those stemming from lack of interest, are common amongst epileptics. Endocrine effects of anti-convulsants, including phenobarbitone, have been recognized (Penovich 2000). These probably stem mainly from enzyme induction effects in the liver that alter the metabolism of steroids and may lead to increased production of sex hormone-binding globulin. Several studies have shown that raised sex hormone-binding globulin levels are common in epileptics taking most types of anti-convulsants and are usually associated with increased total T as well as luteinizing hormone, sometimes to very high levels (Victor et al 1977; Barragry et al 1978; Toone et al 1980). Phenytoin, for example, may cause hirsutism or acne (Hopkins 2000). However, there is evidence that free testosterone is lowered in some cases, in spite of normal or raised total T, and lack of desire or impairment of sleep erections is related to these low free T levels (Toone et al 1983; Fenwick et al 1986). Carbamazepine, an anti-convulsant which does not have this effect on T levels, appears to be relatively free from such adverse sexual effects (see p. 397).

Digoxin

This cardiac glycoside may produce endocrine changes. Raised levels of oestradiol and lowered levels of T and luteinizing hormone have been reported in men taking digoxin (Stoffer et al 1973; Neri et al 1987). In one study, 14 men on long-term digoxin therapy were compared with 12 men of similar age and cardiac functional capacity. The digoxin users had significantly raised oestradiol and lowered T and luteinizing hormone and also reported significantly greater reduction in sexual interest and sexual activity (Neri et al 1980). This was replicated in a further study (Neri et al 1987).

Cimetidine

This drug is a histamine H2 receptor antagonist which is widely used for the treatment of peptic ulceration. Although sexual side effects are played down in the medical literature, there are several reports of such effects (Crenshaw & Goldberg 1996). The endocrine effects of cimetidine are complex and include anti-androgenic activity and an increase in circulating oestradiol, and gynaecomastia occurs in a proportion of subjects (Riley 1980b). In view of the wide use of this drug, it is important that these possible side effects should be properly studied.

Sexual aspects of alcohol and drug addiction

Alcohol and alcoholism

It is widely believed that alcohol enhances sexual pleasure or at least reduces sexual inhibitions. It is also assumed that alcohol increases the likelihood of sexual risk taking and inappropriate or offensive sexual behaviour. There has been a growing literature on the relations between alcohol and sexuality resulting in an increasingly complex picture (George & Stoner 2000).

In the early phase of this research, a series of studies showed that in men, increasing blood levels of alcohol suppressed erectile response to erotic stimuli (e.g. Briddell & Wilson 1976; Farkas & Rosen 1976; Wilson & Lawson 1976a; Wilson et al 1985) and increased the latency to ejaculation (Malatesta et al 1979). More limited evidence from women showed a comparable suppression of vaginal blood flow to erotic stimuli (Wilson & Lawson 1976b, 1978) and increased latency to orgasm (Malatesta et al 1982). These effects have been somewhat taken for granted since, though some more recent studies have suggested that such alcohol suppression is not universal (George & Stoner 2000).

In the second phase, attention turned to experimental studies of expectancy of alcohol effect. Men who believed that they had been given alcohol in the laboratory, whether or not they had, showed greater erectile response and subjective arousal to erotic stimuli. Furthermore, such expectancy also increased the arousal response to deviant stimuli, such as rape scenes.

The impact of expectancy in women has been less well studied, although the straightforward expectancy effects observed in men are less evident in women. An interesting dissociation between subjective arousal and vaginal response was reported by Wilson & Lawson (1976b); increasing blood levels of alcohol in women were associated with increasing subjective arousal but decreasing vaginal blood flow response. This may be a further example of such dissociation between subjective and vaginal response, which has now been identified in a number of ways, and was discussed more closely in Chapter 4 (p. 79).

More recently attention has been paid to the effects of alcohol on cognitive processing. This has been described by Steele & Josephs (1990) as 'alcohol myopia', in which, as a result of the alcohol, attention is focused on the positive, sexually arousing or rewarding aspects of the situation and turned away from appraisal of negative consequences and associated inhibition of arousal. 'Alcohol myopia' is considered as comparable to the impact of sexual arousal on sexual risk taking in Chapter 14 (p. 432). However, the relevance of alcohol to sexual risk taking is not straightforward. In a review of the relevant event-based literature on condom use, as a marker of sexual risk taking, Weinhardt & Carey (2000) concluded that people who use condoms when they are sober tend to use them when they have taken alcohol, and that those who fail to use condoms when drinking, probably also fail to use them when sober. They were not able to reach the same conclusion in relation to other aspects of sexual risk taking (e.g. 'riskiness' of the partner). The implication of their conclusion, particularly for adolescents, is that sexual risk taking is more likely in those who use alcohol (see Chapter 14), as are other 'maladaptive' behaviours (see Chapter 5), but is not a direct consequence of the alcohol. A comparable conclusion, specifically for women, was reached by Beckman & Ackerman (1995).

Chronic alcoholism

Although it is commonly assumed that chronic alcoholics have a high incidence of sexual problems, good evidence to support this is hard to find. The relationship between chronic alcoholism and sexuality is complex. The reasons for abusing alcohol in the first place may be important. In some cases, alcohol is used to cope with socio-sexual anxieties in people who are prone to develop sexual problems for personality reasons. What proportion of alcoholics comes into this category is not known and not easy to establish. The consequences of alcoholism on sexual relationships and marriage are likely to be considerable. Not only may marital and sexual conflict result from heavy drinking, but the development of such conflict will have an adverse effect on the subsequent drinking pattern (Orford et al 1976); alcoholics often drink to cope with the problems produced by their alcoholism. The sexual relationship is bound to suffer in many such cases and marital breakdown is high amongst alcoholics.

Against this background of psychological and interpersonal complexity, we need to consider not only the direct effects of alcohol intoxication on sexual function, but also the more long-term toxic effects of alcohol on the nervous system, liver and endocrine system and their sexual consequences. Neurological conditions such as Wernicke's encephalopathy, Korsakoff syndrome (a form of dementia), alcoholic cerebellar degeneration, autonomic and peripheral neuropathy have been associated with chronic alcoholism (Bruce &

Ritson 1998; Peters 2000). But their prevalence is not well established and it is reasonable to assume that they are rare complications of alcoholism. Liver damage is also considered to be common. According to James (2000) 10–30% of severe chronic alcoholics develop cirrhosis of the liver, although well over 50% have fatty livers. Individual susceptibility, as James (2000) points out, depends on many factors. The earlier literature, reviewed by Van Thiel & Lester (1979), indicated negative effects of alcohol abuse on testicular function, with hypogonadism being a possible consequence, and ovarian atrophy being commonly found at autopsy in the female alcoholic. Female alcoholics may have reduced fertility, and an alteration in the transport and metabolism of oestradiol that is not well understood (Gill 2000; Barbieri 2004).

Male chronic alcoholics were tested by Wilson et al (1978) and were found to show the same susceptibility to erectile failure at higher blood levels of alcohol as non-alcoholics. Tolerance, therefore, does not apparently protect against these negative effects.

Studies comparing ex-alcoholics with non-alcoholic controls have presented a less negative picture. Schiavi et al (1995) compared 20 male alcoholics who had abstained from alcohol for a median of 18 months (range 2–36 months), and their partners, with 20 healthy non-alcoholic controls and their partners. There were no significant differences from the control group in any measure of sexual function, including NPT, although the partners of the ex-alcoholics reported more dissatisfaction with their relationships. Fifteen of the ex-alcoholics reported no sexual problems, three low sexual desire and two erectile problems. Of the five men with problems, four reported that the problem had started since abstaining from alcohol. There were no differences in total or bio-available testosterone or prolactin between the two groups, although the ex-alcoholics showed an increase in LH in the early morning that was not found in the controls. The ex-alcoholics did show significantly more periodic leg movements during sleep, but the neurological significance of this remains uncertain.

In a comparative study of 45 male chronic alcoholics who were still drinking, and 30 non-alcoholic controls, Gumus et al (1998) found the alcoholics to be more likely to lose erections during vaginal intercourse, but did not differ from controls in any other measure of sexual function. They did not differ in testosterone, SHBG or LH levels, but did show significantly higher FSH.

Heiser & Hartmann (1987) compared 55 alcoholic and 54 non-alcoholic women. The alcoholics reported more stressful and conflicted relationships and less sexual desire. It is difficult to conclude to what extent such problems could be a direct rather than indirect effect of the alcoholism.

Although limited, these comparative findings suggest that, except in those with significant hepatic or CNS damage, who were excluded from these two studies, alcoholism does not cause irreversible damage to sexual function in men, and the relevance of the limited endocrine effects are as yet uncertain.

Drugs of addiction

Although the drugs in this category have very varied pharmacological effects, they are considered in this one section because of the lack of clear evidence of their effects and the 'alcohol-like' complex of psycho-social factors, which they all share, which serve to obscure the more direct pharmacological effects. In addition, in contrast with alcohol, the illegal status of these other drugs effectively prevents the controlled experimental evaluation of their effects that we have seen with alcohol, and also means that we are largely dependent on retrospective reports of ex-addicts.

Opiates

The most consistent picture involves the opiates, in particular morphine and heroin. Here the evidence consistently shows a reduction in sexual interest and response (see Pfaus & Gorzalka 1987), with the 'rush' produced by the drug particularly comparing favourably with the pleasure of orgasm (see Chapter 4, p. 89 for further discussion of this comparison). The negative sexual effects are further evident from the often rapid return of sexual interest and response that follows drug withdrawal.

Evidence of endocrine effects of opiate addiction is somewhat conflicting. Some studies have found lowered plasma testosterone and gonadotrophin levels, whilst others have found no such effect (Kolodny et al 1979). Carani et al (1986) reported low free T in young male heroin addicts that could contribute to the loss of sexual desire. In women, amenorrhoea and infertility have been reported as common (Bai et al 1974; Santen et al 1975).

Cocaine

Cocaine is a re-uptake inhibitor of NA and 5HT but most powerfully of DA, an effect which has been demonstrated in the meso-limbic DA system (see Chapter 4, p. 90).

It has a complicated and unusual pharmacological action, combining local anaesthetic and central stimulant properties. Given the three principal neurotransmitter effects, this is not surprising. Increased central NA activity may have a generally arousing effect, assumed to be the basis for the increased mental activity, restlessness and euphoria that cocaine produces. A dopaminergic effect may be involved in pleasure and genital response; a serotonergic effect with inhibition of orgasm and possibly other components of sexual arousal. However, the effects of drugs with relatively single, specific neurotransmitter action are difficult enough to predict because of the variety of mechanisms in which neurotransmitters are involved. Here, that problem is increased at least threefold. We also have to take into account the potential for curvilinear dose–response effects, which were considered in relation to NA in Chapter 4 (see p. 67); low doses producing one effect, high doses the opposite. This might be relevant to the reported tendency for cocaine to have positive sexual effects particularly with early use but negative effects with chronic use, which would be expected to involve some degree of tolerance (Rosen 1991).

Marijuana

Marijuana is commonly regarded as a sexually enhancing drug. The definite association between marijuana use and early onset of sexual activity amongst young people (Goode 1972; Plant 1975), as with alcohol use, is likely to reflect some common determinant, such as a more liberal attitude, than any causal link between the two. As with alcohol, many marijuana users see the drug as enhancing their sexual experiences. In an early *Psychology Today* survey (Athanosiou et al 1970), about 25% of the total sample had experienced intercourse under the influence of marijuana and four-fifths of these reported increased enjoyment. Plant (1975) concluded from his interviews of English drug takers that the main effect reported was a reduction of inhibition. Kolodny et al (1979) reported that of the marijuana users seen at their institute, 83% of men and 81% of women experienced enhanced sexual enjoyment. However, the positive effects described were not increased desire or improved erections or orgasm, but rather 'an increased sense of touch, a greater degree of relaxation (both physically and mentally) and being more in tune with one's partner'. Also, if their partner was not 'high' at the same time, the effect was if anything unpleasant or disruptive. They also found a relatively high incidence of erectile problems (20%) in men using marijuana on a daily basis. Here again we see suggestion of a change of effect from early to chronic use.

On balance, evidence of a pharmacological enhancing effect on sexuality is lacking (Taberner 1985). Long-term adverse effects on sexual function may be related to endocrine changes. Although there is some contradictory evidence, Kolodny et al (1979) reviewed several studies showing lowered testosterone and inhibited spermatogenesis in men and lowered gonadotrophins and altered menstrual cycles in women using marijuana.

Amphetamine and related drugs

The effects of amphetamine addiction on sexuality are not clear. Amphetamine is dopaminergic, but it remains uncertain to what extent its 'sexually enhancing' effect is related to a less specific activation effect rather than a more specific DA effect.

REFERENCES

Abdel-Hamid IA 2004 Phosphodiesterase 5 inhibitors in rapid ejaculation: potential use and possible mechanisms of action. Drug 64: 13–26.

Alexander CL, Sipski ML, Findley TW 1993 Sexual activities, desire and satisfaction in males pre- and post-spinal cord injury. Archives of Sexual Behavior 22: 217–228.

American Cancer Society 2006 What are the key statistics for breast cancer? http://www.cancer.org/docroot/CRI/content/CRI_2_4_1X_What_are _the_key_statistics_for_breast_cancer_5.asp.

Andersen BC 1984 Psychological aspects of gynaecological cancer. In Broome A,Wallace L (eds) Psychology and Gynaecological Problems. Tavistock, London, pp 117–141.

Angst J 1998 Sexual problems in healthy and depressed persons. International Clinical Psychopharmacology 13(Suppl 6): S1–S4.

Araujo AB, Durante R, Feldman HA, Goldstein I, McKinlay JB 1998 The relationship between depressive symptoms and male erectile dysfunction: cross-sectional results from the Massachusetts Male Aging Study. Psychosomatic Medicine 60: 458–465.

Ashton AK, Weinstein W 2006 Tadalafil reversal of sexual dysfunction caused by serotonin enhancing medications in women. Journal of Sex and Marital Therapy 32: 1–4.

Athanosiou R, Shaver P, Tavris C 1970 Sex. Psychology Today 4: 39–52.

Bai J, Greenwald E, Caterini H, Kaminetzky HA 1974 Drug-related menstrual aberrations. Obstetrics and Gynecology 44: 713–719.

Bancroft J 2007 Discussion paper. In Janssen E (ed) Sexual Psychophysiology. Indiana University Press, Bloomington, pp. 57–60.

Bancroft J, Bell C 1985 Simultaneous recording of penile diameter and penile arterial pulse during laboratory based erotic stimulation in normal subjects. Journal of Psychosomatic Research 29: 303–313.

Bancroft J, Smith G 1987 Penile diameter and pulse amplitude change before and after intracavernosal injection of smooth muscle relaxants in men with erectile dysfunction. Paper presented at 13th Annual meeting. International Academy of Sex Research, Tutzing, Germany.

Bancroft J, Bell C, Ewing DJ, McCulloch DK, Warner P, Clarke B 1985 Assessment of erectile function in diabetic and non-diabetic impotence by simultaneous recording of penile diameter and penile arterial pulse. Journal of Psychosomatic Research 29: 315–324.

Barak Y, Achiron A, Elizur A, Gabbay U, Noy S, Sarova-Pinhas I 1996 Sexual dysfunction in relapsing-remitting multiple sclerosis: magnetic resonance imaging, clinical and psychological correlates. Journal of Psychiatry and Neuroscience 21: 255–258.

Barbieri RL 2004 Female infertility. In Strauss III JF, Barbieri RL (eds) Yen and Jaffe's Reproductive Endocrinology, 5th edn. Elsevier Saunders, Philadelphia, pp. 633–668.

Barragry JM, Makin HLJ, Trafford DJH, Scott DF 1978 Effects of anticonvulsants on plasma testosterone and sex-hormone-binding globulin levels. Journal of Neurology, Neurosurgery and Psychiatry 41: 913–914.

Barrat-Connor E, Khaw K-T, Yen SSC 1990 Endogenous sex hormone levels in older adult men with diabetes mellitus. American Journal of Epidemiology 132: 895–901.

Beck AT 1967 Depression. Clinical, Experimental and Theoretical Aspects. Staples Press: London.

Beckman LJ, Ackerman KT 1995 Women, alcohol, and sexuality. Recent developments in Alcoholism 12: 267–285.

Beral V 2000 Cervical cancer and other cancers caused by sexually transmitted infections. In Ledingham JGG, Warrell DA (eds) Concise Oxford Textbook of Medicine. Oxford University Press, Oxford, pp. 1853–1854.

Berger S 1951 The role of sexual impotence in the concept of self of male paraplegics. Dissertation Abstracts International, p. 12.

Bergeron S, Binik YM, Khalife S, Pagidas K, Glazer H 2001 A randomized comparison of group cognitive-behavioral therapy, surface electromyographiuc biofeedback, and vestibulectomy in the treatment of dyspareunia resulting from vulvar vestibulitis. Pain 91: 297–306.

Betancourt-Allbrecht M, Cunningham GR 2003 Hypogonadism and diabetes. International Journal of Impotence Research 15 (Suppl 4): S14–S20.

Binik YM 2005 Should dyspareunia be retained as a sexual dysfunction in DSM-V? A painful classification decision. Archives of Sexual Behavior 34: 11–22.

Bleuler M 1978 The Schizophrenic Disorders. Long-term Patient and Family Studies. Yale University Press, New Haven, CT.

Blumer D 1970 Hypersexual episodes in temporal lobe epilepsy. American Journal of Psychiatry 126: 1099–1106.

Bors E, Comarr AE 1960 Neurological disturbances of sexual function with special reference to 529 patients with spinal cord injury. Urological Survey 10: 191–222.

Bradford A, Meston CM 2006 Hysterectomy and alternative therapies. In Goldstein I, Meston CM, Davis SR, Traish A (eds) Women's Sexual Function and Dysfunction: Study, Diagnosis and Treatment. Taylor & Francis, London, pp. 658–665.

Briddell DW, Wilson GT 1976 The effects of alcohol and expectancy set on male sexual arousal. Journal of Abnormal Psychology 35: 225–234.

Brindley GS 1982 Sexual function and fertility in paraplegic men. In: Hargreave T (ed) Male Infertility. Springer Verlag, Berlin.

Bronner G, Royter V, Korczyn AD, Giladi N 2004 Sexual dysfunction in Parkinson's disease. Journal of Sex and Marital Therapy 30: 95–105.

Bruce M, Ritson B 1998 Substance misuse. In Johnstone ECV, Freeman CPL, Zealley AK (eds) Companion to Psychiatric Studies. Churchill Livingstone, Edinburgh, pp. 329–368.

Buckley PF, Hyde J, Winterich D, Friedman L, Donenwirth K 1997 Sexuality and schizophrenia: behavioral patterns and clinical correlates. Schizophrenia Research 24: 11.

Bulpitt CJ, Dollery C T 1973 Side effects of hypotensive agents evaluated by a self-administered questionnaire. British Medical Journal 3: 485–490.

Bulpitt CJ, Dollery CT, Carne S 1976 Change in symptoms of hypertensive patients after referral to hospital clinics. British Heart Journal 38: 121–128.

Burchardt M, Burchardt T, Anastasiadis AG, Kiss AJ, Baer L, Pawar RV, de la Taille A, Shabisgh A, Ghafar MA, Shabsigh R 2002 Sexual dysfunction is common and overlooked in female patients with hypertension. Journal of Sex and Marital Therapy 28: 17–26.

Burnfield P 1979 Sexual problems and multiple sclerosis. British Journal of Sexual Medicine 6: 33–38.

Buvat J, Lemaire A, Buvat-Herbaut M, Guien J 1985 Comparative investigation of 26 impotent and 26 non-impotent diabetic patients. Journal of Urology 133: 34–38.

Carani C, Zinin D, Caricchioli F et al 1986 Effects of heroin addiction on the endocrine control of sexual function in young men. In Kothari P (ed) Proceedings of the Seventh World Congress of Sexology. IASECT, Bombay, pp. 160–163.

Cassidy WL, Flanagan NB, Spellman M, Cohen ME 1957 Clinical observations in manic depressive disease. Journal of the American Medical Association 164: 1535–1546.

CDC Center for Disease Control 2005 National Diabetes Surveillance System. www.cdc.gov/diabetes/statistics.

Christ GJ, Schwartz CB, Stone BA, Parker M, Janis M, Gondre M, Valcic M, Melman A 1992 Kinetic characteristics of alpha-1 adrenergic contractions in human corpus cavernosum smooth muscle. American Journal of Physiology 263: H15–H19.

Chun J, Richman M, Carson III CC 2001 Peyronie's Disease: history and medical therapy. In Mulcahy JJ (ed) Male Sexual Function: A Guide to Clinical Management. Humana, Totowa, NJ, pp. 307–320.

Clayton PJ, Pitts FN Jr, Winokur G 1965 Affective disorders. IV. Mania. Comprehensive Psychiatry 6: 313–322.

Coderre TJ, Katz J, Vaccarino AL, Melzack R 1993 Contribution of central neuroplasticity to pathological pain: a review of clinical and experimental evidence. Pain 52: 259–285.

Cole T M 1975 Sexuality and physical disabilities. Archives of Sexual Behavior 4: 389–401.

Connolly FH, Gittleson NL 1971 The relationship between delusions of sexual change and olfactory and gustatory hallucinations in schizophrenia. British Journal of Psychiatry 119: 443–444.

Coulter A, Bradlow J, Agass M, Martin-Bases C, Tulloch A 1991 Outcomes of referrals to gynaecologic outpatient clinics for menstrual problems: an audit of general practice records. British Journal of Obstetrics and Gynaecology 98: 789–796.

Craft A (ed) 1994 Practice Issues in Sexuality and Learning Disabilities. Routledge, London.

Craft M, Craft A 1978 Sex and the Mentally Handicapped. Routledge & Kegan Paul, London.

Crenshaw TL, Goldberg JP 1996 Sexual Pharmacology: Drugs that Affect Sexual Functioning. Norton, New York.

Croft H, Settle E, Houser T, Batey SR, Donahue RMJ, Ascher JA 1999 A placebo-controlled comparison of the antidepressant efficacy and effects on sexual functioning of sustained-release bupropion and sertraline. Clinical Therapeutics 21: 643–658.

Croog SH, Levine S, Testa MA, Brown B, Bulpitt CJ, Jenkins CD, Klerman G, Williams GH 1986 The effects of antihypertensive therapy on quality of life. New England Journal of Medicine 314: 1657–1664.

Cyranowski JM, Bromberger J, Youk A, Matthews K, Kravitz HM, Powell LH 2004 Lifetime depression history and sexual function in women at midlife. Archives of Sexual Behavior 33: 539–548.

Dhabuwala CB, Kumar A, Pierce JM 1986 Myocardial infarction and its influence on male sexual function. Archives of Sexual Behavior 15: 499–504.

Dhindsa S, Prabhakar S, Sethi M, Bandyopadhyay A, Chaudhuri A, Dandona P 2004 Frequent occurrence of hypogonadotropic hypogonadism in type-2 diabetes. Journal of Clinical Endocrinology and Metabolism 89: 5462–5468.

Ebrahim S, May M, Ben Shiomo Y, McCorron P, Frankel S, Yamell J, Davey Smith G 2002 Sexual intercourse and risk of ischaemic stroke and coronary heart disease: the Caerphilly study. Journal of Epidemiology and Community Health 56: 99–102.

Ellenberg M 1971 Impotence in diabetes: the neurological factor. Annals of Internal Medicine 75: 213–219.

Ellenberg M 1977 Sexual aspects of the female diabetic. Mount Sinai Journal of Medicine 44: 495–500.

Elliott SL, Krassioukov A 2005 Malignant autonomic dysreflexia following ejaculation in spinal cord injured men. Spinal Cord, Retrieved May 15, 2006, from www.nature.com/sc/journal/vaop/ncurrent/abs/3101847a.html.

Engel J, Kerr J, Schlesinger-Raab A, Sauer H, Holzel D 2004 Quality of life following breast-conserving therapy or mastectomy: results of a 5 year prospective study. The Breast Journal 10: 223–231.

Enzlin P, Mathieu C, Van den Bruel, A, Bosteels J, Vandershueren D, Demyttenaere K 2002 Sexual dysfunction in women with Type 1 diabetes: a controlled study. Diabetes Care 25: 672–677.

Everitt B J 1979 Monoamines and sexual behaviour in non-human primates. In Sex, Hormones and Behaviour. Ciba Foundation Symposium 62 (New Series). Excerpta Medica, Amsterdam, pp. 329–348.

Faerman I, Glocer L, Fox D, Jadzinsky MN, Rapaport M 1974 Impotence and diabetes. Histological studies of the autonomic nervous fibres of the corpora cavernosa in impotent diabetic males. Diabetes 23: 971–976.

Fairburn CG, Wu FCW, McCulloch DK, Borsay DQ, Ewing DJ, Clarke BF, Bancroft J 1982 The clinical features of diabetic impotence: a preliminary study. British Journal of Psychiatry 140: 447–452.

Farkas GM, Rosen RC 1976 The effect of alcohol on elicited male sexual response. Journal of Studies of Alcohol 37: 265–272.

Farquhar CM, Steiner CA 2002 Hysterectomy rates in the United States 1990–1997. Obstetrics and Gynecology 99: 229–234.

Fenwick PBC, Mercer S, Grant R, Wheeler M, Nanjee N, Toone B, Brown D 1986 Nocturnal penile tumescence and serum testosterone levels. Archives of Sexual Behavior 15: 13–22.

Figueira I, Possidente E, Marques C, Hayes K 2001 Sexual dysfunction: a neglected complication of panic disorder and social phobia. Archives of Sexual Behavior 30: 369–377.

Finkel MS, Laghrissi-Thode F, Pollock BG, Rong J 1996 Paroxetine is a novel nitric oxide synthase inhibitor. Psychopharmacology Bulletin 32: 653–658.

Fitting MD, Salisbury S, Davies NH, Mayclin DK 1978 Self concept and sexuality of spinal cord injured women. Archives of Sexual Behavior 7: 143–156.

Francis WH, Jeffcoate TNA 1961 Dyspareunia following vaginal operations. Journal of Obstetrics and Gynaecology of the British Commonwealth 68: 1–10.

Franks S, Jacobs HS 1983 Hyperprolactinaemia. Clinics in Endocrinology and Metabolism 12: 641–668.

Friedman S, Harrison G 1984 Sexual histories, attitudes and behavior of schizophrenic and 'normal' women. Archives of Sexual Behavior 13: 555–568.

Friedrich EG 1987 Vulvar vestibulitis syndrome. Journal of Reproductive Medicine 32: 110–114.

Gastaut H, Collomb H 1954 Etude du comportement sexuel chez les épileptiques psychomoteurs. Annals Medico-Psychologigues 112: 657–696.

Gebhard PH 1973 Sexual behavior of the mentally retarded. In de la Cruz FF, La Veck GD (eds) Human Sexuality and the Mentally Retarded. Brunner-Mazel, New York, pp. 29–49.

Gebhard P, Gagnon J, Pomeroy N, Christenson C 1965 Sex Offenders. Harper Row, New York.

George WH, Stoner SA 2000 Understanding acute alcohol effects on sexual behavior. Annual Review of Sex Research 11: 92–124.

Ghezzi A 1999 Sexuality and multiple sclerosis. Scandinavian Journal of Sexology 2: 125–140.

Gill J 2000 The effects of moderate alcohol consumption on female hormone levels and reproductive function. Alcohol and Alcoholism 35: 417–423.

Gittleson NL, Levine S 1966 Subjective ideas of sexual change in male schizophrenics. British Journal of Psychiatry 112: 779–782.

Gittleson NL, Dawson-Butterworth K 1967 Subjective ideas of sexual change in female schizophrenics. British Journal of Psychiatry 113: 491–494.

Goode E 1972 Drug use and sexual activity on a college campus. American Journal of Psychiatry 128: 1272–1276.

Graziottin TM, Resplande J, Lue T 2001 Surgical treatment of Peyronie's Disease. In Mulcahy JJ (ed) Male Sexual Function: A Guide to Clinical Management. Humana, Totowa NJ, pp. 321–334.

Gregorian RS Jr, Golden KA, Bahce A, Goodman C, Kwong WJ, Khan ZM 2002 Antidepressant-induced sexual dysfunction. Annals of Pharmacotherapy 36: 1577–1589.

Griffith E, Trieschmann RB 1975 Sexual functioning in women with spinal cord injury. Archives of Physical Medicine and Rehabilitation 56: 18–21.

Gumus B, Yigitoglu M, Lekili M, Uyanik B, Muezzinoglu TC 1998 Effect of long-term alcohol abuse on male sexual function and serum gonadal hormone levels. International Urology and Nephrology 30: 755–759.

Hall JE 1975 Sexuality and the mentally retarded. In Green R (ed.) Human Sexuality. A Health Practitioner's Text. Williams & Wilkins, Baltimore, pp. 181–195.

Hanon O, Mounier-Vehier C, Fauvel JP et al 2002 Sexual dysfunction in treated hypertensive patients. Results of a national survey. Cited in Salonia et al 2006.

Harrison WM, Stewart J, Ehrhardt AA, Rabkin J, McGrath P, Liebowitz M, Quitkin FM 1985 A controlled study of the effects of antidepressants on sexual function. Psychopharmacological Bulletin 21: 85–98.

Heiser K, Hartmann U 1987 Disorders of sexual desire in a sample of women alcoholics. Drug and Alcohol Dependency 19: 145–157.

Hellerstein HK, Friedman EH 1970 Sexual activity and the post-coronary patient. Archives of Internal Medicine 125: 987–999.

Herzog AG, Seibel MM, Schomer DL, Vaitukaitis JL, Geschwind N 1986a Reproductive endocrine disorders in women with partial seizures of temporal lobe origin. Archives of Neurology 43: 341–346.

Herzog AG, Seibel MM, Schomer DL, Vaitukaitis JL, Geschwind N 1986b Reproductive endocrine disorders in men with partial seizures of temporal lobe origin. Archives of Neurology 43: 347–350.

Higgins GE 1979 Sexual response in spinal cord injured adults: a review. Archives of Sexual Behavior 8: 173–196.

Hirshkowitz M, Karacan I, Rando KC, Williams RL, Howell JW 1990 Diabetes, erectile dysfunction, and sleep-related erections. Sleep 13: 53–68.

Hoenig J, Hamilton CM 1960 Epilepsy and sexual orgasm. Acta Psychiatrica Neurologica Scandinavica 35: 449–456.

Hopkins AP 2000 Epilepsy in later childhood and adult life. In Ledingham JGG, Warrell DA (eds) Concise Oxford Textbook of Medicine. Oxford University Press, Oxford, pp. 1274–1282.

James OFW 2000 Alcoholi liver disease and non-alcoholic steatosis hepatitis. In Ledingham JGG, Warrell DA (eds) Concise Oxford Textbook of Medicine. Oxford University Press, Oxford, pp. 628–630.

Jensen SB 1981 Diabetic sexual function: a comparative study of 160 insulin treated diabetic men and women and an age-matched control group. Archives of Sexual Behavior 10: 493–504.

Jensen SB 1985 Sexual relationships in couples with a diabetic partner. Journal of Sexual and Marital Therapy 11: 259–270.

Jensen SB 1986 Sexual dysfunction in insulin treated diabetics: a 6 year follow up study of 101 patients. Archives of Sexual Behavior 15: 271–284.

Jensen P, Jensen SB, Sorensen PS, Bjerre BD, Rizzi DA, Sorensen AS, Klysner R, Brinch K, Jespersen B, Nielsen H 1990 Sexual dysfunction in male and female patients with epilepsy: a study of 86 outpatients. Archives of Sexual Behavior 19: 1–14.

Kelly DL, Conley RR 2004 Sexuality and schizophrenia: a review. Schizophrenia Bulletin 30: 767–779.

Kennedy SH, Dickens SE, Eisfeld BS, Bagby RM 1999 Sexual dysfunction before antidepressant therapy in major depression. Journal of Affective Disorders 56: 201–208.

Kinsey AC, Pomeroy WB, Martin CF 1948 Sexual Behavior in the Human Male. Saunders, Philadelphia.

Kinsey AC, Pomeroy WB, Martin CE, Gebhard PH 1953 Sexual Behavior in the Human Female. Saunders, Philadelphia.

Klebanow D, MacLeod J 1960 Semen quality and certain disturbances of reproduction in diabetic men. Fertility and Sterility 11: 255–261.

Knegtering R, Castelein S, Bous H, Van Der Linde J, Bruggeman R, Kluiter H, van den Bosch RJ 2004 A randomized open-label study of the impact of quetiapine versus risperidone on sexual functioning. Journal of Clinical Psychopharmacology 24: 56–61.

Knegtering R, Boks M, Blijd C, Castelein S, van den Bosch RJ, Wiersma D 2006 A randomized open-label comparison of the impact of olanzapine versus risperidone on sexual functioning. Journal of Sex and Marital Therapy 32: 315–326.

Kolarsky A, Freund K, Machek J 1967 Male sexual deviation: association with early temporal lobe damage. Archives of General Psychiatry 17: 735–743.

Koller WC, Vetere-Overfield B, Williamson A, Busenbark K, Nash J, Parrish D 1990 Sexual dysfunction in Parkinson's Disease. Clinical Neuropharmacology 13: 461–463.

Kolodny RC 1971 Sexual dysfunction in diabetic females. Diabetes 20: 557–559.

Kolodny RC, Masters WH, Johnson VE 1979 Textbook of Sexual Medicine. Little, Brown, Boston.

Komisaruk BR, Gerdes C, Whipple B 1997 'Complete' spinal cord injury does not block perceptual responses to genital self-stimulation in women. Archives of Neurology 54: 1513–1520.

Komisaruk BR, Beyer-Flores C, Whipple B 2006 The Science of Orgasm. Johns Hopkins University Press, Baltimore.

Larson JL, McNaughton MW, Ward Kennedy J, Mansfield LW 1980 Heart rate and blood pressure response to sexual activity and a stair climbing test. Heart and Lung 9: 1025–1030.

Lilius HG, Valtonen FJ, Davis FA 1976 Sexual problems in patients suffering from multiple sclerosis. Journal of Chronic Diseases 29: 65–73.

Lilleleht E, Leiblum SR 1993 Schizophrenia and sexuality: a critical review of the literature. Annual Review of Sex Research 4: 247–276.

Lincoln J, Crowe R, Blackley PF, Pryor J 1987 Changes in VIPergic, cholinergic and adrenergic innovation of human penile tissue in diabetic and non-diabetic impotent males. Journal of Urology 137: 1053–1059.

Lindner H 1953 Perceptual sensitisation to sexual phenomena in the chronically physically disabled. Journal of Clinical Psychology 9: 67–68.

Lobel B, Rodriguez A 2003 Chronic prostatitis: what we know, what we do not know, and what we should do! World Journal of Urology 21: 57–63.

Lorrain DS, Matuszewich L, Friedman R, Hull EM 1997 Extracellular serotonin in the lateral hypothalamic area increases during post-ejaculatory interval and impairs copulation in male rats. Journal of Neuroscience 17: 9361–9366.

Lundberg PO 1977 Sexual dysfunction in patients with neurological disorders. In Gemme R, Wheeler CC (eds) Progress in Sexology. Plenum, New York.

Lundberg PO 1980 Sexual dysfunction in women with multiple sclerosis. In Forleo R, Pasini W (eds) Medical Sexology. Elsevier/North Holland, Amsterdam.

Lundberg PO 1992 Sexual dysfunction in patients with neurological disorders. Annual Review of Sex Research 3: 121–150.

Lundberg PO 2006 Neurologic disorders: female neurosexology. In Goldstein I, Meston CM, Davis SR, Traish A (eds) Women's Sexual Function and Dysfunction: Study, Diagnosis and Treatment. Taylor & Francis, London, pp. 650–657.

Maas CP, Weijenborg PTM, ter Kuile MM 2003 The effect of hysterectomy on sexual functioning. Annual Review of Sex Research 14: 83–113.

Malatesta VJ, Pollack RH, Wilbanks WA, Adams HE 1979 Alcohol effects on the orgasmic–ejaculatory response in human males. Journal of Sex Research 15: 101–107.

Malatesta VJ, Pollack RH, Crotty TD, Peacock LJ 1982 Acute alcoholic intoxication and female orgasmic response. Journal of Sex Research 18: 1–17.

Marsden CD 2000 Movement disorders. In Ledingham JGG, Warrell DA (eds) Concise Oxford Textbook of Medicine. Oxford University Press, Oxford, pp. 1320–1332.

Masand PS, Ashton AK, Grupa S, Frank B 2001 Sustained-release bupropion for selective serotonin reuptake inhibitor-induced sexual dysfunction: a randomized, placebo-controlled study of pharmacologic intervention. American Journal of Psychiatry 157: 239–243.

Mathew RJ, Weinman ML 1982 Sexual dysfunction in depression. Archives of Sexual Behavior 11: 323–328.

Mattinson J 1975 Marriage and Mental Handicap, 2nd edn. Tavistock, London.

McCabe MP, McDonald E, Deeks AA, Vowels LM, Conain MJ 1996 The impact of multiple sclerosis on sexuality and relationships. Journal of Sex Research 33: 241–256.

McCulloch DK, Campbell IW, Wu FC, Prescott RJ, Clarke BF 1980 The prevalence of diabetic impotence. Diabetologia 18: 279–283.

McCulloch DK, Young RJ, Prescott RJ, Campbell IW, Clarke BF 1984 The natural history of impotence in diabetic men. Diabetologia 26: 437–440.

McKay M 1993 Dysesthetic ('essential') vulvodynia. Treatment with amitryptiline. Journal of Reproductive Medicine 38: 9–13.

Mease P 2005 Fibromyalgia syndrome: a review of clinical presentation, pathogenesis, outcome measures, and treatment. Journal of Rheumatology Supplement, August, 75: 6–21.

Meston CM 2004 A randomized, placebo-controlled, crossover study of ephedrine for SSRI-induced female sexual dysfunction. Journal of Sex and Marital Therapy 30: 57–68.

Michelson D, Bancroft J, Targum S, Yongman K, Tepner R 2000 Female sexual dysfunction associated with antidepressant administration: a randomized, placebo-controlled study of pharmacologic intervention. American Journal of Psychiatry 157: 239–243.

Michelson D, Kociban K, Tamura R, Morrison MF 2002 Mirtazapine, yohimbine or olansapine augmentation therapy for serotonin reuptake-associated female sexual dysfunction: a randomized, placebo controlled trial. Journal of Psychiatric Research 36: 147–152.

Mickley H 2002 Incidence and treatment of sexual dysfunction in heart disease. Cited in Sumanen et al 2005.

Mitchell W, Falconer MA, Hill D 1954 Epilepsy fetishism relieved by temporal lobectomy. Lancet 2: 626–630.

Modell JG, Katholi CR, Modell JD, DePalma RL 1997 Comparative sexual side effects of bupropion, fluoxetine, paroxetine, and sertraline. Clinical Pharmacology and Therapeutics 61: 476–487.

Money J, Pruce G 1977 Psychomotor epilepsy and sexual function. In Money J, Musaph H (eds) Handbook of Sexology. Excerpta Medica, Amsterdam, pp. 969–977.

Money J, Yankowitz R 1967 The sympathetic inhibiting effects of the drug Ismelin on human male eroticism, with a note on Melleril. Journal of Sex Research 3: 69–82.

Monteiro WO, Noshirvani HF, Marks IM, Leliott PT 1987 Anorgasmia from clomipramine in obsessive compulsive disorder: a controlled trial. British Journal of Psychiatry 151: 107–112.

Montgomery SA, Baldwin DS, Riley A 2002 Antidepressant medications: a review of the evidence for drug-induced sexual dysfunction. Journal of Affective Disorders 69: 119–140.

Morell MJ, Guldner GT 1996 Self-reported sexual function and sexual arousability in women with epilepsy. Epilepsia 37: 1204–1210.

MRC 1981 The Medical Research Council Working Report on Mild to Moderate Hypertension. Adverse reactions to bendroflumethiazide and propanolol for the treatment of mild hypertension. Lancet ii: 539–543.

Mulcahy JJ, Austoni E, Barada JH, Ki Choi H, Hellstrom WJG, Krisnamurti S, Moncada I, Schulteiss D, Wessells H 2004 Implants, mechanical devices and vascular surgery for erectile dysfunction. In Lue TF, Basson R, Rosen R, Giuliano F, Khoury S, Montorsi F (eds) Sexual Medicine: Sexual Dysfunctions in Men and Women. Health Publications 2002, Paris, pp. 469–502.

Nakonezny PA, Byerly MJ, Rush AJ 2007 The relationship between serum prolactin level and sexual functioning among male outpatients with schizophrenia or schizoaffective disorder: a randomized double-blind trial of risperidone vs. quetiapine. Journal of Sex and Marital Therapy 33: 203–216.

Neri A, Aygen M, Zukerman Z, Bahary C 1980 Subjective assessment of sexual dysfunction of patients on long-term administration of digoxin. Archives of Sexual Behavior 9: 343–347.

Neri A, Zukerman Z, Aygen M, Lidor Y, Kaufman H 1987 The effect of long term administration of digoxin on plasma androgen and sexual dysfunction. Journal of Sexual and Marital Therapy 13: 58–63.

Newman AS, Bertelson AD 1986 Sexual dysfunction in diabetic women. Journal of Behavioral Medicine 9: 261–270.

Nofzinger EA, Reynolds CF, Jennings JR, Thase ME, Frank E, Yeager A, Kupfer DJ 1992 Results of nocturnal penile tumescence studies are abnormal in sexually functional diabetic men. Archives of Internal Medicine 152: 114–118.

Nofzinger EA, Thase ME, Reynolds CF, Frank E, Jennings JR, Garamoni GL, Fasiczka AL, Kupfer DJ 1993 Sexual function in depressed men: assessment by self-report, behavioral, and nocturnal penile tumescence measures before and after treatment with cognitive behavior therapy. Archives of General Psychiatry 50: 24–30.

Norton GR, Jehu D 1984 The role of anxiety in sexual dysfunctions: a review. Archives of Sexual Behavior 13: 165–183.

Notley RG 1979 Transurethral resection of the prostate. British Journal of Sexual Medicine 6(55): 10–15 ; 26.

Novak TE, Bivalacqua TJ, Davis R, Hellstrom WJG 2000 Management of erectile dysfunction following radical prostatectomy. In Mulcahy JJ (ed) Male Sexual Function: A Guide to Clinical Management. Humana, Totowa, NJ, pp. 109–122.

Nurnberg HG, Hensley PL, Gelenberg AJ, Fava M, Lauriello J, Paine S 2003 Treatment of antidepressant-associated sexual dysfunction with Sildenafil: a randomized controlled trial. Journal of the American Medical Association 289: 56–64.

Orford J, Oppenheimer E, Egert S, Hensmen C, Guthrie S 1976 The cohesiveness of alcoholism-complicated marriages and its influence on treatment outcome. British Journal of Psychiatry 128: 318–339.

Pearlman CK 1980 Sex and prostatectomy patients. British Journal of Sexual Medicine 7(59): 31–35.

Penovich PE 2000 The effects of epilepsy and its treatment on sexual and reproductive function. Epilepsia 41(S2): S53–S61.

Pentland B, Anderson DA, Critchley JAJH 1981 Failure of ejaculation with indoramin. British Medical Journal 282: 1433–1434.

Peters TJ 2000 Nutritional deficiency syndromes complicating alcohol abuse. In Ledingham JGG, Warrell DA (eds) Concise Oxford Textbook of Medicine. Oxford University Press, Oxford, pp. 1434–1435.

Pfaus JG, Gorzalka BB 1987 Opioids and sexual behavior. Neuroscience and Biobehavioral Reviews 11: 1–34.

Plant MA 1975 Drug Takers in an English Town. Tavistock, London, pp. 188–204.

Pritchard BNC, Johnston AN, Hill ID, Rosenheim ML 1968 Bethanidine, guanethidine and methyldopa in treatment of hypertension: a within-patient comparison. British Medical Journal 1: 135–144.

Pukall CF, Binik YM, Khalife S, Amsel R, Abbott FV 2002 Vestibular tactile and pain thresholds in women with vulvar vestibulitis syndrome. Pain 96: 163–175.

Randolph ME, Reddy DM 2006 Sexual functioning in women with chronic pelvic pain: the impact of depression, support, and abuse. Journal of Sex Research 43: 38–45.

Reed EW, Reed SC 1965 Mental Retardation. Saunders, Philadelphia.

Rendell MS, Rajfer J, Wicker PA, Smith MD for the Sildenafil Diabetes Study Group 1999 Sildenafil for treatment of erectile dysfunction in men with diabetes. Journal of the American Medical Association 281: 421–426.

Riley A 1980a Antihypertensive therapy and sexual function. British Journal of Sexual Medicine 7: 23–27.

Riley A 1980b The sexual side effects of drugs used in the treatment of peptic ulceration and dyspepsia. British Journal of Sexual Medicine 7: 12–16.

Riley AJ, Riley EJ 1983 Cholinergic and adrenergic control of human sexual response. In Wheatley D (ed) Psychopharmacology and Sexual Disorders. Oxford University Press, Oxford, pp. 125–137.

Riley AJ, Riley EJ 1986 The effects of single dose diazepam on female sexual response induced by masturbation. Sexual and Marital Therapy 1: 49–54.

Roose SP, Glassman AH, Walsh BT, Cullen K 1982 Reversible loss of nocturnal penile tumescence during depression: a preliminary report. Neuropsychobiology 8: 284–288.

Rosen RC 1991 Alcohol and drug effects on sexual response: human experimental and clinical studies. Annual Review of Sex Research 2: 119–179.

Rosen RC, Lane RM, Menza M 1999 Effects of SSRIs on sexual function: a critical review. Journal of Clinical Psychopharmacology 19: 67–85.

Rowlands P 1995 Schizophrenia and sexuality. Sexual and Marital Therapy 10: 47–62.

Sacks M, Dermatis H, Looser-Ott S, Burton W, Perry S 1992 Undetected HIV infection among acutely ill psychiatric patients. American Journal of Psychiatry 149: 544–545.

Saenz de Tejada I, Angulo J, Cellek S, Gonzalez-Cadavic N, Heaton, J, Pickard R, Simonsen U 2004 Physiology of erectile function and pathophysiology of erectile dysfunction. In Lue TF, Basson R, Rosen R, Giuliano F, Khoury S, Montorsi F (eds) Sexual Medicine: Sexual Dysfunctions in Men and Women. Health Publications 2002, Paris, pp. 289–343.

Salonia A, Briganti A, Rigatti P, Montorsi F 2006 Medical conditions associated with female sexual dysfunction. In Goldstein I, Meston CM, Davis SR, Traish A (eds) Women's Sexual Function and Dysfunction: Study, Diagnosis and Treatment. Taylor & Francis, London, pp. 263–275.

Sanchez-Ortiz, Broderick GA 2001 Vascular evaluation of erectile dysfunction. In Mulcahy JJ (ed) Male Sexual Function: A Guide to Clinical Management. Humana, Totowa, NJ, pp. 167–202.

Santen RJ, Sofsky J, Bilic N, Lippert R 1975 Mechanism of action of narcotics in the production of menstrual dysfunction in women. Fertility and Sterility 26: 538–548.

Savarimuthu D, Bunnell T 2003 Sexuality and learning disabilities. Nursing Standard 17: 33–35.

Schiavi RC, Fisher C 1982 Assessment of diabetic impotence. Measurement of nocturnal erections. Clinics in Endocrinology and Metabolism 11: 769–784.

Schiavi RC, Fisher C, Quadland M, Glover A 1985 Nocturnal penile tumescence: evaluation of erectile function in insulin dependent diabetic men. Diabetologia 28: 90–94.

Schiavi RC, Stimmel BB, Mandeli J, Rayfield EJ 1993 Diabetes, sleep disorders, and male sexual function. Biological Psychiatry 34: 171–177.

Schiavi RC, Stimmel BB, Mandeli J, White D 1995 Chronic alcoholism and male sexual function. American Journal of Psychiatry 157: 1045–1051.

Schlesinger L 1996 Chronic pain, intimacy and sexuality: a qualitative study of women who live with pain. Journal of Sex Research 33: 249–256.

Schneider H, Wilbrandt K, Ludwig M, Beutel M, Weidner W 2005 Prostate-related pain in men with chronic prostatitis/chronic pelvic pain syndrome. British Journal of Urology 95: 238–243.

Schreiner-Engel P, Schiavi RC 1986 Lifetime psychopathology in individuals with low sexual desire. Journal of Nervous and Mental Diseases 174: 646–651.

Schreiner-Engel P, Schiavi RC, Vietorisz D, Eichel J deS, Smith H 1985 Diabetes and female sexuality: a comparative study of women in relationships. Journal of Sexual and Marital Therapy 11: 165–175.

Schreiner-Engel P, Schiavi RC, Vietorisz D, Smith H 1986 The differential impact of diabetes type on female sexuality. Journal of Psychosomatic Research 31: 23–33.

Seftel A 2007 Testosterone replacement therapy for male hypogonadism: part III. Pharmacologic and clinical profiles, monitoring, safety issues, and potential future agents. International Journal of Impotence Research 19: 2–24.

Segraves RT 1985 Psychiatric drugs and orgasm in the human female. Journal of Psychosomatic Obstetrics and Gynaecology 4: 125–128.

Segraves RT 1998 Psychiatric illness and sexual function. International Journal of Impotence Research 10(Suppl 2): S131–S133.

Sipski ML, Alexander CJ, Rosen R 2001 Sexual arousal and orgasm in women: effects of spinal cord injury. Annals of Neurology 49: 35–44.

Sipski ML, Rosen RC, Alexander CJ, Gomez-Marin O 2004 Sexual responsiveness in women with spinal cord injuries: differential effects of anxiety-eliciting stimulation. Archives of Sexual Behavior 33: 295–302.

Smith KB, Pukall CF, Tripp DA, Nickel JC 2007 Sexual and relationship functioning in men with chronic prostatitis/chronic pelvic pain syndrome and their partners. Archives of Sexual Behavior 36: 301–311.

Smith SM, O'Keane V, Murray R 2002 Sexual dysfunction in patients taking conventional antipsychotic medication. British Journal of Psychiatry 181: 49–55.

Steele CM, Josephs RA 1990 Alcohol myopia, its prized and dangerous effects. American Psychologist 45:921–933.

Stein RA 1977 The effect of exercise training on heart rate during coitus in the post-myocardial infarction patient. Circulation 55: 738–740.

Stewart WFR 1975 Sex and the Physically Handicapped. National Fund for Research in Crippling Diseases, Horsham.

Stoffer SS, Hynes KM, Jiany NS, Ryan RJ 1973 Digoxin and abnormal serum hormone levels. Journal of the American Medical Association 225: 1643–1644.

Stoléru S, Mouras H 2007 Brain functioning imaging studies of sexual desire and arousal in human males. In Janssen E (ed) Sexual Psychophysiology. Indiana University Press, Bloomington, pp. 3–34.

Sumanen M, Ojanlatva A, Koskenvuo M, Mattila K 2005 GPs should discuss sex life issues with coronary heart patients. Sexual and Relationship Therapy 20: 443–452.

Swales JD 2000 Essential hypertension. In Ledingham JGG, Warrell DA (eds) Concise Oxford Textbook of Medicine. Oxford University Press, Oxford, pp. 152–161.

Taberner PV 1985 Aphrodisiacs. The Science and the Myth. Croom Helm, London.

Taylor DC 1969 Sexual behaviour and temporal lobe epilepsy. Archives of Neurology 21: 510–516.

Taylor DC 1972 Psychiatry and sociology in the understanding of epilepsy. In Mandelbrote BM Gelder MG (eds) Psychiatric Aspects of Medical Practice. Staples, London.

Taylor DC, Falconer MA 1968 Clinical, socioeconomic, and psychological changes after temporal lobectomy for epilepsy. British Journal of Psychiatry 114: 1247–1261.

Tennent G, Bancroft J, Cass J 1974 The control of deviant sexual behavior by drugs: a double-blind controlled study of benperidol, chlorpromazine and placebo. Archives of Sexual Behavior 3: 261–271.

Terzian H, Orr GD 1955 Syndrome of Kluver and Bucy reproduced in man by bitemporal removal of the temporal lobes. Neurology 5: 363–380.

Thase ME, Reynolds CF, Glanz LM 1987 Nocturnal penile tumescence in depressed men. American Journal of Psychiatry 144: 89–92.

Toone BK, Wheeler M, Fenwick PBC 1980 Sex hormone changes in male epileptics. Clinical Endocrinology 12: 391–395.

Toone BK, Wheeler M, Nanjee M, Fenwick PBC Grant R 1983 Sex hormones, sexual drive and plasma anticonvulsant levels in male epileptics. Journal of Neurology, Neurosurgery and Psychiatry 46: 824–826.

Tyrer G, Steel JM, Ewing DJ, Bancroft J, Warner P, Clarke BF 1983 Sexual responsiveness in diabetic women. Diabetologia 24: 166–171.

Ueno M 1963 The so-called coition death. Japanese Journal of Legal Medicine 17: 330–340.

Van Minnen A, Kampman M 2000 The interaction between anxiety and sexual functioning: a controlled study of sexual functioning in women with anxiety disorders. Sexual and Relationship Therapy 15: 47–58.

Van Thiel D, Lester R 1979 The effect of chronic alcohol abuse on sexual function. Clinics in Endocrinology and Metabolism 8: 499–510.

Vas C J 1969 Sexual impotence and some autonomic disturbances in men with multiple sclerosis. Acta Neurologica Scandinavica 45: 166–182.

Veening JG, Coolen LM 1998 Neural activation following sexual behavior in the male and female rat brain. Behavioral Brain Research 92:181–193.

Victor A, Lundberg PO, Johansson EDB 1977 Induction of sex-hormone-binding globulin by phenytoin. British Medical Journal ii: 934.

Wabrek AJ, Burchell RC 1980 Male sexual dysfunction associated with coronary heart disease. Archives of Sexual Behavior 9: 69–75.

Walsh PC, Donker PJ 1982 Impotence following radical prostatectomy: insight into etiology and prevention. Journal of Urology 128: 492–497.

Wang CJ, Shen SY, Wu CC, Huang CH, Chiang CP 1993 Penile blood flow study in diabetic impotence. Urology International 50: 209–212.

Ware MR, Emmanuel NP, Johnson MR, Brawman-Mintzer O, Knapp R, Crawford-Harrison M , 1996 Self-reported sexual dysfunctions in anxiety disorder patients. Psychopharmacology Bulletin 32: 530.

Warner P, Bancroft J and members of the Edinburgh Human Sexuality Group 1987 A regional service for sexual problems: a 3-year study. Sexual and Marital Therapy 2: 115–126.

Wassertheil-Smoller S, Blaufax MD, Oberman A, Davis BR, Swencionis C, Kerr MO, Hawkins CM, Langford HG 1991 Effect of antihypertensives on sexual function and quality of life. The TAIM Study. Annals of Internal Medicine 114: 613–620.

Watson JP 1979 Sexual behaviour, relationship and mood. British Journal of Clinical Practice (suppl) 4: 23–26.

Weijmar Schultz WCM, Wijma K, Van de Wiel HBM, Bouma J, Janssen J 1986 Sexual rehabilitation of radical vulvectomy patients. A pilot study. Journal of Psychosomatic Obstetrics and Gynaecology 5: 119–126.

Weijmar Schultz WCM, Van de Wiel HBM, Han DEE, Van Driel MF 1992 Sexuality and cancer in women. Annual Review of Sex Research 3: 151–200.

Weinhardt LS, Carey MP 1996 Prevalence of erectile disorder among men with diabetes mellitus: a comprehensive review, methodological critique, and suggestions for future research. Journal of Sex Research 33: 205–214.

Weinhardt LS, Carey MP 2000 Does alcohol lead to sexual risk behavior? Findings from event-level research. Annual Review of Sex Research 11: 125–157

Welsh M, Hung L, Waters CH 1997 Sexuality in women with Parkinson's disease. Movement Disorders 12: 923–927.

Wessells H 2001 Priapism. In Mulcahy JJ (ed) Male Sexual Function: A Guide to Clinical Management. Humana, Totowa NJ, pp. 335–350.

Whitley MP, Berke P 1984 Sexual response in diabetic women. In Woods NF (ed) Human Sexuality in Health and Illness. CV Mosby, MO, pp. 328–340.

Wilson GT, Lawson DM 1976a Expectancies, alcohol and sexual arousal in male social drinkers. Journal of Abnormal Psychology 85: 587–594.

Wilson GT, Lawson DM 1976b The effects of alcohol on sexual arousal in women. Journal of Abnormal Psychology 85: 489–497.

Wilson GT, Lawson DM 1978 Expectancies, alcohol, and sexual arousal in women. Journal of Abnormal Psychology 87: 358–367.

Wilson GT, Lawson DM, Abrams DB 1978 Effects of alcohol on sexual arousal in male alcoholics. Journal of Abnormal Psychology 87: 609–616.

Wilson GT, Niaura M, Adler JC 1985 Alcohol selective attention and sexual arousal in men. Journal of Studies on Alcohol 46: 107–115.

Wincze J, Albert A, Bansal S 1993 Sexual arousal in diabetic females: physiological and self-report measures. Archives of Sexual Behavior 22: 587–602.

Woodruff RA, Murphy GE, Herjanic M 1967 The natural history of affective disorders: 1. Symptoms of 72 patients at the time of index hospital admission. Journal of Psychiatric Research 5: 255–263.

Wu FCW 2000 Disorders of male reproduction. In Ledingham JGG, Warrell DA (eds) Concise Oxford Textbook of Medicine. Oxford University Press, Oxford, pp. 879–886.

HIV/AIDS and other sexually transmitted infections

Venereal disease: a historical background 413

The story of HIV and AIDS 414

The nature of sexually transmitted infections and associated diseases 414
Bacterial infections 415
Parasitic infections 416
Fungal infections 416
Viral infections 417

The prevalence of sexually transmitted infections in community surveys 419

The HIV/AIDS pandemic 420
The politics of the pandemic 421
Worldwide prevalence 422

The 'feminization' of the pandemic 422

HIV/AIDS prevention programmes 423
Uganda 423
The principles of prevention 423
Some specific aspects 425

Understanding sexual risk taking – the 'individual differences' component 429
Risk appraisal and risk management 429
Relevance of 'individual differences' to HIV/AIDS prevention ... 434

The impact of HIV/AIDS on sexual behaviour 435
The gay communities 435
The heterosexual communities 436

Venereal disease: a historical background

Of the various problems associated with human sexuality, the sexual transmission of disease has a long history, described for several centuries as 'venereal disease', reflecting its association with the 'pursuit of Venus'.

In the 15th century and earlier, gonorrhea and chancroid were probably the most prevalent venereal diseases, though little understood. At the end of the 15th century, syphilis appeared in Europe. Historians are still uncertain whether this was a disease brought from the Americas by Christopher Columbus and his men on their return, or was a new and more virulent version of an earlier infective organism. The 16th century saw a ravaging pandemic of syphilis through most European countries and beyond. As with many infectious diseases, its initial impact was greater, both in terms of infectivity and in terms of intensity of symptoms, but after a while, with the death of the more vulnerable, and the development of some degree of resistance in others, the disease became more chronic, but affecting fewer people, with epidemic episodes occurring in various places for reasons not well understood.

Times of war have been particularly associated with transmission of venereal disease, resulting from the separation of young men from their wives, families and communities, and the disturbance of sexual mores that occur during the chaos of war. Some of the governmental actions to counter venereal diseases have been provoked by concerns about the associated ill health of service men. During World War I, regulated brothels were set up in France for the British troops, to provide them 'safe' sexual release. Not surprisingly, this raised considerable opposition until they were stopped in 1918 (Porter & Hall 1995).

Scientific understanding of the range of sexually transmitted infections (STIs) started in the late 19th century. Following Louis Pasteur's groundbreaking discovery that micro-organisms caused infectious diseases (the 'germ' theory of disease), the gonococcus was identified as the cause of gonorrhoea in 1879, a bacillus as the cause of 'soft chancre' in 1889, and the spirochaete as the cause of syphilis in 1905, followed soon after by the development of the Wasserman blood test to detect syphilitic infection. Attempts at medical treatment of such infections had been very limited, with horrendous accounts of the use of mercury which often caused more suffering than the disease itself, until Salvarsan was introduced by Erhlich, a Prussian scientist, in 1910. This proved to be beneficial in many cases, but did not produce a complete cure. The big breakthrough did not happen until the introduction of penicillin in 1944. This, however, demonstrated the ambivalence of the medical profession about treating venereal disease, which was sixth on the list of priorities for the new antibiotic.

Before we consider the more recent history of HIV and AIDS, it is relevant to identify a number of themes which have recurred or prevailed through this long history, some of which will reverberate with what has been happening in the HIV/AIDS pandemic.

1. Venereal disease, as a manifestation of sex, is God's punishment for the sinner. In 1860, a London surgeon, Samuel Solly, declared syphilis to be 'a blessing, inflicted by the Almighty to act as restraint upon the indulgence of evil passions. Could the disease be exterminated, which he hoped it could not, fornication would ride rampant through the land' (Davenport-Hines 1990, p. 165–166). Although this quotation is an extreme example, variations on that theme have been commonplace. Linked to this, at least through the 19th and early 20th century, was the opposition of the medical profession to any form of help or advice by non-medical therapists. 'Quackery' was, no

doubt, a troubling issue. This led to the Public Health Act of 1917 in the UK, which imposed a penalty of up to 2 years imprisonment for anyone who treated or publically offered to treat or advise on treatment of venereal disease, other than those medically qualified who had also been specially trained for this purpose. This curtailment of non-medical help, however, had to be set against the reluctance by much of the medical profession to provide legitimate alternatives.

2. The stigmatization of the victims of venereal disease led to their being excluded or separated, along the lines of the leper in earlier history.
   In so far as treatment of venereal disease was provided, it resulted in special hospitals that would keep the 'VD' sufferer apart from other patients.

3. Information about sex should not be disseminated to the general public, but should be restricted to the medical and legal professions who can use such information responsibly. This attitude was not only relevant to information about venereal disease, but also accounted for much of the negative reaction to Kinsey's publications in the 1940s and 1950s (Bancroft 2005). But it underlined the earlier reluctance to educate the public about prophylaxis of venereal disease lest it might in some sense encourage them to be sinful without ill consequences. A similar line of reasoning has been apparent in the USA with recent opposition to sex education and research into adolescent sexuality because such education or questioning will 'put ideas in their heads' and encourage young people to be sexual (Bancroft 2004).

4. Counter-balancing the tendency to see the victim of venereal disease as the sinner, has been the attribution of blame to the woman, most obviously the female prostitute. The 1871 Royal Commission on Venereal Diseases made the following statement: 'There is no comparison to be made between prostitutes and the men who consort with them. With the one sex the offence is committed as a matter of gain: with the other it is an irregular indulgence of a natural impulse' (Porter & Hall 1995, p. 137). Such attitudes had led to the Contagious Diseases Act of 1864 in the UK, which required women suspected of being prostitutes to be physically examined, and if they showed any sign of infection they were to be compulsorily detained in a venereal diseases hospital. This inevitably resulted in many working class women, other than prostitutes, being victimized, and understandably generated much opposition, adding to the motivation of the emerging suffragette movement, battling for women's rights to vote. The tendency to see woman as a sexual threat that needs to be contained has been a long-standing theme in patriarchal societies, and has not disappeared (see Chapter 6 for more on historical background).

The story of HIV and AIDS

The literature on HIV and AIDS is now extensive and growing rapidly, and the summary in this chapter does not attempt to provide an exhaustive review. The story started in 1981. Two reports appeared from California and New York of gay men with a rare and lethal form of pneumonia (*Pneumocystis carinii*) and/or Kaposi's sarcoma, a malignant condition of the skin. This was the first indication of what turned out to be a worldwide pandemic, and it became apparent that many people had become infected before 1980. The emerging epidemiological evidence pointed to an infective agent transmitted sexually, by intravenous (IV) drug users sharing needles or by transfusion of infected blood. The variety of unusual infections and other conditions that emerged as associated with this syndrome indicated some abnormality of the immune system.

In 1983 a new retrovirus was isolated which eventually came to be called the human immunodeficiency virus or HIV. As the early victims found to be infected with HIV were gay men, it was initially regarded as a 'gay disease,' echoing earlier attitudes that venereal diseases were God's punishment for sin. Soon other forms of transmission became recognized, and particularly in sub-Saharan Africa, the rapid emergence of an epidemic was clearly due to heterosexual transmission.

Before considering the key issues in dealing with the HIV/AIDS pandemic, let us put HIV infection into context with other STIs.

The nature of sexually transmitted infections and associated diseases

A wide variety of pathogens may be transmitted by sexual activity. The following are the most important:

(i) Bacteria
   Gonococcus (gonorrhoea)
   Treponema pallidum (syphilis)
   Chlamydia trachomatis (pelvic inflammatory disease (PID) and lymphogranuloma venereum (LGV))
   Haemophilus ducreyi (chancroid)
(ii) Parasites
   Trichomonas (trichomoniasis)
(iii) Fungi
   Candida albicans (thrush)
(iv) Viruses
   herpes simplex (genital herpes)
   human papilloma virus (HPV, genital warts)
   hepatitis B
   HIV (HIV/AIDS)

HIV is the least contagious of these various pathogens, although, once transmitted, potentially the most serious. Bacterial, parasitic and fungal infections are all relatively treatable, viral infections much less so, though progress is being made in developing treatments for HIV/AIDS. The non-HIV infections vary in the potential severity of their effects, but they all share the tendency to increase vulnerability to HIV transmission. Conversely, the impairment of the immune system that results from HIV infection increases the likelihood of 'opportunistic' infections of other kinds, which include many STIs. Hence the HIV/AIDS pandemic needs to be considered in association with the epidemiology, diagnosis and treatment of other STIs. Most of these infections can be transmitted from the mother to her infant in utero, at birth or post-natally.

In general, women are more susceptible than men to genital and urethral infections. The shortness of the female urethra and its anatomical position make it vulnerable to ascending infection in women who are sexually active. The normal vagina has a varied bacterial flora, mainly of non-pathogens, and an acidic pH that inhibits the growth of most pathogenic varieties. In an early study of a large number of women attending a family planning clinic, 21% were found to have yeasts or fungi in the vagina, presumably most of them asymptomatically; 1% had Trichomonas present, usually associated with a vaginal discharge. Oral contraceptive users did not have a higher incidence of pathogenic organisms (Goldacre et al 1979), although it remains possible that they have increased vulnerability to such organisms when present.

Organisms causing infection may be normal inhabitants of the bowel or skin which gain access to inappropriate places as a result of sexual activity or become established because of some alteration in the local conditions such as those following the use of broad-spectrum antibiotics.

The impact of the infection may be confined to the genitalia. In women this may result in vaginosis, a condition in which the normal bacterial flora of the vagina is altered with overgrowth of other bacteria. It is usually accompanied by a vaginal discharge, often with an unpleasant odour. There may be burning during urination or itching of the vulva. Although vaginosis can result from sexual transmission, douching or the use of intrauterine contraception can also be the cause. In some cases, this type of vaginal infection is not caused initially by sexual transmission, but is kept going by being passed back and forth between partners within a stable sexual partnership, requiring both partners to be treated.

An increase in the bacterial counts in the urine after sexual intercourse has been reported (Buckley et al 1978). This underlies the condition known as 'honeymoon cystitis', painful and frequent urination that comes on after intercourse, classically in the sexually inexperienced woman. The post-menopausal woman is also particularly prone to this problem, perhaps because, as a result of oestrogen deficiency, her vagina has poor lubrication and does not engorge sufficiently to cushion the urethra against the buffeting of the anterior vaginal wall.

More serious than vaginosis is PID, when the infection spreads internally, and affects the uterus, fallopian tubes or other pelvic structures. Untreated PID can lead to abscess formation, chronic pelvic pain, ectopic pregnancy or infertility. Lesions of the vulva may occur, including genital warts or sores, and may facilitate transmission of further infection, in both directions.

In men, infections are more likely to be asymptomatic, but the most frequent symptoms are urethral discharge and burning on urination. This may lead to epididymitis and, if untreated, infertility.

STIs are not confined to the genitalia. Oral–genital contact may result in pharyngeal infection by organisms from the genital region and vice versa. Similarly, anal intercourse (AI) allows infection of the anal region by genital organisms and vice versa. Both types of cross-infection are particularly important for gay men.

More systemic effects may occur with some types of infection and will be considered in relation to specific organisms.

Bacterial infections

Gonorrhoea

The gonococcus is typically transmitted sexually. It is a sensitive organism that does not flourish in the acidic vaginal environment, hence in women infection is initially in the cervical canal or urethra. Early gonococcal infection in women is usually symptomless, so that a woman may be an active carrier without realizing it. PID occurs in up to 5% of cases, often leading to permanent infertility (Barlow 2000).

In the majority of cases of gonorrhoea in men, the infection is confined to the urethra, causing urethritis with dysuria and purulent discharge. Occasionally, cystitis or prostatitis and generalized infection may occur. In male homosexuals, anorectal infections are common. In general the consequences are more serious for the female than the male, though the initial infection is more obvious in the male. Pharyngeal and rectal gonococcal infections can also occur, although they are typically asymptomatic. Arthritis may occur, sometimes with effusions in larger joints.

The incubation period in men is from 5 to 14 days and sometimes as long as 3 months. Between 1932 and 1990 the mean incubation period increased from 4.9 to 8.3 days and this has been accompanied by a lessening in severity of symptoms (Barlow 2000). Rates of gonorrhoea in the USA increased from the early 1950s to a peak in the mid-1970s of 400–500 cases per 100 000 of the population and declined steadily until around 1995. Since then they have been relatively stable around 100 cases per 100 000 (CDC 2005). In the UK there was a similar pattern, with the annual number of diagnoses peaking at around 60 000 in 1975, falling to around 10 000 in 1995. But since then there has been a further rise and fall, with a peak around 24 000 in 2002, falling to around 18 000 in 2005 (Health Protection Agency (HPA) 2006).

The gonococcus is usually sensitive to antibiotics and hence gonorrhoea, if diagnosed, is highly treatable, usually with a single dose. In some countries, however, antibiotic-resistant strains of gonococcus are increasing.

Syphilis

In the early 20th century, when syphilis was rife, the protean manifestations of the disease, especially as it affected the cardiovascular and central nervous systems, provided much of the more florid pathology of clinical practice. Today AIDS has taken its place in this respect, but syphilis continues to be a serious STI.

The signs and symptoms of syphilis have three stages:

1. *Primary stage:* This is marked by the appearance of a single skin lesion, or chancre, sometimes multiple. This may occur from 10 to 90 days following infection (average 21 days). The chancre is typically firm, round and painless, and usually on the genitalia. It lasts for 3–6 weeks and resolves without treatment.
2. *Secondary stage:* This starts with a rash, which may be generalized on the body and face, but classically involving reddish brown spots on the palms of the hands and soles of the feet. The rash is accompanied by fever, lymphadenopathy, sore throat, headaches, weight loss, muscle aches and fatigue. These symptoms will resolve without treatment, but if untreated, the infection will eventually re-emerge as the tertiary phase.
3. *Tertiary syphilis:* The infection may persist without symptoms for many years. Eventually, gummatous lesions may develop in various parts of the body, and damage will emerge involving the cardiovascular system (classically, aortic aneurysm) and the nervous system, with tabes dorsalis (locomotor ataxia) or 'general paralysis of the insane', a form of dementia, and possibly death. Severe neurological manifestations of syphilis are now quite rare.

Syphilis showed worldwide peaks of incidence associated with World War I and World War II. There was a decline during the 1950s and a further rise in the 1960s in many countries. In the UK, the diagnosis of syphilis in men attending STI clinics increased through the 1960s and 1970s, while the numbers of cases in women remained constant. The male-to-female ratio peaked at 8:1 in 1983, as sex between men became the principal mode of transmission. In the mid-1980s, with the emergence of HIV and the associated increase in safer sex, the rates for syphilis declined in men. However, between 1998 and 2004 rates in males increased by more than 1500%, with a more modest increase in heterosexual women, reflecting a number of localized outbreaks (mainly London; HPA 2006). A comparable pattern has been evident in the USA (CDC 2005).

Syphilis, in the first year of the infection, is readily treatable with a single dose of penicillin or a related antibiotic. For those with longer periods of infection, a more protracted course of antibiotics is needed.

Chlamydia

Chlamydia is possibly the most common STI in the Western world. In 2005, genitourinary clinics diagnosed 109 958 cases in the UK (HPA 2006) and 929 462 cases in the USA (CDC 2005). Most infections with *C. trachomatis* remain undiagnosed, and the CDC estimates that there are around 2.8 million new cases in the USA each year. The reason for its frequently 'hidden' nature is that often it is asymptomatic. However, 10–40% of untreated infected women develop PID, with its potential for ectopic pregnancy and infertility. Untreated infections occasionally cause epididymitis and urethritis in men.

The large majority of infections occur in young women aged 15–24 years. Although the diagnosis rate is much higher for young women than young men, this is in part because the long-term consequences of untreated Chlamydia are much more serious in women, and consequently much more screening of young women is carried out. This does not deal with the asymptomatic infected male as a source of infection, and it is recommended that the male partners of infected women should also be treated. Increasingly, screening for Chlamydia is being recommended as a routine accompaniment to Pap smears.

Specific variants of *C. trachomatis* (serovars L1, L2 and L3) are more invasive and cause a variety of systemic conditions, in particular LGV. This form of Chlamydia is highly prevalent in parts of Africa, Asia and South America and has been unusual in Western Europe for some time. However, since 2003 a series of outbreaks of LGV, all involving the L2 genotype, have occurred in European cities among MSM (HPA 2006).

Chancroid

Genital ulcers caused by the bacillus *H. ducreyi* are known as chancroid. In the USA, the prevalence of chancroid cases declined substantially from the 1980s to 1990s; 4986 cases were reported in 1987 and 143 cases in 1999. Sixty per cent of diagnosed cases have been people aged 35 years or older. However, it is difficult to diagnose without a specific laboratory test, which is not widely available. Chancroid responds to appropriate antibiotic treatment. According to Ronald (2000), all patients with genital ulcers should be treated for both chancroid and syphilis, as clinical diagnosis is inadequate to select specific treatments. It is reasonable to conclude that chancroid is substantially under-diagnosed and under-reported, and its possible association with HIV should be kept in mind (Mertz et al 1998).

Parasitic infections

Trichomonas

This is another common sexually transmitted disease. Trichomonas is a protozoan parasite that typically causes a painful vaginitis and profuse, frothy and offensive discharge, although 10–50% of cases are asymptomatic. This infection seldom extends beyond the external genitalia. Hence it has tended to be regarded as unpleasant but harmless, until the recent recognition that, as with most genital infections, it can facilitate transmission of HIV (Ackers 2000) and may have an adverse effect on pregnancy.

The infection is often asymptomatic in men. The male partner of an infected woman should therefore be treated routinely to prevent recurrent cross-infection within the relationship. Metronidazole (Flagyl) is an effective treatment.

Fungal infections

Candida albicans

C. albicans (previously known as monilia) are commonly present in the vagina and may proliferate when the normal flora is suppressed by broad-spectrum antibiotics. Candida infections are also more common in diabetics, the obese, during pregnancy and when there is immuno-suppression. Hence, it can be an early sign of HIV infection. Oral–pharangeal candida infection is known as 'thrush'.

The main symptom of vaginal candida is an intense burning or itching of the vagina and vulvar region. A thick curd-like discharge may occur. Once again, the partner may harbour the infection. It has been suggested that around 10% of cases are sexually transmitted and in about one-fifth of infected women cure is only obtained if the male partner is also treated (Harris 1977). Fungicides, such as nystatin, can be used, though recurrences are common.

Viral infections

Genital herpes

Human herpes simplex is of two types: HSV1 and HSV2. Type 1 is common around the oral cavity, causing cold sores. Type 2 causes genital herpes; in women, typically a cluster of ulcerating vesicles on the labia and/or the cervix; in men, on the shaft or glans of the penis. Not only may these be very painful, particularly during the first acute outbreak, but also they are notoriously difficult to treat. In a characteristic herpetic fashion, the virus lies dormant in the dermal cells or possibly within the nervous system, breaking out in recurrent vesicles from time to time and often causing serious sexual disability. The primary infection is commonly subclinical. The virus is highly transmissible through sexual contact during the primary acute attack, somewhat less transmissible during recurrences, and much less during the quiescent phases. About 15% of cases involve HSV1, which may have been transmitted by oral–genital contact. The herpes simplex virus has been implicated as a possible causative factor in cervical cancer. Infection of the neonate by active lesions in the mother can also be extremely serious. The presence of genital herpetic vesicles in the latter stages of pregnancy is probably grounds for a Caesarean delivery.

Genital herpes is the most common ulcerative STI in the UK. Between 1971 and 2005, diagnosis of genital herpes increased 5-fold in males and 21-fold in females. In 1972, female-to-male ratio was 0.3:1; in 2005, it had changed to 1.5:1. In 2005, 19 837 new cases were diagnosed in the UK, with highest rates in 20- to 24-year-olds (HPA 2006). In the USA, in 1997, it was estimated that more than one in five Americans were infected with genital herpes, an increase in prevalence of 30% since the late 1970s (Fleming et al 19997). Treatment with antiviral drugs, such as famciclovir or acyclovir, is relatively effective in shortening an attack.

Human papilloma virus

There are more than 100 different HPVs that vary considerably in their potential for causing disease. Many are transmitted sexually. The most important association is with cervical cancer, with HPV-16 and -18 being the most significant in this respect. Women who have been infected with HPV should have cervical screening on a regular basis. Increasing attention is being paid to identifying the specific virus in such screening.

Ano-genital warts, or condyloma are the commonest explicit manifestations of HPV infection, and are most often caused by HPV-6 and HPV-11. They are most often on the vulva of women and the glans penis and foreskin of men. They are unsightly and itch. There is no specific anti-viral treatment for HPV, and infections are usually self-limiting. Localized treatment (e.g. cryotherapy) can be effective in getting rid of warts.

The prevalence of HPV infection is difficult to assess accurately, but estimates in the literature suggest very high levels, particularly among young women. In the UK, between 1972 and 2005, diagnosis of genital warts increased fivefold in men and eightfold in women. It is uncertain how much this reflects increased incidence, greater public awareness or improved diagnosis (HPA 2006). In 2005, more than 80 000 new diagnoses were made in the UK. The highest rates for new cases in males were in the 20- to 24-year-old group, and for females, in the 16- to 19-year-olds; 30% of females with this diagnosis were under 20 years.

In the USA, genital HPV is considered the most common STI (Markowitz et al 2007). In a 3-year study of female college students, around 14% became infected with genital HPV each year (Ho et al 1998). A study of gay and bisexual men in San Francisco found that 60% of HIV negative (HIV−ve) men, and almost all the HIV positive (HIV+ve) men were infected with HPV (Palefsky 1998). Among high-risk women in six cities, 26% of HIV−ve women and 70% of HIV+ve women had HPV (Palefsky 1998). According to Koutsky (1997), an estimated 15% of Americans aged 15–49 were currently infected, whereas an estimated 75% of the population of reproductive age had been infected with sexually transmitted HPV at some stage.

A quadrivalent HPV vaccine was introduced in 2006. This has led to much controversy about how and when it should be used. However, the CDC recommendation is that vaccination, which provides protection againt HPV types, 6–11, 16 and 18, should be given to girls aged 11–12 years (or as young as 9), the idea being to vaccinate before the onset of sexual activity (Markowitz et al 2007).

Hepatitis B virus

There are several viruses causing hepatitis, the most important being A, B and C. Hepatitis B virus (HBV) can be transmitted sexually. Hepatitis C is increased in people who are HIV+ve as a result of their immuno-suppression.

HBV varies in its effects. Some individuals can be asymptomatic, though still capable of infecting others. Others have an acute episode of hepatitis that then resolves, and others end up with chronic liver disease, which can be fatal. Because HBV does not produce genital lesions, it is not normally diagnosed in STI clinics and hence does not appear in the usual STI statistics.

It has been estimated that about 5% of the US population has ever been infected with hepatitis B, with around 200 000 infections occurring each year, 60% of which are believed to result from sexual transmission, mostly among young adults (Coleman et al 1998).

HIV/AIDS

The microbiology of HIV is growing in complexity. The limited overview that follows is largely based on an excellent account by Luzzi et al (2000), which should be consulted for more detail.

HIV-1 and HIV-2 are examples of retroviruses, i.e. their replication is based on the enzyme reverse transcriptase. Viral protease also plays a fundamental part in this replication. Both enzymes are the targets of anti-retroviral (ARV) therapy. CD4 is the surface receptor for HIV. This is found on T-helper lymphocytes, which are a crucial component of the immune system, interacting with and directing other immune cells, hence their title of T-helper. CD4 receptors are also found to a lesser extent on macrophages, Langerhans cells, which are involved in immune reactivity of the skin and mucous membranes, and brain microglial cells, which are crucial to the immune system in the central nervous system. Hence, HIV impacts the immune system, and most of the manifestations of HIV infection are consequences of resulting defects of the immune system.

Infection with HIV results from the exchange of bodily fluids, in particular blood. This may result from sexual interaction between men or between men and women, the sharing of needles or syringes by IV drug users, transfusion of infected blood and by transfer from a mother to her fetus. The susceptibility to infection is increased when other STIs are present, partly because of the associated lesions. This helps to account for the frequent association between HIV infection and other STIs.

The initial infection results in the development of serum antibodies, usually in 2–6 weeks, and in more than 90% of cases within 3 months. This occasional delay may be a reason for repeat testing in high-risk cases. Following sero-conversion, antibodies provide a highly specific test of HIV infection.

Primary syndrome. Once infected with HIV, 50–70% of individuals experience a transient illness after about 2–6 weeks, with fever, myalgia, lymphadenopathy and pharyngitis. In more than half of cases there is also a rash, typically erythematous and maculopapular, on the face and trunk. This illness lasts 1 or 2 weeks, sometimes longer.

The latency period. Following sero-conversion, and the primary syndrome when it occurs, there is usually a long asymptomatic period, which before the introduction of ARV therapy was on average around 10 years, although varying considerably. During this phase, physical examination may be normal, although about one-third have a persistent generalized lymphadenopathy, typically symmetrical and non-tender. The cervical and axillary nodes are most commonly affected.

There are two principal ways of monitoring the course of the infection; the T-helper (CD4) lymphocyte count and the viral load as measured by HIV RNA in the plasma. A higher lymphocyte count and lower HIV RNA level is usually predictive of latency or slow progression. Measurement of these markers early in the infection is advantageous as there is some evidence that early treatment may improve the prognosis. Clearly, there needs to be good grounds for suspecting a new HIV infection to make this regime feasible. Those with moderate-to-poor markers (CD4 count below 200 mm^{-3} and HIV RNA levels above 5000 copies) may have intermittent but relatively mild opportunistic infections (e.g. oral thrush or periodontal disease), and those with the worse levels of marker, are likely to experience more chronic conditions. The distinction between being HIV+ve and having AIDS has become less clear cut with the introduction of ARV therapies, and a 'continuous spectrum' of manifestations of the infection, from asymptomatic to chronically severe, is now considered more appropriate. Early, pre-symptomatic diagnosis raises some complex issues. On the positive side is the potential for early treatment and improvement in prognosis, and reduced likelihood of infecting others. On the negative side are psychological reactions to HIV+ve status plus a range of societal reactions, which can make life insurance, house mortgages, employment and travelling abroad problematic.

The progression to AIDS. The more serious manifestations include respiratory infections, such as bacterial pneumonia (e.g. streptococcus or haemophilus), *P. carinii* pneumonia, less common than it used to be, and tuberculosis (TB), probably the most frequent life-threatening HIV-related disease at present. TB, having declined in frequency over a long period, started to increase in the mid-1980s, after the start of the HIV pandemic. In Central Africa there is a strong association between TB and HIV. In the nervous system, various infections can arise, including cerebral toxoplasmosis and cryptococcal meningitis. Progressive multi-focal leucoencephalopathy, caused by another virus, can occur, with focal neurological deficits, ataxia and personality change. HIV can directly damage the nervous system, and most patients dying of AIDS show evidence of neuronal loss in the brain. In some cases this results in dementia. Neurological changes include slow movement, incoordination, motor weakness and hyper-reflexia, culminating in mutism, inability to walk and incontinence. Such cases lead to death within 2 years or so. Spinal cord damage and peripheral neuropathy can also occur. HIV-related tumours include Kaposi's sarcoma, involving skin or mucous membranes, and non-Hodgkin's lymphoma. Weight loss is a feature of progressive HIV infection, sometimes attributable to HIV-related chronic diarrhoea.

Progress is slowly being made in developing and improving ARV drugs. Zidovudine or AZT was developed quite early in the pandemic, but it soon became apparent that, though it slowed down progression of the disease, resistance to the drug developed. It is now recognized that combination therapy is more effective, usually with two reverse transcriptase inhibitors and a protease inhibitor. This is now known as highly active anti-retroviral therapy (HAART). Drug toxicity is an issue. Nausea, vomiting and diarrhoea are quite common side effects, and interaction with other drugs can be a problem, partly because the ARV drugs can increase the blood levels of other medications. Continuing progress in developing treatment and an effective vaccine is to be hoped.

The prevalence of sexually transmitted infections in community surveys

Most of the evidence of the prevalence and incidence of STIs summarized above is based on analyses of STI or genito-urinary medicine clinic attenders or government accounts of numbers of reported cases. Whilst important, such data does not allow assessment of predictors of STIs that would require comparison with those not affected by STIs. There is a limited amount of relevant information from some of the recent representative community surveys that will be briefly reviewed.

In the USA, NHSLS respondents were asked whether they had ever been told by a doctor that they had one or more of 10 types of STI, and whether they had been told this during the past year (Laumann et al 1994). The list of STIs and the percentages of respondents reporting each as a lifetime infection are shown in Table 14.1. Overall, 15.9% of the men and 17.8% of the women reported at least one lifetime STI. HIV/AIDS was clearly much less prevalent than other STIs. Logistic regression was used to assess the relevance of various possible predictors, including age, race, marital history and number of lifetime sexual partners. Holding other variables constant, men reported fewer STIs than women, African Americans had more bacterial, but fewer viral STIs, and not surprisingly, the strongest predictors for both bacterial and viral STIs were numbers of life time sexual partners. Those reporting 11 or more lifetime partners had rates of STIs that were two to three times as high as those with only one partner.

TABLE 14.2 Rates per 100 000 population of gonorrhoea and syphilis by race/ethnicity in the USA, 1994–98 (CDC 1998, Section 12, Table 12b)

	1994	1995	1996	1997	1998
GONORRHOEA					
White	29.8	29.6	26.1	26.2	28.3
Hispanic	74.0	79.2	66.0	67.4	74.3
Black	1163.0	1045.9	816.8	802.4	861.6
SYPHILIS					
White	1.0	0.8	0.6	0.5	0.5
Hispanic	3.1	2.6	1.8	1.5	1.5
Black	57.2	44.9	29.9	21.8	17.1

The racial difference is of some interest and was examined more closely by Laumann & Youm (2001). The CDC data indicates that African Americans have substantially higher rates of STIs than other ethnic and racial groups in the USA. This is shown in Table 14.2, for gonorrhoea and syphilis, though, as can be seen, the difference lessened somewhat between 1994 and 1998. Hispanics reported higher rates than whites, particularly for gonorrhoea, but their rates were much more similar to whites than to African Americans. The lower rates of viral STIs among African Americans, found in the NHSLS, are not evident in these CDC rates, which were substantially higher for genital herpes and hepatitis B in African Americans than white or Mexican Americans (CDC 2000). The official explanation for this racial contrast in general is that higher rates are related to relative poverty, limited access to good health care, drug use and living in communities with high prevalence of STIs. Laumann & Youm (2001) questioned this explanation, pointing out that Hispanics are closer to African Americans than to whites socio-economically, yet are much closer to whites in terms of STIs. They focused on network factors and concluded that a substantial *intraracial* network effect distinguished African Americans from white and Hispanic Americans. STIs remain within the African American networks because they are highly segregated from other racial/ethnic groups (p. 346–347), but they spread within those groups because other predictors of high STI transmission are prevalent.

The British Natsal I survey found that 3.4% of men and 2.6% of women had attended STD clinics in the past 5 years (Johnson et al 1994). Questions about specific STIs were not asked. Comparison by ethnic group showed similarities with the NHSLS; STD clinic attendance was reported by 3.4% of white, 6.8% of black and 1.6% of Asian men, and 2.5% of white, 9% of black and 0.0% of Asian women. They used a logistic model to assess possible predictors of clinic attendance, including age, marital status, numbers of heterosexual and homosexual partners in the past 5 years and non-prescribed drug injecting (ethnic group was not included, probably because the numbers were too small for the minorities). The adjusted odds ratio for STD clinic attendance for those reporting five or more partners was more than 9 for women and more than 12 for men. For women IV drug use was associated with increased attendance. Men aged 25–44 years and women

TABLE 14.1 Lifetime sexually transmitted infections in men and women with at least one sex partner in their lifetime, shown as cases per 100 (percentage) (from NHSLS; Laumann et al 1994, Table 11.3)

	Men	Women	Total
BACTERIAL INFECTIONS			
Gonorrhoea	9.0	4.7	6.6
Syphilis	0.9	0.7	0.8
Chlamydia	1.9	4.4	3.2
Non-GC urethritis	1.9	NA	1.9
PID	NA	2.2	2.2
Any bacterial	12.1	10.6	11.3
VIRAL INFECTIONS			
Genital warts	3.3	5.9	4.7
Genital herpes	1.2	2.9	2.1
Hepatitis B or C	1.3	0.9	1.1
HIV/AIDS	0.2	0.1	0.1
Any viral	5.4	9.0	7.4

Non-GC urethritis, non-gonococcal urethritis, men only; PID, pelvic inflammatory disease, sexually transmitted, women only aged 16–34 years were more likely to attend STD clinics than other age groups.

In the Natsal II, lifetime experience of being diagnosed with any of a list of nine STIs was assessed (Fenton et al 2001). This included vaginal candidiasis, which as mentioned earlier is probably sexually transmitted in only about 10% of cases. The percentages of men and women reporting lifetime experience of STIs are shown in Table 14.3. Excluding vaginal candidiasis, 10.8% of men and 12.6% of women reported at least one STI. Of the specific STIs, the most frequently reported, by both men and women, were genital warts. For both men and women, STIs were reported more frequently by those living in the Greater London area, compared with the rest of the country.

In this study, a 50% sample of sexually experienced respondents aged 18–44 years were asked to give a urine sample; 71% agreed, resulting in 3569 samples. These were tested for *C. trachomatis*, which as mentioned earlier, is often undiagnosed. Because of some selection biases in those who agreed to give urine samples, the data were weighted. On that basis, 2.2% of men and 1.5% of women tested positive. In men, a positive test was significantly related to at least one new partner in the past year, the number of sexual partners in the past year, and the number with whom no condom had been used. For women, the number of sexual partners in the past year and the number with whom no condoms had been used were the strongest predictors.

In the French ACSF national survey (Spira et al 1994) 2.5% of men and 4.2% of women reported at least one STI in the past 5 years, and 0.6% and 1.4%, respectively, during the past 12 months. However, for 44% of the men and 67% of the women reporting STIs, fungal infections (e.g. candidiasis) were involved, and, as stated above, the majority of such infections are not sexually transmitted. The expected association with number of sexual

partners was apparent; 39% of those reporting and 10% of those not reporting an STI had more than one sexual partner in the previous 5 years.

In the Sex in Australia survey, participants were asked if they had ever been diagnosed with an STI and also whether this had happened in the past 12 months (Grulich et al 2003c). The findings are shown in Table 14.4. Predictors of an STI history in men included homosexual identity (over 20% of those in this sample), managerial/professional occupation, IV drug use, and number of lifetime sexual partners. In women, predictors included bisexual identity, post-secondary education, managerial/professional occupation and IV drug use. HIV testing was reported by 40.7% of the men and 38.9% of the women. The results suggested that, in this sample, 0.13% of men and 0.16% of women were HIV+ve. Of the homosexual men in this sample, 2.5% were HIV+ve.

In comparing the results from these various national surveys, composite rates for 'any STI' are confounded by the variation in specific STIs included. Comparison of rates for specific STIs is more helpful, and in most cases shows similarities across studies. Perhaps the most notable exception is the high rate of lifetime gonorrhoea for men (9%) in the NHSLS. The rates of HIV+ve serostatus are quite similar in the NHSLS and Australian survey. They were not reported for Natsal II.

The HIV/AIDS pandemic

HIV/AIDS has become the fourth most frequent cause of death in the world, and the most frequent in sub-Saharan Africa. An estimated 60 million men, women and children have become infected worldwide. Nearly

TABLE 14.4 Diagnosis of an STI 'ever' or 'in the last 12 months' in 9729 men and 9578 women in the Sex in Australia survey (from Grulich et al 2003c)

	Ever		Last 12 months	
	Men (%)	Women (%)	Men (%)	Women (%)
Any STI	20.2	16.9	2.0	2.2
Public lice or crabs	9.8	4.2	0.3	0.1
Genital warts	4.0	4.4	0.5	0.3
Chlamydia	1.7	3.1	0.2	0.2
Genital herpes	2.1	2.5	0.8	1.1
Syphilis	0.6	0.1	<0.1	0.0
Gonorrhoea	2.2	0.6	<0.1	<0.1
NSU	5.0	—	0.3	—
PID	—	2.3	—	0.2
Bacterial vaginosis	—	1.8	—	0.6
Trichomoniasis	—	0.8	—	<0.1
Candida or thrush*	6.6	57.6	1.3	17.5
Hepatitis B	0.7	0.7	0.0	<0.1

*Not included in the lifetime and 12 month rates for 'any STI'
NSU, non-specific urethritis (males only); PID, pelvic inflammatory disease (females only)

TABLE 14.3 Percentage of those with experience of sexual intercourse who had ever been diagnosed with an STI in the Natsal II (Fenton et al 2001)

	Men*	Women[†]
Any STI (excluding vaginal candidiasis)	10.8	12.6
Genital herpes	1.0	1.3
Trichomoniasis	—	0.8
Gonorrhoea	1.2	0.8
Syphilis	0.3	0.1
Chlamydia	1.4	3.1
NSU or NSGI	3.5	1.3
Genital warts	3.6	4.1
PID	—	2.2
Vaginal candidiasis	—	41.9
Positive urine test[‡] for *Chlamydia trachomatis*	2.2	1.5

Unweighted and weighted *n*:
*4500, 5376
[†]6128, 5232
[‡]3569
NSU, non-specific urethritis; NSGI, non-specific genital infection; PID, pelvic inflammatory disease

half who become infected are under 25 years; most will die before they are 35 years if not treated. By the end of 2000, 22 million people had died of this disease (Piot 2007).

In many badly affected countries, e.g. those in sub-Sarahan Africa, there has been an enormous negative impact on the economy, with reduction of the effective workforce, a disproportionate amount of the budget being used to deal with the epidemic, and health services on the verge of collapse (with more than 60% of hospital beds occupied by HIV+ve patients). This results in a vicious circle; HIV/AIDS reduces economic growth and increases poverty that in turn aggravates the epidemic (De Lay et al 2001).

There is a huge increase in the number of orphaned children as a result of HIV/AIDS. In 1990 16.4% of parental deaths were in this category; the prediction for 2010 is 68% (De Lay et al 2001).

A further major change associated with the pandemic is the increased involvement of women, what has been called the 'feminization' of the HIV/AIDS pandemic. As shown in Table 14.5, almost half of HIV+ve individuals around the world are women and substantially more than half in sub-Saharan Africa. In Kenya, for example, the proportion is 67–68%. This a major change since the early days of the epidemic, and its implications for prevention will be considered more closely later.

The politics of the pandemic

Once it became apparent that this was not an epidemic restricted to gay men or IV drug users, it was not long before there was a strong, worldwide acknowledgement of a need for action. The defining point was a special session of the UN General Assembly on AIDS in June 2001, the first time that two days of the Assembly had been devoted to a specific health issue (Piot 2007).

By then ARV treatments were becoming available, although initially they were exceedingly expensive. For example, in Uganda, in 1998, the cost of such treatment for 1 year for one person was $12 000; by 2002, it was $2000; by 2007, it was $135, what Piot, the Executive Director of UNAIDS, called 'the ultimate expression of

political will' (Piot 2007). In 2007 around $10 billion was budgeted for AIDS worldwide — a third coming from developing countries.

The role of political leaders has been crucial. According to Piot (2007), the leaders of several African countries badly affected by the pandemic were 'in total denial for many years' which effectively delayed the establishment of effective programmes. Uganda was an important exception that is considered more closely below. The 'politics' that have surfaced in this worldwide campaign have been 'good' and 'bad'. 'Good' politics, in Piot's terms, involve activism, science and social reform; 'bad' politics, opposition to sex education in schools for children, opposition to condom promotion, opposition to harm reduction among injecting drug users (for AIDS in particular), homophobia, sexism, not recognizing the gender dimensions, stigma and the discrimination associated with it. A further important issue in the political scene has been a major focus on HIV/AIDS, which has clearly made all politicians, good or bad, stop and think, in contrast to the continuing neglect of other STIs. One important lesson to be learnt from this pandemic is that HIV/AIDS is one of several STIs, which are not independent of each other. Apart from the increased susceptibility to HIV infection caused by other STIs, the damage to the immune system by the HIV virus increases the prevalence of other infections (e.g. herpes). In sub-Saharan Africa, for example, there has been a decline in other STIs that may well have resulted from the impact of HIV/AIDS prevention and treatment programmes. The political attention thus should be on STIs and diseases, including HIV/AIDS.

The clearest and most controversial example of 'mixed' politics in this story is the President's Emergency Plan for AIDS Relief (PEPFAR), implemented by the US President, George W. Bush, in 2003. This assigned $15 billion over 5 years to the ongoing campaigns in developing countries. It carried, however, a number of conditions and restrictions. Initially, 70% was to be used for treatment and palliative care of the HIV infected, 10% for helping orphans and vulnerable children, and 20% for prevention. Of the prevention

TABLE 14.5 Regional HIV and AIDS statistics for women and percentage of HIV+ve individuals who are women (WHO/UNAIDS 2006 AIDS Epidemic Update, Table 2)

	Number of women (aged 15–49) living with HIV		Percentage of HIV+ve who are women	
	2004	2006	2004	2006
Sub-Saharan Africa	12.7 million	13.3 million	59	59
Middle East and North Africa	180 000	200 000	49	48
South and South-East Asia	2.0 million	2.2 million	29	29
East Asia	160 000	210 000	27	29
Latin America	450 000	510 000	30	31
Caribbean	110 000	120 000	50	50
Eastern Europe and Central Asia	410 000	510 000	30	30
Western and Central Europe	190 000	210 000	28	28
North America	300 000	350 000	26	26
Oceania	32 000	36 000	47	47
Total	16.5 million	17.7 million	48	48

money, one-third had to be used for promoting abstinence until marriage (later increased to two-thirds). No more than a third was to be used to promote condom use, and this should be restricted to those individuals already established as high risk and should not be used to promote condom use in the young who were not already high risk. No money should be used to support needle or syringe exchange programmes or provide assistance to any group or organization that does not have a policy explicitly opposing prostitution and sex trafficking. This led to Brazil refusing $40 million of PEPFAR funds in May 2005. The director of Brazil's HIV/AIDS programme explained, 'Brazil has taken this decision to preserve its autonomy on issues related to HIV/AIDS as well as ethical and human rights principles'.

It is clear that, however well intentioned, PEPFAR, in its allocation for prevention, was structured around moral values rather than scientifically-based principles of prevention. Even then, the proposed limitations provoked opposition from some sections of the religious right in the USA who did not want any of the money to be spent on promoting condom use. And there has been widespread opposition and criticism from many in the Global HIV/AIDS programme of such restrictions in the first place, with the Brazilian reaction a particularly cogent example.

Worldwide prevalence

There is considerable variation in prevalence across different regions of the world, as shown in Table 14.5. The highest prevalence is in sub-Saharan Africa, which includes only 11% of the world's population. There are also likely to be considerable variations within any one region, which need to be better understood (e.g. why does South Africa have one of the highest rates in sub-Saharan Africa?). In some cases, such variations reflect the predominant mode of transmission. In East Europe, for example, IV drug use is the most important mode of transmission. That part of Europe has also recently experienced a major epidemic of syphilis for reasons that are not yet clear. In India, IV drug use is the predominant mode in the north east, whereas sexual transmission predominates in the rest of the country (Piot 2007).

The 'feminization' of the pandemic

The increasing involvement of women has produced a variety of reactions. Piot (2007), having stressed the 'underestimated and undervalued burden' of STIs for women, considers it a 'mystery why we are not highlighting this more' (p. 4). Tolan (2005), a young woman who in 2004 worked as a volunteer in South Africa, has written strongly of the vulnerability of married women in that country. South Africa now has one of the highest rates of HIV infection, increasing from 1% of the population in 1990 to more than 26% in 2004. Women in South Africa are 30% more likely to be HIV+ve than men,

married women more than single women. Women interviewed by Tolan indicated that quite often their husbands were reluctant to use condoms. She proposed three factors to account for this situation for married women in South Africa:

1. Migrant labour in a culture which expects male polygamy; many husbands in rural families have to travel to other parts of the country to get paid work, and hence are away from their wives often for long periods, during which they are likely to be sexually active with other women, including sex workers.
2. Lobola, the custom when a man pays a bride price to his wife's family on marriage. This reinforces the husband's sense of ownership of his wife.
3. Gendered economic inequality. Most women, particularly married women, have little opportunity to be independent of male partners.

Tolan (2005) goes on to say that the prevailing HIV/AIDS prevention strategy, the ABC approach (Abstinence, Be faithful, use Condoms), which will be considered further below, is of little value to a married woman in these circumstances. She stresses the importance of establishing a woman-dependent method of prevention such as a microbicide, and this will also be considered further later.

In contrast, Boyce et al (2007) criticize the way that 'African women' have been conceptualized as passive victims. 'This model of women's subjugation simply restates stereotypical relations and archetypal conditions of risk rather than conceiving more complex circumstances of sexual practice...misconceiving the *actual* gendered sexual subjectivities and relations that drive the epidemic' (p. 21). They seem to be arguing that considering patriarchal subjection of women in sexual relationships and marriage is inappropriate and unhelpful in dealing with this pandemic.

The situation of the married South African woman, as described by Tolan (2005), can be contrasted with that of married women in European (and North American) countries. Bajos & Marquet (2000), having compared surveys across a number of European countries, concluded 'The higher the woman's social status, the more women are able to stray from their traditional social roles in the area of sexuality' (p. 1544). However, they found interesting differences between northern and southern Europe, with more evidence of this shift in women's sexuality in the north. How much this can be explained by socio-economic differences between these two parts of Europe and how much reflects long-standing cultural and religious differences, are not clear. The extent to which the repression of women's sexuality has lessened during the 20th century has been considered at various points in this book (e.g. Chapter 6). Clearly this change has varied across cultures, as well as across socio-economic groups, and may be minimal for the married woman in rural South Africa. Cleland & Ali (2006) commented on what was needed to effectively reduce the epidemic in sub-Saharan Africa. In addition to increased access to drug treatment, necessary change will only occur, they concluded, as a result of fundamental changes that reduce poverty and gender inequality.

HIV/AIDS prevention programmes

What have we learnt so far about reducing this horrific epidemic? Overall, in spite of substantial efforts and money spent on an international scale, progress has been modest. Two countries have shown more substantial improvement: Uganda and Thailand (Slutkin et al 2006). Let us consider the Ugandan experience more closely.

Uganda

AIDS was first recognized in 1983 with 900 cases being identified by 1986 and 6000 by 1988. By 1986–1987, 86% of sex workers and 33% of lorry drivers, 14% of blood donors and 15% of antenatal clinic patients in major urban centres were HIV+ve. After 10 years of the prevention programme, the proportion of the population who were HIV+ve declined from 30% to 5–10%. UNAIDS estimated a 67% drop between 1991 and 2001. This change was most evident among youth, who reported a steep decline in the numbers of sexual partners.

Objectives of the Ugandan HIV/AIDS programme included (i) mounting an educational campaign, informing the population about the risks and consequences and how best to avoid them, (ii) checking blood before transfusions and (iii) establishing a careful case surveillance process.

A widespread, extensive information, education and communication programme was initiated, using political speeches, local campaigns, advertising, mass media, public gatherings at district and village levels, and direct connection with high-risk groups. Examples of the intense involvement at district level are given by Slutkin et al (2006). A particular strength of this programme, apart from its connection with all segments of the community, was a continued and increasing political commitment by both the Government and the President, who never failed to mention the programme whenever he spoke in public. The budget for the programme grew from $1 million to $18 million per year in the first 3 years. The programme was well staffed; 45 from the Ministry of Health and 6 from the WHO. The closest number of staff in any other African programme has been 10 from the Ministry of Health and 4 from the WHO.

The main risk-reduction messages were 'stick to one partner', delay first sexual experience, and, to a more limited extent, use condoms when sexually active. Abstinence per se was not promoted apart from advocating delaying onset of sexual activity in those without sexual experience. Church leaders were also involved with about 12% of the population, emphasizing fidelity and monogamy.

There were instances when local district groups decided to challenge some long-standing 'norms', e.g. it was no longer acceptable for policemen or teachers to have sex with young girls. There was presumably an increased openness not only about HIV/AIDS but also about sex, and an accompanying lessening of stigma associated with AIDS.

Delay et al (2001), in summarizing the behavioural impact of this programme, reported a significant increase in condom use, a decreased number of casual partners and the delay of sexual debut by 1 or 2 years. The proportion of girls who had ever had sex declined by almost one-half between 1989 and 1995, and more than half of young, sexually active Ugandans reported condom use at their last encounter (this was close to zero at the start of the programme). HIV+ve rates among 15- to 19-year-old girls declined from 22% in the early 1990s to 8% in 1998. Whether these positive changes are sustained once the intensity of the prevention programme subsides, remains to be seen.

The principles of prevention

Whereas the Ugandan prevention programme can be regarded as effective, it involved a wide range of activities and considerable commitment. It is also likely that its effectiveness depended on certain 'culture specific' components. Important lessons are also being learnt as programmes continue. Delay et al (2001) pointed to the considerable evidence cross-culturally that 'knowledge is not enough'. Knowledge surveys have shown that 95% of the adults in Zimbabwe have learned about AIDS with more than 80% knowing about two or more modes of prevention, yet the epidemic in Zimbabwe is still out of control. A key issue, they conclude, is that many people continue to deny their own danger of becoming infected; AIDS is always someone else's problem. This has led to a 'second generation' of behaviour change tools that include social mobilization, skills building, intensive personal counselling and the addition of HIV testing — having an HIV test often provokes a critical moment of personal awareness' (Delay et al 2001, p. xxi).

ABC approach

The Ugandan programme can be seen as an example of the ABC approach to prevention, which strives for political acceptability across the board. The ABCs of HIV prevention were considered in a report of the UNAID (2002). 'A' stands for abstinence; but this should apply specifically to abstaining from penetrative sexual interaction (vaginal, oral or anal sex) and does not preclude other forms of sexual interaction. This is relevant to the recognized need to delay onset of sexual activity (i.e. penetrative sex). The report points to the evidence of an association between early sexual debut and later sexual risk taking. The hope is that delaying debut will thwart this association. However, the determinants of early onset of sexual activity are complex, as considered in Chapter 5. Nevertheless, this is an appropriate goal.

The 'B' stands for 'be faithful', and here the focus is on at least serial monogamy. The 'C' stands for condom use. Here the report, while acknowledging the fundamental importance of this component, comments on some potential disadvantages. In particular, it points out that in a number of programmes, there has been, over time, a reduced emphasis on the A and B apparently related to increased C promotion. Condom promotion, it was suggested, may inadvertently result in increased behavioural 'disinhibition' (p. 12). In addition is the common assumption of the religious right that condom promotion campaigns may entice young people to become sexually active for the first time. Hence there is the need for ABC approaches to be balanced, with the possible addition of 'D' for delayed onset of sexual activity, making a distinction from abstinence for those who already have had their sexual debut.

In commenting on the Ugandan experience, this UNAIDS (2002) report emphasized the importance of the decline in multiple partners, the enhancement of personal communication networks and the lowering of stigma associated with AIDS. It also underlined the need for 'low-tech' approaches, making use of the mass media, but at the same time, ensuring that messages suitable for North America and Europe should not be 'stamped into African settings without consideration of indigenous culture'. Prevention messages also need to be focused for specific audiences; thus 'condoms and partner reduction' for transport and sex workers; 'partner reduction and delayed sexual debut' for students; 'delayed sexual debut, stigma and discrimination reduction, and fidelity' for church attenders.

Theoretical models of prevention

To what extent can we derive basic principles of relevance to HIV/AIDS and STI prevention more generally? Most of the first generation intervention programmes were based on theoretical models that emphasized rational appraisal of risk and a consequent commitment to risk reduction. Elements from the Health Belief Model (Rosenstock 1974), Social Cognitive Theory (Bandura 1986), the Theory of Reasoned Action (Fishbein & Ajzen 1975) and the Transtheoretical Model of Behavior Change (Prochaska et al 1992) were often used in various combinations. The relevant behaviour in such models was assumed to be under voluntary control, and little or no attention was paid to other aspects of the risk-taking context, in particular the specifically sexual aspects that might make such control more difficult. Ajzen's Theory of Planned Behavior, a modification of the Theory of Reasoned Action, made a move in that direction by introducing the concept of 'perceived behavioural control' (Ajzen 1985). The Health Belief Model considered barriers to action, which could include aspects of sexuality. The AIDS Risk Reduction Model (ARRM) of Catania et al (1990) emphasized the importance of social networks, the role of the sexual partner in making appropriate change possible and the willingness of the individual

to seek help. Affect was considered in terms of distress about the dangers and how this might motivate change. Sexual enjoyment was also considered, though mainly in terms of the perception of what will and will not be enjoyable and the impact that this might have on the commitment to change. But over all sexuality per se did not feature strongly in these approaches.

The individual or the context?

Bajos & Marquet (2000) weighed up the relative importance of individual-oriented approaches and relation-based or contextual approaches. The *individual approach*, from their perspective, was based on how the individual assimilates information about risk, with risks being taken when they have not been evaluated correctly. This approach led to the study of various defining characteristics of the individual to see to what extent they were predictive of risk taking. These included cultural group, socio-economic status, age, alcohol and drug use, knowledge of health guidelines, perceived threat and peer support (Moatti et al 1997). While each of these categories has been shown to have relevance, the failure to 'shed light on the chain of elements leading to a decision' using individual-based variables of this kind has also been apparent.

The *relation-based approach* focuses on the interactive behaviour between the partners in a sexual interaction or relationship and the meanings attributed to such behaviour. In contrast to studying defining characteristics of the individuals involved, characteristics of the relationship are considered in four categories: (i) institutional and macro-social context, (ii) the relationship's close social context, (iii) the interaction between partners and (iv) the intrapersonal level.

As an example of the first category, the crucial nature of a woman's social status in a heterosexual relationship was considered earlier. The second category covered relevant characteristics of the relationship at its onset, and how these might influence a decision to use a condom, e.g. use of a condom is more likely in an interaction with someone not previously involved in that person's social network (school or friends). The third category focused, in particular, on the 'intra-conjugal balance of power', a further issue linked to gender relations. In the fourth category, Bajos & Marquet (2000) used as an example the impact of the breakup, or threatened breakup of a relationship. 'The need for reassurance and/or self esteem or simply the desire to be wrapped in someone's arms is so strong … that the risk of HIV transmission usually takes back seat' (p. 1542). Viewing this as an example of vulnerability, they considered the possibility that the degree of vulnerability might correlate negatively with the degree to which one protects oneself. Here we have some reconsideration of the individual, albeit as a reaction to the relationship.

Bajos & Marquet (2000) concluded that the 'individual' and 'relations-based' approaches are not counteractive, and both need to be taken into account. This, needless to say, presents a considerable challenge. The complexities of human sexuality are clearly apparent, with considerable variation across cultural and subcultural contexts in how sex is experienced and interpreted and what meanings are attributed to it. The history of the campaign against HIV and AIDS has revealed a well intentioned but misleading tendency to apply Western meanings, particularly in structuring the research and surveys used to assess HIV-relevant aspects of a cultural sexual scene. This lesson is being learnt gradually.

Some specific aspects

Condom use and the pursuit of sexual pleasure

Condoms elicit much that is controversial or, for many people, uncomfortable about sex as a topic for education, intervention or policy. Although condoms can be and to some extent are used by married couples, most often as a form of contraception, there has been consistent opposition from sections of the religious right to official promotion of condom use by the unmarried. This has been evident in relation to sex education (see Chapter 5), but also in George W. Bush's controversial PEPFAR, considered earlier, where promotion of condom use was to be severely restricted to those who were already a 'lost cause' from the moral perspective. In spite of these restrictions, the fact that condom promotion could be included in any way in the campaign against HIV/AIDS, generated much criticism from the 'anti-condom' brigade, who are only comfortable with the promotion of abstention. Male condoms raise another key issue, and one that has not been closely researched. It is widely assumed that condoms can reduce sexual pleasure, for either or both partners, but particularly the man wearing the condom. The fact that this has been hinted at implicitly as an obstacle to more effective and widespread condom use, reflects the difficulty that most people planning, funding and implementing intervention programmes have with explicitly acknowledging the importance of sexual pleasure. A welcome break from that trend is an educational organization, based in London, called The Pleasure Project (www.thepleasureproject.org), which works on the principle that it is easier to maintain safe sex if it is at the same time pleasurable. The work of this educational project, in various parts of the world, is convincingly described in two papers by Philpott et al (2006a, b). Although they give some good examples of how the application and use of male condoms can be made more pleasurable, partly by using condoms designed to enhance pleasure for both partners, their description of enhancing pleasure by the use of the female condom was somewhat more persuasive. The female condom is a pouch, typically with a smaller rubber ring at one end (that goes into the vagina) and a larger ring at the other end (that stays outside the vagina), which entirely lines the vaginal wall and cervix and is a protection against pregnancy and STIs. Little attention has been

paid to female condoms in the HIV/AIDS literature. They are now being distributed in some developing countries as part of prevention campaigns, but it remains unclear how female condoms are viewed by women or men, and it is too early to know what part they can play in this campaign.

Prevalence of condom use

Research into the prevalence of condom use and the associated enhancement of safer sex is methodologically challenging. How should one assess the extent of condom use, and of unprotected sex, other than by daily diaries in which each sexual act is chronicled? The pros and cons of different approaches are well reviewed by Graham et al (2005). The variability across studies in the methods used to assess condom use does, however, limit cross-study comparisons.

In the NHSLS (Laumann et al 1994), 16.3% of men and women used a condom on the last occasion of vaginal intercourse; 12.8% of those with no new partners, and 32.8% of those with new partners in the past year. Twelve per cent always used a condom with their primary partner, whereas 35.4% always with a secondary partner. It is of some interest to know to what extent people use condoms as their way of dealing with the threat of HIV/AIDS. Feinleib & Michael (2001), using data from the NHSLS, presented answers to the question 'Have you made any change in your sexual behaviour because of AIDS?' and, if so, 'What have you changed?' Twenty-nine per cent reported making some change; 12% reported fewer partners, 9% used condoms more frequently, 7% were more careful in their choice of partners, and 3% abstained, though the meaning of 'abstain' apparently varied. Such changes were more likely to be reported by young males, blacks, the unmarried, those living in cities and those reporting more lifetime sexual partners. In those reporting changes, 50% also reported condom use on the last occasion of sexual activity, compared with 13% of those who reported no changes. In general, and not surprisingly, those most at risk were most likely to report change. However, there remained 25–30% of those at greatest risk who reported no change, a subgroup of importance to the future of the HIV/AIDS pandemic.

Catania et al (1995) found evidence of increased condom use in the early 1990s, most often in those with higher risk partners. The British Natsal I (Johnson et al 1994) found 19.5% of men and 14.2% of women who had changed their lifestyle because of AIDS; this was more likely in the younger age groups (for men 16–24 years, 36.2%; 45–59 years, 6.2%). Condom use on the last occasion of heterosexual sex was reported by 23.2% of men and 17.5% of women. Again, this was more likely in the younger age groups (for men 16–24 years, 38.9%; 45–59 years, 13.6%). Ten years later, comparing the Natsal II survey with Natsal I (Erens et al 2003), using a condom on *every* occasion in the previous year had increased from 18.2% to 24% in men and 14.9% to 18.0% in women. In the Natsal II, 45.9% of men and 36.7% of women who had a new sexual relationship in the last 4 weeks used a condom on every occasion. However, this left 37.6% of men and 47.7% of women with new relationships who did not use a condom at all.

In the Sex in Australia survey, 90% of those with a regular partner reported no condom use with that partner, and 59% with casual partners reported unprotected vaginal sex (Grulich et al 2003a). Approximately one-third of the men with recent homosexual experience engaged in AI on the last occasion. Of these men, condom use was reported by 46% of those taking the insertive role and by 51% of those taking the receptive role. For those having anal sex with a casual partner, 12% reported no condom use (Grulich et al 2003b).

Predictors of condom use

Many studies have explored possible predictors of male condom use. Sheeran et al (1999) reported a meta-analysis of 121 studies of heterosexual condom use. Inevitably, studies varied considerably in methodology and the variables assessed. They organized their analyses using the ARRM (Catania et al 1990), which describes three *stages* in the process of changing one's condom use behaviour: (i) 'labelling', which covers the recognition that one might be at risk of HIV infection, (ii) 'commitment', the emergence of a commitment to use condoms, and (iii) 'enactment' — putting the condom to use. Overall, correlations between most of the many potentially predictive variables, including those relating to knowledge of the risks involved, were small or absent. The nature of the sexual relationship involved was relevant, however. People were almost twice as likely always to use a condom with a casual, secondary or new partner, compared to a partner in an established or steady relationship. Perception of one's partner's attitude towards condoms was also strongly predictive, particularly among women, and this related to the strongest predictor, the ability and preparedness of two people in a relationship to discuss whether to use condoms — substantially more predictive than their ability to discuss HIV risk. On the basis of these results, Sheeran et al (1999) recommended interventions that increased positive attitudes to condom use, encouraged their use as a method of contraception as well as protection from infection, encouraged communication between partners about condom use, as well as carrying condoms in anticipation of their possible use.

A recent study (Stulhofer et al 2007) is of interest, partly because it was carried out in an East European country, Croatia, which still has a low prevalence of HIV/AIDS, and also because it uses good methodology. In 2005, 1093 men and women aged 18–24 years were interviewed, 85% of whom had experienced sexual intercourse, with the average age of their sexual debut as 17 years for men and 17.6 years for women. In addition to assessing their knowledge of HIV/AIDS and other STIs, and their sexual values and attitudes, three aspects of condom use were assessed: at first experience of vaginal intercourse, at the most recent experience and the proportion of occasions of vaginal intercourse over the last 12 months. Women who had traditional moral values were less likely to have used a condom at first vaginal intercourse. For men, earlier sexual debut was associated with reduced likelihood of condom use, whereas higher parental control increased the likelihood of condom use on the first occasion. The strongest predictor of condom use on the most recent occasion was the use of condoms on the first occasion, particularly for women. One other variable, attitudes to condoms, was predictive for both men and women. Those with negative attitudes to condom use were less likely to use them. Men did not differ in their use of condoms between steady and casual partners, whereas women were more likely to use condoms with casual partners. The predictors of consistent condom use were similar to those of most recent condom use. These findings underline the importance of providing comprehensive sex education to young people before they become sexually active, and support previous research that links early sexual debut to greater sexual risk taking, underlining the importance of encouraging delay in the onset of sexual activity.

Flowers et al (1997) reported a review of the literature involving gay and bisexual men, also organized around the ARRM. In the 'labelling' stage, MSM who did not identify as gay were less likely to be well informed about HIV transmission, but among gay-identified men, such knowledge was not predictive of condom use. Gay men who engaged in unprotected anal intercourse (UAI) tended to underestimate the risk they were taking, perhaps exemplifying 'unique invulnerability'. With the 'commitment' stage, negative attitudes to condoms were predictive of their non-use. Social norms had some significance, though the relevant 'social groups' in the gay community are likely to be variable in their 'norms' about safe sex. As with the heterosexual evidence, the strongest positive association was between 'casual sex' and 'safer sex'. Interestingly, those men with higher numbers of sexual partners were more likely to have safe sex, possibly due to their becoming more competent in their assertion of safer sex. Gay men with poor communication skills or low assertiveness were less likely to have safe sex. The authors concluded that greater theoretical attention needed to be paid to the 'enactment' stage of the ARRM, with more consideration of 'communication, context and culture'. A further review of sexual risk taking among gay men was provided by Hospers & Kok (1995), with broadly similar conclusions.

Little attention has been paid to effects of the sexual process on condom use. An interesting exception was a study by Boldero et al (1992). They assessed subjects' intent to use condoms in the future and then asked them to complete another questionnaire immediately after a subsequent sexual encounter, indicating their intention to use condoms immediately before the encounter, the extent to which they were sexually aroused and communicated with their partner about condom use during the encounter, and whether they actually used a condom. The degree of sexual arousal during the encounter was negatively associated with condom use, whereas intention to use condoms immediately before the encounter and communication with the partner about condom use increased the likelihood that condoms were used. The authors commented, 'The fact that the majority of those changing their intention, shifted from intending to use condoms to having no thoughts of using condoms at the time of the encounter, is suggestive of the influence of arousal'. The relevance of sexual arousal will be considered further below.

Problems with condoms

A consistent finding in the above predictive studies has been the association between negative attitudes about condoms and reluctance to use condoms. Only recently has attention been paid to why negative attitudes might arise, beyond those that are determined by 'traditional values'. A range of problems with condoms used is now apparent, and the relevant literature has been reviewed by Graham et al (2005). Most attention has been paid to breakages and slippages, and practical problems such as the use of oil-based lubricants, which can damage the latex of the condom. Less attention has been paid to incomplete use. Two patterns have been identified: delaying applying the condom until after vaginal intercourse had started, usually an unplanned sequence in casual sexual relationships, and a more planned use of the condom only when ejaculation was expected, more likely to be a negotiated arrangement in a regular relationship (Quirk et al 1998; de Visser 2004). Both patterns suggest a reluctance to use condoms the whole time, either because of reduced sensitivity and hence reduced pleasure, or because of the possibility of losing erection. In the French survey (Spira et al 1994) participants were asked for their opinions on condoms: 45% of condom users and 61% of non-users agreed that condoms lessen sexual pleasure; 46% of users and 57% of non-users agreed that condoms take all the romance out of sex, whereas 27% of users and 45% of non-users agreed that 'when you're in love, you don't need a condom'.

Condoms and erectile failure

In the Kinsey Institute research on high-risk sexual behaviour, reported in the final section of this chapter, we were surprised to find that SIS1, our measure of propensity for sexual inhibition due to fear of performance failure, was, in gay men, positively predictive of number of casual partners and the long-term risk score. It was also negatively related to our measure of 'safe sex assertiveness' (Bancroft et al 2003a). SIS1 is a trait measure that is strongly related to erectile problems, and these findings suggested that lack of confidence in one's erectile function may undermine one's determination or ability to use a condom (see p. 321). In 2003, Richters et al, in a qualitative study of gay men in Australia, reported 'frequent mention of problems with erection, especially in association with condom use ... The inability to gain or maintain an erection while using a condom clearly led to occasional failure to use condoms and for some men abandoning any attempt to use them at all'

(p. 44). A small number of studies have reported erectile loss with condom use (Graham et al 2005). In the most recent study of 278 heterosexual men attending an STI clinic who were asked about the last three occasions of vaginal intercourse, 37.1% reported condom-associated erection loss on at least one occasion. These men also reported more frequent unprotected vaginal sex and were less likely to use condoms consistently (Graham et al 2006a).

Even less attention has been paid to the possible impact of condom-induced reduction in sensation on ejaculation. In our qualitative study of the impact of sexual arousal on risk management (Strong et al 2005; see below), one heterosexual man described how when using a condom he was usually unable to ejaculate, and would take the condom off to make it possible.

A man who lacks confidence about his erectile ability is likely to be reluctant to use a condom because it may aggravate the erectile difficulty. If he is a gay man, he may be more likely to engage in UAI, either as the 'top' without a condom, or as the 'bottom', which is inherently riskier. Clearly, these 'negative' aspects of condom use have to be taken more seriously in both the development of condoms and in the education and prevention messages about condom use. The possibility of losing one's erection as a result of fitting or wearing the condom should be discussed, and ways of dealing with it considered. One possibility that needs to be assessed is that heterosexual men concerned about erection loss may function better using female condoms, the fitting of which does not require an initial or sustained erection. In addition, the suggestions by Philpott et al (2006b) about how to enhance sexual pleasure during the applying and wearing of male condoms should be taken more seriously in prevention programmes, and be on the agenda for individual counselling about risk reduction. A further strategy might be the use of a PDE-5 inhibitor to enhance erection and make condom use less problematic.

The increased attention to problems with condoms, and in particular the fact that they do not provide 100% protection, has been exploited by the religious right anti-condom brigade as further justification for not promoting condom use. On the other hand, it is good that we are becoming more aware of the importance of correct usage, as condoms remain an important part of the campaign against HIV/AIDS and STIs generally, as well as having worthwhile contraceptive efficacy.

Microbicides

At present women can prevent unwanted pregnancy by the use of steroidal contraceptives, but hormonal methods are not without their problems for many women, and they provide no protection against STIs. The relative lack of control that women have over both the safety and the contraceptive implications of their sexual relationship has drawn attention to the need for a woman-controlled method. Work is ongoing to develop suitable vaginal gels and creams that can be applied by the woman before vaginal intercourse and have contraceptive and anti-infection properties, as well as positive lubricant effects. Although it is feasible that such a product will be forthcoming, there are other aspects that have to be taken into consideration. In particular, how will women feel about using such a method and the timing of its application? (Tanner et al, in press) It is nevertheless likely that such a method will be welcomed by a proportion of women and it is to be hoped that it will soon be added to the limited options available to women.

Impact of HIV+ sero-status

One crucial aspect of the HIV/AIDS epidemic is how those who have become infected manage their subsequent sexual behaviour. A number of studies have looked at sexual risk taking in HIV+ve individuals, mainly men, and mainly gay and bisexual men. Hays et al (1997), in a study of young gay or bisexual men, found a higher rate of UAI in the past year in HIV+ve men (59%) than in HIV−ve (35%) or men who did not know their HIV status (28%). This points to the need to help HIV+ve individuals reduce their risk-taking behaviour to avoid infecting others. In this study, similar predictors of UAI were found for HIV+ve and HIV−ve men, including 'sexual impulsivity', substance use and communication problems. Robins et al (1997) studied 156 HIV+ve and 369 HIV−ve gay and bisexual men; here the level of high-risk behaviour in the previous 6 months was somewhat less in the HIV+ve group. However, the correlates of high-risk sexual behaviour were identical in the two groups, and included young age, less education, less distress and greater feelings of mastery, less use of active coping strategies and heavier use of alcohol and amyl nitrate. Reece et al (2001), in a study of HIV+ve men and women, found the men, both gay and heterosexual, to show a pattern of 'sexual compulsivity' associated with UAI, though the explanatory value of the concept of 'sexual compulsivity' in these circumstances is unclear. Van de Ven et al (2002) found reassuring evidence that in sero-discordant regular gay relationships, the HIV+ve partner was more likely to be receptive during AI. Sandfort et al (1995) assessed the use of sexual behaviour in HIV+ve gay men to improve mood, and found that this was related to the number of sexual partners, but not to unsafe sex.

The level of unsafe sex in HIV+ve men clearly varies across samples, and it is obviously difficult to obtain a representative sample of such men. Thus, in a Kinsey Institute study (Bancroft et al 2005b), HIV+ve men were mainly recruited from the Internet, and perhaps for that reason tended to be particularly high risk. In order to explore possible determinants of high-risk sexual behaviour in HIV+ gay men we therefore selected a comparison group of HIV−ve gay men who were matched for their level of sexual risk taking. The two groups were compared using our measure of propensity for sexual excitation and inhibition (SIS/SES; see p. 15), our questionnaire for assessing the relations between negative moods and sexuality (Mood & Sexuality Questionnaire (MSQ); see p. 108), and measures of sensation seeking

(SSS, Form V; Zuckerman 1994), and trait depression (Zemore et al 1990) and anxiety (STAI; Spielberger et al 1970), as well as some specific questions about problems with erection and rapid ejaculation. The only differences we found related to erectile function, and the sexual inhibition subscale, SIS1, which is strongly related to erectile problems. Unfortunately, we did not establish when erectile problems started, and whether they preceded HIV sero-conversion. Given the association between erectile problems and reduced condom use, considered in the previous section, this left us uncertain to what extent the higher prevalence of erectile problems in HIV+ve men was a consequence of the sero-status or its treatment, or a cause of it, because of associated increased risk taking.

An association between HIV status and erectile dysfunction (ED) has been recognized. Tindall & Forde (1994) found ED to be somewhat more likely in HIV+ve men with AIDS than in men with less advanced AIDS-related complex, suggesting a causal relationship. Catalan & Meadows (2000) found examples of psychogenic, organic and 'mixed' ED in HIV+ve gay men. Asboe et al (2007), in a study of 668 gay and heterosexual HIV+ve men from seven European HIV treatment centres, assessed medical history, details of ARV therapy, and ED using the International Index of Erectile Function (Rosen et al 1997). Moderate/severe ED was reported by 33%. The strongest predictors of ED were older age (older than 40 years) and depression. Whereas the quartile with the longest period of ARV therapy reported more ED, there was no linear increase in ED across the other three quartiles. Unfortunately, none of these studies has attempted to establish whether ED, or a tendency to ED, preceded sero-conversion. We are therefore left with uncertainty about the relative importance of four possible explanations for ED in HIV+ve men; a factor increasing the likelihood of UAI and hence sero-conversion, the direct impact of the virus, the possible impact of the ARV therapies on erectile function, or a 'psychogenic' effect of concern about infecting one's partner.

Male circumcision

Male circumcision has re-emerged as a controversial issue with an interesting historical past. The historian Moscucci (1996) has described how, in mid-Victorian Britain, male circumcision was advocated as a cure for masturbation. However, unlike clitoridectomy in the female, recommended for the same reason but which fell from favour, male circumcision remained popular, particularly in higher socio-economic groups. By the 1930s at least two-thirds of British boys attending private schools were circumcised, compared with 10% of working class boys. Moscucci (1996) comments that this 'new mania for circumcision' was remarkable given that it had been unthinkable in Christian countries for centuries. In the 16th and 17th centuries it was believed to diminish male sexual pleasure and hence 'procreative potency'. Subsequently, it was perhaps adopted from the Jewish tradition because Jews were thought to have greater resilience as a result of their circumcisions. It was around the mid-to-late Victorian times that the foreskin became associated with 'filth', and a marker of inferior social status (Moscucci 1996). It is difficult to think of any better reason why the popularity for circumcision has persisted beyond the need to 'treat' masturbation. Interestingly, since the 1950s, a century later, the popularity of circumcision in most of the English-speaking world has declined substantially. In the UK, by 1989, only 7% of males were circumcised. In the USA, however, this has not been the case, and the rate of neonatal circumcision has increased, possibly reflecting the increase in hospital deliveries (Laumann et al 2001). In the NHSLS, 77% of American-born men had been circumcised, compared to 42% of the foreign-born American citizens.

The current controversy is about whether circumcision reduces the likelihood of HIV infection. The idea that circumcision reduces susceptibility to STIs is not new. In the late 19th century, in both the USA and the UK, it was believed to be a protection against syphilis and gonorrhoea. At the end of World War II, Hand (1949), in a study of American service men, found that Jews and circumcised Christians had lower rates of STIs. However, Laumann et al (2001) in their secondary analysis of the NHSLS data, which had been collected in 1992, found that circumcised men were slightly more likely to report a history of STI, and this was particularly noticeable with Chlamydia infections. On the other hand, their uncircumcised respondents were more likely to report sexual problems, and the circumcised men reported more masturbation and a greater preference for fellatio.

In 2000, Szabo & Short proposed that circumcision could be protective against HIV infection, postulating that it is the Langerhans cells (see p. 418) in the inner lining of the foreskin which provide an entry for HIV into the body. They cited experimental evidence from rhesus monkeys to support this hypothesis. They also cited a review of 40 studies (Halperin & Bailey 1999) that led to the conclusion that the circumcised male was two to eight times less likely to become infected with HIV. In addition, other evidence suggests a protection against syphilis and gonorrhoea. Szabo & Short's (2000) article, in the *British Medical Journal*, provoked many critical and negative reactions, demonstrating a continuing reluctance to accept that there are medical grounds for inflicting this surgical procedure on infant males.

By 2007, both the WHO, through UNAIDS (2007), and the CDC (2007) were providing qualified but strong support for circumcision as a prophylactic procedure. Their conclusions had been further strengthened by three randomized, controlled trials in Africa to determine whether circumcision of HIV−ve adult males reduced subsequent sero-conversion. All three trials were stopped prematurely because of clear evidence of benefits from the circumcision. Men who had been randomly assigned to receive circumcision had a 76%, 60% or 55% lower incidence of HIV infection in the South African, Kenyan and Ugandan trials, respectively.

This evidence is becoming persuasive. As yet, it is most convincing in protecting HIV−ve men from infection by HIV+ve women. It may well benefit in the other direction, but as yet we await evidence of its value for MSM. In any case, a strong qualification is that circumcision should not be regarded as a sufficient safeguard, and other methods of prevention should continue.

Understanding sexual risk taking — the 'individual differences' component

Our research at the Kinsey Institute based on the Dual Control model, postulating individual variability in propensities for sexual excitation and inhibition, has been addressed at various points in this book (see Chapters 2 and 6). Having developed a psychometrically sound instrument for measuring such variability, we were interested to see how relevant such concepts might be to high-risk sexual behaviour. This idea was presented at a Kinsey Institute workshop on The Role of Theory in Sex Research, in a session on 'Individual differences in sexual risk taking' (Bancroft 2000a,b). The reactions to this were discussed in Chapter 2 (see p. 7). Thus, in our attempts to explore the relevance of individual differences to understanding high-risk sexual behaviour, we have encountered two forms of opposition. One, 'political correctness', reflects a Foucaultian concern about the abuse of power, and the inappropriate blaming of the individual when it is society that is to blame. The other is an epistemological rejection of 'essentialist science' as responsible for many of our problems, and not to be trusted.

Hopefully such opposition will result in a productive dialectic rather than an obstacle to progress. I strongly agree that we need to take culture and context into account. But I also consider it beyond dispute that underneath our culturally determined sexualities is a neurobiological motivational system, which shows variability across individuals. The origins of this variability are not yet certain, but they are likely to be in part genetically determined and in part the result of learning at some stage in development.

Situational factors, many of which reflect the sociocultural context, are clearly important and are now receiving considerable research attention. Aspects of the personality, on the other hand, could account for the fact that, in the same type of situation, individuals differ in how they respond. Let us assume that any specific explanatory mechanism that relates to the individual will need to be fitted into a multi-factorial model before its heuristic value is evident. On that premise, the theoretical model used in recent Kinsey Institute research on sexual risk taking will be described, and various components of the 'sexual risk-taking process', of possible relevance to risk prevention strategies, considered more closely.

Risk appraisal and risk management

In this approach, a distinction is made between *risk appraisal*, the focus of most of the previous models (how much risk does this type of situation involve?), and *risk management* (how is the risk actually dealt with when the time comes?). Although in real terms there is an overlap between these two processes (e.g. intention to use a condom results from risk appraisal), the distinction is conceptually useful, as risk management focuses attention on both situational factors and personality traits of the individual that influence his or her state of mind *at the time when the risk is either taken or avoided* (e.g. intention is or is not translated into behaviour). This is shown schematically in Fig. 14.1. The appraisal process is influenced by a variety of factors. Basic information about sexual risk may include features such as immediacy and the odds of a risky outcome, and a cost–benefit assessment, of particular importance for HIV risk, when the 'benefit' is likely to be immediate, and the 'cost' is likely to occur, if at all, at some time in the future. Appraisal can be influenced by cultural norms and personal beliefs and attitudes. Cultural norms are of particular importance for adolescents, who are often guided by the norms of their age group. Personality factors may also be relevant to the appraisal process (see below). Risk appraisal may result in misperception of risk, shown in the figure as 'Low (High)', e.g. the false sense of security felt by many adolescents in 'monogamous relationships' (e.g. Hammer et al 1996), or the assumption of low risk when one's sexual partner 'looks healthy' (e.g. Lowy & Ross 1994). Typically, risk appraisal is carried out in advance of a specific sexual interaction. Much of the previous theorizing about high-risk sexual behaviour is most relevant to this 'appraisal of risk' component.

Risk management refers to how the individual uses or does not use that appraisal at the time of the sexual interaction. In particular, if high risk has been appraised, how does that determine what is done, i.e. is the risk avoided or not? An additional component of this model is the potential for risk management to influence subsequent risk appraisal as shown in Figure 14.1 as a feedback loop. In other words, if a situation results in no adverse consequences, in spite of a failure to implement risk avoidance, this may decrease the likelihood of that type of situation being appraised as 'high risk' in the future (Gerrard et al 1996). Interpretation of one's actual experiences (e.g. cautiously or carelessly) may be influenced by personality factors (e.g. conscientiousness or neuroticism; Trobst et al 2002). Central to this theoretical model is consideration of the various factors that can influence and determine risk management. The report of the National Institute of Mental Health (NIMH) Theorists' Workshop (Fishbein et al 1991) concluded that noone performs a given behaviour unless the advantages are seen to outweigh the disadvantages. By risk management we mean the implementation of this tradeoff process, and how it is affected by the state of mind at the time, which is not necessarily a rational process.

Hoyle et al (2000) reported a meta-analysis of 52 studies that related personality factors to sexual risk taking, mostly involving heterosexuals. The one consistent finding was an association between sensation seeking (Zuckerman 1979) and all the aspects of sexual risk taking examined in the meta-analysis (i.e. number

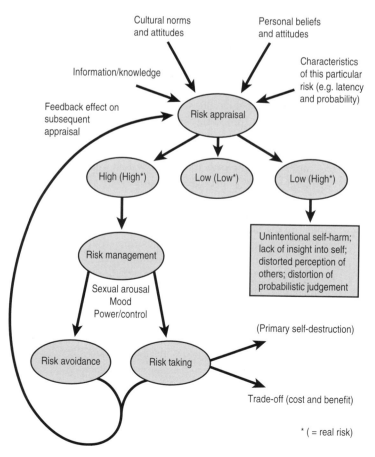

Fig. 14.1 The theoretical model of risk appraisal and risk management (Bancroft 2000a).

of partners, unprotected sex and high-risk situations such as sex with a stranger). High 'sensation seekers', as defined and measured by the Zuckerman scale, also show permissive sexual attitudes and an increased likelihood of engaging in sexual activity. It is not therefore clear in what way this personality construct mediates the risk management process.

Three other factors, related to personality and individual differences, are central to our concept of risk management, sexual arousal, mood and power or control in the relationship.

The impact of sexual arousal

The assumption to be considered here is that in a state of sexual arousal, normal, 'rational' decision making is impaired; sexual arousal, and the need to experience orgasmic release, largely determine how the situation is handled. Thus, a man or woman who recognizes, when not sexually aroused, that a particular form of activity is risky and should be avoided, once aroused feels less concerned about the risk involved (in a way which might happen with substance use). The immediate 'pay-off' or gratification then has an overriding appeal.

Surprisingly late in the evolving literature on HIV/AIDS risk management, the idea that sexual arousal itself may play a special and relatively unique role in influencing sexual risk taking started to emerge. Kelly & Kalichman (1995) stated that 'HIV prevention efforts must more adequately take into account the complexity of sexual behavior', mentioning that 'arousal level' might be a risk-triggering factor. Gerrard et al (1996) commented that 'the unique nature of the sex drive contributes to the fact that decisions about sex are oftentimes made in the heat of the moment — when the person is emotionally and physically aroused — rather than after careful, or even rational, deliberation' (p. 400). Canin et al (1999) commented that sexual arousal and desire for sexual satisfaction impose a sense of urgency that can distort judgement. Gold & Skinner (1997) looked at the 'self-justifications' that gay men use to explain UAI. They concluded that in many cases the decision to withdraw before ejaculating is most often taken 'in the heat of the moment' rather than as a premeditated plan. In a later commentary, Gold (2000) proposed that such 'heat of the moment' self-justifications could be explained as a consequence of the sexual arousal, tipping the balance towards UAI.

If sexual arousal can have this effect on sexual risk management how do any of us avoid sexual risk? The concept that individuals vary in their likelihood of becoming or remaining sexually aroused when faced by threats, such as the risk of STI, did not emerge in this literature, but is now central to the Kinsey Institute's Dual Control model, and the associated research programme on high-risk sexual behaviour. Propensities for sexual excitation and sexual inhibition have been measured in men using the SIS/SES (Janssen et al 2002; see Chapter 6, p. 229) and in women using the SESII-W (Graham et al 2006b). The relation of these propensities to sexual risk taking have been explored in large samples of heterosexual men and gay men and, to a more limited

extent, in heterosexual women, and the findings from these studies will be briefly reviewed.

Heterosexual men

Bancroft et al (2004) studied 879 men who self-identified as heterosexual. Their mean age was 25.2 years. Included in their questionnaire assessment were three questions: With how many different partners have you had sex (sexual intercourse) (i) in the past year, (ii) during the past 3 years with whom no condom was used and (iii) on one and only one occasion in your life time (one-night stands)? The SIS/SES questionnaire, used in this study, provides a measure of propensity for sexual arousal (SES) and two sexual inhibition subscales: SIS1, a measure of propensity for sexual inhibition due to the threat of performance failure, and SIS2, propensity for sexual inhibition due to threat of performance consequences, which includes consequences such as sexually transmitted infection and unwanted pregnancy. Other measures used in this study included trait anxiety (STAI; Spielberger et al 1970) and a two-question assessment of 'safer sex assertiveness (SSA)' (see below).

Controlling for age, SIS2 was strongly and negatively predictive of number of partners in the past 3 years with whom no condoms were used ($p = 0.008$), and also the lifetime number of one-night stands ($p = 0.001$). The fact that SIS2 was a significant predictor but not SES points to the importance of inhibition in limiting sexual risk taking, at least of some types.

Gay men

Most of the literature on sexual risk among gay men focuses on AI unprotected by condom use (UAI) because it is the single most important factor in HIV transmission between gay men and has become seen as such within the gay community. AI itself has a complex relationship to risk. Thus, it is not only important whether the AI is unprotected, but also whether the subject is usually the insertor or the recipient, which have different significance, both in terms of HIV transmission and also of control over the sexual act and implementation of safe sex procedures.

Apart from anal sex, other factors relating to the individual's sexual behaviour can be seen as relevant to a 'risk-taking tendency' in men who have sex with men. Number of partners, experience of unprotected oral sex, tendencies to visit gay bars, bathhouses, parks or public toilets for the purpose of finding sexual partners (Binson et al 2002), and substance use (Leigh & Stall 1993) are all relevant, to varying degrees, to a sexual risk-taking tendency.

Bancroft et al (2003a) studied 589 men who self-identified as gay; their mean age was 35.7 years. A more detailed assessment of sexual risking taking was used than in the study of heterosexual men described above, and distinguished between risk taking in the past 6 months (recent) and longer term. Recent risk assessment covered two aspects of specific sexual activity, UAI and oral sex, and two patterns of sexual contact, casual sex and cruising. A fifth assessment used the same three questions as in the study of heterosexual men described above, combined to give a 'long-term risk' score. For each of the five risk assessments, participants were distributed in five ordinal categories, which were then compared for possible predictors of sexual risk taking. The two 'sexual activity' variables, UAI and oral sex both showed significant negative associations with SIS2. SIS2 was significantly lower in the high-frequency UAI ($p = 0.004$) and oral sex ($p = 0.006$) categories. Different associations were found for the two patterns of sexual contact; both were associated with negative mood, which will be considered in the next section. In addition, the number of casual partners was significantly higher in those with high SES scores ($p < 0.001$), but also high SIS1 ($p = 0.04$). Cruising was not associated with SES, SIS1 or SIS2. Long-term risk was associated with low SIS2 ($p = 0.002$) and high SES ($p = 0.05$), but also with high SIS1 ($p = 0.01$).

Thus, as predicted, low propensity for sexual inhibition in sexually threatening situations (i.e. low SIS2) or, to put it another way, those whose sexual arousal was least likely to be reduced in a risky situation, were more likely to report high-risk sexual activity, in particular UAI. This pattern was more predictable using the measure of propensity for inhibition (SIS2) than for excitation or arousabiity (SES). The *positive* associations between SIS1, number of casual sex partners and long-term risk, however, were not predicted. We had not expected SIS1 to show associations in the opposite direction to SIS2; these two variables are positively correlated ($r = 0.283$, $p < 0.01$ in this study). In other studies SIS1 has been strongly related to ED (e.g. Bancroft et al 2005a). In this study, we found a difference between the highest and lowest long-term risk categories, with the highest reporting more erectile problems in the past, but no clear ordinal relationship across the categories. The relevance of this to condom use was considered earlier (p. 427). Thus, this is further evidence that a tendency to lose one's erection may influence a man's risk management adversely. This is not likely to be a general effect in all men with erectile problems; many such men probably avoid sexual interactions because of anticipation of erectile failure.

Heterosexual women

There is as yet more limited data relevant to sexual risk taking in women. In a sample of heterosexual women with a mean age of 33.7 years ($n = 540$; 38% married), the SESII-W was used to predict propensity for casual sex (Simpson & Gangestad 1991), number of lifetime sexual partners and condom use during the previous year. These variables are related to but are not direct measures of sexual risk taking. The SESII-W has higher-order factors for sexual excitation (SE) and for inhibition (SI) and several lower-order factors in each case (see Chapter 2, p. 17). Using multiple regression, and controlling for age, SE and an SE subscale, 'excitability' were positive predictors ($p < 0.04$ and < 0.009, respectively) and 'relationship importance', a subscale of the inhibition factor, a negative predictor ($p < 0.0001$) of propensity for casual sex. In a similar way, and controlling for age, number of lifetime partners was predicted positively by SE ($p < 0.003$) and negatively by two SI subfactors, 'relationship importance' ($p < 0.0001$) and 'risk of getting caught' ($p < 0.04$). Frequency of condom use was not predicted by SE or SI or any of their subfactors.

These early studies suggest that propensity for sexual inhibition is an important source of variability in sexual risk taking. What the evidence does not tell us is how the impact of inhibition, or the lack of it, is experienced. This is of potential importance for the application of these findings to prevention programmes. To explore this issue a qualitative study was carried out with 34 gay and 51 heterosexual men (Strong et al 2005). During the course of an interview, each participant was asked to recall a sexual episode that either at the time or later he regretted. A detailed narrative of that episode was then obtained, in the course of which the subject was asked to comment on the relevance of sexual arousal, mood and interpersonal control. This was followed by a series of open-ended questions about the general relevance of sexual arousal to sexual risk taking. Three patterns emerged from these interviews. Some participants described how their risk management is impaired by sexual arousal on some if not all occasions; some have recognized this problem and have learnt to 'plan ahead' (e.g. by making sure in advance that they have a condom with them), some have not found that sexual arousal interferes with their risk management. It is not possible from this study to assess the prevalence of these three patterns, and other patterns may exist which were not apparent in this study, e.g. the tendency to become more sexually aroused because of the risk involved. Other points of interest that emerged in this study included (i) the impact of the relationship, with risk management being more difficult in a loving relationship than a casual encounter, (ii) the negative impact of using a condom, which was considered earlier (see p. 425), and (iii) the striking impact of the immediate post-ejaculatory interval (see p. 90 for the physiological basis) in distinguishing between episodes which were followed by good feelings and closeness to the partner, and others followed by an immediate feeling of regret. This demonstration of the stark contrast between sexual arousal before ejaculation and non-arousal immediately after ejaculation warrants further attention, as it may prove to be a useful model for individuals to predict the outcome of a sexual interaction (e.g. 'How am I likely to feel immediately after I ejaculate?'), with potential for enhancing risk management.

There is, therefore, support for the idea that the persistence of sexual arousal in a high-risk situation can undermine risk management. How is this effect mediated? Our theoretical model postulates a process by which appraisal of a situation as dangerous results in increased inhibition of sexual arousal. However, this raises a number of as yet unanswered questions. Is the increase in inhibitory tone (or the failure of reduction of inhibitory tone; see p. 104) an automatic or implicit mechanism that does not require explicit or controlled information processing (see p. 106) and occurs adaptively in some but not all individuals? Or is more explicit, controlled information processing involved, which would allow a range of personality or situational factors to interact? And in those cases where inhibition of arousal is insufficient, in what way does the prevailing sexual arousal interfere with risk management? In our qualitative study, some participants described a lessening of perceived risk when aroused; for others, risk goes 'out of mind' when aroused. Does sexual arousal operate in the same way as alcohol? Steele & Josephs (1990) have formulated this as the 'alcohol myopia theory', which postulates that alcohol, by causing a restriction in attentional capacity, shifts the emphasis from inhibiting cues (those that emphasize risk) to impelling cues (those that emphasize the benefits). MacDonald et al (2000) reported an interesting experimental study that led them to conclude that sexual arousal interacts with alcohol to increase sexual risk taking. But we remain uncertain whether sexual arousal is acting in a similar way to alcohol or contributing to the process in a more specific way.

The issue of implicit appraisal of risk may be relevant to the impact of the relationship with the sexual partner or the distinction between 'making love' and 'having sex'. There is a growing literature addressing this issue (e.g. Flowers et al 1997 Elford et al 2001), although it is unusual for the interaction between intimacy and sexual arousal to be considered. Is it that an implicit appraisal of the intimacy and exclusiveness of the relationship lowers the perception of threat or risk and, hence, lessens the inhibitory component, even though the possibility of risk remains? Or is it simply that such situations are more arousing, with excitation overwhelming inhibition? Is it a combination of both, or are there other relevant mechanisms not dependent on excitation and inhibition, such as the motivation to demonstrate one's commitment by taking the risk? This important aspect of sexual risk taking deserves closer study.

The impact of negative mood

In conventional wisdom, it is assumed that sexual interest and, to some extent, sexual responsiveness are reduced in states of negative mood such as depression or anxiety. If that were always the case one would expect less sexual risk taking in negative mood states. However, in Chapter 4 (p. 106) we considered evidence of individual variability in this respect. In studies of heterosexual men (Bancroft et al 2003b), gay men (Bancroft et al 2003c) and heterosexual college women (Lykins et al 2006), a substantial minority, somewhat larger in men than in women, reported an increase in sexual interest and/or responsiveness when in negative mood states. In heterosexual men, this paradoxical mood–sexuality pattern was more frequent in younger men. A simple instrument, the MSQ (see p. 108) was developed to measure this trait. What is the possible relevance of this paradoxical pattern to sexual risk taking?

There is a substantial literature showing that affect or mood can influence judgement and decision making (e.g. Gerrard et al 1993). Two studies reported an association between sexual risk taking and the use of sex to reduce tension or cope with stress (McKusick et al 1991 Folkman et al 1992). In their comprehensive review, Canin et al (1999) commented:

'Affective states have an impact on cognitions, self-perception, behavior and inter-personal dynamics. They may interfere with recall of information relevant to self-protection and accurate risk appraisal, impede problem solving, contribute to the perpetuation of self-defeating behavior and diminish the likelihood of establishing and maintaining the types of relationship that encourage self-change and protective behaviour. In addition, negative mood can engender hopelessness.'

(p. 345)

Crepaz & Marks (2001), in contrast, carried out a meta-analysis of 25 studies in which the relation between mood and sexual risk taking was assessed. The effect sizes varied considerably and in both directions, leading these authors to conclude that there is 'no compelling support for the hypothesis that negative affect is associated with increased sexual risk behavior' (p. 297). Neither in this paper, nor in a commentary on it by Kalichman & Weinhardt (2001), was any consideration given to the possibility that negative affect could have different effects on sexual risk taking in different people. A tendency for negative affect to increase sexual risk taking in some individuals and reduce it in others would result in the overall 'nil effect' found in this meta-analysis. A risk-enhancing effect of negative mood would either depend on an 'excitation transfer' effect (see p. 111) most apparent with highly aroused states such as anxiety or a lack of inhibition of sexual arousal, which thus allows sexual interaction to occur with risk management altered by the negative mood.

In our study of gay men (Bancroft et al 2003a), we found that the trait measure of anxiety (STAI; Spielberger et al 1970) was negatively related to UAI ($p = 0.002$) and unprotected oral sex ($p = 0.004$); those men more prone to anxiety were less likely to engage in these two forms of high-risk sexual activity. More striking, however, was a strong association between increased sexuality in negative mood states, as measured by our MSQ, and higher numbers of casual partners ($p < 0.001$) or more frequent cruising behaviour ($p = 0.006$). This paradoxical mood–sexuality pattern was relevant to 'patterns of sexual contact' but not to the type of sexual activity during such contacts.

When we consider the three questions used to assess risk in our study of heterosexual men (see p. 431) and combined to assess long-term risk in our study of gay men, we can make a direct comparison between gay and straight men (Bancroft et al 2004). In both groups, excluding those in exclusive relationships, we found that men who reported increased sexual interest when depressed (high MS1 scores) reported significantly more sexual partners, though the effect was stronger in the gay men. Data from the qualitative interview study (with findings for mood reported in Bancroft et al 2003b, c) showed depression to have a more varied impact on sexuality than anxiety. The increase in sexual interest in states of anxiety or stress is probably explainable as an 'excitation transfer' effect when the sexual activity is driven by the need for the arousal-reducing and calming effect of the post-orgasmic state. This has been reported most clearly in 'out of control' patterns of masturbation (Bancroft & Vukadinovic 2004; see p. 330) and is of less certain relevance to sexual risk taking. The effects of depression are more complex, with sexual activity when depressed serving a range of purposes, including the pursuit of intimacy, and self-validation, in addition to a simple 'mood-enhancing' effect. An alteration of the significance of risk, as described by Canin et al (1999), or caring less about the consequences when depressed, was more often reported by the gay men than the straight men in our studies, described by one gay man as 'What the heck'. As yet we have no comparable data for women.

In a recent study using daily diary data from 155 MSM, Mustanski (2007) was able to assess the relevance of both trait and state measures of positive and negative affect to sexual risk taking. He found that state-positive affect had a negative association, whereas neither state- nor trait-negative affect had any association with sexual risk taking. Unfortunately, he did not attempt to assess whether this lack of association reflected individual variability in trait mood–sexuality relationships, as shown by our MSQ. However, his findings with anxiety are of relevance. Trait anxiety interacted with state anxiety in influencing sexual risk taking. In those men with high trait anxiety, state anxiety was negatively related to sexual risk taking, whereas in those with low trait anxiety, state anxiety was positively related. This suggests that the 'excitation transfer' effect of anxiety can augment the effects of sexual arousal in increasing risky behaviour in those who are not usually anxious. Those who have high trait anxiety have presumably developed more negative attitudes to sexual risk taking. It would be interesting to compare the effects of anxiety on masturbation, which is unassociated with risk, and partnered sex, in high and low trait anxiety individuals.

Power or control in the sexual interaction

Unfortunately, we did not attempt to assess this aspect of sexual activity in our study of gay men. For the heterosexual men we had a simple assessment of SSA based on two items: 'If I wanted to practice 'safe sex' with someone, I would insist on doing so' and 'I would ask about STDs before having sex with someone' (Bancroft et al 2004). (The correlation between these two items was $r = 0.37$.) This two-item variable was strongly predictive of number of partners in the past year and also number of partners, in the past 3 years, with whom no condoms had been used; it was marginally significant for number of one-night stands. This variable, which can be regarded as a measure of intention to practise safer sex as well as assertiveness in implementing that intention, appears to be relevant to more than condom use. Respondents scoring high on SSA reported fewer sexual partners; this is suggestive of sexual attitudes or values, which relate to more than safe sex. The associations between this variable and our personality trait measures, however, were of considerable interest. Using multiple linear regression, SIS1 was negatively predictive ($p < 0.001$); SIS2 ($p < 0.001$) and SES ($p = 0.02$) were both positively predictive of SSA. These findings raise the possibility that behavioural

intentions of the kind that feature greatly in interventions to reduce HRSB may themselves be reflective of the propensities for sexual inhibition and excitation measured by our SIS/SES instrument. Thus, SIS1 (inhibition due to the threat of performance failure), which is strongly related to erectile problems, was negatively associated with SSA; this suggests that confidence in ones' erectile response is important for asserting safer sex. In contrast, SIS2 (inhibition due to the threat of performance consequences), was positively associated, suggesting that those who are likely to be less aroused in the face of risk find it easier to assert safer sex. STAI, the trait measure of propensity for anxiety, was also predictive in a negative direction ($p = 0.01$); the higher the propensity for anxiety the lower the SSA. Together these findings are consistent with the idea that confidence in one's capacity for sexual response, particularly in a low-risk situation, is necessary for a clear determination to practice safer sex, perhaps particularly condom use. Interestingly, disinhibition, a subscale of sensation seeking, was negatively, but only marginally predictive of SSA ($p = 0.046$).

Relevance of 'individual differences' to HIV/AIDS prevention

Carey & Lewis (1999), while acknowledging the relevance of personality characteristics to the motivation to change high-risk behaviour, regarded them as less important than situational factors mainly because they reflect genetic determinants and early learning, and are therefore not easy to change. This notion of 'why study personality factors when you can't change them' seems to be widespread, leading to a tendency to ignore them. Jaccard & Wilson (1991), on the other hand, considered at some length how personality factors might influence interventions, and pointed to the need to focus on aspects of personality that are more specific to sexual behaviour and in particular to relatively enduring patterns of sexual behaviour. In the preceding section a number of studies that meet those requirements were reviewed. To what extent are their findings of relevance to HIV/AIDS prevention programmes?

There are at least four reasons for taking relevant personality factors into consideration in prevention programmes.

1. In the 'second phase' of interventions, described by Delay et al (2001), there has been a shift to include intensive individual counselling. Personality characteristics of the kind considered in the previous section may play a crucial role in counselling of that kind. Thus, for example, with individuals who have a tendency to take sexual risks when depressed or who use sex as a form of mood regulator, an initial behavioural analysis of the relationship between mood and sexual behaviour (e.g. using daily diaries) would help to confront the individual with this pattern and to focus motivation for change, followed by a cognitive-behavioural approach to develop and maintain alternative methods of mood regulation.

Our data suggest that this approach is particularly relevant to those gay men who cruise for casual sexual partners. As the negative mood in such men is driving them to go out and look for partners, interventions should focus on redirecting that sequence early, before the contact with a partner is made.

Clearly, some men deal with the arousal problem by planning ahead in a determined fashion. This strategy can be proposed to those men whose arousability appears to be unimpeded by risk. Pointing out such individual differences may serve to motivate the individual to see this not as just general common sense advice, but of particular relevance to him. Gold (2000) makes the point that interventions which focus on how the individual thinks 'in the heat of the moment', confronting the subject with his arousal-related thought processes which allow the unsafe behaviour to occur, can be effective in reducing unsafe sex.

Encouraging the self-discipline of contemplating the likely post-ejaculatory reaction sufficiently early in an encounter has already been mentioned, and can be added to the interventionist's agenda as one possible way of increasing the salience of inhibitory cues. On the other hand, the contrast between the romantic or committed and non-romantic, uncommitted situation is likely to be manifested in the subjective reaction immediately following ejaculation — the anticipated feeling of closeness and intimacy in the first compared with the regret, or alarm about possible consequences, or a need to escape from the situation, in the second. This emphasizes the importance of developing alternative intervention strategies to deal with potential risk in committed relationships. The impact of the relationship on risk management is a major factor for both straight and gay men and deserves careful research scrutiny in its own right.

2. Personality characteristics are likely to be important prognostic factors or mediators in determining the response to any intervention programme. Such crucial sources of variance in the outcome need to be controlled to assess interventions effectively (Warner & Bancroft 1986).
3. Personality characteristics should be considered when deciding what kind of message is going to be most effective in any intervention campaign, such as those involving the media. Donohew et al (1994) have pointed out that high-sensation seekers are likely to respond to styles of communication that would be ineffective or even counterproductive in low-sensation seekers. This evidence might encourage the use of more than one type of message.
4. Given the relative stability of relevant personality characteristics, there is the potential to identify young people who are not yet engaging in high-risk sexual behaviour but who are likely to do so in the future. This is well illustrated by a longitudinal study of a birth cohort followed up to their early 20s (Caspi et al 1997). These authors found that evidence

at the age of 3 years of 'under-controlled' behaviour predicted high 'negative emotionality' and low 'constraint' from the Tellegen personality profile (Tellegen & Waller 1985) at the age of 18 years, which in turn predicted a range of high-risk behaviours, including sexual behaviour at the age of 21 years. In a similar vein, Bates et al (2003) found externalizing behavioural tendencies in kindergarten-aged children to be predictive of number of sexual partners at the age of 16 and 17 years.

The impact of HIV/AIDS on sexual behaviour

The gay communities

When the last edition of this book was written we were seeing a major impact of HIV/AIDS on the gay communities in the Western world. In areas such as California or New York, where the epidemic was first established, bereavement of lovers and friends was a recurring experience comparable to wartime. Added to such losses was the fear of developing the disease and the often protracted and unique problem of living with and trying to support an AIDS sufferer who will surely die.

There was already evidence that in gay communities sexual behaviour was changing as a result of the epidemic. McKusick et al (1985) surveyed 655 gay men in San Francisco regarding their sexual practices during the previous month and the same month 1 year previously. They were recruited from gay bathhouses, gay bars and through gay organizations. The bathhouse group, probably those at highest risk, reported little change in their number of sexual partners. The other groups showed substantial reductions in casual sexual contacts, whereas men in monogamous relationships showed little change in sexual behaviour within their relationships. Martin (1987) assessed a cohort of 745 initially AIDS-free gay men in New York, assessing their behaviour both before and after they became aware of the AIDS epidemic. Knowledge of AIDS was associated with a substantial reduction in the number of sexual partners and certain forms of sexual activity, in particular ingestion of semen (anally or orally), anal genital sex oral–anal sex and number of sexual partners. There was even a 50% reduction in sexual kissing.

Then came the introduction of HAART and in many treated cases substantial reduction in viral load. This has raised the issue of whether the introduction of effective therapy has reduced the concern about HIV/AIDS and led to an increase in high-risk sexual behaviour among MSM. In 1999, the CDC reported increases in unsafe sex and rectal gonorrhoea in MSM in San Francisco between 1994 and 1997 (CDC 1999). In the UK, Dodds et al (2000) reported a comparable increase in London. Reporting from a prospective four-centre cohort study of homosexual men in the USA, Ostrow et al (2002) found that less concern about HIV transmission as a result of HAART was strongly associated with sexual risk taking. Crepaz et al (2004) reported a meta-analysis of 25 English language studies, mostly involving MSM, which had examined the relationship between receiving HAART, or having an undetectable viral load on HAART, or beliefs about HAART, viral load and the risks of HIV transmission. They found no consistent difference in sexual risk taking in HIV+ve individuals between those taking and those not taking HAART, nor any difference between those who had an detectable and an undetectable viral load. They did find, however, that those who believed that HAART or an undetectable viral load would protect against HIV transmission and those who had reduced concerns about unsafe sex because of the availability of HAART, were more likely to engage in unsafe sex. They therefore emphasized the importance of communicating the fact that neither HAART nor an undetectable viral load eliminated the risk of HIV transmission.

The heterosexual communities

The impact of the AIDS epidemic on the heterosexual community is more difficult to assess. In both the USA and the UK, campaigns to promote safe sex have been aimed at the heterosexual as well as the homosexual populations. But, as considered earlier, the prevalence of HIV+ve status in heterosexuals is still fairly low in Western countries. Obviously in the areas of high heterosexual transmission, such as sub-Saharan Africa, the threat is much more significant, and it is unclear to what extent heterosexual behaviour has changed as a result, apart from the limited evidence of reduction of the number of partners and increased condom use among the young achieved in Uganda. The key problem appears to be the tendency among heterosexuals to see HIV/AIDS as 'other people's problems'.

We should, in any case, expect relevant individual differences in how people, whether heterosexual or homosexual, react to the threat of HIV/AIDS, and how they interpret the availability of treatment in relation to the need for safer sexual behaviour.

REFERENCES

Ackers JP 2000 Trichomoniasis. In Ledingham JGG, Warrell DA (eds) Concise Oxford Textbook of Medicine. Oxford University Press, Oxford, Chapter 16.95.

Ajzen I 1985 From intentions to action: a theory of planned behavior. In Kuhl J, Beckmann J (eds) Action Control: From Cognition to Behavior. Springer-Verlag, New York, pp. 11–39.

Asboe D, Catalan JM, Mandalia S, Dedes N, Florence E, Schrooten W, Noestlinger C, Colebunders R 2007 Sexual dysfunction in HIV-positive men is multi-factorial: a study of prevalence and associated factors. AIDS Care 19: 955–965.

Bajos N, Marquet J 2000 Research on HIV sexual risk: social relations-based approach in a cross-cultural perspective. Social Science and Medicine 50: 1533–1546.

Bancroft J 2000a Individual differences in sexual risk taking. In Bancroft J (ed) The Role of Theory in Sex Research. Indiana University Press, Bloomington, pp. 177–209.

Bancroft J (ed) 2000b The Role of Theory in Sex Research. Indiana University Press, Bloomington.

Bancroft J 2004 Kinsey and the politics of sex research. Annual Review of Sex Research 15: 1–39.

Bancroft J 2005 The history of sexual medicine in the United Kingdom. Journal of Sexual Medicine 2: 569–574.

Bancroft J, Vukadinovic Z 2004 Sexual addiction, sexual compulsivity, sexual impulsivity or what? Towards a theoretical model. The Journal of Sex Research 41: 225–234.

Bancroft J, Janssen E, Strong D, Carnes L, Vukadinovic Z, Long JS 2003a Sexual risk-taking in gay men: the relevance of sexual arousability, mood and sensation seeking. Archives of Sexual Behavior 32: 555–572.

Bancroft J, Janssen E, Strong D, Carnes LC, Vukadinovic Z, Long JS 2003b The relationship between mood and sexuality in heterosexual men. Archives Sexual Behavior 32: 217–230.

Bancroft J, Janssen E, Strong D, Vukadinovic Z 2003c The relationship between mood and sexuality in gay men. Archives Sexual Behavior 31: 231–242.

Bancroft J, Janssen E, Carnes L, Goodrich D, Strong D 2004 Sexual activity and risk taking in young heterosexual men: the relevance of sexual arousability, mood, and sensation seeking. Journal of Sex Research 41: 181–192.

Bancroft J, Herbenick D, Barnes T, Hallam-Jones R, Wylie K, Janssen E and members of BASRT 2005a The relevance of the dual control model to male sexual dysfunction: The Kinsey Institute/BASRT Collaborative Project. Sexual and Relationship Therapy 20: 13–30.

Bancroft J, Carnes L, Janssen E 2005b Unprotected anal intercourse in HIV-positive and HIV-negative gay men: the relevance of sexual arousability, mood, sensation seeking and erectile problems. Archives of Sexual Behavior 34: 299–305.

Bandura A 1986 Social Foundations of Thought and Action: A Social Cognitive Theory. Prentice Hall, Englewood Cliffs, NJ.

Barlow D 2000 Neisseria gonorrhoeae. In Ledingham JGG, Warrell DA (eds) Concise Oxford Textbook of Medicine. Oxford University Press, Oxford, Chapter 16.42.

Bates JE, Alexander DB, Oberlande SF, Dodge KA, Pettit GS 2003 Antecedents of sexual activity at ages 16 and 17 in a community sample followed from age 5. In Bancroft J (ed) Sexual Development in Childhood. Indiana University Press, Bloomington, pp. 206–238.

Binson D, Woods WJ, Pollack L, Paul J, Stall R, Catania JA 2002 Differential HIV risk in bathhouses and public cruising areas. American Journal of Public Health 91: 1482–1486.

Boldero J, Moore S, Rosenthal D 1992 Intention, context, and safe sex: Australian adolescents' responses to AIDS. Journal of Applied Social Psychology 22: 1374–1396.

Boyce P, Huang Soo Lee M, Jenkins C, Mohamed S, Overs C, Paiva V, Reid E, Tan M, Aggleton P 2007 Putting sexuality (back) into HIV/AIDS: issues, theory and practice. Global Public Health 2: 1–34.

Buckley RM Jr, McGuckin M, MacGregor RR 1978 Urine bacterial counts after sexual intercourse. New England Journal of Medicine 298: 321–324.

Canin L, Dolcini MM, Adler NE 1999 Barriers to and facilitators of HIV-STD behavior change intrapersonal and relationship-based factors. Review of General Psychology 3: 338–371.

Carey MP, Lewis BP 1999 Motivational strategies can enhance HIV risk reduction programs. AIDS and Behavior 3: 269–276.

Caspi A, Begg D, Dickson N, Harrington HL, Langley J, Moffitt TE 1997 Personality differences predict health-risk behaviors in young adulthood: evidence from a longitudinal study. Journal of Personality and Social Psychology 73: 1052–1063.

Catalan J, Meadows J 2000 Sexual dysfunction in gay and bisexual men with HIV infection: evaluation, treatment and implications. AIDS Care 12: 279–286.

Catania JA, Kegeles SM, Coates TJ 1990 Towards an understanding of risk behavior: an AIDS risk reduction model (ARRM). Health Education Quarterly 17: 53–72.

Catania JA, Binson D, Dolcini MM, Stall R, Choi K-H, Pollack LM, Hudes ES Canchola J, Philips K, Moskawitz JT, Coates TJ 1995 Risk factors for HIV and other sexually transmitted diseases and prevention practices among US heterosexual adults: changes from 1990 to 1992. American Journal of Public Health 85: 1492–1499.

CDC 1999 Increases in unsafe sexed rectal gonorrhoea among men who have sex with men — San Francisco, California 1994–1997. Journal of the American Medical Association 281: 696–697.

CDC 2000 Tracking the hidden epidemics. Trends in STDs in the United States 2000. http://www.cdc.gov/nchstp/dstd/Stats_Trends/Trends2000.pdf.

CDC 2005 Trends in reportable sexually transmitted diseases in the United States, 2005. http://www.cdc.gov/std/stat/trends2005.htm.

CDC 2007 Male circumcision and risk for HIV transmission and other health conditions: implications for the United States. http://www.cdc.gov/hiv/resources/factsheets/circumcision.htm

Cleland J, Ali MM 2006 Sexual abstinence, contraception, and condom use by young African women: a secondary analysis of survey data. Lancet 368: 1788–1793.

Coleman PJ, McQuillan GM, Moyer LA, et al 1998 Incidence of Hepatitis B virus infection in the United States, 1976–1994: estimates from the National Health and Nutrition Examination Surveys. Journal Infectious Diseases 178: 954–960.

Crepaz N, Marks G 2001 Are negative affective states associated with HIV sexual risk behaviors? A meta-analytic review. Health Psychology 20: 291–299.

Crepaz N, Hart TA, Marks G 2004 Highly active antiretroviral therapy and sexual risk behavior. Journal of the American Medical Association 292: 224–236.

Davenport-Hines R 1990 Sex, Death and Punishment. Attitudes to Sex and Sexuality in Britain since the Renaissance. Collins, London.

Delay PR, Stanecki K, Emberg G 2001 Introduction. In Lamptey PR, Gayle HD (eds) HIV/AIDS Prevention and Care in Resource-constrained Settings. A Handbook for the Design and Management of Programs. Family Health International, Arlington, VA.

de Visser R 2004 Delayed application of condoms, withdrawal and negotiation of safe sex among heterosexual young adults. AIDS Care 16: 315–322.

Dodds JP, Nardone A, Mercey DE, Johnson AM 2000 Increase in high risk sexual behaviour among homosexual men, London 1996–8. British Medical Journal 320: 1510–1511.

Donohew L, Palmgren P, Lorch EP 1994 Attention, need for sensation and health communication campaigns. American Behavioral Scientist 38: 310–332.

Elford J, Bolding G, Maguire M, Sherr L 2001 Gay men, risk and relationships. AIDS 15: 1053–1055.

Erens B, McManus S, Prescott, Field J, Johnson AM, Wellings K, Fenton K, Mercer C, Macdowell W, Copas AJ, Nanchahal K 2003 National Survey of Sexual Attitudes and Lifestyles II: reference tables and summary report. National Centre for Social Research, London.

Feinleib JA, Michael RT 2001 Reported changes in sexual behavior in response to AIDS in the United States. In Laumann EO, Michael RT (eds) Sex, Love and Health in America: Private Choices and Public Policies. University of Chicago Press, Chicago, pp. 302–326.

Fenton KA, Korovessis C, Johnson AM, McCadden A, McManus S, Welklings K, Mercer CH, Carder C, Copas AJ, Nanchahal K, Macdowall W, Ridgway G 2001 Sexual behaviour in Britain: reported sexually transmitted infections and prevalent genital *Chlamydia trachomatis* infection. Lancet 358: 1851–1854.

Fishbein M, Ajzen I 1975 Belief, attitude, intention and behavior: an introduction to theory and research. Addison-Wesley, Reading, MA.

Fishbein M, Bandura A, Triandis HC, Kanfer FH, Becker MH, Middlestadt SE 1991 Factors influencing behavior change: Final report. Paper presented at NIMH Workshop, 1991 (October), Washington, DC.

Fleming DT, McQuillan GM, Johnson RE, Nahmias AJ, Aral SO, Lee FK, St Louis ME 1997 Herpes Simplex Virus Type 2 in the United States, 1976 to 1994. New England Journal of Medicine 337: 1105–1111.

Flowers P, Smith JA, Sheeran P, Beail N 1997 Health and romance: understanding unprotected sex in relationships between gay men. British Journal of Health Psychology 2, 73–86.

Folkman S, Chesney MA, Pollack L, Phillips C 1992 Stress, coping, and high-risk sexual behavior. Health Psychology 11: 218–222.

Gerrard M, Gibbons FX, McCoy SB 1993 Emotional inhibition of effective contraception. Anxiety, Stress and Coping 6: 73–88.

Gerrard M, Gibbons FX, Bushman BJ 1996 Relation between perceived vulnerability to HIV and precautionary sexual behavior. Psychological Bulletin 119: 390–409.

Gold RS 2000 AIDS education for gay men: towards a more cognitive approach. AIDS Care 12: 267–272.

Gold RS, Skinner MJ 1997 Unprotected anal intercourse in gay men: the resolution to withdraw before ejaculating. Psychological Reports 81: 496–498.

Goldacre MJ, Watt B, Loudon N, Milne LJR, Louden JDO, Vessey MP 1979 Vaginal microbial flora in normal young women. British Medical Journal 1: 1450–1453.

Graham CA, Crosby RA, Sanders SA, Yarber WL 2005 Assessment of condom use in men and women. Annual Review of Sex Research 16: 20–52.

Graham CA, Crosby RA, Yarber WL, Sanders SA, McBride K, Milhausen RR, Arno JN 2006a Erection loss in association with condom use among young men attending a public STI clinic: potential correlates and implications for risk behaviour. Sexual Health 3: 1–6.

Graham CA, Sanders SA, Milhausen RR 2006b The Sexual Excitation/Sexual Inhibition Inventory for women: psychometric properties. Archives of Sexual Behavior 35: 397–409.

Grulich AE, de Visser RO, Smith AMA, Rissel CE 2003a Sex in Australia: injecting and sexual risk behaviour in a representative sample of adults. Australian and New Zealand Journal of Public Health 27: 242–250.

Grulich AE, de Visser RO, Smith AMA, Rissel CE, Richters J 2003b Sex in Australia: homosexual experience and recent homosexual encounters. Australian and New Zealand Journal of Public Health 27: 155–163.

Grulich AE, de Visser RO, Smith AMA, Rissel CE, Richters J 2003c Sex in Australia: Sexually transmissible infection and blood-borne virus history in a representative sample of adults. Australian and New Zealand Journal of Public Health 27: 234–241.

Halperin DT, Bailey RC 1999 Male circumcision and HIV infection: 10 years and counting. Lancet 354: 1813–1815.

Hammer JC, Fisher JD, Fitzgerald P, Fisher WA 1996 When two heads aren't better than one: AIDS risk behavior in college-age couples. Journal of Applied Social Psychology 26: 375–397.

Hand EA 1949 Circumcision and venereal disease. Archive of Dermatology and Syphilology 60: 341.

Harris JRW 1977 Other sexually transmitted disease. In Money J, Musaph H (eds) Handbook of Sexology. Excerpta Medica, Amsterdam, pp. 1023–1036.

Hays RB, Paul J, Ekstrand M, Kegeles SM, Stall R, Coates TJ 1997 Actual versus perceived HIV status, sexual behaviors and predictors of unprotected sex among young gay and bisexual men who identify as HIV-negative, HIV-positive and untested. AIDS 11: 1495–1502.

Ho GYF, Bierman R, Beardsley L, Chang CJ, Burk RD 1998 Natural history of cervicovaginal papillomavirus infection in young women. New England Journal of Medicine 338: 423–428.

Hospers HJ, Kok G 1995 Determinants of safe and risk-taking sexual behavior among gay men: a review. AIDS Education and Prevention 7: 74–95.

Hoyle RH, Fejfar MC, Miller JD 2000 Personality and sexual risk taking: a quantitative review. Journal of Personality 68: 1203–1231.

HPA Health Protection Agency 2006 Sexually Transmitted Infections http://www.hpa.org.uk/infections/topics_az/hiv_and_sti/stidefault.htm.

Jaccard J, Wilson T 1991 Personality factors influencing risk behaviors. In Wasserheit JN, Aral SO, Holmes KK (eds) Research Issues in Human Behavior and Sexually Transmitted Diseases in the AIDS Era. American Society for Microbiology, Washington, DC, pp. 177–200.

Janssen E, Vorst H, Finn P, Bancroft J 2002 The Sexual Inhibition (SIS) and Sexual Excitation (SES) Scales: I. Measuring sexual inhibition and excitation proneness in men. Journal of Sex Research 39: 114–126.

Johnson AM, Wadsworth J, Wellings K, Field J 1994 Sexual Attitudes and Lifestyles. Blackwell, Oxford.

Kalichman SC, Weinhardt L 2001 Negative affect and sexual risk behavior: comment on Crepaz and Marks (2001). Health Psychology 20: 300–301.

Kelly JA, Kalichman SC 1995 Increased attention to human sexuality can improve HIV-AIDS prevention efforts: key research issues and directions. Journal of Consulting and Clinical Psychology 63: 907–918.

Koutsky L 1997 Epidemiology of genital human papillomavirus infection. American Journal Medicine 102(suppl 5A): 3–8.

Laumann EO, Youm Y 2001 Racial/ethnic group differences in the prevalence of sexually transmitted diseases in the United States: a network explanation. In Laumann EO, Michael RT (eds) Sex, Love and Health in America: Private Choices and Public Policies. University of Chicago Press, Chicago, pp. 327–351.

Laumann EO, Gagnon JH, Michael RT, Michaels S 1994 The social organization of sexuality: sexual practices in the United States. University of Chicago Press, Chicago.

Laumann EO, Masi CM, Zuckerman EW 2001 Circumcision in the United States: prevalence, prophylactic effects, and sexual practice. In Laumann EO, Michael RT (eds) Sex, Love and Health in America: Private Choices and Public Policies. University of Chicago Press, Chicago, pp. 277–301.

Leigh BD, Stall R 1993 Substance use and risky sexual behavior for exposure to HIV: issues in methodology, interpretation, and prevention. American Psychologist 48: 1035–1045.

Lowy E, Ross MW 1994 'It'll never happen to me': gay men's beliefs, perceptions and folk constructions of sexual risk. AIDS Education and Prevention 6: 467–482.

Luzzi GA, Weiss RA, Conion CP 2000 HIV infection and AIDS. In Ledingham JGG, Warrell DA (eds) Concise Oxford Textbook of Medicine. Oxford University Press, Chapter 16.35.

Lykins AD, Janssen E, Graham CA 2006 The relationship between negative mood and sexuality in heterosexual college women and men. Journal of Sex Research 43: 136–143.

MacDonald TK, MacDonald G, Zanna MF, Fong GT 2000 Alcohol, sexual arousal, and intentions to use condoms in young men: applying Alcohol Myopia Theory to risky sexual behavior. Health Psychology 19: 290–298.

Markowitz LE, Dunne EF, Saraiya M, Lawson HW, Chesson H, Unger ER 2007 Quadrivalent human papillomavirus vaccine. Recommendations of the Advisory Committee on Immunization Practices (ACIP). http://www.cdc.gov/mmwrhtml/rr5602a1.htm.

Martin JL 1987 The impact of AIDS on gay male sexual behavior patterns in New York City. American Journal of Public Health 77: 578–581.

McKusick L, Horstman W, Coates TJ 1985 AIDS and sexual behaviour reported by gay men in San Francisco. American Journal of Public Health 75: 493–496.

McKusick L, Hoff CC, Stall R, Coates TJ 1991 Tailoring AIDS prevention: differences in behavioral strategies among heterosexual and gay bar patrons in San Francisco. AIDS Education and Prevention 3: 1–9.

Mertz KJ, Trees D, Levine WC, Lewis JS and members of the Genital Ulcer Disease Surveillance Group 1998 Etiology of genital ulcers and prevalence of human immunodeficiency virus co-infection in 10 US cities. Journal of Infectious Diseases 178: 1795–1798.

Moatti JP, Hausser D, Agrafiotis D 1997 Understanding HIV risk-related behaviour: a critical overview of current model. In Van Campenhoudt L, Cohen M, Guizzardi G, Hausser D (eds) Sexual Interaction and HIV Risk. New Conceptual Perspectives in European Research. Taylor & Francis, London, pp. 100–126.

Moscucci O 1996 Clitoridectomy, circumcision and the politics of sexual pleasure in Mid-Victorian Britain. In Miller AH, Adams JE (eds) Sexualities in Victorian Britain. Indiana University Press, Bloomington, IN, pp. 60–78.

Mustanski B 2007 The influence of state and trait affect on HIV risk behaviours: a daily diary study of MSM. Health Psychology 26: 618–626.

Ostrow DE, Fox KJ, Chmiel JS, Silvestre A, Visscher BR, Vanable PA, Jacobson LP, Strathdee SA 2002 Attitudes towards highly active antiretroviral therapy are associated with sexual risk taking among HIV-infected and uninfected homosexual men. AIDS 16: 775–780.

Palefsky JM 1998 Human papillomavirus infection and anogenital neoplasia in human immunodeficiency virus-positive men and women. Monographs of National Cancer Institute 23: 15–20.

Philpott A, Knerr W, Maher D 2006a Promoting protection and pleasure: amplifying the effectiveness of barriers against sexually transmitted infections and pregnancy. Lancet 368: 2028–2031.

Philpott A, Knerr W, Boydell V 2006b Pleasure and prevention: when good sex is safer sex. Reproductive Health Matters 14: 23–31.

Piot P 2007 STI's and HIV: learning from each other for the long-term response? Speech at 17th Annual Meeting of International Society for Sexually Transmitted Diseases Research, Seattle, July.

Porter R, Hall L 1995 The Facts of Life. The Creation of Sexual Knowledge in Britain, 1650–1950. Yale University Press, NH.

Prochaska JO, DiClemente CC, Norcross JC 1992 In search of how people change: applications to addictive behaviors. American Psychologist 47: 1102–1114.

Quirk A, Rhodes T, Stimson GV 1998 'Unsafe protected sex': qualitative insights on measures of sexual risk. AIDS Care 10: 105–114.

Reece M, Plate PL, Daughtry M 2001 HIV prevention and sexual compulsivity: the need for an integrated strategy of public health and mental health. Sexual Addiction and Compulsivity 8: 157–167.

Richters J, Hendry O, Kippax S 2003 When safe sex isn't safe. Culture, Health and Sexuality 5: 37–52.

Robins AG, Dew AM, Kingsley LA, Becker JT 1997 Do homosexual and bisexual men who place others at potential risk for HIV have unique psychosocial profiles? AIDS Education and Prevention 9: 239–251.

Ronald A 2000 Haemophilus ducreyi and chancroid. In Ledingham JGG, Warrell DA (eds) Concise Oxford Textbook of Medicine. Oxford University Press, Oxford, Chapter 16.48.

Rosen RC, Riley A, Wagner G, Osterloh IH, Kirkpatrick J, Mishra A 1997 The international index of erectile function (IIEF): a multidimensional scale for assessment of erectile dysfunction. Urology 49: 822–830.

Rosenstock IM 1974 The health belief model and preventive health behavior. Health Education Monographs 2: 354–385.

Sandfort TGM, Clement U, Knobel J, Keet R, De Vroome EMM 1995 Sexualization in the coping process of HIV-infected gay men. Clinical Psychology and Psychotherapy 2: 220–226.

Simpson JA, Gangestad SW 1991 Individual differences in socio-sexuality: evidence for convergent and discriminant validity. Journal of Personality and Social Psychology 60: 870–883.

Sheeran P, Abraham C, Orbell S 1999 Psychosocial correlates of heterosexual condom use: a meta-analysis. Psychological Bulletin 125: 90–132.

Slutkin G, Okware S, Naamara W, Sutherland D, Flannagan D, Carael M, Blas E, Delay P, Tarantola D 2006 How Uganda reversed its HIV epidemic. AIDS Behavior 10: 351–361.

Spielberger CD, Gorsuch RL, Lushene RE 1970 STAI Manual for the State Trait Anxiety Inventory. Consulting Psychologists Press, Palo Alto, CA.

Spira A, Bajos N and the ACSF group 1994 Sexual behaviour and AIDS. Aldershot, Avebury.

Steele CM, Josephs RA 1990 Alcohol myopia: its prized and dangerous effects. American Psychologist 45: 921–933.

Strong DA, Bancroft J, Carnes LA, Davis LA, Kennedy J 2005 The impact of sexual arousal on sexual risk taking: a qualitative study. Journal of Sex Research 42: 185–191.

Stulhofer A, Graham C, Bozicevic I, Kufrin K, Ajdukovic D 2007 HIV/AIDS-related knowledge, attitudes and sexual behaviors as predictors of condom use among young adults in Croatia. International Famiiy Planning Perspectives 33: 58–65.

Szabo R, Short RV 2000 How does male circumcision protect against HIV infection? British Medical Journal 320: 1592–1594.

Tanner A, in press Young women's use of a microbicide surrogate: the role of internal and contextual factors. Archives of Sexual Behavior (under review).

Tellegen A, Waller NG 1985 Exploring personality through test construction: development of a multidimensional personality questionnaire. In Briggs SR, Cheek JM (eds) Personality Measures: Development and Evaluation. Jai Press, Greenwich, CT, Vol. 1, pp. XX.

Tindall B, Forde S 1994 Sexual dysfunction in advanced HIV disease. AIDS Care 6: 105–108.

Tolan J 2005 Married women and AIDS vulnerability. http://surj.Stanford.edu/2005/pdfs/Jenny.pdf.

Trobst KK, Herbst JH, Masters HL III, Costa PT Jr 2002 Personality pathways to unsafe sex: personality, condom use and HIV risk behaviors. Journal of Research in Personality 36: 117–133.

UNAIDS 2002 The 'ABCs' of HIV Prevention. Report of a USAID technical meeting on behavior change approaches to primary prevention of HIV/AIDS. September 17, 2002. http://phnip.com/portfolio/pub_examples/abc.pdf.

UNAIDS 2007 New data on male circumcision and HIV prevention: policy and program implications. http://data.unaids.org/pub/Report/2007/mc_recommendations_en.pdf.

Van De Ven P, Kippax S, Crawford J, Rawstorne P, Prestage G, Grulich A, Murphy D 2002 In a minority of gay men, sexual risk practice indicates strategic positioning for perceived risk reduction rather than unbridled sex. AIDS Care 14: 471–480.

Warner P, Bancroft J 1986 Sex therapy outcome research: a reappraisal of methodology. II. Methodological considerations. Psychological Medicine 16: 855–863.

Zemore R, Fischer DG, Garratt LS, Miller C 1990 The Depression Proneness Rating Scale: reliability, validity, and factor structure. Current Psychology: Research and Reviews 9: 255–263.

Zuckerman M 1979 Sensation seeking; beyond the optimal level of arousal. Erlbaum, Hillsdale, NJ.

Zuckerman M 1994 Behavioral expressions and biosocial bases of sensation seeking. Cambridge University Press, Cambridge.

Sexual aspects of fertility, fertility control and infertility

15

Pregnancy and the post-partum period........................... 439
Socio-cultural factors 440
Concerns about harming the fetus............................... 440
The impact of pregnancy on the couple's
relationship 440
Post-partum dyspareunia 440
Negative mood changes — maternity blues 441
Post-natal depression 441
Post-partum fatigue.. 441
Breastfeeding 441

Fertility control and contraception 442
The need for fertility control 442
Socio-cultural attitudes to contraception 442
Contraceptive use 443

Hormonal contraception... 445
The effects of hormonal contraceptives on sexual
behaviour 446
Long-acting reversible methods.................................. 452
Hormonal contraception in the male........................... 453
Barrier methods.. 454
'Natural' methods 454

Sterilization 454
Female sterilization... 455
Male sterilization.. 456

Induced abortion 457

Infertility... 458
Infertility and sexual function...................................... 459

The most important consequence of heterosexual activity is pregnancy. What effect does pregnancy have on the sexual relationship? The avoidance of unwanted pregnancy is crucial if the non-reproductive benefits of human sexuality are to be exploited. For health professionals, their involvement in the provision of fertility control provides one of the main opportunities for discussing the sexual problems of their clients and patients. In addition, sexual problems may arise as a consequence of fertility control. There is therefore a fundamental need to understand the sexual implications and consequences of fertility regulation. It is an unfortunate fact that of the huge sums of money that have been spent on developing and evaluating methods of fertility control, a negligible proportion has gone on appraising their effects on sexual behaviour. This was the case when the last edition of this book was written, and it remains the case today, nearly 20 years later. This is surprising considering that were it not for sexual activity, fertility control would be unnecessary; also surprising when the major obstacle to world population control lies not in a lack of suitable technology but in the low level of acceptance of the various effective methods that are already available. And yet we know virtually nothing about the importance of sexual factors in producing this low acceptance and usage. In this chapter we will consider fertility control under three headings: contraception, sterilization and induced abortion. Avoidance of unwanted pregnancy is not the only issue, however. Inability to conceive is a source of much distress for many would-be parents and high rates of infertility are a cause of social concern in certain parts of the world. We will therefore close the chapter by considering the sexual aspects of infertility. But first let us consider pregnancy.

Pregnancy and the post-partum period

The complex and markedly different hormonal state that characterizes pregnancy was considered in Chapter 3. It is physiologically different from the non-pregnant state mainly because of the impact of the placenta, which produces large amounts of reproductive hormones, especially progesterone, and is not under normal feedback control.

The literature is reasonably consistent in finding a decline in sexual activity and sexual interest of the woman during the third trimester of pregnancy. There is somewhat less consistency about changes in the first and second trimester. This may reflect the variable degree of nausea commonly experienced towards the end of the first trimester, and in some women there may be a return to more normal pre-pregnancy levels of sexual interest and response in the second trimester. Sexual responsiveness may continue relatively unchanged, at least until the latter part of the third trimester. Orgasm may be associated with uncomfortable pelvic spasm by the third trimester.

Studies of sexual interest and the resumption of sexual activity post-partum show more variability. In the post-partum period, Robson et al (1981) found that nearly all women had resumed sexual intercourse by the 12th week, and a third had done so by the 6th week. Grudzinskas & Atkinson (1984) found 51% of 328 women had resumed intercourse, when interviewed between 5 and 7 weeks post-partum. In the most comprehensive study to date, Hyde et al (1996) assessed 570 women and their husbands/partners at the fifth month of pregnancy, and also at 1, 4 and 12 months post-partum. At the assessment during pregnancy, 89% of women reported sexual intercourse in the previous month, at 1 month post-partum only 17%, increasing to 89% at 4 months and 92% at 12 months post-partum. Sexual interest is typically less in the first 3–4 months post-partum than it was before the pregnancy, but in the later post-partum stages there is considerable variability across women, and to some extent among their male partners also (Von Sydow 2006).

In understanding the impact of pregnancy and post-partum on the sexuality of the parental couple, a range of factors need to be considered: (i) the socio-cultural values about sex during pregnancy, (ii) fears about possible harm of sexual activity to the fetus, (iii) alterations in the relationship between partners resulting from pregnancy, (v) damage to the vulva from tears or episiotomies during delivery, causing dyspareunia, (vi) negative mood change and fatigue in the pregnant and post partum woman and its impact on sexual interest, and, as a more fundamental component of the reproductive process, (vii) the impact of breastfeeding.

Socio-cultural factors

Ford & Beach (1952) showed how taboos against sex during pregnancy were widespread across cultures, though varying in severity and extent. Various reasons for such taboos were suggested, principally fear of harming the fetus.

Concerns about harming the fetus

Such fears are common, though not institutionalized in our own culture, and, in the absence of medical reassurance to the contrary, understandable. Von Sydow (2006) points out the fairly general reluctance of medical practitioners and obstetricians to discuss sexual aspects of pregnancy with their patients. There are grounds for caution in some instances. Women who have a tendency to abort towards the end of the first trimester should avoid orgasm until that phase has passed. Vaginal intercourse and orgasm should be avoided in the second trimester in women with evidence of cervical incompetence, at least until the defect has been surgically corrected, and avoided in the third trimester in women with obvious obstetric complications such as bleeding, ruptured membranes, premature dilatation of the cervix or the threat of premature labour (White & Reamy 1982; Von Sydow 2006). In the absence of clear contraindications, the couple should feel free to continue, change or discontinue their sexual interactions in ways that suit them both.

The impact of pregnancy on the couple's relationship

This varies considerably, as one would expect. For many couples, particularly with the first pregnancy, the joy of anticipating their first wanted child can enhance intimacy.

In other cases, there may be some withdrawal of the woman from the intimacy of the relationship, and this may be more noticeable in second and subsequent pregnancies. Post-partum is a challenging time for the relationship, with many adjustments required to accommodate the new family member, and a considerable increase in demands on both parents' time. De Judicibus & McCabe (2002) reported from their study of couples having their first child that relationship satisfaction reached a low point at 12 weeks post-partum. However, most women remained moderately satisfied with their relationships.

Post-partum dyspareunia

An important factor influencing the quality of the early post-partum sexual experience is pain, particularly in those women who have had an episiotomy — a procedure for cutting the perineum so as to avoid uncontrolled tearing during delivery. This is commonly done, especially for women undergoing their first delivery. In an early study, Beischer (1967) assessed the effects of this procedure and its subsequent repair on sexual function. In one Australian hospital, episiotomies were performed in 30% of deliveries. Ninety per cent of these were repaired by medical students. Post-partum, 39% of the women with episiotomies had experienced dyspareunia, persisting 3 months after delivery in 23%. In 6% the dyspareunia was severe and in those cases there was usually some narrowing of the vaginal introitus or the creation of a skin bridge due to inappropriate repair. Garner (1982) studied 204 women following their second delivery in an English maternity hospital. Thirty per cent of the women with episiotomies and 30% of those with perineal tears reported interference with their sex lives. Of interest was the finding that these sequelae were less common in women who had forceps deliveries. This was attributed to the involvement of more skilled personnel at the repair stage in such cases. Some attention has also been paid to the positioning of episiotomies, with suggestions that midline episiotomies cause fewer problems subsequently than the more usual mediolateral incisions (Reamy & White 1987). The midline incision is usually avoided, however, in case it extends into a third degree tear involving the anal sphincter.

In the UK, a survey of 101 NHS hospitals was carried out in 1993. Some form of perineal trauma was experienced by 83% of women following childbirth; 40% had an episiotomy only, 6% had an episiotomy and a perineal tear, and 37% had tears without episiotomy. There was considerable variation across the hospitals and regions surveyed in the rates of episiotomy, suggesting lack of uniformity in the indications for this procedure (Williams et al 1998). In the USA, in the 1980s, episiotomy was carried out in about two-thirds of deliveries (Reamy & White 1987). From 1980 through to 1998 the episiotomy rate dropped by 39%. The incidence of first- and second-degree perineal tears increased for women without episiotomies, but the more severe third- and fourth-degree lacerations remained more frequent for women with episiotomies. Women with episiotomies were more likely to have forceps-assisted deliveries or vacuum extractions. Despite this decline, episiotomy remains one of the most frequent surgical procedures performed on women in the USA (Weeks & Kozak 2001). Clearly these almost routine procedures and the manner in which they are repaired require careful reappraisal.

Negative mood changes — maternity blues

Transient mood change, starting most often around day 5 post-partum and lasting for 12–14 days, is very common, with prevalence rates ranging from 30 to 80% across studies (Scott & Jenkins 1998). This is usually called 'post-partum blues' or 'maternity blues'. This pattern is often preceded by negative mood change during the third trimester, also quite common. The causes of such mood changes are not well understood. They occur cross-culturally and are relatively specific to childbirth (e.g. the same pattern does not occur after surgery). They have often been attributed to the major changes in hormone levels following delivery, but as yet there has been little evidence to support this hypothesis (Heidrich et al 1994).

Post-natal depression

This is a clinically more significant affective disorder that typically starts around the fourth week post-partum, and occurs in 10–15% of post-partum women. Although this prevalence is not markedly higher than the prevalence for depression for women in general, there is some evidence that in many such cases the depression is a specific reaction to the changes occurring post-partum, with an increased likelihood of recurrence with subsequent pregnancies (Cooper & Murray 1995). On the other hand, there are other women who are more generally vulnerable to depression and who experience it post-partum as well as at other times. Post-natal depression is important in that it can have negative effects on the evolving mother–infant relationship. Treatment is also complicated in those women who breastfeed by the possibility of medication being absorbed by the infant through the breast milk. Efforts are therefore made to treat the problem with cognitive therapy as far as possible (Scott & Jenkins 1998). Negative mood changes are clearly an important cause of low sexual interest in the post-partum period.

Post-partum fatigue

Fatigue and weakness are commonly given by women as reasons for loss of sexual desire in late pregnancy and post-partum (De Judicibus & McCabe 2002). Hyde et al (1998) found that this impact of fatigue was less apparent by 4 months post-partum, when they found depression to be a more important predictor of low sexual interest.

Breastfeeding

It is generally agreed that breastfeeding has a number of advantages for the infant over other methods, particularly in developing countries. In the UK, in 2005, 76% of mothers initiated breastfeeding with their infants (IC.NHS 2005). This had been 71% in the 2000 Infant Feeding Survey with a steady increase since 1990. There are clearly socio-cultural factors that influence breastfeeding. In the USA, the rates of breastfeeding are overall lower (58% in 1994), and substantially lower in African Americans (27%) than in white (61%) or Hispanic (67%) mothers (Hyde & DeLamater 2003). It is probably easier for a mother in the UK to breastfeed her baby in public without being stared at disapprovingly, than for a mother in the USA.

Mothers vary substantially in the period of time they continue breastfeeding. Some stop quickly because of problems with providing enough milk. Some continue for 2 years or more. A typical duration is around 6 months. The effectiveness of the breastfeeding, the emotional rewards to the mother and the attitudes of both parents are all factors that influence this process.

There is consistent evidence that breastfeeding mothers are less sexually active and have less sexual interest than bottle-feeding mothers (Von Sydow 2006). This was shown in a study of 60 breastfeeding and 31 bottle-feeding mothers (Alder & Bancroft 1988). Hyde et al (1996), in their study of 570 women progressing through pregnancy and the post-partum period, found that 68% initiated breastfeeding. The non-breastfeeders were significantly more likely to have resumed sexual intercourse at 1 month post-partum, and the breastfeeders were more likely to report lack of sexual desire. These differences were still evident at 4 months post-partum. By 1 year post-partum, however, only 12% of mothers were still breastfeeding, and differences between the two groups were no longer significant.

The main determinant of the hormonal status of the woman in the puerperium is her method of infant feeding. The fully breastfeeding woman is likely to have ovarian suppression, raised prolactin levels and relative oestrogen (E) deficiency. The raised prolactin may be directly associated with reduced sexual interest (see p. 129) and the low E with lack of vaginal lubrication and resulting dyspareunia. In a small study of 14 breastfeeding women (Alder et al 1986), we found that five women reported low sexual interest, and they had significantly lower testosterone (T) levels than the other nine women (Fig. 15.1). Given the more recent evidence of variability in the importance of T for sexual desire in women (see Chapter 4, p. 114) the findings from this study warrant replication.

Apart from hormonal impact of lactation, however, there are obviously other factors to be taken into account. Breastfeeding is associated with more disrupted sleep for the mother and hence greater fatigue. The psychological implications of breastfeeding for both the mother and her partner are complex and may be important. For some mothers there is an erotic aspect to

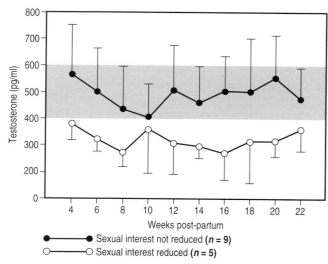

Fig. 15.1 Levels of total plasma testosterone in 14 breastfeeding women for 22 weeks post-partum. The women are divided into two groups according to whether or not they reported loss of sexual interest. The shaded area represents the range of testosterone levels in normal women (analysis of variance $p < 0.05$). (From Alder et al 1986.)

TABLE 15.1	The current world use (percentage) of different contraceptive methods, comparing the developed and developing worlds, and 1987 with 1998. (Van Look 2000)					
	World		More developed regions		Less developed regions	
	1987	1998	1987	1998	1987	1998
Sterilization						
Female	29	33	11	12	37	39
Male	8	7	6	7	9	8
OC	14	14	20	24	11	11
Injectables	2	3	–	<1	2	4
IUD	20	22	8	9	25	26
Condom	9	8	18	19	5	4
Vaginal barrier	1	1	3	3	1	<1
Rhythm	7	5	13	9	4	4
Withdrawal	8	7	19	17	4	4
Others	2	1	2	1	2	1

breastfeeding. For some, such a reaction makes them feel uncomfortable and may lead to their giving up breastfeeding. Some men are disturbed by the sight of their partner breastfeeding (Reamy & White 1987). Full breastfeeding may make it difficult for the mother to carry out all her other usual commitments, leading in some cases to tension or resentment in the spouse or other family members. The emotional involvement of the mother in the breastfeeding process may also be at the expense of her usual level of involvement and intimacy with her partner. Hyde et al (1996) found that their breastfeeding and non-breastfeeding mothers did not differ at 1 month or 4 months post-partum in their level of sexual satisfaction, but, in terms of how rewarding the sexual relationship was, the non-breastfeeding women rated significantly higher at both 1 and 4 months. In terms of how much physical affection the woman received from the relationship, breastfeeding and non-breastfeeding women did not differ at 1 month, but non-breastfeeding women reported more physical affection at 4 months. The male partners of the non-breastfeeding women, on the other hand, reported significantly higher sexual satisfaction, sexual reward and physical affection than the partners of breastfeeding women, at both time points.

Fertility control and contraception

The need for fertility control

During the 20th century the world population increased from 1.65 billion to 6 billion, with the increase from 5 to 6 billion taking only 12 years. Current projections are that the world population will stabilize around 10 billion after 2200 (Van Look 2000). In the last four decades there has been a substantial rise in the use of fertility control. In 1998, this applied to 58% of all married couples. However, there remain substantial differences between the

developed and the developing world in the methods used. These differences are shown in Table 15.1. This is most noticeable in female sterilization and intrauterine devices (IUD)s, which are more frequently used in the developing world, and oral contraceptives (OCs) and condoms, which are more frequently used in the developed world. The evidence clearly indicates, however, that fertility control is a long way from being sufficient; around 46 million unwanted pregnancies are terminated each year, about 20 million carried out in unsafe conditions, with around 78 000 women dying as a result each year (Van Look 2000).

Socio-cultural attitudes to contraception

D'Emilio & Freedman (1988) documented how, in the 1920s and 1930s, societal reaction to sexual change focused on contraception, and the dissociation of sex from reproduction that it implies. Whereas in the 1920s and early 1930s this issue was closely related to women's rights, with the economic crises of the 1930s contraception started to be seen as a way of protecting the family from getting too large; children, once regarded as an economic asset, were increasingly regarded as additional expense. Then came World War II, following which the impact of the 'baby boom' complicated the situation further. But concerns about contraception, and its potential for reducing social control of women's sexuality, a long-standing mainstay of patriarchy, flared up again with the introduction of 'the pill' (Marks 2001; Watkins 1998).

In the developing world a major difference in the proportion of sterilizations that involve women rather than men can only be understood in terms of socio-cultural attitudes to gender and sexuality, and this will be considered further in the section on sterilization.

Of considerable importance is the morality of contraception. The Roman Catholic Church, in particular, deems any artificial method of avoiding conception to be immoral (Humanae Vitae 1968), a dictate that continues to be strongly reinforced by the Vatican. In the face of changing modern attitudes, and the inescapable fact of world over-population, an increasing number of Catholics are rejecting this particular part of the Church's teaching. In the USA, this has resulted in a serious divide between the Church and the Catholic laity, and a split in the Catholic clergy, a story well documented by Tentler (2004). Orthodox Jewry also opposes contraception, though with the constant threats to the survival of the Jewish race this is perhaps more understandable (Parrinder 1987). One hopes that the price that rebellious Catholics pay in terms of religious conflict and guilt is small in comparison with the consequences that so many, particularly women and their children, suffer as a result of unwanted pregnancies or the fear of them. The basic reproductive function of sex became combined with a non-reproductive role for sex in relationships at an early stage of human evolution. However, the idea that sex is only acceptable as a means of reproduction is still fostered by such religious beliefs and goes deep in many individuals (see Chapter 6). Thus for some, most commonly women, sex requires at least the possibility of conception for it to be fully enjoyed. Methods of contraception that are foolproof, such as steroidal contraceptives, or irreversible, such as sterilization, may thus be unacceptable. For others, the associated conflict may make it difficult for the individual to take active responsibility for contraception, particularly those methods that have to be repeatedly exercised, such as taking a pill each day or inserting a diaphragm. In such cases, medical methods, such as IUDs, the fitting of which is the responsibility of the doctor, may hold special appeal. On the other hand, there are others who need the security of foolproof contraception to be able to enjoy sex fully.

Problems may reflect difficulties in male/female relationships. Thus conflict may lead to reluctance in one or other partner to take responsibility. A woman may decline oral contraception because she resents her partner's failure or refusal to take a share of responsibility. Barrier methods, such as the condom or diaphragm, are disliked by some because of their interference with the spontaneity of love-making or the physical barrier they present between partners. For others, this same barrier may be an added attraction; the man or woman who dislikes mess may prefer ejaculate to be captured in a sheath rather than allowed to run free. The protection afforded by the sheath against sexually transmitted disease is one increasingly important consideration, and is considered closely in Chapter 14. Any method of contraception that substantially alters the enjoyment or interest of the user may cause repercussions in the sexual relationship. A woman established on secure contraception may find herself under increased pressure for sex from her partner. Conversely, a woman whose sexuality has been inhibited for years by fear of pregnancy, once started on effective contraception may find that her sexual awakening leads to anxieties or sexual failure in her partner, who cannot cope with the apparent increase in sexual demands upon him.

It is difficult to dispute the idea that modern methods of fertility control have contributed to the changing status of women, who can now decide whether or not to have children and, to some extent, when. They are much less likely to be trapped in traditional female roles by unplanned pregnancies. The social impact of this is, and will continue to be, considerable. And yet, for some individuals, such freedom can be threatening. In its most extreme form, this threat may be linked with a fear of losing one's female identity or of becoming promiscuous. In the case of oral contraception, this can be compounded by a fear of anything that changes one's internal chemistry and hence one's behaviour. Some people dislike taking any kind of drug that alters their internal state in an unpredictable way. Women with such personalities may find OCs difficult to tolerate.

Contraceptive use

Oral contraceptives became available in the 1960s, and there has been a general increase in availability and use of various methods of contraception since. From the 1970s there was increased interest in surgical methods of sterilization, and since the late 1980s, as a result of the HIV/AIDS pandemic, an increased attention to the use of condoms, sometimes combined with steroidal methods.

The use of different methods varies considerably from one culture to another, and to a lesser extent within cultures according to age and social class. A consistent finding is that single women are nearly twice as likely to use oral contraception as married or co-habiting women.

Figures for married women in the UK for the years 1970, 1975 (Bone 1978) and 1983 (General Household Survey 1983) are given in Table 15.2, showing that in 1975 and 1983 oral contraception was the most widely used method in the UK, whereas barrier methods, such as the diaphragm and condom, were being used less.

These earlier figures can be compared to figures from the UK Natsal I (1990) and Natsal II (2000) surveys. The use of different methods of contraception in the past year, reported by men and women who had at least one heterosexual partner in that year, are shown in Table 15.3 for the total for Natsal I (Johnson et al 1994) and also by age group for Natsal II (Erens et al 2003).

TABLE 15.2	Contraceptive use in the UK amongst fertile married women, not pregnant and not trying to conceive		
Current method	1970[*] (n=1895) (%)	1975 (n=1655) (%)	1983[†] (n=1917) (%)
Withdrawal	19	7	10
Pill	25	42	40
IUD	5	9	12
Diaphragm	6	3	3
Condom	36	25	28
Safe period	6	1	3
None	7	11	8

[*]Figures for 1970 and 1975 are for women aged under 41 (Bone 1978)
[†]Figures for 1983 are for women aged under 44 (General Household Survey 1983)

TABLE 15.3 Contraceptive methods used in the last year, age and gender in the UK in 2000 for all with at least one heterosexual partner in the last year (from Natsal II (2000); Erens et al 2003; total also from Natsal I (1990); Johnson et al 1994)

	16–17*		18–19		20–24		25–34		35–44		Total		Total (Natsal I)	
	M	F	M	F	M	F	M	F	M	F	M	F	M	F
	%	%	%	%	%	%	%	%	%	%	%	%	%	%
METHOD														
OC (pill)	35.6	54.7	52.3	69.8	51.6	62.0	47.1	43.7	21.8	16.8	**38.2**	**38.2**	40.2	38.3
Condom	88.2	82.2	87.0	68.8	79.7	56.7	51.1	36.9	32.0	26.3	**51.3**	**39.2**	43.2	30.6
IUD	2.4	0.5	0.2	0.4	0.9	2.5	4.0	6.9	5.9	7.9	**4.0**	**6.1**	5.3	7.3
Natural method	7.7	3.7	9.9	8.4	10.9	7.5	13.0	10.5	9.2	7.2	**10.9**	**8.5**	9.6	6.4
Injectables	1.9	6.4	3.1	6.2	2.6	8.6	3.1	4.5	1.4	1.6	**2.4**	**4**	n.a	n.a
Other methods	6.5	4.8	6.2	10.5	7.0	5.5	3.1	3.9	3.2	2.7	**4.0**	**4.1**	3.2	4.2
None	3.7	3.2	4.5	6.2	3.8	7.0	10.4	11.3	16.0	16.8	**11.0**	**12.1**	11.2	12.7
SURGICAL METHOD														
Vasectomy	—	—	—	0.4	0.2	0.6	3.3	6.3	19.7	18.7	**8.7**	**9.5**	9.6	11.5
Female sterilization	—	—	—	—	—	—	3.0	4.9	8.8	14.9	**4.5**	**7.4**	7.0	8.8

*Age in years
M, male; F, female

This suggests a slight decrease in the proportion of OC users from 1975 to 2000, and a more substantial increase in condom use, which probably reflects the impact of the HIV/AIDS pandemic.

Johnson et al (1994) used logistic regression to assess the relationship between socioeconomic and other variables and contraceptive use. Controlling for the other variables, non-use of contraception increased with age, whereas use of OCs decreased with age more markedly in women than men. Whereas number of sexual partners was predictive of contraceptive use, this was more marked in men than women. Men with more than one sexual partner in the past year were four times more likely to report contraceptive use than those with one partner. Men in non-manual social class groups were twice as likely to report contraceptive use as those in manual groups; this effect was apparent but less strong in women.

Methods of fertility control used by women aged 15–44 years in the USA for the years 1982, 1995 and 2002 are shown in Table 15.4. Of those currently using some form of fertility control, the percentages predominantly using each method are shown. Comparable data for women users in Australia in 2000–2002 are shown in Table 15.5. One needs to be cautious in making direct comparisons of such data across countries, as there are a number of subtle differences in the ways contraceptive users are defined. However, broadly speaking there are more similarities than differences in the UK, USA and Australian data.

Contraceptive use amongst teenagers is often inconsistent, particularly for the first few years of sexual activity. Some factors influencing contraceptive use among teenagers were considered in Chapter 5 (see p. 158). Lindemann (1977) suggested three stages of birth control behaviour: the 'natural stage' when no contraceptives are used, the 'peer stage', when methods learned from peers are used, and the 'expert stage', when experts or professionals are consulted. In the natural stage, she suggested, 'the very nature of sexual activity is not

TABLE 15.4 Women aged 15–44 in the USA using fertility control in 1982, 1995 and 2002 (percentage distribution by current method) (Mosher et al 2004, Table 5)

	1982	1995	2002
STERILIZATION			
Female	23.2	27.8	27.0
Male	10.9	10.9	9.2
HORMONAL			
OC	28.0	26.9	30.6
Implant/patch	—	1.3	1.2
DMPA	—	3.0	5.3
IUD	7.1	0.8	2.0
Diaphragms	8.1	1.9	0.3
Condoms	12.0	20.4	18.0
Rhythm/natural	3.9	2.3	1.6
Withdrawal	2.0	3.1	4.0
Other	1.3	1.7	0.9

TABLE 15.5 Contraceptive methods chosen by women using contraception in Australia in 2001–2002 (Sex in Australia Survey; Richters et al 2003)

Method	% (n=6278)
STERILIZATION	
Female	22.5
Male	19.3
HORMONAL	
OC	33.6
Progestogen injection	1.5
Progestogen implant	1.1
BARRIER METHODS	
Male condom	21.4
Female condom	<0.01
Diaphragm or cervical cap	0.9
IUD	1.2
Spermicides	0.2
Withdrawal	4.5
Safe periods	4.4

conducive to the use of contraceptives'. Intercourse is unplanned, and hence unpredictable and, at this stage, usually infrequent. Spontaneous sex is seen as natural — contraception as artificial. There is, in any case, a generally low level of awareness of the possibility of pregnancy that may be reinforced by the experience of sexual activity that does not lead to pregnancy. To some extent this may be less unrealistic than it seems for the young adolescent girl who may still be in a phase of relative adolescent infertility, although this is less relevant than it used to be because of the earlier age of menarche. At some point, determined by such factors as a delayed period, or pregnancy of a friend, awareness of the need for contraception develops. We know little about how sex education affects this process. Knowledge may be acquired, but it is not seen to be of personal relevance.

A disturbing fact is that we remain largely ignorant of this crucial stage of sexual development. Research has predominantly focused on when teenagers start to have sexual intercourse and whether they get pregnant. What precedes the onset of sexual intercourse (e.g. non-penetrative sexual activity) and how adolescents typically negotiate that sequence and the subsequent frequency of intercourse, and what information they need to do so appropriately, remain obscure. In part this is because of the reluctance to ask adolescents questions about sex which might possibly put 'ideas into their heads', a reluctance that persists in spite of the fact that the average age of onset of vaginal intercourse has lessened substantially (Ehrhardt 1996). In Chapter 5, several developmental patterns were considered; 'the parent vs peer group' pattern (see p. 158) is of particular relevance. Parental influences are important, particularly for girls, but depend on the quality of the parent–child relationship. Peer group influences are also important, particularly for those lacking close parent–child relationships. The peer group impact relevant to contraception requires an understanding of normal fertility and how this relates to the menstrual cycle, particularly if artificial methods of contraception are seen to be inaccessible.

Two other contrasting themes of potential relevance were considered in Chapter 6. These are early socio-cultural patterns that have become somewhat obscured in the modern Western world. The 'fertility factor', characteristic of early Northern European hunter–gatherer societies, had a typical sequence of betrothal and marriage once fertility was demonstrated by pregnancy (the 'bundling' system, see p. 191), a pattern related to the relatively long period of adolescent infertility typical of such societies. The 'virginity ethic', more characteristic of early Mediterranean agricultural societies, in which adolescent infertility was less marked, was influenced by the property status of the young wife and hence the importance of virginity (see p. 191). It is possible that remnants of these two patterns continue to contribute to the cross-cultural variability of adolescent sexual development.

For a girl, to take the decision to use contraception, particularly methods such as the pill, which imply long-term needs, may be much more difficult than her becoming involved periodically and 'in the heat of the moment' in unprotected sexual activity. More attention has been paid recently to fostering responsibility for contraception in the adolescent male, and it is possible that this is having some effect. Parental attitudes are highly relevant in this respect. The double standard prevalent in parental attitudes encourages boys to see the responsibility for contraception as being with the girl. As considered in Chapter 6, there is evidence of an increase in contraceptive use among teenagers but, of particular relevance, a shift from using OCs to using condoms (Grunbaum et al 2002). The decision to use OCs, requiring a daily pill, may pose a particular challenge for some teenage girls, who might be concerned about how this 'commitment to sexual activity' would be interpreted by her partner.

Certainly we can conclude that contraceptive use amongst adolescents is far from being a straightforward matter of availability and common sense. We have more questions than answers about how young people incorporate fertility control into their emerging sexuality, and there is a clear need to combine appropriate information about fertility with the message that the potential for fertility, and the creation of another human being, poses one of the greatest responsibilities that we face throughout life, for males as well as females. The messages contained in the Surgeon General's *Call to Action to Promote Sexual Health and Responsible Sexual Behavior* (Satcher 2001), discussed further in Chapter 1, should be part of normal sex education, important for all of us.

With these general considerations in mind, let us look at the various methods of fertility control in more detail.

Hormonal contraception

Most steroidal contraceptives are taken orally. Oral contraceptives are of three main types: combined, sequential and progestagen only. Combined pills contain both E (usually ethinyloestradiol) and progestagen (usually norethindrone, levonorgestrel (LN) or one of its derivatives, desogestrel, norgestimate or gestodene). They are taken for 21 days, followed by 7 pill-free days during which there is a monthly withdrawal bleed. There are now several versions of sequential pill, most of them triphasic. Typically a fixed dose of E is combined with a low dose of progestagen for the first 7 days, a slightly higher dose for the next 7 days and the highest dose for the last 7 days (e.g. Ortho Tri-Cyclen: ethinyl oestradiol 35 µg, norgestimate 0.18, 0.215 and 0.25 mg). There are then the usual 7 pill-free days.

Both combined and sequential types are believed to work by suppressing ovulation, though other effects on the cervical mucus, reducing sperm penetration, and elsewhere on the reproductive tract, may also inhibit fertility. The progestagen-only pills are less predictable in inhibiting ovulation and rely primarily on their endometrial effects (Hawkins & Elder 1979). Whereas the combined and sequential pills are taken cyclically, leading to predictable withdrawal bleeds, the progestagen-only preparations are taken continuously and menstrual bleeding may be irregular or 'breakthrough' bleeding may occur. This affects the acceptability of the method for many women.

The injectable forms of steroidal contraceptives have mainly contained progestagen only, e.g. medroxy-progesterone acetate (Depo-Provera). They have the advantage of long-term efficacy. Vaginal rings or intra-uterine systems (IUS) containing slowly released pro-gestagens are now available. For the breastfeeding mother, progestagen contraception is probably the method of choice, as oestrogens are likely to inhibit lactation. However, injectable progestagens are more likely to appear in the milk and oral preparations are therefore to be preferred.

The effects of hormonal contraceptives on sexual behaviour

Oral contraceptives

Although the literature on OCs and their various potential negative effects is now extensive, little attention has been paid to their effects on women's sexuality. This is starting to change. Two recent reviews (Schaffir 2006; Davis & Castano 2006) succeeded in conveying the confusion and inconsistencies that have prevailed in the relevant literature, without providing much guidance on how this might be resolved. Both reviews play down negative sexual effects of OCs. Schaffir (2006) concludes that 'on the basis of the literature that is currently available, clinicians can continue to prescribe hormonal contraception with the security that adverse (sexual) effects are likely to be minimal and experienced in an idiosyncratic fashion by a minority of users' (p. 391). Davis & Castano (2006) advise that 'providers must be cautious in attributing negative experiences to oral contraceptives, and be willing to explore other explanations for the common experience of decreased libido' (p. 295). The authoritative texts on contraception certainly minimize the negative sexual effects of OCs. In the comprehensive chapter on contraception by Mishell (2004) there is no mention of sexual interest or any other aspect of sexuality. Hatcher et al (2004), in their *Contraceptive Technology*, the gold standard in this field, provide a reasonable, though brief, comment. They point to the need to consider the coexistence of low libido and depression, but acknowledge that OCs may reduce libido as a consequence of dyspareunia caused by lowered oestradiol and impaired vaginal lubrication, or more directly by lowering testosterone.

In spite of the unresolved issues in this specific aspect of oral contraception, there has been little or no support for research from either government or industry. The World Health Organization (WHO) has a somewhat different record in this respect. In the late 1980s, I was asked by the Safety & Efficacy Task Force of the Human Reproduction Program at the WHO to work with Norman Sartorius, then a member of the WHO Division of Mental Health, and together review the literature on the effects of OCs on well-being and sexuality (Bancroft & Sartorius 1990). On the basis of this review, we recommended a series of research studies. The Task Force agreed to fund a study that is considered below (Graham et al 1995). This is the most substantial placebo-controlled study in this field and had the added advantage of comparing women from two contrasting cultures. The results pointed to a negative effect of OCs on sexuality in a significant minority of women. By the time we had completed and written up this study, and submitted it to the Task Force for their approval for publication, external members of the Task Force had changed, and the new members did not want it published. The study was too small, we were told, and could be misleadingly negative in its effects. The WHO staff, fortunately, did not take this view and the study was published. However, we failed to obtain external funding for the next research step (from the WHO, NIH, private foundations or the pharmaceutical industry), which was to look at predictors of discontinuation in women starting on OCs. We ended up carrying out a small study based on Kinsey Institute departmental funds. This is also considered below (Sanders et al 2001). The results from this were sufficiently convincing that we were able to get partial support from Ortho-McNeill for a further study examining the effects of OCs on T and sexuality (Graham et al 2007).

As we shall see, the issue of negative effects of OCs on the sexuality of women is complex, and this may account for the prevailing tendency therefore to dismiss it as unimportant. But one can confidently conclude that no such dismissal would occur if one was considering potential negative effects of steroidal contraception on men's sexuality (e.g. Martin et al 2000). It can also be argued that improving our understanding of these complex effects would not only enable better clinical management of oral contraception and possibly further improvements in the methods, but would also increase our understanding of women's sexuality in general. The following section identifies several crucial issues and briefly considers the limited relevant evidence that is available.

Reasons for discontinuation

Discontinuation of oral contraception is common: 11% within the first month of use, 28% by 6 months and by 1 year from 33 to 50% (Hatcher & Nelson 2004). To a large extent, the reasons for discontinuation are not well understood, and most studies that have explored this have paid little attention to sexual explanations. An early exception was a study by Herzberg et al (1971), who carefully assessed depression, headaches and libido prior to starting contraception in 218 women using OCs and 54 using an IUD. Of the OC users, 25% discontinued during the first year. These women were more likely to have been depressed before starting OCs and to have a tendency to premenstrual mood changes. They also tended to show a decline in libido while using the OC. Of the IUD users, breakthrough bleeding was the most common reason for discontinuation. A number of studies have found an association between a tendency to premenstrual mood changes and discontinuation of OCs (e.g. Sanders et al 1983; Dennerstein et al 1984), whereas Kutner & Brown (1972) found a comparable association with past history of post-natal depression.

A more recent study, designed to assess predictors and correlates of discontinuation, and unusual in its systematic attention to mood and sexuality variables, was reported by Sanders et al (2001). As mentioned earlier, this was a small study because of the failure to obtain external funding. Seventy-nine women completed the study; 38% were still on the same OC at the end of 12 months, 47% had discontinued OCs and 14% had switched to another pill. When asked the reasons for discontinuing or switching OCs, the spontaneously cited reasons included physical side effects (37%), emotional side effects (33%), bleeding problems (18%), relationship ended (18%) and sexual side effects (8%). The sexuality of these women was assessed before starting OCs, and at 3, 6 and 12 months or shortly after discontinuation, using two established methods, Interview Ratings of Sexual Function (IRSF; e.g. Tyrer et al 1983; Cawood & Bancroft 1996) and the Sexual Experience Scale (SES; Frenken & Vennix 1981). Although physical side effects were the most frequent reasons given spontaneously, they were reported almost as frequently by those who did not discontinue (27 and 20%, respectively) and they did not figure in the logistic regression model that was the best predictor of discontinuation. Three variables were significant in this model: the frequency of sexual thoughts (IRSF; $p = 0.029$), the SES2 scale from SES, which measures sexual arousability ($p = 0.032$), and the emotional side effect score ($p = 0.031$). This small study involved young women, the majority unmarried students, and these findings may not be equally relevant to older married women. But they do illustrate an important point. Asking for reasons for discontinuation may result in socially acceptable explanations, such as physical side effects, and it is clearly important, in addition to asking for such explanations, to assess systematically changes in mood and sexuality. An early study showed clearly that side effects of OCs are more prevalent when they are systematically assessed (Talwar & Berger 1979). This is particularly important with adverse changes in mood and sexuality.

The limitations of cross-sectional studies
Given the high rate of discontinuation, mostly within the first few months of OC use, cross-sectional studies of OC users cannot be used to study adverse effects of OC use, as most women experiencing such effects will have selected themselves out by discontinuing. Studies of established OC users are of interest for other reasons. An example is the McGill study of students (Bancroft et al 1991a), in which established OC users were compared with women using other methods of contraception. The OC group showed not only more sexual activity than the non-OC group, but also more liberal and less inhibited attitudes about sex. Thus, it is likely that they were more sexually active before starting on OCs, this being one of the reasons for choosing OCs.

The impact of the menstrual cycle on women's sexuality was considered in Chapter 4. Cyclical variations in both mood and sexual interest are experienced by many women, though not all, with the cyclical patterns also varying somewhat, but with peaks of interest most commonly occurring during the post-menstrual week. Given the impact of OCs on the woman's hormonal cycle, with most suppressing ovulation, it is of some interest to compare OC users and non-users for their cyclical pattern of sexual interest and mood. In a large-scale retrospective study, readers of a monthly women's magazine completed a questionnaire about menstrual health (Warner & Bancroft 1988). They were asked, amongst other things, to indicate when in their last cycle their well-being and their sexual interest were at their highest and lowest. They could choose between 'week before period', 'during period', 'week after period', 'other times' or 'never'. There were 860 women who had been using OCs for more than 6 months and 3252 women not using OCs. The distributions of the highs and lows for pill-using and non-pill-using women are shown in Figure 15.2. There was a strong association between well-being and sexual interest in both groups, with the week after the period being the best time for both groups and both variables. But the two groups did differ significantly from each other: the pill-using women were less likely to report either highs or lows, and more likely to report high sexual interest either during menstruation or *the week before*. This difference between the groups in the timing of sexual interest could not be attributed to differences in the timing of highs and lows of well-being. The pill appeared to be having a direct effect on sexuality, independently of its effects on mood. We then compared low dose combined ($n = 369$) with triphasic ($n = 295$) OC users in this sample. The triphasic group came midway between the low-dose combined OC and the non-OC groups in their distribution of highs and lows of both sexuality and mood, distributions that were significantly different.

These findings were based on retrospective assessments of 'highs' and 'lows'. We then examined the cyclical patterns further in a prospective study in which three groups of women (triphasic, combined and non-OC groups, matched for age and parity) completed daily ratings of mood, sexuality and other changes for three consecutive cycles (Walker & Bancroft 1990). Most striking

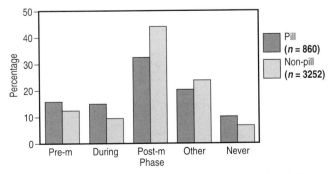

Fig. 15.2 Timing of high sex interest during the menstrual cycle by pill and non-pill users. Women were asked to indicate the week before the period (pre-m), during the period, the week after the period (post-m) or at other times. (From Warner & Bancroft 1988.)

was the degree of similarity of the three groups, raising the question of how important a normal ovulatory cycle is for the perimenstrual changes that women commonly experience.

Sexuality and mood were closely related to each other in all three groups, and the groups did not differ significantly from each other in either variable. The one variable to show clear differences was cyclical breast changes; the non-pill and triphasic users were indistinguishable in this respect, whereas the combined pill users reported significantly fewer breast changes (Fig. 15.3). The differences between groups, which had been found to be significant in the larger retrospective study, were noticeable in this prospective study but were not large enough to reach statistical significance.

The apparent differences between this retrospective study and the prospective study raise questions of methodology and interpretation. The prospective data, while showing hints of non-significant patterns comparable to those in the retrospective data, were most convincing in showing no differences (except for breast tenderness). The retrospective method asked women about their last menstrual cycle, but the answers may have been influenced by the pattern, if any, that each woman had come to recognize as typical of her cycles.

Other examples of studies that compare established OC users and non-users are reviewed in Bancroft & Sartorius (1990).

The need for placebo-controlled prospective evaluation of OCs

Since the introduction of OCs in the 1960s there have been five placebo-controlled studies of the effects of OCs on women's sexuality. Two of these involved small samples (Grounds et al 1970; Leeton et al 1978) and are reviewed briefly in Bancroft & Sartorius (1990). Graham & Sherwin's (1993) study focused on the treatment of pre-menstrual syndrome (PMS) and was mentioned in the previous section. A basic issue in such studies is the need to avoid unplanned pregnancy during placebo administration. Cullberg (1972) achieved this by asking his subjects to continue with their usual non-steroidal contraception, and to participate in a study to assess the effects of hormone administration on their menstruation. The 322 women who participated were randomly assigned to one of four groups, one receiving placebo, the other three an E/progestagen combination, with a set dose of 50 µg ethinyl oestradiol, and one of three doses of norgestrel, 1.0, 0.05 or 0.06 mg. These were taken for two menstrual cycles with a treatment-free fourth week in each cycle. The women were divided into two groups according to their level of pre-menstrual irritability before treatment. Those with higher levels of pre-menstrual irritability showed more negative mood change with the low progestagen dosage. Conversely, those with little or no pre-menstrual irritability showed more negative mood change with the high progestogen dosage. Negative effects on sexuality were infrequent and, in Cullberg's view, secondary to negative mood changes. The main limitation of this study is in the methods of assessment, particularly of sexual aspects; after the two treatment cycles, women were asked if they had experienced any changes, positive or negative, in their sexual interest or sexual satisfaction during the 2 months of medication. No attempt was made to assess levels at baseline.

Graham et al (1995), in the WHO funded study mentioned earlier, recruited women in Edinburgh, Scotland,

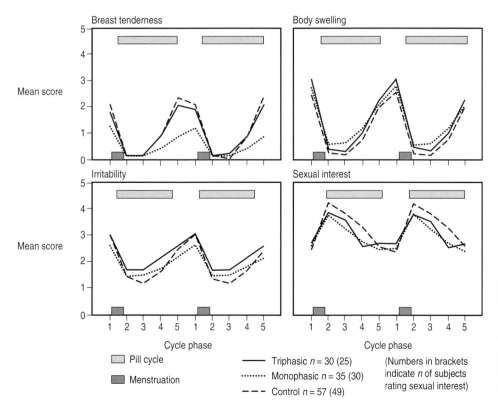

Fig. 15.3 The timing of four changes, breast tenderness, body swelling, irritability and sexual interest, through two menstrual cycles in three groups of women: triphasic pill users, monophasic (combined) pill users and non-pill controls. Each cycle is divided into five phases according to the varying dose levels of the triphasic pill regime. Only breast tenderness showed a significant difference between the groups. (From Walker & Bancroft 1990.)

and in Manila, the Philippines, who had either been sterilized or whose partners had been vasectomized. This not only allowed the use of placebo, it also meant that the effects studied were independent of any concerns about the need for contraception. A double-blind, parallel group design was used, with random assignment to one of three treatment groups, a combined OC (COC; Microgynon; 30 μg ethinylestradiol (EE) and 0.15 mg LN), a progestogen-only pill (POP, Microlut; LN 0.03 mg daily) or placebo. Each treatment was for four cycles. Assessment included IRSF carried out four times, twice at baseline (before and at the end of the baseline month), and after 2 and 4 months of treatment. Beck Depression Inventories (BDIs) covering the pre- and post-menstrual weeks were completed during the baseline and the third treatment cycle. Daily diaries were completed, rating various aspects of mood and sexuality. Fifty women were in each group, 25 from each country, a total of 150. A significant minority of women on the COC reported a decline in sexual interest and enjoyment compared to placebo, an effect not observed with the progestogen-only method. Interestingly, this was evident in the Scottish women, but not in the Filipino women. It is noteworthy that, during the baseline month, the Filipino women, although their frequency of partner-initiated sexual activity was higher, reported lower sexual interest than the Scottish women and showed no significant further decline during the treatment cycles. The effect of the COC on the sexuality of the Scottish women, therefore, was to make them more similar to the Filipino women. Both Scottish and Filipino women reported some worsening of mood on the COC, but not on the POP.

What are the possible explanations for these findings? Given that the negative mood change that occurred in both Scottish and Filipino women was less marked than the decline in sexual interest in the Scottish group and was not associated with a decline in sexual interest in the Filipino group, it is unlikely that the adverse sexual effects observed were secondary to mood change. The differences in sexuality at baseline are likely to be important. The Scottish women were much more positive about their sexuality and hence had much more scope for negative change. On the other hand, we should keep in mind that, even though the Filipino interviewers were trained to use the method of assessment, our measures may not have been culturally appropriate in the Philippines. In further studies of this kind, more cross-cultural piloting of assessment methods should be carried out.

The lack of negative effect of the POP, apart from its expected disruption of the bleeding pattern, was striking. However, in considering the possible role of the progestogen, the dose of LN was five times higher in the COC than the POP, for the 21 days in the cycle that it was taken. The possibility that the COC effects were due to reduced free T will be considered later.

Other comparative prospective studies assessing sexuality

Bancroft et al (1987) studied women starting on OCs who were randomly assigned to a monophasic OC (Microgynon; EE 30 μg, LN 150 μg) or a triphasic OC (Logynon; EE 30 μg, LN 50 μg 6 days/EE 40 μg, LN 75 μg 5 days/EE 30 μg, LN 125 μg 10 days). Assessment included daily diaries for the first two pill cycles. We assessed the women's degree of cyclical mood change before starting on the pill and divided them into two groups: those with and those without pre-menstrual mood change. We then found that for the women with no history of pre-menstrual mood change, the type of pill made no difference to how they felt. But for the other group, with previous pre-menstrual mood change, those taking the triphasic pill showed significantly more lowering of mood than those on the combined preparation. This was also reflected in the daily sexual interest ratings, but this could have been secondary to the mood effect. These findings are consistent with the evidence from Cullberg's (1972) study, mentioned earlier.

Martin-Loeches et al (2003), in a Spanish study, assessed 760 women starting on OCs and 313 who were fitted with an IUD, at 3, 6 and 12 months of use. The Female Sexual Function Index (FSFI; Rosen et al 2000) was used to assess sexual desire. About 10% of women with both methods reported a decrease in sexual desire. This is a large study, but apart from not involving randomization to treatment method, the report of the findings is difficult to follow and evaluate. The only data presented are from a logistic regression analysis, and the finding that reduced sexual desire was less with longer duration of OC use was not clarified in terms of the numbers who discontinued. In a study from Thailand, Oranratanaphan & Taneepanichskul (2006) compared two COCs; Yasmin (EE 30 μg, drospirenone 3 mg) and Meliane (EE 20 μg, gestodene 75 μg). Eighty-six women were randomly assigned to one of these OCs and assessed using the FSFI to measure sexual variables, and blood sampling to measure the free androgen index (FAI). After 3 months of OC use, both groups of women showed significant improvement in sexual interest and sexual satisfaction, and neither group showed significant reduction in FAI. Meliane is not currently used in North America or Europe. Yasmin is an OC with a newly developed progestogen, drospirenone. Both progestogens in this study are reported to have anti-androgenic properties.

Two recent studies from Italy are of relevance to this Thai study, although they did not involve direct comparison of different OCs. Caruso et al (2005) used the Personal Experience Questionnaire (Dennerstein et al 1997) to assess the effects on sexuality of women starting Yasmin. They found a significant improvement in sexual enjoyment and orgasmic frequency from the third month onwards. In an earlier study (Caruso et al 2004) they had used the same methodology to assess a monophasic OC containing 15 μg EE and 60 μg gestodene, similar but with slightly lower dosages than Meliane in the Thai study. Here they found a significant *decrease* in sexual arousal and sexual enjoyment by the third month, and of sexual desire and frequency of sexual activity by the ninth month of use. The lack of direct comparison of these two OCs and the absence of any hormonal assessment limit the value of these two studies.

Greco et al (2007) compared two triphasic OCs with the same progestogen (norgestimate, 0.18, 0.215 and 0.25 mg) but differing in the E level: Ortho-Tricyclen (OTC), with 35 µg EE and Ortho-Tricyclen-Lo (OTC-Lo), with 25 µg EE. Mood and sexual interest were assessed, before starting the OC and again after 3 months of use, with the BDI and the Sexual Desire Inventory (SDI; Spector et al 1996). Blood samples were taken pre-OC and during the third OC cycle to assay levels of free T. Sexual interest scores did not change significantly from baseline with either OC, although there was considerable variability, with many women showing either an increase or a decrease. Women on OTC-Lo were significantly more likely to show improvement in premenstrual mood than those on OTC. OTC-Lo also produced significantly less reduction in free T than OTC. However, there was no correlation between the change in pre-menstrual mood and change in free T, and their causal relationship is therefore uncertain.

The impact of hormonal variability on mood

More attention has been paid to the effects of OCs on mood than on sexuality. In the first phase of OC use, when pills with relatively high E levels were used, there was concern that the prevalence of depressive illness might be increased, particularly in those vulnerable to depression (Kay 1984). With the predominant use of lower E levels (35 µg or less) in the second and third phase of OC use, this concern has lessened. However, mood change, which is not sufficient to be diagnosed as a depressive illness but which is relevant to quality of life, is still an issue, and its impact on sexual interest and response, as well as discontinuation, relevant. The available literature suggests a variable impact of OCs on mood: some women experience improved mood, some worse mood and the majority no change (Bancroft & Sartorius 1990; Oinonen & Mazmanian 2002). The evidence for the effect of OCs on pre-menstrual mood change is also variable, suggesting that some women experience a worsening of pre-menstrual mood and others an improvement. It would clearly be helpful to have a better understanding of this individual variability.

I have previously proposed (Bancroft 1993) a three-factor model to account for variability in how women react to their menstrual cycles: a timing factor imposed by the ovarian hormonal cycle and possibly linked to cyclical changes in CNS neurotransmitter activity, a menstruation factor by which the processes involved in the build up and shedding of the endometrium may affect how women feel during both the pre-menstruum and menstruation, and the vulnerability factor, covering a variety of characteristics, psychosocial as well as biological, which are not functions of the menstrual cycle per se, but which may influence how vulnerable a woman is to the first two factors. This helps us to explain the paradox that some women with PMS report improvement on OCs whereas others find their pre-menstrual mood changes are worse and discontinue OCs for that reason. The second group of women may be those whose vulnerability is to the timing factor and whose cyclical mood change is aggravated by the artificial cycle imposed by the OC. The first group of women may be those whose vulnerability is to the menstruation factor, who benefit from the substantial modification of menstruation induced by OCs.

Whether the hormones in OCs, particularly the progestogens, have a direct negative effect on mood apart from the cyclical component remains to be demonstrated. It was noticeable, however, that the women in Graham et al's (1995) study who took a continuous low-dose progestogen had no negative mood changes. A continuous high-dose progestagen may have been a different story. An interesting single case study also raises the possibility that the progestogen may have an inhibitory effect in cyclical OCs until the pill-free week, when the woman can escape from this effect. A typical cycle from this woman is shown in Figure 15.4. She was using Ovranette (EE 30 µg/LN 150 µg) and complained that she only felt sexually interested and responsive for a few days each month, starting 2–3 days after stopping the pill and continuing for 2–3 days into the next pill cycle. Daily recording of sexual interest and activity, as shown in Figure 15.4, coincided with the peaks of both oestradiol 17β and T. However, increasing her oestradiol (with micronized oestradiol) or T (with

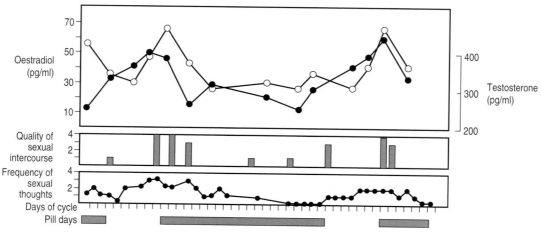

Fig. 15.4 The effects of an OC (Ovranette) on a 32-year-old woman. Her sexual interest and activity increased during the pill-free week at the same time as her endogenous oestradiol and testosterone were rising. (From Bancroft et al 1980.)

sublingual T) had no effect on the behavioural pattern. When she finally stopped using the OC, there was a dramatic improvement throughout the month.

The relationship between mood and sexuality

A recurring theme in this limited literature is that negative sexual effects are secondary to negative mood effects. There is convincing evidence of a link between negative mood and lowered sexual interest and response (see Chapter 4, p. 106). However, we should not assume that if OC use results in worsening of mood and reduction of sexual interest, the latter is necessarily a consequence of the former. And it is also clear that reduction of sexual interest during OC use can occur without negative mood change. Graham & Sherwin (1993) reported a study in which a triphasic OC was compared with placebo in the treatment of PMS, using a double-blind randomized design. Pre-menstrual mood improved in both the OC and the placebo group, whereas there was a significant reduction in sexual interest in the OC group only. Both mood and sexuality need to be carefully assessed in research on the effects of OCs on women's quality of life.

Oral contraceptive-induced reduction in free testosterone

It has been known for some time that OCs reduce free T (Jung-Hoffman & Kuhl 1987; Van der Vange et al 1990; Janaud et al 1992; Darney 1995; Thorneycroft et al 1999; Boyd et al 2001). This was considered in Chapter 4 (see p. 117) and is the most common iatrogenic cause for lowered T in women. Two principal mechanisms are involved: the mid-cycle rises in T and androstenedione (A) are blocked by suppression of ovulation and the associated pattern of gonadal steroid change, and the E in the OC increases SHBG levels and hence reduces the free T available. There is more limited evidence of a reduction in DHEA and DHEA-S (Coenen et al 1996; Graham et al 2007). Given these predictable hormonal effects, what happens to sexual arousability in COC users? Very little attention has been paid to this potentially important issue (Bancroft & Sartorius 1990), which is in striking contrast to the much greater interest in the androgenic effects of some progestagens used in OCs (e.g. Mishell 2004), with associated side effects such as acne. As Coenen et al (1996) pointed out, any androgenic effect of the progestagen used in an OC is negligible when compared to the reduction of endogenous androgens. Given the currently intense interest in the role of T in the sexuality of women, considered in Chapter 4, it is obviously relevant to ask whether OC-induced reduction in free T has any adverse effects of women's sexuality. Here again, the evidence presents a complex picture.

In an early study (Bancroft et al 1980) we compared 20 established OC users complaining of sexual problems that they attributed to the OC, with 20 OC users without sexual problems, matched for OC and age. The total T levels were low in both groups (free T was not estimated) and not significantly different. When we correlated our measure of sexual interest with the T level we found a significant correlation in the 'no problem' group ($r = 0.65$; $p < 0.01$) but not in the 'problem' group ($r = 0.02$; not significant). In general, as with men, plasma T or free T levels have not predictably correlated with measures of sexuality in women. The most substantial demonstration of lack of association between levels of plasma T and sexuality in women was in a large community survey in Australia (Davis et al 2005). However, a significant correlation between plasma T and sexual interest was found in two other studies of OC users (Bancroft et al 1991b; Alexander & Sherwin 1993). Therefore, a predictable association between T level and sexual interest in women has so far only been observed in women on OCs, whose T levels are in the lower part of the physiological range. This led Alexander & Sherwin (1993) to postulate a 'threshold' effect in women, comparable to that in men, but at a much lower level of plasma T, i.e. correlations between plasma T level and measures of sexual interest will only become apparent when the T levels are around this threshold level, which is presumably in the lower part of the normal range. This is an interesting idea, but somewhat difficult to reconcile with the evidence, reviewed in Chapter 4, that supraphysiological levels of T following T administration can have beneficial sexual effects, at least in some women.

What can we learn from the lack of correlation in the OC users with sexual problems, mentioned above (Bancroft et al 1980)? One possibility is that once a sexual problem becomes established in a woman, with all of the interpersonal and intrapersonal repercussions that tend to result, the subtle relationship between T and sexual interest becomes obscured. If so, we would be more likely to observe a correlation in women without sexual problems.

Recently, results from the first study to measure change in free T *and* in measures of sexuality and mood in women starting on OCs were reported (Graham et al 2007). Sixty-one women were involved, starting on OTC, OTC-Lo, or Ortho-Cyclen (a monophasic equivalent of OTC).

Sexuality was assessed by IRSF, and mood by the BDI. The expected, highly significant reductions in free T and DHEA-S were found, though there was considerable individual variability in the degree of reduction. As in previous studies, there was considerable variability in the measures of sexuality and mood. Thus the 'frequency of sexual thoughts', our principal measure of sexual interest, increased in 33% of women and decreased in 23%, the remainder showing no change. The BDI, while showing on average very little change, had 39% of women showing improvement in mood and 29% worsening. We found some support for the hypothesis that reduction in sexual interest (and other sexuality measures) would be related to the reduction in free T. Direct correlations between the change scores for behavioural and hormonal measures were not significant. But when we correlated change in hormonal measure with the actual level of sexuality after 3 months on OC, we found a significant correlation for free T and frequency of sexual thoughts ($r = 0.35$; $p = 0.006$), and percentage of occasions of sexual activity with partner when the woman felt sexually aroused or excited

($r = 0.28$; $p = 0.03$). We found no correlations with other aspects of sexual enjoyment or response, no correlations with change in DHEA-S, and no correlations between hormonal change and mood scores. What was clearly evident from this data was that though some women showed the association between hormonal change and sexual interest, sufficient to produce a significant correlation in the whole group, there were other women who experienced a substantial decline in free T and no apparent reduction of sexual interest, or even an increase in sexual interest. These findings are consistent with the desensitization hypothesis considered elsewhere in this book (see Chapters 4 and 6, p. 127) that postulates a considerable variation among women in their behavioural responsiveness to T. This would predict that a subgroup of T sensitive women, the other characteristics of which remain to be identified, will be affected by the OC-induced reduction in free T, whereas the majority of women will not be.

If OC-induced reduction of free T causes reduction of sexual interest in some women, would those women benefit from T replacement together with the OC? As yet, only one study involving controlled evaluation of such an intervention has been reported. In our early study (Bancroft et al 1980) we used a placebo-controlled, double-blind cross-over study to evaluate the effect of oral A administration in 15 of the OC users who presented with sexual problems. At that time suitable methods of T administration for women were less available, and we were able to show that administration of A substantially increased plasma levels of T. However, in the 15 women involved, only one showed an improvement sexually (though in her case it was clear-cut and reproducible). Further research should be done to replicate this study.

Conclusions

The evidence undoubtedly presents a complex picture. But there are several points that, if kept in mind, may help us to reduce the uncertainty as we proceed with further research. First, minimal group changes in either sexuality or mood measures often conceal a considerable variability. There is sufficient evidence across studies of significant proportions of women who show either positive or negative change in mood and/or sexuality after starting on OCs. The tendency has been to assume that this is 'noise' in the data, reflecting recent survey data showing that transient negative changes in sexuality are common among women in any case (see Chapter 11, p. 310). Future research needs to address this possibility (e.g. to what extent are there other current explanations for these positive and negative changes), and if they are not found to a sufficient extent, then we need to know what distinguishes women who have positive from those who have negative reaction to OCs.

Three specific mechanisms contributing to this variability warrant further study. First, a direct effect of OC-induced negative mood on sexuality. In Chapter 4 we consider the considerable individual variability of the relationship between negative mood and sexuality. Some women may be particularly likely to experience reduced sexual interest in negative mood states.

Second, the possibility that a substantial minority of women are dependent sexually on T and experience negative sexual changes, particularly in sexual interest, because of the OC-induced reduction in free T, is supported by the limited evidence. If this is a valid assumption, we need to know how such T-dependent women can be identified *before* they start on OCs. In other words, are there predictors of this negative effect? The different patterns of women's sexuality, considered in Chapters 4 and 6, may be relevant here. I would be surprised, for example, if a woman fitting the basic pattern, but not the superadded pattern, as described on p. 131, would be T dependent in her sexuality. In addition, those women who experience a clear mid-cycle peak of spontaneous sexual interest, at the time when their T levels are also peaking, may prove to be T sensitive.

The third potential mechanism is a direct effect of the progestagen, independent of the OC-induced reduction in free T. If the positive effects on women's sexuality of OCs containing the progestogen, drospirenone, reported in two studies so far (Caruso et al 2005; Oranratanaphan & Taneepanichskul 2006) are found to be consistent, then a closer look at this progestogen and how it differs from other progestogens will be warranted. Here again, it may be necessary to distinguish between direct progestogenic effects on sexuality, and direct effects on mood, which then affect sexuality secondarily.

Long-acting reversible methods

Since the last edition of this book there have been a number of developments in contraceptive technology. Intra-uterine devices have become smaller, either releasing copper (e.g. Cu T 380A) or LN, when they are called intrauterine systems (IUS) (e.g. LNG-IUS). The copper device works by impairing sperm function and preventing fertilization. The LNG-IUS works in a number of ways, mainly localized to the reproductive tract: thickening the cervical mucus, inhibiting sperm capacitation and survival, and suppressing the endometrium. In some women, systemic absorption is sufficient to inhibit ovulation (Grimes 2004). The amount of LN released daily is about 10% that of an OC containing 150 µg LN.

Systemic long-acting use of progestogens is by implant (Norplant, releasing LN; Implanon, releasing etonogestrel) or by injection (Depo-Provera; depot medroxyprogesterone acetate, DMPA; 150 mg intramuscularly every 3 months). With these methods the progestogen inhibits ovulation. DMPA does this by suppressing gonadotrophin release.

In 2005, in the UK, the National Institute for Health and Clinical Excellence (NIHCE) commissioned a report on long-acting reversible contraception (NIHCE 2005). In the section on IUDs and IUS, increased bleeding problems and dysmenorrhoea were reported to be associated with IUD use. Although one randomized control trial found higher rates of discontinuation because of depression after 5 years of IUS use compared with IUD use, the report's conclusion was that 'women should be informed that any changes in mood and libido are similar whether using IUD or IUS, and that changes are small' (p. 50). This may not be unreasonable, though the small amount of systemic absorption of the progestogen from the IUS might have adverse effects in some vulnerable women, and when they say that 'changes are small' they are presumably referring to the small prevalence, rather than the degree of change in individuals.

The two most widely used implants for long-acting contraception have been Norplant and Implanon. Norplant releases LN for 5 years, around 85 µg/day during the first month, reducing to 25–30 µg/day. Implanon releases etonogestrel sufficient to suppress ovulation for 3 years. Both require to be inserted under the skin of the upper arm. The NIHCE (2005) report starts this section by stating that Norplant has not been marketed in the UK since 1999. As there is much more research evidence on the effects of Norplant, this is used to augment the more limited evidence about Implanon. The fact that Norplant was withdrawn in the UK and the USA following class action suits by women claiming major adverse effects is not mentioned. A Norplant Action Group was set up in 1995, with women claiming that the implant had left some of them with endless periods and others with no periods at all, and had caused skin problems, hair loss, mood swings and other side effects (Lattimer 1999). There were also problems with its surgical implantation and its removal, mainly due to the fact the Norplant consisted of six separate rods, taking about 20 minutes to implant and up to an hour to remove. However, it is still in use in developing countries.

In one British study reviewed by NIHCE (2005), 11% of women reported mood changes associated with Implanon, and in 9% these were severe enough to require removal. A meta-analysis of a number of studies showed that in Implanon users 4.9% reported emotional lability and 3.3% loss of libido; in Norplant users the rates were 7.6% and 5.4%, respectively. However, the NIHCE report concludes that less than 2% of Implanon users have loss of libido, and they recommend that 'women should be informed that Implanon use is not associated with changes in weight, mood, libido or headaches' (p. 103).

Although both the sections on IUDs and implants contained short paragraphs on mood and libido change, in the section on DMPA there was no mention of either. Of all these long-acting methods, DMPA is probably the most likely to have adverse effects on sexuality and mood. DMPA suppresses levels of FSH and LH, and, as the pituitary gland remains responsive to gonadotrophin-releasing hormones, DMPA is probably acting directly on the hypothalamus. DMPA is used in the USA to control male sex offenders (see Chapter 16, p. 502). In these circumstances, it is extraordinary that this official report is recommending the use of DMPA, a long-acting method for long-term contraception, with no mention of its possible impact on sexuality or mood. Two studies have given some relevant information about DMPA (Paul et al 1997; Westhoff et al 1998). Both were cited in the NIHCE report, but neither was referred to in the section on DMPA. Paul et al (1997) recorded reasons for discontinuation of DMPA; at 3 months, 12% of

women gave depression and 6% loss of libido as their reason. Westhoff et al (1998) reported a multicentre prospective study in which mood (but not sexuality) was assessed at baseline using six questions relevant to depression from the Mental Health Inventory (Veit & Ware 1983). Women were reassessed after 12 months. Of the 495 women starting on DMPA, 21% were lost to follow-up, and the effects of the DMPA were not known. Of those followed up, 56% had discontinued DMPA. These women reported significantly higher depression scores at baseline, but on average they were no higher when assessed at follow-up; their depression scores before discontinuing were not known. This study provides an example of varied changes in mood with some women improving and some getting worse, and with an overall insignificant mean change. The authors comment that 'although the lack of change in average scores over the course of 1 year is generally reassuring, a large adverse change in a small subgroup may be more clinically relevant' (p. 239). This issue was considered earlier in relation to OCs. Hatcher (2004) commented 'Depression becomes a particular concern when it occurs in a woman following a Depo-Provera (DMPA) injection because it is not possible to discontinue Depo-Provera immediately' (p. 470). He recommends a trial period of oral MPA in women with a vulnerability to depression, before moving to the Depo method.

With one or two exceptions relating to mood, the evidence of side effects from long-acting injectables have apparently depended on spontaneous reporting by the women, or, at best, unstructured questions about whether there had been 'adverse events'. A fair amount of attention is paid to the impact of the method on bleeding patterns, but no consideration was given to how this might affect the woman's enjoyment of sex or her sexual relationship. In a WHO-sponsored study of patterns of menstruation in 10 countries, Snowden & Christian (1983) found that almost all respondents believed that sexual intercourse should be avoided during menstruation.

Hormonal contraception in the male

The possibility of using reversible hormonal methods to suppress fertility in men has been receiving attention in the past decade (Wu 2006). The most feasible way to do this is to suppress spermatogenesis by inhibiting LH and FSH. However, it is not possible to do this without, at the same time, suppressing T production. Where men are concerned, no one would consider this because of the likely adverse effect on the man's sexuality. Suppression of LH and FSH would therefore have to be accompanied by administration of T. Exogenous T administration is not without its problems, particularly in relation to the prostate (see Chapter 4). Anderson et al (1999) reported an investigation of a new T substitute (MENT) in hypogonadal men in Scotland and Hong Kong, with its use in male contraception in mind. Various progestagens have been explored. A range of studies have been carried out comparing different progestagens, and Martin et al (2000) assessed men's attitudes to using a 'contraceptive pill' in four different cultures, Scotland, South Africa, China and Hong Kong, finding a fair amount of interest in such methods, reflecting in part a widespread view that condoms reduced sexual pleasure.

In a review of the mainly small controlled evaluation studies, Grimes et al (2004) concluded that no male contraceptive was yet ready for use. This is perhaps mainly because of uncertainties about the predictability of adequate suppression of spermatogenesis. In the female, suppression of ovulation is by comparison straightforward. You either suppress ovulation in a cycle or you do not. With spermatogenesis, it is a question of how much the sperm count has to be lowered to ensure infertility. There are some indications that the pharmaceutical industry is currently withdrawing from further involvement. It remains to be seen what happens in this respect.

Barrier methods

Male condoms

Issues concerning the acceptability of male condoms and hence their reliable usage were considered closely in Chapter 14. They are clearly important in combining contraceptive effect with a barrier to sexually transmitted infections. Contraceptive failure when condoms are used consistently is around 2% (Warner et al 2004).

Female barrier methods

The two main methods in current use are the diaphragm, which has a long history, and the female condom, which is relatively new. Both require careful application to achieve effectiveness contraceptively; the failure rate with 'perfect use' is 6% for the diaphragm and 5% for the female condom (Cates & Stewart 2004). These rates may be slightly improved with the added use of a spermicide. Various aspects of the female condom, and its potential for pleasure, were considered in Chapter 14.

Some women, however, dislike the handling of the genitalia which is required, and the potential interference with spontaneity. Occasionally, the male partner finds the presence of the diaphragm uncomfortable during intercourse or, if the diaphragm is too large, the woman may find that her sexual enjoyment is impaired.

'Natural' methods

The various rhythm methods that avoid conception by avoiding intercourse during the fertile period of the woman's cycle are the only methods of fertility control acceptable to the Roman Catholic Church. The ovulation method involves taking a daily temperature and identifying the day of ovulation by the rise in temperature, or the woman learning to observe the nature of her cervical mucus and, by this means, to recognize when she is getting close to ovulation (Billings & Billings 1973). Intercourse is then avoided until the safe period is reached. Unfortunately, this method has an unacceptably high failure rate and in a five-centre WHO study there was an annual rate of 19.4 pregnancies per 100 women years, though according to the WHO report this was mainly due to a failure to abstain, rather than failure to recognize the fertile period (WHO 1978). With 'perfect' use of the ovulation method, the failure rate has been estimated as 3.2% (Trussell & Gummer-Strawn 1990).

The extent of abstinence required is considerable; in the first half of the cycle, intercourse has to be avoided on alternate days so that the partner's semen does not obscure the mucus changes. Then, with the change in consistency of the mucus, abstinence may be required for 7–14 days before the next safe period prior to menstruation is reached. It is notable that the instructions on this method distributed by Catholic agencies seem to be as much concerned with the spiritually uplifting effects of self-imposed abstinence as on the avoidance of conception. There is no suggestion that other forms of sexual stimulation, such as oral or manual, leading to orgasm with ejaculation well away from the vagina, might be used instead of vaginal intercourse. It may well be that for such reasons this method has not been adequately explored. According to the evidence presented in Chapter 4, there is no obvious peak of female desire around ovulation in most women, so that limitation of sexual activity around this time may not be as physiologically contradictory as it first seems. As it is, such methods may hold appeal for couples whose level of sexual appetite is modest and who may welcome a good reason for restricting their sexual activity.

Post-partum contraception

The infertility associated with breastfeeding is probably the most natural method of birth spacing. Whilst breastfeeding is by no means a foolproof contraceptive, there is little doubt that reduction of breastfeeding and increased use of artificial methods of feeding have led to reduced birth intervals in many parts of the world (Short 1976). The contraceptive effect may depend on the nutritional status of the mother. There is some evidence that if the mother is undernourished, her prolactin levels will be higher as part of a process of ensuring adequate nutrition in the breast milk for the infant. These higher prolactin levels have the added biological advantage of preventing ovulation. If the mother is well nourished, the prolactin levels are not so high and inhibition of ovulation is less certain. As discussed in Chapter 3, the suckling frequency is also relevant; ovulation becomes more likely if the frequency of suckling declines and supplementary feeds are introduced.

Other alternatives for breastfeeding mothers should not involve oestrogens as they decrease the milk supply; barrier methods or POPs are acceptable (Kennedy & Trussell 2004).

Sterilization

Surgical methods of contraceptive sterilization are now well established. In the female, various techniques have been employed to cut or obstruct the fallopian tubes (tubal ligation), most frequently by means of laparoscopy. In the male, vasectomy is normally carried out under local anaesthetic and is a relatively simple and quick surgical procedure.

The use of elective sterilization increased markedly in the 1970s and 1980s. In the UK, in 1970, in 4% of couples where the wife was aged under 41 years, one of the couple had been electively sterilized. By 1973, the figure had risen to 13% (Bone 1978). In the General Household Survey of 1983, around 21% of couples (with the female partner aged 18–44 years) had been sterilized: 11% of the women and 10% of the men. There was also an increasing tendency for younger couples with fewer children to elect for sterilization. This increase was noted in many countries. According to Population Reports (1978) there were an estimated 3.4 million surgical sterilizations worldwide in 1950, 20 million in 1970 and 65 million in 1975. By 1983 the estimated figure was 135 million (95 million females and 40 million males (Population Reports 1985). Since then, the situation appears to have stabilized.

A striking aspect of the use of elective sterilization is the extent to which it is the female or male who is sterilized. As indicated above, this has been fairly equally divided in the UK, although in recent years, as shown by the Natsal I and II data in Table 15.3, there is now a predominance of male sterilization (female:male around 0.8). However, in most parts of the world, female sterilization is more common than male, and this contrast is particularly large in the developing countries. As shown in Table 15.1, the percentage of fertility control based on female sterilization is much higher than in the developed countries, whereas the proportion using male sterilization is fairly similar. The ratio of female to male sterilization in several different countries is shown in Table 15.6. Four countries in this list show a predominance of male sterilization: the UK, New Zealand, The Netherlands and Bhutan (a small, interesting country in the Himalayas, between India and China). In Australia (not shown in Table 15.6) male exceeded female sterilization in 1974, with the female:male ratio 0.8. In 2002, however, it was 1.17 (see Table 15.5). France is an interesting

contrast to the UK and The Netherlands, with a ratio of 15.6. This reflects the fact that until 2001, both female and male sterilization were against the law, though prosecutions for this 'offence' had not occurred for many years. In the circumstances, illicit sterilization was much more likely to be carried out in women. In the USA there has been some modest increase in the female:male ratio between 1982 (ratio 2.1:1) and 2002 (ratio 2.9:1; see Table 15.4). Within the USA, however, there are noteworthy ethnic differences in this respect. In 1970, black Americans showed a female:male ratio of 22.5:1 in their use of sterilization; in 1976, this had reduced to 6.4:1 (Hollerbach & Nortman 1984). In 2002, the ratio for white Americans was 2.1:1, for Hispanic Americans, 7.6:1 and for black Americans, 15.9:1 (Mosher et al 2004). Socioeconomic factors are relevant, however. Vasectomy is more likely to be chosen by men from higher socioeconomic groups or higher education groups (Mosher et al 2004).

Female sterilization, while a safe surgical procedure if done properly, is nevertheless more complex than vasectomy and has greater potential for post-operative complications. It requires a general anaesthetic and is substantially more expensive than the male method. The chances of reversal, for those who change their minds about permanent infertility, are small with both female and male procedures, but somewhat greater, and surgically less demanding, in the male. Given these differences, what is the explanation for the striking predominance of female over male sterilization in so many parts of the world? It is difficult to escape the conclusion that, to a large extent, this reflects a patriarchal tendency to see the woman as responsible for fertility and its regulation, and to attach less importance to the sexual well-being of the woman compared to the man. This pattern has already been considered in relation to the relative denial of the impact on women's sexuality in assessing the acceptability of different contraceptive methods. There have also been well-entrenched beliefs in many cultures that vasectomy will somehow undermine a man's masculinity as well as his sexuality, and these are considered further below. Of possible relevance is an awareness that women's fertility is only available until the menopause, whereas a man should remain fertile until old age.

TABLE 15.6	Ratio of female to male sterilization, by country (year data collected) (Engender Health 2002)
Country	**Female:male**
UK (1993)	0.8
New Zealand (1995)	0.8
The Netherlands (1993)	0.4
France (1994)	15.6
Brazil (1996)	15.4
Columbia (1995)	37.1
Nicaragua (1998)	52.3
Bahrain (1995)	6.0
Iran (1992)	8.4
South Africa (1998)	7.5
Zimbabwe (1994)	12.3
Bhutan (1994)	0.4
India (1992–93)	8.0
China (1992)	3.5
Thailand (1993)	7.1

Female sterilization

Before the marked increase in the use of female sterilization in the 1970s, the procedure was often recommended on medical grounds or as a condition of termination of pregnancy. With the clear increase in women self-selecting sterilization for contraceptive purposes, negative psychological repercussions have been less prevalent. The number of women who subsequently regret being sterilized has been small, and it is uncertain how many of them would actually choose to have the operation reversed if they had the opportunity. One of the most obvious reasons for regret is marital breakdown and the wish for further children with a new partner (Alder

1984). Given the steady increase of marital breakdown (see Chapter 6), this issue is likely to be of growing importance and may help to explain why the earlier increases in popularity of this method levelled off after the 1980s.

There were earlier concerns that tubal ligation may in some way alter ovarian function and lead to adverse changes in the menstrual bleeding pattern and menstrual pain (e.g. Kasonde & Bonnar 1976; Noble 1978). More recent evidence has not supported these concerns. For example, in a prospective comparison of women who had been sterilized with women whose partners had been vasectomized, assessed over 5 years following sterilization, no evidence of worsening of menstrual patterns in the female sterilized group was found. In fact, there was some evidence that they were more likely to have beneficial changes, with decreased bleeding and menstrual pain, and an increased likelihood of less regular cycles (Peterson et al 2000).

There is also no reason to believe that female sterilization procedures have any direct effect on sexual function. Adverse effects, when they occur, are more likely to stem from psychological reactions to the sterilization, either in the woman or in her spouse. These may reflect the need to link sex with potential reproduction or conversely, the freedom from the fear of pregnancy may increase the woman's enjoyment and interest in sex and put pressure on the husband who reacts adversely. Most studies were done in the 1970s or early 1980s. In these early studies, the majority of women reported no change in their sexual relationships; improvement was relatively common and deterioration usually occurred in no more than 3–5%. (Smith 1979; Bean et al 1980; Rönnau 1980; Cliquet et al 1981; Cooper et al, 1982). More recently, Costello et al (2002), in a study of more than 4000 women, found that the majority reported no change in sexual interest or enjoyment after sterilization, and those reporting change were more likely to experience positive than negative change. The authors concluded that such positive changes were likely to be indirect, in particular resulting from reduced worry about pregnancy or stopping a method of contraception (e.g. OCs) that may have been having negative sexual effects.

Male sterilization

Given widespread beliefs in the importance of semen as a source of energy and vitality, and the associated concerns about losing semen (see Chapter 6, p. 184), it is not surprising that vasectomy would be feared in many cultures as a threat. A common belief in South Asia, for example, is that vasectomy leads to both impotence and physical weakness (Caldwell et al 1987; Khan & Patel 1997). Even in the West, before vasectomy was so widespread, opinions about the psychologically castrating effects of vasectomy were often expressed (Wolfers 1970) and there was a tendency to be suspicious about the type of man who asked for the operation (Rodgers et al 1967). Negative attitudes have even been evident among health professionals. In Kenya, men posing as potential vasectomy clients in various family planning clinics encountered ridicule, inadequate information and bias against vasectomy among clinic staff (Wilkinson et al 1996).

As with tubal ligation, there were early concerns, based on animal studies, that vasectomy could have negative health effects, in particular long-term impairment of cardiovascular function. These have also been laid to rest. Massey et al (1983) administered a comprehensive health questionnaire to more than 10 000 vasectomized men and an equal number of matched controls and found no difference in the incidence of cardiovascular disease (see also Linnet et al 1982; Petitti et al 1982a,b).

From the earliest studies, evidence about the effects of vasectomy on men's sexuality has been reassuring. The Simon Population Trust (1969) followed up 1092 vasectomized men with questionnaires and obtained a 93% response: 73% reported an improvement in their sexual lives, 79% an improvement for their wives. In 25% of the men and 20% of the women there was no change; 1.5% and 0.5%, respectively, reported a deterioration. The Margaret Pyke Centre (1973) also reported on 1000 vasectomies studied prospectively: 460 men were sent follow-up questionnaires 1 year after the operation and 271 replied (60% response rate). Of those replying, 62% reported an improvement in their sexual life, 34% no change and 4% some deterioration. Other reassuring findings were reported by Hart & Deane (1980) and Newman & Leavesley (1980).

In an early study, Howard (1978) reported on the reasons given by men for seeking vasectomy. Prevention of further pregnancies because of completed family size and protection of the wife from the health hazards of other contraceptive methods, from the dangers of childbearing or from the fears of pregnancy, were the principal reasons. However, many couples added that they hoped for an improvement in their sex life, and in some cases this was the principal reason. This was particularly so in couples aged 35 years and over. Also of interest was the finding that most of the men had small families and had tended to use male methods of contraception in the past.

In a recent Brazilian study, 64 men were assessed before vasectomy, using the IIEF (Rosen et al 2002), and again 90 days after surgery. No man developed erectile problems, and the IIEF scores for erectile function, sexual desire and sexual satisfaction all showed significant improvement (Bertero et al 2005).

How health professionals advise men and women who are considering sterilization is important. Alder et al (1981) compared a small but representative sample of sterilized women with the wives of vasectomized men, matched for age and social class. It was noticeable that whereas most of the vasectomy couples had been counselled before the decision to carry out vasectomy was finalized, for most of the sterilized women discussion had been minimal and the husband was hardly involved in the decision-making. It was thus of interest to find that the sterilized women reported a significantly lower frequency of sexual intercourse and more sexual problems than the wives of the vasectomized men. It was not clear whether this reflected a difference in the quality of the sexual and marital relationships before the operation, a consequence of the different methods of sterilization or a reaction of the women to how the decision had been taken. The results did suggest, however, that in the marriages of the sterilized women, the wife's responsibility for fertility control was more likely to be taken for granted, whereas with the vasectomy couples the husband was more involved in sharing responsibility. The differing qualities of relationship implicated may have accounted for the sexual differences in the two groups. This interpretation is similar to that reached by Bean et al (1980). In general it would seem desirable to encourage couples to consider carefully the advantages and disadvantages of male and female methods of sterilization before making their decision, and the policy of discussing these issues with both partners together should be followed, whether it is female sterilization or vasectomy that is being considered.

Induced abortion

During the 19th century, concerns about declining birth rates led to induced abortion and contraception being made illegal. Not until the mid-20th century was there a move to legalize both contraception and abortion, starting in Scandinavia in 1930s, in Japan in 1948, the Soviet Union and some Soviet bloc countries in the 1950s. In the late 1960s, Great Britain and Canada revised their laws, followed in the 1970s by Austria, France, Germany, Italy and the USA, and Belgium in the early 1990s. By then, legal abortion services were available in all industrialized countries except Ireland, and reforms were gradually emerging in the developing world (Henshaw 1994). This process of liberalization has met with considerable resistance, most notably from the 'pro-life' movement in the USA. To some extent such resistance, mainly driven by more fundamentalist religion-based groups, has resulted in some modifications, but for the most part abortion within the first trimester is legal, with increasing restrictions for later in pregnancy.

Characteristics of those who obtain induced abortions were reviewed for women from 56 different countries (Bankole et al 1999). Some findings from this survey, from a selection of 18 countries, ordered by region (or by British Commonwealth) are shown in Table 15.7. In general abortion rates by age showed an inverted U-shaped pattern, with highest rates among women aged 20–29 years. There were two contrasting patterns, with one or other being evident in many of the countries reviewed, and apparent from the data in Table 15.7. One pattern shows abortions predominantly in unmarried, nulliparous women, as evident in the British Commonwealth and Western European countries. The other pattern is mainly in women who are married and have already had enough children or wish to space their childbearing; this is notable in the Eastern European countries, but also in other parts of the world. In the USA there were clear differences between ethnic groups. The 1995 US abortion rate was much higher for black

TABLE 15.7	Induced abortion in 18 countries: total abortion rate* marital status and nulliparity for 1995–1996[†] (from Bankole et al 1999)		
Country	Total abortion rate	Abortions in unmarried (%)	Abortions in nulliparous (%)
Australia	0.67	na	na
England and Wales	0.43	78.6	53.8
New Zealand	0.49	70.8	47.7
Belgium	0.19	65.6	47.0
Denmark	0.48	na	45.9
Germany	0.17	47.6	36.5
Netherlands	0.16	49.8	48.9
Spain	0.16	67.2	54.0
USA	0.73	83.8	45.0
Israel	0.43	53.6	4.4
Bulgaria	1.52	25.3	na
Estonia	1.63	30.3	22.8
Hungary	1.07	47.8	na
Romania	3.40	na	7.8
Russia	2.36	na	na
Kazakhstan	1.70	12.0	4.5
Cuba	1.44	na	na
Japan	0.40	na	na

*Number of abortions an average women has in her lifetime
[†]Data for Cuba are from 1990
na, not available

American (56 per 1000) than white American women (17 per 1000).

Explanations for socio-cultural differences are likely to be complex and varied. The first pattern is evident in societies in which women are more likely to pursue a career and marry at a later age. The second pattern is more likely in societies where women are expected to marry at an earlier age and have children early in marriage, and where there is more limited availability of contraception once they have achieved the desired number of children. Evidence of the second pattern in Eastern European countries reflects a previous tendency for Communist countries to be pro-natalist and to rely less on contraception. In Table 15.7, Romania stands out as having the highest total abortion rate. Djerassi (1979) gave an interesting account of how this situation unfolded in Romania. Until 1966, this country had the highest number of legal abortions anywhere in the world: nearly four for each live birth. The Romanian Government, concerned about the rapidly failing birth rate, introduced a very restrictive abortion law, following which the birth rate rose dramatically by 150% in 1 year. Thereafter the Romanian population apparently adjusted to the changed circumstances with an increased use of other methods of fertility control and since then there has been a further continuing decline in the birth rate. A salutary lesson from the Romanian experience is that the restriction of legal abortion was followed by an increased use of illegal abortion and a substantial rise in maternal deaths from abortion.

Communist China, where an ideologically based pro-natalist policy was pursued for some time in spite of enormous overpopulation problems has, in more recent years, adopted an active and so far moderately successful anti-natalist strategy. Legal abortion, it would appear, is one part of this broadly based programme.

As with sterilization, earlier reports were full of gloom about the psychiatric and sexual consequences of abortion (Simon & Senturia 1966). It is of course difficult to distinguish between the effects of the abortion per se and the impact of an unwanted pregnancy. Early follow-up studies, however, consistently failed to find evidence of adverse psychiatric consequences (e.g. Pare & Raven 1970; Hamill & Ingram 1974; Greer et al 1976; Brewer 1977), though short-lived emotional reactions were not unusual (Ashton 1980; Broome 1984). Bradshaw & Slade (2003) reviewed the relevant literature since 1990. Their conclusions were that following discovery of pregnancy and before abortion, 40–45% of women experienced significant anxiety and around 20% depression. These negative moods tended to decline following termination of the pregnancy, though around 30% were still experiencing some anxiety and/or depression at 1 month. However, they concluded that, in the longer term, women do no worse following induced abortion than following a live birth.

Unfortunately, very little information is available about the sexual consequences. Greer et al (1976) interviewed 360 women shortly before legal abortion. Whereas 91% were contacted 3 months later, this dropped to 60% at the final follow-up, 15 months to 2 years after the abortion. The proportion of women whose sexual adjustment was rated as satisfactory rose from 59% before the abortion to 74% 3 months later, and improvement was maintained up to 2 years after termination. Ashton (1980) interviewed 64 women 8 weeks after abortion. Of those with a continuing sexual relationship, 61% reported no change in the quality of their sexual fulfilment, 36% improvement and 19% worsening. Some 12% attributed sexual deterioration to the abortion. In a recent study, Bradshaw & Slade (2005) assessed women who were about to have an abortion, and again 2 months after the termination, and compared them with a control group of non-pregnant women. They found some increase in sexual problems in the period between discovering the pregnancy and being assessed for abortion, but these returned to their pre-pregnancy levels by the 2-month follow-up.

The available evidence of the effects of induced abortion, whilst mostly reassuring, is nevertheless very limited. It is not unusual to find a woman presenting at a sexual problem clinic for whom an earlier abortion had been followed by some sexual difficulties. It remains a possibility that for some women, the experience of abortion leads to some problematic changes in their sexual self-image. One should not necessarily attribute this to the abortion itself; it is difficult to know what the sexual consequences would have been if the pregnancy had continued, and they may have been much worse. But the whole experience, occurring at a time when the young woman's sexual self-esteem is still precarious, would have been best avoided. It is to be hoped that more attention will be paid to the sexual consequences of legal abortion in future studies. In the meantime, we can continue to use this procedure with no particular fear that psychological harm will follow. But we should not lessen our attempts to avoid unwanted pregnancies in the first place by doing our best to ensure that if sexual activity occurs, it is protected by appropriate contraception.

Infertility

The average time required for pregnancy to occur in normal couples not using contraception is 5.3 months. After 1 month of unprotected intercourse, 25% will have conceived; after 6 months, 63% and after 1 year, 80%. After 1 year of unsuccessful attempts to conceive, therefore, a couple may be regarded as potentially infertile. Between 10 and 15% of couples of fertile age remain unable to have children (Nelson & Marshall 2004). For many such couples the infertility is a cause of considerable distress.

In order to appreciate the psychological and sexual significance of infertility, we first need to understand why people have children. Motivation for parenthood has received limited attention from behavioural or social scientists (Bell et al 1985; Langdridge et al 2005). This in part reflects a general tendency to assume that having children is the norm; there is little need to question it (McCormick et al 1977). It is often assumed that the desire for children is innate, biologically determined. In fact, with the possible exception of self-protection against physical harm, it is difficult to think of any other behavioural pattern which is more 'biologically' driven than the tendency, at least when the socially prescribed circumstances are right, to have children. It is an interesting question to what extent this results from rational decision-making, as distinct from a post hoc rational justification for a 'natural' choice. But in the face of changing circumstances this exceedingly important question is now receiving more attention. It is perhaps more appropriate to consider rational decision making in the process of avoiding or delaying having children. The dramatic changes in birth rate and family size that have occurred over the past two centuries indicate how susceptible to social factors this process is. More recently, the general shift towards a preference for two-children families has been accompanied by an increase in voluntary childlessness. People now question whether it is pathological not to want any children. Economic factors are probably important. Whereas in the past, children were often seen as a material resource, they are now widely regarded as a major expense. Whereas the rewards of parenthood may have increased to some extent, particularly for fathers, the costs of having children are rising steadily and inexorably. The benefits of children are therefore receiving closer scrutiny by would-be parents. But also involved, and germane to our subject, is the increased availability of alternative roles for the woman. Whereas being a mother has figured largely in the expectations and ambitions of most women in the past, it is now competing with other potentially rewarding roles. Such changes are not universal, however, and in many situations motherhood still presents one of the most powerful sources of self-esteem for women. In societies where the opportunities for women are improving, it may be easier for a woman to accept infertility with little distress. However, mechanisms relevant to fertility are so fundamental to a woman's experience of her body, it would not be surprising if women would prefer to *choose* not to have children, rather than have infertility thrust upon them. For men, the importance of fatherhood, particularly in those not yet fathers, seems to vary considerably for reasons not well understood. For some men, fatherhood is clearly important for their sense of masculinity (Humphrey 1977). The sense of immortality that parents derive from having children is important for some and may be manifested in the pressure that older parents put on their adult children to give them grandchildren. Men do not have the same intensive awareness of reproductive processes through their experience of their bodies and, perhaps for that reason, it is easier for a man to have ambitions which are not dependent on fatherhood. On the other hand, as discussed in Chapter 6, the threat of cuckoldry has a powerful effect on many men, underlining the more detached and less obvious role that the father plays in the biology of reproduction (p. 212). Until recently, less attention was paid to the contribution of the male to infertility, and for a man to discover that he lacks fertile sperm, whereas his wife is reproductively normal, can be damaging to his self-esteem.

Attention has been paid to the impact of infertility on the relationship (Leiblum 1993) and clearly many couples discovering that they are infertile experience understandable distress. In general, for reasons already discussed, women are more likely to be distressed by infertility than men. There has been a notable lack of attention in the relevant literature to assessing the relative importance of infertility which results from the woman's reproductive status, and that which results from the man's. What has been recognized is that many infertile couples weather the initial stress of infertility and emerge with their relationship in some sense strengthened. Schmidt et al (2005) assessed a large cohort of couples beginning fertility treatment and again 12 months later. A third of these couples remained infertile. Of these, 26% of the women and 21% of the men reported that their marital relationship had benefited from the experience. Among the men, a non-avoidant coping style (e.g. letting feelings out and asking others for advice) was predictive of marital improvement. None of the variables studies were predictive in the women.

Infertility and sexual function

Infertility may be a consequence of earlier sexual behaviour and sexually transmitted infections (see Chapter 14), with tubal obstruction resulting from pelvic inflammatory disease in women, and azospermia following urethral infection in men.

Sexual difficulties are common amongst infertile couples. Steele (1976) reported sexual or marital problems in 37% of 500 couples attending an infertility clinic. Mai et al (1972) found infertile women to have more disturbances of sexual identity and problems of sexual adjustment. Rubinstein (1980) found that 50% of couples with primary infertility had 'a fearful approach to sex which caused a problem in marital relations'.

In a proportion of cases the infertility is likely to be a direct consequence of the sexual problem. Dubin & Amelar (1972) concluded that in 5.5% of their series of infertile couples a sexual difficulty was a primary cause of the infertility. Any problem that interferes with the deposition of semen in the vagina will obviously impair, if not entirely prevent, fertility. Non-consummation, vaginismus or erectile dysfunction, inability to ejaculate inside the vagina and severe premature ejaculation occurring usually before vaginal entry are obvious examples. The role of more subtle changes in sexual response is not so clear. The frequency of sexual intercourse is relevant. Too frequent intercourse or ejaculation may lead to a reduction in sperm count. Intervals between ejaculation of less than 12 h or greater than 7 days result in reduced fertility of the ejaculate (Eliasson 1965; Mortimer et al 1982), even to the extent of reducing sperm penetration (Rogers et al 1983). Macleod & Gold (1953) estimated that within a 6-month period, the relationship between coital frequency and conception would be 84% conception for a frequency of four times or more per week, 32% for once but less than twice per week, and 17% for less than weekly. Obviously reduced frequency, if otherwise unrelated to the timing of ovulation, will reduce the likelihood of intercourse occurring during the fertile period.

Does the coital frequency influence the woman's fertility? In a series of studies, Cutler and her colleagues have proposed that it does and that if intercourse is less than once weekly the likelihood of ovulatory cycles is reduced (Cutler et al 1979, 1980, 1985). Their evidence is suggestive but not conclusive. What is lacking is evidence that by changing coital frequency, the ovarian cycle is affected. Without such evidence one is left with the possibility that the coital frequency is in some way a *consequence* of the woman's reproductive physiology rather than a cause of it (Bancroft 1987).

The importance of the female orgasm to fertility has also been much discussed and was considered closely in Chapter 4. At present there is no clear evidence that a woman's orgasm influences her fertility, and no evidence that women who have difficulty or are unable to experience orgasm are more likely to be infertile.

It is a common clinical impression that when stress, which might be associated with a sexual problem, declines, conception occurs. There is some evidence that ovulation can be delayed by stress of various kinds (Peyser et al 1973), but the importance of such a mechanism to infertility remains very uncertain. If it is relevant, then one might expect to find conception occurring in some couples when their general sexual relationship improves. It is therefore of interest that in Rubinstein's study (1980), 32 of the 40 couples with sexual anxieties felt more relaxed and enjoyed sex more after sexual counselling and 18 of the women conceived.

The adverse effects of infertility on the sexual relationship also have to be taken into consideration. The potential importance of fertility to one's gender identity has already been mentioned. Berger (1980) interviewed 16 married couples after the diagnosis of azoospermia had been made. Ten of the men suffered a period of erectile failure, usually starting within 1 week of being informed of the diagnosis. Hostility and guilt were also quite common in the wives. Humphrey (1984) was unable to replicate these rather negative findings. But it would not be surprising if the discovery that one's partner is sterile leads to tensions that in turn have adverse effects on the sexual relationship. It is commonplace to find that infertile couples, once they have started to strive to conceive, find that their sexual enjoyment is impaired. This can be particularly marked if the couple are concentrating on the fertile period, producing the 'this is the night' syndrome (Kaufman 1969). This problem may come to light when arranging post-coital tests, which find the man unable to respond or to ejaculate at the appropriate time. Certainly, any tendency to sexual dysfunction in either partner is likely to be aggravated by following such a timetable of 'optimal coitus'. This should be taken into consideration when recommending such an approach to the infertile couple.

AID, or artificial insemination using the semen of a donor, is the principal method for dealing with male infertility. This procedure has been controversial, although in spite of the initial very negative attitudes of the Church and medical profession, acceptance of this method has grown (Snowden & Mitchell 1980). The ethical issues have been highlighted in the controversy over the use of AID for lesbian women who wish to be mothers. The legal complexities remain unresolved; the child of an AID conception is illegitimate. With all this ethical uncertainty, it would not be surprising to find that some couples making use of AID experience psychological or sexual repercussions. Clearly, the decision to use this method should be taken by both partners. So far the limited evidence is reassuring. Short-term adverse effects on the marital and sexual relationship may occur, but it is not always clear whether this stems from the AID or the infertility itself (Alder 1984).

When the cause of the infertility lies with the woman, in vitro fertilization (IVF) is most often used. While not without its ethical complexities, this procedure has been less controversial. Leiblum et al (1998) compared three groups of infertile couples receiving IVF. In one group, IVF was successful, in the second group IVF was not successful and the couple adopted a child, and in the third group IVF was unsuccessful and the couple remained childless. They found that the women in the first group, who became biological mothers through IVF, were significantly more satisfied with their lives than women in the third group who remained childless. The third group reported that the infertility had a significantly greater negative impact on their marriages compared to the other two groups. However, there were no significant differences between the three groups on standardized measures of marital and sexual satisfaction. The authors concluded

that 'most couples successfully survive infertility treatment without undue negative effects on their marital and sexual relationship' (p. 3574).

Whilst infertility and the attempts to treat it may be challenging and stressful for many couples, we should not assume that such effects will necessarily be permanent. Some marriages may break up as a consequence. Others will eventually work through this crisis and may end up with their relationship strengthened. The weight of evidence suggests that in the long term childless couples are physically and psychologically as well off, if not better off, than couples with children (Humphrey 1975).

REFERENCES

Alder E 1984 Psychological Aspects of AID. In Emery AEH & Pullen IM (eds) Psychological Aspects of Genetic Counseling. Academic, London, pp. 187–199.

Alder E, Bancroft J 1988 The relationship between breast feeding persistence, sexuality and mood in the post-partum woman. Psychological Medicine 18: 389–396.

Alder E, Cook A, Gray J, Tyrer G, Warner P, Bancroft J, Loudon N, Loudon J 1981 The effects of sterilisation: a comparison of sterilised women with the wives of vasectomised men. Contraception 23: 45–54.

Alder E, Cook A, Davidson D, West C, Bancroft J 1986 Hormones, mood and sexuality in lactating women. British Journal of Psychiatry 148: 74–79.

Alexander GM, Sherwin BB 1993 Sex steroids, sexual behavior, and selection attention for erotic stimuli in women using oral contraceptives. Psychoneuroendocrinology 18: 91–102.

Anderson RA, Martin CW, Kung A, Everington D, Pun TC, Tan KCB, Bancroft J, Sundaram K, Moo-Young AJ, Baird DT 1999 7α-Methyl-19-Nortestosterone (MENT) maintains sexual behavior and mood in hypogonadal men. Journal of Clinical Endocrinology & Metabolism 84: 3556–3562.

Ashton JR 1980 The psychosocial outcome of induced abortion. British Journal of Obstetrics and Gynaecology 87: 1115–1122.

Bancroft J 1987 Hormones, sexuality and fertility in women. Journal of Zoology (London) 213: 445–454.

Bancroft J 1993 The premenstrual syndrome — a reappraisal of the concept and the evidence. Psychological Medicine Monographs 24 (Suppl): 1–47.

Bancroft J, Sartorius N 1990 The effects of oral contraceptives on well-being and sexuality. Oxford Reviews of Reproductive Biology 12: 57–92.

Bancroft J, Davidson DW, Warner P, Tyrer G 1980 Androgens and sexual behaviour in women using oral contraceptives. Clinical Endocrinology 12: 327–340.

Bancroft J, Sanders D, Warner P, Loudon N 1987 The effects of oral contraceptives on mood and sexuality: a comparison of triphasic and combined preparations. Journal of Psychosomatic Obstetrics and Gynaecology 7: 1–8.

Bancroft J, Sherwin B, Alexander GM, Davidson DW, Walker A 1991a Oral contraceptives, androgens, and the sexuality of young women. I. A comparison of sexual experience, sexual attitudes, and gender role in oral contraceptive users and nonusers. Archives of Sexual Behavior 20: 105–120.

Bancroft J, Sherwin B, Alexander GM, Davidson DW, Walker A 1991b Oral contraceptives, androgens, and the sexuality of young women. II. The role of androgens. Archives of Sexual Behavior 20: 121–135.

Bankole A, Singh S, Haas T 1999 Characteristics of women who obtain induced abortion: a worldwide review. International Family Planning Perspectives 25: 68–77.

Bean FD, Clark MP, South S, et al 1980 Change in sexual desire after voluntary sterilisation. Social Biology 27: 186–193.

Beischer NA 1967 The anatomical and functional results of mediolateral episiotomy. Medical Journal of Australia 2: 189–195.

Bell JS, Bancroft J, Philip A 1985 Motivation for parenthood: a factor analytic study of attitudes towards having children. Journal of Comparative Family Studies 16: 111–119.

Berger DM 1980 Impotence following the discovery of azoospermia. Fertility and Sterility 34: 154–156.

Bertero E, Hallak J, Gromatzky C, Lucon AM, Arap S 2005 Assessment of sexual function in patients undergoing vasectomy using the International Index of Erectile Function. International Brazilian Journal of Urology 31: 452–458.

Billings J, Billings EL 1973 Determination of fertile and infertile days by the mucus pattern: development of the ovulation method. In Urrichio WA, Williams MK (eds) Natural Family Planning. The Human Life Foundation, Washington, DC.

Bone M 1978 The Family Planning Services: Changes and Effects. OPCS Social Survey Division. HMSO, London.

Boyd RA, Zegarac EA, Posvar EL, Flack MR 2001 Minimal androgenic activity of a new oral contraceptive containing norethindrone acetate and graduated doses of ethinyl estradiol. Contraception 63: 71–76.

Bradshaw Z, Slade P 2003 The effects of induced abortion on emotional experiences and relationships: a critical review of the literature. Clinical Psychology Review 23: 929–958.

Bradshaw Z, Slade P 2005 The relationships between induced abortion, attitudes towards sexuality and sexual problems. Sexual and Relationship Therapy 20: 391–406.

Brewer C 1977 Incidence of post-abortion psychosis: a prospective study. British Medical Journal i: 476–477.

Broome A 1984 Termination of pregnancy. In Broome A, Wallace L (eds) Psychology and Gynaecological Problems. Tavistock, London, pp. 60–76.

Caldwell J, Gaminiratne K, Caldwell P, de Silva S, Caldwell B, Silva P 1987 The role of traditional fertility regulation in Sri Lanka. Studies in Family Planning 18: 1–21.

Caruso S, Agnello C, Intelisano G, Farina M, Di Mari L, Cianci A 2004 Sexual behavior of women taking low-dose contraceptive containing 15 μg ethinyl-estradiol/60 μg gestodene. Contraception 69: 237–240.

Caruso S, Agnello C, Intelisano G, Farina M, Di Mari L, Cianci A 2005 A prospective study on sexual behavior of women using 30 μg ethinylestradiol and 3 mg drospirenone oral contraceptive. Contraception 72: 19–23.

Cates W Jr, Stewart FH 2004 Vaginal barriers: the female condom, diaphragm, contraceptive sponge, cervical cap, Lea's Shield and FemCap. In Hatcher RA, Trussell J, Stewart FH, Nelson AL, Cates W Jr, Guest F, Kowal D (eds) Contraceptive Technology, 18th edition. Ardent Media, New York, pp. 365–390.

Cawood EHH, Bancroft J 1996 Steroid hormones, the menopause, sexuality and the wellbeing of women. Psychological Medicine 26: 925–936.

Cliquet RL, Thiery M, Stailens R, Lambert G 1981 Voluntary sterilisation in Flanders. Journal of Biosocial Science 13: 47–67.

Coenen CMH, Thomas CMG, Borm GF, Hollanders JMG, Rolland R 1996 Changes in androgens during treatment with four low-dose contraceptives. Contraception 53: 171–176.

Cooper PJ, Murray L 1995 Course and recurrence of postnatal depression. Evidence for the specificity of the diagnostic concept. British Journal of Psychiatry 166: 191–195.

Cooper P, Gath D, Rose N, Fieldsend R 1982 Psychological sequelae to elective sterilisation in women: a prospective study. British Medical Journal 284: 461–464.

Costello C, Hillis SD, Marchbanks PA, Jamieson DJ, Peterson HB for the US Collaborative Review of Sterilization Working Group 2002 The effect of interval tubal sterilization on sexual interest and pleasure. Obstetrics & Gynecology 100: 511–517.

Cullberg J 1972 Mood changes and menstrual symptoms with different gestagen/estrogen combinations. Acta Psychiatrica Scandinavica (Suppl) 236: 1–86.

Cutler WB, Garcia CR, Krieger AM 1979 Luteal phases defects: a possible relationship between short hyperthermic phase and sporadic sexual behaviour in women. Hormones and Behavior 13: 214–218.

Cutler WB, Garcia CR, Krieger AM 1980 Sporadic sexual behaviour and menstrual cycle length in women. Hormones and Behavior 14: 163–172.

Cutler WB, Preti G, Huggins GR, Erickson B, Garcia CR 1985 Sexual behavior frequency and biphasic ovulatory type menstrual cycles. Physiology and Behavior 34: 805–810.

Darney PD 1995 The androgenicity of progestins. American Journal of Medicine 98(Suppl 1A): 104S–110S.

Davis AR, Castano PM 2006 Oral contraceptives and sexuality. In Goldstein I, Meston S, Davis S, Traish A (eds) Women's Sexual Function and Dysfunction: Study, Diagnosis and Treatment. Taylor & Francis, London, pp. 290–296.

Davis SR, Davison SL, Donath S, Bell RJ 2005 Circulating androgen levels and self-reported sexual function in women. Journal of the American Medical Association 294: 91–96.

De Judicibus MA, McCabe MP 2002 Psychological factors and the sexuality of pregnant and postpartum women. Journal of Sex Research 39: 94–103.

D'Emilio J, Freedman EB 1988 Intimate Matters. A History of Sexuality in America. Harper & Row, New York.

Dennerstein L, Soencer-Gardner C, Brown JB, Smith MA, Burrows GD 1984 Premenstrual tension: hormonal profiles. Journal of Psychosomatic Obstetrics and Gynaecology 3: 37–51.

Dennerstein L, Dudley EC, Hopper JL, Burger H 1997 Sexuality, hormones and the menopausal transition. Maturitas 26: 83–93.

Djerassi IC 1979 The Politics of Contraception, Vol. 1, The Present. The Portable Stanford, Stanford Alumni Association, Stanford, CA.

Dubin L, Amelar RD 1972 Sexual causes of male infertility. Fertility and Sterility 23: 579–582.

Ehrhardt AA 1996 Our view on adolescent sexuality- a focus on risk behavior without the developmental context [editorial]. American Journal of Public Health 86: 1523–1525.

Eliasson R 1965 Effect of frequent ejaculation on the composition of the human seminal plasma. Journal of Reproduction and Fertility 9: 331–336.

Erens B, McManus S, Prescott, Field J, Johnson, AM, Wellings K, Fenton K, Mercer C, Macdowell W, Copas AJ, Nanchahal K 2003 National Survey of Sexual Attitudes and Lifestyles II: reference tables and summary report. National Centre for Social Research.

Ford CS, Beach FA 1952 Patterns of Sexual Behaviour. Eyre & Spottiswoode, London.

Frenken J, Vennix P 1981 Sexuality Experience Scales manual. Swets & Zietlinger, Lisse, The Netherlands.

Garner P 1982 Dyspareunia after episiotomy. British Journal of Sexual Medicine 9(86): 11–12.

General Household Survey 1983, 1985. OPCS. HMSO, London.

Graham CA, Sherwin BB 1993 The relationship between mood and sexuality in women using an oral contraceptive as a treatment for premenstrual symptoms. Psychoneuroendocrinology 18: 273–281.

Graham CA, Ramos R, Bancroft J, Maglaya C, Farley TMM 1995 The effects of steroidal contraceptives on the well-being and sexuality of women: a double blind, placebo-controlled, two-center study of combined and progestogen-only methods. Contraception 52: 363–369.

Graham CA, Bancroft J, Doll HA, Greco T, Tanner A 2007 Does oral-contraceptive-induced reduction in free testosterone adversely affect the sexuality or mood of women? Psychoneuroendocrinology 32: 246–255.

Greco T, Graham CA, Bancroft J, Tanner A, Doll HA 2007 The effects of oral contraceptives on androgen levels and their relevance to premenstrual mood and sexual interest: a comparison of two triphasic formulations containing norgestimate and either 35 μg or 25 μg of ethinyl estradiol. Contraception 76: 8–17.

Greer HS, Lal S, Lewis SC, Belsey EM, Beard RW 1976 Psychosocial consequences of therapeutic abortion. Kings termination study III. British Journal of Psychiatry 128: 74–79.

Grimes DA 2004 Intrauterine devices (IUDs) In Hatcher RA, Trussell J, Stewart FH, Nelson AL, Cates W Jr, Guest F, Kowal D (eds) Contraceptive Technology, 18th edition. Ardent Media, New York, pp. 495–530.

Grimes DA, Lopez LM, Gallo MF, Halpern V, Nanda K, Schulz KF 2004 Steroid hormones for contraception in men. Cochrane Database Systematic Reviews CD004316.

Grounds D, Davies B, Mowbray R 1970 The contraceptive pill, side effects and personality: a report of a controlled double-blind trial. British Journal of Psychiatry 116: 169–172.

Grudzinskas JC, Atkinson L 1984 Sexual function during the puerperium. Archives of Sexual Behavior 13: 85–92.

Grunbaum JA, Kann L, Kinchen, SA, Williams B, Ross JG, Lowry R, Kolbe L 2002 Youth Risk Behavior Surveillance - United States, 2001. MMWR Surveillance Summaries SS04: 1–64.

Hamill E, Ingram IM 1974 Psychiatric and social factors in the abortion decision. British Medical Journal i: 229–232.

Hart AJL, Deane RF 1980 A retrospective study of 100 vasectomies carried out at the FPA. British Journal of Sexual Medicine 7(67): 10–14.

Hatcher RA 2004 Depo-Provera injections, implants, and progestin-only pills (Minipills). In Hatcher RA, Trussell J, Stewart FH, Nelson AL, Cates W Jr, Guest F, Kowal D (eds) Contraceptive Technology, 18th edition. Ardent Media, New York, pp. 461–494.

Hatcher RA, Nelson AL 2004 Combined hormonal contraceptive methods. In Hatcher RA, Trussell J, Stewart FH, Nelson AL, Cates W Jr, Guest F, Kowal D (eds) Contraceptive Technology, 18th edition. Ardent Media, New York, pp. 391–460.

Hatcher RA, Trussell J, Stewart FH, Nelson AL, Cates W Jr, Guest F, Kowal D 2004 Contraceptive Technology, 18th edition. Ardent Media, New York.

Hawkins DF, Elder MG 1979 Human Fertility Control, Theory and Practice. Butterworth, London, p. 98.

Heidrich A, Schleyer M, Springler H, Albert P, Knoche M, Fritze J, Lanczik M 1994 Postpartum blues: relationship between non-protein bound steroid hormones in plasma and postpartum mood changes. Journal of Affective Disorders 30: 93–98.

Henshaw SK 1994 Recent trends in the legal status of induced abortion. Journal of Public Health Policy 15: 165–172.

Herzberg BN, Draper KC, Johnson AL, Nicol GC 1971 Oral contraceptives, depression and libido. British Medical Journal 3: 495–500.

Hollerbach PE, Nortman DL 1984 Sterilisation. In Emery AEH, Pullen IM (eds) Psychological Aspects of Genetic Counseling. Academic, London, pp. 169–186.

Howard G 1978 Motivation for vasectomy. Lancet i: 546–548.

Humphrey M 1975 The effect of children upon the marriage relationship. British Journal of Medical Psychology 48: 273–279.

Humphrey M 1977 Sex differences in attitude to parenthood. Human Relations 30: 737–749.

Humphrey M 1984 Infertility and alternative parenting. In Broome A, Wallace L (eds) Psychology and Gynaecological Problems. Tavistock, London, pp. 77–94.

Hyde JS, DeLamater JD 2003 Understanding Human Sexuality, 8th edition. McGraw Hill, Boston.

Hyde JS, DeLamater JD, Plant EA, Byrd JM 1996 Sexuality during pregnancy and the year postpartum. Journal of Sex Research 33: 143–151.

Hyde JS, DeLamater JD, Hewitt EC 1998 Sexuality and the dual earner couple: multiple roles and sexual functioning. Journal of Family Psychology 12: 354–368.

IC.NHS 2005 Infant feeding survey 2005: early results. http://www.ic.nhs.uk/pubs/breastfeed2005.

Janaud A, Rouffy J, Upmalis D, Dain M-P 1992 A comparison of lipid and androgen metabolism with triphasic oral contraceptive formations containing norgestimate or levonorgestrel. Acta Obstetrica Gynecologica Scandinavica Suppl 156: 33–38.

Johnson AM, Wadsworth J, Wellings K, Field J 1994 Sexual Attitudes and Lifestyles. Oxford, Blackwell.

Jung-Hoffman C, Kuhl H 1987 Divergent effects of two low-dose oral contraceptives on sex hormone-binding globulin and free testosterone. American Journal of Obstetrics & Gynecology 156: 199–203.

Kasonde JM, Bonnar J 1976 Effect of sterilization on menstrual blood loss. British Journal of Obstetrics & Gynaecology 83: 572–575.

Kaufman SA 1969 Impact of infertility on the marital and sexual relationship. Fertility and Sterility 20: 380–383.

Kay CR 1984 The Royal College of General Practitioners' oral contraception study: some recent observations. Clinics in Obstetrics and Gynaecology 11: 759–786.

Kennedy KI, Trussell J 2004 Postpartum contraception and lactation. In Hatcher RA, Trussell J, Stewart FH, Nelson AL, Cates W Jr, Guest F, Kowal D (eds) Contraceptive Technology, 18th edition. Ardent Media, New York, pp. 575–600.

Khan ME, Patel BC 1997 Male Involvement in Family Planning: A Knowledge, Attitude, Behaviour, and Practice Survey of Agra District. Project Report. Population Council, Delhi, India.

Kutner SJ, Brown SL 1972 Types of oral contraceptives, depression and premenstrual symptoms. Journal of Nervous and Mental Disorders 115: 153–162.

Langdridge D, Sheeran P, Connolly K 2005 Understanding the reasons for parenthood. Journal of Reproductive and Infant Psychology 23: 121–134.

Lattimer M 1999 Norplant contraceptive implant withdrawn. http://www.prochoiceforum.org.uk/comm9.asp.

Leeton J, McMaster R, Worsley A 1978 The effects of sexual response and mood after sterilization of women taking long term oral contraceptives: results of a double-blind cross-over study. Australian and New Zealand Journal of Obstetrics and Gynecology 18: 194–197.

Leiblum SR 1993 The impact of infertility on sexual and marital satisfaction. Annual Review of Sex Research 4: 99–120.

Leiblum SR, Aviv A, Hamer R 1998 Life after infertility treatment: a long-term investigation of marital and sexual function. Human Reproduction 13: 3569–3574.

Lindemann C 1977 Factors affecting the use of contraceptives in the non-marital context. In Gemme R, Wheeler CC (eds) Progress in Sexology. Plenum, New York, pp. 397–408.

Linnet L, Moller NP, Bernth-Petersen P, Ehlers N, Brandslund I, Svehag SE 1982 No increase in arteriosclerotic retinopathy or activity in tests for circulating immune complex 5 years after vasectomy. Fertility and Sterility 37: 798–806.

Macleod J, Gold RZ 1953 The male factor in fertility and sterility. Fertility and Sterility 4: 10–14.

Mai FMM, Munday RN, Rump EE 1972 Psychiatric interview comparisons between infertile and fertile couples. Psychosomatic Medicine 34: 431–440.

Margaret Pyke Centre 1973 One thousand vasectomies. British Medical Journal 4: 216–221.

Marks LV 2001 Sexual Chemistry: a History of the Contraceptive Pill. Yale University Press, New Haven.

Martin CW, Anderson RA, Cheng L, Ho PC, van der Spuy Z, Smith KB, Glasier AF, Everington D, Baird DT 2000 Potential impact of hormonal male contraception: cross-cultural implications for development of novel preparations. Human Reproduction 15: 637–645.

Martin-Loeches M, Orti RM, Monfort M, Ortega E, Rius J 2003 A comparative analysis of the modification of sexual desire of users of oral hormonal contraceptives and intrauterine contraceptive devices. European Journal of Contraception and Reproductive Health Care 8: 129–134.

Massey FJ Jr, Bernstein GS, Schuman LM, O'Fallon WM 1983 The effects of vasectomy on the health status of American men. Fertility and Sterility 40: 414–415.

McCormick EP, Johnson RL, Friedman HL, David HP 1977 Psychosocial aspects of fertility regulation. In: Money J, Musaph H (eds) Handbook of Sexology. Elsevier/North Holland, Amsterdam, pp. 621–653.

Mishell DR Jr 2004 Contraception. In Strauss JF III, Barbieri RL (eds) Yen & Jaffe's Reproductive Endocrinology, 5th edition. Elsevier Saunders, Philadelphia, pp. 899–938.

Mortimer D, Templeton AA, Lenton EA, Coleman RA 1982 Influence of abstinence and ejaculation-to-analysis delay on semen analysis parameters of suspected infertile men. Archives of Andrology 8: 251–256.

Mosher WD, Martinez GM, Chandra A, Abma JC, Willson SJ 2004 Use of contraception and use of family planning services in the United States: 1982-2002. Advance Data from Vital Health Statistics, Number 350. December 10, 2004.

Nelson AL, Marshall JR 2004 Impaired fertility. In Hatcher RA, Trussell J, Stewart FH, Nelson AL, Cates W Jr, Guest F, Kowal D (eds) Contraceptive Technology, 18th edition. Ardent Media, New York, pp. 651–671.

Newman P, Leavesley JH 1980 Medicine in Australia – a review of vasectomy in general practice. British Journal of Sexual Medicine 7(64): 48–56.

NIHCE 2005 Long-Acting Reversible Contraception: the Effective and Appropriate Use of Long-Acting Reversible Contraception. National Institute for Health and Clinical Excellence. RCOG Press, London.

Noble AD 1978 Female sterilization: long term effects. In Sciarra JJ, Zatuchni GI, Speridel JJ (eds) Risks, Benefits and Controversies in Fertility Control. Harper & Row, Maryland.

Oinonen KA, Mazmanian D 2002 To what extent do oral contraceptives influence mood and affect? Journal of Affective Disorders 70: 229–240.

Oranratanaphan S, Taneepanichskul S 2006 A double-blind randomized control trial comparing effect of Drospirenone and Gestodene on sexual desire and libido. Journal of Medical Association of Thailand 89(Suppl 4): S17–S21.

Pare CMB, Raven H 1970 Follow up of patients referred for termination of pregnancy. Lancet i: 635–638.

Parrinder G 1987 A theological approach. In Geer JH, O'Donohue WT (eds) Theories of Human Sexuality. Plenum, New York, pp. 21–48.

Paul C, Skegg DCG, Williams S 1997 Depot Medroxyprogesterone acetate: patterns of use and reasons for discontinuation. Contraception 56: 209–214.

Peterson HB, Jeng G, Folger SG, Hillis SA, Marchbanks PA, Wilcox LS for the US Collaborative Review of Sterilization Working Group. 2000 The risk of menstrual abnormalities after tubal sterilization. New England Journal of Medicine 343: 1681–1687.

Petitti D, Klein R, Kipp H, Kahn W, Siegelaub AB, Friedman GD 1982a A survey of personal habits, symptoms of illness and histories of disease in men with and without vasectomies. American Journal of Public Health 72: 476–480.

Petitti D, Klein R, Kipp H, Kahn W, Siegelaub AB, Friedman GD 1982b Physiologic measures in men with and without vasectomies. Fertility and Sterility 37: 438–440.

Peyser MR, Ayalon D, Harell A, Toaff M, Cordova T 1973 Stress-induced delay of ovulation. Obstetrics and Gynecology 42: 667–671.

Population Reports 1978 M/F Sterilization. Special Topic Monograph No 2. Department of Medical and Public Affairs, Washington, DC.

Population Reports 1985 Female sterilization. Series C, No 9. Johns Hopkins University, Baltimore.

Reamy KJ, White SE 1987 Sexuality in the puerperium: a review. Archives of Sexual Behavior 16: 165–186.

Richters J, Grulich AE, de Visser RO, Smith AMA, Rissel CE 2003 Sex in Australia: contraceptive practices among a representative sample of women. Australian & New Zealand Journal of Public Health 27: 210–216.

Robson KM, Brant HA, Kumar R 1981 Maternal sexuality during first pregnancy and after childbirth. British Journal of Obstetrics and Gynaecology 88: 882–889.

Rodgers DA, Ziegler FJ, Levy N 1967 Prevailing cultural attitudes about vasectomy: a possible explanation of post-operative psychological response. Psychosomatic Medicine 29:367–375.

Rogers BJ, Perreault SD, Bentwood BJ, McCarville C, Hale RW, Soderdahl DW 1983 Variability in the human-hamster in-vitro assay for fertility evaluation. Fertility and Sterility 39: 204–211.

Rönnau HJ 1980 The psychologic influence of female sterilisation on sexology and family structure. In Forleo R, Pasini W (eds) Medical Sexology. Elsevier/North Holland, Amsterdam, pp. 378–380.

Rosen R, Brown C, Heiman J, et al 2000 The Female Sexual Function Index (FSFI): a multidimensional self-report instrument for the assessment of sexual function. Journal of Sex & Marital Therapy 26: 191–208.

Rosen RC, Cappelleri JC, Gendrano N III 2002 The International Index of Erectile Function (IIEF): a state-of-the-science review. International Journal of Impotence Research 14: 226–244.

Rubinstein I 1980 Sterility caused by sexual disturbance. In Forleo R, Pasini W (eds) Medical Sexology. Elsevier/North Holland, Amsterdam, pp. 364–366.

Sanders D, Warner P, Backstrom T, Bancroft J 1983 Mood, sexuality, hormones and the menstrual cycle. I. Changes in mood and physical state: description of subjects and method. Psychosomatic Medicine 45: 487–501.

Sanders SA, Graham CA, Bass JL, Bancroft J 2001 A prospective study of the effects of contraception of sexuality and well-being and their relationship to discontinuation. Contraception 64: 51–58.

Satcher D 2001 A Call to Action to promote sexual health and responsible sexual behavior. www.surgeongeneral.gov/library/sexualhealth.

Schaffir J 2006 Hormonal contraception and sexual desire: a critical review. Journal of Sex and Marital Therapy 32: 305–314.

Schmidt L, Holstein B, Christensen U, Boivin J 2005 Does infertility cause marital benefit? An epidemiological study of 2250 women and men in fertility treatment. Patient education and counselling. Special issue. Social and Cultural Factors in Fertility 59: 244–251.

Scott J, Jenkins R 1998 Psychiatric disorders specific to women. In Johnstone EC, Freeman CPL, Zealley AK (eds) Companion to Psychiatric Studies, 6th edition. Churchill Livingstone, Edinburgh, pp. 551–564.

Short RV 1976 The evolution of human reproduction. In Short RV, Baird DT (eds) Contraceptives of the Future. Royal Society, London.

Simon NM, Senturia AG 1966 Psychiatric sequelae of abortion: review of the literature 1935-1964. Archives of General Psychiatry 15: 278–289.

Simon Population Trust 1969 Vasectomy: Follow up of 1000 Cases. Simon Population Trust, Cambridge.

Smith AHW 1979 Psychiatric aspects of sterilisation: a prospective study. British Journal of Psychiatry 135: 304–309.

Snowden R, Christian B 1983 Patterns and Perceptions of Menstruation. A WHO International Study. Croom Helm, London.

Snowden R, Mitchell GD 1980 A sociological view of artificial insemination by donor. British Journal of Family Planning 6: 45–49.

Spector IP, Carey MP, Steinberg L 1996 The Sexual Desire Inventory: development, factor structure and evidence of reliability. Journal of Sex & Marital Therapy 22: 175–190.

Steele SJ 1976 Sexual problems related to contraception and family planning. In Crown S (ed) Psychosexual Problems. Academic Press, London, pp. 383–401.

Talwar OO, Berger GS 1979 A prospective randomized study of oral contraceptives: the effect of study design on reported rates of symptoms. Contraception 20: 329–337.

Tentler LW 2004 Catholics and Contraception: an American History. Cornell University Press, Ithaca.

Thorneycroft IH, Stanczyk FZ, Bradshaw KD, Ballagh SA, Nichols M, Weber ME 1999 Effect of low-dose oral contraceptives on androgenic markers and acne. Contraception 60: 255–262.

Trussell J, Gummer-Strawn L 1990 Contraceptive failure of the ovulation method of periodic abstinence. Family Planning Perspectives 22: 65–75.

Tyrer G, Steel JM, Ewing DJ, Bancroft J, Warner P, Clark BR 1983. Sexual response in diabetic women. Diabetologia 24: 166–171.

Van der Vange N, Blankenstein MA, Kloosterboer HJ, Haspels AA, Thijssen JH 1990 Effects of seven low-dose combined oral contraceptives on sex hormone binding globulin, corticosteroid binding globulin, total and free testosterone. Contraception 41: 345–352.

Van Look PFA 2000 Contraceptives of the future. In Glasier A, Gebbie A (eds) Handbook of Family Planning and Reproductive Health Care. Churchill Livingstone, London, pp. 395–416.

Veit CT, Ware JE Jr 1983 The structure of psychological distress and well-being in general populations. Journal of Consulting and Clinical Psychology 51: 703–742.

Von Sydow K 2006 Pregnancy, childbirth and the postpartum period. In Goldstein I, Meston S, Davis S, Traish A (eds) Women's Sexual Function and Dysfunction: Study, Diagnosis and Treatment. Taylor & Francis, London, pp. 282–289.

Walker A, Bancroft J 1990 The relationship between premenstrual symptoms and oral contraceptive use: a controlled study. Psychosomatic Medicine 52: 86–96.

Warner P, Bancroft J 1988 Mood, sexuality, oral contraceptives and the menstrual cycle. Journal of Psychosomatic Research 32: 417–427.

Warner L, Hatcher RA, Steiner MJ 2004 Male condoms. In Hatcher RA, Trussell J, Stewart FH, Nelson AL, Cates W Jr, Guest F, Kowal D (eds) Contraceptive Technology, 18th edition. Ardent Media, New York.

Watkins ES 1998 On the Pill: a Social History of Oral Contraceptives, 1950-1970. Johns Hopkins University Press, Baltimore.

Weeks JD, Kozak LJ 2001 Trends in the use of episiotomy in the United States: 1980-1998. Birth 28: 152–160.

Westhoff C, Truman C, Kalmuss D, Cushman L, Davidson A, Rulin M, Heartwell S 1998 Depressive symptoms and Depo-Provera. Contraception 57: 237–240.

White SE, Reamy KJ 1982 Sexuality and pregnancy: a review. Archives of Sexual Behavior 11: 429–444.

WHO 1978 World Health Organization Special program of research, development and research training in human reproduction, 7th annual report. November 1978.

Williams FLR, Florey C duV, Mires GJ, Ogston SA 1998 Episiotomy and perineal tears in low-risk UK primigravidae. Journal of Public Health 20: 422–427.

Wilkinson D, Wegner MN, Mwangi N, Lynam P 1996 Improving vasectomy services in Kenya: lessons from a mystery client study. Reproductive Health Matters 7: 115–121.

Wolfers H 1970 Psychological aspects of vasectomy. British Medical Journal 4: 297–300.

Wu FC 2006 Hormonal approaches to male contraception: approaching reality. Molecular & Cell Endocrinology 250: 2–7.

Sexual offences

Introduction...464

Sexual offences as defined in the UK............................465

What is the true incidence of sexual offences?..............468
The UK...468
How does the USA compare?...470
Methodological issues in recalling earlier experiences
of sexual assault or abuse...471

The socio-cultural context of sexual offending...............471
Rape and sexual assault..471
Sexual exploitation and abuse of children.......................473
Incest...476
Indecent exposure or exhibitionism...................................478

The sexual offender...478
Determinants of sexual offences in general.....................478

Re-offending..482
Rape and sexual assault..482
Sexual offences against children.......................................483
Exhibitionism and voyeurism..486
Sexual offences by females..488

The victims of sexual offences..489
Rape...489
The victim of child sexual abuse..492

The management of sex offenders....................................501
Hormonal reduction of sexual interest..............................501
Pharmacological reduction of sexual interest...................502
Surgical methods of control...503
Psychological methods of treatment..................................503

Conclusions..505

Introduction

The one common factor in the variety of sexual offences is breaking the law. The law can be seen to have three functions in this respect: first, to protect the individual, second, to avoid social disruption caused by explicit sex in public places and, third, the 'declarative' function, or the discouragement of certain forms of behaviour, considered for one reason or another to be undesirable.

Protection of the individual is concerned not only with assault, the use of physical force or the threat of it to achieve sexual ends, but also with exploitation. Protection against assault is in itself not controversial. The main problems are associated with evidence, particularly in cases of rape. Protection against exploitation raises more disputes. It is accepted in principle, but the definition of exploitation poses many problems, most notably in relation to age of consent.

The second function, avoidance of social disruption, is likely to continue in some form. The imposition of social constraints on public sexuality appears to be a universal of human societies, though there have been certain exceptions when public orgies were allowed on specific days.

It is the third, 'declarative' function that is the most controversial and which has shown and will continue to show the most change. There has been long-standing controversy over the use of the law in this way. John Stewart Mill (1859) considered that 'the only purpose for which power can be rightfully exercised over any member of a civilised community against his will, is to prevent harm to others'. Many years later, in a similar vein, the Wolfenden (1957) Committee asserted: 'it is not the duty of the law to concern itself with immorality as such ... it should confine itself to those activities which offend against public order and decency, or expose the ordinary citizen to what is offensive or injurious'. These views, needless to say, have not been the prevailing ones (Freeman 1979). In fact both the Church, through the ecclesiastical courts of earlier times and the more recent legal system, have consistently punished immorality, though what constitutes punishable immorality has changed dramatically, often reflecting the prevailing norms of the establishment. Adultery or fornication has in the past been punishable in Western societies and still remains proscribed in some states of the USA. Though such law is seldom, if ever, used in Christian countries, there are still some cultures, e.g. Islamic, where it is applied with considerable severity. The most recent example of such a change in the Western world concerns homosexuality and this is considered in Chapter 8. The law involving sexual obscenity and the purveying of pornography has provided some of the more striking inconsistencies of the system at the present time, and the advent of the Internet has added a large dimension, confronting us with new and extremely difficult legal and moral challenges.

Legal proscription of certain forms of sexual behaviour on the grounds of immorality also has indirect consequences that are undesirable. When the proscribed behaviour is a source of pleasure, a 'black market' develops based on organized crime. Not infrequently, the sexually deviant individual becomes involved in an escalation of deviant activities, described as secondary or amplified deviance (Lemert 1967). Thus in weighing up the pros and cons of legislation against immorality, we have to consider the extension of other criminal behaviour that may result. Also, as much of the behaviour proscribed on grounds of immorality rather than the protection of others does not involve a victim or a complainant, the police are more likely to resort to entrapment techniques. These are themselves of very dubious morality and bring discredit to the legal and police systems.

When considering those acts that, in my view, are unequivocally the proper concern of the law — the protection of the victim against sexual assault or exploitation — we are faced with some interesting challenges, most notably whether such offences are driven by sexual or other motives. The importance of sexual reward in determining sexually offensive behaviour is variable and often obscure, and we will consider this more closely when dealing with some of the specific types of sexual offence.

Sexual offences as defined in the UK

Sexual offences are defined by the legal process and vary in detail from country to country and, within the USA, to some extent between states.

When the last edition of this book was published (1989), there was much concern in the UK about the legal process concerning sexual offences, in particular rape and sexual assault. There was widespread recognition, not just in the UK, that the majority of women who suffered rape or sexual assault did not report this to the police. The reasons for this were well recognized. The victims often received very unsympathetic, if not humiliating, treatment at the hands of the police and the courts, and not infrequently felt stigmatized by the experience in the eyes of their spouses or families. Chambers & Millar (1983) carried out an in-depth study of the police methods of investigating sexual assaults in Scotland. They found grounds for criticism of police methods on a number of counts. The collection of evidence was often carried out insensitively at a time of considerable emotional distress. This tended to be justified or at least defended on the grounds that the first priority was to catch the offender. Some CID officers clearly saw it as their job to challenge the truth of the victim's story as a way of testing its validity, little realizing that they were probably reducing its validity in the process, an approach which, in any case, would seldom be used with the victims of other types of crime. Police officers were often unaware of the up-to-date interpretations of the law on rape, and there was a tendency to apply stricter standards of evidence than were actually required to prove a case. Almost one-quarter of the cases studied were 'no-crimed' by the police. This involves amending the initial crime report after a judgement has been made that no crime has been committed. Such cases do not appear in the official statistics of crimes reported to the police. Decisions to 'no-crime' a case were often taken by relatively junior or inexperienced officers. The 'no-crime' rate for sexual offences found by Chambers &

Millar (1983) was considerably higher than that reported for crime in general. Other studies have found comparable 'no-crime' rates for sexual assault, e.g. 24% in England and 20% in the USA.

Investigation by the police is only one of the deterrents to reporting. The legal process is another off-putting experience. As Chambers & Millar (1986) found in Scotland, one-third of cases reported to the Procurator Fiscal were not prosecuted, the principal reason being the lack of independent third-party evidence. To have one's case turned down for lack of such evidence must be extremely distressing for genuine victims. Rules about corroboration of evidence are more stringent in Scotland than in England.

Most women were not only anxious about going to court, they also found the experience worse than they had expected. This was due in particular to the cross-examination, which often made the complainant feel that her own character was on trial. The defence often used tactics to discredit the complainant and rarely did the judge intervene to protect the complainant from such lines of questioning. In general, women were inadequately prepared for the experience in court. The 1976 Sexual Offence Act made evidence of the previous sexual history of the complainant with other men inadmissible in the course of a rape trial, except with the leave of the trial judge. This was intended to reduce the extent that the woman rather than the defendant was being put on trial. But Chambers & Millar (1986) and others have concluded that this Act did little to reduce the humiliation of rape victims by the judicial procedure.

To some extent this highly unsatisfactory situation for the victims of rape stems from the potential severity of the sentence if the defendant is convicted. The maximum sentence for rape is life imprisonment, though the average sentence is 3–4 years. Occasionally false accusations of rape are made. There is therefore an understandable desire on the part of the police and judiciary to ensure that no one is unjustly convicted, and an undue tendency not to prosecute if the evidence is not 'cast-iron'.

Another cause of concern at that time was the fact that a husband could not be charged with rape of his wife, an exemption that applied in England and Wales, but not in Scotland. The underlying principle that a man was entitled to sex with his wife and she had no right to refuse is horrendous by any standards. There was also concern about different ages of consent for sex between two males (21 years) and between a male and a female (16 years), reflecting continuing homophobic values in the legal system.

Many of these concerns have since been addressed. The Sexual Offences Act 2003 came into force in 2004. It repealed almost all of the existing statute law in relation to sexual offences, in order to strengthen and modernize the law on sexual offences, whilst improving preventative measures (Crown Prosecution Service 2006). These changes will be briefly reviewed, and their benefits discussed. It is too soon, however, to know the extent that these changes have reduced the obstacles to reporting such offences.

Sexual assault

There are now three categories of sexual assault, the first two are considered 'serious', the third 'less serious'.

1. *Rape.* This involves penetration of the vagina, anus or mouth with a penis, without the complainant's consent, and without reasonable grounds for the defendant to believe that the act was consensual. This is an indictable offence (i.e. has to be tried in a Crown Court with a jury) with a maximum penalty of life imprisonment. It is no longer the case that a man cannot, in legal terms, rape his wife. Rape now includes penetration of the anus or mouth, which are both considered to be as potentially traumatic as penetration of the vagina. Rape can be carried out by one man on another, when anal or oral insertion is involved. The issue of consent has been redefined on the grounds that the 'penetrator' has little to lose if his wish to penetrate is not granted, whereas the person who is penetrated has a great deal to lose if this is done against his or her wishes. The new law thus places emphasis on the defendant's justification for the belief that the act was consensual, and the 'reasonable' grounds for reaching that conclusion, rather than the complainant having to justify the claim that the act was carried out without the complainant's consent. Thus, for example, having sex with a woman who is intoxicated to the extent that she is unable to judge properly her wish to participate would preclude 'reasonable' grounds for believing that she had consented. This hopefully will go some way to reducing the trauma of the legal process for the victim, and further studies, like that reported by Walmsley & White (1979), are awaited with interest.

2. *Sexual assault by penetration.* The previous offence of indecent assault under the Sexual Offences Act 1956 covered a very wide range of offending behaviour, which the 2003 Act broke down into two clearly defined offences of 'assault by penetration' and the 'lesser offence of sexual assault'. Assault by penetration involves sexual penetration of the vagina or anus (not the mouth) by a body part (e.g. finger or tongue) other than the penis, or some object (e.g. a bottle). The issue of consent is the same as for rape. This offence can be committed by either gender. It may be charged if there is insufficient evidence that rape has occurred (e.g. uncertainty whether the penetration was by a penis). As with rape, it is indictable with a maximum penalty of life imprisonment.

3. *Less serious sexual assault (without penetration).* This lesser form of sexual assault, which can be committed by men or women, has a minimum threshold that the event caused 'fear, alarm or distress'. There are three sub-categories:

   (i) *Sexual touching without consent.* 'Touching' may be with any part of the body, or with an object, and can be through clothing, and would include penetration of the mouth (as with kissing). This offence can be indicted but may also be tried in a Magistrate's court. Maximum penalty in the Crown Court is 10 years' imprisonment. The seriousness of such an offence will be influenced by the exact nature of the sexual touching, e.g. at one extreme, using one's naked genitalia to stroke, rub, press or touch the naked genitalia of another person, and at the other, lower, end of the scale, patting someone on the bottom through clothing.

   (ii) *Indecent exposure* or flashing, which prior to 2000, was not listed as a sexual offence.

   (iii) *Sexual threats* (e.g. demanding sex in a threatening manner; following or cornering the victim in a threatening way). In most cases, such threats are not legally designated a crime.

Factors that may make the act more serious, in legal terms, include abuse of one's position (employer or teacher), use of force or coercion and repeated offending.

Causing sexual activity without consent

In this case, the offence is to intentionally cause another person to engage in some form of sexual activity, without that person's consent. The activity may not involve contact with the offender, e.g. coercing someone to masturbate or forcing someone to have sex with a third person, who may or may not consent. It may involve forcing or coercing someone to have sex with you, e.g. a woman forcing a man to penetrate her sexually. One of the principal reasons for establishing this category of offence was to provide a female version of rape, which carries the same legal consequences as the male version.

Sexual offences against children

The 2003 Act defines three categories of offences against children according to the child's age.

1. *Offences against children under 13.* Each of the earlier categories of 'sexual assault' and 'causing sexual activity' apply to this category, with the important difference that consent is irrelevant. A child under 13 does not, under any circumstances, have the legal capacity to consent to any form of sexual activity. The prosecution in such cases has to prove only two facts: first, the intentional sexual activity and, second, the age of the complainant at the date of the sexual activity.

2. *Offences against children under 16.* The 2003 Act provides that the age of consent is 16 years. This now applies whether it is opposite- or same-sex sexual interaction. Thus any sexual activity involving consenting children under 16 is unlawful. This includes (i) sexual activity with a child, (ii) causing or inciting a child to engage in sexual activity, (iii) engaging in sexual activity in the presence of a child and (iv) causing a child to watch a sexual act, when the purpose of the offender is to obtain sexual gratification. In each of these, an additional condition is that there is no 'reasonable' belief that the child is 16 years or older.

It is an offence if a person under 18 does anything which would be an offence against children defined above, although the severity of the penalty is likely to be less than with an offender over 18.

When children who engage in sexual activity with each other are of the same or similar age, and where the activity is truly consensual and there are no aggravating features, such as coercion or corruption, it is unusual to prosecute. Instead, emphasis is on providing education for the children and young people and providing them and their families with access to advisory and counselling services.

3. *Other related offences against children under 16.*

Arranging and facilitating a child sex offence. This is aimed to prevent people from making it possible for a child under 16 to be sexually abused and is of particular relevance to 'sex tourism' and other forms of sexual exploitation of children considered on p. 473.

Meeting a child following sexual grooming. This category is intended to protect children from adults who communicate (not restricted to online communications) with them and then arrange to meet them with the intention of committing a sexual offence against them, either at that meeting or subsequently. The offence is committed when the offender meets the child or travels with the intention of meeting the child.

4. *Offences against children under 18.* This category is primarily concerned with a 16–18-year-old child giving ostensible consent to sexual activity with an adult who is in a position of trust or authority with the young person in a *community* setting (e.g. an educational establishment or residential setting) or *familial* setting (i.e. living within the same household as a child and assuming a position of trust or authority over that child, as well as relationships defined by blood ties, adoption, fostering, marriage or living together as partners). (Incestuous relationships between adult blood relatives are not included in this category.) Offences include sexual activity with the child and inciting the child to engage in sexual activity.

In determining the seriousness of the offences the following factors may be taken into consideration: the nature of the sexual activity, the age and degree of vulnerability of the victim, the age gap between the victim and the offender, and the breach of trust arising from the community or family relationship.

Abuse of children through prostitution or pornography

The law relating to child prostitution and pornography now includes children aged from 16 to 18.

The related offences include paying for sexual services of a child, causing or inciting child prostitution or pornography, controlling a child prostitute or a child involved in pornography and arranging or facilitating child prostitution or pornography. Consent is not relevant. A person is involved in pornography if an image of the child is recorded.

Sexual offences against persons with a mental disorder

This legislation focuses on the impact of the mental disorder on an individual's ability to give appropriate consent. A distinction is made between (i) those whose mental disorder is sufficiently severe that they are 'unable to refuse', (ii) those who have the capacity to consent to sexual activity but whose mental disorder makes them vulnerable to inducement, threat or deception and (iii) those who have the capacity to consent to sexual activity but whose mental disorder puts them in a position of dependency on the person who sexually interacts with them. Individuals with learning disabilities are included within this category of mental disorder, which is defined in Section 1 of the Mental Health Act 1983.

Incest

In English law until recently, a man committed incest if he had or attempted to have sexual intercourse (i.e. vaginal intercourse) with a female he knew to be his daughter, sister, half-sister, granddaughter or mother. If the female involved was over 16, she also committed an offence (Freeman 1979).

In Scotland, the law against incest dates from 1567 and the offence was punishable by death until 1887. In England and Wales, incest (between parent and child, brother and sister) has only been a criminal offence since 1908. In the past it was punished by the ecclesiastical courts. From the early or mid-19th century until the 1908 Act, it was probably dealt with as rape or unlawful sexual intercourse. Some legal systems today, such as the French, Dutch and Belgian, do not have a specific crime of incest (Freeman 1979).

In the 1970s, in the UK, The National Council for Civil Liberties (NCCL 1976), in their evidence to the Criminal Law Revision Committee (CLRC), recommended that the crime of incest should be abolished. They believed the law as it governed assault and intercourse with minors would provide adequate protection, as is the case in some other countries in Europe. The British Medical Association and Royal College of Psychiatrists, on the other hand, advised maintaining the legal status quo on the grounds of greater genetic risks associated with incest (CLRC 1980). The CLRC discussed the various arguments in their report but found themselves divided, principally on whether to recommend a minimum age of say 18 or even 21, above which incest would not be a criminal offence (CLRC 1980). However, in the Sexual Offences Act 2003, the crime of incest was replaced with a new offence of *familial* sexual abuse, to cover not just assaults by blood relatives, but also by foster and adoptive parents and live-in partners (PCS 2006). This would protect those aged 18 and younger.

The comprehensive revision of the law relating to sexual offences in the 2003 Act included reducing the age of consent for sex between males to 16, making it the same as for heterosexual sex. There is a new offence of voyeurism, which protects against the installation of cameras in public changing areas, and being spied on inside a building that had an expectation of privacy. However, there remain a number of inconsistencies or anomalies in the law. For example, the acts of gross indecency, buggery and soliciting by men (i.e. 'cottaging' or 'cruising'), and group sex involving men are no longer listed as illegal. However, it remains illegal for two men to engage in sex in a public toilet. Prostitution per se is not illegal, but many of the activities associated with it, e.g. importuning, organizing, as in a brothel, and living off the proceeds, remain illegal.

What is the true incidence of sexual offences?

The UK

The use of national crime statistics, in the UK or elsewhere, to assess the incidence of sexual offences, and how it changes over time, is fraught with difficulty for three principal reasons. First is the long-standing reluctance for victims of sexual crimes to report them. The reasons for this, in the case of rape, were discussed above. In the case of sexual offences against children, the legal process is very demanding, and the impact on the child of such processes has not been well studied but is unlikely to be trivial, hence a reluctance of many parents to report an act of child sexual abuse (CSA). Sexual abuse within the family is likely to have major effects on the family structure, often breaking up the family, so that many cases are kept hidden. However, such unreported incidents of sexual offence may well be reported in subsequent surveys. A second reason is that various factors influence whether an offence reported to the police is included in the official crime statistics. 'No-criming' of incidents by the police has already been mentioned, and local police forces vary in how they deal with such issues (Grubin 1998). Third, definitions of sexual offence have changed, particularly with the inclusion of 'indecent exposure' as a sexual offence. There is an added problem with offences against children in that the official statistics do not state the age of the victim, so that the crucial distinction between abuse of children under 10 and those over 14 is not possible. Throughout this chapter, and indeed throughout the literature on sexual offences, we are limited by uncertainties concerning incidence, although there are good reasons for believing that the official statistics, across the world, seriously underestimate the extent of sexual offences, more so than most other types of offence.

With these provisos, we will compare and contrast official crime statistics with figures from surveys of police records and community samples. This will be followed by a brief overview of evidence from the USA.

The following trends in sexual crime statistics in the UK can be noted. In 2004/2005, in England and Wales there were 60 946 recorded sexual offences overall, an increase of 17% from the previous year, and almost twice as many as in 1993, and 12 867 reported cases of 'rape of a female', an increase of 4% from the previous year, and an approximately 300% increase since 1993. For 'sexual assault on a female', there were 24 120 reported cases in 2004/2005, a 10% *decrease* from the previous year, and an approximately 140% increase from 1993. For 'other sexual offences', the numbers have remained relatively stable, around 9000, from 1993 to 2001/2002, when they started to rise, showing an 84% increase from 2003/2004 to 2004/2005 to a total of 23 959. This large increase in 1 year can be mainly accounted for by the inclusion of 'indecent exposure' as a sexual offence (Home Office 2006). This apparent increase in sexual assault of women contrasts with a tendency for less frequent convictions for sexual offences against children. Table 16.1 compares such convictions in 1985 and 1995, indicating a marked reduction in relation to the most common offences. According to Grubin (1998), this could be attributed to the fact that the age of child victims is now being recorded less often, resulting in the true figure being even more masked than previously. Alternative explanations are that such cases are increasingly dealt with in ways other than prosecution, or the criteria determining when to prosecute have hardened, or there is a real decrease in sex offending against children.

Figures for convictions and cautions in the courts can be compared to the numbers of notifications of offences to the police. Notifications of gross indecency with children 14 and under, of either sex, more than doubled from 633 to 1287 between 1985 and 1995, contrasting with an around 30% reduction in cautions or convictions for this offence. In a Home Office survey of the records of 28 police forces between 1990 and 1994 (Home Office 1997), 26% of all females recorded as alleged victims of rape were under the age of 16, and girls between the ages of 10 and 15 were at the highest risk of all females of being the reported victims of rape. Both females and males between the ages of 10 and 15 are at greatest risk of indecent assault, about two and a half times greater than the 16–24 age group (Grubin 1998).

TABLE 16.1	Number of convictions or cautions in England and Wales for the six most common sexual offences against children in 1985 and 1995 (from Grubin 1998)		
	1985	**1995**	**Percentage change**
Indecent assault on female <16	2416	2116	−12
Unlawful sexual intercourse with girl <16	1550	603	−61
Indecent assault on male <16	674	476	−29
Gross indecency* with girls <14	206	129	−37
Unlawful sexual intercourse with girl <13	168	122	−27
Gross indecency* with boy <14	122	84	−31
Total	5136	3530	−31

*Gross indecency relates to behaviour that is against public propriety but does not amount to an assault, e.g. a man getting a child to touch him sexually

TABLE 16.2   The percentage of women and men in the British Crime Survey 2001 (Walby & Allen 2004) who reported being victims of sexual assault or abuse

	Women (n = 13 551)			Men (n = 11 375)		
	Ever	Since age 16	Past 12 months	Ever	Since age 16	Past 12 months
ANY SEXUAL ASSAULT (INCLUDING ATTEMPTS)	24.1	16.6	2.1	4.7	2.1	0.2
Rape (2001 definition)	4.4	3.1	0.2	0.7	0.2	0
Penetration (not rape)	2.2	1.2	0.2	0.3	0.1	0
LESS SERIOUS SEXUAL ASSAULT	22.3	15.3	1.9	3.9	1.8	0.2
Indecent exposure	12.8	8.0	0.5	1.2	0.5	0.1
Touching	10.7	7.0	1.1	2.3	1.1	0.1
Threatening*	4.9	3.8	0.6	0.8	0.4	<0.1

*In most cases this is not legally categorized as a crime

These figures of sexual crimes reported to the police can then be compared with the results from British Crime Surveys (BCS). The most recent BCS was carried out in 2001 (Walby & Allen 2004). With a response rate of 66%, a representative sample of 11 375 men and 13 551 women, aged 16–59, living in households, completed a computer-based questionnaire about domestic violence, sexual assault and stalking. Experience of being sexually assaulted, at least once, was assessed for lifetime, at any time since age 16, and during the past year. The percentages of women and men with such experiences are shown in Table 16.2. We can deduce from these figures that 7.5% of women and 2.6% of men experienced some form of sexual assault before the age of 16. However, these surveys do not focus on CSA per se. Comparison with earlier BCS surveys suggests that, if anything, the percentage of women who say they have been raped (based on the 1994 definition of rape) since the age of 16 has declined (6.3% in 1994, 4.9% in 2000 and 3.6% in 2001). There are methodological differences between these earlier BCS surveys and the recent 2001 survey, but these findings certainly do not suggest an increase in rape and sexual assault, as is suggested by the reported crime statistics. This is consistent with there being an increase in the proportion of sexual assaults reported to the police.

The only British study to assess the national prevalence of CSA in the general population was carried out by Market Opinion and Research International (MORI; Baker & Duncan 1985), involving a probability sample of 2019 individuals. Twelve per cent of women and 8% of men reported that they had been sexually abused before the age of 16. In two-thirds, only one incident was involved, and in about half of the incidents no physical contact occurred (mainly indecent exposure by a stranger). The age when this happened was significantly younger in females (10.7 years vs. 12 years for males). In about half the cases, the abuser was known to the victim, and in 14% this was an incestuous relationship.

The true incidence of CSA in the UK remains uncertain from these variable findings. It is the police reports that show the highest rates, and Grubin (1998) has recommended that these be studied in more detail on a nationwide basis. It is reasonable to conclude, however, that it is more common than indicated by the official crime statistics, though not showing any obvious signs of increasing.

The number of offenders convicted of incest in England and Wales was reported for the years 1990–2000 (Criminal Statistics 2001) and showed a decline. For 1990, there were 181 convictions, in 1993 there were 127, in 1996 there were 62, in 1999 there were 42 and in 2000 there were 50. A more detailed analysis of incest offending was reported by Walmsley & White (1979) for the year 1973. (A more recent analysis for the UK has not been found.) There were 129 convictions for incest in 1973; the majority (65%) involved girls aged 10–15. The type of relationship is shown in Table 16.3. Almost half of the liaisons involving paternal incest listed in this table lasted for a year and only a quarter consisted of isolated incidents. By contrast, the majority of the sibling cases were isolated incidents. It is not clear why the number of convictions fell between 1990 and 2000, but we should now expect the reported figures to reflect the recent recategorization of incest to 'familial abuse'.

Indecent exposure

The number of convictions for indecent exposure in England and Wales declined from 1990 to 2000 (Criminal Statistics 2001). In 1990 the number was 1294, in 1993 it was 1014, in 1996 it was 740, in 1999 it was 649 and in 2000 it was 553. Earlier, Rooth (1972) had examined the conviction rates from 1948 to 1970. These had shown an increase over that time period. Between 1948 and 1957 the average annual rate was 2198; in 1970 it was 2839. Although the large majority of offenders were over 21 years, he found a proportionately greater increase among young teenagers (14–17 years) with an approximate doubling of their number, which Rooth linked to a general increase in juvenile delinquency over that period.

TABLE 16.3   Type of relationship in incest cases for 1973 (Walmsley & White 1979)

	Percentage of total convicted	Person convicted
Grandpaternal	1	1 grandfather
Paternal	72	91 fathers, 2 daughters
Sibling	24	30 brothers, 1 sister
Maternal	3	2 sons, 2 mothers
Total		124 males, 5 females

The above figures indicate convictions for this offence in 2000 were around 20% of what they had been in 1970. Little attention has been paid to this decline, and the reasons for it are not yet apparent. However, Maletzky (1991) reported a decline in the proportion of offenders attending his treatment clinic who were exhibitionists. Between 1973 and 1978, 57% of his clinic attenders were exhibitionists; from 1978 to 1990 this reduced to 15%. It could reflect a change in how seriously this offence is regarded, leading to a reduction in the proportion of reported cases that are convicted, or referred for treatment, or a reduction in the number of incidents that are reported. Alternatively it could mean a reduction in the behaviour itself.

Voyeurism

Until 2003, voyeurism did not have a separate offence category, coming under the heading of 'breach of the peace' or, if a number of victims were involved, 'being a public nuisance'. Hence, the statistics of this type of offence were difficult to come by. Now that voyeurism has been established as a separate category it will become possible to assess its prevalence.

How does the USA compare?

A substantial proportion of sex offenders in the USA are adolescents. Davis & Leitenberg (1987) estimated that 30–50% of sex offences against children in the 1980s were committed by adolescents. In the 1990s, about 15% of males charged with rape were under 18 years of age (Ryan et al 1996).

Kilpatrick et al (1985), in a survey of women in South Carolina, found 15% who reported one or more attempted or complete sexual assaults; a third of these women described the assault as rape, and close to a third as attempted rape. Russell (1984), in a sample of 930 married women in San Francisco, found 24% who reported one or more incidents of forced sexual intercourse. Laumann et al's (1994) National Health and Social Life Survey (NHSLS) involved a representative sample of 1748 women, who were asked 'After puberty, did a male force you to do anything sexually that you didn't want to do?' Twenty-two per cent of the women answered yes; of these, 9% indicated that the man forcing them was their husband, 46% indicated it was someone they were in love with, 22% said it was someone they knew well and only 4% said it was a stranger.

Substantial changes in the laws relating to rape and sexual assault, similar in their intentions to those described above for the UK, took place in the USA earlier than in the UK, though implemented at a state level, and varying in detail from state to state. Prior to these changes, non-reporting of rape was a major factor, making assessment of its frequency difficult. Some attention has been paid to the impact that these changes have had on the reporting of rape. The National Crime Victimization Survey (NCVS) is the US equivalent of the BCS. This annual survey has shown a substantial reduction in crimes of violence, including rape and sexual assault between 1973 and 2005, the most notable and consistent decline being since 1994 (Catalano 2006). However, the form of questioning used by the NCVS, with its focus on acts regarded by the woman as criminal, has been criticized for resulting in seriously underestimating the prevalence of rape and sexual assault. Clay-Warner & Burt (2005) used the National Violence against Women Survey, which they considered less problematic in this respect than the NCVS, to assess the extent to which reporting of rape and sexual assault to the police had increased since the changes in the law. They found that rapes committed after 1990 were more likely to be reported than those occurring before 1974. However, reporting continues to be more likely in cases of 'aggravated rape' (i.e. involving a stranger, more than one rapist or the use of weapons), than with 'simple rape' (which applies to the majority). Hence, they concluded that changes in the laws had only been partially successful.

In the Kinsey survey, 24% of women reported prepubertal sexual experience with post-pubertal males (systematic questions were not asked of their male subjects; Gebhard & Johnson 1979). In a study of parents, asked by questionnaire about their own childhood, 15% of women and 6% of men reported sexual abuse during their childhood (Finkelhor 1984). In Russell's (1983) San Francisco study of women, using a broad definition of sexual abuse (i.e. including non-contact abuse such as genital exposure and verbal solicitation), 48% had had such experiences by the age of 14 and 54% by 18. For contact abuse, 12% had experienced at least one such experience involving a family member before the age of 14, and 16% before the age of 18. The percentages for extra-familial abuse were 20% and 31%, respectively. Thus, combining intra- and extra-familial situations, 28% before the age of 14 and 38% before the age of 18 were affected. However, it is striking that only 2% of intra-familial and 6% of extra-familial incidents were reported to the police. In a further California study of women, Wyatt (1985) found 62% recalling some form of abuse before the age of 18, with 47% experiencing contact abuse.

Feldman et al (1991) compared rates in a number of North American studies published in the 1980s with those reported in the major study of sexual behaviour in the USA carried out by Kinsey and colleagues (Kinsey et al 1948, 1953). They found that in spite of increased rates of reporting, overall prevalence rates of CSA appeared to be similar in the 1980s to those described by Kinsey 30–40 years earlier.

In the NHSLS (Laumann et al 1994), about 17% of the women and 12% of the men reported that they had been sexually touched when they were younger than 14. This incidence did not vary across the age groups, suggesting that there had not been any marked variation over time. The girls were mainly touched by men, most of whom were aged over 18; the boys were most often touched by teenage girls, but also by males.

There is some information on incest from studies in the USA, though not recent. In Finkelhor's study (1980), whereas 75% of incidents involved an older person known to the child, in 6% it was the father or stepfather. Some 15% of females and 10% of males reported some type of sexual experience involving a sibling, most commonly genital touching and fondling. In Russell's (1983) study, 44 (4.7%) of 930 women had had an incestuous relationship with their fathers. For 27 it was the biological father, for 15 the stepfather, 1 the foster father and 1 the adoptive father. A total of 46 had sexual involvement with an uncle, 19 with a brother, 8 with a grandfather, 3 with a sister and 1 woman with her mother. In terms of the seriousness of the abuse, the stepfathers were the worst offenders.

Finkelhor (1980) estimated that some form of father–daughter sexual interaction might occur in about 1.5% of families, though coitus would seldom be involved. (It is important to distinguish between the legal definition of incest given above and the psychosocial meaning which emphasizes the relationship rather than the precise sexual act involved.)

Methodological issues in recalling earlier experiences of sexual assault or abuse

A variety of factors might contribute to the varying prevalence rates in the earlier studies. Thus higher figures would result from taking an upper age of 18 (as in Russell & Wyatt's studies, compared with 17 in Finkelhor's studies) and by the inclusion of abuse by peers, though such cases were only included if the experience was unwanted. Graham (2003) reviewed methodological issues related to adult recall of childhood sexual abuse, pointing out much uncertainty about reasons for poor recall. Some argue that experiences are more easily forgotten if they had little impact initially; others argue that forgetting is actually repression, which is more likely with traumatic experiences. Both explanations may be relevant. Finkelhor (2003b), who has probably done the most research in this area, has become discouraged about retrospective recall methodology in this area and no longer uses it.

The socio-cultural context of sexual offending

Most of the literature of sexual offending has focused on the individual offender and reasons why that particular individual might be prone to such behaviour. Much less attention has been paid to socio-cultural factors that might increase or decrease the likelihood of such behaviour, or whether such behaviour is reported. Let us consider such factors in relation to the two main categories of sexual offence: rape and sexual assault, and sexual abuse of children.

Rape and sexual assault

The large majority of rapes and sexual assaults are perpetrated by men on women. To what extent does the prevailing cultural 'norm' of male–female interactions influence this? And what can we learn by looking at sexual aggression and how it relates to male dominance in primitive societies? Both Broude & Greene (1980) and Sanday (1981) examined the evidence from the Human Relations Area Files, initiated by Murdock (1967) and others, which archived anthropological data from a large number of societies. In Broude & Greene's analysis of evidence from 65 pre-industrial societies, they found 41% in which rape was common and 24% in which it was virtually absent. Sanday analysed evidence from 156 societies and concluded that 47% were rape-free and 18% rape-prone. A rape-prone culture characteristically promoted male–female antagonism, whereas rape-free societies showed sexual equality, women were highly valued and, perhaps of greater relevance, there were generally low levels of interpersonal violence. Grubin (1992), in reviewing these studies, considered it reasonable to conclude that in male dominated and aggressive primitive societies rape is more common.

We are, if anything, less well placed when trying to make cross-cultural comparison of modern societies. Once again we are faced with differences in legal definitions. Baron et al (1988), however, in what can be considered a comparison of local cultures in the multicultured USA, assessed the 50 states for their reported frequency of rape. An index of the acceptance of violence (e.g. corporal punishment, hunting animals and viewing of violent television programmes) was significantly related to the frequency of rape, but the strongest predictor of rape was the proportion of divorced men in the state. Although Baron et al (1988) argued that the level of divorce is related to the extent to which the culture supports violence, this association between divorce and rape has not yet been convincingly explained (Grubin 1992).

Russell (1982) described the USA as a 'rape-supportive culture'. Burt (1980) found that more than a half of an American sample agreed with the statement 'a woman who goes to the home or apartment of a man on the first date implies she is willing to have sex'. Howells et al (1984) found that British men who held stereotyped views about women's roles were more likely to blame the victim for the assault. It is not clear to what extent these cultural patterns have changed in the past 25 years.

There are many men with aggressive and criminal tendencies; only a proportion of them rape. There are many men with doubts about their masculinity; very few of them rape. It is difficult, as we shall see in the next section, to identify a meaningful stereotype of the typical rapist. An alternative view is to see most men as potential rapists, or the rapist as a relatively normal male who, as a result of socially learned attitudes to women, is likely to rape in certain circumstances. Some feminist writers have taken this view. Brownmiller (1975) presented an appalling catalogue of rape carried out in war conditions by men, most of whom presumably would not rape in normal circumstances. Probably no particular nationality is free from blame in this respect, though some may be more culpable than others. The most ghastly example in the second half of the 20th century was the mass rape of Bengali women during the

Bangladesh war of independence. Accounts of rape by both American and South Vietnamese soldiers during the Vietnam war also make gruesome reading. The dehumanizing effect of war obviously plays an important part and Brownmiller gave a convincing account of how much of this rape is an extension of the violence of war in which women become the particular victims. It may be those soldiers who have the least reason to feel proud as a result of the more conventional violence who assert their masculinity in this way (Brownmiller 1975). Horrific accounts continue into the 21st century, the most recent being from Darfur. This not only highlights the upsurge of rape during war conditions, which is not confined to rape by enemy soldiers, but a seemingly general increase of rape by those who should be protecting the women and children, including policemen (Nieuwoudt 2006). One of the most horrendous aspects of the mass rape of Bengali women was the stigmatization they suffered, not so much from society at large as from their husbands, who were likely to disown them. By tradition, no Muslim husband takes back a wife who has been touched by another man, even if she is subdued by force. The Bangladesh government attempted to counter this trend by declaring that the rape victims were 'national heroines', but with little effect (Brownmiller 1975). Such reactions are less likely in Christian countries but do occur (Katz & Mazur 1979). On the other hand, less extreme attitudes that view the raped woman as 'defiled' or spoiled in some way are probably widespread in most modern cultures and play a significant part in the traumatic consequences of rape (see p. 489).

Muehlenhard et al (1992) looked at the cultural context from a different perspective; the accounts of the scientific and academic community. For the period from 1927 to 1972 they could find only 17 scientific articles on rape. From 1973 there was a steady increase each year, peaking at 102 during 1988. Between 1973 and 1991 they found 858 articles on rape, attributing this change to the second wave of the feminist movement. This underlines the importance of the political climate to the attention paid to sexual assault and rape.

Muehlenhard and her colleagues (1992) considered different theoretical approaches to the explanation of rape. Most of the earlier literature in the time period they examined was psychoanalytic, revealing a tendency to attribute rape, in one way or another, to the woman's behaviour. But the literature, in a more general sense, points to periodic shifts of socio-cultural emphasis in relation to sex which, in the case of rape, resulted in long periods when it was relatively ignored or attributed, to a disturbing extent, to false accusations by women, or to their provocatively seductive behaviour. There has been less attention to rape in the psychoanalytic literature since the early 1970s, but those articles that have appeared tend to focus on women's masochism and desire to be raped.

Muehlenhard et al (1992) went on to consider psychopathological theories of rape and sexual assault. Here the emphasis is on identifying psychopathological mechanisms in the individual offender, which could explain the offender's rape behaviour. This approach continues to dominate the literature on sexual offending and is considered quite extensively in this chapter. The problem here, for Muehlenhard and her colleagues, is the tendency to ignore the possible impact of the prevailing culture as it relates to male–female relationships and sex. They drew attention to the fact that in the USA, at least until recently, marital rape is a lesser crime than stranger rape, or is only criminal in certain circumstances. And they cited a particularly forceful example of how prejudicial attitudes and values have impacted socio-cultural reactions to rape: the rape of white women by black men has been treated more seriously than rape of black women or rape by white men. In any case, focusing on the individual, and looking for ways to stop that individual from re-offending, diverts attention from considering ways in which socio-cultural factors could be changed to make rape less likely in the first place. I will return to this point in the conclusions to this chapter.

Muehlenhard et al (1992) then considered evolutionary theories. Here they pointed out the various arguments that men, for evolutionary reasons, are designed to mate with as many women as possible, to enhance their likelihood of having offspring, whereas women are designed to select mates who either show signs of 'evolutionary strength' or offer the chance of support for child rearing. Apart from an apparent lack of any evidence that men who rape father more children, and there are a range of reasons why such theorizing should be questioned on scientific grounds (see Chapter 2), their concern was that 'biological determinism' of this kind fosters acceptance of the status quo and impedes attempts to bring about relevant socio-cultural change that would make rape and sexual assault less likely.

Feminist theories, on the other hand, have focused on how societal change might reduce the likelihood of rape. Muehlenhard et al (1992) discussed two themes in the feminist literature: the function of rape in perpetuating male dominance and the issue of whether rape should be regarded as sexual or violent behaviour. Relevant to male dominance are traditional gender role socialization, adult gender roles and rape myths: ' . . . girls are taught to be passive and submissive; boys are taught to be active and aggressive. Girls are taught to be uninterested in sex, even when they desire it, so as not to appear "easy"; boys are taught that girls will refuse even when they want to have sex, and thus they are justified in disregarding girls' refusals, especially if a girl's dress or demeanour suggests to them that she desires sex. Both boys and girls are taught that rape is justified under certain circumstances — that women are "asking for it" if they engage in certain "unladylike" behaviors' (p. 235). The more liberal feminists, they suggest, consider that what is needed is for these 'lessons' to cease, and different ones to be taught. More radical feminists, on the other hand, see these lessons as part of a more general pattern of male dominance, 'keeping women in their place', which men are not likely to let go, and which therefore requires a more fundamental reorganization of society.

The controversy about whether rape should be seen as sex or violence raises some interesting issues, addressed by Muehlenhard et al (1992). On the one hand, the focus on rape as an act of violence was regarded as important in order to shift emphasis from rape as a sexual act. In doing so, rape is more likely to be seen as terrifying and humiliating rather than sexually arousing for the victim. It is less likely to be trivialized, especially when perpetrated by someone known to the victim. The victim is less likely to be blamed because of her provocative clothing or flirtatious behaviour. Also, by focusing on the violence rather than the sex, feminists could be anti-rape without being anti-sex, which they are sometimes accused of being. There are also disadvantages, however. If rape is seen as a form of violence rather than sexually driven, it is less likely to be prosecuted if it involves coercion but not violence, which is the case in the majority of rapes. Muehlenhard and her colleagues concluded this discussion by suggesting that the crucial issue should not be one of sex versus violence, but of control, and that women should be free to control their own sexuality, a conclusion with which I wholeheartedly agree. However, both the sexuality and the violence or force involved in rape are relevant to understanding this behaviour. The extent to which sexuality and aggression can become linked so that in some individuals being coercive or forceful, or even violent, may augment the sexually arousing nature of the experience is considered later (p. 480). But it is important to recognize that this pattern is more likely to become established and acted on in a society which promotes male dominance and the sexual possession of women by men.

Given that a substantial proportion of sexual assault occurs in established sexual relationships, it is also important to consider carefully the role of other forms of violence in such relationships. Buntin et al (2004) report on intimate partner violence and forced sexual activity in intimate relationships from the Chicago Health & Life Survey. They found that 29% of women and 22% of men in the Cook County sample (which includes Chicago) reported at least one incident of moderate or severe violence in their intimate relationship in the previous year. This did not mean, however, that the violence was perpetrated only by the male partners; 7% of the women said that it was only their partner who was violent, whereas 11% said that it was they themselves who were the only ones violent; the remainder reported both partners being violent. Participants in this study were also asked whether they had been forced to do something sexual since the age of 13 years. Fourteen per cent of the women and 2% of the men answered yes; 4% of the women indicated this had happened at least twice. Reporting on this incident or the most recent, if there had been more than one, 35% said it was with their intimate partner, 32% with an acquaintance or friend and only 10% with a stranger. Unfortunately, we are not told to what extent there is overlap between forced sex and non-sexual violence in this sample. It is conceivable that some men, provoked in some way in their primary relationship, may find it easier to express anger by forcing their partner to have sex, rather than assaulting her non-sexually. A woman, on the other hand, does not have the option of forcing sex on her partner when angry with him, or at least, only to a limited extent.

Sexual exploitation and abuse of children

From historical records there are indications that sexual activity with young boys was widespread in ancient Greece and accepted in various parts of the world during the 18th century (Grubin 1992). Ford & Beach (1952) gave examples from pre-industrial societies in North Africa and Central Australia. Sexual activity with young girls in ancient Rome is also well documented. Roman law required that girls should be no younger than 12 and boys 14 before they could marry. Apparently marriages were not infrequently arranged with girls younger than 12, with the rule that sexual activity would not begin before that age. But the rule was sometimes broken and, if made public, the penalties were severe (Lascaratos & Poulakou-Rebelakou 2000). Ritualized sexual activity with children, either boys or girls, has featured in some early societies, and examples from Melanesian societies were discussed in Chapter 5.

The only cross-cultural study of CSA in modern societies was reported by Finkelhor (1994), who reviewed incidence rates from studies in 21 countries. Seven of these were English-speaking (the USA, Canada, the UK, Ireland, Australia, New Zealand and South Africa), twelve were European and two were South American (Costa Rica and Dominican Republic). Rates of CSA varied from 7% to 36% for women and from 3% to 16% for men. The proportion of such cases which were intra-family also varied substantially: for women, ranging from 14% in the UK to 36% in Switzerland; for men, from 0% in Switzerland to 25% in Denmark. This marked variability probably reflects the methodological complexities, which we have already considered, making interpretation of differences in cultural terms inappropriate. The issue of how childhood is defined socioculturally is crucial, and this will be considered more closely below. Nevertheless, Finkelhor (1994) concluded that this evidence confirmed that CSA was an international problem.

Sexual exploitation of children across the world has been well reviewed by Levesque (1999), who regards much of this global pattern as driven by commercial interests. Hence it is not only the adults who buy the child's sexual participation who are a cause for concern, but also the adults, often families, who knowingly benefit from the commercial aspect. Needless to say, this commercialization, to a large extent, involves children who live in poverty, or who are 'street children', and their exploitation is by adults who are by comparison wealthy. This is mainly manifested in the form of 'sex tourism', reminding us that there are various intermediaries, apart from the child's family, who benefit financially.

As with most aspects of sexual offence behaviour, it is difficult to be confident about the prevalence of child prostitution. The United Nations, in its 1993 report on contemporary forms of slavery, estimated that, for example, more than 800 000 children in Thailand, 400 000 in India and 250 000 in Brazil are involved in prostitution. UNICEF estimated 20 000 child prostitutes in the Philippines, two-thirds of whom are street children. This is not just a Third World phenomenon: Jenkins (2003) suggests that socio-cultural conditions highly likely to facilitate sexual exploitation of children prevailed in urban areas of the USA between about 1880 and 1930; 'both social investigators and moral crusaders cited sexual abuse as one of the principal evils arising from catastrophic poverty' (p. 9). But the problem has not gone away in the USA; recent government figures estimated that around 600 000 girls and 300 000 boys were involved in prostitution (Flowers 1994). We have less certain evidence about this problem in the UK. A National Commission of Inquiry estimated that there were more than 5000 children under 16 involved in prostitution, but this could have been a serious underestimate (Childhood Matters 1996). Today, worldwide, several million children are exploited in a $10-billion-a-year, global child sex market (Levesque 1999).

Apart from the impact of poverty, there are some cultural factors that may influence this. Levesque (1999) gives the example of an ancient religious practice in certain parts of India which, in spite of being outlawed, continues to some extent, with tens of thousands of girls pledging themselves to the goddess Renuka at puberty and then, with the full knowledge of their parents, being shunted off to brothels. Levesque (1999) also considers closely cultural practices such as child marriages and genital circumcision, which do not break the law in the societies involved, but which certainly override the rights of the child. World Health Organization estimates suggest that more than 130 million women in the world have been subjected to some form of 'circumcision', which varies in precise detail according to the culture. In so far as these practices are justified by the culture, it is usually on the grounds of protecting and ensuring the recognition of the girl's virginity in preparation for marriage. Although the procedures vary in extent, they are all likely to impair the girl's and subsequently the woman's capacity for genital pleasure. In addition to reinforcing the property status of women in such cultures, it is also possible that they have become entrenched because they are seen as methods to contain women's sexuality, consistent with the idea that sexual pleasure is the man's prerogative, and that 'sexually driven' women are a threat to patriarchal societies. Presumably motivated by concerns about such practices, the United Nations added to the International Bill of Rights, in 1989, the Convention on the Rights of the Child. This 'Children's Convention', which asserts that all children have the right to participate in decisions affecting them, has been almost universally ratified, with one interesting exception being the USA. The principle that the child's individual rights can over-ride the rights of the child's family, although motivated by the extent that families can exploit their children, has certainly been controversial (Levesque 1999).

The concept of childhood

It is, however, important, both when making cross-cultural comparisons and when striving to understand child sexual exploitation and abuse, to consider how 'childhood' is defined. As Levesque (1999) points out, there are important cultural differences in this respect, with age not always being the marker of transition for child to adult. And the concept of 'adolescence' may be meaningless outside Western societies (Dowsett 2000), although I would argue that, in terms of emerging hormonal and brain mechanisms, the concept of adolescence is crucial to understanding sexual development and how the individual reacts to the cultural norms in any culture (see Chapter 5). In this present context we are focusing on sexual behaviour that breaks the law. The law in the UK and the USA, for example, imposes arbitrary 'cut offs' between a child and a non-child in the legal sense, which are mainly based on age. Thus a girl over 16 can consent to sexual intercourse; a girl under 16, in the eyes of the law, cannot. There is also the issue of the sexual attractiveness of a 'child'. Whereas there is general agreement that a child should be protected from sexual exploitation by adults and that it is a matter of responsibility for an adult not to sexually exploit children, there is an important distinction to be made between 'children' who are sexually appealing to a 'normal' adult because they have many of the physical characteristics of a sexually attractive adult, and those who are not 'because they are children'. A key variable, in terms of the sexual appeal of a 'child' is whether and to what stage that child has progressed through puberty. Here we are faced with something of a paradox. The age at puberty has fallen, particularly for girls, over the past century in most parts of the world, yet in the Western industrialized societies, the age of consent, in legal terms, has increased, confronting us with the contrast between definitions of childhood based on age, and those found in many less industrialized societies, which are still based on pubertal stage. Whereas the moral values that most modern societies purport to maintain would emphasize the importance of protecting the young adolescent from exploitation by older people, the signals that contribute to a mature adult, particularly a male, being sexually attracted and becoming sexually aroused, may be very evident in such a young female (or male) adolescent. This then takes us to how the 'mature adult' fits those sexual attributes into the concept of an 'appropriate sexual partner', and what other factors should be taken into account. If that does not limit the adult's attraction, then the crucial issue is the adult's ability to behave in a responsible manner, which will, to some extent, be influenced by cultural norms.

When we consider sexual involvement with a prepubertal child, then we are probably dealing with a fundamentally different set of sexual signals. Sexual exploitation or abuse of such a child then more appropriately raises the issue of 'deviant' sexual preference, and why that arises. This issue is considered more closely below.

The cycle of concern about child sexual abuse

Although we remain uncertain about the true prevalence of CSA, the evidence points to it being a long-standing issue, with no clear indication that it has increased or reduced over time. Public reactions to CSA, on the other hand, have changed dramatically, at least since the latter part of the 19th century. In the section on rape and sexual assault we considered how social attitudes to rape had seemingly changed over time, with the most notable change brought about by the vigorous political campaigning of the second feminist movement. With CSA we have another pattern of change.

Freud started off attributing much of neurosis to sexual trauma during childhood. Then, around the end of the 19th century, he changed his opinion; the 'sexual trauma' was in fact a wish-fulfilling fantasy. Since then, at least for many years, anyone revealing CSA within the family to a psychoanalyst was likely to be told that it was, in fact, a fantasy. This would certainly have contributed to the widespread reluctance to reveal such experiences. Masson (1984) links this radical change in psychoanalytic thinking to a wider reaction within Europe in the late 19th century. Public opinion at that time, particularly in France, was confronted by increasing evidence of sexual abuse of children, much of it from the mortuary. Then, in some mysterious way, the problem seemed to disappear. This pattern of high concern followed by a period of relative lack of concern has been documented as a repeated cycle through the 20th century by Jenkins (1998, 2003). Peaks of concern about CSA, which Jenkins describes as 'moral panic', were apparent in 1915, 1950 and 1985 — what seemed like a 35-year pattern. In between the peaks concern would gradually go down to a 'trough', where very different reactions of both the scientific community and the public to such abuse would be evident. Jenkins (2003) exemplified this contrast with two episodes. In 1931, during a 'trough', an 11-year-old girl was brought before a juvenile court following repeated sexual intercourse with a 60-year-old man. The man was acquitted, and the girl was considered the offender because of her 'moral depravity'. Such 'trough' reactions tended to see the young person as inappropriately seductive, but in addition, there was less concern about the long-term effects of such interactions. Contrasting with this was Jenkin's example of 'moral panic', a widespread reaction of outrage to a scientific paper. In 1998, Rind et al published, in *Psychological Bulletin*, a highly reputable journal, a meta-analysis of 59 studies of college students in which sexual abuse experiences during childhood were related to subsequent adjustment. The authors concluded that, when other factors during childhood (e.g. negative family environment) were controlled for, the effect of childhood sexual abuse seemed to be small for the majority, especially boys. This paper was condemned as an endorsement of paedophilia. A resolution condemning the paper was passed unanimously by the House of Representatives in Washington, DC (12 July 1999), a political act probably without precedent. Following that, a number of academics who either supported Rind and his colleagues against this attack or in some way questioned the assumption that victims of childhood sexual abuse are invariably seriously traumatized have been accused in public of being pro-paedophile.

The Rind et al's (1998) meta-analysis is not beyond criticism (for a critical appraisal and further discussion, see Hyde 2003 and p. 495), but it was a serious scientific study. It is doubtful that many, if any, of the representatives who voted to condemn this scientific paper had actually read it. But it is also understandable that, in the current climate of opinion about CSA and childhood sexuality, no politician could afford to take the risk of voting against the resolution. The intense negative reaction to this meta-analysis paper tells us that, in the public mind, CSA is bad, regardless of what form it takes. One might have expected reassurance that a child is not necessarily damaged by such experiences, which should come as a big relief to many parents of sexually abused children.

Both of these examples of the cyclical pattern are disturbing and, furthermore, Jenkins' 35-year cycle appears to have been de-railed. Since the peak in the mid-1980s there has been little sign of retreat from 'moral panic'. To what extent can we explain or understand these extreme positions? This is not an easy question to answer. One possible factor contributing to the 'moral panic' is the difficulty many people have in accepting that children can in any way be sexual. But it remains difficult to understand why there is this tendency to assume that the child has been permanently damaged, regardless of what actually happened. Perhaps there is need to see the child as permanently damaged, as more importance is attached to demonizing the child abuser than helping the child deal with the experience. This explanation certainly fits the extraordinary reaction to the Rind et al (1998) paper. The general concern about sexual offending, particularly against children, has led to changes in the law relating to sex offenders after release from prison. This has become known as 'Megan's law' as it followed the sexual murder of a 7-year-old girl named Megan. In effect, this law, which is now widespread in the USA, requires not only registration of sex offenders with local law enforcement agencies, but also notification of neighbours and community organizations such as schools, of the presence of an ex-offender in their neighbourhood. As Jenkins (1998) pointed out, there has been no other equivalent of this form of community control 'since the days when thieves, adulterers, and blasphemers were branded or otherwise mutilated in order that they be identifiable by their crimes' (p. 199). Sample & Bray (2006) reviewed the evidence of recidivism among sex offenders and pointed out that Megan's law was indiscriminately applied to sex offenders, regardless of the nature of their offence, or the likelihood of their re-offending. They pointed out that the negative consequences not only included a violation of human rights but also the risk of unnecessarily increasing the public's fear of the likelihood of sexual violence, and the inappropriate use of public funds to monitor sex offenders, the large majority of whom are not likely to re-offend. They advocated a modification of this law so that it is used selectively to monitor those with a likelihood of re-offending.

All of this indicates a social climate that makes genuine and unbiased research into the effects of childhood sexual abuse hazardous. It has also produced a situation where human rights have been undermined. The tendency has been to assume that anyone accused of sexual involvement with a child is guilty until proved innocent. There have been some extremely disturbing examples of miscarriage of justice resulting from this, well documented by Rabinowitz (2003). What is clearly needed is a relatively stable state of public opinion which comes some way in between the extremes of this cycle, which takes CSA seriously, aims to protect children from it, but without assuming that any child who is abused is seriously damaged thereafter. Only in this way can we expect to understand not only why such abuse occurs in the first place, but how best to deal with it when it does. (For further consideration of the political implications see Bancroft 2004.)

Pornography and the Internet

The implications of pornography for human sexuality and its problems are numerous and were considered more closely in Chapter 6. Here we will focus on pornography depicting children, which usually means depictions of children engaged in some form of sexual activity with or without an adult involved. Child pornography qualifies as an offence on several grounds: it involves participation of the child, legally unable to give consent, in the activities portrayed and captured by the photography, there is evidence that child pornography increases the likelihood of the viewer actually abusing a child (Marshall 1988), and it encourages abusers to see children as seductive and able to enjoy sexual stimulation. Although Kutchinsky (1985) reported that availability of child pornography in Denmark was associated with a reduction in the number of offences against children, subsequent studies, at least in North America, have failed to support that conclusion (Levesque 1999).

As with child prostitution, the production of child pornography reveals a global process on a huge scale, with the commercialized aspects being a multi-billion-dollar industry. The Department of Justice in the USA estimates the market to range between $2 and $3 billion a year and that pornographers have recorded the abuse of more than a million children in the USA alone. However, presumably because of the growing concern about this industry, there has been an increasing move towards using children from the developing world (Levesque 1999). The law against child pornography raises interesting issues. Making the use of adult pornography illegal has been resisted because to do so is invading an individual's privacy. But invading that privacy to prevent use of child pornography is considered differently. However, in most countries, the law focuses on the production and distribution of child pornography. In the USA, this varies from state to state, and around half the states have passed laws making it illegal to possess such pornography. US Federal law compromises and deems it illegal to have three or more copies of any item of child pornography.

A major challenge to the legal system is the availability of child pornography on the Internet. Although attempts have been made to place legal restrictions on this, they have so far proved unsuccessful (Levesque 1999) and illustrate the major problems for social control that the Internet is posing in several respects. The use of computerized imaging to create images of child pornography, which are not actual photographs, also presents a challenge. Whereas in most countries these are excluded from legal restriction, the law was changed in the UK in 1994 to include computer-generated pornography along with photographic pornography. This is a time of much uncertainty about how to deal with the impact of modern technology, especially the Internet, on sexuality (see p. 226 for further discussion).

Incest

The taboo against incest is so universal that it has generated a great deal of debate and speculation about its origins. The precise forms of kinships for which sexual activity is proscribed vary from culture to culture. The taboo against mother–son incest is more or less universal; with father–daughter and brother–sister relationships there are exceptions. The strength of the taboos and the sanctions associated with them also vary considerably across cultures (Fox 1967). In some instances royalty has been exempt to allow them to maintain the sanctity of royal blood; ancient Egypt and the Inca aristocracy are well-known examples from the past. Restrictions on sexual relationships beyond the nuclear family vary enormously, reflecting the extent to which rules of descent are matrilineal or patrilineal. It is important to distinguish between rules concerning incest and those governing marriage, or exogamy. If a relationship is deemed incestuous then it will not be considered marriageable. But a man, whilst not allowed to marry his grandmother, his father's, son's, grandfather's or grandson's wife, his wife's mother, daughter, grandmother or granddaughter, is not legally prohibited in our society from having sex with them (Honoré 1978).

The various theories that have been put forward to account for the incest taboo can be considered under two headings: social and biological. Levi-Strauss (1969) was one of the main proponents of social determination. He saw the incest taboo as an important step in the socialization of the human primate by which the male retains his 'own' (i.e. his daughters) as something to exchange with others, the primal basis of most social structure. As Fox (1980) pointed out, Levi-Strauss' explanation is better suited to explain exogamy than incest avoidance. A man could presumably have sex with his daughter and still be in a position to 'exchange' her in his dealings with others. Implicit in this kind of theory is the assumption that taboos are necessary to control a behaviour that would otherwise be likely to occur. This view was central to Freud's theory. But the contrasting and more biological explanation was that put forward by Westermark in his *Short History of Marriage* (Westermark 1926). He suggested that there was a marked lack of erotic feeling between people who lived closely together from childhood, leading to little or no inclination for incestuous behaviour. This view was attacked by Freud and Sir James Frazer in the 1920s and lost favour until two interesting sources of evidence emerged to support it: that children brought up together in Israeli kibbutzim are most unlikely to fall in love and marry one another (Shepher 1971) and the strange custom in Taiwan of marrying children to each other when they are as young as 3 years, a pattern associated with a high incidence of sexual difficulty and marital breakdown in adulthood (Wolf 1970). But why, it is often asked, is there a need for an incest taboo if there is no inclination to behave incestuously? As Westermark himself cogently argued in his rebuttal of Freud and Frazer's criticism, one does not only have laws forbidding behaviour that we are all inclined to commit. In other words there is no need for incest taboos for most of us but there is for some. And as we have seen earlier in this chapter, incestuous relationships are far from rare, particularly when young members of a family are involved. Fox (1980), in attempting to reconcile these two apparently conflicting theoretical models, pointed out how cultures vary considerably in the degree of propinquity that exists between opposite-sex siblings during childhood. He described some societies where the degree of segregation between brother and sister may actually mystify and hence enhance the erotic potential of the incestuous relationship — certainly very different to the typical kibbutzim experience of boys and girls. It should, however, be stressed, rather more than Fox did, that this argument relates to brother–sister, but rather less well to parent–child incest. It is not necessarily irrelevant, however. As we shall see, the likelihood of incest involving a stepfather is substantially greater than that involving a father, who will have lived in relatively close proximity with the child since the child's birth.

Perhaps the most important part of Fox's analysis was his consideration of the cross-species comparative evidence, particularly from primates. Levi-Strauss (1969) saw incest taboo, or more precisely exogamy, as one of the attributes that distinguish humans from other animals: 'The important point on which human marriage and animal mating differs is that man became the exogamous animal. The exogamic rule, that we should find mates outside one's own social unit, is at the basis of all human social organisation.' This assertion was obviously made in ignorance of animal behaviour. Bischof (1975) reviewed the comparative evidence of incest avoidance and found it to be widespread, though manifested in a variety of ways, and possibly serving a variety of purposes. In a more recent and extensive review, Bixler (1992) considered the variety of negative outcomes of inbreeding or incest, which sooner or later reduce reproductive success, what he called 'inbreeding depression'. He was able to find only a few species where there was no evidence of 'inbreeding depression', but these were very much the exceptions. He also found extensive evidence in other species of failure of individuals to find sexually attractive those whom they intimately associate with, while either or both are immature, what he described as 'one of the best established principles of sexual behaviour' (p. 315).

It therefore seems inescapable that across species there is a basic genetic disadvantage to inbreeding, which has resulted in 'incest avoidance' in almost all species studied, including humans. We can wonder how this 'incest avoidance' has become established, and it seems unlikely that humans (or other species) have avoided it because of awareness of the negative genetic outcomes. However, we can speculate that a variety of social structures have emerged, whose survival will depend in part on their establishment of incest avoidance. We can consider this in other primates where there are a variety of different social structures and mating strategies, i.e. the promiscuous, multi-male pattern (e.g. chimpanzee), polygamous (e.g. gorilla), monogamous (e.g. gibbon) and solitary (e.g. orang-utan). Incest avoidance can be observed in all of these situations. Other mating patterns may have existed in the past but did not survive because of inbreeding depression. The monogamous pattern is of particular relevance to humans. The gibbon lives in family groups consisting of a monogamous parental pair and their young, but the group only survives one generation as the father drives the sons away when they reach maturity, and the mother the daughters. A similar pattern is seen in monogamous marmosets, though it is common for three or four sets of offspring to be retained within the family group. The onset of puberty may be delayed in such circumstances and those reaching reproductive maturity either leave or are driven away from the family group. Fox (1980) pointed out that in all the various primate mating strategies, the established senior males aim to monopolize the females, and the young or unsuccessful males are excluded. With the baboon, which, Fox suggested, provides the best primate model for early hominid social groups, the powerful males each collect a harem of females but move around together with the other families to form a troop. Obviously there are more females than males in these troops; the remaining males, the young and less powerful, remain on the fringe of the troop in 'all-male' groups. Occasionally, one of these males will be able to take over a harem from an ageing senior or manage to start one of his own. Fox drew a parallel between this primate model and the primitive human system that Freud (1918) described in *Totem and Taboo*, emphasizing the crucial significance of the competition between the older (father) male and the younger males in the all-male group. He proposed that the determinants of exogamy and the incest taboos evolved from this basis. An alternative interpretation is that this pattern, which may have been determined by other social group factors, survived because it avoided inbreeding depression. Similarly, female–female rivalry in the monogamous primate family group, expressed by the mother driving the daughter away as soon as there is any evidence of father–daughter sexual interaction, may have survived because it also avoided inbreeding depression, even if it served other adaptive purposes. Perhaps the incest taboo against mother–son sex, which is certainly the most universal in human societies, derives from the male–male rivalry model, whereas the taboo against father–daughter sex, which is less strong in many cultures, derives from the family group model. And perhaps the propinquity mechanism of Westermark (1926) has helped to reduce negative consequences of sibling incest. This of course is all very speculative, but it is certainly appropriate to take the primate evidence into account.

In the human, the evidence clearly indicates the need for an incest taboo, particularly in controlling sexual interaction between parents or other adult family members and children who have reached or are approaching sexual maturity. The incest taboo, on the other hand, was probably not designed to deal with sexual interaction between adult and young child, which is of a different order and requires different explanations.

Indecent exposure or exhibitionism

Although indecent exposure is widely recognized throughout Europe, Britain is the only country to allocate this behaviour to a separate offence category, which has recently been included in the general category of sexual offence. Most countries include it under some broad heading, such as 'offences against public morality'. Comparative statistics are therefore difficult to establish. When Rooth (1973b) carried out a cross-cultural assessment, however, he found this behaviour to be uncommon outside western Europe and the USA, and particularly uncommon in African countries. It was also uncommon in Japan, suggesting that the difference is not related to industrialization. It would be interesting to have more up-to-date information on this issue, particularly in view of the apparent decline in convictions for this offence over the past 30 years in the UK.

The sexual offender

Determinants of sexual offences in general

Let us first consider the variety of mechanisms and developmental factors that may be of *general* relevance to sexual offending. There is consensus in the sexual offender literature that we are dealing with a multi-factorial process, which has so far proved challenging for those striving to identify causal factors modifiable by interventions or treatment. A variety of explanatory theoretical models have appeared, often overlapping with each other, and some of these will be briefly reviewed. As we shall see, the three-strand model of sexual development (see Chapter 5) and the Dual Control model (see Chapter 2, p. 15) with its application to understanding the relation between mood and sexuality (see Chapter 4, p. 106) are of particular relevance to this chapter and will enable us to maintain some conceptual continuity with the rest of this book in what otherwise readily becomes conceptually confusing.

The developmental process

Adolescents may be responsible for up to a third of all sexual offences (Horne et al 1991; Vizard et al 1995). In many cases, although the offence is against a child, the difference in age between offender and victim is small, and in such cases the sexual interest of the offender can be seen as 'age appropriate'. Adolescent sex offenders are as heterogeneous as their adult counterparts, and showing similar types of offence behaviour. Many adult sex offenders first offended in adolescence, but only a small minority of adolescent sex offenders continue to sexually offend as adults (Grubin 1998). The process of sexual development is therefore clearly central to understanding much of sexual offending.

The three strands model, described in Chapter 5 (see p. 145), sees sexual responsiveness, gender identity and the capacity for forming dyadic relationships as relatively separate developmental strands during childhood, which start to integrate as the child approaches puberty, to form the sexual adult. There are at least three ways, relevant to later sexual offending, in which this process can go wrong:

1. The establishment of sexual preferences which, for most individuals, leads to a sexual identity, can be derailed during this developmental phase, particularly in those who are not well integrated with their peer group, leading to various patterns of deviant sexual responsiveness. Here we have a highly relevant gender difference. Males go through a stage of learning, not well understood, which results in establishment of the 'sexually desirable person', sexual orientation and sexual identity. It is possible that this involves a characteristically male 'critical period' involving gender specific aspects of brain development around puberty, but as yet we can only speculate on this issue. The female, as described in Chapter 4, does not show the same sequence of sexual identity formation but develops with an emphasis on attraction to a particular type of relationship rather than a particular type of person. Thus, for the female, the 'object of desire' is determined by how the 'object' behaves, which is not the case for the male. This goes some way to explaining the gender difference in sexual offending. Deviant thoughts leading to an offence by a male do not require the 'victim' to behave in a particular way. This gender difference is well illustrated by the example of fetishism: being sexually aroused by an object or part of a person's body (also known as partialism), or wearing the clothes of the opposite sex (fetishistic transvestism). These 'sexual preferences', which sometimes dominate an individual's sexual life, are rarely found in women. The possible brain mechanisms involved in the establishment of fetishism are considered more closely in Chapter 9. Deviant patterns are more likely in males who are relatively isolated from their peer group during this developmental phase (see Chapter 5) and who hence lack the 'normalizing' influence of their peer culture.
2. Problems during childhood with the 'dyadic relationship' strand, most commonly a consequence of negative parent–child relationships, result in barriers to intimacy and the incorporation of one's sexuality into a dyadic sexual relationship. Other traumatic experiences, including being sexually abused, may contribute to these barriers.

3. Maladaptive patterns of behaviour, often evident from early childhood, lead to various types of delinquency during adolescence and early adulthood (see Chapter 5, p. 158). 'Delinquent' sexual behaviour, in terms of both sexual risk taking and inappropriate or coercive sexual behaviour, is often part of this maladaptive adolescent pattern. Precisely what underlies this maladaptive tendency is not well understood, although some personality factors have been identified as relevant, but its relatively non-specific nature contributes to the overlap between sexual and non-sexual offending, which has been well documented. Later in this chapter we will consider the consequences of CSA and the effects on the 'victim' and will see that much of the evidence points to a 'sexualizing' effect; children who have been sexually abused are more likely to show sexualized as well as other maladaptive behaviour, during both childhood and adolescence, including promiscuity and sexual aggression (Beitchman et al 1991). Furthermore, the literature indicates that a proportion of sexual offenders who abuse male children report being abused themselves during childhood (Barbaree & Langton 2006). Hence the 'abused' may become the 'abuser'. However, this pattern should not be overemphasized; a history of sexual abuse as a child is neither necessary nor sufficient to lead to adult sexual offending (Grubin 1998).

Marshall & Marshall (2000) emphasize the fundamental importance of parent–child attachments in the developmental process leading to sexual offending. Children with secure attachment to their parents are effective in establishing relationships outside the family (i.e. the 'dyadic relationship' strand), and they are emotionally resilient. The child who is left anxious and ambivalent by the relationship with the parent has low self-esteem, a need for closeness with others, while being fearful of closeness for fear of rejection. Parents who are cold and distant have children with an 'avoidant style' who see others as untrustworthy. Both of these inadequate coping styles, according to Marshall & Marshall (2000), leave the child readily responsive to the attention of others, increasing the likelihood of being sexually abused. Being sexually abused, they suggest, leads to early onset of masturbation, and the use of sex as a coping strategy, which in turn predicts adult sexual aggression. The sexual offender literature, however, is somewhat inconsistent in this respect. Marshall et al (2000), for example, compared child molesters, non-sexual offenders and non-offenders recruited from a local employment agency. The groups were small ($n = 30$, 24 and 29, respectively), and they found no difference between them in types of parent–child attachments, either with mother or with father. In addition, the links between these developmental stages, proposed by Marshall & Marshall (2000), are to some extent questionable. Early masturbation, for example, is not necessarily associated with maladaptive sexual patterns in adolescence and later. In a study using age of onset of masturbation as a marker of sexual development (Bancroft et al 2003a), we found no support for an association between early onset of masturbation and experience of being sexually abused. The early masturbators among the boys were, however, somewhat more likely to be isolated from their peer groups in childhood. It will also be interesting, in future research, to assess whether the paradoxical relationship between negative mood and sex, which may lead to sex (or masturbation) being used as a coping strategy, and which, from our own studies (see Chapter 4, p. 108), is far from rare in men and women, is associated with a history of sexual abuse as a child.

There is, however, a general point to be made. Early childhood experiences do not necessarily have a direct and sustained effect on the outcome of later adolescent development. This issue was discussed at a Kinsey Institute workshop on sexual development in childhood (Bancroft 2003). Browning & Laumann (2003) drew the distinction between 'psychogenic' theoretical explanations, and a 'life-course perspective'. The psychogenic perspective, which features in much of the literature on the effects of early abuse and trauma, sees the original trauma and its severity as the key determinants of the final outcome of development. The life-course perspective adopts a more sequential approach in which an early negative experience may influence the next stage of development, which then interacts with other factors to determine the next stage, and so on. In other words, the original trauma does not predetermine the final outcome, but alters the developmental sequence, depending on other interacting factors, before the final outcome is determined. A possibly relevant distinction between these two theoretical approaches is that the first psychogenic perspective has evolved from studies of people with negative outcomes; the life-course perspective, in contrast, emerges from community-based survey data, such as that reported by Browning & Laumann (2003), in which CSA experiences are not necessarily associated with negative long-term outcomes. Obviously, the severity and duration of the initial trauma need to be taken into account; abusive experiences, which are repeated over long periods, are likely to have a more dominant effect on subsequent development. Such long-term experiences, however, most often occur within families, with the likelihood of other family factors having negative effects on development. In discussion, Finkelhor (2003a) proposed that both the psychogenic and the life-course perspectives were relevant and complimented each other. The conclusion at this point is that we should keep in mind that specific childhood experiences may contribute to the developmental process without necessarily determining its outcome. Children vary in their resilience as well as the adverse experiences that they encounter. We will return to this issue when reviewing some of the related literature.

Sexual excitation and sexual inhibition

The concept of inhibition has received a fair amount of attention in the sexual offence literature. Two questions which have understandably recurred are 'How is it possible to behave sexually when the consequences could be disastrous?' and 'Could a "normal" man become sexually aroused and respond sexually in such negative circumstances?'. The implication of such questions is that, in the normal individual, sexual arousal in such circumstances would be inhibited. Are those who sexually offend lacking in such inhibition?

The Dual Control model, described in Chapter 2 (p. 15), postulates that the occurrence of sexual arousal depends on a balance between sexual excitation and inhibition in the brain, which involves relatively discrete response systems. Furthermore, the model postulates that individuals vary in their propensity for both sexual excitation and sexual inhibition, and the SIS/SES scales (Janssen et al 2002) have been established to measure these propensities in men, showing a relatively normal distribution in non-clinical samples (see p. 230). It is assumed that the middle part of the range for both excitation and inhibition propensity reflects adaptive response patterns. Thus, the 'normal' range for SIS2, which measures 'inhibition due to threat of performance consequences', reflects adaptive inhibitory responses, which prevent or reduce the likelihood of sexual arousal developing in inappropriate circumstances. We have already shown that individuals with low SIS2 scores, particularly when combined with high SES (high propensity for sexual excitation), are more likely to take sexual risks. In other words, in such individuals, sexual arousal develops even when the consequences of sexual response and behaviour are likely to be negative and even disastrous. The assumption is that the role of inhibition of sexual arousal is normally adaptive. If, however, sexual arousal occurs in inappropriate circumstances, this results in an altered emotional state (see p. 429), which is assumed to adversely affect normal 'risk management', in a manner analogous to alcohol intoxication (Bancroft 2000).

So far, SIS/SES scales have not been used with sexual offenders. However, they offer an obvious way to assess this aspect of sexual offending, with the proviso that sexual offenders may have an increased likelihood to give 'socially desirable' answers.

In Chapter 4, when mechanisms of information processing were considered, the question arose whether an inhibitory response was relatively 'automatic' or resulted from conscious processing. The evidence from brain-imaging studies suggests that a variety of mechanisms, involving different parts of the brain, could contribute to inhibition of sexual arousal, including a pre-existing 'inhibitory tone', which needs to be actively reduced if sexual arousal is to occur. We should therefore be open to the idea that both automatic and conscious processing could be involved, perhaps varying in importance across individuals but also across situations. In the sexual offence literature, a number of studies, using non-rapists as participants, have experimentally manipulated cognitive appraisal in various ways (reviewed by Barbaree & Marshall 1991). In one study, participants were told that being sexually aroused by a rape scene was normal and not an indication of the individual's rape proclivities. This resulted in 'disinhibition' and an enhanced arousal response to rape sequences (Barbaree & Marshall 1991). In another study, the amount of sexual arousal in response

to rape sequences depended on whether the victim was aroused by the experience (Malamuth & Check 1980). In a further study, more arousal was shown to rape sequences when there were indicators that the victim was in some sense blameworthy (e.g. in her style of dress) (Sundberg et al 1991). Studies found greater arousal to rape scenes when the participant had been led to believe that he had taken alcohol in the experimental context, whereas actual alcohol ingestion did not affect the response (Bridell et al 1978). Although there are some inconsistencies in this literature, it nevertheless indicates that, to some extent, inhibition can be lessened by cognitive manipulations, an explanatory mechanism that features commonly in the literature on sexual offences. Wright & Schneider (1997), for example, suggested that sexual offenders progressively incorporate elements into their sexual fantasies that bolster their self-esteem and at the same time justify their deviant interests. However, it is not clear to what extent such manipulations involve conscious rather than automatic processing, and none of these studies of rapists or non-rapists has considered the possibility that there could be individual variability in the propensity for inhibition and, in a related way, the likelihood of such inhibition being manipulated cognitively. Future research needs to take this aspect into consideration, as it could prove to be crucial.

The impact of mood on sexual response

As discussed in Chapter 4 (p. 108), the relationship between negative mood states and sexual arousability, as measured by the Mood and Sexuality Questionnaire (MSQ), varies across individuals. Whereas in states of depression or anxiety, the majority report a reduction or no change, a minority report increased sexual interest or arousability. This 'paradoxical' mood/sexuality pattern has been shown to be related to some aspects of high-risk sexual behaviour (e.g. number of casual partners or 'one-night stands') in both heterosexual and gay men (Bancroft et al 2003c, d). In one small study of self-defined 'sex addicts', there was a strong association between this paradoxical pattern and 'out of control' sexual behaviour (Bancroft & Vukadinovic 2004).

This paradoxical pattern is likely to be highly relevant to sexual offence behaviour. There are frequent references in the sexual offender literature to such concepts as 'emotional dysregulation' (Ward & Siegert 2000), 'emotional state augmentation' (Barbaree & Marshall 1991) and the use of sex as a coping strategy (Marshall & Marshall 2000), and there is some evidence that allows a more direct comparison to our 'paradoxical pattern'. The measure in this literature closest to the MSQ is the Coping Using Sex Inventory (CUSI), reported by Cortoni & Marshall (2001), which asks 'how much you engage in these types of activities when you encounter a difficult, stressful or upsetting situation', followed by a series of sexual behaviours, fantasized or real, or involving use of pornography. In addition to a total score, three sub-scales were identified, 'consenting', 'rape' and 'child' to describe the content of the fantasy or behaviour. Four groups of incarcerated offenders were compared: rapists, child molesters, violent non-sexual offenders and general,

TABLE 16.4 Coping Use Sex Inventory (CUSI) scores in four group of offenders (Cortoni & Marshall 2001)				
n =	Rapists 54	Child molesters 56	Violent 57	General 27
Total (16–80)*	32.0 (±11.9)[†]	34.2 (±9.3)[†]	24.5 (±6.4)[‡]	24.5 (±5.6)[‡]
Consent (6–30)	14.5 (±5.7)[†]	15.4 (±5.3)[†]	12.2 (±5.7)[‡]	11.8 (±4.5)[‡]
Rape (6–30)	10.2 (±5.6)[†]	8.9 (±4.1)[†]	6.2 (±0.7)[‡]	6.4 (±1.6)[‡]
Child (4–20)	4.4 (±2.2)[†]	7.6 (±3.8)[‡]	4.0 (±0.3)[†]	4.1 (±0.8)[†]

*The range for each scale or subscale, with each item scored from 1 (not at all) to 5 (very much)
[†]Is significantly different to[‡]

non-violent offenders. The total and sub-scale CUSI scores from these groups are shown in Table 16.4.

This shows that rapists and child molesters are similar in most aspects of this measure, including their scores for 'rape', while differing from the two non-sexual offender groups. The child molesters differ from rapists and the rest on the 'child' scale. However, the scores are low, given that the lowest score in each range indicates 'not at all', and it would be helpful to have distributions presented. It is also difficult to know precisely what these scores indicate, given that fantasies and overt behaviours are combined. These findings are compatible with a paradoxical relationship between negative mood and sexual arousal, somewhat more evident in the sexual than in the non-sexual offenders, and, interestingly, more evident for the 'consent' subscale than the other two. However, Cortoni & Marshall's (2001) conclusions that 'sexual offenders make extensive use of sex as a way of coping with distress or problems' and that sex is a 'coping strategy used by all their participants' (p. 40) are less clearly justified.

Obviously one of the most important negative moods relevant to sexual offending is anger or hostility, and it is not clear whether this is relevant to the CUSI scores. As yet, apart from a limited literature on the effects of inducing anger in the laboratory and finding that it can augment sexual response (and vice versa) (Yates et al 1984; see Chapters 4, p. 108, and 11, p. 318), we have no evidence of how much individual variability there is in this respect, in the non-offender or offender populations.

Proulx et al (1996) asked incarcerated sex offenders to complete a computerized 'fantasy report' every 2 days over a 2-month period. First the respondents assessed the frequency of both deviant and non-deviant fantasies (on a five-point 'much more than to much less than usual' scale). They were then asked if they had masturbated during these fantasies (yes or no). Next, they rated their mood over the 2 days, using the same five-point scale. Finally, they were asked whether they had 'interpersonal conflicts' during the 2 days, and if so what emotions were aroused by those: humiliation, oppression, rejection, anger, feeling of inadequacy or loneliness. Of the 39 offenders in this study, 19 were rapists, 12 heterosexual paedophiles and 8 homosexual paedophiles. In the rapists and heterosexual paedophiles, negative moods and interpersonal conflicts coincided with increased deviant fantasies and associated masturbation. For the homosexual paedophiles, negative moods and conflict were associated with increased deviant fantasies,

but not masturbation. The emotions most frequently following the conflicts were anger, loneliness and humiliation for the rapists, loneliness and humiliation for the heterosexual paedophiles, and loneliness for the homosexual paedophiles. These findings are of interest and are compatible with negative mood leading to deviant fantasies and masturbation. But we should keep in mind that these experiences occurred while in prison for the sexual offence. The nature of the interpersonal conflicts was not reported, though it is likely that quite often they would involve criticism of the sexual offence by other inmates (child molesters in particular are heavily stigmatized by other prisoners). This leaves us less certain how relevant these associations are to mood and sexuality when the offender is not incarcerated.

Pithers et al (1988) asked 136 paedophiles and 64 rapists about their mood immediately before their recent offence. Among the rapists, 88% reported anger, whereas of the paedophiles, 46% reported anxiety and 38% depression. These were retrospective reports, relating to only one episode and may be distorted by a need to rationalize or excuse the behaviour. This issue, of course, is a problem for any method of studying sex offenders using self-report. However, the role of negative mood in sexual offending might be better understood if more qualitative studies were carried out, comparable to those used with non-offending heterosexual (Bancroft et al 2003c) and gay men (Bancroft et al 2003d).

The concept of 'coping' in interpreting paradoxical mood/sexuality relationships warrants closer consideration. Marshall & Marshall (2000) postulated that the comfort and relief from negative moods or stress that result from masturbating act as a negative reinforcer, hence conditioning the pattern of masturbation and the particular fantasies used. The role of conditioning in the development of sexual preferences, both normal and deviant, was considered in Chapter 4 (p. 104), and over all, the evidence in favour of typical conditioning processes (i.e. classical or operant) being involved is weak or inconsistent. Here the suggestion is that negative reinforcement is involved. Marshall & Marshall (2000) illustrate the principle of negative reinforcement with the example of someone who develops a panic attack while in a lift (elevator) and leaves the lift at the next floor. The reduction in fear on getting out of the lift reinforces the fear response on getting into a lift subsequently. However, the parallel with masturbating when in a negative mood state is not a straightforward one. For example, if the individual with a phobia of lifts masturbates when in a lift, the sexual response and associated pleasure might temporarily relieve the fear of the lift. However, that effect is transient and fairly quickly he would realize he was still in the lift. Men with 'out of control' patterns of sexual behaviour, which are considered more closely in Chapter 11 (p. 330), often fit Endler & Parker's (1990) description of an 'emotion-focused' coping style, with the tendency to dwell on the negative emotion, but with the added effect that focusing on their negative emotion, for reasons which are not yet fully understood, leads to the development of sexual arousal. This then motivates the individual to masturbate to orgasm. But soon after, the realization that the same 'out of control' behaviour has reoccurred leads to a return of negative mood, and a reinforced sense of failure of control (Bancroft & Vukadinovic 2004). Thus, rather than seeing the sexual behaviour as an 'attempt to regulate emotional distress' (Marshall et al 2000), it may be more helpful to focus on behaviour driven by potentially problematic sexual arousal, which is either initiated or augmented by negative mood, not exactly a 'coping strategy'.

Neuropsychological factors

Sexual offenders on average have a lower IQ than non-sexual offenders (Blanchard et al 2006). Anomalies of neurodevelopment, including left handedness, and brain injuries during childhood have been associated with paedophilia, although the mediating mechanisms are not as yet understood. The very limited evidence from brain-imaging studies of sexual offenders is as yet inconclusive (Blanchard et al 2006). Further research on such factors could be important, particularly in helping us to understand how brain mechanisms normally influence development of sexual preferences and related inhibitory or control mechanisms.

Re-offending

Hanson & Bussiere (1998) carried out a meta-analysis of 61 follow-up studies, involving nearly 29 000 sexual offenders. On average the recidivism rate for further sexual offences was low (13.4%) compared with rates for non-sexual offenders. Less than 10% of first offenders were reconvicted within 5 years of prison release, compared with a recidivism rate of over 30% for those with any previous sex offence convictions. The best predictors of re-offending, apart from previous offending, were young age and evidence of deviant sexual preferences. The strongest single predictor was in child molesters, with phallometric evidence of sexual responsiveness to children. Hanson & Morton-Bourgon (2004) updated their meta-analysis to include a total of 95 studies, and more than 31 000 sexual offenders. The recidivism rate remained similar (13.7%). Deviant sexual preferences remained strong predictors together with antisocial orientation. Phallometric evidence of sexual responsiveness to children in child molesters became less strongly predictive.

Let us now consider how these various determinants may relate to specific types of sexual offence.

Rape and sexual assault

Most of the literature on rape attempts to explain it as a deviant sexual act, varying in the extent to which anger or hostility is involved. An alternative approach sees the rape of women by men as primarily an act of hostility or humiliation, or an expression of power over women (e.g. Groth 1979). We will consider both approaches.

Various multi-factorial models have been presented to account for rape and different types of rapist. Prentky & Knight's (1991) model first distinguishes between two levels of aggression: 'low', which means that only enough force to ensure compliance is involved, and 'high', where extreme force is used. If aggression is 'high', then a distinction should be made between 'explosive anger', which gets out of control, and 'sadism', in which hurting or humiliating the victim is sexually arousing. If the aggression is 'low', are there other indicators of 'antisocial personality', with sexual assault being one manifestation of a wider antisocial pattern? If not, is the sexual assault 'sexualized', i.e. is forcing someone to have sex particularly sexually arousing? If there is no indication of 'sexualization', is there evidence that the offender was under stress, had a more general need to exert power or dominate or had more extreme 'double-standard' attitudes, such as women being intended for sexual use by men? Two additional components emerged as relevant at each level, whether or not there was 'impulsivity', and the general level of social competence. The authors commented that distinct identifiable developmental paths may lead to different expressions of violence. However, application of this model to produce a taxonomy of rapists proved difficult, and Prentky & Knight (1991) concluded that 'extensive work remains before the enigmatic complexity of sexual aggression is deciphered' (p. 659).

Barbaree & Marshall (1991) proposed six different models of the relation between aggression during rape and sexual response. They described two '*response control*' models:

1. Sexually aggressive men differ from non-sexually aggressive men in being less able to suppress sexual arousal.
2. Rapists differ from non-rapists in being able to be aggressive and sexually responsive at the same time; in the 'normal man' the two responses are mutually inhibitory.

Their other four models were listed under '*stimulus control*':

3. 'Excitation', when force and violence have an excitatory effect; this seems similar to their second 'response control' model, but with the added feature that forcing the victim or expressing violence is itself sexually arousing.
4. 'Inhibition', when rapists show less inhibition; it is not clear how this differs from their first 'response control' model. Malamuth (1981) had earlier suggested that the 'likelihood of raping' was a continuum among the general male population,

although he did not distinguish between a continuum of inhibition proneness and a continuum of how the concept of rape was appraised cognitively and attitudinally.

5. 'Disinhibition', which covers the extent to which cognitive mechanisms, as discussed earlier, can reduce the inhibitory response. Anger was seen as operating in a similar way, although it is not clear whether this results from the 'arousing' effect of anger, or its effects on the cognitive appraisal process leading to inhibition. Alcohol intoxication is widely regarded as a 'disinhibitor', and as many as 50% of sexual offenders have been intoxicated at the time of the offence (Marshall & Marshall 2000). Interestingly, whereas alcohol may disinhibit one's behavioural intentions, it also tends to reduce sexual arousability (see p. 405).

6. 'Emotional state augmentation', by which non-sexual emotional states modulate the strength of the sexual response.

Although there appears to be overlap between these six theoretical models of Barbaree & Marshall, it is striking how much they anticipate the Dual Control model, and the mood/sexuality model described earlier, in spite of the fact that these more recent models were not developed to account for sexual offending.

The alternative approach sees rape as primarily an act of aggression rather than a sexual act; if a man has a need to hurt or humiliate a woman, or women in general, then sexual assault may be a preferred method as it carries the dubious justification, or at least excuse, that the act was sexually motivated, and men cannot be entirely responsible for their sexual behaviour (or so it might be believed by such individuals). Groth who regards rape as 'pseudo-sexual' in this way, in a report on 170 rapists found that about a third were sexually dysfunctional during the assault; 16% had some degree of erectile failure, 15% had difficulty ejaculating and 3% had premature ejaculation (Groth et al 1977). Premature ejaculation, in such circumstances, is compatible with high sexual arousal. Erectile and ejaculatory difficulties, on the other hand, are suggestive of increased inhibition. It is noteworthy how little attention has been paid to this aspect in the rape literature. It is possible that such individuals may have been sexually aroused initially and then became more inhibited once they started to assault the victim. In such cases, the failure to respond could intensify the anger and associated violence. Alternatively, the assault may not have been sexually motivated in the first place but driven by the need to hurt or humiliate the victim. Such individuals would not need to be characterized by Barbaree & Marshall's (1991) six models. It would be interesting to know to what extent such dysfunctional rapists were under the influence of alcohol.

Sexual offences against children

Between 60% and 70% of child molesters abuse only girls, about 20–33% boys, and about 10% children of either sex. In the majority of cases the child is known to them, and around 80% of offences take place in the home of either the offender or the victim. Sex offenders against children are convicted of non-sexual crimes to a slightly greater extent than in the male population in general. This contrasts with rapists and those convicted of other kinds of sexual assault, who tend to have a relatively high rate of non-sexual offending.

The Kinsey Institute study of sexual offenders incarcerated in prison or state hospital (Gebhard et al 1965) involved 496 offenders against children and 499 against minors. They covered a broad age range but tended to be older than other sex offenders. The median age at first conviction was 34.5 years for offenders against girls and 30.2 years for offenders against boys. The majority of them were married, and although marital breakdown and remarriage were common, more happy marriages were reported than in most other groups of offenders. Other studies, however, have emphasized the problems sex offenders against children have in establishing satisfactory adult relationships, possibly encouraging their resort to relationships with children (Mohr et al 1964; Pacht & Cowden 1974). Marshall (1997) has emphasized lack of intimacy and marked loneliness resulting from an inadequate attachment style, itself the consequence of impaired parent–child relationships, though the evidence for this particular pattern is not consistent. A meta-analysis of 14 studies reported by Dreznick (2003) assessed 'heterosocial competence', which was defined as 'the ability to competently interact with members of the other sex'. Child molesters showed significantly less heterosocial competence than rapists and non-sex offenders. However, it is not entirely clear what 'heterosocial competence' actually means as it was based on the combination of a variety of measures. It is also not clear to what extent this effect was characteristic of child molesters in general or just those who had been convicted and imprisoned. No consistent picture of sexual offenders against children emerges in terms of personality characteristics (Levin & Stava 1987), although clear evidence of psychopathology is less apparent in this group when compared to other types of offender. However, not surprisingly, there is a subgroup of such offenders whose offences are more serious and where such abnormalities are more likely to be present (Marshall 1997).

There are some relevant differences between extra- and intra-familial (incest) offenders. Extra-familial offenders are more likely than incest offenders to report a sexual interest in children before the age of 18 years. Extra-familial offenders tend to show more sexual arousal to images of children than other sex offenders or controls; there is some evidence that intra-familial offenders do not differ from other groups in this respect, but the evidence is not consistent (Marshall 1997). Such findings do point to paedophilia as a preference (see below) being more likely in extra-familial offenders.

Around 30% of sexual offenders against children report intoxication with alcohol or drugs at the time of the offence, though it is not always clear to what extent the behaviour was made more likely by the intoxication or the intoxication was induced to make the behaviour easier to enact (Marshall 1997).

There has been little recent attention paid to the incest offender, as distinct from the child molester, and no clear picture of the characteristics emerges from the literature. Weinberg (1976) suggested three categories: (i) the 'endogamic' man (in this context someone who confines his social and sexual interest to within his family), (ii) the indiscriminately promiscuous personality and (iii) the paedophile, who may be interested in young children apart from his own. He did not present any evidence of the relative frequency of these types.

Gebhard et al (1965) drew some distinction between those who offended against children (i.e. under 12 years of age) and those against adults within the family, usually their teenage daughters, aged 17–18. The first type was described as 'a rather ineffectual, non-aggressive dependent sort of man who drinks heavily, works sporadically and is preoccupied with sexual matters'. The other type was less preoccupied sexually and generally more inhibited. He was described as 'conservative, moralistic, restrained, religiously devout, traditional and uneducated'. He sounds comparable, in some respects, to the men in Weinberg's 'endogamic' group.

Later literature on incest reflected the relatively new interest of child protection agencies and the women's movement (Finkelhor 1982). The former tended to emphasize the family unit as a cause of the problem but also as something that should be kept together if at all possible. Those in the women's movement tended to concentrate on the male perpetrator, seeing CSA as an extension of the sexual exploitation of women by men, and seeking the removal and usually punishment of the male offender. Two accounts exemplifying these two contrasting viewpoints are those of Porter (1984) and Ash (1984). Porter edited a working party report sponsored by the Ciba Foundation. This was very much based on the family approach and rather surprisingly, more attention was paid to the characteristics of the mother of the incest victim than of the father or perpetrator. Ash's account was very much in the feminist mould and strongly criticized the tendency to blame the mother who, it was stated, can seldom be seen to hold any responsibility for what happened, the man always being the culprit. Neither view seems to be sufficiently balanced. Clearly the family is likely to be important. It is also of interest that women who have been sexually abused themselves during childhood are more likely to have children who are sexually abused.

Incest families studied have often been crisis-ridden and characterized by discord, lax sexual morality and illegitimate births. The sexual relationship of the parents was often unsatisfactory. The number of children tended to be higher than average and the mother was away from home more than usual, often because of ill-health (Ash 1984).

Furniss (1985) described two types of sexually abusive family. In one the sexual abuse served to avoid open conflict between the parents (the conflict-avoiding family). The mother, it was suggested, set the rules for emotional relationships and the pattern of communication about sexual and emotional matters. In the second type more open parental conflict existed; the mother provided little support to the children and a child was 'sacrificed' to stop the conflict leading to family breakdown (the conflict-regulating family). The emphasis placed on the mother in both these descriptions is noteworthy.

Much attention has been paid to the 'abused becomes abuser' hypothesis. Given the link between CSA and other problems in the child's family and childhood, which will be considered more closely in the next section, it is not surprising that there is a less specific association between CSA and subsequent offending in general. A more specific link with subsequent sexual offending is most apparent in those who themselves offend against children (Freund & Kuban 1993; Seto 2004).

Explanatory models of child sexual abuse

Finkelhor (1984) proposed a model in which there are four preconditions for CSA to occur.

1. There is *motivation to sexually interact with a child*. Three examples of motivation are given: (i) *'emotional congruence'* because sexual interaction with a child satisfies some important emotional need. This, in turn, may reflect a variety of predisposing factors, including arrested emotional development, which may result in a need to be powerful or controlling, reflecting socio-cultural influences that masculinity requires dominance and power in sexual relationships. Re-enactment of childhood trauma may be used 'to undo the hurt' or, more simply, there may be 'narcissistic identification with self as a young child'. (ii) *'Sexual arousal'* — the child is sexually arousing, possibly resulting from powerful sexual experiences in the offender's own childhood, or in some cases because of brain abnormalities. This factor may have been strengthened by exposure to child pornography. (iii) *'Blockage'* — alternative sources of sexual gratification are not available or are less satisfying, maybe because of abnormal developmental experiences.
2. The second precondition is that there are factors that *'counteract internal inhibitors'*. These include alcohol, psychotic illness, impulse disorder or a family background that has not reinforced 'incest inhibition'. This equates to the 'disinhibition' factor cited in other models (e.g. Barbaree & Marshall 1991).
3. The third precondition is that there are factors *'overcoming external inhibitors'*. These refer to circumstances in which the child victim is more accessible to the abuser: a mother who is absent, not close or inadequately supervising the child, unusual sleeping arrangements or other unusual opportunities to be alone with the child.
4. The fourth precondition is that there are factors reducing the child's resistance to abuse. This may be because the child is emotionally insecure or deprived, or insufficiently informed about the possibilities of being abused, because of a position of unusual trust between the child and the abuser, or the use of coercion.

Ward & Siegert (2000) reviewed Finkelhor's precondition model, and also Hall & Hirschman's (1992) quadripartite model and Marshall & Barbaree's (1990) integrated theory, and attempted to integrate what they considered the best features of these models into their 'pathways model'. This postulates four clusters of problems: (i) emotional regulation problems, (ii) intimacy and social skill deficits, (iii) deviant sexual arousal or 'sexual scripts', and (iv) cognitive distortions. Deficits in empathizing are subsumed under (i) and (iv).

Emotional dysregulation may be manifested as a need to avoid expressing or experiencing emotions, or as poorly modulated affective states. Intimacy and social skill deficits may result from insecure attachment as children and, together with emotional dysregulation, may result in problems with mood management, impaired problem solving, low self-esteem, reduced autonomy, low self-efficacy and avoidance of close relationships for fear of rejection. Early abuse may have led to inappropriate sexual scripts before the individual was cognitively and emotionally ready to process them. Cognitive distortions reflect maladaptive beliefs and attitudes. However, they may simply represent rationalizations designed to excuse the abuser's 'morally reprehensible actions'. The pathways model goes on to postulate that each of the above four problem clusters is relevant to every CSA offence. However, the 'different pathways' concept indicates that one of the clusters predominates in each pathway and interacts with the other three clusters. Thus, in Pathway 1, intimacy deficits predominate, leading to children becoming substitutes for adults. In Pathway 2, deviant sexual scripts predominate. This may not mean a sexual preference for children, but the confusion of sex with intimacy, i.e. interpreting cues indicating the need for emotional closeness, with cues that indicate desire for sex. Pathway 3 has emotional dysregulation as the predominant factor, with a range of patterns: inability to modulate negative emotions, problems controlling anger, strong negative emotions leading to loss of control in other ways, use of sex as a soothing strategy and masturbation as a mood regulator. Pathway 4 centres around antisocial cognitions and tendencies. Pathway 5 involves 'multiple dysfunctional mechanisms'. To illustrate the complexity of this model it is proposed that biological factors exert differential effects depending on the particular pathway. Ward & Beech (2006) went on to report 'a *first attempt* to provide an integrated framework to explain the onset, development and maintenance of sexual offending' which they called 'an integrated theory of sexual offending' (ITSO). This mainly differs from the Ward & Siegert (2000) model by suggesting what brain systems (i.e. the 'motivation/emotion' system, the 'action selection and control' system and the 'perception and memory' system) are involved in the various 'problem clusters', as well as proposing that the model is of general relevance to sexual offending.

The above examples of explanatory models, both for rape and assault and for CSA, exemplify the struggle that has prevailed in attempting to account for sexual offence behaviour. This, in part, has been driven by a need to establish a taxonomy of sexual offenders relevant to choice of methods of intervention to reduce re-offending.

The concept of paedophilia

Where does the concept of paedophilia fit in our attempt to understand CSA? 'Paedophilia', according to the DSM IV (American Psychiatric Association 1994), indicates the presence of 'recurrent, intense sexually arousing fantasies, sexual urges, or behaviours involving sexual activity with a prepubescent child or children (generally aged 13 or younger)'. The question of whether paedophilia should be regarded as a mental disorder, as implied by its inclusion in DSM-IV, has generated vigorous debate (Green 2002; Schmidt 2002; and see ensuing commentaries on these two papers in the same issue of *Archives of Sexual Behavior*). Although we should keep in mind the possibility that in some cases, which are probably rare, paedophilia results from some pathological brain condition, we are more likely to understand it by considering psychobiological developmental processes and their interaction with socio-cultural factors (see Chapter 5). We have already acknowledged that with many of the offences against children, the 'child' involved is a young teenager who may well be sexually attractive, at least in some respects, to most adults. The issue is then one principally of lack of responsibility and exploitation of the young person rather than a deviant sexual preference. But as we go down the age range, this blending with appropriate adult sexual attractiveness diminishes substantially or stops. This change is probably most obvious around the developmental transition through puberty. Does it then become more appropriate to think of 'deviant' sexual interest, when the object of attraction is pre-pubertal?

This distinction between pre- and post-pubertal objects of attraction confronts us with another gap in our understanding of normal sexual development. If we return to the idea of a 'critical period' of male sexual learning, discussed in Chapter 5, during which certain types of individual (or more impersonal stimuli, such as fetishes) acquire sexual attractiveness, and if we assume that for most males that happens around puberty, then the issue of the age of the sexually attractive person becomes relevant. Does the 12- or 13-year-old boy, destined to be heterosexual, find his sexual attraction focusing on girls of around the same age? And if so, how does this age-related attractiveness change as the male gets older, leading to attraction to more mature females? This may be related to the issue of *specificity vs novelty* discussed on p. 105. This addresses the fact that some individuals establish very specific sexual preferences, which change little over time. An extreme example of this is the fetish. At the other extreme are those who require novelty, at least in terms of different partners or types of sexual activity, to be sexually aroused. Most of us come somewhere in between. This type of variability has not yet been explained but seems to involve varying degrees of plasticity in what is sexually arousing. This concept is probably much more relevant to males than females. Is the paedophile showing less plasticity, becoming fixated on what is learnt early in this process, i.e. attraction to similar-aged peri-pubertal boys or girls?

There are other relevant questions potentially more answerable. For example, what are the key differences in sexual attractiveness between a 14- and an 18-year-old female? To what extent is attractiveness determined by visual appearances and to what extent by the individual's behaviour? How many of these 'key features' might be found in a 10–11-year-old girl? Are there some men who would find sexual interaction with a 14-year-old girl appealing, and others who would require other features of the female, related to more mature age? And if so, what determines this difference between men? This is a matter of 'sex appeal' and does not necessarily relate to responsibility in responding to the 'appeal'. But it does raise the possibility of a learning process underlying sexual attraction, which as yet we know little about, which could go wrong or become arrested in certain situations. There is limited evidence relevant to these questions. Freund et al (1972) assessed penile volume change in 40 non-offending heterosexual men (mean age 24.5 years) to images of males and female of varying ages (from age 6 to adulthood). They found the greatest erectile response to post-pubertal and adult women, but the responses to pre-pubertal girls were greater than the responses to the males in any age group. Interestingly, with images of the pre-pubertal children, only those showing the pubic region, and to-some extent the buttocks, elicited obvious erectile responses. In a further study of 'normal' men (Quinsey et al 1975) erections to images of pubescent and pre-pubertal girls averaged 70% and 50%, respectively, of the erectile responses to adult women. Such findings are consistent with the idea that most males start off with sexual attraction to females of about the same age, and that as sexual development proceeds and the male gets older, the age of the sexually attractive female also increases. If that is the case, then one would expect variability in this process.

The impact of the culture could also be important; a 'normal' progression through this learning process may be influenced by cultural norms of acceptable age for a sexual partner. What determines that in some individuals this age increase is minimal or does not happen becomes the crucial question that we cannot yet answer (see Seto 2004 for further consideration of this issue).

In this respect the concept of paedophilia, defined as a sexual *preference* for pre-pubertal children, has some importance. However, this only applies to a proportion of those who sexually abuse children. Seto (2004) concluded, on reviewing a number of studies, that a paedophilic preference of this kind is evident in about 30% of adolescent sexual offenders, and 40–50% of adult offenders. This difference is in itself interesting; as Seto (2004) points out, adolescents with paedophilic preferences may be more likely to continue to offend than other adolescents and hence would form a larger proportion of the older sex offender group. Gebhard et al (1965) divided their sexual offenders into those offending against adults, minors (aged 12–15) and children (aged less than 12). However, they did not distinguish between those who had a preference for children over minors or adults. Marshall (1997) pointed out that in

his clinical work the paedophilia concept would only apply to around 40% of non-familial child molesters, and less than 25% of incest offenders. He thus questioned its usefulness and expressed his preference for using the more general term 'child molester'. In much of the literature the term 'paedophile' is used to describe any offender against children, whether or not the child is pre-pubertal or the offender has a preference for pre-pubertal children.

The disturbing evidence about the worldwide sexual exploitation of children and the huge commercial aspect of it, considered earlier, strongly indicate that sexual attraction to children is much more common than the incidence of reported sexual offences would suggest. At the same time, the cross-cultural variation in how childhood is defined and the tendency in the developed world not to distinguish between pre- and post-pubertal children when reporting their sexual exploitation serve to obscure the prevalence of sexual *preference* for pre-pubertal children.

In striving to understand this preference we should be cautious in confining our attention to those who are convicted or charged with the offence. In one early American study of practising paedophiles who were interviewed, only 1% had ever been arrested (Rossman 1979). What evidence is there of the prevalence of paedophilic preferences among non-offenders? Probably the majority of paedophiles are never convicted; they are either extremely cautious or they confine their attentions to those children who are clearly seeking such encounters and are therefore less likely to report them. And there may be many who are sufficiently responsible that they restrict their expression of paedophilia to solitary masturbation with or without child pornography.

We clearly need to understand more about why this type of sexual preference emerges. To what extent is it attributable to individual or family-specific patterns of abnormal sexual development, but also, to what extent does this pattern reflect socio-cultural factors? Such factors are not likely to directly encourage paedophilic preferences, as they do with rape of adult women, but they may have indirect effects, increasing the likelihood of paedophilic preference by discouraging or obstructing more appropriate and socially acceptable sexual development? I agree with Seto (2004) that more research focus on the concept of paedophilia is needed. However, the assessment of such preference is not easy; given the intense stigma that is associated with CSA at the present time, we should not expect those with such preferences to reveal them unless they have already been convicted.

Exhibitionism and voyeurism

Together with the decline in the prevalence of 'indecent exposure', little attention has been paid to these two behaviours in recent years, and most of the evidence comes from early studies. However, in a recent Swedish national survey on sexuality and health, a representative sample of 1279 men and 1171 women (59% response rate) was asked two questions relevant to exhibitionism and voyeurism, not in terms of who had encountered such behaviour, but who had enacted it: 'Have you ever exposed your genitals to a stranger and become sexually aroused by this?' and 'Have you ever spied on what other people are doing sexually and become sexually aroused by this?' (Langstrom & Seto 2006). For the exhibitionistic question, 4.1% of men and 2.1% of women answered yes. For the voyeuristic question, 11.5% of men and 3.9% of women answered yes. There was an increased likelihood of participants responding positively to one of these questions also doing so for the other question, suggesting a link between the two behaviours. Possible predictors and correlates of these two responses were examined. Apart from being more common in men, both were associated with having more psychological problems, lower satisfaction with life, greater alcohol and drug use, and greater sexual interest and activity in general. The positive respondents were also more likely to report other atypical sexual behaviour (i.e. sadomasochistic or cross-dressing behaviour). While these are unique and valuable data, it is important to keep in mind its limitations. Only two questions were asked; there is no indication of when or how often such behaviours had occurred and, most notably with the voyeuristic question, no information on the circumstances of the act. Of the two behaviours, the voyeuristic one is not only reported more frequently but also is less clearly abnormal. There must be many people who are not sexually unusual, who have by chance observed others engaged in sexual activity and watched them with interest. The term 'spied on' could be interpreted in various ways. What is particularly noteworthy, however, is the number of women who responded positively, given that it is extremely unusual for women to be convicted of either of these offences.

Exhibitionism

Returning to the earlier evidence, Radzinowicz (1957) estimated that at least 80% of people convicted of indecent exposure are exhibitionists, i.e. people for whom genital display to members of the opposite sex is an end in itself. The remainder have a variety of other reasons for exposing themselves. Gebhard et al (1965) found that after the exhibitionist, the commonest offenders were those who exposed themselves when drunk for no very clear reason, except possibly disorganized solicitation, drunken humour, or an expression of hostility. These men usually denied that they intended to expose. The third most common type was the mentally defective who exposes in the belief or hope that the female will be sexually excited; it is thus a form of sexual approach or solicitation in such individuals.

Gebhard et al (1965) found an early onset of the behaviour in most of their subjects. The majority of indecent exposers are only charged once; the court appearance seems to have a strong deterrent effect. However, the chance of re-conviction increases markedly with a second conviction, particularly for men previously convicted for non-sexual offences. In the Cambridge study (Radzinowicz 1957) the overall recidivism rate was 18.6% over 4 years. Forty per cent of re-convictions occurred within the first year after conviction. Convictions

tend to become less frequent after the age of 40 (Rooth 1971). However, Marshall et al (1991), in a group of 44 exhibitionists, found re-offending in 39% of those receiving treatment and 57% of those untreated. There is, however, a need for caution in comparing studies for recidivism, as the reasons for involvement in a study are often crucial.

The exhibitionist group is difficult to classify further (Rooth 1971). However, there are a number of variables probably crucial to understanding the different types of exhibitionism:

1. *The age of the victim.* A minority of exhibitionists expose persistently to pre-pubertal girls and in some of them this behaviour may lead on eventually to more direct sexual contact with children (Rooth 1973a). The commonest age of the victim is at, or around, puberty.
2. *The nature of the act.* The exposure may be clearly sexual, associated with an erect penis, sexual excitement and masturbation either during the exposure or shortly afterwards. In some cases, the penis is flaccid and there is no obvious sexual arousal. The reaction of the female is often important and an exhibitionist may go on exposing until he produces the desired response. Rooth (1971) describes a typical example of an ideal exposure as 'one of dominance and mastery. The exhibitionist, usually timid and unassertive with women, suddenly challenges one with his penis, briefly occupies her full attention and conjures up in her some powerful emotion such as fear and disgust, or sexual curiosity and arousal .... He experiences a moment of intense involvement in a situation in which he is in control. The reaction that he most dislikes is indifference. '
3. *The frequency of exposing behaviour.* In some exhibitionists, urges to expose occur occasionally, possibly at times of crisis or emotional distress. In between these episodes, exposure holds no particular appeal. For others, the idea of exposing is always sexually stimulating and may feature in masturbation fantasies. Such men experience the urge to expose frequently. For them the behaviour has become a well-established form of sexual stimulation that they may find difficult to control.
4. *Risk-taking.* Some exhibitionists are careful to avoid being caught or recognized. Others appear to behave in a way to *ensure* that they are caught. They may, for example, repeatedly expose from their car, so that their car registration number leads readily to their arrest.

Exhibitionists show a fairly normal range of intelligence and social class, though there is some evidence that they are underachievers. There does not appear to be any specific personality type or pattern of psychological problems that characterizes the exhibitionist (Murphy 1997). There is also no consistent evidence of a specific pattern of deviant responsiveness. Several studies have compared exhibitionists' erectile response to images that portray exhibitionistic scenes as well as more typical visual erotic stimuli. Whereas the exhibitionists did show greater erectile response to the exhibitionistic images than either non-exhibitionist offenders or non-offending controls, their responses to the 'normal' erotic stimuli were substantially greater than to the exhibitionistic stimuli (Murphy 1997).

The association between exhibitionism, and voyeurism, sado-masochism and cross-dressing, found in the Swedish population survey (Langstrom & Seto 2006), is consistent with a number of studies of offenders showing an overlap between exhibitionism, voyeurism, frotteurism and rape. This has been taken to indicate that exhibitionism or voyeurism is often one manifestation of a more general 'paraphilic' pattern of sexuality, as well as associated with a tendency to non-sexual offending, suggesting an antisocial component (Murphy 1997).

However, of the various common types of sexual offence, exhibitionism is probably the most difficult to understand. We are faced with the problem of distinguishing between sexual and non-sexual determinants. In certain circumstances, genital display does have a simple sexual significance. It is the most common form of sexual interaction amongst children (see Chapter 5) and may precede sexual activity between adults. With the exception of exposure by the mentally handicapped, the characteristics and circumstances of most of these acts do not suggest that they are aimed at establishing further sexual contact with the 'victim'. The theme of mastery and insult, which is much more noticeable, suggests that this is genital display as an expression of hostility. Such display is common amongst many species of primates, especially the males. It may therefore represent a primitive form of communication, though it remains a mystery why it should be expressed in a small proportion of men, often in a somewhat compulsive fashion.

Other secondary determinants stem from the social consequences of the act. Not only is the offender likely to be punished, but his wife and family will also probably feel humiliated. In many cases, one is struck by the apparent need of the exhibitionist to provoke these reactions. In such cases, one wonders to what extent the behaviour is reinforced by being criminalized. If exhibitionism was no longer regarded as an offence, would it be more or less likely to occur?

Certainly for the vast majority of exhibitionists, their behaviour should be seen as harmless, if unseemly and transiently unpleasant for the 'victim'. A substantial number of women must have witnessed such acts. Gittelson et al (1978) found that 44% of a group of nurses had had this experience, usually in their early teens. Though their initial reactions were often unpleasant, any continuing reaction seemed to be unusual.

Voyeurism

Until recently, voyeurism did not have its own offence category, coming under the heading of 'breach of the peace' or, if a number of victims were involved, 'being a public nuisance'. Hence the statistics of this type of offence up till now are difficult to come by. Voyeurism, or scopophilia as it is sometimes called, is of theoretical interest beyond its forensic implications. First, there is a tendency for most people to look at sexually interesting scenes. In some, looking is preferred to actually participating, presumably because real contact is too threatening for one reason or another. This voyeuristic element is sometimes revealed in people's fantasies, in which they look at other people rather than participate themselves. This can be an important clue to their basic sexual problem.

There is even less information about the characteristics of voyeurs, or 'peeping toms' as they are often called, than about exhibitionists. Gebhard et al (1965) interviewed a series of 56 'peepers' in their study of sex offenders. The average age at first conviction for this offence was 23.8 years. Relatively few were married, compared with other types of offender. Perhaps most important was the tendency for many of them to be socio-sexually underdeveloped, having had less experience than is usual for their age, being shy with females and having marked feelings of inferiority.

Typically the voyeur peeps at a stranger, usually from outside the building. Voyeurs usually take care not to be seen. Occasionally they enter a building in order to peep, or alternatively they peep in the course of pursuing some other crime, such as burglary. Occasionally they draw attention to themselves, e.g. by tapping on the window. Gebhard and his colleagues believed that it is the peeper who enters buildings and draws attention to himself who is most likely to progress from peeping to sexual assault, but for the majority, assault is unlikely. However, given the tendency for the coexistence of what Freund (1990) calls 'courtship disorders', there may be a tendency for voyeurism to be one of the first paraphilic behaviours to be manifested, leading on to exhibitionism and occasionally sexual assault of some kind (Kaplan & Krueger 1997).

The most obvious explanation for this type of behaviour is that it provides a form of sexual stimulus without the threat of sexual contact or rejection. The peeper usually masturbates whilst peeping and is likely to be easily aroused by looking at women. Hence the pattern becomes sexualized. It can thus be seen as an extension of the general tendency to look, in those who are too frightened to participate. But other factors are presumably involved. The risk and its associated excitement may be a further incentive. For those who draw attention to themselves, the fear that their behaviour induces in the victim may indicate that expression of hostility or, as with the exhibitionist, the momentary feeling of power may be a determinant. In this respect, peeping has something in common with the obscene telephone call, an exploitation of modern technology, which is probably on the increase. Whereas the sexuality of the telephone call may be a sufficient determinant in some cases, the hostile and sadistic element seems common and may be a further example of the expression of 'power through sex' that has recurred throughout this chapter.

Sexual offences by females

The large majority of the literature on sexual offending concerns male offenders. This in part reflects the comparatively small number of women or girls known to have sexually offended, and in part a prevailing attitude which sees sexual assault in particular as a male-type behaviour. However, the number of known female sex offenders is apparently increasing and more attention is now being paid to them. Finkelhor (1984), in his book on CSA, pointed out various inconsistencies in the literature and came to the conclusion that the proportion of sexual abusers of children who were female was indeed small, around 5% in the case of girls and 20% in the case of boys. He commented, however, on the recent increased attention to the possibility that these figures were underestimates and considered various reasons why that might be so. Finkelhor and colleagues later carried out a national telephone survey of more than 2600 respondents in the USA. Of the 27% of women and 16% of men who reported having been sexually abused in some way during childhood, 1% of the women and 17% of the men said their abuser had been female (Finkelhor et al 1990).

In 2001, according to the Federal Bureau of Investigation, 98% of individuals arrested for forcible rape were male and 1.2% female. Of those arrested for other sexual offences (excluding forcible rape and prostitution) 8% were female (Hunter et al 2006). Finkelhor (1984) drew attention to an interesting enigma. There is evidence in males that being sexually abused as a child increases the likelihood of becoming a child sexual abuser when an adolescent or adult. But given the fact that a majority of victims of CSA are girls, why is this particular 'sexualizing' effect apparently restricted to males? We will return to the gender aspects of 'sexualization' later in this chapter when considering the impact of sexual abuse on the victim. In general, however, it is of interest to see to what extent gender differences in sexually offensive behaviour throw light on their determinants.

Hunter et al (2006) described three types of juvenile female sex offender:

1. 'Naïve experimenters'. These are girls who have engaged in limited sexual offending, not usually involving force or coercion, but often exploitation of the context, e.g. when acting as a babysitter. This type of offender does not show major psychopathology or other manifestations of antisocial behaviour, is unlikely to reoffend and is described as 'somewhat fearful or anxious about sexuality and primarily motivated by curiosity' (p. 154).
2. Adolescent girls who have engaged in more extensive sexual acting out with one or more children, over a period of time, often several months. These girls typically have a history of being themselves sexually abused as children, and in many cases their abusive behaviour parallels their own experience as the abused victim. This group shows some degree of psychopathology, often a history of depression or a background of a troubled or dysfunctional family. Nevertheless, according to Hunter et al (2006), their prognosis is generally good.
3. Adolescent girls with more serious and pervasive sexual problems and related psychopathology. Their abuse of children is more likely to involve force, and

their own developmental histories reveal high levels of sexual and physical trauma, exposure to violence and family upheaval. Many of them meet the diagnostic criteria for post-traumatic stress disorder (PTSD) or major affective disorders. Some of them experience recurrent sexual and aggressive impulses, and given their difficulties with mood regulation, reoffending is likely. Psychotic manifestations may arise, and suicidal or self-harm behaviour is relatively common.

Hunter et al (2006) do not indicate the comparative prevalence of these three types.

Adult women who commit sexual offences are considered by Hunter & Mathews (1997). Here again they describe three types of offender:

1. Women who co-offend with a male, who tend to be influenced by a fear of the male co-offender and an emotional dependence on him. At least in their early offences they appear to be more passive than active as a participant in the offence. They usually have long-standing emotional insecurity, low self-esteem and social isolation, and most of them have been sexually, physically or emotionally abused themselves as children.
2. Women who abuse pre-pubescent children; this group also come from dysfunctional families with experience of being physically or sexually abused as children. They are described as re-enacting the trauma they themselves experienced. Some of these women show patterns of deviant sexual interest comparable to those of male sex offenders.
3. Women who sexually interact with teenage males show the least evidence of childhood trauma of the three groups. Their involvement with teenage males is, however, often associated with dissatisfaction or dysfunction in their adult or marital relationships, Many such women see their involvement with the young post-pubertal male as an 'affair' rather than sexual exploitation, reflecting different social attitudes to sexual involvement with a teenage boy than with a teenage girl.

Less than 5% of sex offences against children are known to have been committed by women, often in association with men, but population surveys suggest higher rates of offending by females. The damage caused by female abusers appears to be similar to that caused by males.

Overall, there are more similarities than differences, it would seem, between female and male sexual offenders. Two interesting differences are less likelihood of the female offender being involved in non-sexual offences and their being less likely to identify sexual arousal as a major motivator of their offence behaviour than male offenders.

The victims of sexual offences

Rape

Most rape victims are teenagers or young adult women, though no age group is immune. In the USA, 43% of rape victims are aged 16–19 years, 16% are 12–15 and 13% are

20–24. Black women are twice as likely as white women, and women from households with annual incomes less than $7500 are more than twice as likely as those with higher incomes, to be raped (Catalano 2006). The characteristics of the typical rape victim are therefore very similar to those of the typical victim of non-sexual violence, except that the latter is more often male.

Rape is an exceedingly traumatic experience for most women. Hence it is not surprising that substantial psychological after-effects commonly occur. However, there are many factors that may interact to influence the impact of such experiences, including the personality and resilience of the rape victim before the event, characteristics of the rape and the victim's reactions during it, the level of support following the experience, and the effect, on those who report it, of being involved in the legal process. Not surprisingly, the outcomes of rape are variable. Resick (1993), in a useful review of the literature, concluded that, nevertheless, there was reasonable consistency across studies. Most rape victims experience a strong acute reaction that may last several months. By 3 months after the rape, the emotional reaction has started to subside for most women, but for some, chronic problems become established for an indefinite period. Such problems include fear and PTSD, depression, loss of self-esteem, social adjustment problems, sexual problems and anxiety disorders (Resick 1993).

Resnick (1997), who has studied the reactions of rape victims seen at the emergency room, found that nearly 90% met the criteria for a panic attack at the time of the rape. Other types of reaction have been reported; Galliano et al (1993) found that 37% of women retrospectively reported responses consistent with a 'tonic immobility reaction', characterized by freezing or feeling immobilized even though there had been no physical constraint. Rothbaum et al (1992) assessed 99 rape victims at weekly intervals for 3 months. After 1 week, 94% showed symptoms of PTSD or depression; after 3 months this had reduced to 47%. Kilpatrick et al (1992) reported on a community survey of 4008 women; 507 (12.6%) had previously been raped at least once. Thirty-one per cent had developed PTSD at some stage since the rape and 11% still showed symptoms. Several retrospective and prospective studies have found that a majority of rape victims develop PTSD, which may persist in some for a year or more (Van Berlo & Ensink 2000).

A number of earlier studies had reported on the prevalence of depression following rape. In a study of 34 rape victims, 23% were moderately and 21% severely depressed, as measured by the Beck Depression Inventory (BDI; Frank et al 1979). In a study of 178 rape victims and 50 controls, 51% of the victims reported depressive symptoms compared with 8% of the controls. Many of the victims were experiencing depression several years after the assault (Becker et al 1984). In Kilpatrick et al's (1992) survey, 30% had suffered at least one episode of major depression since the rape, and 21% were still depressed. This compared with 10% and 6%, respectively, for women who had not been raped.

Sexual problems are common following rape, most often experienced as a need for avoidance of sexual activity and an impairment of sexual arousal when sexual activity does occur (van Berlo & Ensink 2000). Becker et al (1986), for example, found sexual problems in 59% of survivors of sexual assault compared with 17% in a control group. Whilst for most women these reactions will eventually subside, in some they may continue for years. Interestingly, there is no evidence that rape is followed by the development of vaginismus (Pukall et al 2006).

There has been disagreement about the relevance of the circumstances of the rape to the psychological after-effects. In one report it was concluded that the 'stranger' rape was the most traumatic whereas, in another, victims who were raped by persons known to them were seen to face more difficulties. Frank et al (1980) found no association between the circumstances of the rape and the psychological reactions, except that those who suffered physical injury or who were threatened by a weapon reported fewer problems in their post-rape relationship with their families, presumably because their rape was taken more seriously.

Becker et al (1984) found depression to be more common in women whose rape had involved a threatening weapon, suggesting that the life-threatening quality of the rape experience and the associated feeling of no control over one's own life are of particular importance in causing post-assault depression. Resick (1993) found that the occurrence of confusion or disorientation during the rape experience was a strong predictor of subsequent PTSD.

Given the attention that has been paid in the legal process to the sexual experience of rape victims prior to the assault, it is noteworthy that there is no clear evidence on this issue. Whereas most studies show the majority of adolescent victims to be sexually experienced, there are no appropriately controlled data to indicate whether they are more so than would be expected by chance. Yet this has been relevant to one of the most controversial issues concerning rape — victim precipitation. In cases of rape by a complete stranger, or where there is clear evidence of premeditation by the rapist, the victim is unlikely to be considered in any way responsible. But in those cases where rape occurs between friends or casual acquaintances, the victim has been likely to find herself under suspicion or held to be responsible to a greater or lesser extent. As discussed earlier (p. 470) changes in the law in the USA, and subsequently in the UK, have shifted the emphasis on consent, so that it is now the accused who has to give 'reasonable grounds' for believing that the complainant had consented, rather than the complainant proving her case that she had not. This is a change in the right direction, but it is still too early to know how much difference this is going to make, and as mentioned previously, this has had more impact on 'aggravated rape' than 'simple rape'. The issue of consent has been, and probably still is, a major factor in the humiliation that rape victims experience after reporting the rape. Thus if a girl allowed herself to get involved in limited love-making but refused to go 'all the way', she may have found it difficult to have her charge of rape taken seriously. This remarkable fact stems from an almost universal attitude about male/female sexuality — that if a female allows a male to become sexually aroused in her presence, there comes a time when his arousal goes beyond the point of control and he can no longer be held responsible for his actions. Such a belief is by no means of recent origin. It is also linked to the idea that if a young woman dresses in a sexually provocative way, she is 'asking for it' or 'deserves what she gets'. The problem for the woman is further compounded by the social significance of being raped, which prevails to a greater or lesser extent in most cultures. The raped woman is seen as 'defiled' and 'spoiled', a reflection of her 'property status' (see p. 471 for further discussion of this).

The universality and long-standing nature of these attitudes may tempt one to believe that they are inevitable because of our biological natures. But apart from the fact that there is no physiological basis to account for the assumed sex difference in sexual control, the implications that this value system has for the nature of male/ female relationships are profound and extend far beyond the problem of rape. The woman is seen as the responsible person and 'the property to be taken' at one and the same time. In societies where such abdication of interpersonal responsibility is more or less institutionalized, one should not be surprised to find other examples of man's inhumanity to man as well as to woman. These issues will be considered further at the end of this chapter.

Not surprisingly, therefore, many women are reluctant to reveal that they have been raped. In some instances they are frightened of reprisals from the rapist but more often fear the stigmatization that follows and being put on trial themselves in order to convince people that they were not responsible for the assault. This is a unique position for any victim of crime to find him- or herself in.

A further aspect of evidence in rape cases is the reaction of the woman to the rape. If she screams, actually resists, or is seen to be physically injured, her story is more likely to be believed. Probably the over-riding emotional experience for most victims is 'a fear of death' (Katz & Mazur 1979). In those circumstances, one should expect a variety of reactions, not necessarily rational. Burnett et al (1985) found that a woman who normally harboured high anxiety about death was less likely to put up physical resistance to rape. Clearly, for many women rape or the threat of rape is a threat to life. Also, many women show minimal physical resistance because of an understandable fear that by doing so they are more likely to be hurt or disfigured. Such relative passivity leads some rapists to conclude that the women were consenting, a form of deceit that becomes more understandable when prevailing social attitudes about female passivity and masochism are taken into account. Some women try to flatter or help the rapist in the hope that this will diffuse his aggression. In such cases the man may believe them to the extent of trying to arrange another meeting (West et al 1978) or of raping someone else (Gibbens et al 1977). It is nevertheless difficult for a woman to know how best to react, even assuming she is in a position to choose. Some rapists are likely to be discouraged by the act of resistance whilst others may be further aroused by it. It is not surprising that rape is such a traumatic experience with often lasting adverse effects for many women.

Helping the victim of rape

The victim of rape is likely to require help at three stages: first, immediately following the rape, second, in the aftermath, during the next few days and weeks, and, third, coping with long-term consequences. Foa et al (1993) reviewed studies attempting to evaluate different treatment approaches. Not surprisingly no sufficiently comprehensive study was found, with appropriate, randomly assigned 'no treatment' control groups, and with treatment postponed until after a period of time to allow spontaneous improvement. Various cognitive behavioural techniques (CBTs) have been used, in particular to deal with the anxiety symptoms. At present, given the extent of trauma involved, I consider it appropriate and ethical to provide some form of 'crisis intervention' until alternative methods have been clearly shown to be superior.

Immediately following the rape

Two types of support are required at this stage.

Various procedures need to be gone through once the rape has been reported to the police and are more to do with investigating the offence and finding the offender than with helping the victim. As discussed earlier, these procedures can be handled very insensitively by police and police doctors, adding substantially to the trauma. The victim clearly needs support whilst going through these procedures, and various ways in which the police could help have been described by Chambers & Millar (1983). A chapter by O'Reilly (1984), who for many years led the Sex Crimes Analysis Unit in New York City, should be required reading for any police officer involved with rape victims. It is an admirable combination of compassion and common sense, with an understanding of the difficulties the police have to face in these circumstances.

The physical examination is a crucial part of the procedure, and whilst it is of some relevance to the victim's management, it is largely determined by the need for evidence. The doctor involved has considerable scope for making this part of the process more or less traumatic. A useful account of how to deal with the examination together with a description of the other practical procedures that are more or less obligatory (e.g. collecting specimens, blood tests for pregnancy, sexually transmitted disease and prophylactic treatment for sexually transmitted infections) is given by Silverman & Apfel (1983).

Rape crisis centres often provide experienced women to accompany the victim to the police station or hospital to support them through this phase.

The aftermath

In helping the victim to cope with the aftermath of rape the general principles of crisis intervention apply. These have been described in detail elsewhere (Graham &

Bancroft 2006) and will only be outlined here. Intervention may involve 'intensive care', when the person is so distressed or shocked that she is not able to look after herself and, for a short time at least, others have to take over the responsibilities of her day-to-day living. A judgement of whether or not this takeover of responsibility is necessary has to be made in each case. Implementing 'intensive care' usually means someone remaining with the victim until she has started to settle down. This type of care can be provided in hospital but more often it is arranged in the home of the victim, relative or friend. At this stage the woman may be in a state of mute shock, in which case some effort should be made to initiate more normal communication. Alternatively she may be uncontrollably agitated or distressed. The principal objective of intervention in such circumstances is to help her return to a less disorganized emotional state in which she can start to look usefully at what had happened and also to ensure that she obtains a reasonable amount of sleep. In crisis states, lack of sleep simply adds to the individual's decompensation and inability to cope. Once the initial shock phase is beginning to pass, intervention can move into crisis counselling. The objectives then are to deal appropriately with the emotional reaction and eventually, when the emotional state allows, to adopt problem-solving strategies to enable her to reorganize and re-enter normal living.

The crisis precipitated by rape is close to that produced by bereavement or loss (Hopkins & Thompson 1984) and once the initial shock phase is passed, the proper working through or mourning of this loss is a crucial part of recovery which can be greatly aided by sensitive counselling. As with other forms of loss there is a predictable sequence of reactions. After the shock comes the denial, anger and guilt. Denial often shows itself as an assumption of the victim that she has got over the rape and is back to normal. Anger is usually an understandable fury towards the assailant, and sometimes at others. Guilt often shows itself as self-blame for having allowed the incident to happen. Each of these reactions must be acknowledged and dealt with.

The principal losses following rape are of trust (e.g. no longer able to trust men), freedom (no longer able to go out or stay at home alone) and, possibly most important, of identity (I am no longer the person I was). There is often a sense of being 'spoiled' by the rape, of no longer being as attractive or acceptable as a person or as an appropriate recipient of other people's love or affection. Often the woman feels that the incident has made her disgusting, so much so that she fears that the doctor, who examines her, will be offended by her defiled body.

The counsellor has several important tasks: first, to deal with the emotional reaction and sense of loss. As with other forms of bereavement, there is a crucial need for the victim to share her feelings with someone who can empathize. As with bereavement, relatives and friends often find this difficult to do, taking the view that 'the less said about it the better', which is usually their way of dealing with their own difficulties in coping with this situation. In addition to sharing, acknowledging and validating the emotional experience, the counsellor can positively affirm various aspects of the victim's behaviour at the time of the rape — commending her for how she coped, how sensible or brave she was, etc (Silverman & Apfel 1983). The victim's assumptions about her culpability should be repeatedly and consistently challenged and resisted, the counsellor making it absolutely clear that there was no possible justification or excuse for the behaviour of the assailant. It is often necessary to consider how the victim should best deal with her anger. The inability to express her fury to the rapist can be intensely frustrating.

Although in the initial stages it is the post-traumatic aspect that is most important, the sexual implications of the assault should not be ignored. As a high proportion of victims develop sexual problems following rape, at an appropriate stage the sexual feelings and anxieties of the victim should be explored.

A further important role for the counsellor is to work with the partner or family of the victim. They may not be only affected by feelings of guilt for having allowed it to happen but also be influenced by the common myths and prejudices surrounding rape. These can lead to negative feelings towards the victim, as already mentioned. Silverman & Apfel (1983) stress the importance of not being judgemental in such circumstances, but rather spending time with the relatives, apart from the victim, to help them come to terms with these feelings.

The counsellor should also be on the look-out for other post-rape problems, which may require specialized help. Depression, which is a common feature, may only become apparent some time after the rape. The incident may bring to the surface pre-existing problems in the family or marriage, which then require help in their own right.

Long-term consequences

It is not unusual for victims to experience adverse reactions years after the assault. Often this is because they did not adequately work through their feelings at the time (sometimes they told no one about it at the time). The unresolved feelings are then reactivated by some subsequent event — it may be the rape of a friend. Some delayed 'mourning' may then be required.

The victim of child sexual abuse

Since the last edition of this book there has not only been a substantial amount of research and literature on the effects of CSA, there has also been the change in public attitudes, referred to earlier, associated with the 'moral panic' described by Jenkins (1998). As a consequence, some of what I wrote in the second edition now looks 'politically incorrect' rather than simply out of date. I shall strive, in revising and updating this section, to retain what seems informative about the earlier research, while reviewing, briefly, the extensive literature that has appeared in the past 15 years and aim to integrate my earlier review with the more recent one. I do not think I have encountered a comparable challenge in any other part of this book. I have used the term 'CSA' throughout this chapter on the grounds that, whatever the nature of the interaction, sexual exploitation of a child by someone older is morally unacceptable. However, as we shall see, this does not mean that a child is necessarily harmed by the experience, and in some circumstances may even find the experience pleasurable. It is this aspect of the issue which is most clearly 'politically incorrect'.

We are faced with a number of crucial issues, which need to be taken into account. Probably the most crucial is (i) the age and developmental stage of the child when first abused, but also (ii) the gender of the child, (iii) whether the effects of CSA are assessed shortly after the abuse, or at least in childhood, or whether they are based on retrospective recall of the childhood experiences by adults, (iv) the considerable diversity of abusive sexual experiences that have to be considered, which range from 'indecent exposure' by a stranger to a prolonged period of repeated sexual intercourse with an older family member, (v) the differential effects of extra- and intra-familial CSA, (vi) the factors which determine whether an incident of CSA is reported and hence contributes to follow up studies of known cases, (vii) the need to distinguish between the effects of the sexual abuse per se, and the effects of other negative family factors which frequently exist in such cases, and finally (viii) the need to grapple with and reconcile the evidence of negative emotional effects, such as depression, with the evidence that a substantial proportion of victims of CSA show what has become known as 'sexualization', with a range of sexual consequences such as early onset of voluntary sexual activity, and sexual risk taking.

What are the effects of CSA on the child shortly after the abuse? Kendall-Tackett et al (1993) reviewed 45 relevant studies in which all subjects were less than 18 years at the time of assessment. Ages of the victims when abused ranged from preschool to adolescence. Studies varied in terms of comparison groups; some included non-abused controls, others compared sexually abused children with children presenting for psychiatric or psychological treatment; nearly half the studies had no comparison group. A wide range of symptoms were reported, including anxiety or fear, PTSD, depression, low self-esteem, aggression, 'sexualized' behaviour, behavioural problems and combinations fitting the description of both 'internalizing' and 'externalizing' behaviours. All of these symptom patterns were more likely in the abused than in the non-abused controls. They did not, however, combine to present any 'syndrome', which could be regarded as characteristic of CSA. The sexualized behaviours were most unique in this respect, but these were by no means evident in all CSA cases and were found to some extent in non-abused children. Sexualized behaviours and PTSD were, however, the only patterns that were more common in the CSA groups than in the clinical comparison groups. This is not surprising, given that the clinical comparison group consisted of children undergoing treatment for psychological problems of one kind or another, whereas the CSA group had only been assessed following their

abuse experience. The symptom profile, however, did vary with age. Thus, for preschoolers, the most common symptoms were anxiety, PTSD, internalizing and externalizing and sexually inappropriate behaviour. For school-age children, fear, aggression, school problems, hyperactivity and regressive behaviour were most common. For adolescents, depression, withdrawn, suicidal or self-injurious behaviour, somatic complaints, illegal acts, running away and substance abuse were the most common. This age pattern makes sense when one considers the developmental stage at which the abuse occurred.

Eleven longitudinal studies were reviewed by Kendall-Tackett et al (1993), most of them following up abused children for 12–18 months, two of them for 2–5 years. Most of these studies found a majority, around two-thirds, in whom the symptoms abated, but with 10–20% getting worse (some of these had been asymptomatic at first assessment). Overall, anxiety-related symptoms tended to abate, whereas aggressive behaviour patterns tended to persist or get worse. A number of mediating variables were considered. Strong family support, particularly maternal, enhanced recovery. Although most of the studies reviewed did not distinguish between intra- and extra-familial abuse, the evidence indicated that a perpetrator who was 'close' to the victim would cause more serious effects than one less close. Apparently, 'closeness' was not used consistently across studies. Involvement in court proceedings had mixed effects, leading Kendall-Tackett et al (1993) to conclude that involvement in such proceedings impairs recovery from the traumatic experience, at least in the short term. But they also concluded that such negative effects could be mitigated by not requiring the child to give repeated testimony, and by not having a frightened child confronted by the defendant. They therefore did not consider there were grounds for avoiding criminal prosecution.

However, the emotional status and the family background may well have a bearing on which cases are reported. Because the consequences of reporting these incidents to the police can have traumatic effects on the child, in part because of the emotional impact of the legal procedure, it is likely that in well-integrated and supportive families parents will protect their child from further trauma by not reporting the incident, particularly if the offender is not seen as vicious. The disturbed family, on the other hand, will not only find it more difficult to cope with such a crisis without outside support but may also project their own guilt in their reactions to the episode, and their determination to punish the offender at all costs.

It is noteworthy that in reporting the percentages of children with specific symptoms, most of these studies reviewed by Kendall-Tackett et al (1993) gave no indication of the percentage that were symptom free, 'perhaps out of concern that such figures might be misinterpreted or misused' (p. 168). They cited four studies, however, which did report on this; the percentage of children who were asymptomatic at the time of assessment ranged from 21% to 49%. The reviewers went on to consider possible explanations; perhaps appropriate symptoms were not always measured; perhaps they were assessed before the symptoms had become manifest, either because of suppression of symptoms by the child or because of a genuine delay in the impact of the abuse. Finally, they acknowledged that 'perhaps asymptomatic children are truly less affected' (p. 170), either because they suffered the least damaging abuse or because they were more resilient. This account contrasts strikingly with earlier reports, both in how the abusive experiences and the children's reactions to them are described. For example, in the Kinsey survey (Kinsey et al 1953), 24% (i.e. *n* = 1075) of the female sample had been approached when they were preadolescent by adult males (i.e. at least 15 years old), 'who appeared to be making sexual advances, or who had made sexual contacts with the child' (p. 117). In 62% of these cases the 'sexual approach' was only verbal or involved genital exposure; in 3% coitus occurred. Around 80% of these 1075 women said they were upset or frightened at the time, 'a small proportion had been seriously disturbed, but in most instances the reported fright was nearer the level that children will show when they see insects, spiders or other objects against which they have been adversely conditioned' (p. 121). On the other hand 5% had been sexually aroused by the experience and 1% experienced orgasm. Here we see an example of how the 'peaks and troughs of moral panic' affect scientific reporting on this issue. We also need to consider possible gender differences in the impact of CSA.

A large proportion of the relevant literature has, until recently, focused on female victims. More attention is now being paid to male victims (Bauserman & Rind 1997; Holmes & Slap 1998). It is apparent that CSA without a negative short-term impact or long-term consequences is more likely when a boy is abused than a girl. A 14-year-old boy who interacts sexually with an adult woman is less likely to see the interaction as negative, than in the case of a 14-year-old girl. A proportion of boys who are abused by older males may find the experience positive because it is not coercive and they are sexually attracted to males more than females (Stanley et al 2004). There is less evidence that a boy becomes homosexual as a result of sexual abuse by a female, and more evidence that the reverse occurs. This in part reflects the gender difference in the development of sexual identity considered in Chapter 5, with the greater impact of relational issues in female development. But we should continue to keep an open mind about the explanations for the observed gender difference in CSA effects, while also keeping in mind that many males have very negative consequences of CSA.

There is now an extensive literature, involving both clinical and community-based samples, where adults are asked to recall CSA experiences, and those who report such experiences are compared with those who do not in their current problems. Mullen et al (1996) elicited histories of physical and emotional abuse as well as sexual abuse during childhood. There were more similarities than differences in the associations between these three types of childhood abuse and adult adjustment. However, sexual abuse was more likely to be associated with subsequent sexual problems, emotional abuse with low self-esteem and physical abuse with marital breakdown. Multivariate analyses indicated that some, but not all of the adult problems could be attributed to the 'matrix of childhood disadvantage from which abuse so often emerged' (p. 8).

There is a consistent literature showing a relationship between CSA and depression in adulthood. The evidence that this is more likely in women than in men who have been abused is somewhat inconsistent, but Weiss et al (1999), in reviewing this literature, pointed out that both CSA and depression were more common in females. They raised the possibility that potentially irreversible effects of CSA-related acute stress on the hypothalamo-pituitary-adrenal axis could result in an increased vulnerability to subsequent depression, and that this effect may be more likely in women.

Spataro et al (2004), in an Australian study, identified 1327 females and 285 males who had been medically assessed following CSA before the age of 16, listed in the Victorian Institute of Forensic Medicine, and then linked this sample with cases registered on the Victorian Psychiatric Case Register, which records all contacts with public in-patient and community mental health services in that state. The mean age when examined following the alleged sexual abuse was 9.4 years (SD 4.1); 90.8% of the females and 63.2% of the males had been judged, on the basis of the medical examination, to have experienced penetrative abuse. In comparison with the population controls born within the same time period, the CSA cases were significantly more likely to be diagnosed with childhood mental disorders, major affective disorders, anxiety and acute stress disorders and personality disorders. The male victims were significantly more likely than the female victims to have received psychiatric treatment since the abuse. These authors estimated that the percentage of CSA that involves penetration is around 5%. This review therefore shows a clear association between more severe and clearly traumatic CSA and subsequent psychiatric problems. It does not allow for control for other potential risk factors in these cases.

The issue of whether the long-term adverse consequences are a direct effect of the CSA or are associated with other factors, mainly family related, that may also increase the likelihood of CSA, has remained in contention. Early studies showed that children who were sexually involved with adults had disturbed family backgrounds: broken homes, inadequate parents, child neglect, illegitimacy and generally poor relationships amongst family members (Katz & Mazur 1979). Finkelhor (1980) assessed factors that might increase the likelihood of CSA. Several of these involved the family, e.g. (i) low income family, (ii) social isolation of the child, (iii) presence of a stepfather (though it was not necessarily the stepfather who abused), (iv) conservative 'family' values held by the father, (v) little physical affection shown by the father, (vi) absent mother, (vii) detached mother, (viii) mother never finished high school and (ix) mother with punitive attitudes towards sexual matters. Finkelhor combined these variables to form a sex abuse risk factor scale. In his subjects with none of these risk factors, sexual abuse was almost non-existent. If five or more factors were present, two-thirds of the subjects had suffered abuse.

Recent attempts to resolve the issue of background family factors have mainly relied on twin studies. Using the Australian Twin Register, Nelson et al (2002) compared those with a history of CSA to their twins who had no such history, but who would have experienced largely the same family background. They found that whereas family background factors were associated with adverse outcomes, the association was stronger in those who had also been sexually abused. The adverse outcomes included major depression, attempted suicide, conduct disorder, alcohol dependence, social anxiety, rape after the age of 18 and divorce. Overall the associations were stronger in females than males, particularly when penetrative abuse had been involved. Unfortunately, this does not help us to assess the extent that family background factors increased the likelihood of CSA. Comparable findings had been reported from an earlier US twin study of women (Kendler et al 2000).

In 1997, Rind & Tromovitch (1997) reported a meta-analysis of seven national community-based representative surveys, from the USA, Canada, Great Britain and Spain, concluding that only a small proportion of individuals who have experienced CSA are permanently harmed by it and that such harm is more likely to affect females than males. This paper did not receive much attention. The following year, Rind et al (1998) published the paper in *Psychological Bulletin* that caused the firestorm mentioned earlier, leading to unanimous condemnation by the House of Representatives in Washington DC. In both of these papers, Rind and his colleagues criticized the literature on the effects of CSA on various grounds, including the focus on clinical and legal samples and the relative neglect of individuals who had experienced CSA but had not reported it. In the second paper, long and difficult to read, they reported a meta-analysis of 59 studies of university students. Definitions of CSA varied across studies, but most studies defined sexual experience as CSA if there was a sizeable age discrepancy (at least 5 years) between the child and perpetrator, and most studies included both contact and non-contact (e.g. exhibitionism) sexual experiences. It is not clear what proportion of CSA acts were reported at the time they occurred. Rind et al (1998) concluded that long-term adverse effects of CSA on later adjustment were of small size, in meta-analytic terms, and when the effects of other confounding variables, such as family environment, were controlled for, the causal relationship between CSA and psychological adjustment largely disappeared. Females were more likely than males to report negative emotional reactions in the short term. This was related to there being more non-consensual and intra-familial CSA among the females than the males. Reactions were most negative when the CSA involved force or incestuous relationships, and intra-familial CSA was unusual in these college samples.

Because of the extraordinary public and political reaction to this paper, it was carefully scrutinized by Hyde (2003). She concluded that the meta-analysis was generally well conducted, but she had reservations about the authors' interpretation of their results. Focusing on college students would select out those who had been more seriously affected. There were, nevertheless, significant effects in both the national (Rind & Tromovitch 1997) and college student analyses (Rind et al 1998), which, though small, probably reflected a large effect for some and little or no effect for the majority. The fact that a wide range of sexual experiences were included, many of which (e.g. exhibitionism) would be unlikely to be more than transiently unpleasant, would contribute to this picture. In Hyde's opinion, studies that examined the effects of force, duration of the abuse and incest were too few to allow Rind et al (1998) to validly assess the moderators. She also suggested that in the first paper (Rind & Tromovich 1997) the magnitude of effect may have been underestimated because of the very limited questions used in these surveys, all of which had a much wider objective than assessing CSA.

If we accept Hyde's evaluation we are faced with an extensive literature which focuses on the more serious forms of CSA and the literature meta-analysed by Rind et al (1998) which focuses predominantly on the less severe forms.

Models of the impact of child sexual abuse

A recurring theme in this literature is the apparent surprise that the consequences of CSA are so variable, involving a wide range of psychological sequelae, and obviously substantial individual variability in response patterns. When one considers the substantial variation in the nature of CSA, the differing ages at which it occurs, varying degrees of 'closeness' to the perpetrator, ranging from a complete stranger to one's father, variability in responses to stress and coping strategies used, as well as the level of support available to the young person, this variability of CSA effects seems hardly surprising. However, the tendency to see CSA as a 'unitary' phenomenon leads to an expectation of a predictable 'unitary' response pattern. The closest that the evidence gets to indicating a characteristic CSA response pattern is in the development of 'sexualized' behaviours and the relative frequency of PTSD.

Various models have been proposed to account for the sequelae of CSA. Two will be considered here. The particular difficulties that follow sexual abuse of a child by a family member, and which place the child in a seemingly impossible position, were well described by Summit (1983). He used the term 'child sexual abuse accommodation syndrome' to describe a reaction 'which allows for the immediate survival of the child within the family but which tends to isolate the child from eventual acceptance, credibility or empathy within the larger society'. There are five components to this syndrome:

1. *Secrecy*. The child, following abuse, is readily caught in a web of secrecy. 'You mustn't tell anyone or ...' and a variety of alarming consequences may be spelt out, including the perpetrator being sent to prison, the family breaking up, the mother being

heartbroken, etc. The need for secrecy makes it clear that what has happened is *bad,* whilst the maintenance of secrecy seems to be the only safe escape route to follow.

2. *Helplessness.* The need for secrecy plus the natural tendency for a child to be influenced by an adult in a position of authority results in a sense of helplessness and the likelihood of acquiescence to further and continuing sexual abuse. 'The child has no choice but to submit quietly and to keep the secret ... The threat of loss of love and loss of family is more frightening to the child than any threat of violence'. The resulting feeling of having allowed the abuse to occur then leads to self-condemnation and self-hate.

3. *Entrapment and accommodation.* Once the child becomes entrapped in this helpless situation, accommodation to the continuing abuse may result in a variety of maladaptive or pathological patterns of survival, which may lead to long-term behavioural and personality problems. These include pathological dependency, self-punishment, self-mutilation, 'selective restructuring of reality and multiple personalities'. It is difficult for a child to accept the conclusion that a parent is ruthless and self-centred — 'this is tantamount to abandonment'. The only acceptable conclusion for the child is to believe that the child has provoked the painful encounter. The potential for distortion of reality and self-reproach in such a situation was well described by Summit: 'She may fight with both parents but her greatest rage is likely to focus on her mother whom she blames for driving the father into her bed'. A child in these circumstances is given the power to destroy the family and hence the responsibility for holding it together — a demand which reinforces the sense of entrapment.

4. *Delayed, conflicted and unconvincing disclosure.* Disclosure either does not occur at all or often at a much later date when the child is locked in destructive battle with one or other parent which results from the chronic tension and unresolved resentment. Frequently therefore the child makes the disclosure at the time when the child is least likely to be believed. According to Summit, most mothers are unaware of ongoing sexual abuse in the family. Faced with the child's disclosure there is an understandable tendency in many mothers to believe the father — 'to accept the alternative means annihilation of the family and a large piece of her own identity'.

5. *Retraction.* 'Whatever a child says about sexual abuse, she is likely to reverse it. ... In the chaotic aftermath of disclosure the child discovers that the threats underlying the secrecy are true'. The split in the family looms large, the child may be disowned by other family members — and perhaps most unjust of all, the child is the one most likely to be removed from the home, the father left unscathed because of the difficulties of mounting sufficient evidence against him. The rejection of the child's pleas for help may be the most traumatic aspect of the whole experience. It is not surprising that faced with the cataclysmic consequences of disclosure the child ends up retracting the complaint.

Summit's account is plausible and makes psychological sense, yet it has been largely ignored in the recent literature.

Finkelhor & Browne (1986) proposed that the experience of CSA, in more general terms, can be analysed in terms of four trauma-causing factors, what they called 'traumagenic dynamics': traumatic sexualization, betrayal, powerlessness and stigmatization. 'Traumatic sexualization' is considered further below. Betrayal relates to the sense that one has been exploited by someone one had previously trusted. Powerlessness refers to the process in which the child's will, desires and sense of efficacy are continually overruled. Such 'entrapment' is not confined to the use of force or threat; a child can feel trapped simply because of awareness of the consequences of disclosing the abuse. Stigmatization involves the various ways that the child may feel bad, guilty or ashamed, which may result from the ways that others react to the abuse. It should also be considered that such guilt may be engendered in a child who has experienced some sexual pleasure from the abuse experience, when confronted by the 'official' view that children are asexual. Finkelhor & Browne (1986) regarded these broad categories as useful for organizing and categorizing our understanding of the effects of CSA. There are obviously a number of overlaps with Summits' model, though this four-factor model is of more general relevance to CSA. Both models are examples of 'organizing models' as described in Chapter 2 (see p. 17); they do not lead to testable hypotheses, but they do help us to organize how we think about complex interactive patterns of reaction, in ways which are of clinical value.

Barker-Collo & Read (2003) reviewed a number of other models aimed at linking CSA to later adjustment problems. In these models the interaction between factors specific to the CSA experience, interactions with others following the abuse, and individual coping patterns were explored using path analysis. Although the explained portion of the variance varied according to which mediators and moderators were entered in each model, and some explanatory value may have resulted, there is, as yet, no clear evidence that such post hoc modelling is of clinical value when working with victims of CSA, at whatever age.

The effects of child sexual abuse on sexual development

In addition to this pervasive tendency to see any form of sexual involvement with a child as damaging, another contrast with the earlier literature is apparent. Part of the current reaction to CSA involves a need to see any child, however defined, as asexual. Thus it is not currently acceptable to even consider whether a child (i.e. any one under 16) may have consented to a sexual interaction, or in any way found it pleasurable, even though evidence of consent may influence the legal sentencing, as considered at the start of this chapter. Whereas the issue of consent in no way affects the moral and legal unacceptability of an older person exploiting the child sexually, it could have a considerable bearing on how the child reacts to the experience, and how best the child should be helped to deal with it. The relevance of this to the vexed issue of 'sexualization' will be considered later. This issue of consent was, however, addressed in the earlier literature. In those cases that came before the courts, it was usually considered difficult to establish the extent to which the child consented, particularly when below the age of 10. Walmsley & White (1979), however, concluded that with victims of indecent assault, about one-fifth of girls aged 10–12, one-third of girls aged 13–15, about one-fifth of boys aged 10–13 and about two-fifths of boys aged 14–15 consented. In Gebhard et al's study 1965, 16% of the girls under 12 and 86% of girls aged 12–15 were said to be 'encouraging' to the offender, whilst the percentages for the boys were 52% for the under 12 and 70% for those aged 12–15. These figures were based on evidence in the records; the percentages were, needless to say, higher according to the offenders themselves. It is perfectly possible that a child could be encouraging yet end up being frightened or disturbed by the experience. But we should also accept the possibility that in a proportion of cases the child gains some emotional reward from the experience, although this is much less likely when the abuser is a family member. However, this confronts us with the crucial issue of the extent to which the sexual abuse experience was, at least at the time it occurred, sexually arousing and in some sense pleasurable, or predominantly distressing, or a mixture of the two.

In so far as CSA is traumatic, it is not difficult to understand the various emotional and cognitive adverse reactions, both short and long term, which have been considered above. The variability not only reflects varying degrees of trauma, but also the varied family and social reactions as well as marked individual variability in coping with trauma and stress. However, it is conceivable that, in some cases, the major psychological trauma evolves later as the child comes to terms with what has happened. Hence, the initial experience may have been sexually pleasurable, or at least 'neutral', but was followed by a negative psychological reaction. However, understanding how subsequent behaviour becomes 'sexualized', probably the most predictable consequence of CSA, presents us with a formidable challenge, and it is probably fair to say that no adequate explanation has yet emerged. Much of the literature points to a 'polarization' with some individuals experiencing negative effects on their sexuality, leading to subsequent varieties of 'sexual dysfunction' or 'sexual aversion' and others showing 'sexualization' in the sense of increased or enhanced sexuality, though typically maladaptive or inappropriate in some respect. Overall, there is much more evidence on this issue relating to women than to men.

The literature on the adverse effects of CSA on sexual function during adolescence and adulthood is not only extensive but also confusing and inconsistent (e.g. see reviews by Loeb et al 2002; Ahmad 2006). This, to a large extent, results from inconsistencies in how both CSA and sexual function were defined or assessed, and varying types of samples, mostly clinical and, in several cases, involving individuals who have presented with complaints of sexual problems. Of particular importance is variability in the age range for when CSA occurred. If we are to understand the impact of CSA on sexual development, we should pay particular attention to the stage of sexual development at which it occurred, or at least started. As considered earlier, Kendall-Tackett et al (1993) in their review concluded that one of the characteristic reactions of the sexually abused preschool child is sexually inappropriate behaviour, less evident in school-age children. The developmental sequence elaborated in Chapter 5 should be kept in mind; in particular, Friedrich's finding that such behaviour that had hitherto been considered evidence of CSA, occurred in a proportion of unabused young children (Friedrich et al 1991; see p. 148). Such explicit behaviours are more likely to be observed by parents of preschool children before the child learns that such behaviours are taboo, and should be kept private — in what used to be called the 'latency period'. However, the pre-pubertal school-aged child, while having started to attribute 'sexual meanings', may not have started to adopt any age-appropriate 'sexual script', and may not have even experienced 'sexual arousal'. The young person in mid-adolescence will not only be more likely to be familiar with sexual response and arousal but will have, in most cases, adopted age-appropriate sexual scripts. We then have to consider what impact CSA might have at these very different stages of sexual development.

The limited evidence from community-based samples of the relationship between a history of CSA and sexual problems or dysfunction in adulthood suggest that some recover from the CSA with little long-term disruption of their sexual function, whereas others end up with sexual problems. The NHSLS survey asked questions about CSA, restricting attention to CSA before puberty (or the age of 12; Laumann et al 1994). Limited questions were also asked about sexual response. In assessing predictors of what they called 'sexual dysfunction' they found that being 'sexually touched before puberty' was, in women, associated with an increased likelihood of sexual arousal problems, but not low sexual desire or sexual pain; in men it was associated with an increased likelihood of premature ejaculation, erectile dysfunction and low sexual desire (Laumann et al 1999). Najman et al (2005), on the other hand, in a community sample of Australian men and women, and using the same questions about 'sexual dysfunction' as in the NHSLS, found stronger association between CSA and sexual problems in women than in men. The results from both these studies should be treated with caution because of the method of assessing sexual dysfunction. This is discussed more fully in Chapter 11 (see p. 310).

The evidence of 'sexualization' is paradoxically more consistent. Women with a history of CSA, in comparison with women without such history, show earlier onset of 'voluntary' sexual intercourse, and by age 18 years, more sexual partners, more unprotected sex, a higher pregnancy rate, more STDs and more sexual revictimization (e.g. Browning & Laumann 1997; Fergusson et al 1997). Men with a history of CSA are more likely to engage in high-risk sexual behaviour as adolescents and adults, to have more sexual partners and to become victimizers themselves (Dhaliwal et al 1996). They are also more likely to end up with a homosexual identity (Laumann et al 2003; Paul et al 2003). This has raised the vexed question of whether or not the CSA influenced their sexual identity development. Gender identity confusion may occur as a result of the abusive experiences undermining the boy's sense of masculinity (Gill & Tutty 1999). It is also possible, however, that gender non-conformity during childhood, which pre-empted the emergence of their homosexual identity, made them more likely to be sexually abused.

The study reported by Paul et al (2003), which focused on adult homosexual males who had clearly been coerced sexually before the age of 17, showed that their increased likelihood of high-risk sexual behaviour was more likely to involve unprotected *insertive* than unprotected *receptive* anal intercourse, which as the authors comment, contrasts with the more receptive risk taking of sexually abused women, pointing to a gender difference in the impact of CSA on sexuality. It is possible, however, that this pattern in homosexual males who have been abused reflects some identification with their abusers who were insertive with them (Paul et al 2003), a pattern that is not relevant to a female who has been abused.

An important longitudinal study of intra-familial sexual abuse of female children, reported by Noll et al (2003), warrants close consideration. Girls who had been sexually abused were recruited, together with their principal carer (usually mother) from protective service agencies in Washington DC. They were aged 6–16 and had experienced sexual abuse by a family member involving genital contact and/or penetration. They were all assessed within 6 months of disclosure of their abuse. A control group of non-abused girls, matched for age and other demographics was also recruited. Childhood sexual behaviour problems were assessed using the Child Sexual Behavior Inventory (Friedrich et al 1992) completed by the principal carer. After the initial assessment, four further follow-up assessments were carried out over the next 10 years; age at final assessment ranged from 13.3 to 28.3 years, with 77 in the abused and 89 in the control group. Using a measure of sexual activities and attitudes, four factors were assessed at follow up: 'sexual permissiveness', 'sexual preoccupation', 'negative attitude towards sex' and 'pressure to engage in sex'. Established measures of depression and trait anxiety were used together with a measure of 'childhood dissociation', an area of particular interest to one of the authors (Putnam 1997).

In comparing the abused and non-abused control groups for the factor scores on the sexual activity and attitudes measure, only 'sexual pre-occupation' was significantly but modestly higher in the abused group ($p = 0.04$). However, the abused group reported a significantly younger age at first sexual intercourse ($p = 0.0002$), endorsed significantly lower birth control efficacy ($p = 0.0008$), significantly more teenage births ($p = 0.0001$) and younger age at birth of first child ($p = 0.0004$). CSA remained a significant predictor of 'sexual preoccupation' at final follow-up, after controlling for depression, pathological dissociation and sexual behaviour problems at earlier assessments. In addition, trait anxiety, as measured at the third follow-up, was predictive of 'sexual preoccupation' at final follow-up ($p < 0.05$). Interestingly, childhood sexual behaviour problems (e.g. public displays of sexualized behaviour, inappropriate sex play and excessive masturbation) were predictive of later 'sexual aversion', but only in the abused group.

Using criteria from a previous study, the abused group were divided into three subgroups: a single perpetrator (SP) subgroup ($n = 34$), abused by one person, not their biological father, with relatively short duration of abuse, and violence infrequent; multiple perpetrator (MP) subgroup ($n = 23$), abused by more than one person, not their biological father, over a relatively short period but with physical violence relatively frequent; and a biological father (BF) subgroup ($n = 20$), abused by their biological father over a long period, beginning at a relatively young age, with a low occurrence of violence. Comparison of these three subgroups showed that only the SP subgroup scored significantly higher than the control group for 'sexual preoccupation'; the BF subgroup scored significantly higher than the SP subgroup and the controls for 'sexual aversion'. A 'sexual ambivalence' score was derived by combining the 'sexual preoccupation' and 'sexual aversion' factors scores. This 'sexual ambivalence' score was significantly higher in the BF subgroup than both the SP and the MP subgroups and the controls.

In discussing these findings Noll et al (2003) speculated that the association between CSA and early motherhood may result from an expectation that having a child might compensate for feelings of inadequacy and loneliness. The BF subgroup can, perhaps, be regarded as the most seriously abused group, given that it was their biological father abusing them over a long time period. As the authors pointed out, the absence of physical force in this subgroup does not detract from the large power differential in such abuse. But at the same time, the continuing compliance in the absence of force may lead to greater self-blame subsequently. It is therefore of particular interest that this subgroup were most likely to show 'sexual aversion'. Equally interesting is the greater tendency for the SP subgroup, who can be regarded as experiencing the least severe or traumatic abuse of the three subgroups, to show later 'sexual preoccupation'. The authors suggested that this might be an indication of 'unexpressed or internalized sexual compulsions'.

How might we explain the 'polarized' effects of CSA on adolescent and adult sexuality? Browning & Laumann (1997, 2003), in comparing the relative merits of their life-course perspective and the more conventional psychogenic perspective in explaining long-term consequences of CSA (see p. 479), challenged the 'polarizing' assumption in much of the psychogenic literature, i.e. victims of CSA end up with either sexual avoidance or 'sexualization'. They used data from the NHSLS and the Chicago HSLS to show that 'sexualization' was clearly evident, but sexual avoidance was not. This was based on the apparent lack of association between history of CSA and sexual inactivity, in contrast to the association with early onset of sexual intercourse, more partners, more sexual risk taking, etc. However, they did, as mentioned above, find some associations with impaired sexual function. Hence a polarizing effect may distinguish between 'hypersexuality' and 'impaired sexual response or interest'. In some respects it may be possible to get some degree of both in the same individual. It is also possible that individuals who react to CSA with sexual avoidance, or 'sexual aversion', such as those identified by Noll et al (2003; see above), may be less likely to report a history of CSA in community surveys (for discussion of this issue, see Bancroft 2003; pp. 375–379).

Leonard & Follette (2002), in their review, commented that the literature on the effects of CSA 'continues to be overrun by correlational data. There is a significant lag in research that would actually support any theoretical position' (p. 362). They went on to consider two explanatory models for sexual avoidance or aversion, although, needless to say, neither with supportive evidence. They pointed to 'avoidance' as a recurring theme in the literature, and considered more closely Polusny & Follette's (1995) 'experiential avoidance' model. 'Experiential avoidance ... includes an unwillingness to experience painful thoughts, feelings or memories associated with abuse or other traumatic events' (p. 363). However, in spite of the avoidance of negative affective states that result, this pattern is considered to be part of less effective coping. They suggest that this avoidance mechanism could contribute to avoidance of sexual activity per se, but also to 'compulsive' patterns of sexuality of the kind referred to above as 'sexualization', presumably because the avoidance excludes proper consideration of the consequences. No indication is given as to why this 'experiential avoidance' leads to sexual avoidance in some and 'sexualized' behaviour in others. They go on to consider Greenberg's 'emotion theory' (e.g. Greenberg et al 1993), which includes the concept of 'emotion schemes,' which contain complex cognitive, affective motivational and relational action components. Such 'schemes', when evoked, involve the whole response complex. Negative emotional experiences, such as CSA, might result in the development of maladaptive 'emotion schemes' that may be activated inappropriately, e.g. by the partner's intimate physical touching in an adult relationship, resulting in sexual relationship problems. Leonard & Follette (2002) point out that such models overlap with other theoretical models. It may be particularly relevant to consider the overlap between 'experiential avoidance' and 'denial'. This defence against painful reality has been described as evident from early childhood, becoming less evident as the child matures (Paulhus et al 1997). It may therefore be a coping strategy, which becomes established with early CSA and persists in a maladaptive fashion.

Is the Dual Control model, conceptualizing individual differences in the propensity for sexual excitation and inhibition, a recurring theme throughout this book, of any relevance to the impact of CSA on sexual development? Recent research on these concepts in men and women has shown a range of factors that inhibit sexual response with considerable individual variability in the propensity for such inhibition (Janssen et al 2002; Graham et al 2006). There are similarities but also differences between men and women in the types of situation or thought that inhibit sexual response. It is not yet clear to what extent these propensities are learnt or are more innate, although there is evidence from a twin study of a genetic contribution to inhibition proneness in men (Varjonen et al 2007). This has not yet been assessed in women. Of particular interest in women is the factor labelled 'arousal contingency', involving items such as 'unless everything is just right I have difficulty becoming sexually aroused' and 'the slightest thing can turn me off'. This factor is strongly related to sexual problems in women. As yet such instruments have not been used to assess victims of CSA. However, it is possible that men or women with a high propensity for sexual inhibition are particularly susceptible to the negative effects of CSA. Future research should examine more closely sexual inhibition and excitation proneness in men and women with and without a history of CSA, and at the same time explore the potentially inhibiting thoughts that such individuals have in sexual situations, keeping in mind that there may be important gender differences.

What mechanisms may account for 'sexualization'? This is particularly difficult to answer when conceptualized as 'traumatic sexualization'. If we put the traumatic aspect on one side for a moment, we can more easily ask whether or not, at least in some cases, CSA produces early sexual arousal and pleasure which may then be further pursued by the child, in ways which are usually inappropriate. This confronts us once again with the 'political incorrectness' of considering sexual pleasure in a child, particularly resulting from interaction with someone older. It is the reluctance in the more recent literature to explicitly explore this possibility that may have contributed to the prevailing confusion. In contrast, Browning & Laumann (1997), in elaborating their life-course perspective, explicitly considered the possibility that the adult–child sexual experience eroticizes the child, albeit resulting in adoption of age-inappropriate sexual scripts leading to problematic sexual behaviour. Much earlier, Gagnon & Simon (1973) suggested that for some preadolescent girls, less likely for boys, the impact of the adult–child sexual contact is less determined by any resulting sexual arousal or pleasure and more by 'an instrumental use of sexuality to achieve non-sexual goals and gratifications' (p. 37). If we accept these accounts then we can start our list of explanations of 'sexualization' with (i) early activation of sexual pleasure as a motivation for subsequent behaviour and (ii) early discovery that engagement in sexual interaction may result in non-sexual rewards. It is difficult from the existing literature to assess how often these two types of 'sexualization' occur, but it is reasonable to conclude that they are more likely when there is some degree of consent by the child and when the adult's behaviour is not frightening, threatening or physically painful. Such cases, therefore, are less likely to feature in case studies involving clinical or legal interventions, which account for much of the literature. A third pattern, mentioned earlier, is that the initial adult–child sexual experience is sexually pleasant or rewarding for the child but is followed by awareness of the implications of the adult–child experience, leading to various kinds of negative emotional response. This may be particularly likely if the child finds that after the first involvement the adult expects repeated involvement, resulting in a sense of powerlessness in the child. This is one aspect of the models of negative reaction by Summitt (1983) and Finkelhor & Browne (1986), considered above. This may overlap with a fourth pattern, what Noll et al (2003) called 'unexpressed or internalized sexual compulsions' (see above). The concept of 'sexual compulsivity' is problematic. However, if we instead use the concept of sexual behaviour which is in some sense 'out of control, often called 'sexual compulsivity' or 'sexual addiction', then a paradoxical relation between negative mood and sexual arousability is of considerable importance for both men and women (Bancroft & Vukadinovic 2004, and see p. 330 for further discussion). This raises the potentially crucial possibility that early abusive sexual experiences, which result in a mixture of sexual arousal or pleasure and negative mood, such as anxiety or depression, could lead to such paradoxical mood–sexuality relationships, shown in men to be not only relevant to 'out of control' sexual behaviour, but also to sexual risk taking (Bancroft et al 2003b, 2004; Bancroft & Vukadinovic 2004). Given that in men they have found to be negatively correlated to age (this association has not yet been assessed in women), it remains a possibility that there may be a 'critical period' during early sexual development when such paradoxical mood–sexuality relationships may be established. As the evidence points to 'sexualized' behaviour being a more common consequence of CSA than 'sexual avoidance', it should be possible to establish in community-based samples of younger adults, whether these paradoxical mood–sexuality relationships, found in around 15% of men (Bancroft et al 2003c,d) and 19% of college women (Lykins et al 2006), are more common in those with a history of CSA, and if so what pattern of CSA they are most associated with. Schloredt & Heiman (2003) have made a start; they compared 70 women with a history of CSA, 44 of whom also experienced physical abuse, with 78 women with no abuse histories. The abused group reported more negative affect during sexual arousal (in particular, anger or 'unpleasant excitement'). The Dual Control model may also be relevant here; these paradoxical patterns are more likely in men with high propensity for sexual excitation and low propensity for sexual inhibition, and in women with high propensity for sexual excitation (Bancroft et al 2003c,d; Lykins et al 2006).

Helping the victims of child sexual abuse

Once sexual abuse has been established or suspected, the style of intervention varies according to the nature of the abuse. When children have been abused by strangers, there is a particular need to work with the family, as the reactions of family members, especially parents, may be important in determining whether the child suffers long-term consequences. The parents should be helped to deal with the child in a supportive way, encouraging open discussion of what happened rather than maintaining a collusive silence, which serves to reinforce the 'badness' of what happened. Such incidents provide an opportunity for parents to have more open discussions of sexual matters, which help to place the abuse incident into perspective, whilst also having a generally beneficial educational effect.

When abuse involves an acquaintance, and even more a family member, intervention becomes much more problematic. There is likely to be a need for individual support for the child. It is of paramount importance to ensure that the child has *someone* who believes the story and who repeatedly affirms the child's fundamental innocence (whatever the circumstances) in a consistent fashion. It is not always possible to achieve that, especially in those cases where the abuse is denied by the alleged perpetrator, there is no corroborative evidence and the family closes ranks to prevent contact with the child. Clearly there is also likely to be a need for counselling and support for the parents. Many workers advocate family therapy and report success in keeping many families together, which might otherwise disintegrate in such circumstances. The Ciba working party on the subject (Porter 1984) made recommendations for family involvement, as well as guidelines for general management of such cases, based on the work of the NSPCC Special Unit and Family Centre.

Treatment of sexual problems in adults with a history of CSA was considered by Leonard & Follette (2002). In particular, they discussed the use of acceptance and commitment therapy (ACT) based on the theory of experiential avoidance, and emotion-focused therapy, based on emotion theory and attachment theory. These approaches address some of the key issues that may be involved in the sexual aftermath of CSA. Group therapy may be helpful in dealing with the emotional consequences. Kessler et al (2003) reviewed 13 outcome studies of group therapy, 7 of which had some form of control. They concluded that, while variable, there was evidence of benefits, particularly in those less severely traumatized. When dealing with the negative sexual consequences, the principles outlined can be incorporated into the model of sex therapy which is described in Chapter 12, and by Hall (2007) where examples are given of how to proceed when issues relating to CSA arise. The value of this sex therapy approach is that it provides a behavioural framework that, stage by stage, elicits key issues relevant to impairment of sexual interest and response. Once issues are elicited in this way, a variety of psychotherapeutic strategies, including cognitive behavioural therapy, can be employed to deal with them.

Helping the individual with 'sexualization' as a consequence of CSA presents, in some respects, a more complex challenge. In those cases where there is evidence of sex being used as a mood regulator, as with many forms of 'out of control' sexual behaviour, cognitive behaviour therapy (CBT), focusing on the sequence typically leading from negative mood to sexual 'acting out', can pave the way for behavioural change. There is also a place for the use of pharmacological agents, especially serotonin selective reuptake inhibitors (SSRIs) in such cases. Group methods are also used, particularly for those with 'out of control' sexuality and there are obvious advantages to the group format in this context; it can be particularly helpful to have a number of women with similar experiences who can share their feelings and validate each other's reactions. These treatment approaches are also considered more closely in Chapter 12.

Overall, however, we remain with little empirical evidence of the effectiveness of any of these treatment approaches, particularly in dealing with the sexual consequences of CSA. As with helping the rape victim, considered earlier, until we have a clear evidence base for how to proceed in such cases, it is appropriate and ethical to apply more general principles of counselling and sex therapy.

The management of sex offenders

There is little doubt that the most effective method of discouraging sexual offences is the threat of legal sanctions. The large majority of first-time convicted sex offenders (around 86%; see above) are not re-convicted of sexual offences. There is nevertheless a small minority of recidivists who may present considerable problems both to themselves and to society. Ironically, it is the sex offender who is most likely to benefit from psychological treatment or counselling who is also the one most effectively deterred by the threat of re-conviction. The recidivist, on the other hand, usually presents a formidable treatment problem. It therefore remains an issue of some importance that we find methods of intervention that reduce re-offending, which if effective, might also have value in reducing offending in the first place, at least in those potential offenders who are motivated to seek help.

In practice, the opportunities for helpful interventions are largely restricted to when an offender is incarcerated in prison or hospital, or occasionally as a condition of probation. Two types of intervention will be considered: the use of pharmacological or hormonal agents and psychological methods of inducing behaviour change. Each has its own particular challenges.

The use of pharmacological or hormonal agents raises a major ethical issue. It is essential, from the ethical point of view, to distinguish between social control, which is control of the offender for the benefit of society, and treatment aimed at helping the offender. The normal methods of social control, such as custodial sentences, are subject to the normal rigors of the legal process and are consequently not problematic in this sense. On the other hand, drugs or hormones (or in the past surgical castration or psychosurgery), because of their medical connotations, can be imposed without the full surveillance of the legal process.

Drugs that lower sexual drive can be used as part of genuine medical treatment and do have a place in that respect. But their use in the management of offenders, particularly those in custody, makes it difficult, if not impossible, to ensure consent free from coercion. The offender may end up receiving social control without the safeguards that accompany the usual legal sanctions, justified on the grounds that it is 'medical treatment' and in the offender's own interest. Such use presents a troubling precedent. One can see how drugs could eventually be used for other types of offence, e.g. to control aggressive behaviour — the thin end of a particularly worrying medico-political wedge. I continue to hold the view that if such methods are to be used, they should only be used under the public scrutiny of the court, and not only according to the personal judgement of a forensic physician or psychiatrist. Some attempt to safeguard against such a development was introduced in the 1983 Mental Health Act, where, under Section 57, the administration of libido-reducing hormone preparations by means of surgical implant required not only the formal consent of the offender but also the concurring opinion of a member of the Mental Health Act Commission.

With this major qualification about their use, let us therefore consider the effects of such pharmacological and hormonal methods before passing on to psychological methods of treatment and counselling, and the particular challenges that they pose.

Hormonal reduction of sexual interest

In Chapter 4, we discussed the evidence for hormonal and biochemical determinants of human sexuality and concluded that sexual appetite or interest, and some central aspects of sexual arousal are androgen dependent in the majority of males. It is thus feasible that unwanted sexual drive can be reduced by lowering androgens or in some way blocking their action. Whether such an approach is useful in managing a particular sex offender obviously depends on the extent to which the offender's criminal behaviour is determined by the sexual drive. As we have seen throughout this chapter, this is not a straightforward matter. But in a proportion of cases, such an approach is likely to be effective.

Oestrogens were used for this purpose for many years (Scott 1964). The precise mechanism of action was never clearly established but probably involved a combination of an anti-gonadotrophic effect resulting in a reduction of circulating androgen levels, and some more direct anti-androgenic effect at the target organ. As discussed in Chapter 4, such anti-androgenic effects of oestrogens are somewhat paradoxical, given the extent to which androgen effects in the brain depend on aromatization to oestrogen. In any case, estrogens are unpleasant hormones for men to take. Nausea is common and gynaecomastia develops in the majority of cases. Malignant change in the resulting breast tissue and thrombotic complications elsewhere may occasionally occur.

Progestagens have also been used, although their effects in reducing sexual drive in men are also complex, involving both anti-gonadotrophic and other more direct antiandrogenic effects. Medroxyprogesterone acetate (MPA) has been used in the USA for this purpose for many years (Walker 1978). Once again, the mechanism of action is not fully understood. MPA reduces plasma T by about 80%, whereas luteinizing hormone (LH) is reduced by only 30% and follicle stimulating hormone is unaffected, raising questions about other direct effects on testosterone (T) synthesis or metabolism (Meyer et al 1985). However, the T suppression can be reversed by human chorionic gonadotrophin (Kirschner & Schneider 1972). Other direct progestational effects may also be involved. Use of MPA for reducing relevant patterns of sexual interest and response in sexual offenders has been reviewed by Bradford & Greenberg (1996). There is reasonably consistent evidence of a beneficial effect, although little placebo-controlled evaluation has been reported and long-term use appears to be necessary to be effective. Side effects are probably less troublesome than with oestrogens; however, diabetes mellitus, increased blood pressure and gallstones have all been reported with long-term MPA use (Meyer et al 1985).

The preparation that has been most widely used outside the USA is cyproterone acetate (CPA), an antiandrogen that combines a specific blocking of androgen effects at the androgen receptor with an anti-gonadotrophic progestagenic action. Its effectiveness in controlling a variety of sexual offence behaviour was reported in early studies (Laschet & Laschet 1969; Davies 1974). In an early controlled study, CPA was found to be similar to ethinyloestradiol in short-term effects (5 weeks), each reducing both self-reported sexual interest and activity (Bancroft et al 1974). There was no consistent effect of either compound on erectile response to erotic stimuli. A placebo-controlled evaluation of CPA taken over a longer period (total of 6 months of CPA and 6 months of placebo) was reported by Bradford & Paulak (1993). This also showed a significant effect of CPA on measures of sexual interest and behaviour, and subjective ratings of arousal in response to erotic stimuli, but not erectile response to erotic stimuli. These discrepant findings between subjective and erectile response in these early studies need to be reconsidered in the light of more recent evidence of the effects of T deficiency discussed in Chapter 4 (see p. 112). Early studies of hypogonadal men, relying on measurement of maximum penile circumference increase to erotic stimuli, concluded that erectile response was not T dependent. More recent studies have shown this to be an artefact of the method of assessing erectile response; if rigidity of erection, as well as duration of erectile response beyond withdrawal of the erotic stimulus, is assessed, then T replacement is shown to enhance erectile response.

There have also been a series of studies showing that long-term CPA administration reduces re-offending in offenders with previously high recidivism rates (for review see Bradford & Greenberg 1996). Side effects of CPA are relatively minor, but significant depression sometimes occurs and there is a 20% likelihood of gynaecomastia. There is also suppression of spermatogenesis, but this is probably reversible.

Increasing attention is being paid to the use of luteinizing hormone releasing hormone (LHRH) agonists or antagonists to manage sexual offenders. (Agonists initially stimulate androgen production but quickly pass on to reduce it by receptor down-regulation.) In Chapter 4, recent studies were reviewed showing that lowering of T by such agonists or antagonists produces a reversible decline in sexual interest in normal eugonadal young men (Bagatell et al 1994; see p. 113). There is, as yet, limited evidence of their use in the management of sexual offenders. Rosler & Witztum (1998) reported an open study of 30 sex offenders (25 paedophiles). Of the 25 men who continued treatment for 12 months, all reported virtual elimination of deviant fantasies and interests. Comparable results were reported by Thibaut et al (1996). In a recent study, Schober et al (2005) assessed the combination of CBT and leuprolide acetate, an LHRH agonist in five paedophiles, all previously imprisoned for sex offences. The subjects were all informed that they would be randomly assigned to either active drug or placebo, and the therapists and researchers assessing them were also blind. In fact, they were all given 3-monthly depot injections of active drug for a year, followed by a year of placebo injections. Their assessment included 'lie detection' by polygraphy. The combination of CBT and active injections reduced their sexual interest and erectile responsiveness but did not eliminate a paedophilic preference. Active injections reduced T to castrate levels. Polygraphy indicated that deceptive answers to assessment questions were given during the placebo period, but not during the active treatment. Further evaluation of long-term use of LHRH agonists/antagonists is clearly required, but these early results are promising.

Pharmacological reduction of sexual interest

Various tranquillizers and psychotropic drugs have been tried for this purpose (Bartholomew 1968), and a butyrophenone, benperidol was marketed as having specific libido-reducing effects (Sterkmans & Geerts 1966). The mechanism of action of such a drug is not known and the endocrine effects are not the same as those produced by CPA or oestrogens (Murray et al 1975). In one controlled study, benperidol was found to be significantly more effective than chlorpromazine or placebo in reducing sexual interest, though the effect on sexual activity was not significant and over all the effects were modest (Tennent et al 1974). Benperidol has sedative as well as extrapyramidal side effects.

More recently considerable attention has been paid to the effects of SSRIs in the management of paraphilic sexuality. This was considered more closely in Chapter 12 in relation to treatment of 'out of control' sexual behaviour. Evidence of the benefits of SSRIs in the management of sexual offenders is so far limited. Bradford and colleagues (cited in Bradford & Federoff 2006) reported a 12-week open-label dose-titrated study of sertraline in the treatment of paedophilia. A significant decrease in 'the severity of paedophilia' was found. For some reason this report has not been published. Because of these potential benefits of SSRIs, and observations that decrease in paraphilic interest can occur without impairment of 'non-paraphilic' sexual response, paedophilia and other illegal paraphilias are being considered as obsessive–compulsive phenomena. As yet the published evidence does not warrant such an assumption. The effects of SSRIs are likely to be complex. Relatively specific inhibition of sexual response, particularly orgasm and ejaculation, is a common side effect in both men and women (Rosen et al 1999). SSRIs are also effective in improving mood. The possibility that much of the beneficial effects of SSRIs in relation to unwanted sexuality relate to the underlying paradoxical relationship between negative mood and sexuality, discussed earlier, is considered in Chapter 12 (p. 376).

The use of pharmacological and hormonal agents to control sexual offences is therefore still of uncertain value. This is of particular relevance when using them for social control, when it is important to be confident of the effects before using such agents as an alternative to imprisonment. A further problem is to ensure that the drugs are taken. The availability of injectable CPA, MPA and LHRH agonists is a partial solution to that problem.

The use of such drugs as part of genuine medical treatment is less problematic. They are then used at the request of the patient, who carries the responsibility for whether he takes them or not. Similarly, he can decide whether to run the risks of side effects once they have been fully explained to him. Some individuals may find that the reduction of problematic sexual interest is a considerable relief and drug administration can be usefully combined with other psychological methods of treatment.

Surgical methods of control

Far more controversial than pharmacological methods of control was the earlier use of irreversible surgical procedures, notably castration and psychosurgery. Castration was used to obtain substantial reduction of androgens. Helm & Hursch (1979) reviewed the principal follow-up studies of surgical castration for sexual offenders. Although there were a proportion of men, ranging from 10% to 34%, who continued to be sexually active indefinitely after the operation, the majority in each study showed a rapid decline in sexual interest with others showing a more gradual decline. Helm & Hursch (1979) rightly pointed out the methodological problems in evaluating the outcome in such cases, most of which were comparable to those affecting uncontrolled drug studies. But they rather overstated the case when claiming that there is no scientific basis for the operation. They also objected to the operation on ethical grounds, about which there can be little argument. It is difficult

to see how this operation, which is not only irreversible but also physically and psychologically mutilating, can be justified even in the face of unequivocal proof of its efficacy in reducing sexual offences.

Similar considerations apply to the past use of psychosurgery to control sexual offenders. Stereotaxic hypothalamotomy, aimed at ablating the ventromedial nucleus on one side, was advocated as a specific method of controlling unwanted sexual behaviour. Needless to say, a good scientific rationale of such a procedure was not presented and the ethical objections are insurmountable. This approach, which was largely confined to West Germany, was strongly criticized on both scientific and ethical grounds by Rieber & Sigusch (1979).

Psychological methods of treatment

Psychological treatment is less problematic from the ethical point of view. Change is only likely to occur if it is desired and actively sought by the offender. However, the use of such treatment confronts us with other, rather different challenges. First, effective treatment depends on an appropriate therapist–client relationship of the type described in Chapter 12. This is of 'adult–adult' type, as between a teacher and his adult pupil; the responsibility for change must lie with the pupil, however much the teacher provides guidance. Unfortunately, it is difficult to achieve such a relationship when the offender is either confined in prison or under pressure from the legal system to be compliant (Bancroft 1979). However, it is such a therapeutic relationship that is required if offenders are to be helped, at least on an individual basis. Group therapy may have advantages in dealing with this issue within prison (West et al 1978). Participants can use other group members to reflect their own problems and confront them with their need to accept responsibility for their actions. But here also lack of security and fear that one's release may be jeopardized may inhibit offenders from revealing all their fears and concerns.

Whereas in the early days of behaviour therapy for modifying deviant sexual behaviour, there was a tendency to prescribe specific and rather limited techniques such as aversion therapy, a more broad-spectrum and flexible approach emerged, designed to fit the needs of the individual case (Abel et al 1978). Before embarking on such treatment, it is therefore necessary to make a careful assessment of what Abel and his colleagues called the 'excesses and deficits' in each case. In many respects these are similar in the different categories of sexual offenders, as will have become apparent in this chapter. Certain aspects are more specific to particular kinds of offence, such as the sexually arousing effect of force or aggression in many rapists. The problem areas on which to focus in treatment and counselling can be considered under the following headings:

1. Problems in establishing satisfactory sexual relationships
2. Problems in established relationships of a sexual or general kind

3. Problems of lowered self-esteem, lack of assertiveness or lack of rewarding activities
4. Inadequate sexual arousal to normal sexual stimuli.
5. Problems of self-control and inappropriate sexual arousal to deviant stimuli

Whenever possible, it is desirable and more effective to take a constructive, positive approach to treatment, to help the individual build up or reinforce new and more adaptive behaviours rather than simply to eliminate old, undesirable ones. Sociosexual difficulties in establishing relationships can be tackled by means of social skills training on either a group or individual basis. The individual offender's methods of social interaction are analysed and fed back to him by means of video or audio recordings and appropriate comments. New ways of behaving are modelled and rehearsed. Methods of self-assertion are practised. Role-playing of relevant social situations using female subjects is often used, and both non-verbal and verbal skills are addressed (Pacht et al 1962; Abel et al 1978; Crawford & Allen 1979).

Individual counselling may have similar goals, particularly in offenders outside institutions. Thus specific target behaviours, such as a limited approach to a particular sexual partner, may be agreed and the offender sent away to try them out. The offender's attempts are then discussed with the therapist and possible reasons for failure considered and alternative approaches planned (Bancroft 1977).

In those men with established relationships, sexual problems are common, and counselling with the couple, as described in Chapter 12, is often appropriate once the offender is out of prison. The basic assumption is that if 'normal' sexuality becomes more rewarding, there will be less need for the antisocial forms of sex. The relevant problem in the relationship may not be sexual, however, and general marital counselling may be indicated.

General counselling or psychotherapy may also be helpful in those whose sexual offences are reflections of generally low self-esteem. In what ways can this individual reorganize his life to bolster his self-respect and provide greater personal rewards? Does he need special help with educational deficits? Would he benefit from some re-training, etc.?

Inadequate sexual responsiveness to appropriate stimuli may also be the focus of treatment, relevant to some individuals who have no current sexual partner. Exploration of sexual fantasies may be helpful, as discussed in Chapter 12, and systematic modification of fantasies during masturbation may be used (Bancroft 1974, 1977).

Most obvious as a goal of treatment is the improvement of self-control over antisocial sexual urges or, alternatively, a reduction in the strength of those urges. It is in this area of self-control that responsibility must be unequivocally placed with the offender. In both group and individual therapies, the open statement of a commitment to self-control can be helpful, making it more difficult for the offender to engage in self-deception. For this reason, periodic but regular contact between offender and therapist can be beneficial with little more involved than 'keeping an eye' on the offender and reiterating his commitment to self-control. At the same time, the therapeutic relationship can be maintained and the channels of communication kept open so that they can be used at times of crisis.

There are also more direct methods of enhancing self-control. In those cases where offences occur in a specific situation, as at the end of a predictable sequence of events, plans can be made to interrupt the sequence at an early stage and introduce some alternative, well-rehearsed behaviour. Thus if an exhibitionist tends to visit a particular place to expose himself, an early point on the route to that place should be identified and linked clearly with an alternative response (e.g. whenever you find yourself walking up X road, stop at the telephone box and phone up the hospital, asking to speak to the therapist). Such an approach requires not only a predictable sequence of behaviour for it to be easily applied but also a fair level of motivation. But there are cases that benefit from such tactics. Such self-management methods were described in more detail by Kanfer (1975).

Aversive techniques of one kind or another may still have a place in this context. A stimulus that would typically provoke antisocial behaviour is associated, either in imagination or in reality, with a noxious stimulus, such as an electric shock or an imagined traumatic event. This 'pairing' is carried out repeatedly, either in the presence of the therapist or by the subject on his own. Whereas the original rationale of such aversive techniques was based on principles of aversive learning or conditioning, there is no evidence that any clear-cut classical or operant learning is involved or, if it is, that it is relevant to the change that follows (Bancroft 1974). Nor is it clear whether aversion leads directly to a reduction in the arousing properties of deviant stimuli, or whether the greater control of behaviour that follows is based on some cognitive mediating process. It may be, for example, that recall of the aversive experience is effective in blocking the arousal that might otherwise occur. It could well be this mechanism that makes the threat or the past experience of legal sanctions effective in so many cases. The would-be offender, on the verge of offending, conjures up the thought of the legal consequences and this is sufficient to deter the offender from taking the action. Similarly, the person who has experienced aversion therapy may recall the aversive experiences in the same way, hence blocking or reducing sexual arousal that might otherwise occur. Because of this basic uncertainty about the underlying process of change, aversive techniques should be seen as empirical. Also, because of their inherent unpleasantness, they are challenging to the patient–therapist relationship, which could be of particular importance when attempting to treat offenders who are incarcerated, and should be used cautiously.

As an alternative, the judicious use of libido-lowering drugs can be combined with these other counselling approaches. By reducing the strength of deviant urges, it may be more feasible for the sex offender to begin to build up a more appropriate repertoire of alternative behaviours. It is nevertheless important to ensure that the use of drugs, by suggesting a more medical type of treatment, does not undermine the offender's sense of responsibility for his own behaviour, or foster an attitude of passive dependence.

The above section on psychological treatment of the offender is much as it appeared in the last edition of this book (1989). Since then the history of such treatment has been an interesting one. In the 1980s increasing interest was shown in applying the range of CBTs that then prevailed, as described above. In addition, there was the emergence of 'relapse prevention' techniques, along the lines used for preventing relapse among alcoholics (Pithers et al 1983). Skepticism about the effectiveness of these approaches, as applied to sex offenders, was expressed by Furby et al (1989) in their review of 42 studies of such methods. In spite of this, programmes continued to evolve, and some more optimistic appraisal of effectiveness started to appear. Hanson et al (2002) reported a meta-analysis of 43 studies, with a combined n of 9454. The average recidivism rate for treatment groups was 12.3% compared with 16.8% for untreated comparison groups, a modest difference. Focusing on CBT, the impact was somewhat better; 9.9% vs 17.4%. Not deterred, Marshall and his colleagues continued to provide a comprehensive rolling programme of treatment for prison inmates, covering the full range of issues listed earlier, using CBT principles in a predominantly group format. A book describing this programme in considerable detail was published in 2006 (Marshall et al 2006). In this the authors considered the literature on treatment effectiveness. Marshall & Barbaree (1988) reported results from a community-based treatment clinic for child molesters. They compared 68 treated patients with a comparison group of 58 untreated individuals. For extra-familial offenders the recidivism rate was 13% of the treated compared to 43% of the untreated group. For incest offenders the rates were 8% and 22%, respectively. They also reported preliminary findings from an ongoing evaluation of 614 offenders who had entered their prison treatment programme. They have yet to report the follow-up for their untreated comparison group. However, for an average of 5.2 years follow-up, their treated offenders showed a 3.2% recidivism rate, compared to an estimated 16.8% recidivism rate for the relevant offender population in Canada.

The methodological problems affecting such studies are not trivial, however. One long-running study uniquely involved random assignment to an inpatient CBT 'relapse prevention' treatment and comparison with two untreated prison groups. The results were finally published in 2005 (Marques et al 2005). No difference in recidivism rates were found between the three groups, which included both rapists and child molesters. There was some suggestion, however, that those in the treated group who met the treatment goals, were less likely to reoffend — a mixed message, encouraging attempts to improve rather than abandon such methods.

Challenges to this treatment approach continue. Petrosino & Soydan (2005) reported a meta-analysis of 300 randomized field trials of individually focused crime reduction, including some studies involving sex offenders. They found that studies in which the evaluators of outcome were heavily involved in the development and implementation of the treatment found substantially larger effect sizes than in those where relatively uninvolved evaluators were used. They left the reader to choose between a 'cynical' and 'high fidelity' conclusion, the former pointing to a 'conflict of interest' and the latter to much more informed and hence valid assessment by those deeply involved!

In my view, it is of considerable importance to continue to improve these methods rather than abandon them, and the government of each country should take responsibility for carrying out appropriate evaluations of such programmes.

Conclusions

Two themes have recurred through this chapter. First, the difficulty in explaining why some people commit sexual offences and to what extent they are different from non-offenders. Second, in what ways do socio-cultural factors increase the likelihood of sexual offending? In the first case, we need better understanding in order to improve methods of prevention and treatment aimed at the individual. In the second case, we need to consider what types of social change might improve the situation.

In the case of rape and sexual assault, there are strong grounds for concluding that social attitudes about gender power differences and the 'property status' of women have an enhancing effect. Clearly, such factors vary in importance across modern societies, but there are few, if any, where they are no longer relevant. This certainly applies to the UK and the USA. Particularly disturbing is the tendency to see women as the sexual property of men and, at the same time, the responsible person in sexual interactions, coupled with the belief that a sexually aroused man cannot be held responsible for his actions. Such attitudes are of much wider relevance than the impact on rape and sexual assault. And there is an important need to vigorously challenge them in whatever way is possible. The US Surgeon General, Dr David Satcher's *Call to Action to Promote Sexual Health and Responsible Sexual Behaviour* (Satcher 2001) is an important step in that direction which has not been shown the continuing government support that it deserves. This has been considered at various points in this book. The basic message is that both men and women should be equally responsible in their sexual lives.

In the case of sexual abuse of children, we remain with an important need to better our understanding of how and why paedophilic preferences become established. The need for socio-cultural intervention is less straightforward than is the case with rape and sexual assault of adults. There is no obvious, direct way that the prevailing moral panic about CSA increases the likelihood of it happening. But we should consider closely the possibility that the prevailing 'sex negativism' increases the likelihood of paedophilic preferences developing in some individuals, perhaps because of some, as yet ill–understood, obstacle to normal sexual development. The prevailing political climate of moral panic, and the need to assert the asexuality of children, certainly makes it more difficult to understand both why the abuse occurs and how the abused child should best be helped. The apparent need to see the abused child as permanently damaged is particularly disturbing. The extent of ignorance about normal sexual development, considered in Chapter 5, is a more general consequence of this political climate. For a range of reasons, therefore, we need a society in which the emerging sexuality of the child is not denied, but rather better understood. At the same time, we need the clear unqualified principle that children should not be exploited for the sexual benefit of someone older.

All of these aims are compatible with the establishment of a society with genuine gender equality, in which sexuality is regarded as a positive feature of close relationships when enacted responsibly.

REFERENCES

Abel GG, Blanchard EH, Becker JV 1978 An integrated treatment program for rapists. In Rada R (ed) Clinical Aspects of the Rapist. Grune & Stratton, New York.

Ahmad S 2006 Adult psychosexual dysfunction as a sequela of child sexual abuse. Sexual & Relationship Therapy 21: 405–418.

American Psychiatric Association 1994 Diagnostic and Statistical Manual of Mental Disorders, 4th edn. American Psychiatric Association, Washington DC.

Ash A 1984 Father–daughter Sexual Abuse: the Abuse of Paternal Authority. Social Theory and Institutions, Bangor.

Bagatell CJ, Heiman JR, Rivier JE, Bremner WJ 1994 Effects of endogenous testosterone and estradiol on sexual behavior in normal young men. Journal of Clinical Endocrinology and Metabolism 78: 711–716.

Baker AW, Duncan SP 1985 Child sexual abuse: a study of prevalence in Great Britain. Child Abuse and Neglect 9: 457–467.

Bancroft J 1974 Deviant Sexual Behaviour: Modification and Assessment. Clarendon Press: Oxford.

Bancroft J 1977 The behavioural approach to treatment. In Money J, Musaph H (eds) Handbook of Sexology. Excerpta Medica, Amsterdam, pp. 1197–1226.

Bancroft J 1979 The nature of the patient–therapist relationship: its relevance to behaviour modification of offenders. British Journal of Criminology 19: 416–419.

Bancroft J 2000 Individual differences in sexual risk taking by men: a psycho-socio-biological approach. In Bancroft J (ed) The Role of Theory in Sex Research. Indiana University Press, Bloomington, pp. 177–212.

Bancroft J (ed) 2003 Sexual Development in Childhood. Indiana University Press, Bloomington.

Bancroft J 2004 Alfred C Kinsey and the politics of sex research. Annual Review of Sex Research 15: 1–39.

Bancroft J, Vukadinovic Z 2004 Sexual addiction, sexual compulsivity, sexual impulse disorder or what? Towards a theoretical model. Journal of Sex Research 41: 225–234.

Bancroft J, Tennent TG, Loucas K, Cass J 1974 Control of deviant sexual behaviour by drugs: behavioural effects of oestrogens and anti-androgens. British Journal of Psychiatry 125: 310–315.

Bancroft J, Herbenick D, Reynolds M 2003a Masturbation as a marker of sexual development. In Bancroft J (ed) Sexual Development in Childhood. Indiana University Press, Bloomington, pp. 156–185.

Bancroft J, Janssen E, Strong D, Carnes L, Long JS 2003b Sexual risk taking in gay men: the relevance of sexual arousability, mood, and sensation seeking. Archives of Sexual Behavior 32: 555–572.

Bancroft J, Janssen E, Strong D, Vukadinovic Z, Long JS 2003c The relation between mood and sexuality in heterosexual men. Archives of Sexual Behavior 32: 217–230.

Bancroft J, Janssen E, Strong D, Vukadinovic Z 2003d The relation between mood and sexuality in gay men. Archives of Sexual Behavior 32: 231–242.

Bancroft J, Janssen E, Carnes L, Strong DA, Goodrich D, Long JS 2004 Sexual activity and risk taking in young heterosexual men: the relevance of personality factors. Journal of Sex Research 41: 181–192.

Barbaree HE, Langton CM 2006 The effects of child sexual abuse and family environment. In Barbaree HE, Marshall WL (eds) The Juvenile Sex Offender, 2nd edn. Guilford, New York, pp. 58–76.

Barbaree HE, Marshall WL 1991 The role of male sexual arousal in rape: six models. Journal of Consulting and Clinical Psychology 59: 621–630.

Barker-Collo S, Read J 2003 Models of response to childhood sexual abuse. Trauma, Violence & Abuse 4: 95–111.

Baron L, Straus MA, Jaffee D 1988 Legitimate violence, violent attitudes, and rape: a test of the cultural spillover. Annals of the New York Academy of Science 528: 79–110.

Bartholomew AA 1968 A long acting phenothiazine as a possible agent to control deviant sexual behavior. American Journal of Psychiatry 124: 917–923.

Bauserman R, Rind B 1997 Psychological correlates of male child and adolescent sexual experiences with adults: a review of the non-clinical literature. Archives of Sexual Behavior 26: 105–141.

Becker JV, Skinner LJ, Abel GG, Axelrod R, Treacy EC 1984 Depressive symptoms associated with sexual assault. Journal of Sexual and Marital Therapy 10: 185–192.

Becker JV, Skinner LJ, Abel GG, Cichon J 1986 Level of post assault sexual functioning in rape and incest victims. Archives of Sexual Behavior 15: 37–49.

Beitchman JH, Zucker KJ, Hood JE, da Costa GA, Akman D 1991 A review of the short-term effects of childhood sexual abuse. Child Abuse & Neglect 15: 537–556.

Bischof N 1975 The comparative ethology of incest avoidance. In Fox R (ed) Biosocial Anthropology. Malaby Press, London.

Bixler RH 1992 Why littermates don't: the avoidance of inbreeding depression. Annual Review of Sex Research 3: 291–328.

Blanchard R, Cantor JM, Robichaud LK 2006 Biological factors in the development of sexual deviance and aggression in males. In Barbaree HE, Marshall WL (eds) The Juvenile Sex Offender, 2nd edn. Guilford Press, New York, pp. 77–104.

Bradford JMW, Greenberg DM 1996 Pharmacological treatment of deviant sexual behavior. Annual Review of Sex Research 7: 283–306.

Bradford JMW, Federoff P 2006 Pharmacological treatment of the juvenile offender. In Barbaree HE, Marshall WL (eds) The Juvenile Sex Offender, 2nd edn. Guilford, New York, pp. 358–382.

Bradford JMW, Paulak A 1993 Double-blind placebo crossover study of cyproterone acetate in the treatment of paraphilias. Archives of Sexual Behavior 22: 383–402.

Bridell DW, Rimm DC, Caddy GR, Krawitz G, Sholis D, Wunderlin RJ 1978 Effects of alcohol and cognitive set on sexual arousal to deviant stimuli. Journal of Abnormal Psychology 87: 418–430.

Broude GJ, Greene SJ 1980 Cross cultural codes on 20 sexual attitudes and practices. In Barry H III, Schlegel A (eds) Cross Cultural Samples and Codes. University of Pittsburgh Press, Pittsburgh, pp. 313–333.

Browning CR, Laumann EO 1997 Sexual contact between children and adults: a life course perspective. American Sociological Review 62: 540–560.

Browning CR, Laumann EO 2003 The social context of adaptation to childhood sexual maltreatment: a life course perspective. In Bancroft J (ed) Sexual Development in Childhood. Indiana University Press, Bloomington, pp. 383–403.

Brownmiller S 1975 Against Our Will. Men, Women and Rape. Simon Schuster, New York.

Buntin JT, Lechtman Z, Laumann EO 2004 Violence and sexuality: examining intimate-partner violence and forced sexual activity. In Laumann EO, Ellingson S, Mahay J, Paik A, Youm Y (eds) The Sexual Organization of the City. University of Chicago Press, Chicago, pp. 226–263.

Burnett RC, Templer DI, Barker PC 1985 Personality variables and circumstances of sexual assault predictive of a women's resistance. Archives of Sexual Behavior 14: 183–188.

Burt MR 1980 Cultural myths and supports for rape. Journal of Personality and Social Psychology 38: 217–230.

Catalano SM 2006 Criminal Victimization 2005. Bureau of Justice Statistics Bulletin, September 2006.

Chambers G, Millar A 1983 Investigating Sexual Assaults. HMSO, Edinburgh.

Chambers G, Millar A 1986 Prosecuting Sexual Assaults. HMSO, Edinburgh.

Childhood Matters 1996 Report of the National Commission of Inquiry into the Prevention of Child Abuse. Stationery Office, London.

Clay-Warner J, Burt CH 2005 Rape reporting after reforms. Have times really changed? Violence Against Women 11: 150–176.

CLRC 1980 Working Paper on Sexual Offence. HMSO, London.

Cortoni F, Marshall WL 2001 Sex as a coping strategy and its relationship to juvenile sexual history and intimacy in sexual offenders. Sexual Abuse: A Journal of Research and Treatment 13: 27–43.

Crawford DA, Allen JV 1979 A social skills training programme with sex offenders. In Cook M, Wilson G (eds) Love and Attraction. Pergamon, Oxford, pp. 503–508.

Criminal Statistics 2001 Criminal Statistics for England & Wales 2000. HMSO, Norwich.

Crown Prosecution Service 2006 Sexual Offences Act 2003. www.cps.gov.uk/legal/section7/chapter_a.html#01.

Davis G, Leitenberg H 1987 Adolescent sex offenders. Psychological Bulletin 101: 417–427.

Davies TS 1974 Cyproterone acetate for male hypersexuality. Journal of International Medical Research 2: 159–163.

Dhaliwal GK, Gauzas L, Antonowicz DH, Ross RR 1996 Adult male survivors of childhood sexual abuse: prevalence, sexual abuse characteristics, and long term effects. Clinical Psychology Review 16: 619–639.

Dowsett G 2000 Discussant. In Bancroft J (ed) The Role of Theory in Sex Research. Indiana University Press, Bloomington, pp. 294–295.

Dreznick MT 2003 Heterosocial competence of rapists and child molesters: a meta-analysis. The Journal of Sex Research 40: 170–178.

Endler NS, Parker JDA 1990 Multidimensional assessment of coping: a critical evaluation. Journal of Personality and Social Psychology 58: 844–854.

Feldman W, Feldman E, Goodman JT, McGrath J, Pless RP, Corsini L, Bennett S 1991 Is childhood sexual abuse really increasing in prevalence? An analysis of the evidence. Pediatrics 88: 29–33.

Fergusson DM, Horwood LJ, Lynskey M 1997 Childhood sexual abuse, adolescent sexual behaviors, and sexual revictimization. Child Abuse and Neglect 21: 789–803.

Finkelhor D 1980 Sex among siblings: a survey on prevalence, variety and effects. Archives of Sexual Behavior 9: 171–194.

Finkelhor D 1982 Sexual abuse — a sociological perspective. Child Abuse and Neglect 6: 95–102.

Finkelhor D 1984 Child Sexual Abuse: New Theory and Research. The Free Press, New York.

Finkelhor D 1994 The international epidemiology of child sexual abuse. Child Abuse & Neglect 5: 409–417.

Finkelhor D 2003a Discussion paper. In Bancroft J (ed) Sexual Development in Childhood. Indiana University Press, Bloomington, pp. 370–372.

Finkelhor D 2003b Discussion. In Bancroft J (ed) Sexual Development in Childhood. Indiana University Press, Bloomington, pp. 98–99.

Finkelhor D, Browne A 1986 Initial and long-term effects: a conceptual framework. In Finkelhor D (ed) A Sourcebook on Child Sexual Abuse. Sage, Beverly Hills, CA, pp. 180–198.

Finkelhor D, Hotaling G, Lewis IA, Smith C 1990 Sexual abuse in a national survey of adult men and women: prevalence, characteristics, and risk factors. Child Abuse and Neglect 14: 19–28.

Flowers RB 1994 The Victimization and Exploitation of Women and Children. McFarland, Jefferson, NC.

Foa EB, Rothbaum BO, Styeketee GS 1993 Treatment of rape victims. Journal of Interpersonal Violence 8: 256–276.

Ford CS, Beach FA 1952 Patterns of Sexual Behaviour. Eyre & Spottiswoode, London.

Fox R 1967 Kinship and Marriage. Penguin, London.

Fox R 1980 The Red Lamp of Incest. Hutchinson, London.

Frank E, Turner S M, Duffy B 1979 Depressive symptoms in rape victims. Journal of Affective Disorders 1: 269–277.

Frank E, Turner SM, Duffy B 1980 Initial response to rape: the impact of factors within the rape situation. Journal of Behavioural Assessment 2: 39–53.

Freeman MDA 1979 The law and sexual deviation. In Rosen I (ed) Sexual Deviation, 2nd edn. Oxford University Press, Oxford, pp. 376–440.

Freud S 1918 Totem and Taboo. Norton, New York.

Freund K 1990 Courtship disorder. In Marshall WL, Laws DR, Barbaree HE (eds) Handbook of Sexual Assault: Issues, Theories and Treatment of the Offender. Plenum Press, New York, pp. 195–207.

Freund K, Kuban M 1993 Toward a testable developmental model of pedophilia: the development of erotic age preference. Child Abuse & Neglect 17: 315–324.

Freund K, McKnight CK, Langevin R, Cibiri S 1972 The female child as a surrogate object. Archives of Sexual Behavior 2: 119–133.

Friedrich WN, Grambsch P, Broughton D, Kuiper J, Beilke RL 1991 Normative sexual behavior in children. Pediatrics 88: 456–464.

Friedrich WN, Grambsch P, Damon L, et al 1992 Child Sexual Behavior Inventory: normative and clinical comparisons. Psychological Assessment 4: 303–311.

Furby L, Weinrott MR, Blackshaw L 1989 Sex offender recidivism: a review. Psychological Bulletin 105: 3–30.

Furniss T 1985 Conflict-avoiding and conflict regulating patterns in incest and child sexual abuse. Acta Paediopsychiatrica 50: 299–313.

Gagnon JH, Simon W 1973 Sexual Conduct: the Sources of Human Sexuality. Aldine: Chicago.

Galliano G, Noble LM, Travis LA, Puechi C 1993 Victim reactions during rape/assault. A preliminary study of the immobility response and its correlates. Journal of Interpersonal Violence 8: 109–114.

Gebhard PH, Johnson AB 1979 The Kinsey Data: Marginal Tabulations of the 1938–1963 Interviews Conducted by the Institute for Sex Research. Saunders, Philadelphia.

Gebhard P, Gagnon J, Pomeroy N, Christenson C 1965 Sex Offenders. Harper Row, New York.

Gibbens TCN, Way C, Soothill KL 1977 Behavioural types of rape. British Journal of Psychiatry 130: 32–42.

Gill M, Tutty LM 1999 Male survivors of childhood sexual abuse: a qualitative study and issues for clinical consideration. Journal of Child Sexual Abuse 7: 19–33.

Gittelson NL, Eacott SE, Mehta BM 1978 Victims of indecent exposure. British Journal of Psychiatry 132: 61–66.

Graham CA 2003 Methodological issues involved in adult recall of childhood sexual experiences. In Bancroft J (ed) Sexual Development in Childhood. Indiana University Press, Bloomington, pp. 67–76.

Graham CA, Bancroft J 2006 Crisis intervention. In Bloch S (ed) An Introduction to the Psychotherapies, 4th edn. Oxford University Press, Oxford, pp. 197–214.

Graham CA, Sanders SA, Milhausen RR 2006 The Sexual Excitation/Sexual Inhibition Inventory for women: psychometric properties. Archives of Sexual Behavior 35: 397–410.

Green R 2002 Is pedophilia a mental disorder? Archives of Sexual Behavior 31: 467–471.

Greenberg LS, Rice LN, Elliott R 1993 Facilitating Emotional Change: the Moment-by-Moment Process. Guilford, New York.

Groth AN 1979 Men Who Rape; the Psychology of the Offender. Plenum, New York.

Groth AN, Burgess AW, Holmstrom LL 1977 Rape: power, anger and sexuality. American Journal of Psychiatry 134: 1239–1243.

Grubin D 1992 Sexual offending: a cross-cultural comparison. Annual Review of Sex Research 3: 201–217.

Grubin D 1998 Sex Offending against Children: Understanding the Risk. Police Research Series, Paper 99. Research, Development and Statistics Directorate, Home Office, London.

Hall K 2007 Sexual dysfunction and childhood sexual abuse: gender differences and treatment implications. In Leiblum SR (ed) Principles and Practice of Sex Therapy, 4th edn. Guilford, New York, pp. 350–378.

Hall GCN, Hirschman R 1992 Sexual aggression against children: a conceptual perspective of etiology. Criminal Justice and Behaviour 19: 8–23.

Hanson RK, Bussiere MT 1998 Predicting relapse: a meta-analysis of sexual recidivism studies. Journal of Consulting and Clinical Psychology 66: 348–362.

Hanson RK, Gordon A, Harris AJR, Marques JK, Murphy WD, Quinsey VL, Seto MC 2002 First report of the collaborative outcome data project on the effectiveness of psychological treatment of sex offenders. Sexual Abuse: A Journal of Research and Treatment 14: 169–195.

Hanson RK, Morton-Bourgon K 2004 Predictors of Sexual Recidivism: an Updated Meta-analysis. Public Safety and Emergency Preparedness, Canada.

Helm N, Hursch CJ 1979 Castration for sex offenders: treatment or punishment? A review and critique of recent European literature. Archives of Sexual Behavior 8: 281–304.

Holmes WC, Slap GB 1998 Sexual abuse of boys: definition, prevalence, correlates, sequelae and management. Journal of the American Medical Association 280: 1855–1862.

Home Office 1997 Aspects of Crime: Children as Victims. Crime and Criminal Justice Unit, Research and Statistics Directorate. Home Office, London.

Home Office 2006 Crime statistics for England and Wales. www. crimestatistics.org.uk/output/page29.asp.

Honoré T 1978 Sex Law. Duckworth: London.

Hopkins J, Thompson EH 1984 Loss and mourning in victims of rape and sexual assault. In Hopkins J (ed) Perspectives on Rape and Sexual Assault. Harper & Row, London.

Horne L, Glasgow D, Cox A, Calam R 1991 Sexual abuse of children by children. Journal of Child Law 3: 147–151.

Howells K, Shaw F, Greasley M, Robertson J, Gloster D 1984 Perceptions of rape in a British sample: effects of relationship, victim status, sex and attitudes to women. British Journal of Social Psychology 23: 35–40.

Hunter JA, Mathews R 1997 Sexual deviance in females. In Laws DR, O'Donohue W (eds) Sexual Deviance: Theory, Assessment and Treatment. Guilford, New York, pp. 465–480.

Hunter JA, Becker JV, Lexier LJ 2006 The female juvenile sex offender. In Barbaree HE, Marshall WL (eds) The Juvenile Sex Offender, 2nd edn. Guilford, New York, pp. 148–165.

Hyde JS 2003 The use of meta-analysis in understanding the effects of child sexual abuse. In Bancroft J (ed) Sexual Development in Childhood. Indiana University Press, Bloomington, pp. 82–91.

Janssen E, Vorst H, Finn P, Bancroft J 2002 The Sexual Inhibition (SIS) and Sexual Excitation (SES) Scales: II. Predicting psychophysiological response patterns. Journal of Sex Research 39: 127–132.

Jenkins P 1998 Moral Panic: Changing Concepts of the Child Molester in Modern America. Yale University Press, New Haven.

Jenkins P 2003 Watching the research pendulum. In Bancroft J (ed) Sexual Development in Childhood. Indiana University Press, Bloomington, pp. 3–20.

Kanfer FH 1975 Self-management methods. In Kanfer FH, Goldstein AP (eds) Helping People Change. Pergamon, New York, pp. 309–355.

Kaplan MS, Krueger RB 1997 Voyeurism: psychopathology and theory. In Laws DR, O'Donohue W (eds) Sexual Deviance: Theory, Assessment, and Treatment. New York, Guilford Press, pp. 297–310.

Katz S, Mazur MA 1979 Understanding Rape Victims: a Synthesis of Research Findings. Wiley, New York.

Kendall-Tackett KA, Williams LM, Finkelhor D 1993 Impact of sexual abuse on children: a review and synthesis of recent empirical studies. Psychological Bulletin 113: 164–180.

Kendler KS, Bulick CM, Silberg J, Hettema JM, Myers J, Prescott CA 2000 Childhood sexual abuse and adult psychiatric and substance abuse disorders in women. An epidemiological and co-twin control analysis. Archives of General Psychiatry 57: 953–959.

Kessler MRH, White MB, Nelson BS 2003 Group treatments for women sexually abused as children: a review of the literature and recommendations for future outcome research. Child Abuse & Neglect 27: 1045–1061.

Kilpatrick DG, Best CL, Veronen LJ, Amick AE, Villeponteaux LA, Ruff GA 1985 Mental health correlates of criminal victimization: a random community survey. Journal of Consulting and Clinical Psychology 53: 866–873.

Kilpatrick DG, Edmunds CN, Seymour AK 1992 Rape in America: a Report to the Nation. National Victim Center, Arlington, VA.

Kinsey AC, Pomeroy WB, Martin CE 1948 Sexual Behavior in the Human Male. Saunders, Philadelphia.

Kinsey AC, Pomeroy WB, Martin CE, Gebhard PH 1953 Sexual Behavior in the Human Female. Saunders, Philadelphia.

Kirschner MA, Schneider G 1972 Suppression of the pituitary-Leydig cell axis and sebum production in normal men by medroxyprogesterone acetate (Provera). Acta Endocrinologica 69: 385–393.

Kutchinsky B 1985 Pornography and its effects in Denmark and the United States. Comparative Social Research 8: 301–330.

Langstrom N, Seto MC 2006 Exhibitionistic and voyeuristic behavior in a Swedish National Population Survey. Archives of Sexual Behavior 35: 427–436.

Lascaratos J, Poulakou-Rebelakou E 2000 Child sexual abuse: historical cases in the Byzantine Empire (324–1453 AD). Child Abuse and Neglect 24: 1085–1090.

Laschet V, Laschet L 1969 Anti-androgens in the treatment of sexual deviations of men. Journal of Steroid Biochemistry 6: 821–826.

Laumann EO, Gagnon JH, Michael RT, Michaels S 1994 The Social Organization of Sexuality: Sexual Practices in the United States. University of Chicago Press, Chicago.

Laumann EO, Paik A, Rosen RC 1999 Sexual dysfunction in the United States: prevalence and predictors. Journal of the American Medical Association 281: 537–544.

Laumann EO, Browning CR, van de Rijt A, Gatzeva M 2003 Sexual contact between children and adults: a life course perspective. In Bancroft J (ed) Sexual Development in Childhood. Indiana University Press, Bloomington, pp. 293–326.

Lemert E 1967 Human Deviance, Social Problems and Social Control. Englewood Cliffs, New Jersey.

Leonard LM, Follette VM 2002 Sex functioning in women reporting a history of child sexual abuse: clinical and empirical considerations. Annual Review of Sex Research 13: 346–388.

Levesque RJR 1999 Sexual Abuse of Children: a Human Rights Perspective. Indiana University Press, Bloomington.

Levin SM, Stava L 1987 Personality characteristics of sex offenders: a review. Archives of Sexual Behavior 16: 57–80.

Levi-Strauss C 1969 The Elementary Structures of Kinship. Beacon: Boston.

Loeb TB, Williams JK, Carmona JV, Rivkin I, Wyatt GE, Chin D, Asuan-O'Brien A 2002 Child sexual abuse: associations with the sexual functioning of adolescents and adults. Annual Review of Sex Research 13: 307–345.

Lykins AD, Janssen E, Graham CA 2006 The relationship between negative mood and sexuality in heterosexual college women and men. Journal of Sex Research 43: 136–143.

Malamuth NM 1981 Rape proclivity among males. Journal of Social Issues 37: 138–156.

Malamuth NM, Check JVP 1980 Penile tumescence and perceptual responses to rape as a function of victim's perceived reactions. Journal of Applied Social Psychology 10: 528–547.

Maletzky BM 1991 Treating the Sexual Offender. Sage, Newbury Park, CA.

Marques JK, Weideranders M, Day DM, Nelson C, van Ommeren A 2005 Effects of a relapse prevention program on sexual recidivism: final results from California's Sexual Offender and Evaluation Project (SOTEP). Sexual Abuse: A Journal of Research and Treatment 17: 79–107.

Marshall WL 1988 The use of sexually explicit stimuli by rapists, child molesters, and non-offenders. Journal of Sex Research 25: 267–288.

Marshall WL 1997 Pedophilia: psychopathology and theory. In Laws DR, O'Donohue W (eds) Sexual Deviance: Theory, Assessment, and Treatment. Guilford, New York, pp. 152–174.

Marshall WL, Barbaree HE 1988 The long term evaluation of a behavioral treatment program for child molesters. Behaviour Research and Therapy 26: 499–511.

Marshall WL, Barbaree HE 1990 An integrated theory of the etiology of sexual offending. In Marshall WL, Laws DR, Barbaree HE (eds) Handbook of Sexual Assault: Issues, Theories, and Treatment of the Offender. Plenum, New York, pp. 257–275.

Marshall WL, Marshall LE 2000 The origins of sexual offending. Trauma, Violence & Abuse 1: 250–263.

Marshall WL, Payne K, Barbaree HE, Eccles A 1991 The treatment of exhibitionists: a focus on sexual deviance versus cognitive and relationship features. Behaviour Research and Therapy 29: 37–40.

Marshall WL, Serran GA, Cortoni FA 2000 Childhood attachments, sexual abuse, and their relationship to adult coping in child molesters. Sexual Abuse: A Journal of Research and Treatment 12: 17–26.

Marshall WL, Marshall LE, Serran GA, Fernandez YM 2006 Treating Sexual Offenders: an Integrated Approach. Routledge, New York.

Masson JM 1984 The Assault on Truth: Freud's Suppression of the Seduction Theory. Farrar, Straus & Giroux: New York.

Meyer WJ, Walker PA, Emory LE, Smith ER 1985 Physical, metabolic, and hormonal effects on men of long-term therapy with medroxyprogesterone acetate. Fertility and Sterility 43: 102–109.

Mill JS 1859 On Liberty. Ticknor and Fields, Boston.

Mohr JW, Turner RE, Jerry MB 1964 Pedophilia and Exhibitionism. University of Toronto Press, Toronto.

Muehlenhard CL, Harney PA, Jones JM 1992 From 'victim-precipitated rape' to 'date rape': how far have we come? Annual Review of Sex Research 3: 219–253.

Mullen PE, Martin JL, Anderson JC, Romans SE, Herbison GP 1996 The long term impact of physical, emotional and sexual abuse of children; a community study. Child Abuse and Neglect 20: 7–21.

Murdock GP 1967 Ethnographic Atlas. University of Pittsburgh Press, Pittsburgh.

Murphy WD 1997 Exhibitionism: psychopathology and theory. In Laws DR, O'Donohue W (eds) Sexual Deviance: Theory, Assessment, and Treatment. Guilford, New York, pp. 22–39.

Murray MAF, Bancroft J, Anderson DC, Tennent TG, Carr PJ 1975 Endocrine changes in male sexual deviants after treatment with anti-androgens, oestrogens or tranquillisers. Journal of Endocrinology 67: 179–188.

Najman JM, Dunne MP, Purdie DM, Boyle FM, Coxeter PD 2005 Sexual abuse in childhood and sexual dysfunction in adulthood: an Australian population-based study. Archives of Sexual Behavior 34: 517–526.

NCCL 1976 Sexual offences; evidence to the Criminal Law Revision Committee. Report no 13. NCCL, London.

Nelson EC, Heath AC, Madden PAF, Cooper ML, Dinwiddie SH, Bucholz KK, Glowinski A, McLaughlin T, Dunne MP, Statham DJ, Martin NG 2002 Association between self-reported childhood sexual abuse and adverse psychosocial outcomes. Archives of General Psychiatry 59: 139–145.

Nieuwoudt S 2006 No justice for Dafur rape victims. Institute for War and Peace Reporting. Africa Reports iwpr.net 23 November 2006.

Noll JG, Trickett PK, Putnam FW 2003 A prospective investigation of the impact of childhood sexual abuse on the development of sexuality. Journal of Consulting and Clinical Psychology 71: 575–586.

O'Reilly HJ 1984 Crisis intervention with victims of forcible rape: a police perspective. In Hopkins J (ed) Perspectives on Rape and Sexual Assault. Harper & Row, London.

Pacht AR, Cowden JE 1974 An exploratory study of 500 sex offenders. Criminal Justice and Behavior 1: 13–20.

Pacht AR, Halleck SL, Ehrmann JC 1962 Diagnosis and treatment of the sex offender: a 9 year study. American Journal of Psychiatry 118: 802–808.

Paul JP, Catania JA, Pollack LM 2003 Childhood/Adolescent sexual coercion among men who have sex with men. In Bancroft J (ed) Sexual Development in Childhood. Indiana University Press, Bloomington, pp. 327–358.

Paulhus DL, Fridhandler B, Hayes S 1997 Psychological defense: contemporary theory and research In Hogan R, Johnson J, Briggs S (eds) Handbook of Personality Psychology. Academic Press, San Diego, pp. 546–547.

PCS 2006 Guide to the Sexual Offences Act. PCS Equality, Health and Safety Department. http://www.pcsproud.org.uk/SexualOffencesGuide.pdf.

Petrosino A, Soydan H 2005 The impact of program developers as evaluators on criminal recidivism: results from meta-analyses of experimental and quasi-experimental research. Journal of Experimental Criminology 1: 435–450.

Pithers WD, Marques JK, Gibat CC, Marlatt GA 1983 Relapse prevention with sexual aggressives: a self-control model of treatment and maintenance of change. In Greer JG, Stuart IR (eds) The Sexual Aggressor: Current Perspectives on Treatment. Van Nostrand Reinhart, New York, pp. 214–239.

Pithers WD, Kashima KM, Cumming GF, Beal LS, Buell MM 1988 Relapse prevention of sexual aggression. In Prentky RA, Quinsey VL (eds) Human Sexual Aggression: Current Perspectives. New York Academy of Sciences, New York, pp. 244–260.

Polusny MA, Follette VM 1995 Long-term correlates of childhood sexual abuse: theory and review of the empirical literature. Applied and Preventive Psychology 4: 143–166.

Porter R (ed) 1984 Child Sexual Abuse within the Family. Ciba Foundation Report. Tavistock, London.

Prentky RA, Knight RA 1991 Identifying critical dimensions for discriminating among rapists. Journal of Consulting and Clinical Psychology 59: 643–661.

Proulx J, McKibbon A, Lusignan R 1996 Relationships between affective components and sexual behavior in sexual aggressors. Sexual Abuse: A Journal of Research and Treatment 8: 279–289.

Pukall CF, Lahaie M-A, Binik YM 2006 Sexual pain disorders: pathophysiologic factors. In Goldstein I, Meston CM, Davis SR, Traish AM (eds) Women's Sexual Function and Dysfunction: Study, Diagnosis and Treatment. Taylor & Francis, London, pp. 529–538.

Putnam FW 1997 Dissociation in children and adolescents: a developmental perspective. Guildford, New York.

Quinsey VL, Steinman CM, Bergersen SG, Holmes TF 1975 Penile circumference, skin conductance, and ranking responses of child molesters and 'normals' to sexual and non-sexual visual stimuli. Behavior Therapy 6: 213–219.

Rabinowitz D 2003 No Crueler Tyrannies: Accusation, False Witness and Other Terrors of Our Time. Wall Street Journal Books, New York.

Radzinowicz L 1957 Sexual Offences. MacMillan, London.

Resick PA 1993 The psychological impact of rape. Journal of Interpersonal Violence 8: 223–255.

Resnick H 1997 Acute panic reactions among rape victims: implications for prevention of post-rape psychopathology. NCP Clinical Quarterly 7 (3): 41–45.

Rieber I, Sigusch V 1979 Psychosurgery in sex offenders and sexual deviants in West Germany. Archives of Sexual Behavior 8: 523–528.

Rind B, Tromovitch P 1997 A meta-analytic review of findings from national samples of psychological correlates of child sexual abuse. Journal of Sex Research 34: 237–255.

Rind B, Tromovitch P, Bauserman T 1998 A meta-analytic examination of assumed properties of child sexual abuse using college samples. Psychological Bulletin 124: 22–53.

Rooth FG 1971 Indecent exposure and exhibitionism. British Journal of Hospital Medicine April: 521–533.

Rooth FG 1972 Changes in the conviction rate for indecent exposure. British Journal of Psychiatry 121: 89–94.

Rooth FG 1973a Exhibitionism, sexual violence and paedophilia. British Journal of Psychiatry 122: 705–710.

Rooth FG 1973b Exhibitionism outside Europe and America. Archives of Sexual Behavior 2: 351–363.

Rosen RC, Lane RM, Menza M 1999 Effects of SSRI's on sexual function: a critical review. Journal of Clinical Psychopharmacology 19: 67–85.

Rosler A, Witztum, E 1998 Treatment of men with paraphilia with a long acting analogue of gonadotrophin-releasing hormone. New England Journal of Medicine 338: 416–465.

Rothbaum BO, Foa EB, Murdock T, Riggs DS, Walsh W 1992 A prospective examination of post-traumatic stress disorder in rape victims. Journal of Traumatic Stress 5: 455–475.

Rossman GP 1979 Sexual Experience between Men and Boys: Exploring the Pederast Underground. Temple Smith, London.

Russell DEH 1982 Rape in Marriage. MacMillan, New York.

Russell DEH 1983 The incidence and prevalence of intrafamilial and extrafamilial sexual abuse of female children. Child Abuse and Neglect 7: 133–146.

Russell DEH 1984 Sexual Exploitation: Rape, Child Sexual Abuse, and Workplace Harassment. Sage, Thousand Oaks, CA.

Ryan G, Miyoshi TJ, Metzner JL, Krugman RD, Fryer GE 1996 Trends in a national sample of sexually abusive youths. Journal of the American Academy of Child and Adolescent Psychiatry 5: 17–25.

Sample LL, Bray TM 2006 Are sex offenders different? An examination of re-arrest patterns. Criminal Justice Policy Review 17: 83–102.

Sanday PR 1981 The socio-cultural context of rape: a cross-cultural study. Journal of Social Issues 37: 5–27.

Satcher D 2001 The Surgeon General's Call to Action to Promote Sexual Health and Responsible Sexual Behaviour. http://www.surgeongeneral.gov/library/sexualhealth.

Schloredt KA, Heiman JR 2003 Perceptions of sexuality as related to sexual functioning and sexual risk in women with different types of child abuse histories. Journal of Traumatic Stress 16: 275–284.

Schmidt G 2002 The dilemma of the male pedophile. Archives of Sexual Behavior 31: 473–477.

Schober JM, Kuhn P, Kovacs PG, Earle JH, Byrne PM, Fries RA 2005 Leuprolide acetate suppresses pedophilic urges and arousability. Archives of Sexual Behavior 34: 691–706.

Scott PD 1964 Definition, classification, prognosis and treatment. In Rosen I (ed) Pathology and Treatment of Sexual Deviation. Oxford University Press, Oxford.

Seto MC 2004 Pedophilia and sexual offences against children. Annual Review of Sex Research 15: 321–361.

Shepher J 1971 Mate selection among second generation kibbutz adolescents and adults: incest avoidance and negative imprinting. Archives of Sexual Behavior 1: 293–307.

Silverman DC, Apfel RJ 1983 Caring for the victims of rape. In Nadelson CC, Marcotte DB (eds) Treatment Interventions in Human Sexuality. Plenum, New York.

Spataro J, Mullen PE, Burgess, PM, Wells DL, Moss SA 2004 Impact of child sexual abuse on mental health. British Journal of Psychiatry 184: 416–421.

Stanley JL, Bartholomew K, Oram D 2004 Gay and bisexual men's age discrepant childhood sexual experiences. Journal of Sex Research 41: 381–389.

Sterkmans P, Geerts F 1966 Is benperidol (RF504) the specific drug for the treatment of excessive and disinhibited sexual behaviour? Acta Neurologica et Psychiatrica Belgica 66: 1030–1040.

Summit R 1983 The child sexual abuse accommodation syndrome. Child Sexual Abuse & Neglect 7: 177–193.

Sundberg SL, Barbaree HE, Marshall WL 1991 Victim blame and disinhibition of sexual arousal to rape vignettes. Violence and Victims 6: 103–120.

Tennent G, Bancroft J, Cass J 1974 The control of deviant sexual behavior by drugs: a double-blind controlled study of benperidol, chlorpromazine and placebo. Archives of Sexual Behavior 3: 261–271.

Thibaut F, Cordier B, Kuhn J-M 1996 Gonadotrophin hormone releasing hormone agonist in cases of severe paraphilia: a lifetime treatment? Psychoneuroendocrinology 21: 411–419.

Van Berlo W, Ensink B 2000 Problems with sexuality after sexual assault. Annual Review of Sex Research 11: 235–257.

Varjonen M, Santtila P, Hoglund M, Jern P, Johansson A, Wager I, Witting K, Algars M, Sandnabba NK 2007 Genetic and environmental effects of sexual excitation and sexual inhibition in men. Journal of Sex Research 44: 359–369.

Vizard E, Monck E, Misch P 1995 Child and adolescent sex abuse perpetrators: a review of the research literature. Journal of Child Psychology and Psychiatry 36: 731–756.

Walby S, Allen J 2004 Domestic Violence, Sexual Assault and Stalking: Findings from the British Crime Survey, Home Office Research Study 276. Research, Development and Statistics Directorate, London.

Walker PA 1978 The role of antiandrogens in the treatment of sex offenders. In Qualls CB, Wincze JP, Barlow DH (eds) The Prevention of Sexual Disorders. Plenum, New York, pp. 117–136.

Walmsley R, White K 1979 Sexual Offences, Consent and Sentencing. Home Office Research Study no 54. HMSO, London.

Ward T, Beech A 2006 An integrated theory of sexual offending. Aggression and Violent Behavior 11: 44–63.

Ward T, Siegert RJ 2000 Toward a comprehensive theory of child sexual abuse: a theory knitting perspective. Psychology, Crime and Law 8: 319–351.

Weinberg SK 1976 Incest Behavior. Citadel, New York.

Weiss EL, Longhurst JG, Mazure CM 1999 Childhood sexual abuse as a risk factor for depression in women: psychosocial and neurobiological correlates. American Journal of Psychiatry 156: 816–828.

West DJ, Roy C, Nichols FL 1978 Understanding Sexual Attacks. Heinemann, London.

Westermark E 1926 A Short History of Marriage. MacMillan, New York.

Wolf AP 1970 Childhood association and sexual attraction: a further test of the Westermark hypothesis. American Anthropologist 72: 503–515.

Wolfenden J 1957 Report on Homosexual Offences and Prostitution. HMSO, London.

Wright RC, Schneider SL 1997 Deviant sexual fantasies as motivated self-deception. In Schwartz BK, Cellini HR (eds) The Sex Offender: New Insights, Treatment Motivations and Legal Developments, vol. 2. Civic Research Institute, Kingston, NJ, pp. 8.1–8.14.

Wyatt GE 1985 The sexual abuse of Afro-American and white American women in childhood. Child Abuse and Neglect 9: 507–519.

Yates E, Barbaree HE, Marshall WL 1984 Anger and deviant sexual arousal. Behavior Therapy 15: 287–294.

Glossary of abbreviations

5-ARD	5-alpha-reductase deficiency
5-HT	5-hydroxytryptamine
17-βHSD	17-β hydroxysteroid dehydrogenase deficiency
A	adrenaline
A	agreableness
A	androstenedione
AARP	American Association for Retired Persons
ABC approach	Abstinence, Be faithful, use Condoms
ACC	anterior cingulate cortex
ACh	acetylcholine
ACSF	Analyse des Comportements Sexuels en France
ACTH	adrenocorticotropic hormone
AEA	autoerotic asphyxia
AGI	Alan Guttmacher Institute
AH/POA	anterior hypothalamic/preoptic area
AI	anal intercourse
AID	artificial insemination by donor
AIS	androgen insensitivity syndrome
α-MSH	alpha-melanocyte-stimulating hormone
AND	4,16-androstadien-3-one
AR	androgen receptor
ARRM	AIDS risk reduction model
ARV	antiretroviral therapy
ASHR	Australian Study of Health and Relationships
ATP	adenosine triphosphate
ATS	American Teenage Survey
BAS	behavioural activation system (or scale)
BCS	British Crime Survey
BDI	Beck Depression Inventory
BIS	behavioural inhibition system (or scale)
BMI	body-mass index
BNST	bed nucleus of the stria terminalis
BOLD	blood-oxygen level-dependent contrast
C	conscientiousness
CAH	congenital adrenal hyperplasia
CAIS	complete androgen insensitivity syndrome
cAMP	cyclic adenosine monophosphate
CASI	computer assisted self interview
CBCL	Child Behavior Check List
CBT	cognitive behaviour therapy
CC	corpus callosum
cGMP	cyclic guanosine monophosphate
CHSLS	Chicago Health and Social Life Survey
CLRC	Criminal Law Revision Committee
CLS	Companionate Love Scale
CMV	magnetic equivalent of contingent negative variation (CNV)
COC	combined oral contraceptive
CPA	cyproterone acetate
CPPS	chronic pelvic pain syndrome
CSA	child sexual abuse
CSBI	Child Sexual Behavior Inventory
CSEP	childhood sexual experience with peers
CUSI	Coping Using Sex Inventory
DA	dopaminergic or dopamine
DHEA	dehydroepiandrosterone
DHEAS	dehydroepiandrosterone sulphate
DHSS	Department of Health and Social Security
DHT	dihydrotestosterone
DM	diabetes mellitus
DSM-IV	Diagnostic and Statistical Manual – IV
DZ	dizygotic
E	estrogen, oestrogen, oestradiol
E	extraversion/introversion
ED	erectile dysfunction
EE	ethinyl oestradiol
EEA	environment of evolutionary adaptiveness
ERP	event-related potential
ESRC	Economic and Social Research Council
FAI	free androgen index
fMRI	functional magnetic resonance imaging
FSAD	female sexual arousal disorder
FSFI	Female Sexual Function Inventory
FSH	follicle-stimulating hormone
GABA	gamma-aminobutyric acid
GD	gender diagnosticity
GID	gender identity discordance
GnRH	gonadotrophin releasing hormone
GRISS	Golombok-Rust Inventory of Sexual Satisfaction
GSS	General Social Survey
GSSAB	Global Study of Sexual Attitudes and Behavior

HAART	highly active anti-retroviral therapy		O	openness to experience
HBIGDA	Harry Benjamin International Gender Dysphoria Association		OC	oral contraceptive
			OR	odds ratio
HBV	hepatitis B virus		OT	oxytocin
HIV	human immunodeficiency virus		P	toughmindedness
HPA	Health Protection Agency		PAIS	partial androgen insensitivity syndrome
HPV	human papilloma virus			
HR	hormone replacement		PANAS	Positive and Negative Affect Scales
HRSB	high risk sexual behaviour		PD	Parkinson's disease
HRT	hormone replacement therapy (or treatment)		PDE-5	phosphodiesterase-5
			PE	premature ejaculation
HSDD	Hypoactive Sexual Desire Disorder		PEPFAR	President's Emergency Plan for AIDS relief
HSV	herpes simplex virus			
ICI	intra-cavernosal injection		PET	positron emission tomography
IHD	ischaemic heart disease		PFSF	Profile of Female Sexual Function
INAH 1-4	interstitial nuclei of the anterior hypothalamus 1-4		PGE1	prostaglandin E1
			PID	pelvic inflammatory disease
IRSF	interview ratings of sexual function		PLS	Passionate Love Scale
IUD	intrauterine device		PMS	premenstrual syndrome
IUS	intrauterine system		PNS	parasympathetic nervous system
IV	intravenous		POA	preoptic area
IVF	in vitro fertilization		POP	progestogen-only pill
KO	'knock out' mice		PRC	People's Republic of China
l.c.	locus coeruleus		PRL	prolactin
LD	learning disability		PTSD	posttraumatic stress disorder
LGV	lymphogranuloma venereum		PVN	paraventricular nucleus
LH	luteinizing hormone		rCBF	regional cerebral blood flow
LHRH	luteinizing hormone releasing hormone		RDD	random digit dialing
LMN	lateral mamillary nucleus		REM	rapid eye movement phase of sleep
LN	levonorgestrel		RNA	ribonucleic acid
LSD	lysergic acid diethylamide		SADI	Sexual Arousal and Desire Inventory
MEG	magnetoencephalography		SAI	Sexual Arousal Inventory
MI	myocardial infarction		SC	skin conductance
MIF	Mullerian inhibiting factor		SCI	spinal cord injury
MMAS	Massachusets Male Aging Study		SCID	sexual content-induced delay
MMN	medial mamillary nucleus		SDI	Sexual Desire Inventory
MOFC	medial orbito-frontal cortex		SDN	sexually dimorphic nucleus
MPA	medroxyprogesterone acetate		SE	sexual excitation (SESII-W)
MPOA	medial preoptic area		SES	sexual excitation system (or scale)
MRI	magnetic resonance imaging		SESII-W	sexual excitation/sexual inhibition inventory for women
MS	multiple sclerosis			
MSM	men who have sex with men		SHBG	sex hormone binding globulin
MZ	monozygotic		SI	sexual inhibition (SESII-W)
N	neuroticism		SIDI-F	Sexual Interest and Desire Inventory for Women
NA	noradrenaline			
NANC	nonadrenergic-noncholinergic neuro-effector system		SIS	sexual inhibition system
			SIS1	sexual inhibition scale 1 – inhibition due to threat of performance failure
NATSAL	National Survey of Sexual Attitudes and Lifestyles			
			SIS2	sexual inhibition scale 2 – inhibition due to threat of performance consequences
NCCL	National Council for Civil Liberties			
NCVS	National Crime Victimization Survey			
NHS	National Health Service		SNS	sympathetic nervous system
NHSLS	National Health and Social Life Survey		SOS	Sexual Opinion Survey
NICHD	National Institute of Child Health and Development		SPF	subparafascicular nucleus
			SRY	testis determining factor
NIH	National Institute of Health		SSA	safer sex assertiveness
NIMH	National Institute of Mental Health		SSRI	selective serotonin reuptake inhibitor
NO	nitric oxide		SST	Sexual Strategy Theory
NPT	nocturnal penile tumescence		STD	sexually transmitted disease
NSAM	National Survey of Adolescent Males		STI	sexually transmitted infection
NSFG	National Survey of Family Growth		SV	simple virilising (variant of CAH)

SW	salt wasting (variant of CAH)	VEF	visual evoked field
SWAN	Study of Women's Health Across the Nation	VIP	vasoactive intestinal polypeptide
		VPA	vaginal pulse amplitude
T	testosterone	VS	vaginal stimulation
TB	tuberculosis	VSS	visual sexual stimuli
TRH	thyrotrophin-releasing hormone	VTA	ventral tegmental area
UAI	unprotected anal intercourse	VVS	vulvar vestibulitis syndrome
VBF	vaginal blood flow	WHO	World Health Organization
VCD	vacuum constriction device	WHR	waist-to-hip ratio
VCS	vaginal and cervical stimulation	YRSB	Youth Risk Behavior Survey

Index of referenced authors

A

Aalsma, M.C., 147–148
Abbott, E., 282
Abdelgadir, S.E., 126
Abdel-Hamid, I.A., 363–364, 404
Abdo, C., 367
Abel, G.G., 503–504
Abma, J.C., 155
Abrahamson, D.J., 98
Abramowitz, S.I., 297
Abramson, P.R., 5, 8
Abruzzo, M., 45
Achenbach, T.M., 147, 148
Ackerman, K.T., 406
Ackers, J.P., 416
Adler, N.T., 65, 132
Ahmad, S., 497
Ahmadi, N., 217–218
Ajzen, I., 424
Akers, J.S., 165
Alder, E., 441, 455, 456, 460
Alexander, C.L., 400
Alexander, G.M., 113, 451
Alexander, J.L., 247
Ali, M.M., 422
Allen, J., 469
Allen, J.V., 504
Allen, L.S., 60
Allgeier, E.R., 9
Alonso, A., 132
Althof, S.E., 343, 366, 367
Altman, A.M., 246
Altman, D., 260
Amarel, D.G., 57
Amelar, R.D., 459
Andersen, B.C., 386–387
Anderson, R., 200
Anderson, R.A., 112–113, 453
Andersson, K.E., 68
Angier, N., 24
Angst, J., 107, 387–388
Apfel, R.J., 491–492
Appelt, H., 117
Araujo, A.B., 241, 387
Arentewicz, G., 357
Argiolas, A., 67, 93, 128, 129
Arlt, W., 23–24
Arnold, M.B., 61
Aron, A., 73
Asayama, S., 193
Asboe, D., 428
Ash, A., 484
Ashton, A.K., 404

Ashton, J.R., 458
Athanosiou, R., 407
Atkinson, L., 439
Auchus, R.J., 111, 125
Avis, N.E.R., 218, 244, 250, 306
Aziz, A., 118

B

Babb, P., 206, 212, 238
Babula, O., 326
Bach, A.K., 101
Bachmann, G.A., 23, 115, 246
Backstrom, T., 116
Bacon, C.G., 241
Bagatell, C.J., 113, 502
Bagemihl, B., 165–166
Bai, J., 407
Bailey, J.M., 160, 163, 291, 294–295
Bailey, J.V., 270
Bailey, R.C., 429
Baird, A.A., 61
Bajos, N., 422, 424
Baker, A.W., 469
Baker, R.R., 94
Bakwin, H., 148
Balint, M., 345
Bancroft, J., 46
    ageing and, 242, 243, 244–245
    assessment/treatment, 345, 356, 358–359,
        360, 361, 363, 373, 376
    excitation/inhibition and, 64, 67, 68,
        69–70
    fertility and, 441, 446, 447, 448, 449, 450,
        451, 459
    genital response and, 75, 76
    heterosexuality and, 185, 214, 216,
        221–222, 225, 232
        marriage, 201, 209, 211
        sex surveys, 177, 179, 180, 181–182
    homosexuality and, 255–256, 257, 268,
        270, 271, 272, 274
    hormones and, 111, 114, 115, 116, 117,
        119, 120, 127–128, 131
    information processing and, 96, 104,
        108, 110
    medical practice and, 392–393
    orgasm and, 85, 91, 96
    patient-therapist relationship, 353
    problematic sexuality and, 304, 305,
        309, 310, 330–333, 336
        reduced interest, 319, 322, 324,
        329

    sexual development and, 151–153, 154,
        156–157, 159
    sexual offences and, 476, 492, 499–500
        offenders, 479, 480, 481–482, 502,
        503–504
    sexual variations and, 280, 284
    sexually transmitted diseases and, 414,
        431–432, 433–434, 434, 435
        HIV/AIDS, 427, 428, 429
    theory, role of and, 5, 7, 8, 13, 15
    transgender/transvestism and, 290, 292,
        296
Bandura, A., 424
Bankole, A., 457
Barak, Y., 398
Barbaree, H.E., 479, 480, 482–483, 484–485,
    505
Barbarino, A., 46
Barbieri, R.L., 42, 406
Barclay, A.M., 108
Bard, P., 75
Barfield, R.J., 65, 91
Barker-Collo, S., 496
Barlow, D., 415
Barlow, D.H., 100, 101, 107, 110
Baron, L., 471
Barragry, J.M., 405
Barrat-Connor, E., 392
Barry, H. III, 174, 187
Bartels, A., 73, 205
Barth, R.J., 330
Bartholomew, A.A., 502
Basson, R., 338, 365
Bates, J.E., 148, 159, 435
Bateson, P.P.G., 165
Baumeister, R.F., 220, 331, 332
Bauserman, R., 494
Beach, F.A., 65–66, 91, 165, 174, 265, 440,
    473
    marriage and, 201, 212
    premarital sex and, 186, 188, 191
Beam, L., 175–176, 257
Bean, F.D., 456, 457
Bearman, P.S., 158
Beaumont, T., 287, 296
Bechara, A., 104, 366
Beck, A.T., 387
Beck, J.G., 64, 81, 96, 98, 107–108, 222
Becker, J.V., 490
Becker, M.A., 106
Beckman, L.J., 406
Beech, A., 485
Beggs, V.E., 107

515

Beischer, N.A., 440
Beitchman, J.H., 479
Bell, A.P., 178, 271, 273–275
Bell, C., 96, 392
Bell, J.S., 458
Bell, R.J., 116
Bell, R.R., 192–193, 212
Bellard, H.S., 99
Bellerose, S.B., 117
Bellis, M.A., 94
Bem, D.J., 167
Bem, S.L., 272
Benjamin, H., 294
Benson, G.S., 75
Bentler, P.M., 87, 295
Beral, V., 386
Berg, P., 360
Berg, R., 51
Berger, D.M., 460
Berger, G.S., 447
Berger, S., 401
Bergeron, S., 359, 385
Berke, P., 393–394
Berlowitz, A., 216
Berman, J.R., 80
Bern, S.L., 229
Berridge, K.C., 63, 333
Berscheid, E., 222
Bertelson, A.D., 394
Betancourt-Allbrecht, M., 392
Bieber, I., 256
Billings, E.L., 454
Billings, J., 454
Billy, J.O.G., 178
Binik, Y.M., 84, 86, 117, 324–326, 336, 385
Binson, D., 268, 431
Biron, C., 97
Bischof, N., 477
Bitran, D., 67, 68–69
Bixler, R.H., 477
Bixo, M., 126
Bjorklund, D.F., 65, 133
Black, D.W., 107, 330, 333
Black, S.L., 97
Blackwood, E., 265
Blaicher, W., 93, 129
Blanchard, R., 287, 290–291, 334, 482
Blander, D.S., 373
Bleuler, M., 388
Blinn, K., 372
Blumer, D., 397
Blumstein, P.W., 160, 207, 208, 275
Bocher, M., 72
Bochinski, D., 68
Bocklandt, S., 163
Bogaert, A.F., 167, 282
Bogart, L.M., 155
Bohlen, J.G., 85
Bohm-Starke, N., 326
Boime, I., 22
Boldero, J., 426
Bole-Feysot, C., 129
Bolin, A., 290
Bone, M., 193, 443, 455
Bonnar, J., 42, 456
Boolell, M., 78
Boonstra, H., 198
Borneman, E., 148
Bors, E., 75, 372, 400
Boswell, J., 254
Both, S., 100
Boulton, A.J., 361
Bowlby, J., 145

Boxer, A., 160
Boyce, P., 422
Boyd, R.A., 451
Boyle, M., 329
Boz, M., 181
Bozman, A.W., 107–108
Bozon, M., 207–208, 208
Bradford, A., 81–82, 327, 386
Bradford, J.M.W., 502, 503
Bradley, S.J., 44, 167, 293
Bradshaw, Z., 458
Brauer, M., 80, 325
Braunstein, G.D., 121
Bray, T.M., 475
Breiter, H.C., 333
Bremner, W.J., 241
Breslow, N., 286
Brewer, C., 458
Briddell, D.W., 405, 480
Briere, J., 224
Brindley, G.S., 75, 362, 401
Brinkman, P.D., 176
Brock, G.B., 68
Brockman, B., 357
Brockman, F.S., 175
Broderick, C.B., 154
Broderick, G.A., 384
Brody, S., 87, 93
Bronner, G., 399
Broome, A., 458
Brotto, L.A., 81, 101, 217, 218, 365
Broude, G.J., 174, 212, 265, 471
Brown, J.B., 29
Brown, S.L., 447
Browne, A., 496, 500
Browning, C.R., 145, 479, 498–499
Brownmiller, S., 471–472
Bruce, M., 406
Brückner, H., 158
Brust, J.C.M., 335
Buckley, P.F., 389
Buckley, R.M. Jr, 415
Buena, F., 113–114
Buhrich, N., 287, 296
Bullough, V.L., 184, 210, 254, 255, 289
Bulpitt, C.J., 396, 402
Bunnell, T., 390
Buntin, J.T., 473
Burchardt, M., 396
Burchell, R.C., 395
Burger, H.G., 119, 244
Burgess, E.W., 175, 203
Burnett, R.C., 491
Burnfield, P., 398
Burt, C.H., 470
Burt, M.R., 471
Bury, J., 191–192, 199
Buss, D.M., 8, 9, 201, 204, 226
Buster, J.E., 121
Buvat, J., 24, 121, 242, 372, 393
Byard, R.W., 334
Byrne, D., 100, 106, 214, 229

C

Cacioppo, J.T., 74
Cain, V.S., 218
Caldwell, J., 456
Caldwell, J.D., 125, 129
Call, V., 208
Cameron, J., 28
Canale, D., 130
Canin, L., 431, 434

Cantor, J.M., 128
Cantor, J.R., 82
Caplow, T., 192, 205, 206
Carani, C., 112–114, 129, 242, 407
Carballo, M., 183
Carey, M.P., 107, 310, 391, 406, 434
Carillo, H., 271
Carmichael, M.S., 93, 128
Carney, A., 118, 358
Carrier, J.M., 265
Carroll, R.A., 297, 300, 377
Carson, R.C., 336
Carter, C.S., 129
Caruso, S., 365, 449, 452
Carver, C.S., 16
Caspi, A., 148, 159, 435
Cass, V.C., 260–261
Cassidy, W.L., 387
Castano, P.M., 446
Catalan, J.P., 315, 326, 352, 359–360, 428
Catalano, S.M., 470, 490
Catania, J.A., 178, 180, 181, 424, 425, 426
Cates, W. Jr, 454
Cawood, E.H.H., 116, 232, 244–245, 447
Chahl, L.A., 90
Chakravarti, S., 246
Chalkley, A.J., 284
Chambers, G., 465, 491
Chambless, D.L., 85
Chang, L., 181
Charney, D.S., 70
Chaskes, J.B., 193
Check, J.V.P., 480
Chesser, E., 256
Chivers, M., 333
Christ, G.J., 243, 392
Christensen, H.R., 193
Christenson, C.V., 249
Christian, B., 210, 453
Christian, J.J., 66
Chun, J., 382
Chung, W.C., 295
Clark, B.J., 20, 22
Clark, R.A., 108
Clayton, A.H., 222
Clayton, P.J., 388
Clay-Warner, J., 470
Cleland, J., 422
Clement, U., 192, 193, 194
Cliquet, R.L., 456
Coakley, M., 151
Coates, S.W., 167
Cochran, S.D., 273
Coderre, T.J., 385
Coenen, C.M.H., 451
Cohen, H.D., 88
Cohen-Kettenis, P.T., 49–50, 294, 296
Colapinto, J., 44
Cole, T.M., 399–400, 401
Coleman, E., 332
Coleman, P.J., 418
Coles, L., 315, 356
Collaer, M.L., 45, 51
Collins, J.K., 214
Collomb, H., 397
Comarr, A.E., 75, 400
Conley, R.R., 389
Connolly, F.H., 389
Conoway, C.H., 165
Conti, C.R., 361
Coolen, L.M., 89, 404
Cooper, A., 227, 330
Cooper, A.J., 323, 360

Cooper, P.J., 441, 456
Cornog, M., 182, 184
Correa, M., 64
Cortoni, F., 480–481
Costa, M., 102
Costa, P.T., 228
Costello, C., 456
Cottrell, L.S., 175
Coulter, A., 385
Couzinet, B., 245
Cove, J., 329
Cowden, J.E., 483
Craft, A., 389–390
Craft, M., 389–390
Cranston-Cuebas, M.A., 100, 101, 107
Crawford, D.A., 504
Crawford, M., 156
Creasey, H., 241
Crenshaw, T.L., 69, 362, 402, 403, 405
Crepaz, N., 433, 436
Crilley, R.G., 244
Crocker, J., 216
Croft, H., 403
Crompton, L., 253–254
Croog, S.H., 402
Crouch, J., 212
Crowe, M., 315
Csillag, E.R., 98
Cullberg, J., 448–449
Cunningham, G.R., 392
Cupach, W.R., 231
Cuthbert, B.N., 101, 101–102
Cutler, W.B., 97, 459
Cyranowski, J.M., 106, 111, 387

D

Dacakis, G., 299
Daker-White, G., 373
Daly, M., 191
Daneback, K., 227
Darney, P.D., 451
Darroch, J.E., 197
Darvishpour, M., 218
D'Augelli, A.R., 161
Davenport, A.E., 360
Davenport-Hines, R., 413
Davidson, J., 49
Davies, T.S., 502
Davis, A.R., 446
Davis, G., 470
Davis, G.C., 240
Davis, K.B., 175–176
Davis, S.R., 115–116, 120, 121, 125, 451
Davison, S.L., 244
Daw, S.F., 29
Dawson-Butterworth, K., 388–389
De Graaf, R., 274
De Judicibus, M.A., 440, 441
de Keizer, M., 328–329, 376
de Visser, R., 427
DeAmicis, L.A., 357
Dean, K.E., 225
Deane, R.F., 456
DeCecco, J.P., 261
Deenen, A.A., 276
Dekker, A., 185, 186
Dekker, J., 98, 357
DeLamater, J.D., 5, 177, 239, 441
Delancey, J.O.L., 33
Delay, P.R., 421, 423, 434
Deldon-Saltin, D.M., 246

Deliganis, A.V., 78–79
D'Emilio, J., 442
Dennerstein, L., 179, 306, 447, 449
    ageing and, 243–244, 245, 246, 250
Derogatis, L.R., 115, 373
Dessens, A.B., 50, 295
Devor, H., 284, 294
Deysach, L.J., 75
Dhabuwala, C.B., 396
Dhindsa, S., 392
Diamond, L.E., 130, 131, 362, 366
Diamond, L.M., 159, 205, 261, 264
Diamond, M., 44, 46
Dickinson, R.L., 75, 175–176, 257
Dietz, P.E., 335
Dillon, J.S., 24
Dinsmore, W.W., 360
Dion, K., 201, 203
Dittus, P.J., 158
Dixson, A.F., 66, 75, 89, 95, 132, 184, 201
Djerassi, I.C., 456
Dodds, J.P., 435
Dollery, C.T., 402
Donatucci, C.F., 366
Donker, P.J., 383
Donohew, L., 435
Dopke, C.A., 287
Dörner, G., 161–162
Doty, R.L., 97
Dow, M.G.T., 118, 358
Dowsett, G., 474
Draper, K., 345
Dreilinger, A., 94
Dreznick, M.T., 483
Dryfoos, J.G., 197
Dubin, L., 459
Duddle, C.M., 345, 356
Dufy, B., 21
Dugger, K., 216
Dula, E., 362
Duncan, B., 7
Duncan, S.P., 469
Dunn, K.M., 95, 181, 312, 327
Dunn, M.E., 90
Dunne, M.P., 157, 158, 180
Dupree, M.G., 164

E

Eardley, I., 362
Easton, D., 174
Eaton, D.K., 195
Ebrahim, S., 396
Edwards, A.E., 242
Egli, M., 128
Ehrenberg, M., 284
Ehrhardt, A.A., 12, 122, 123, 159, 210, 445
    sexual differentiation and, 44, 45, 47, 48, 50
Ekman, P., 320
Elder, M.G., 445
Elford, J., 433
Elias, J., 147, 150
Eliasson, R., 459
Ellenberg, M., 392, 394
Elliott, S.L., 400
Ellis, H., 184, 255–256, 262, 334, 335
Elterman, I., 373
Elwin, V., 187
Endler, N.S., 482
Engel, J., 387
Ensink, B., 490

Enzlin, P., 394
Eplov, L., 181, 221
Erens, B., 180, 212, 213, 269–270, 425, 443
Ericksen, J.A., 174–175, 177
Erikson, E.H., 145
Ernst, C., 179
Erwin, J., 166
Escoffier, J., 6
Evans, H., 219–220
Evans, M., 356
Everaerd, W., 80, 99, 101, 106, 132, 357
Everitt, B.J., 63, 67, 68, 90, 131, 404
Exner, M., 175
Exton, M.S., 90, 92–93, 130
Eysenck, H.J., 106, 180, 202, 228
Eysenck, S.B.G., 106

F

Faerman, I., 392
Fairburn, C.G., 391
Falconer, M.A., 397
Falk, G., 286
Farkas, G.M., 100, 106, 405
Farley, F., 228
Farman-Farmaian, S., 190
Farquhar, C.M., 118, 385
Farrell, C., 192
Fausto-Sterling, A., 24, 30, 60, 253, 290
Federoff, J.P., 330, 503
Feinleib, J.A., 425
Feldman, H.A., 241
Feldman, M.P., 256
Feldman, W., 470
Fenton, K.A., 181
Fenwick, P.B.C., 405
Fergusson, D.M., 110, 148, 273
Fernandez-Guasti, A., 91, 126
Fessler, D.M.T., 283
Fields, J.M., 212, 215
Figueira, I., 387
Finer, L.B., 198
Finkel, M.S., 404
Finkelhor, D., 145, 151
    sexual offences and, 470–471, 473, 479, 484, 494, 496, 500
Finkelstein, J.W., 157
Finley, S.K., 126
Fiorino, D.F., 92
Fishbein, M., 424, 430
Fisher, C., 391
Fisher, S., 87, 96, 321
Fisher, W.A., 99, 214, 228, 229, 264, 361, 373
Fitting, M.D., 400
Fleming, D.T., 297, 417
Flowers, P., 7, 426, 433
Flowers, R.B., 474
Foa, E.B., 491
Folkman, S., 433
Follette, V.M., 499–500
Follingstad, D.R., 224
Ford, C.S., 174, 201, 212, 265, 440, 473
    premarital sex and, 186, 188, 191
Forde, S., 428
Forest, H.G., 156
Fortenberry, J.D., 147–148
Foster, D.L., 28
Foucault, M., 259
Fox, B., 86, 87
Fox, C.A., 86, 87
Fox, G.L., 199
Fox, R., 476, 477

Francis, W.H., 386
Frank, E., 490
Franken, J., 113
Franks, S., 129, 384
Freedman, E.B., 442
Freedman, J.L., 66
Freeman, M.D.A., 464, 467
Freeman, M.E., 129
Frenken, J., 228, 232, 244, 447
Freud, S., 82, 255, 286
Freund, K., 271, 287, 484, 486, 488
Friedman, E.H., 396
Friedman, S., 388
Friedrich, E.G., 385
Friedrich, W.N., 147, 148–149, 334, 497–498
Frisch, M., 276
Frohlich, P., 106, 110, 111
Fugl-Meyer, A.R., 221, 246, 310, 312
Fugl-Meyer, K.S., 221, 246, 310, 312
Fuhr, R., 100
Furby, L., 505
Furniss, T., 484
Futterweit, W., 296

G

Gagnon, J.H., 7, 10–12, 131, 178, 191, 197, 249, 499
   homosexuality and, 266, 268, 271
   sexual development and, 145, 155, 159
   sexual deviance and, 280
Galenson, E., 148
Gallagher, J., 118
Galliano, G., 490
Galton, F., 201
Gamman, L., 284
Gamson, J., 261
Gangestad, S.W., 264, 432
Garcia-Velasco, J., 97
Garde, K., 133, 223, 244, 249
Garfinkel, B.D., 334
Garner, P., 440
Gastaut, H., 397
Gathorne-Hardy, J., 175
Gay, J., 266
Gebhard, P.H., 37, 94, 147, 150, 268, 285
   heterosexuality and, 185, 186, 208–209, 210, 215
   sexual offences and, 389, 470, 483–484, 486, 487–488, 497
Geer, J.H., 99, 100, 106
Geerts, F., 502
Geertz, C., 6
Gelder, M.G., 256
Gelfand, M.M., 120
George, W.H., 405
Gerber, P.N., 334
Gerrard, M., 430, 431, 433
Gerressu, M., 184–185, 231
Ghezzi, A., 398
Gibbens, T.C.N., 491
Gill, J., 406
Gill, M., 498
Gillis, J.R., 187–189, 199, 203–204
Gillman, M., 90
Gilman, D.P., 132
Gilman, S.E., 273
Giraldi, A., 35, 80
Gittleson, N.L., 388–389, 488
Giuliano, F., 80, 361
Gladue, B.A., 162
Glass, D.V., 206

Glass, S.J., 256
Glover, J., 359
Gold, R.S., 431, 435
Gold, R.Z., 459
Gold, S.N., 330
Goldacre, M.J., 415
Goldberg, J.P., 69, 362, 402, 403, 405
Goldfoot, D., 165–166
Goldman, J., 147, 149–150, 293
Goldman, J.E., 241
Goldman, R., 147, 149–150, 293
Goldstat, R., 119
Goldstein, I., 362
Golombok, S., 122
Gonzalez, L., 212
Gonzalez-Cadavid, N.F., 363
Goodall, J., 66
Goode, E., 407
Goodman, A., 331, 333
Goody, J.R., 189, 217
Goodyer, I.M., 24
Gooren, L.J.G., 46, 60, 114, 125, 364
   sexual development and, 157, 162
   transgender issues and, 294, 296, 299
Gorski, R.A., 51, 59–60
Gorzalka, B.B., 80–82, 101, 107, 129, 407
Gosselin, C., 281, 284, 285, 287
Goy, R.W., 165–166
Graber, B., 35, 85, 88
Graber, J.A., 155
Grafenberg, E., 82
Graham, C.A., 16, 97, 132, 147, 282, 310, 431
   fertility and, 446, 448, 450, 451, 455
   heterosexuality and, 181, 200–201, 222, 226, 229
   HIV/AIDS and, 425, 427
   sexual offences and, 471, 491, 499
Gramsci, A., 6
Granata, A., 304
Granot, M., 326
Gray, J.A., 7, 16, 63, 64, 66, 68
Gray, J.P., 208
Graziottin, T.M., 382
Greco, T., 450
Green, R., 48, 160, 163–164, 178, 260, 286, 485
   transgender issues and, 293–294, 295, 297
Green, V., 151
Greenberg, D.M., 502
Greenberg, L.S., 499
Greene, J.G., 249
Greene, S.J., 174, 186, 212, 265, 471
Greer, H.S., 458
Gregg, C.F., 193
Gregorian, R.S. Jr, 403
Gremaux, R., 289
Griffith, E., 401
Grimes, D.A., 452, 454
Grino, P.B., 49
Groth, A.N., 482–483
Grounds, D., 448
Grubin, D., 468–469, 471, 473, 478–479
Grudzinskas, J.C., 439
Grulich, A.E., 269, 270, 420, 426
Grumbach, M.M., 111, 125
Grunbaum, J.A., 196, 199, 445
Guldner, G.T., 397
Gummer-Strawn, L., 454
Gumus, B., 406
Gur, M., 158

H

Haavio-Mannila, E., 156, 185
Haber, R.N., 108
Hager, J.L., 164
Hajjar, R.R., 242
Halbreich, U., 92–93
Haldeman, D.C., 256
Hale, V.E., 107
Hall, G.C.N., 484
Hall, J.E., 21, 389
Hall, K., 500
Hall, L., 413–414
Hallstrom, T., 243–244, 249
Halperin, D.T., 429
Halpern, C.J.T., 114, 115, 147, 157, 158
Hamann, S., 72, 89
Hamer, D.H., 161, 163
Hamill, E., 458
Hamilton, C.M., 397
Hammer, J.C., 430
Hampson, E., 116
Hand, E.A., 429
Hanon, O., 396
Hansen, C.H., 99
Hansen, R.D., 99
Hanson, R.K., 482, 505
Hariton, E.B., 225
Harlow, H.F., 166
Harris, G., 338
Harris, J.R.W., 417
Harris, M., 6, 13–14
Harrison, G., 388
Harrison, W.M., 404
Harry, J., 271
Hart, A.J.L., 456
Hart, B.L., 97
Hartmann, U., 406
Hassold, T.J., 45
Hastings, D.W., 344
Hatcher, R.A., 446, 453
Hatfield, E., 65, 203, 205
Hatzichristou, D., 346
Haugaard, J.J., 151
Hawkins, D.F., 445
Hawton, K., 243, 244, 326, 352, 356–357, 359–360
Hay, A.G., 249
Hayes, R., 243
Hays, R.B., 428
Hayward, A.H.S., 66
Hazan, C., 204
Hazelwood, R.R., 334
Heath, R.G., 88
Heatherton, T.F., 331, 332
Heaton, J.P.W., 67, 69, 362
Hebb, D.O., 7
Hedricks, C.A., 116
Heffner, C.L., 330
Hegeler, S., 240
Heidrich, A., 441
Heiman, J.R., 145, 249, 355, 356, 360, 500
   sexual arousal and, 70, 78–79, 80, 82, 98, 108
Heiser, K., 406
Heisler, J., 356, 357
Hellerstein, H.K., 396
Helm, N., 503
Hems, S.A., 315
Hendricks, C.A., 210
Heninger, G.R., 70
Henning, K., 224, 225
Henry, G.W., 256, 257, 281

Henshaw, S.K., 198, 457
Henson, D.E., 96
Herbert, J., 21, 62, 129
Herdt, G.H., 5, 8, 13, 49, 174, 187, 266
   sexual development and, 156, 160, 161,
      164–165, 168
Herek, G., 268
Herrell, R., 274
Hershberger, S.L., 161
Hertoft, P., 187
Herzberg, B.N., 446
Herzog, A.G., 397
Hess, E.H., 202
Heston, L.L., 163
Hewison, M., 23–24
Hicks, T.V., 224
Higgins, G.E., 74, 399
Hilliges, M., 83
Hines, M., 45, 47, 51, 60, 72, 162
Hines, T.M., 83
Hirschfeld, M., 161, 253, 255, 257, 334
Hirschman, R., 484
Hirshkowitz, M., 393
Hirst, J.F., 315
Hite, S., 87, 176, 186
Ho, G.Y.F., 417
Hobsbawm, E., 155
Hodgson, R., 284
Hoenig, J., 295, 397
Hofferth, S.L., 193, 215
Hoffman, H., 105
Hoffman, M., 260
Holden, C., 333
Hollerbach, P.E., 455
Holmes, W.C., 494
Holstege, G., 88, 89
Honoré, T., 476
Hooker, E., 256, 260
Hoon, E.F., 229, 282, 373
Hoon, P.W., 98, 107
Hoopes, J.E., 300
Hopkins, A.P., 405
Hopkins, J., 492
Hopwood, N.J., 28
Horne, L., 478
Horowitz, S.M., 274
Hospers, H.J., 426
Hotvedt, M.E., 187, 265–266
Houston, L.N., 216
Howard, G., 456
Howells, K., 471
Howie, P.N., 42
Hoyle, R.H., 430
Hoyt, R.F., 83
Hrdy, S.B., 10, 191, 199
Hu, S., 163
Hucker, S.J., 286, 334
Huffman, J.W., 93
Hull, E.M., 67, 68–69
Humphrey, M., 459, 460
Hunter, J.A., 489
Hursch, C.J., 503
Husted, J.R., 242
Hviid, A., 276
Hyde, J.S., 5, 30, 439, 441–442, 475, 495

I

Iervolin, A.C., 31
Ignarro, L.J., 76
Imperato-McGinley, J., 49
Inazu, J.K., 199
Ineichen, B., 203

Ingram, I.M., 458
Insel, T.R., 73, 128
Iversen, S., 62, 67

J

Jaccard, J., 158, 434
Jacklin, C.N., 31
Jacobs, H.S., 129, 384
Jaffe, R.B., 41, 45, 47, 49, 50
Jaffe, Y., 108
James, O.F.W., 406
Janaud, A., 451
Jannini, E.A., 82
Janssen, E., 15–16, 64, 116, 243, 272, 282, 431
   assessment/treatment and, 363, 373
   heterosexuality and, 226, 227
   information processing and, 96, 99, 100,
      101
   sexual offences and, 480, 499
Jay, D., 282
Jay, K., 296
Jeffcoate, T.N.A., 386
Jehu, D., 388
Jenkins, A.R., 334
Jenkins, P., 254, 474, 475, 492
Jenkins, R., 441
Jensen, G.D., 90
Jensen, P., 397–398
Jensen, S.B., 391, 393–394
Johnson, A.B., 37, 94, 470
   heterosexuality and, 185, 186, 208, 210,
      215
Johnson, A.M., 282, 419, 425, 443–444
   heterosexuality and, 183, 196, 213, 214
     marriage, 203, 207–208, 209, 212
     sex surveys, 179, 180, 182
   homosexuality and, 268–269, 270
Johnson, J., 345
Johnson, R., 256
Johnson, V.E., 247, 256, 262
   assessment/treatment and, 345–346, 347,
     349, 352, 356–358, 359
   information processing and, 98
   orgasm and, 85, 86–87, 90
   problematic sexuality and, 304, 306, 323,
     328–329, 337
   sexual arousal and, 74, 78–79, 79, 82
Jones, E.F., 193, 197
Jorm, A.F., 274
Josephs, R.A., 406, 433
Jost, A., 6, 24
Joyner, K., 195, 199, 203, 215
Junge, A., 297
Jung-Hoffman, C., 451
Junginger, J., 284

K

Kafka, M.P., 330–331, 376
Kagan, J., 148, 154, 167
Kahr, B., 225
Kalichman, S.C., 110, 431, 433
Kallman, F.J., 163
Kampman, M., 387
Kandel, E.R., 56–57
Kanfer, F.H., 504
Kantner, J.F., 193, 199
Kaplan, H.S., 337, 346, 349
Kaplan, M.S., 488
Karacan, I., 151
Karama, S., 72

Kasonde, J.M., 456
Katz, S., 472, 491, 494
Katzenstein, L., 78
Kaufman, S.A., 460
Kay, C.R., 450
Kelly, D.D., 126
Kelly, D.L., 389
Kelly, J.A., 431
Kelly, J.P., 62–63
Kendall, K., 266
Kendall-Tackett, K.A., 493, 497
Kendell, R., 336
Kendler, K.S., 495
Kenna, J.C., 295
Kennedy, H.C., 260
Kennedy, K.I., 454
Kennedy, S.H., 387
Kenney, M.J., 81
Kenyon, F.E., 273
Kessler, M.R.H., 500
Keverne, E.B., 66, 96–97, 163–164
Khan, M.E., 456
Khan, S., 268
Kilpatrick, A., 151
Kilpatrick, D.G., 470, 490
Kim, J., 205
Kinder, B.N., 330
King, M., 313
Kinnish, K.K., 159, 264
Kinsey, A.C., 7, 9, 65, 82, 238, 323, 390
   epilepsy and, 397
   heterosexuality and, 175–177, 209, 215,
     220–221, 225
     premarital sex, 189, 191, 192, 197
   homosexuality and, 258, 260, 261, 268
   hormones and, 115
   orgasm and, 84–85, 86–87, 88, 90–91, 94
   sexual development and, 147, 150,
     152–153, 155, 157
   sexual offences and, 470, 494
   sexual variations and, 281, 284, 286–287
Kinsman, S.B., 158
Kipp, K., 65, 133
Kirby, D., 182
Kirk, K.M., 163
Kirschner, M.A., 502
Klassen, A.D., 178, 255
Klebanow, D., 391
Klein, F., 262, 264
Kleinplatz, P.J., 286, 287
Kline-Graber, G., 35, 85
Klosterman, S., 126
Knafo, A., 31
Knauft, B.M., 266
Knegtering, R., 404–405
Knight, R.A., 482
Knoblauch, H., 295
Kohlberg, L., 31, 144
Kok, G., 426
Kolarsky, A., 397
Kolata, G.B., 191
Koller, W.C., 399
Kolodny, R.C., 91, 383, 393, 401, 402, 407
Komisaruk, B.R., 66, 83, 88–89, 95, 128, 400
Kon, I.S., 185, 190
Kontula, O., 156, 185
Korenchevsky, V., 94
Koster, A., 244, 249
Koukanas, E., 105
Koutsky, L., 417
Kozak, L.J., 441
Kraft-Ebbing, R. von, 255, 283, 284
Krantz, K.E., 39, 79

Krassioukov, A., 400
Kreider, R.M., 212, 215
Kritzer, M.F., 126
Krosnik, J.A., 181
Krueger, R.B., 488
Krüger, T.H.C., 87, 90, 92–93, 128, 130
Kruijver, F.P.M., 295
Ku, L., 178
Kuban, M., 484
Kuffel, S.W., 108
Kuhl, H., 451
Kuhn, R.A., 75
Kuhn, T.S., 8
Kupfermann, I., 128
Kurtz, R.G., 65
Kutchinsky, B., 476
Kutner, S.J., 447

L

La Torre, R., 285
Laan, E., 80, 132, 226, 248–249, 325
Labrie, F., 23, 116
Lalumiere, M.L., 105
Lamb, S., 151
Landolt, M.A., 275, 276
Lang, P.J., 100
Langdridge, D., 458
Langfeldt, T., 148
Langstrom, N., 291, 487, 488
Langton, C.M., 479
Langworthy, O.R., 87–88
Lansky, M.R., 360
Larson, J.L., 396
Larsson, K., 166
Lascaratos, J., 473
Laschet, L., 502
Laschet, V., 502
Lattimer, M., 453
Lau, M.P., 219–220
Laumann, E.O., 11–12, 84–85
  ageing and, 240, 246, 250
  heterosexuality and, 203, 214, 215–216,
    221
    marriage, 209, 210, 213
    masturbation, 183, 185
    premarital sex, 195, 196, 199
    sex surveys, 178–179, 180, 182
  HIV/AIDS and, 419, 425, 429
  homosexuality and, 268, 270
  problematic sexuality and, 305, 306,
    310–311
  sexual development and, 145, 159, 167
  sexual offences and, 470, 479, 497–499
Lawrence, A.A., 283, 295, 297
Laws, D.R., 96
Lawson, D.M., 405
Lazarus, A.A., 345
Lazarus, R.S., 320
Leavesley, J.H., 456
LeBoeuf, B.J., 165
LeDoux, J., 62, 99
Lee, J.A., 204
Leedy, M.G., 97
Leeton, J., 448
Lehert, P., 250, 306
Leiblum, S.R., 12, 227, 245, 246, 389
  assessment/treatment and, 343, 360, 361
  infertility and, 459, 460
  problematic sexuality and, 309, 332–333
Leitenberg, H., 151, 224, 225, 470
Lemaire, A., 242, 372
Lemert, E., 464

Leonard, L.M., 499–500
Leridon, H., 208
Lesch, K.P., 332
Leshner, A.I., 179
Lester, R., 406
LeTourneau, E.J., 105
Levesque, R.J.R., 473–474, 476
Levi, L., 71
Levin, R.J., 35, 39, 75, 79–80, 83, 85, 87, 88,
    94, 133, 323
Levin, S.M., 483
Levine, L.A., 373
Levine, R., 204
Levine, S., 388–389
Levi-Strauss, C., 476–477
Levitt, E.E., 255
Lev-Ran, A., 50
Lewis, B.P., 434
Lewis, R.W., 114, 366
Lichtigfield, F., 90
Lilius, H.G., 398
Lilleleht, E., 389
Lillie, F.R., 6
Lincoln, J., 392
Lindemann, C., 444
Lindner, H., 401
Lingiardi, V., 267–268
Linnet, L., 456
Lippa, R.A., 264, 272
Littler, W.A., 85
Littlewood, B., 189
Liu, D., 24, 220
Lloyd, E.A., 10, 94–96, 209
Lobel, B., 383
Lobo, R.A., 42
Lock, M., 249
Lockerd, L.K., 224
Lockhart, A.B., 66
Loeb, T.B., 497
Loewenstein, J., 345
Longford, Lord, 225
Lorrain, D.S., 69, 71, 91, 404
Lottman, P.E., 367
Lowe, K., 180
Lowy, E., 430
Luker, K., 192
Lundberg, P.O., 74, 397, 398, 399
Lunde, I., 133, 223
Luzzi, G.A., 308, 418
Lykins, A.D., 108, 272, 433, 500

M

Maas, C.P., 386
McCabe, M.P., 214, 330, 398, 440, 441
McCall, K., 223
McCarthy, P., 358
McClintock, M.K., 97, 132, 156, 161, 168
Maccoby, E.E., 31
McConaghy, N., 256, 285, 296
McCord, C., 335
McCormick, E.P., 458
McCormick, N.B., 11–12
MacCorquodale, P., 177
McCulloch, D.K., 390–391, 392
McCullough, A.R., 363
MacCullough, M.J., 256
MacDonald, T.K., 433
McEwan, B.S., 51
McEwan, L., 300
McFall, R., 7
McGrew, W.C., 97
McGuire, R.J., 284

McHorney, C.A., 245
MacIan, P., 226
McIntosh, T.K., 91
McKay, M., 385
Macke, J.P., 164
McKenna, K.E., 67, 68, 69, 360–361
McKusick, L., 433, 435
MacLeod, J., 391, 459
MacMahon, B., 28
McMahon, C.G., 364
McNeely, C., 158
McWhirter, D.P., 261, 276
Mah, K., 84, 86
Mahay, J., 10–11, 215–217, 218, 219
Mai, F.M.M., 459
Maines, R.P., 305
Makinen, M., 284
Malamuth, N.M., 225, 480, 482
Malatesta, V.J., 405
Maletzky, B.M., 470
Malinowski, B., 174
Mancia, G., 69
Maple, T., 166
Maravilla, K.R., 78–79, 83, 84, 249
Marazziti, D., 130
Margesson, L.J., 370
Markowitz, L.E., 417
Marks, G., 433
Marks, I.M., 104, 256, 283
Marks, L.V., 305, 442
Marques, J.K., 505
Marquet, J., 422, 424
Marsden, C.D., 398–399
Marshall, D.S., 174
Marshall, E.A., 28, 29
Marshall, J.R., 458
Marshall, L.E., 479, 480–481, 483
Marshall, W.L., 479, 480–482, 482–483,
    484–485, 486–487, 505
Marson, L., 69
Martin, C.E., 240, 249
Martin, C.W., 446, 453
Martin, J.L., 435
Martin-Alguacil, N., 97
Martin-Loeches, M., 449
Mas, M., 91
Masand, P.S., 404
Mason, F.L., 286
Massey, F.J. Jr, 456
Masson, J.M., 475
Masters, W.H., 247, 256, 262
  assessment/treatment and, 345–346, 347,
    349, 352, 356–358, 359
  information processing and, 98
  orgasm and, 85, 86–87, 90
  problematic sexuality and, 304, 306, 323,
    328–329, 337
  sexual arousal and, 74, 78–79, 79, 82
Mathers, N., 345
Mathew, R.J., 107, 387–388
Mathews, A.M., 96, 118, 201, 356, 359–360
Mathews, R., 489
Mattinson, J., 390
Mattison, A.M., 261, 276
Mays, V.M., 273
Mazmanian, D., 450
Mazur, M.A., 472, 491, 494
Mazur, T., 47, 49
Mead, M., 174, 203
Meadows, J., 428
Mease, P., 385
Meisel, R.L., 93
Meisler, A.W., 107

Melis, M.R., 67, 93
Melman, A., 78, 363
Melnick, T., 367
Melton, J.S., 99
Mercer, C.H., 245, 270, 310–311
Mertz, K.J., 416
Mesiano, S., 41
Meston, C.M., 218, 223, 356, 360, 373
  medical practice and, 386, 404
  orgasm and, 85, 88, 96
  sexual arousal and, 70–71, 80–82, 106,
      110, 111
Metts, S., 231
Meuleman, E., 360
Meyer, W.J., 502
Meyer-Bahlburg, H.F.L., 48, 50, 51, 123
  sexual development and, 147, 148–149,
      161, 167
Meyerowitz, J., 290
Michael, R.P., 97, 125–126
Michael, R.T., 178, 425
Michaels, S., 178, 182
Michelson, D., 404
Mickley, H., 395
Milhausen, R., 17
Millar, A., 465, 491
Miller, K., 119
Miller, L., 158
Miller, P.Y., 145
Miller, W.B., 157
Miller, W.I., 320
Mills, T.M., 114, 243
Milne, H.B., 356
Milne, J.S., 287
Ming Chow, K., 335
Minto, C.L., 47, 122
Minton, H.L., 256, 257
Mischel, W., 144
Mishell, D.R. Jr, 446, 451
Mishkin, M., 71
Mitchell, G.D., 460
Mitchell, W., 285, 397
Mitchell, W.B., 107
Moatti, J.P., 424
Modell, J.G., 403
Mohr, J.W., 483
Molitch, M.E., 364
Moll, A., 148, 256
Möller, A., 300
Mondragon, M., 97
Money, J., 87, 122, 164, 281, 283, 334–335
  medical practice and, 397, 402
  sexual differentiation and, 44, 45, 48, 50
Monteiro, W.O., 403
Montgomery, M.J., 154
Montgomery, S.A., 71, 403
Montorsi, F., 114, 243
Moon, D., 261
Moore, M.M., 132
Morales, A.J., 121, 242
Moreault, D., 224
Morell, M.J., 397
Morgan, A.J., 299
Morokoff, P.J., 80
Morris, N.M., 97
Morris, S., 147
Morrison, A.R., 112
Mortensen, M., 240
Mortimer, D., 459
Morton-Bourgon, K., 482
Moscucci, O., 428–429
Moser, C., 281, 286, 287
Mosher, D.L., 226, 229

Mosher, W.D., 195, 197, 455
Mosovich, A., 88
Moss, H.A., 148, 154, 167
Moulier, V.G., 102
Mouras, H., 56, 60, 71, 72, 102, 397
Moxham, J., 335
Muehlenhard, C.L., 472–473
Muir, H., 267
Mulcahy, J.J., 366, 384
Mullan, B., 200
Mullen, P.E., 494
Munoz, M., 70, 242
Murdock, G.P., 200, 471
Murnen, S.K., 226
Murphy, M.R., 93, 128
Murphy, W.D., 487–488
Murray, L., 441
Murray, M.A.F., 502
Mushayandebvu, T., 244
Mustanski, B.S., 69, 111, 157, 162–163,
      163–164, 226, 434
Myers, L.S., 120

N

Najman, J.M., 497
Nakamura, Y., 81
Nakonezny, P.A., 405
Nanda, S., 289
Nathan, S.G., 309
Nathanson, C.A., 182, 192, 215
Nathorst-Böös, J., 117, 247
Nazareth, I., 180, 181
Nelson, A.L., 446, 458
Nelson, E.C., 495
Neri, A., 405
Newcomer, S.F., 155, 197
Newman, A.S., 394
Newman, P., 456
Newton, N., 250
Nichols, M., 329, 376
Nieuwoudt, S., 472
Nijland, E., 364–365
Nishimori, K., 21, 128
Njikam Savage, O.M., 189–190
Noble, A.D., 456
Noe, J., 300
Nofzinger, E.A., 107, 111, 388, 391
Noll, J.G., 498–500
Northman, D.L., 455
Norton, G.R., 388
Notley, R.G., 383
Novak, T.E., 383
Nurnberg, H.G., 404

O

Oates, J.M., 299
O'Carroll, R., 242
O'Carroll, T., 281
O'Connell, H.E., 33–34, 82
O'Connor, D.B., 113
O'Donohue, W., 104–105
Oettel, M., 114, 243
Oggins, J., 216–217
Oinonen, K.A., 450
Okami, P., 5
Olsson, S.-E., 300
Opie, I., 32
Opie, P., 32
O'Rahilly, R., 25
Oranratanaphan, S., 449, 452

Orbuch, T.L., 216
O'Reilly, H.J., 491
Orenstein, P., 156
Orentreich, N., 244
Orford, J., 329, 406
Oriel, J.D., 66
Orr, G.D., 397
Ortiz-Torres, B., 11–12
Ortner, S.B., 6, 174
Osborn, M., 312
Ostovich, J.M., 157, 160–161, 167–168
Ostrow, D.E., 435
O'sullivan, L.F., 147
Ottesen, B., 75, 80
Ottosson, D., 267
Over, R., 105

P

Pacht, A.R., 483, 504
Padavic, I., 217
Padma-Nathan, H., 361, 366
Paff, B.A., 329
Paik, A., 310
Palace, E.M., 107
Palefsky, J.M., 417
Pan, S., 190
Parades, R.G., 132
Pare, C.M.B., 458
Park, K., 72, 126
Parker, J.D.A., 482
Parker, R., 174, 182
Parmeggana, P.L., 112
Parrinder, G., 443
Parsons, W.A., 165–166
Patel, B.C., 456
Paton, J.F.R., 81
Pattatucci, A.M.L., 161, 163
Paul, C., 453
Paul, J.P., 498
Paulak, A., 502
Paulhus, D.L., 499
Pauly, I.B., 294, 295
Pearcey, S.M., 162
Pearlman, C.K., 383
Pearlstein, S., 335
Peeler, W.H., 87
Pendleton, L., 5
Penev, P.D., 241
Penovich, P.E., 398, 405
Pentland, B., 403
Peplau, L.A., 159–160, 162, 167
Perimenis, P., 362
Perper, T., 164, 202, 208
Perry, J.D., 82
Peters, T.J., 406
Peterson, H.B., 456
Petitti, D., 456
Petrosino, A., 505
Peyser, M.R., 459
Pfaff, D.W., 132
Pfafflin, F., 297
Pfaus, J.G., 56, 129, 130, 131, 222–223, 407
Pfeiffer, E., 240
Pfrang, H., 228
Phelps, J.S., 367
Philpott, A., 425, 427
Phinney, V.G., 154
Pietropinto, A., 210
Pillard, R.C., 163, 272
Pinello, D.R., 259
Pinkerton, S.D., 5
Piot, P., 421, 422

Pithers, W.D., 481, 505
Plant, M.A., 407
Plant, T.M., 29, 191, 215
Plaud, J.J., 104
Plummer, K., 281
Polani, P.E., 46, 48
Pollen, J.J., 94
Polusny, M.A., 499
Pomerantz, S.M., 362
Popp, D., 156
Popper, K.R., 5, 6, 8, 12
Porst, H., 361
Porter, R., 413–414, 484, 500
Posner, M.I., 99
Potts, A., 305, 361
Poulakou-Rebelakou, E., 473
Powell, G.E., 284
Powell, K., 61
Prause, N., 282
Prentky, R.A., 482
Preti, G., 97
Price, K.P., 98
Pritchard, B.N.C., 402
Prochaska, J.O., 424
Proulx, J., 481
Pruce, G., 397
Przybyla, D.P.J., 100
Pukall, C.F., 326, 385, 490
Putnam, F.W., 498
Puts, D.A., 94–95
Puy, L., 126

Q

Quadland, M.C., 330
Quinsey, V.L., 105, 486
Quirk, A., 427

R

Rabinowitz, D., 476
Raboch, J., 46
Rachman, S., 104, 284
Rademakers, J., 147, 149
Radzinowicz, L., 487
Rainwater, L., 177
Ramirez-Valles, 158
Ramsey, G.V., 111, 147, 159
Randolph, M.E., 385
Rao, S.P., 81
Rapoport, S.I., 241
Rapson, R.L., 65, 203
Ratcliffe, S.G., 46
Raven, H., 458
Raviv, M., 330
Read, J., 496
Ream, G.L., 167
Reamy, K.J., 440, 442
Rechtschaffen, A., 69
Reddy, D.M., 385
Redouté, J., 72, 103–104, 126, 332
Reece, M., 428
Reed, E.W., 390
Reed, S.C., 390
Regan, P.C., 222
Reinisch, J.M., 155, 295
Reiss, I.L., 177, 192, 217
Rejman, J., 78
Remafedi, G., 161, 274
Remez, G.V., 155
Renaud, C., 190
Rendell, M.S., 361, 393

Resick, P.A., 490
Resko, J.A., 125, 126
Reynolds, M.A., 150, 154, 160
Rhodes, J.C., 118
Richfield, E.K., 104
Richters, J., 185, 227, 310–311
Rieber, I., 503
Rieger, G., 264
Riley, A.J., 67, 70, 116, 361, 402–403, 403, 405
Riley, E.J., 116, 403
Riley, J.W., 177
Rind, B., 475, 494, 495
Rinehart, N.J., 330
Ritson, B., 406
Robbins, M.B., 90
Robbins, T.W., 63, 90
Roberts, A., 216
Robie, W.F., 175
Robins, A.G., 428
Robins, E., 273–274
Robinson, B.W., 71
Robinson, P., 258
Robinson, T.E., 63, 333
Robson, K.M., 439
Rodgers, D.A., 456
Rodgers, J.L., 157
Rodriguez, A., 383
Rodriguez-Manzo, G., 91
Roger, M., 244
Rogers, B.J., 459
Rogers, S.M., 268
Roiphe, H., 148
Role, L.W., 62–63
Ronald, A., 416
Rönnau, H.J., 456
Roose, S.P., 110, 388
Root, W.S., 75
Rooth, F.G., 469, 478, 487
Roselli, C.E., 126
Rosen, I., 344
Rosen, R.C., 304, 327, 428, 449, 456, 503
    assessment/treatment and, 343, 360–361, 362, 363, 365, 366, 373
    medical practice and, 403, 405, 407
    sexual arousal and, 64, 70, 81, 96, 98
Rosenblatt, P., 200
Rosenstock, I.M., 424
Rosler, A., 502
Ross, M.W., 291, 430
Rosser, B.R.S., 329
Rossman, G.P., 486
Rothbaum, B.O., 490
Rowland, D.L., 98, 129, 242, 323–324
Rowlands, P., 388–389
Roy, J., 316
Ruan, F.-F., 219–220
Rubin, H.B., 96
Rubinstein, I., 459
Ruble, D.N., 30–31
Russell, D.E.H., 470–471
Rust, J., 122
Ryan, G., 470
Ryder, A.G., 217
Ryder, N.M., 177

S

Sabini, J., 157, 160–161, 167–168, 201
Sabogal, F., 218
Sachs, B.D., 65, 91, 93, 152
Sacks, M., 389
Sadd, C., 176
Saenz de Tejada, I., 70, 392

Saghir, M.T., 273–274
Sahheim, D.K., 98
Sai, F.A., 190
Sala, M., 67–68, 70
Salamone, J.D., 64
Salemink, E., 100
Salkovskis, P.M., 333
Sample, L.L., 475
Samuelsson, S., 244
Sanchez, R.A., 361
Sanchez-Ortiz, R.F., 384
Sanday, P.R., 471
Sandberg, D.E., 51
Sanders, D., 108, 270, 447
Sanders, S.A., 155, 264, 272, 295, 446
Sandfort, T.G.M., 110, 271, 273–274, 328–329, 376, 428
Sandnabba, N.K., 286
Sanjeevan, K.V., 82
Sansone, G., 66, 128
Santelli, J., 155, 182, 194–195, 199, 215
Santen, R.J., 407
Saper, C.B., 62–63
Sarrel, P.M., 34, 249
Sarrieau, A., 126
Sartorius, N., 446, 448, 450, 451
Satcher, D., 186, 258, 445, 505
Savarimuthu, D., 390
Savic, I., 162
Savin-Williams, R.C., 159, 167
Schaffir, J., 446
Schatzberg, A.F., 271
Schenk, J., 228
Schiavi, R.C., 46, 114, 387, 391, 406
    ageing and, 241, 242, 243
Schlegel, A., 174, 187
Schlesinger, L., 385
Schloredt, K.A., 500
Schmidt, G., 266, 269, 357, 485
    heterosexuality and, 185, 186, 189, 213, 225
Schmidt, L., 459
Schmidt, P.J., 121
Schmitt, D.P., 8
Schneider, G., 502
Schneider, H., 383
Schneider, S.L., 480
Schober, J.M., 502
Schofield, M., 154, 155, 192–193, 199, 213
Schoof-Tams, K., 148, 150, 154, 156
Schreiner-Engel, P., 116, 387, 393–394
Schrenck-Notzing, A. von, 256, 344
Schreurs, K.M.G., 159, 276
Schuhrke, B., 147
Schulte, L., 229
Schultz, J.H., 344
Schupp, H.T., 101
Schwartz, I.M., 155
Schwartz, P., 160, 207, 208, 275
Scott, J., 441
Scott, P.D., 501
Seal, D.W., 12
Seals, D.R., 81
Seftel, A., 384
Segal, N.L., 295
Segraves, R.T., 362, 366, 388, 404
Seligman, M.E.P., 164
Sell, L.A., 89
Semans, J., 323, 344, 355
Semans, J.H., 87–88
Senturia, A.G., 458
Seto, M.C., 484, 486, 487, 488
Seyler, L.E., 296

Shabsigh, R., 363
Shah, F.K., 193–194
Shapira, N.A., 333
Shaver, P., 204
Sheehan, W., 334
Sheeran, P., 426
Shepher, J., 477
Shernoff, M., 329, 376
Sherwin, B.B., 120–121, 247, 364, 448, 451
Shields, J., 163
Shifren, J.L., 120–121, 125
Shlamovitz, G.Z., 335
Short, R.V., 29, 191, 429, 454
Shorter, E., 188–189, 199
Siegel, J., 69
Siegelman, M., 161, 167, 256, 271, 273
Siegert, R.J., 480, 484–485
Sieving, R., 158
Sigusch, V., 213, 503
Sill, M., 239
Silverman, D.C., 491–492
Simenauer, J., 210
Simon, J., 121
Simon, N.M., 458
Simon, W., 7, 10–12, 131, 177, 499
    homosexuality and, 266, 268, 271
    premarital sex and, 191, 197
    sexual development and, 145, 155
    sexual deviance and, 280
Simons, J.S., 310
Simonsen, U., 71
Simpson, E.R., 125
Simpson, J.A., 264, 432
Singer, I., 86, 87
Singer, J.L., 225
Singh, D., 162
Sipova, I., 296
Sipski, M.L., 88, 400
Sisk, C.L., 28, 59, 61
Skidmore, W.C., 271, 275
Skinner, M.J., 431
Skuse, D.H., 163
Slade, P., 458
Slap, G.B., 494
Slutkin, G., 423
Smith, A.H.W., 456
Smith, A.M.A., 269, 274–275, 282
Smith, E.R., 231
Smith, G., 393
Smith, K.B., 383
Smith, S.M., 404
Smithwick, R.H., 87
Snowden, R., 210, 453, 460
Snyder, D.K., 360
Somers, V.K., 69
Sonenstein, F.L., 155
Sorell, G.T., 154
Soules, M.R., 42
Soydan, H., 505
Spataro, J., 494
Spector, I.P., 222–223, 282, 450
Speiser, P.W., 50
Spielberger, C.D., 274, 428, 431
Spiering, M., 99, 106
Spira, A., 179, 180, 203, 209, 210, 312, 420, 427
Spitzer, R.L., 258–259
Sprecher, S., 203, 204, 205
Stahl, S.M., 69, 90
Stanley, J.L., 494
Staples, R., 214
Starka, L., 296
Stava, L., 483

Steel, J.L., 147, 148
Steele, C.M., 406, 433
Steele, S.J., 459
Steers, W.D., 60, 68
Stein, D.J., 330, 333
Stein, E.A., 89, 90
Stein, R.A., 396
Steiner, C.A., 385
Steinman, J.L., 83
Stekel, W., 281
Sterk-Elifson, C., 214
Sterkmans, P., 502
Sternberg, R.J., 205
Stewart, C.S., 193
Stewart, E.G., 370
Stewart, F.H., 454
Stewart, W.F.R., 382
Stief, C., 362
Stockton, M., 226
Stoffer, S.S., 405
Stoléru, S., 332, 397
    sexual arousal and, 56, 60, 71, 72, 98, 102–104
Stoller, R., 30
Stone, L., 187–188, 199, 203–204, 255
Stoner, S.A., 405
Storms, M.D., 167, 272
Strassberg, D.S., 107, 180, 224
Strauss, B., 117
Strauss, J.F., 22
Strong, D.A., 427, 432
Stuart, F.M., 116
Stulhofer, A., 426
Suggs, R.C., 174
Suh, D.D., 32, 33, 247–248, 249
Sulcová, J., 244
Sumanen, M., 395
Summit, R., 495–496, 500
Sundberg, S.L., 480
Swales, J.D., 402–403
Symons, D., 10, 95, 160, 200–202
Szabo, R., 429

Taberner, P.V., 345, 407
Tallafero, A., 88
Talwar, O.O., 447
Taneepanichskul, S., 449, 452
Tannahill, R., 184
Tanner, A., 428
Tanner, J.M., 28, 29
Tavris, C., 176
Taylor, D.C., 397
Tchombe, T.M., 189–190
Tellegen, A., 159, 435
Tennent, G., 411, 502
Tennov, D., 203
Tenover, J.L., 241
Tentler, L.W., 443
Teplin, V., 118
Terman, L., 175
Terzian, H., 397
Thase, M.E., 388
Thibaut, F., 502
Thigpen, J.W., 151
Thompson, E.H., 492
Thompson, L., 305
Thorburn, M., 358
Thorneycroft, I.H., 451
Thornton, J.W., 23
Tiefer, L., 338
Tilhonen, J., 88–89

Tilly, C., 151
Tindall, B., 428
Titta, M., 367
Tolan, J., 422
Toledano, R., 222–223
Tolman, D.L., 156
Tomlinson, J., 361
Toone, B.K., 405
Toran-Allerand, C.D., 51
Tovee, M.J., 201–202, 217
Travison, T.G., 242
Trieschmann, R.B., 401
Trobst, K.K., 430
Tromovitch, P., 495
Trost, J.E., 90
Truitt , W.A., 89
Trumbach, R., 254
Trussell, J., 454
Tsitouras, P.D., 241
Tuiten, A., 119, 125
Tunnadine, P., 345
Turner, C.F., 148, 180, 268
Turner, W.J., 163
Tutty, L.M., 498
Tuzin, D., 5, 7
Twenge, J.M., 216
Tyler, P.A., 165
Tyrer, G., 393–394, 447

U
Uckert, S., 362, 366
Udry, J.R., 155, 157, 178, 197, 204
    sexual arousal and, 97, 114, 115
Ueno, M., 396
Ugarte, F., 362
Uva, J.L., 334

V
Vague, 122–123
Van Anders, S.M., 116
van Beijsterveldt, C.E.M., 31
Van Berlo, W., 490
Van de Ven, P., 428
van den Houte, M.A., 100
Van der Ploeg, L.H.T., 130
Van der Vange, N., 451
Van Houten, T., 34, 35
Van Lankveld, J.J.D.M., 100, 359
Van Look, P.F.A., 442
van Lunsen, R.H.W., 248, 249, 325
Van Minnen, A., 387
Van Thiel, D., 406
Vance, C.S., 174
Vance, E.B., 86
Varjonen, M., 17, 323, 499
Vas, C.J., 398
Vasey, P.L., 165–166
Veening, J.G., 404
Veit, C.T., 453
Veith, I., 305
Veith, J., 97
Velasco, J., 97
Veldhuis, J.D., 241
Vellucci, S.Y., 66
Vener, A.M., 193
Vennix, P., 113, 232, 244, 447
Vermeulen, A., 241–242
Verwoerdt, G.C., 240
Vestergaard, P., 246
Victor, A., 405

Viitanen, T., 212
Vilain, E., 24–25
Vincent, J.D., 21
Virag, R., 75
Visotsky, H.M., 217
Vizard, E., 478
Voeller, B., 260
Volbert, R., 147, 149
Von Sydow, K., 440, 441
Vroude, G.J., 186
Vukadinovic, Z., 330, 332, 376, 434, 480, 482, 500

W

Wabrek, A.J., 395
Wagner, G., 75, 80, 85
Wagner, N.N., 86
Waite, L.J., 203
Walby, S., 469
Waldinger, M.D., 323–324
Walker, A., 447
Walker, P.A., 502
Wallen, K., 31, 165–166
Waller, N.G., 159, 435
Wallin, P., 175, 203
Walmsley, R., 466, 469, 497
Walsh, P.C., 383
Walster, E., 212
Walster, G.W., 203
Wang, C.J., 392
Wang, R., 366
Ward, T., 480, 484–485
Ware, J.E. Jr, 453
Ware, M.R., 387
Warne, G., 52
Warner, L., 454
Warner, P., 108, 249, 313, 315, 382, 447
    assessment/treatment and, 344, 356, 359, 360
Warwick, H.M.C., 333
Wasserheit, J.N., 210
Wassertheil-Smoller, S., 402
Watkins, E.S., 305, 442
Watson, J.P., 357, 387
Watson, L.A., 46
Weeden, J., 201
Weeks, J., 259, 261
Weeks, J.D., 441
Weijmar Schultz, W.C.M., 387
Wein, A.J., 75
Weinberg, M.S., 178, 214, 215, 284, 285
    homosexuality and, 262–264, 267, 271, 273–275
Weinberg, S.K., 484
Weinberg, T.S., 286, 287

Weinberger, D.R., 60–61, 158, 159
Weinhardt, L., 433
Weinhardt, L.S., 406
Weinman, M.L., 107, 387–388
Weinrich, J.D., 160, 262
Weinstein, W., 404
Weis, D.L., 5, 12
Weisberg, R.B., 101
Weiss, E.L., 494
Wellings, K., 190, 198, 199, 200
Wellings, L., 206
Welsh, M., 399
Wessells, H., 362, 383
West, D.J., 491, 503
West-Eberhard, M.J., 94
Westbrook, W.H., 132
Westermark, E., 476–477
Westfall, M.P., 271
Westhoff, C., 453
Westoff, C.F., 177
Westphal, S.P., 223
Westrom, L.V., 326
Whipple, B., 82, 83, 89
White, K., 466, 469, 497
White, M., 177
White, P.C., 50
White, S.E., 440, 442
White, T.L., 16
Whitehead, A., 359–360
Whitehead, H., 6, 174
Whitehead, M.I., 249
Whitelaw, G.P., 87
Whitley, M.P., 393–394
Whyte, M.K., 186, 200, 210
Widom, C.S., 147
Wiederman, M.W., 9
Wiegel, M., 101, 110
Wiener, J., 178
Wienhardt, L.S., 391
Wikberg, J.E.S., 130
Wiklund, I., 247
Wilkinson, D., 456
Willen, R., 326
Williams, B., 225
Williams, C.J., 178, 214, 215, 267, 273
Williams, F.L.R., 440
Williams, L.M., 147
Williams, M.R.I., 24
Wilson, C.A., 68
Wilson, E.O., 66
Wilson, G.D., 202, 281, 284, 285, 286, 287
Wilson, G.T., 405, 406
Wilson, J.D., 49
Wilson, M., 191
Wilson, T., 434
Wincze, J., 394

Winn, R.L., 250
Winters, S.J., 20, 22
Wisniewski, A.B., 122
Witchel, S.F., 29, 191, 215
Witztum, E., 502
Wllings, K., 195–196
Wolchick, S.A., 107
Wolf, A.P., 477
Wolfe, S.M., 167
Wolfenden, Lord, 259
Wolfers, H., 456
Wolpe, J., 345
Wonnacott, S., 90
Woodruff, R.A., 387
Worcel, M., 71
Wouda, J., 80, 325
Wright, D., 361
Wright, R.C., 480
Wu, F.C.W., 384, 453
Wyatt, G.E., 199, 470, 471
Wylie, K.R., 367
Wynne-Edwards, V.C., 66
Wysocki, C.J., 97

Y

Yaffe, M., 225
Yankowitz, R., 87, 402
Yardley, K.M., 299
Yates, E., 481
Yates, W.R., 113
Yen, S.S.C., 23–24
Yost, M.R., 224–225
Youm, Y., 419
Young, A., 296
Young, W.S., 21, 128

Z

Zeki, S., 73, 205
Zelnick, M., 193–194, 199
Zemore, R., 274, 428
Zerhouni, E.A., 179
Zhou, J., 60, 295
Zilbergeld, B., 304, 356
Zillman, D., 82, 111, 159, 331
Zimmer-Gembeck, M.J., 155
Zitzman, M., 46
Zucker, K.J., 44, 49, 51, 160, 167, 291, 293, 294–295
Zuckerman, M., 428, 430
Zumoff, B., 244
Zurbriggen, E.L., 224–225

Index

NB: Page numbers in **bold** refer to figures and tables

A

ABC (Abstinence, Be faithful, use Condoms) approach, 422, 423–424
Abortion
  induced, 457–458, **457**
  legality of, 457–458
  spontaneous, 395
  teenage, 197–198, **198**, 199
Abstinence, 158, 454
  HIV/AIDS and, 423
  PEPFAR and, 422
Abuse see Child sexual abuse (CSA)
Acceptance and commitment therapy (ACT), 500
Acculturation, 202, 217–218
Acebutolol, 402
Acetylcholine (ACh), 63, 68, 76, 78
ACSF (Analyse des Comportements Sexuels en France) survey, 208, 209, 210, 221, 312, 420, 427
Acyclovir, 417
Adaptations, 131
  adaptionists, 133
  evolutionary, 94–96
'Adaptive perception' process, 293
Add Health survey, 155, 158, 167, 178
Addiction
  drugs of see Drugs of addiction
  mood disorders and, 107
  'out of control' behaviour as, 333
  sexual, 110, 330, 480, 500
Addisonian crises, 50
Adenosine triphosphate (ATP), 63
Adolescence
  autoerotic asphyxia (AEA) and, 334–335
  brain development, 60–61
  computers and, 148
  concept of, 474
  contraception and, 182, 192, 199
  delinquency, 479
  family influence, 199
  genital operations, 187
  hanging deaths and, 334
  hormone levels, 25–30
  infertility during, 191–192
  initiation ceremonies, 186–187
  internet and, 227
  maladaptive pattern, 32, 156, 158–159
  masturbation and, 175, 219–220
  paedophilic preferences and, 486

parents vs peer group pattern, 158
  peri-pubertal pattern, 156–158
  same-sex interaction, 266–267, 269
  sex offenders, 470, 478
    female, 489
  sex surveys, 181–182, 192–193, 194–195
  sexual activity, 155
    non-coital, 197
  sexual learning, 285, 296
  sexual revolution and, 177
  social class and, 214
  transgender issues, 296, 299–300
  transition from childhood, 154–159, **154**
  see also Development, sexual; Teenagers
Adrenal medulla, 58
Adrenaline (A), 58, 92
Adrenarche, hormone levels and, 28, 153, 156–157
Adrenergic neurone-blocking drugs, 402
Adrenocorticotropic hormone (ACTH), 28, 130
Adrenogenital syndrome see Congenital adrenal hyperplasia (CAH)
Adultery, 212–213, 319, 329–330, 396, 464
Affection, 177
Affective disorders, 328, 489, 494
'Agape' love, 204
Age
  mood, sexuality and, 108, 110
  sexual activity and, 208
  victims, child sexual abuse (CSA), 493
Ageing, 238–250
  hypogonadism and, 392
  mechanisms, 241–243
  refractory period and, 91
  sexual behaviour changes, 238–240
    in female, 243–250, 311, 327–328
    in male, 114, 240–243, 311, 327
  tactile sensitivity, 242
Aggression
  child sexual abuse (CSA) victims and, 493
  juvenile female sex offenders and, 489
  rape and, 482–483
Agoraphobia, 387
Agricultural societies, 65, 187, 202, 265–267
AIDS see HIV/AIDS pandemic
Akinesia, 398–399
Alan Guttmacher Institute (AGI), 182, 198
Alcohol, 332, 368, 405–406
  cerebellar degeneration and, 406
  child sexual abuse (CSA) and, 483, 495

chronic alcoholism, 406
  disinhibitory effects of, 483, 484
  exhibitionism and, 487
  'myopia', 406
  sexual activity and, 396
  sexual arousal and, 480
  sexual effects of, 368
  vascular impairment and, 392
Aliphatic acids, 97
Alpha1 adrenergic agonists, 383
Alpha1 adrenergic antagonists, 363
Alpha2 adrenergic antagonists, 363
Alpha2 agonists, 402
Alpha1 antagonists, 366, 403
Alpha2 antagonists, 70, 242, 361, 366, 404
Alpha1 receptors, 361–362
5Alpha-reductase 2 deficiency (5-ARD), 49
7Alpha-methyl–19-nortestosterone (MENT), 453
Alprostadil, 363
Ambivalence, sexual, 498
Amenorrhoea, opiates and, 407
American Association for the Advancement of Science, 179
American Association for Retired Persons (AARP), 238–239
American Cancer Society, 387
American Psychiatric Association (APA), 257, 333, 337, 360, 485
American Psychological Association, 179
American Sociological Association, 179
American Teenage Study (ATS), 178, 182
Amitryptyline, 403
Amputees, female, 283–284
Amygdala, 57, 72, 89, 99
  activation/deactivation, 89
Anal intercourse (AI), 209, **209**, 270, 271, 329, 415, 426
  unprotected (UAI), 426, 427, 428, 431, 432
Androgen insensitivity syndrome (AIS), 47–49
  complete see Complete androgen insensitivity syndrome (CAIS)
  partial (PAIS), 49
Androgens, 22–23, 29, 59
  ageing and, 241–242, 244–245
  alpha adrenoceptor antagonists, 69, 70
  female and, 114–124, 153
    adrenal, replacement of, 121
    development aspects, 115
    effects, 118–123, 127–128, 156–157

Androgens (Continued)
  endogenous levels, 115–116
  hormone replacement of, 121
  iatrogenic level lowering, 117–118
  insufficiency, 115
  menstrual cycle, 116–117, **116**, **117**
  pharmacological effects, 123
  placebo effect, 121
  sexual desire, 116
  threshold effect, 123–124
  homosexuality and, 161, 162
  male and, 111–114, **112**, **113**
    ageing, 114
    developmental aspects, 114
    effects, 127–128, 156–157, 501
    mode of action, 124–126
    organizational effects, 59
    ovarian, 42
    receptors (AR), 125–126, 296
    role of, 29
    sensitivity to, 365
  see also Androstenedione;
      Dehydroepiandrosterone (DHEA);
      Dihydrotestosterone (DHT);
      Testosterone (T); developmental
      aspects
Andrology, 382–384
Androstenedione (A), 23, 28, 121,
    244–245, 246
Androstenol, 97
Aneuploidies, sex chromosome, 44–47
Anger
  rape and, 482, 492
  in relationships, 318, 473
  sexual interest and, 108, 111, 483
  sexual offending and, 481
Angina, 396
Angiography, colour Doppler, 383
Angiotensin-converting enzyme (ACE)
    inhibitor, 402–403
Annual Review of Sex Research, 11
Ano-genital warts (condyloma), 417
Anorectal infections, 415
Anorgasmia, 80, 315–316, 354–355, 360, 398
Anterior cingulate cortex (ACC), 71, 73
Anterior hypothalamic/pre-optic area
    (AH/POA), 60
Anterior pituitary-adrenal cortex
    system, 21
Anterior pituitary-gonadal system, 21,
    22, **22**
Anthropological data, 174
Anti-adrenergic drugs, 87, 361–362
Anti-androgen drugs, 117, 376
  gender reassignment and, 292, 299
Anticipation of reward, 90
Anti-convulsant drugs, 295, 397–398, 405
Anti-depressant drugs, 366, 403, 403–404
  side effects, sexual, 363, 403
Anti-hypertensive drugs, side effects,
    sexual, 328, 402
Anti-psychotic drugs, 404–405
  side-effects of, 399
Anti-retroviral (ARV) therapy, 418–419, 421
Anxiety
  child sexual abuse (CSA) victims and,
      493, 494, 495, 498, 500
  cognitive behavioural techniques (CBT)
      and, 491
  diabetes mellitus (DM) and, 391
  disorders, 330, 490
  low sexual interest and, 107, 108–110, **109**,
      330–331, 387–388

multiple sclerosis (MS) and, 398
Oedipal, 320
orgasm and, 87
'out of control' behaviour and, 376
performance, 175, 307, 329, 347,
    350–351, 388
selective serotonin re-uptake inhibitors
    (SSRIs) and, 305
sex offenders and, 480
systematic desensitization of, 358
Aphrodisiacs, 345
Apomorphine, 67, 69, 362, 363, 366
Apoptosis, 59
Appetitive behaviour, 64, 89, 220
Appropriations Bill (HHS), 179
Aquinas, St Thomas, 184, 254
Archives of Sexual Behavior, 258, 324, 485
Arcuate nucleus, 129
L-Argenine, 71
Aromatase, 125, 126, 296
Arousal Contingency, 499
  sub-scale of SEII-W, 327
Arousal, general, 63
  central arousal system, 327
Arousal, sexual
  age of onset, 154, **154**
  central component, 361
  central system, 327
  child sexual abuse (CSA) and
      deviant, 485
  clitoral response, 84
  fear and, 111
  female, 80–82
  as motivation, child sexual abuse
      (CSA), 484
  oral contraceptives and decrease in, 449
  pain and, 308
  problems, 365
  rape sequences and, 480
  risk taking, impact of, 431
  role of inhibition, 480
  sexual desire and, 64–65, 220
  see also Genital response
Arousal, specific, 63
Arterial disease, 395
Arthritis, 415
Artificial insemination, donor (AID), 460
Asexuality, 223, 275, **275**, 281–283
  sexual problems and, 321, 324, 338
Asian community
  American, 218
  female, 218–219
Assault, sexual, 286, 464, 465, 482–483
  categories of, 466
  recalling, 471
  socio-cultural context, 471–473
  in United States (US), 470
Assessment, sexual problems, 367–374
  by angiography, 383
  interviews, 367–368
  psychometric, 373–374
  three windows approach, 306–307,
      316–328, 338, 343, 346, 373–374
Association therapy, 256
Asthma, 334–335
Ataxia, 418
Atenolol, 402
Atomage correspondence club, 284
Atropine, **68**, 75
Attachment, 73, 167
  mothers, 'close binding intimate', 161
  parent-child, 445, 479, 483
  problems, 276, 483

theory, 145, 500
types, 204
'Attentional' bias, 99
Attitude Towards Women Scale, 224
Attitudes, sexual
  child sexual abuse (CSA) and public, 492
  double-standard see Double standards
  extramarital sex, 212
  female body and, 369
  masturbation, 183–184, 354
  measures of, 228–229, 239
  negative, 320–321, 346, 354, 456, 460, 498
    'sex negativism', 176, 185, 255, 280, 505
  premarital sex, 186, **186**
  rape and prejudicial, 472, 491
  restrictive, 332
  'sex positivism', 280, 282
  sexual assault, 489
  sexual problems, 368
  treatment and, 348, 368
  unmarried, 177
  see also Catholicism; Christian culture;
      Islamic culture; Jewish tradition;
      Protestantism; Religion
Attraction, sexual, 154–155, **154**, 200–202
Attractiveness, puberty and, 485–486
Australian Study of Health and
    Relationships (ASHR), 310–311
Australian Twin Register, 495
Autoerotic asphyxia (AEA), 334–335
Autogynephilia, 290–291, 297
Autonomic dysreflexia, 400
Autonomic nervous system, 39, **40**, 57–58,
    63, 385, 398
'Autonomic storms', 69
Autoradiography, 125
AVEN (Asexual Visibility and Education
    Network), 282
Aversion, sexual, 387, 498–499
  child sexual abuse (CSA) and, 497
  disorder, 337
Aversion therapy, 503
Aversive techniques, 256, 504
  conditioning, 345
Avoidance, sexual, child sexual abuse
    (CSA) victims and, 499–500
Azoospermia, 459, 460

B
'Baby boom', 177, 442
Bacterial infections, 414–415, 415–416, 418
Balanitis, 372
Baltimore Longitudinal Aging Study, 240
Barbiturates, 295
Barrier methods, contraceptive, 443, 454
Bartholin's glands, 34
Basal ganglia, 57
Basic pattern, sexuality, 327
  female, 131–132, 186, 232
  male, 131–132, 232, 249
BBC Internet survey, 264
BDSM (bondage, discipline, sadism and
    masochism), 286
Beaumont Society for Transvestites and
    Transsexuals, 284
Beck Depression Inventory (BDI), 106, 108,
    119, 449–450, 451, 490
Bed nucleus of solitary tract (BNST), 295
Bed nucleus of stria terminalis (BST), 59–60,
    73, 89, 125–126, 404
Behaviour therapy, 344–345, 346, 503

Behavioural Activation Scales (BAS), 16
Behavioural approach system (BAS), 63
Behavioural Inhibition Scales (BIS), 16
Behavioural inhibition system (BIS), 63
Behaviours, sexual
  ageing and *see under* Ageing
  appetitive, 64, 89
  childhood/adolescence transition,
      154–159, **154**
  coital frequency, 208
  complementarity, 165
  consummatory, 64
  contraception, effects on, 446–452,
      447, 448
  evidence sources, 146–148
  externalizing, 149, 156, 159, 493
  functions of, 146
  HIV/AIDS, impact on, 435–436
  internalizing, 493
  maladaptive, 32, 156, 158–159, 479
  pre-pubertal child, 148–153, **149**
  problems in, 329–335, 376
  proceptive, female, 132
  relevant, 154–155
  risk taking *see* Risk taking, sexual
  same-sex *see* Homosexuality
  taboos *see* Taboos
  see also 'Out of control' sexual behaviour
Beliefs, negative, 320–321
Bendroflumethiazide, 402
Benefits, sexual, barriers to, 338–339
Benperidol, 405, 502
Benzodiazepines, 403
Bergin, Allen E., 356
Beta adrenergic blockers, 402–403
Beta-blockers, 402–403
Beta-endorphin, 67, 90, 129
17Beta-hydroxysteroid dehydrogenase
      deficiency (17betaHSD), 49–50
Bethanidine, 402
Bibliotherapy, 359
Biological determinism, 472
Birth control *see* Contraception
Birth Control Federation of America, 177
Birth rate
  amongst teenagers, 197–198, **198**
  declining, 177
  increasing, 187
  sex surveys and, 175
Bisexual Center (San Francisco), 262
Bisexual Forum (New York), 262
Bisexuality, 255–256, 266
  gender differences, 264
  practices, same-sex interaction, 270
  prevalence of, 268–270, **269**, 274
  sexual identity and, 260, 261–264,
      263, 335
    development, 159, 161, 165–166, 169
  sexual problems and, 328–329
  types of, 262–263
Black community
  African Americans, 214–215, **215**, 419,
      441, 455, 457
  female, 177, 185, 194, 211, 215–217,
      218–219, 311
    rape victims, 490
  male, 193, 215, **215**
Bladder dysfunction, 392, 398, 400
'Blockage', motivation for child sexual
      abuse (CSA), 484
Blood flow
  pelvic abnormalities, 384
  penile, 384

regional cerebral (rCBF), 56, 71, 72, 104
  vaginal (VBF), 79–82, 107, 130, 325,
      333, 405
Blood pressure, 393, **394**, 396
Blood-oxygen level-dependent (BOLD)
      contrast, 56, 102
Body image, 32
Body mass index (BMI), 201, 216
Body shape changes, 156
'Bolsters', concept of, 75
Bondage, 286
Bonding
  emotional cues, 223
  pair, 205
Bowel dysfunction, 398, 400
Brain, 56–65
  abnormalities, 328
    fetishism and, 285
  androgen receptors (AR), 125–126
  androgen/oestrogen mode of action,
      124–126
  childhood/adolescence development,
      60–61
  emotional, 21, 61–64
  function decline with ageing, 241
  gonadal steroid receptors, 125
  inhibitory signals *see* Inhibitory
      mechanisms
  injuries, 398, 482
  masculinization, abnormal, 161–163
  orgasm and, 88–89, 398
  'problem clusters' and, 485
  sexual differentiation of, 59–60, **60**
  structure, 57–59, **58, 59**, 162
  temporal lobe disorders, 305–306
  tumours, 328
  see also Information processing
Brain imaging, 88
  addiction and, 333
  functional imaging, 56
  gonadal steroid activity, 126
  impaired inhibition and, 332
  magnetic resonance imaging (MRI),
      78–79, 83–84, 398
    functional (fMRI), 56, 61, 72, 89,
        102, 126
  regional cerebral flow (rCBF), 56, 71,
      72, 104
  romantic love, 73–74
  sexual stimulation, 71–73, 102–104, **103**
Brainstem, 57
  abnormalities, 398
Breast development, 191
Breast-conserving therapy (BCT), 387
Breastfeeding, 42, 441–442, **442**
  infertility and, 454
  lactation, 41–42, **43**, 446
  post-natal depression and, 441
Bremelanotide (PT141), 130, 131,
      362–363, 366
Brief Inventory of Sexual Function
      (BSFIW), 120–121
British Crime Survey (BCS), 469
British Medical Association, 255, 467
British Medical Journal, 429
Brodmann's area 10, 88
Bromocriptine, 364
Buddhism, 219
Buggery, 468
Bulbocavernosus muscle, 59, 84
Bulbocavernosus reflex, 372, 393
Bulbospongiosus muscle, 76, 84
'Bundling' system, 187, 189, 191, 445

Bupropion, 366, 403–404
Burke, Kenneth, 10
Bush, President George W., 421, 425
Buspirone, 404
Butyrophenones, 405, 502
By-product explanation, 10, 131, 133

C

Cabergoline, 364
Calcium channel blockers, 75, 399, 403
*Call to Action to Promote Sexual Health and
      Responsible Sexual Behavior*
      (Satcher), 8, 258, 445, 505
Cancer
  breast, 387
  cervical, 386, 417
  endometrial, 386
  gynaecological malignancy, 386–387, 502
  Kaposi's sarcoma, 414, 418
  non-Hodgkin's lymphoma, 418
  ovarian, 385
  prostate, 383
  uterine, 385
Candida albicans (thrush), 326, 371, 372, 414,
      416–417
Captopril, 402–403
Carbamazepine, 398, 405
Cardiovascular disease, 311, 395–396
Cardiovascular system
  exercise, sexual response, 81
  responses, in orgasm, 85–86
  syphilis and, 415
Castration, 503
Catholicism, 195, 208, 218–219, 267, 282,
      442–443, 454
Caudate nucleus, 57, 73, 104
Cauldwell, David O., 290
Caverject, 363
Celibacy, 282
Cellular connectionism, 57
Center for Disease Control (CDC), 415, 416,
      417, 419, 429, 435
Central autonomic dysregulation, 391–392
Central nervous system (CNS), **58**, 62, 63,
      114, 125, 415, 450
Cerebellum, 57
Cerebral hemispheres, 57
Cerebral toxoplasmosis, 418
Cervical fluid, 79
Cervix, 79
  cancer of, 386, 417
  vaginal/cervical stimulation (VCS), 79,
      89, 128
Chancroid, 414, 416
Charing Cross Gender Identity Clinic, 295
Chemotherapy, 387
Chicago Health and Social Life Study
      (CHSLS), 182, 473, 499
  'sex markets' and, 203
Child Behavior Checklist (CBCL), 147,
      148–149, 293
Child protection agencies, incest and, 484
Child sexual abuse (CSA)
  'abused becomes abuser' hypothesis,
      484, 489
  accommodation syndrome, 495–496
  asymptomatic victims, 493–494
  betrayal and, 496
  child molesters, 480–481, 482,
      483–484, 486
  cycle of concern, 474–476

Child sexual abuse (CSA) *(Continued)*
  depression in adulthood and, 494
  exploitation and, 473–476
    commercial interests, 473, 486
  family factors, 494–495
  'force' fantasies and, 224
  historical perspective, 473–476
  models, 499–500
    explanatory, 484–485
    of impact, 495–496
  offenders and, 483–486
    female, 489
  paedophilia, concept of, 485–486
  peak and trough reactions, 475
  pornography, internet and, 467, 473–474, 476
  prostitution and, 467, 473–474
  recalling, 306, 471
  reporting, 493, 495
  sex abuse risk factor scale, 494–495
  sexual development and, 111, 145, 147–148, 159, 496–500
  Sexual Offences Act (2003) and, 466–467
  sexual problems and, 315, 331, 369
  statistics, 468–469
  victims, 321, 492–501
    counselling, 500–501
Child Sexual Behavior Inventory (CSBI), 147, 148–149, 498
Childhood
  /adolescence transition, 154–159, **154**
  brain development, 60–61
  concept of, 474
  consent and, 466
  dissociation, 498
  exhibitionism and, 488
  gender identity discordance (GID), 293–295
  hormone levels, 25–30
  mental disorders and, 494
  orphans, 421
  pre-pubertal, 148–153, **149**
  rejection, 275
  sexual experiences, 91
    with peers (CSEP), 150, 151
  sexual response in, 151–153
  sexual trauma in, 111, 321, 335, 493, 497
  street children, 473
  see also Child sexual abuse (CSA)
Childhood Matters (National Commission of Inquiry), 474
China, 219–220
  birth control programme, 219
Chlamydia, 416, 429
Chlamydia trachomatis, 414, 416, 419
Chlordiazepoxide, 403
Chlorpromazine, 405, 502
Chlorthalidone, 402
'Choking game', 334
Cholinergic (ACh) system, 63
'Chordee' (bending of penis), 384
Christian culture, 464
  artificial insemination and, 460
  circumcision and, 428–429
  heterosexuality and, 187, 200, 217, 219
  homosexuality and, 253–254
  rape and, 472
  sexual variations and, 280–289
  see also Catholicism
Chromosomal gender, 24–25
Chromosome aneuploidies, sex, 44–47
Chronic pelvic pain syndrome (CPPS), 308, 383

Cialis, 361
Ciba Foundation, 484, 500
Cimetidine, 405
Cingulate cortex, 61
Circumcision, 187, 428–429
  historical perspective, 428–429
Cirrhosis of liver, 406
Civil Partnership Act, 259
Civil rights movement, 257
Civil unions (gay marriage), 259, 267, 275, 276
Class *see* Social class
Claustrum, 72
Clinics
  Edinburgh, 313, 344, 358, 382
  Guys Hospital Sexual Problem Clinic, 315
  Kinsey Institute Sexual Health Clinic, 324, 336, 344, 355
  Maudsley Hospital Psychosexual Dysfunction Clinic, 284, 315
  Oxford Sexual Problems, 315, 356, 358, 360
  sexual health, 313–316, **314**, **315**, 344
    HIV/AIDS and, 419–420
    medical practice, 382, 387, 395
Clinton, President Bill, 155, 183
Clitoral-vaginal transfer, 86
Clitoridectomy, 187, 305
Clitoris, 33–34, **33**, **34**
  ageing and, 247, 248
  orgasm and, 82, 86–87
  removal, 387
  response, 78–79, 82–83, 83–84, 247
  retraction process, 78, 247
  stimulation, 122, 133
Cloacal exstrophy, 51, 52
Clomipramine, 404
Clonidine, **68**, 71, 82, 402
Clozapine, 389
Cognitive behavioural technique (CBT), 359, 385, 491
  mood regulation and, 434
  sex offender management and, 500–501, 502, 505
Cognitive factors
  learning, 144
  processing, 406
Cognitive manipulations, 99–101
  distortions, child sexual abuse (CSA) and, 485
  distraction effects, 100–101
  false feedback, 101
  misattribution/misinformation, 101
  sexual content-induced delay (SCID), 99–101
  subliminal priming, 100
Co-habitation *see* Marriage/cohabitation
Coitus reservus, 184
Collective denial, 260, 268
Collectivism, 204, 205
Combined oral contraceptives (COC), 449
Commercial interests, child sexual abuse (CSA) and, 473, 486
Commission on Obscenity and Pornography, 225
Committee on Nomenclature (APA), 257
Committee for the Study of Sex Variants, 257, 281
Common sense, 6
Communication
  with children, for grooming, 467
  methods, 318
  patterns, set, 484

physical handicap and, 382
pleasure and, 316, 347, 349, 369
poor, 319, 348, 360
Community
  sexual offences against children in, 467
  sexual problems in, 310–313, **310**, **312**
  sexualization and, 321
  sexually transmitted infections (STIs) in, 419–420, **419**, **420**
Co-morbidity, 330
Companionate love, 65, 203, 205
Companionate Love Scale (CLS), 205
Companionate marriage, 175
Compensation hypothesis, 285
Competence
  heterosocial, 483
  sexual, 31
Complementarity of sexual behaviour, 165
Complete androgen insensitivity syndrome (CAIS), 47–49, **47**
  gender identity and, 47
  hypothalamus, positive feedback response, 60
  sexual orientation and, 47
  sexuality and, 49, 122–123
  study of, unpublished, 47–48
Compulsion, sexual, 110, 330, 428, 499, 500
Conditioning, 104–105
  aversive, 345
  childhood, 283
  conditioned stimulus (CS), 105
  of erections, 284
  fetishism and, 296
  processes, 481
  sexual learning and, 164
  unconditional stimulus (US), 105
Condoms
  ABC approach, 422, 423–424
  attitudes towards, 426
  contraceptive failure and, 454
  female, 425, 427, 454
  HIV/AIDS and, 423, 424, 425–427, 443
  negative impact of, 432
  PEPFAR and, 422
  pleasure and, 425
  problems with, 427
  sexually transmitted infections (STIs) and, 317, 454
  traditional moral values and, 426
  use, prevalence of, 425–427
    teenage, 198–199
    in United Kingdom, 443–444
    in World, **442**
Condyloma, 417
Conflict-avoiding family, 484
Conflict-regulating family, 484
Confrontational political activism, 257
Confucianism, 219
Congenital adrenal hyperplasia (CAH), 50, 123, 295
  salt-wasting (SW) form, 50, 123
  simple virilizing (SV) form, 50
Congress of Sexology, 356
Conscious processing, 99
Consent
  age of, 465
  causing sexual activity without, 466
  children and, 466, 467, 496–497
  learning disabled (LD) and, 390
  legal changes, 490
  use of drugs, treatment, 501
Consistency, sexual response cycle, 308, 309
Consummatory behaviour, 64

Contagious Diseases Act 1864 (UK), 414
Contingent magnetic variation (CMV), 102
Contingent negative variation (CNV), 102
Contraception, 177, 192
  barrier methods, 443, 454
  bleeding problems, 446, 452
  condoms see Condoms
  diaphragm, 443, 454
  fertility control and, 442–454, **442**
  hormonal, 445–446
    effects on sexual behaviour, 446–452,
      447, **448**
    male, 453–454
  intrauterine see Intrauterine
    contraception
  for learning disabled, 390
  long-acting reversible methods, 198, 390,
    452–453
  microbicides, 427–428
  natural methods, 454
  opposition to, 317
  oral see Oral contraceptives (OC)
  post-partum period, 454
  reappraisal, 368
  spinal cord injuries (SCI) and, 401
  sterilization, 454–457, **455**
  steroidal see Steroidal contraceptives
  for teenagers, 182, 192, 198–199, 444–445
  use, methods of, 443–445, **443**, **444**
Contraceptive Technology (Hatcher), 446
Control
  'letting go', 316, 317, 321, 348
  safe sex and, 434
  self-, 320–321, 330
  sexuality, own, 473
Convention on the Rights of the Child
  (UN), 474
Conversion therapy, 256
Coping strategy
  'emotion-focused', 482
  masturbation as, 481
  sex as, 479, 480, 485
Coping Using Sex Inventory (CUSI),
  480–481, **481**
Copper, intrauterine devices (IUDs) and,
  425
Corpora cavernosa (CC), 75–78, **76**, **77**, 382,
  383, 384
  intracavernosal injections(ICI), 304, 361,
    363, 366, 383, 393
Corpus callosum, 57, 60
Corpus spongiosum, 74
Corticosteroids, 382
Co-therapy, 352–353
'Cottaging', 468
Counselling
  before vasectomy, 456
  cardiovascular disease and, 396
  child sexual abuse (CSA) victims and,
    500–501
  clinics and, 315–316
  communication and, 318
  crisis, 491, 492
  directed practice and, 358
  erectile dysfunction (ED) and, 355
  gynaecological malignancy and, 387
  HIV/AIDS and, 434
  physical handicap and, 382
  prostatectomy and, 383
  schizophrenia and, 389
  sex offenders and, 501, 504
  spinal injuries and, 401
  testosterone (T) therapy and, 118

Coupled genetic oscillators, 66
Couples
  contraception for disabled, 390
  therapy for, 346–353, 355–360, **356**,
    357, 359
  treatment for same-sex, 375–376
Courts
  ecclesiastical, 464, 467
  proceedings in, 465, 493
Courtship, 187–188, 202
  'disorders', 488
Cowper's glands, 37, 94
Cranial nerve, 10th, 58
Crime
  reporting, 465, 468, 470, 491, 493, 495
  sadistic violent, 286
  statistics, 468–471
  see also Offences, sexual
Criminal Law Revision Committee
  (CLRC), 467
Crisis counselling, rape victims and,
  491, 492
Cross-gender behaviour, 265
  cross-dressing, 290, 291, 296, 487, 488
  see also Transvestism
Crown Prosecution Service, 465
'Cruising', 432, 468
Cryotherapy, 417
Cryptococcal meningitis, 418
'Cuckoldry', 212–213
Cultural factors, 164–165
  acculturation, 217–218
  cross-cultural comparisons, 174, 183
  cultural influence model, 174
  heritage, 217
  homosexuality and, 265–268
  indigenous, 219–220
  initiation of sex and, 208
  mainstream, 217
  masturbation and, 184–185
  North America/Europe, 214–220, **215**
  premarital sex and, 186–190, **186**,
    188, **190**
  romantic love and, 204–205
  sexual attraction and, 201
  sexual identity and, 164–165
  sexual intercourse, age at first and, **190**,
    191–199
  transsexuals and, 291
  see also Catholicism; Christian culture;
    Islamic culture; Jewish tradition;
    Protestantism; Religion; Socio-
    cultural factors
Cultural materialism, 6, 13–15, 187
'Cyber sex', 226
Cyclic adenosine monophosphate (cAMP),
  78
Cyclic guanesine monophosphate (cGMP),
  76, 78
Cyproterone acetate (CPA), 117, 124, 299,
  376, 502, 503
Cystitis, 415
Cystometrogram, 393

D

Dannemeyer, William, 178
Darwin, Charles, 10
Death
  during sexual activity, 396
  fear of, 395
  hanging, 334

HIV/AIDS and, 418, 421
  lesbian 'bed', 376
'Declarative' function of law, 464
Dehydroepiandrosterone (DHEA), 23–24,
  28, 121, 123, 127, 156, 451
  sulphate (DHEAS), 23–24, 28, 115–116,
    123, 127, 130, 244, 451–452
Delequamine, 69, 361
Delinquency, in adolescence, 479
Delivery hypothesis, brain oestrogens
  and, 51
Delusions, 389
Dementia, 328, 406, 416
Denial
  child sexual abuse (CSA) victims
    and, 499
  collective, 260, 268
  rape victims and, 492
Department of Health and Social Security
  (DHSS) (UK), 179
Depo-Provera, 446, 452–453
Depot medroxyprogesterone acetate
  (DMPA), 452–453
Depression
  ageing and, 249
  child sexual abuse (CSA) victims and,
    493, 495, 498, 500
    in adulthood, 494
  clinical, 307
  depot medroxyprogesterone acetate
    (DMPA) and, 453
  diabetic mellitus (DM) and, 394
  erectile dysfunction (ED) and, 387
  female, 317
  homosexuality and, 110, 272, 273, 274
  induction of, 107–108
  low sexual interest and, 330–331,
    387, 441
  masturbation and, 110
  medical practice and, 387–388
  menopause and, 327
  multiple sclerosis (MS) and, 398
  nocturnal penile tumescence (NPT) and,
    304
  'out of control' behaviour and, 333, 376
  pain and, 385
  post-natal, 441, 447
  rape victims and, 490, 492
  selective serotonin re-uptake inhibitors
    (SSRIs) and, 305
  sex offenders and, 480
  sexual desire and, 388
  sexual risk taking and, 110
  sexuality and, 108–110, **109**
Derogatis Interview for Sexual Function,
  119
Desensitization hypothesis, 127, 345
'Design, good', 200
Desire/interest, sexual
  ageing and, 239, 240, 243, 245, 246
  androgens and, 116
  child sexual abuse (CSA) and low, 497
  gender differences, 231–232
  heterosexual, 220–223, **221**
  hypoactive sexual, 387
  increased, depression and, 388
  lack of, 219, 307–308, 308–309, 353–354,
    358
  low, 80, 313–316, **314**, 324, 364, 366
    assessment, 371–372
    depression and, 330–331, 387, 441
  mood and, 124
  pharmacological reduction of, 502–503

Desire/interest, sexual (Continued)
  pregnancy and, 439
  reduced, 307–310
    hormonal, 501–502
    see also Treatment, sexual problems
  romantic/implicit cues, 223
  sexual arousal and, 64–65
  spontaneity and, 223
  surgical control, 503
  vasectomy and, 456
  visual/proximity cues, 223
Desogestrel, 445
Development, sexual, 144–170
  appropriate, 155–156
  child sexual abuse (CSA) and, 496–500
  discontinuous, 165, 168, 169, 266
  gender identity and, 30–32
  hormone levels and, 25–30
    testosterone (T), 25–26, 27, 28
  interactional model, 145–146, 146
  latency period, 150
  learning, sexual, 285, 296
  process of, 144–146
  psychoanalytic model, 145
  psychogenic approach, 145
  sex offenders and, 478–479
  sexual behaviour/relationships, 146–159
    evidence sources, 146–148
    pre-pubertal child, 148–153
  sexual identity and, 159–169
  sexual meaning, 149–150
  stages of, 37
  see also Three-strand model
Developmental calibration of psychological
      mechanism, 9
Deviance, sexual, 280–281, 345
  secondary/amplified, 464
  types of, 280
Dextromoramide, 68
Diabetes mellitus (DM), 240, 390–395
  aetiological mechanisms and, 391–393
  candida infections and, 417
  erectile dysfunction (ED) and, 343, 381
  hypogonadism and, 384
  laboratory tests, 372
  male sexual problems and, 305, 390–391,
      391–393, 391, 393
  neuropathy, 87
  sexual interest and, 328
Diagnostic classification, 316
Diagnostic procedures, 304
Diagnostic and Statistical Manual of Mental
      Disorders (DSM), 336–337
Diarrhoea, chronic, 418
Diazepam, 358, 403
Diencephalon, 57
Diethyl dithiocarbamate (DDC), 91
Diethylstilboestrol (DES), 51, 162
Differentiation see Sexual differentiation,
      anatomical
Digoxin, 405
Dihydrotestosterone (DHT), 23, 25, 49, 125
Dilators, vaginal, 344, 349, 354, 359
Directed practice, 358
Discipline
  parental, 199
  personal, 255
Disclosure, child sexual abuse (CSA)
      accommodation syndrome,
      495–496
Discontinuous sexual development, 165,
      168, 169, 266
Disease, 'germ' theory of, 413

Disgust, 320
'Disinhibition' model, 480, 483, 484
Distraction, 81, 82
  effects of, 100–101
Distress, 312–313, 337, 391
Diuretics, 402
Diurnal rhythm, 40
Divorce, 175, 212–213, 215
  age at, 212
  child sexual abuse (CSA) victims and,
      495
Divorce Reform Act, 205
Dizygotic (DZ) twins, 157, 163
DNA, 163, 164, 363
Dominance, male
  exhibitionism and, 487, 488
  hierarchy, 66
  homosexuality and, 265
  in marriage, 200, 208
  rape and, 472, 482
  sadomasochism and, 286
  and submission, patterns of, 286–287
  voyeurism and, 488
Dopamine and dopaminergic (DA) system
  agonists, 362, 366
  antagonists, 389, 404–405
    side effects, sexual, 399
  meso-limbic system, 407
  pathways, 61
  sexual arousal and, 62–64, 67–73 passim,
      88–93 passim, 129, 399
Doppler wave-form analysis, 80, 383, 384,
      393
'Dormitory' environment, 187, 266
Dose-response relationships, 67–68, 407
'Double role' pattern, transvestism,
      293, 299
Double standards, 189, 200, 212, 219, 337,
      445, 482
Dowry systems, 189, 191
Drospirenone, 452
Drugs of addiction, 63, 89–90, 407
  amphetamines, 362, 407
  child sexual abuse (CSA) and, 483
  cocaine, 90, 362, 407
  exchange programmes, PEPFAR and, 422
  exhibitionism and, 487
  heroin, 90
  marijuana, 407
  needle sharing, 414, 418
  nicotine, 89–90
  opiates, 407
  'out of control' behaviour and, 333
  'rush' of, 89–90
  sexual effects of, 368
'Dry-run' orgasm, 87, 308, 371, 391
DSM system of classification, 336–337
Dual Control model, 7, 15–17
  ageing and, 243
  child sexual abuse (CSA) victims and,
      499–500
  erectile dysfunction (ED) and, 243
  female and, 131, 133
  high-risk sexual behaviour (HRSB) and,
      429, 431
  homosexuality and, 272
  information processing and, 105–106
  negative mood and, 330
  personality and, 229–231
  refractory period and, 91
  sex therapy and, 346
  sexual offences and, 478
  sexual problems and, 305–306, 332

sexual response and
    control models, 483
    patterns, 63, 64
  sexual risk taking and, 480
Dyadic relationships, 161, 264, 336, 478–479
  sexual learning and, 285
Dyadic scale, 222
Dysfunction, sexual, defined, 306
Dysmenorrhoea, 452
Dyspareunia, 80, 309, 324–326
  breastfeeding and, 441
  community, sexual problems and, 312
  epilepsy and, 397
  hysterectomy and, 386
  medical practice and, 383–384, 385, 394
  outcome studies, 358
  pelvic pathologies and, 370–371
  post-menopausal, 315
  post-partum, 440–441
Dysthymia, 387
Dysuria, 383, 415

E
Economic choice theory, 182–183
Economic and Social Research Council
      (ESRC) (UK), 179
'Ecstasy', 84
Ectomorphs, 201
Edinburgh clinics, 313, 344, 358, 382
Education, sex, 150, 175, 192, 196
  learning disabled (LD) and, 390
EEG (electroencephalography) studies, 88,
      101–102
Effeminacy, 271, 273, 289, 294
'Ego-dystonic homosexuality', 257
Ehrlich, Paul, 413
Ejaculation
  alpha1 antagonists and, 403
  bladder dysfunction and, 392
  capacity, spinal cord injuries (SCI) and,
      399–400
  delayed/absent (DE), 87, 308, 315, 324
    hypertension medication and, 402
    schizophrenia and, 404
    treatment, 355, 358, 364, 371
  fear of, 384
  female, 93–94
  inevitability of, 85, 88
  in marriage, 209
  mechanisms underlying, 87–90
  multiple sclerosis (MS) and, 398
  pain with, 372
  premature see Premature ejaculation (PE)
  rape and, 483
  retrograde, 87, 391
  spinal cord centre for, 87
  see also Orgasm
Elders, Jocelyn, 183
Electrodes, heated oxygen, 80
Eli Lilly, 362
'Emic' knowledge, 6
Emotional factors
  abuse, low self-esteem and, 494
  anger, 318
  bonding cues, 223
  brain, 21, 55, 61–64
  'congruence', child sexual abuse (CSA)
      and, 484
  'dysregulation', 480
  'emotion schemes' concept, 499
  emotion-focused therapy, 482, 500

excitation and inhibition, 63
insecurity, female sex offenders and, 489
intimacy, homosexual, 276
'negative emotionality', 435
regulation, child sexual abuse (CSA) and, 485
response systems, 100
self-control and, 320
sex therapy and, 352
theory, 500
Emotional state augmentation model, 480, 483
Endocrine disorders, 119, 328
'Endogamic' man, incest and, 484
Endometriosis, 309, 324, 328, 370, 385
Endometrium, cancer of, 386
Endomorphs, 201
Endothelial cell dysfunction, 392
Endothelin, 78
Enteric division, autonomic nervous system, 58
Entrapment, child sexual abuse (CSA) accommodation syndrome, 495–496
Environment of evolutionary adaptiveness (EEA), 9, 200, 202
Ephedrine, 70, 82, 404
Epididymis, 35, 85
Epididymitis, 372, 415
Epilepsy, 397–398, 405
temporal lobe, 285, 397
Episiotomy, 440–441
scarring, 324
Erectile dysfunction (ED), 70, 72, 78
ageing and, 240–241, 242, 243
assessment, 371–372, 372, 373
azoospermia and, 460
child sexual abuse (CSA) and, 497
clinical problems and, 382, 382
condoms and, 427
delequamine and, 361
depressive symptoms and, 387
diabetes mellitus (DM) and, 381, 390–391, 391, 392–393
distraction and, 100
feedback and, 98
HIV status and, 428
homosexual, 328–329
hormones and, 114
hypertension and, 396, 402
infertility and, 459
ischaemic heart disease (IHD) and, 395
marijuana and, 407
multiple sclerosis (MS) and, 97, 398
nocturnal penile tumescence (NPT) and, 373
outcome studies, 356, 358, 360, 365
Parkinson's disease (PD) and, 399
penile blood flow and, 384
personality and, 241
physical disease and, 382
psychological mechanisms and, 392
rape and, 483
schizophrenia and, 404
sexual desire, low and, 307, 321–322, 322, 364
Sexual Inhibition Scale (SIS1) and, 432
treatment, 343, 355, 360–363
clinics and, 313, 314, 315–316
in diabetics, 393
integrated, 366–367
surgical, 304, 345, 373
vascular impairment and, 345, 392

Erection, penile, 68, 74–76, 76, 77
conditioning of, 284
psychogenic, 399
reflexive, 399
smooth muscle responsiveness, 392
'Eros' love, 204
Erotica
blood pressure response, 394
erotic/explicit cues, 223
films, 71, 97, 100, 101, 107, 226
heterosexual response to, 225–226
Erotophobia-erotophilia, 228–229, 231, 264, 373
'Escalation points', 202
Essentialism, 5–6, 429
Estraderm 50, 247
Ethical issues
Kinsey Institute and, 181–182
reparative therapy and, 258
surgical methods of control, 503
Ethinylestradiol (EE), 124, 299, 445, 449–450
'Etic' knowledge, 6
Etonogestrel, 452–453
Eulenspiegel Society (New York), 286
Event-related potential (ERP), 101
Evolutionary perspective, 200, 202, 205
adaptation, 94–96
psychology, 9, 213
theories, 472
Examination, physical, 321, 325, 369–371, 372–373, 491
'Excesses and deficits', sex offender, 503
Excitation, sexual, 305–306
central control, 65
cognitive component, 72
emotional, 63
excitatory tone, 112, 304
model of, 72–73, 482
see also Dual Control model
'transfer', 82, 105, 111, 159, 167, 331, 434
see also Arousal, sexual
Exercise
effects
female genital response, 81–82
sexual activity, 396
pelvic floor, Kegel's, 354, 366
relaxation, 354
vaginal dilatation, 354
Exhaustion, sexual, 91
Exhibitionism, 330, 470, 478, 486–488
social class and, 487
Exogamy, 476–477
Exotic-Becomes-Erotic theory, 167
'Expectancy' system, emotional response, 100
Expectations, 316
altered, 101
inappropriate, 348
traditional, 318
Experiential avoidance theory, 499, 500
Exploitation, sexual, 321, 464, 473–476
commercial interests, 473, 486
historical perspective, 473–476
'Explosive anger', 482
External genitalia, 25, 26, 27, 32, 33, 35–37, 37
Externalizing behaviours, 149, 156, 159, 493
Extramarital affairs, 212–213, 319, 329–330, 396, 464
Eye contact, 202, 203
Eysenck Personality Inventory, 106, 284

F
'Face-in-the-crowd' effect, 99
Fakery, sexual, 329
Fallopian tubes, 35–36, 35, 454
Famciclovir, 417
Family influence, 199, 467, 469
Family Planning Association, 345
Fantasy, sexual
categories of, 224
'force', 224
heterosexual, 223–225
onset of, 154, 154
'report', mood and, 481
same-sex, 160
sex offenders and, 504
sexual arousal/response and, 85, 97, 105, 112, 122
stability of, 264–265, 265
training, 359
Fatherhood, 459
Fatigue, 332
post-partum period, 441
Fear
child sexual abuse (CSA) victims and, 493
memory system, 99
phobic, 352
rape victims and, 490
sexual arousal and, 111
Federal Bureau of Investigation, 489
Feedback
effects, 98
false, 101
negative, 296
positive, 60, 296
Female
ageing, 327–328
physiological response, 247–248, 248
psychophysiological evidence, 248–249
psychosocial factors, 249–250
sexual behaviour changes, 243–250
androgens and, 114–124, 153, 156–157
assessment for treatment, 368–371, 373–374
autoerotic asphyxia (AEA), 334
BDSM and, 286
beta-endorphin effects, 129
black see under Black community
brain imaging, 72
Chinese, 220
circumcision, 474
condoms, 425, 427, 454
contraception see Contraception
courtship, 202
diabetes mellitus (DM) and, 393–395
exercise, 81–82
facial attraction, 201
gender identity discordance (GID), 294–295
genital anatomy, adult, 25, 26, 27, 32–35, 32, 33, 34, 35
genital response, 78–84, 85
gonadal steroid effects, 127–128
'gradual disinvestment', 208
gynaecology, 385–387
infertility, 415
inhibition, 232
love and, 231
maladaptive behaviour in, 32
masturbation, 175, 184–185, 216, 231
melanocortin effects, 130
menopause see Menopause

Female *(Continued)*
  menstruation *see* Menstruation
  noradrenaline (NA) systems, 70–71
  oestrogens (E) and, 29–30, 97, 124, 127, 128
  offenders and child sexual abuse (CSA), 489
  orgasm, 231
    by-product, explanation of, 95–96
    ejaculation, 93–94
    importance of, 175, 176, 209, **211, 212**
    mechanisms underlying, 88
    multiple, 152
    premature, 311
    problems, 309, 358, 365, 393, 404
    types of, 86–87
  oxytocin (OT) effects, 89, 128–129
  peptide effects, 128–130
  power, 208
  proceptive behaviours, 132
  prolactin (PRL) effects, 87, 129–130
  puberty, 28–29
  relationship, importance of, 303–304
  reproductive organs, internal, 25, **26,** 34–35, **35**
  self-esteem, 459
  sex offenders, 488–489
  sexual arousal, 80–82, 432–433
  sexual identity in, 159–165, 261
  sexual intercourse, age at first, 231
  sexual interest, 231–232
  sexual problems, 305, 308–310, 324–327, 354–355
    diabetics and, 393–395
  sexual well-being and, 210–212, **211, 212**
  sexuality
    basic patterns, 131–132, 186, 232
    development pattern, 169
    superadded component, 133, 169, 186, 232, 249, 376
  sexually transmitted infections (STIs) and, 415
  spinal cord injuries and, 400–401
  status, 190, 200, 254–255, 424, 443, 474
  sterilization, 442, 455–456
  testosterone (T) and, 115–117, 118–119, 120–121, 124, 127–128, 133, 364–365
  treatments, 364–366
  venereal disease (VD), blame and, 414
  see also Lesbianism; Gender differences
Female sexual arousal disorder (FSAD), 249, 337
Female Sexual Function Index (FSFI), 327, 449
Femininity, 271–272
Feminist theories, 257
  on incest, 484
  on rape, 471, 472
Feminization
  of HIV/AIDS, 421, 422–423
  of testes, 47
Fenton's operation, 345
Fertility
  age at, 191
  control *see* Contraception
  culture, impact on, 217
  diabetes mellitus (DM) and, 395
  poor working class and, 189
  regulation, 17
  role of, 191–192

  sexual arousal and, 66, 95, 133
  spinal injuries and, 401
  surveys, 177
  see also Infertility
Fetishism, 104, 164, 283–286
  abnormal learning, 285–286
  concept of, 283
  conditioning and, 296
  determinants of, 284
  dyadic relationships, sexual learning and, 285
  Female Fetishism (Gamman & Makinen), 284
  homosexuality and, 256
  inanimate body extensions, 284
  partialism, 283–284
  sex offenders and, 478
  textures, specific, 284
  transvestic, 290, 292–293, 295, 296, 297
Fibroids, 385
Fibromyalgia, 385
Fight/flight system (F/FLS), 63
Finger length ratio, 163
First International Conference on Psychosexual Medicine, 345
Flagyl, 416
Flirting, 132
Fluoxetine, 403
Foetus
  oestrogens (E) in, 25
  sexual interaction and, 440
Follicle stimulating hormone (FSH)
  alcohol and, 406
  aromatase deficiency and, 125
  childhood/adolescence levels, 25, 28, 29
  depot medroxyprogesterone acetate (DMPA) and, 453
  intersex conditions and, 45, 46
  menopause and, 42
  menstrual cycle and, 40
  passionate love and, 130
  progestogens and, 502
  role of, 21, 22
Food and Drug Administration (FDA) (US), 121, 363
Foot fetishists, 285
Foot Fraternity, 284
Forebrain, 57
Foreskin, 36, 372, 384, 429
Formicophilia, 281
Fornication, 212–213, 319, 329–330, 396, 464
Foucault, Michel, 7, 429
Fragrance, mood and, 97
Frazer, Sir James, incest and, 476–477
Free androgen index (FAI), 449
Free association, 344
Freedom, loss of, 492
Frenken Sexual Experience Scales, 232, 244
Freud, Sigmund, 10, 86–87, 175, 224
  adolescence and, 145, 148
  sexual trauma and, 475
  taboos and, 476–477
Frigidity, 175, 304, 337
Frotteurism, 488
Functional cerebral asymmetry, 162
Functional magnetic resonance imaging (fMRI), 56, 61, 72, 89, 102, 126, 249
Fundamentalism, 254
Fungal infections, 414–415, 416–417

G
'G spot', 82–83, 87
Gamma-aminobutyric acid (GABA), 61, 63, 69, 92
Ganglion blockers, 402
Gay, Jan, 257
Gay community
  gay lesbian bisexual transgender (GLBT), 290
  Gay Liberation Movement, 178
  gay marriage, 259, 267, 275, 276
  gay rights movement, 256, 258, 260, 261, 336
  see also Homosexuality; Lesbianism
Gender
  chromosomal, 24–25
  dysphoria, 289–290, 297, 299
  'gender diagnosticity' (GD), 272
  'gender similarities' hypothesis, 30
  stereotyping, 31–32, 271, 289, 290, 291
  see also Female; Male; Sexual differentiation, anatomical
Gender differences
  basic pattern and superadded components, 131–133
  bisexuality and, 264
  explanatory model of, 131–133
  fetishism and, 287
  heterosexuality and, 231–232
  impact of child sexual abuse (CSA) and, 494
  information processing and, 130–133
  refractory period and, 316
  same-sex and, 269
  sexual fantasy and, 224–225
  sexual identity and, 261
  sexual offences and, 489
  sexual response and, 283
    to erotica, 225–226
  socio-cultural factors, 133, 214
Gender identity
  change of, 49
  confusion, 498
  core, 30, 31, 289
  development of, 30–32, 160
  homosexuality and, 270–272
  problems, 336
  role behaviour *see* Behaviours, sexual
  sexual identity and, 260–261, 292
  socio-cultural factors, 289–291
  treatment, problems, 377
Gender identity discordance (GID), 291, 293–295
Gender identity disorder (GID), 160, 167, 290
Gender reassignment, 162, 290–291, 296–300
  alternatives to, 299
  assessment/selection, 293, 297–300
  care, standards of, 300–301
  contract, initial, 298
  female-to-male, 297, 298–299
  historical perspective 290z
  hormone treatment, 299
  male-to-female, 297, 298–299
  management, 296–300
  outcomes, 297
  practical steps, 298–299
  surgery, 300
General Household Survey (UK), 443, 455
General medicine, 390–396
General Social Survey (GSS), 30, 213, 227, 268

Genetic factors
  gene therapy, 363
  sexual development and, 157–158
  sexual identity and, 163–164
Genital anatomy
  congenital abnormalities, 51–52
  differentiation of, 24–25, **26**, **27**
  examination, 369–371, 372
  female, 32–35, **32**, **33**, **34**, **35**
    blood supply, 35
  male, 36–38, **36**, **37**, **38**, **39**
    blood supply, 37–38, **39**
    stages of development, **37**
  nerve supply, 38–39, **40**
Genital factors
  contact, sex therapy and, 348–350
  herpes, 417
  infections, 328
  operations, 187
  sores, 415
  warts, 414–415, 417
Genital response, 74–84
  decline in, 247
  female, 78–84, 85
  male, 74–78, **76**, **77**, 84–85
    fluid secretion survey and, 38
  orgasm see Orgasm
  to sexual stimuli, 96–98
'Germ' theory of disease, 413
Gestodene, 445, 449
Global Study of Sexual Attitudes and
        Behaviors (GSSAB), 239, 246, 250
Globus pallidus, 57, 73
Golden Notebook (Lessing), 87
Golombok-Rust Inventory of Sexual
        Satisfaction (GRISS), 122
Gonadal dysgenesis (45-X0), 25, 45, **45**,
        163–164
Gonadal steroids, 111–114, **112**, **113**,
        126–127
  male/female effects, 127–128
  receptors, 125
Gonadotrophin-releasing hormone (GnRH),
        22, 28, 113, 384
  Gonadotrophins, 22, 246, 372, 384, 407
  see also Follicle stimulating hormone
        (FSH); Luteinizing hormone (LH)
  Gonads, 25
  see also Ovaries; Testes
Gonococcus, 413, 414, 415
  infections of, 415
Gonorrhoea, 413, 414, 415, 429
G-protein
  coupling, 125
  decoupling, 129
Graham, Rev. Billy, 176
Grant Projects (HHS), 179
Grooming, sexual, 467
Gross indecency, 468
Group therapy, 359, 500–501, 503
Growth of American Families
        study, 177
Growth hormone, 28
Guanethidine, **68**, 402
Guave-doce (penis at 12), 49
Guilt
  child sexual abuse (CSA) and,
        321, 496
  childhood, 335
  Christian culture and, 217
  dominance and, 286
  'force' fantasies and, 224
  lack of, 224, 225

masturbation and, 216, 331
  adolescent, 175, 183
'out of control' behaviour and, 333
rape victims and, 492
restrictive attitudes and, 332
sex-, measures, 229
Guy's Hospital Sexual Problem Clinic
        (London), 315
Gynaecological conditions, 328
Gynaecology, 385–387
Gynaecomastia, 405
  oestrogens (E) and, 95, 501

H
Habituation, 105
Haemophilus, 418
Haemophilus ducreyi, 414, 416
Halban's fascia, 83
Hallucinations, 389
Halperidol, 405
Handedness, right/left, 162, 482
Handicap
  learning disabled (LD), 389–390, 467
  physical, 381–382
  sexual activity and, 389
Harry Benjamin International Gender
        Dysphoria Association (HBIGDA),
        standards of care, 299, 300–301
Health
  good, 200, 202
  masturbation, threat to, 184
  mental, 211, 246, 273–275, 313
  physical, 313
  problems, 328
Health Belief Model, 424
Health Education Authority (UK), 179
Health Protection Agency (HPA), 415,
        416, 417
Heart Disease, 240
Heart rate, orgasm and, 396
Heller, State Representative, 176
Helms, Jessie, 178
Helplessness, child sexual abuse (CSA)
        accommodation syndrome,
        495–496
Hepatitis B virus (HBV), 414, 417–418
Heritable alternative strategies, 9
Heritable calibration of psychological
        mechanisms, 9
Hermaphroditism, 261
Herpes simplex virus (HSV), 372, 414, 417
Heterosexuality, 174–232
  cultural influences, 214–220, **215**
  erotica, sexual response to, 225–226
  fetishistic transvestism and, 290
  gender differences, 231–232
  HIV/AIDS impact, 436
  information sources, sex surveys, 174–183
  internet, sex and, 226–228
  marriage/co-habitation, 200–213
  masturbation and, 183–186
  personality/individuality in, 228–231
  premarital sex, 186–199
  sexual desire and, 220–223, **221**
  sexual fantasy and, 223–225
  sexual identity and, 335
  social class and, 213–214
Heterosocial competence, 483
Hexamethonium, 402
Highly-active anti-retroviral therapy
        (HAART), 418, 435–436

Hindbrain, 57
Hippocampus, 57, 61, 62, 68, 99
Hirschfeld, Magnus, 289
Hispanic Americans, 218
  breastfeeding and, 441
  female, 218–219, 311
  male, 311
  sexually transmitted infections (STIs)
        and, 419
  sterilization and, 455
Histamine, 68
  H2 receptor antagonist, 405
  histaminergic system, 63
History taking, 368, 370, 372, 465
Hite Report (Hite), 176
HIV/AIDS pandemic, 420–423, **421**
  AIDS Risk Reduction Model (ARRM),
        424, 426
  altered sexual response and, 328–329
  anti-retroviral drugs and, 421
  community surveys and, 419–420
  effects on condom use, 443
  feminization of, 421, 422–423
  as 'gay disease', 261, 435
  historical perspective, 414
  impact, sexual behaviour, 435–436
  latency period, sexual development and,
        418
  lymphocyte count, T-helper (CD4), 418
  nature of, 414–415, 416, 418–419
  orphaned children and, 421
  politics of, 421–422
  prevention
    ABC approach, 423–424
    circumcision and, 428–429
    condoms and, 425–427
    individual
      differences and, **430**, 434–435
      vs relation-based approach, 424–425
    microbicides and, 427–428
    principles of, 423–425
    programmes, 421, 423–429, 434
    in Uganda, 423
  ribonucleic acid (RNA), latency period
        and, 418
  schizophrenia and, 389
  sex surveys and, 175, 178–179, 180, 182
  sexual risk taking and, 428, 431, 434–435
  transmission, 8, 183, 192, 197, 208, 431
  UNAIDS, 421, 423, 424, 429
  World AIDS day, 183
  worldwide prevalence, 422
Home Office survey, sexual offence
        notifications, 468
Homophile movement, 256
Homophobia, 254, 255, 267
Homosexual Law Reform Society Report,
        267
Homosexuality
  in animals, 165
  brain masculinization and, 161–163
  characteristics of male/female, 270–275
  child sexual abuse (CSA) and, 498
  conversion to heterosexuals, 335–336
  cross-cultural comparisons, 265–268
  depathologization, 336
  depression and, 110
  effeminacy and, 271, 273
  fetishism and, 284, 296
  genetic factors, 163
  historical perspective, 253–259
  HIV/AIDS impact, 261, 435–436
  institutionalized, 266

Homosexuality *(Continued)*
  learning disabled (LD) and, 389
  legal status of, 259, 267–268
  morality and, 159
  negative mood and, **109**
  paedophiles and, 481
  persecution and, 255
  prevalence of, 268–269, **269**
  relationships
    six stages, 276
    status of, 275–277, **275**, **276**
  ritualized, 266
  sex surveys and, 178
  sexual arousal, impact of, 431–432
  sexual identity and, 159–161, 167,
      258–265, **263**, **265**, 335–336
  sexual practices in, 270
  sexual problems and, 328–329
    treatment, 375–376
  stereotyping, 271
  transsexualism and, 290–291
  typology of, 275, **275**
  see also Bisexuality; Gay community
Homosocial sexuality, 191
'Honeymoon cystitis', 415
Hooker, Evelyn, 178
Hormonal contraception, 445–446
  effects on sexual behaviour, 446–452, **447**,
      448
  male, 453–454
  mood and, 450–451, **450**
Hormonal treatments, 360–366
  gender reassignment, 299
  'out of control' behaviour and, 376
  for sex offenders, 501–502
Hormone replacement therapy (HRT), 45,
    48, 118, 119, 120, 246, 365
Hormones
  measurement of, 372
  see also Androgens; Oestradiol;
      Oestrogens (E); Testosterone (T)
Hostility
  exhibitionism and, 488
  indecent exposure and, 487
  rape and, 482
  sexual offending and, 481
  voyeurism and, 488
House of Representatives (US), 475
Human chorionic gonadotrophin (HCG),
    25, 28, 41
Human immunodeficiency virus (HIV)
    see HIV/AIDS pandemic
Human papilloma virus (HPV), 386–387,
    414, 417
Human Relations Area File (HRAF), 174,
    186–187, 208, 250, 265, 471
Human Reproduction Program (WHO), 446
Human Sex Anatomy (Dickinson), 75
Human Sexual Inadequacy (Masters &
    Johnson), 345
Human sexuality, defined, 18
Humiliation, 286, 287, 481, 482, 488
Hunter-gatherer societies, 65, 187, 191, 202,
    266, 445
Hydralazine, **68**
Hymen, 34
Hyperactivity, child sexual abuse (CSA)
    victims and, 493
Hypercapnia, acute, 335
Hypergonadotrophic hypogonadism, 384
Hypermasculinity, 286, 287
Hyperprolactinaemia, 129, 328, 373,
    384, 404

Hypersexuality, 281, 329, 330, 397, 499
Hypertension, 240, 311, 361, 392, 396,
    399, 402
Hypnosis, 256, 344
Hypnotic drugs, 403
Hypoactive sexual desire disorder (HSDD),
    72, 98, 103–104, **103**, 222–223,
    281, 337
  DSM IV criteria, 120, 220, 245
  outcome studies, 359
Hypogonadism, 111, 114, 307, 384, 392
  alcohol abuse and, 406
  laboratory tests, 372
  treatment, 374
Hypomania, 307, 388
Hyposexuality, 281, 397
Hypospadias, 51–52, 384
Hypothalamo-pituitary-adrenal
      axis, 494
Hypothalamus, 22, 57–62 *passim*, **59**, **60**,
      71–72, 130, 162
Hypoxia, acute, 335
Hypoxyphilia, 334–335
Hysterectomy, 120–121, 300, 385–386

I

Idazoxan, 67, **68**, 70, 242
Identity
    rape victims' loss of, 492
    separate, 155–156
Identity, sexual, 159–169
    concept of, 259–265, **263**, **265**
    cultural factors, 164–165
    gender differences, 261
    genetic factors, 163–164
    homosexuality and, 159–161, 167, 258,
        259–265, **263**, **265**
    interactive processes, 166–169
    personality and, 260–261
    problems, 335–336
    sex offenders, 478
    six stages of, 261
    stability of, 264–265, **265**
    transgender identity and, 295
    treatment, problems, 377
    see also Gender identity
Illegitimacy, 187, 188, **188**
Imipramine, **68**, 403, 404
Immigrant groups, 214, 218–219
    Immorality, 184, 280, 464–465
    see also Moral values
Immune system, HIV and, 418
Immuno-suppression, candida infections
        and, 417
Implanon, 452–453
Implants
    contraceptive release, 452–453
    penile, 304, 345, 366
Impotence, 304, 337, 345, 456
Impulse disorders, 330
    as counter to inhibitors, child sexual
        abuse (CSA), 484
Impulsivity, 482
In vitro fertilization (IVF), 460
INAH3 nerve cells, 162
'Inbreeding depression', 477
Incentive and reward, 64–65, 333
    incentive motivation system, 72, 307,
        309
Incerto-hypothalamic (A14) periventricular
        system, 62, 67

Incest, 467–468, 469, **469**
    avoidance, 66, 477
    inhibition, in family, 484
    offenders, 483–484, 486
    socio-cultural context and, 476–478
    US statistics, 470–471
Indecent exposure, 466, 468, 469–470, 476,
        486, 487
Index fingers, 163
Individual
    differences, HIV/AIDS and, **430**, 434–435
    protection of, 464
    vs society, 7–8, 14
    see also Personality
Individualism, 204, 217, 260
Industrial societies, homosexuality and,
        267–268
Industrialization, 189
Infections
    genital, 328
    hypogonadism and, 384
    vaginal, 395
    vulvar, 324
    yeast, 385
    see also Sexually transmitted infections
        (STIs)
Infertility, 458–460
    breastfeeding and, 454
    coital frequency and, 459
    hypogonadism and, 384
    in men, 415
    opiates and, 407
    pelvic inflammatory disease (PID) and,
        415
    sexual function and, 459–460
Infidelity, 212–213
Inflammation, chronic, 385
Inflammation, genital, 325
Information about sex
    control of, 176, 226, 414
    ignorance, 351
    lack of, 316–317, 348
    learning disabled (LD) and, 390
    sex surveys, 174–183
    sources of, 56, 174
    therapist and, 348
    see also Internet
Information processing, 55, 96–111
    automatic vs attentional, 99, 100
    brain imaging, 102–104
    conditioning/learning/habituation,
        104–105
    EEG studies, 88, 101–102
    gender differences and, 130–133
    inhibition, role of, 105–106
    inhibitory response and, 480
    misattribution/misinformation, 101
    models of, 98–101
    mood and, 106–111, **109**
    personality influence, 106
    physiological responses to, 100
    reflex enhancement, 100
    sexual fantasy and, 105
    sexual stimuli,sexual response to, 96–98
Infrastructural determinism, 13–15
Inheritance, landed property, 189
Inhibin, 21
Inhibited child syndrome, 167
Inhibitory mechanisms
    adaptive, 305–306, 480
    'automatic', 332–333, 480
    central control of, 65
    emotional excitation and, 63

evidence of
   animal, 67–69
   human, 69–71, 72
female propensity, 326–327, **326**
functions of, 66–67
gender differences, 232
impaired, 331–332
information processing and, 105–106
inhibitory tone, 72, 305, 332, 346, 392, 399
models of, 73, 482–483
see also Dual Control model
need for, 65–67
reactive, 319, 346, 347
refractory period and, 91
role of, 305–307
sex therapy and, 353–354
Initiation
   ceremonies, 186–187
   of sexual activity, 208, 339, 347, 348, 351, 376
Insecurity, 318, 348
Institute for Advanced Study of Human Sexuality, 262
Institute of Medicine, 178
Institute of Psychosexual Medicine, 345
Institute for Sexual Science, 289
Insula, 73, 103
Insulin, 28
Insulin-like growth factor (IGF-I), 28
Integrated theory
   child sexual abuse (CSA), 485
   of sexual offending (ITSO), 485
'Intensive care', rape victims and, 492
Interest, sexual *see* Desire/interest, sexual
Internal organs, female, 25, **26**, 34–35, **35**
Internalizing behaviour, 493
International Bill of Rights (UN), 474
International Classification of Diseases (ICD), 313, 336
International Consensus Development Conference on Female Sexual Dysfunction: Definitions and Classifications, 336
International Index of Erectile Function (IIEF), 360, 456
Internet, 32, 226–228
   alternative sex forums, 284
   BBC survey, 264
   homosexuality and, 255, 260
   Kinsey Institute study, 428
   law and, 464
   'out of control' use, 227–228
   panels, sex surveys, 181
   pornography and, 225, 476
   sexual deviance and, 281
   transgender support groups and, 297
Intersex conditions, 44–52, 253, 255, 261, 290
Intersex Societies, 44, 52, 261
Interstitial cells of ovary, 244–245
Interstitial nuclei of anterior hypothalamus (INAH 1–4), 60
Interview Ratings of Sexual Function (IRSF), 447, 449, 451
Intimacy
   barriers to, 321
   capacity for, 145, 355
   homosexual, 276
   lack of, child sexual abuse (CSA) and, 483, 485
   mothers, 'close binding', 161
   pregnancy and, 440
   retreat from, 186
   suspension of disgust, 320

Intracavernosal injections (ICI), 67–68, **68**, 304, 361, 363, 366, 383, 393
Intraconjugal balance of power, 424
Intracrine processes, 111, 116
Intramuscular injections, 364, 452
Intrauterine contraception
   devices (IUDs), 425, 442, 443, 446, 452–453
   systems (IUS), 446, 452–453
   vaginosis and, 415
Ischaemic heart disease (IHD), 381, 395
Ischiocavernosus muscle, 76
Islamic culture, 187, 219, 464, 472
   principle of 'unity', 217
Isolation, social, female sex offenders and, 489
Isosexual group studies, 166

J

Jackson, Hughlings, 57
James-Lange approach, 61
Jewish tradition
   circumcision and, 428–429
   contraception and Orthodox, 443
Jorgensen, George/Christine, 290
Journal of the American Medical Association, 305
Journal of Bisexuality, 262
Journal of Sex and Marital Therapy, 336
Journal of Sex Research, 5, 8

K

Kahn, Fritz, 75
Kallman's syndrome, 384
Kaposi's sarcoma, 414, 418
Kegel's exercises, 354, 366
Kinsey, Alfred C.
   impact of, 226, 290
   Thomas Painter and, 257
Kinsey Institute research, 160
   ageing and, 245
   anal sex, 209
   asexuality, 282
   Dual Control model and, 429
   ejaculation, fluid discharge before, 37
   ethics and, 181–182
   gender differences and, 214
   grants to, 178
   high-risk sexual behaviour, 427
   on incarcerated sex offenders, 483
   internet and, 226–227, 428
   kissing, 208
   oral contraceptives and sexuality, 446
   sexual assault, 470
   sexual problems, 312–313, 329
   sexual risk taking, 183
   survey of men, 268
   survey of women, 211, 216, 249
   white college educated males, study, 213
   workshops
      Role of Theory in Sex Research, 5, 7, 8, 13, 159, 429
      Sexual Development in Childhood, 479
Kinsey Institute Sexual Health Clinic, 324, 336, 344, 355
Kinsey Scale, 262, 264
Kissing, 208
Klein Sexuality Orientation Grid, 262

Klinefelter's syndrome (47-XXY), 45–46, **46**, 384
Klismaphilia, 281
Kluver-Bucy syndrome, 397
Knowledge Networks, 181
Korsakoff syndrome, 406

L

Labetolol, 402
Labia
   majora, 32, **32**, **33**, 247
   minora, 33, **33**, 34, 247, 248
   'pouting of', 78–79
Lactation, 41–42, **43**, 446
Langerhans cells, 429
Laparoscopy, 455
Lashley, Karl Spencer, 57
Latency period, sexual development, 150, 418, 497
L-dopa, sexual desire and, 399
Learning disabled (LD), 389–390, 467
Learning, sexual, 104–105, 285, 296
   early, 164
   models, 144
Legal matters
   abortion, 457–458
   artificial insemination, donor (AID), 460
   consent and, 490, 496–497
   divorce, 205, 212
   gender reassignment, 298
   homosexuality and, 254, 259, 267–268
   marriage, 207, 219
   sex surveys and, 181
   sexual risk taking consequences, 330
   Spanner case (UK), 286
   sterilization and, 455
   see also Offences, sexual
Lesbianism, 257, 260, 265
   artificial insemination, donor (AID), 460
   'bed deaths', 376
   'butch/femme' concepts, 271
   cross-cultural comparisons, 265–268
   gender reassignment and, 292
   genetic factors, 163
   legal status, 259, 267–268
   mental health and, 273
   personality and, 272
   recognition of, 267
   relationships, status of, 275–277, **275**, **276**
   sexual identity and, 160–161, 162, 335
   sexual practices in, 270
   treatment, sexual problems, 375–376
   typology of, 275, **275**
   see also Gay community
Lessing, Doris, 87
Leuprolide acetate, 502
Levitra, 361
Levonorgestrel (LN), 445, 449, 452–453
Leydig cells, 25, 37, 42
Libido, 228
   -lowering drugs, 504–505
   see also Desire/interest, sexual
Lie detection, 502
Lie scale, 106
Life course approaches, 145, 479
Lignocaine, **68**
Limbic function, impairment of, 397
Limerence, 160, 203, 262, 264
Listening tasks, dichotic, 100
Liver damage, 406
Local hormones, 20
Locus coeruleus (l.c.), 59, 68, 112

Logynon, 449
Lombroso, Cesare, 253
Loneliness, 481, 483
Longford, Lord, 225
Lordosis, 59, 95, 132
Love, 203–205
    bisexuality and, 262
    companionate, 65, 203, 205
    gender differences and, 231
    learning disabled (LD), capacity for, 390
    passionate, 65, 130, 203, 205
    types of, 204
    see also Romantic love
Lubrication see Vaginal dryness
'Ludus' love, 204
Lumpectomy, 387
Lust, 160, 264, 291
Luteal phase, 79
Luteinizing hormone (LH)
    ageing and, 114, 241, 245, 246
    alcohol and, 406
    anti-convulsants and, 405
    aromatase deficiency and, 125
    beta-endorphin and, 129
    childhood/adolescence and, 25, 28, 29
    depot medroxyprogesterone acetate (DMPA) and, 453
    digoxin and, 405
    homosexuality and, 161–162
    hypogonadism and, 392
    intersex conditions and, 45, 46
    menopause and, 42
    menstrual cycle and, 40
    ovariectomy and, 117
    pregnancy and, 41
    progestogens and, 502
    role of, 22, 23
Luteinizing hormone-releasing hormone (LHRH), 129, 502, 503
Lymphogranuloma venereum (LGV), 414, 416

M

McGill University, study of contraceptive use, 447
Mackintosh Society, 284
Magnetic resonance imaging (MRI)
    brain imaging, 78–79, 83–84, 398
    female genitalia, 247, **248**
    functional (fMRI), 56, 61, 72, 89, 102, 126, 249
Magnetoencephalography (MEG), 102
Major depressive disorder (MDD), 106
Maladaptive behaviours, 32, 156, 158–159
Male
    ageing, sexual behaviour changes, 114, 240–243, 311, 327
    androgens and, 111–114, **112, 113,** 156–157
    andrology, 382–384
    assessment for treatment, 371–373, 373–374
    autoerotic asphyxia (AEA), 334
    beta-endorphin effects, 129
    black, 193, 215, **215**
    contraception, hormonal, 453–454
    see also Condoms
    dominance see Dominance, male
    gender identity discordance (GID), 293–294

genital anatomy, adult, 25, **26, 27,** 36–38, **36, 37, 38, 39**
genital response, 74–78, **76, 77,** 84–85
gonadal steroid effects, 127–128
index fingers, 163
inhibition, 232
love and, 231
masturbation, 184–185, 231
melanocortin effects, 130
noradrenaline (NA) systems, 69–70
oestrogens (E) and, 29, 30, 124, 127
orgasm, 176, 231
    /seminal emission/ejaculation distinction, 87–88
oxytocin (OT) effects, 89, 128–129
peptide effects, 128–130
prolactin (PRL) effects, 87, 129–130
puberty, 28–29
relationships and, 304
sexual arousal, impact of, 431–432
sexual identity, 159–165, 261
sexual intercourse, age at first, 231
sexual interest, 231–232
sexual problems, 304–305, 307–308, 321–324, 355
    diabetics and, 390–391, 391–393, **391, 393**
sexuality
    basic pattern, 131–132, 232, 249
    development pattern, 169
sexually transmitted infections (STIs) and, 415
sildenafil, erectile dysfunction and, 393
spinal cord injuries and, 399–400, 401
sterilization, 456–457
superiority, 289
testosterone (T) effects, 111–114, **112,** 127
treatments for, 360–364, 366, 393
see also Gender differences; Homosexuality
Malignancy see Cancer
Man who would be Queen: Science of Gender Bending and Transsexualism (Bailey), 291
Mania, 388
    love, 204
Margaret Pyke Centre, 456
Marital rape, 472
Market Opinion and Research International (MORI), on child sexual abuse (CSA), 469
Marriage Law (China), 219
Marriage/co-habitation, 200–213
    adapting to, 318–319
    age at first, 187, **188,** 190, **190,** 200, 205–206, **206**
    age gap, 190, **190,** 200
    arranged, 200, 204
    bartering approach to, 318
    breakdown, 212–213, 319, 406
        infertility and, 460
        physical abuse and, 494
        sex offenders and, 483
        sterilization and, 455–456
    chronic alcoholism and, 406
    companionate, 175
    courses, 175
    gay, 259, 267, 275, 276
    incidence of, 205, **205, 206**
    learning disabled (LD) and, 390
    sex surveys and, 175

sexual activity in, 207–210, **207, 208**
    initiation of, 208, 339
    sexual well-being and, 176, 210–212, **211, 212**
Marx, Karl, 13
Masculinity, 271–272
    doubts about, 471
    fatherhood and, 459
Masochism, 334, 491
    see also Sadomasochism
Mass rape, 471–472
Massachusetts Male Aging Study (MMAS), 240, 243, 387
Massachusetts Women's Health Study, 244
Mastectomy, 300, 387
Masturbation
    adolescent, 175, 219–220
    age of onset, 151–153, **152–153,** 185, 479
    ageing and, 239, 240
    attitudes to
        negative, 354
        social, 183–184
    Big Book of Masturbation (Cornog), 183
    black Americans and, 215
    children, young and, 148
    circumcision and, 429
    cross-cultural comparisons, 184–185
    cross-dressing and, 296
    depression and, 110
    female, 122
    frequency of, 210–211
    gender differences, 231
    heterosexuality and, 183–186
    immigrant groups and, 219
    learning disabled (LD) and, 389
    mood regulation and, 106, 485
    orgasm and, 87
    'out of control', 330, 433–434
    physical handicap and, 382
    prevalence of, 184–185
    public display of, 389
    sex surveys and, 175, 183
    sexual development and, 115
    social class and, 213–214
    techniques, 186
Mate selection, 104, 202–203, 477
Maudsley Hospital Psychosexual Dysfunction Clinic (London), 284, 315
Meaning, sexual, 149–150, 497
Mechanical devices, sexual problems and, 345
Media, 32, 260, 290
Medial orbitofrontal cortex (MOFC), 72, 73, 98, 104
    deactivation, 98
Medial pre-optic area (MPOA), of hypothalamus, 59, 67, 69, 89, 126, 129, 162
Medical conditions
    impact of, 343
    sexual effects of, 381
Medical practice, 381–407
    andrology, 382–384
    general medicine, 390–396
    gynaecology, 385–387
    medical/psychological, integrated treatments, 366–367
    medication, sexual side effects, 307, 328, 381–382, 396, 401–405
    neurology, 397–401
    principles, 381–382
    psychiatry, 387–390

Medical profession
  gender reassignment and, 290–291,
      296–300, 300–301
  historical perspective, 303
  initial attitude to artificial insemination,
      460
  sex negativism and, 255–257, 280
  sexual problems and, 304–305
  venereal disease (VD), ambivalence to,
      413
Medical Research Council (MRC), 179, 402
Medications, sexual side effects, 307, 328,
      381–382, 396, 401–405
Medroxyprogesterone acetate (MPA), 376,
      446, 502, 503
Medulla, 57
'Megan's law', 475
Melanocortin agonists, 362–363
Melanocortins, 130
Melanotan-II, 362
Melatonin receptor agonists, 366
Melbourne Women's Midlife Health
      Project, 179, 244
Meliane, 449
Memory, 147
  explicit vs implicit, 99
Men who have sex with men (MSM), 258,
      261, 270
  sexually transmitted infections (STIs)
      and, 416, 426, 429, 431, 434, 435
  see also Homosexuality
Menarche, age at, 154, 191, 282
Menninger, Karl, 336
Menopause, 42, 44
  changes and, 244–245, 249–250, 327–328
  depression and, 249
  in diabetic women, 394
  natural, 119–120
  surgical, 120–121
Menorrhagia, 385
Menstruation, 40, 41
  androgens and, 116–117, 116, 117
  assessment, 369
  hygiene, learning disabled (LD) and, 390
  impact of, 210
  irregularities, 296
  mood change and, 108, 449–450
  patterns, 447–448, 447, 448
  sexual intercourse during, 453
  spinal cord injuries (SCI) and, 401
  synchronization, 97
  taboos, 210
Mental health, 211, 246
  disorders, sexual offences and,
      467–468, 487
  homosexuality and, 273–275
  measure of (MSC12), 313
Mental Health Act (1983), 467, 501
Mental Health Inventory, 453
Mercury, 413
Mesenteric ganglion, 58
Mesocortical system, 62
Meso-limbic DA system, 62, 67, 88, 404, 407
Mesomorphs, 201
Meso-striatal system, 62
Metabolism, inborn errors of, 47–50, 121
Metaraminol, 68
Methodology of Sex Research
      (conference), 178
Methyldopa, 402
Methyltestosterone, 364
Metronidazole, 416
Meyer, Adolph, 336

Microbicides, 427–428
Microgynon, 449
Microlut, 449
Midbrain, 57
Migration, 190
Mill, John Stuart, 464
Mind-body dualism, 306
Minnesota Adolescent Health Survey, 274
Minnesota Multiphasic Personality
      Inventory, 393
Minorities, sexual, 280
Mirror-neuron system, 102
Mirtazapine, 404
Models, 8–17
  AIDS Risk Reduction (ARRM), 424, 426
  biopsychosocial, of sexual dysfunction,
      366
  child sexual abuse (CSA), 484–485,
      499–500
    impact of, 495–496
  cultural influence, 174
  cultural materialism, 13–15
  'disinhibition', 480, 483, 484
  Dual Control see Dual Control model
  emotional state augmentation, 480, 483
  erectile response, 76
  excitation and inhibition, 72–73, 482
  explanatory, 6–7, 9
  gender differences, 131–133
  health belief, 424
  information processing, 98–101
  of learning, 144
  mood/sexuality, 108, 109, 110, 483
  negative reaction, 500
  pathways, child sexual abuse (CSA), 485
  of prevention, 424
  psychoanalytic, 145
  Psychosomatic Circle of Sex, 17, 55–56,
      56
  quadripartite, child sexual abuse (CSA),
      485
  response control, 482
  risk appraisal/risk management,
      429–434, 430, 435
  sexual development see Three-strand
      model
  sexual response, linear, 364
  sexual scripting theory, 10–13
  sexual strategy theory (SST), 8–10
  traumagenic dynamics, 145
Modern learning theory, 104
Monitoring, 332, 333
Monoamine oxidase inhibitors (MAOIs),
      403–404
Monoamines, 62, 67–69
Monogamy, 200, 477
Monozygotic twins (MZ), 157, 163
Mood, 106–111, 109
  disorders, 106–107, 272, 330
  experimental manipulation and, 107–108
  fragrance and, 97
  hormonal variability and, 450–451, 450
  long acting reversible contraception and,
      453
  mediating mechanisms, 110–111
  menstrual cycle and, 449
  negative, 348, 432, 434, 500
  non-clinical variations of, 108–110
  passionate love and, 205
  regulation, 106, 321, 331, 434, 485, 489
  sex offenders and, 480–482, 481
  sexual desire and, 124, 451
  sexual risk taking and, 111

  sexual well being and, 210–212, 211,
      212
  /sexuality model, 108, 109, 110, 483
  see also Negative mood
Mood and Sexuality Questionnaire (MSQ),
      108–111, 109, 331, 428, 433, 480
Moral values, 159, 189, 192, 332
  contraception and, 442
  exploitation, child, 493, 496
  homosexuality and, 257
  immorality, 184, 280, 464–465
  imposition of, 258
  judgement, sex surveys and, 181
  moral panic, 506
    child sexual abuse and, 475, 492, 494
  PEPFAR, 422
  repugnance, 320
  sexual offences and, 474
  traditional, 156, 207, 426, 427
Morphine, 68
Motherhood
  'close binding intimate', 161
  self-esteem and, 459
  spinal cord injuries (SCI) and, 401
Motivation, sexual, 114
MSM see Men who have sex with men
      (MSM)
Müllerian differentiation, 95
Müllerian duct, 25
Müllerian-inhibiting factor, 25
Multi-cultured societies, 214
Multiple sclerosis (MS), 97, 398
Multivariant sexuality, 287
Murder, sadistic sexual, 286
Myocardial infarction (MI), 395, 396

N

Naftidrofuryl oxalate, 68
'Naive experimenters', female sex
      offenders, 489
NalGlu, 113
Naloxone, 70
Narcissists, 256
National AIDS Behavioral Surveys, 178
National Association for Research and
      Therapy in Homosexuality
      (NARTH), 258
National Campaign to Prevent Teenage
      Pregnancy, 179
National Commission of Inquiry into the
      Prevention of Child Abuse, 474
National Comorbidity Survey, 273
National Council for Civil Liberties
      (NCCL), 467
National Crime Victimization Survey
      (NCVS) (US), 470
National Family Opinion Research, 238
National Fertility Study (NFS), 177
National Health Service (NHS), 298
  clinics, 316
  hospitals survey, 440
  Information Centre (IC.NHS), 441
National Health and Social Life Survey
      (NHSLS) (US), 11, 178
  age at puberty and, 167
  child sexual abuse and, 497, 499
  circumcision and, 429
  community, sexual problems and,
      310–312
  condom use and, 425
  extramarital sex and, 213

National Health and Social Life Survey
(NHSLS) (US) *(Continued)*
  female sexual dysfunction and, 305
  homosexuality and, 268
  masturbation and, 183, 184, 216
  Mexican Americans and, 218
  onset of sexual intercourse and, 215
  orgasm and, 209, 210
  premarital sex and, 195, 199
  sexual assault and, 470
  sexually transmitted diseases and,
    419–420
  social networks and, 203
National Household Survey of Drug Abuse,
  273
National Institute of Child Health and
  Human Development (NICHD),
  177, 178, 179
National Institute for Health and Clinical
  Excellence (NIHCE), 452–453
National Institute of Mental Health (NIMH)
  Task Force on Homosexuality, 178
  Theorists' Workshop, 430
National Institutes of Health (NIH),
  177–179, 446
National Longitudinal Study of Adolescent
  Health (Add Health), 155, 158,
  167178
National Marriage Guidance Council,
  358
National Opinion Research Center, 274
National Research Council, 176
National Survey of Adolescent Males
  (NSAM), 155, 194–195, **195**, 196
National Survey of Families and
  Households, 207
National Survey of Family Growth (NSFG),
  155, 193, 194–195, **195**, **196**, 197
National Survey of Sexual Attitudes and
  Lifestyles (UK), 182
  NATSAL I (1990)
    asexuality and, 282
    condom use and, 425
    contraceptive use and, 443
    homosexuality and, 268–269, 270
    marriage and, 207–208, 209, 212, 213
    masturbation and, 183
    premarital sex and, 196, **197**
    sexual desire and, 221
    sexually transmitted infections (STIs)
      and, 419–420
    sterilization and, 455
  NATSAL II (2000)
    ageing and, 245
    community, sexual problems and,
      310–312
    condom use and, 425–426
    contraceptive use and, 443
    homosexuality and, 269, 270
    marriage and, 203, 208, 209, 212, 213
    masturbation and, 184–185
    premarital sex and, 195, 196, **197**, 198,
      199
    sexual desire and, 221
    sexually transmitted infections (STIs)
      and, 420
    sterilization and, 455
National Violence against Women Survey
  (US), 470
NATSAL *see* National Survey of Sexual
  Attitudes and Lifestyles (UK)
Natural methods, contraceptive, 454
Nature-nurture divide, 159

Nausea, 439
  oestrogens and, 501
Necrophilia, 281
Nefadazone, 403
Negative mood
  maternity blues, 441
  'negative emotionality', 435
  post-natal depression, 441
  relationships and, 348
  sexual response and, 275, 317, 330
  sexual risk taking and, 433–434, 435
Negative reaction models, 500
Negative reinforcement, principle of, 481
Neostigmine, **68**
'Nerve sparing' procedures, prostatectomy,
  383
Nesbit's operation, 382
Networks, sexual, 182–183
Neurobiological basis of sexual
  responsiveness, 15
Neurological disorders, 74, 328
Neurology, 397–401
Neuropathy, 303, 393, 406
  autonomic, 394
  diabetes mellitus (DM) and, 390–391,
    392
  peripheral autonomic/non-autonomic,
    391–392
Neuropeptide Y, 63, 80
Neuroticism, 228, 273
Neurotransmitters, 332, 407
Nicotine, 89–90
Nicotinic receptors, 63
Nitrazepam, 403
Nitric oxide (NO), 63, 71, 76, 78, 243
NO synthesase (NOS), 392, 404
'No-crime' cases, sexual offences and,
  465, 468
Nocturnal penile tumescence (NPT), 69, 151
  ageing and, 242
  androgens and, 112–114, **113**
  assessment, 373
  delequamine and, 361
  depression and, 110, 388
  diabetes mellitus (DM) and, 391
  diagnosis and, 304
Nonadrenergic-noncholinergic
  neuroeffector system (NANC), 78
Non-coital sex, 197, 208–209
Non-consummation, infertility and, 459
Non-Hodgkin's lymphoma, 418
Non-judgemental approach, rape victims
  and, 492
Noradrenaline and noradrenergic (NA)
  systems
  ageing and, 242, 243
  cocaine and, 407
  noradrenergic receptors, 62, 67, 68
  sexual arousal/response, 58, 62, 63,
    67–68, 90, 91–92
    female, 70–71, 80
    male, 69–70, 76, 78, 81, 112, 392
Norepinephrine *see* Noradrenaline and
  noradrenergic (NA) systems
Norethindrone, 445
Norgestimate, 445, 450
L-Norgestrel, 124
Norms, 176
Norplant, 452–453
Norplant Action Group, 453
NSPCC Special Unit and Family Centre, 500
'Nubility', 200–201
Nucleus accumbens, 57

Nucleus paragigantocellularis, 62, 71, 404
Nucleus prepositus hypoglossi, 62
Nucleus of solitary tract, 59
Nymphomania, 330
Nystatin, 417

O

Obesity
  candida infections and, 417
  hypogonadism and, 384, 392
Obscenity, 464
  telephone calls, 488
Obsessive-compulsive disorder, 307, 333,
  503
Odour *see* Smell
Oedipal anxieties, 320
Oestradiol, 245, 246–247, 405, 450
  alcohol abuse and, 406
Oestradiol–17beta, 23
Oestrogen-like steroids (EST), 162
Oestrogens (E), 22–23, 95
  ageing and, 245, 246
  aromatization from testosterone, 125
  brain activity and, 59, 60, 126
  conversion from androstenedione, 121
  deficiency, 325, 365, 441
  female effects, 29–30, 97, 124, 127, 128
  foetal, 25
  gender reassignment and, 292, 299
  gynaecomastia and, 95, 501
  homosexuality and, 161–162
  lactation and, 446, 454
  levels, post-natal, 25
  male effects, 29, 30, 124, 127
  menopause and, 44
  mode of action, 124–126
  mood and, 450
  pregnancy and, 41
  receptors (ER), 111, 125, 296
  replacement, 119–120, 247
  role of, 29–30
  sex offenders, management and, 501–502
  sexual interest, reduction, 502
  sexual response and, 122–123
  synthetic, 50
Oestrone, 23, 29
Oestrous pattern, 66
Offences, sexual, 464–506
  adolescents and, 478
  against children, 467
  defined (UK), 465–468
  gender differences, 478
  incidence of (UK/US), 468–471, **468**, **469**
  learning disabled (LD) and, 389
  'no-crime' decisions, 465, 468
  offenders *see* Offenders, sex
  socio-cultural context of, 471–478
  victims, 489–501
  see also Child sexual abuse (CSA)
Offenders, sex, 478–489
  brain-imaging studies, 482
  child sexual abuse and, 479, 489
  determinants, offences, 478–482
  female, 488–489
  incest, 483–484
  management of, 501–505
  neuropsychological factors, 482
  registration of, 475
  re-offending, 482
  self-esteem, low and, 504
  sexual fantasies and, 480

Olanzapine, 404
Olfactory stimuli, 96–97
Onanism or *Treatise upon the Disorder of Masturbation* (Tissot), 184
Onuf's nucleus, 60
Oocytes, 25
Oophorectomy, 300, 385–386
'Open gender schema', 263
Opioids
  endogenous, 21
  opiates, 407
    antagonists, 90
  orgasmic pleasure effect, 90
Oral contraceptives (OC), 442, **442**
  comparative studies on sexuality and, 449–450
  fertility control and, 446–452
  learning disabled (LD) and, 390
  medical practice and, 385
  pathogenic organisms and, 415
  placebo-controlled prospective evaluation, 448
  premarital sex and, 198–199
  sexual arousal and, 119
  sexual desire, low and, 446
  sexual problems and, 305
  use in United Kingdom (UK), 444
Oral hypoglycaemic drugs, 390
Oral incorporation, disgust and, 320
Oral sex, 155, 432
  homosexuality and, 266, 270, 271
  in marriage, 208–209, **209**
  social class and, 213–214
  unmarried, 197
Orchidectomy, 300
'Organic' dysfunction, 304, 306
Orgasm, 84–96
  ageing and, 240, 243
  altered consciousness and, 84, 86
  brain effects, 88–89
  cardiovascular/respiratory responses, 85–86
  carpo-pedal spasm, 86
  cross-dressing and, 296
  definitions, 84
  delayed/absent, 364
  'dry-run', 87, 308, 371, 391
  epilepsy and, 88
  female *see under Female*
  foetus and, 440
  frequency of, 209, 210
  functions of, 94
  gender differences, 176, 231
  genetic factors, 95
  genital/pelvic responses, 84–85
  key components of, 84
  mechanisms underlying, 87–90
  muscular responses, 85
  pelvic spasm and, 439
  'platform', 79, 85, 247
  pleasure, source of, 89–90
  problems, 337
    brain damage and, 398
    epilepsy and, 397
    schizophrenia and, 404
  prolactin (PRL) levels and, 92–93, **92**
  psychological components, 86
  refractory period, 55, **56**, 66, 84, 90–93, 152, 153
  seminal emission and, 55, 87–88
  somatic sensations, 86
  spinal cord injuries (SCI) and, 400
  thought-induced, 89
  'total sexual outlet', 176, 209, 220–221
  uterine, 87
  vaginal/cervical stimulation (VCS) and, 89
Orientation disturbance, sexual, 257
Ortho-Cyclen, 451
Ortho-McNeill, 446
Ortho-Tricyclen (OTC), 450, 451
Ortho-Tricyclen-Lo (OTC-Lo), 450, 451
'Out of control', sexual behaviour, 500–501
  as addiction, 333, 480
  depression and, 272
  inhibition, impaired and, 331–332
  internet and, 227–228
  masturbation, patterns, 330, 433–434
  negative mood and, 330–331
  as obsessive-compulsive disorder, 333
  selective serotonin re-uptake inhibitors (SSRIs) and, 502–503
  sex offenders and, 482
  sexual problems and, 330–333
  three windows approach and, 307
  treatment, 376
Ovarian steroids, 245
Ovariectomy, 117–118, 120–121, 365
Ovaries, 35–36, **35**
  activity
    return post-partum, **43**
    suppression, 441
  androgens and, 42
  atrophy of, alcohol abuse and, 406
  cancer of, 385, 386
  hysterectomy and, 386
  interstitial cells of, 244–245
  prolapsed, 385
Ovranette, 450
Ovulation, 97, 454
Oxford Sexual Problems clinic, 315, 356, 358, 360
Oxytocin (OT), 21, 73, 93
  male/female effects, 89, 128–129
  pain-reducing mechanisms and, 66
  prolactin (PRL) production and, 130
  sexual excitation system and, 67

P

Pacific Center for Gays and Lesbians, 262
Paedophilia, 330, 475, 481, 482, 483
  concept of, 485–486
  incest and, 484
  setraline and, 503
  socio-cultural factors and, 486
Paedophilia Information Exchange (PIE), 281
Pain
  assessment, 372
  depression and, 385
  disorders, 324–325
  ejaculation and, 372
  genital disorders and, 385
  history, 370
  orgasm and, 287
  oxytocin (OT) and, 66
  pelvic *see* Pelvic pain
  penile, 363
  reduction, vaginal stimulation, 83, 325
  sexual activity *see* Dyspareunia
  sexual response and, 308
  thresholds, 95, 325, 385
Painter, Thomas, 257
Pair bonding, 205
Panic disorder, 387–388
  rape victims and, 490
'Pap smears' (Papanicolaou), 386
Papaverine, **68**, 75, 361, 363
Paradoxical sleep, 69
Parametritis, 370
Paraphilias, 281, 290
Paraphimosis, 372
Parasitic infections, 414, 416
Parasympathetic nervous system (PNS), 39, 58–59, 75, 81
Paraventricular nucleus (PVN), 67, 89, 127, 129, 130
Parental influences
  conflict, open, 484
  discipline, 199
  gender identity discordance (GID) and, 293–294
  mothers, 'close binding intimate', 161
  parent-child attachment, 445, 479, 483
  parents vs peer group pattern, 158, 445
  rejection, 275
  reports, 147
Parenthood, 318–319
  sexual barriers to, 338
Parietal lobe, 104
Parkinson's disease (PD), 67, 398–399
Paroxetine, 403
Partial Androgen Deficiency in Aging Men (PADAM), 241
Partial androgen insensitivity syndrome (PAIS), 47, 48, 49
Partialism, 283–284
Parturition, 41–42
Passionate love, 65, 130, 203, 205
Passionate Love Scale (PLS), 203, 205
Pasteur, Louis, 413
PATH Through Life Project, 274
'Pathways model', child sexual abuse (CSA), 485
Patient-therapist relationship, 343, 347–348, 349, 353, 503
Patterns of Sexual Behaviour (Ford & Beach), 265
PDE-5 inhibitors *see* Phosphodiesterase-5 inhibitors (PDE-5)
'Peeping toms', 488
Peer group
  acceptance, 167
  composition, 167–168
  stigmatization, 299
  vs parents pattern, 158, 445
Pelvic blood flow abnormalities, 384
Pelvic floor
  exercises, 354, 366
  muscles, 34–35, **35**, 309, 325, 326, 385, 386
Pelvic inflammatory disease (PID), 370, 385, 414–415, 416, 459
Pelvic pain, 383–384
  chronic, 308, 383, 385, 415
  spasm, orgasm and, 439
Pelvic pathologies, 324, 370–371
Pelvic steal syndrome, 371
Penectomy, 300
Penicillin, 413, 416
Penile arteriography, 384
Penile pulse amplitude response, 392
Penis, 36–37, **36**, **37**, **38**, **39**
  agenesis of, 51
  bending of (chordee), 384

Penis (Continued)
  blood flow abnormalities, 384
  erection, **68**, 74–76, **76**, **77**, 151
  see also Erectile dysfunction (ED);
      Nocturnal penile tumescence
      (NPT)
  implants for, 304, 366
  inflammation of, 384
  medical problems, 382–383
  rings for, 345
  splints for, 345
  tactile sensitivity, 242
  vacuum devices for, 304
Pentolinium, 402
PEPFAR (President's Emergency Plan for
    AIDS Relief) (US), 421–422, 425
Peptides, 20–21, 21–22, 62, 67
  male/female effects, 128–130
Performance
  anxiety, 175, 307, 329, 347, 350–351, 388
  demand, 98, 355
Pergolide, 364
Perineal trauma, 440
Peripheral autonomic neuropathy, 392
Peripheral response mechanisms, ageing
    and, 242–243
Peri-pubertal boys, 254
Peri-pubertal pattern, 155–156, 156–158,
    167–168
Permissive societies, 186, 191
Permissiveness, 177, 188, 214, 217
Persistent genital arousal disorder (PGAD),
    309, 332–333
Personal Distress Scale, 245
Personal Experience Questionnaire, 449
Personality, 200, 228–231
  antisocial, 482
  change, HIV/AIDS and, 418
  disorders, 344, 494
  Dual Control model and, 229–231
  HIV/AIDS prevention programmes and,
      434
  homosexuality and, 256, 272
  inhibition and, 305
  principle factors, 228
  sexual attitudes, measures, 228–229
  sexual identity and, 260
  sexual problems and, 353, 406
  sexual response and, 106
  sexual risk taking and, 429, 432
  submissive, 243
Perversion, sexual, 281
Peyronie's disease, 371, 372, 382
Pfizer Inc., 78
Phalloplasty, 300
Pharmacological treatments, 303, 360–366,
    402–403
  sex offenders, 502–503
Pharyngeal gonococcal infections, 415
Phenelzine, 403, 404
Phenobarbitone, 405
Phenothiazines, 405
Phenoxybenzamine, **68**, 75
Phentolamine, **68**, 361–362, 363, 366
Phenylephrine, 383
Phenytoin, 398
Pheromones, 96–97
Phobic anxiety, 256, 352
Phosphodiesterase-5 inhibitors (PDE-5),
    77, 393, 404, 427
  sexual interest, impaired and, 343,
      360–361, 364–365, 373
Photography, 226

Phrenology, 56
Physical abuse, marital breakdown and,
    494
Physical examination, 321, 325, 369–371,
    372–373, 491
Physical health, measure of (PCS12), 313
Piaget, Jean, 144
Planned Behavior, Theory of, 424
Planned Parenthood Federation of America,
    177
Plateau phase, 78
Pleasure Project, 425
Pleasure, sexual, 79
  barriers to, 339
  condoms and, 427
  fear of, 320
  from touching, 347, 348
  orgasmic, source of, 89–90
Plummer, Ken, 8
Pneumocystis carinii, 414, 418
Pneumonia, 414, 418
'Polarization', child sexual abuse (CSA)
    and, 497–498
Political correctness, 7, 337–338, 429,
    492–493, 499
Politics
  activism, 257
  child sexual abuse (CSA) and, 475
Polycystic ovarian disease, 296
Polygamy, 265, 477
  'polygamous play', 187
  polygamous societies, 200
Polygraphy, 502
Pons, 57
Population factors, 14
  density, 66
  falling, 192
  homeostatic control of, 65
  over-, 219, 458
Population Reports (US), 455
Pornography, 225–226, 227, 464
  internet and, 476
Positive and Negative Affect Scale
    (PANAS), 205
Positron emission tomography (PET), 56,
    72, 88, 126
Posterio-medial bed nucleus, ejaculation
    and, 404
Post-natal period, 25–26, 28, **28**
  depression, 441, 447
Post-partum period, 439–442
  'blues', 441
  contraception, 454
  dyspareunia, 440–441
  fatigue, 441
Post-pubertal development, androgens
    and, 115
Post-traumatic stress disorder (PTSD)
  child sex abuse (CSA) victims and,
      493
  juvenile female sex offenders and, 489
  rape victims and, 490
Poverty
  children and, 473–474
  teenage motherhood and, 192
  working class, 188–189
Power
  female, 208
  intraconjugal balance of, 424
  powerlessness, child sexual abuse (CSA)
      and, 496
  see also Dominance, male
'Preattentional' automatic processing, 99

Preferences, sexual, 146, 159–169
  in animals, 165–166
  for pre-pubertal children, 486
'Prefigured gestalt', 164
Pregnancy, 40–41
  candida infections and, 417
  child sexual abuse (CSA) and, 497
  concerns, 317
  ectopic, 415
  fear of, 443, 456
  maternity blues, 441
  methyldopa and, 402
  post-partum period and, 439–442
  prenuptial, 187–188, **188**
  relationship, impact on, 440
  socio-cultural factors and, 440
  trichomonas and, 416
  unwanted, 329, 427, 439
  see also Teenagers
Pre-hormones, 20
Premarin, 124
Premarital sex, 186–199
  cross-cultural aspects, 186–190, **186**, **188**,
      190
  family influence, 199
  frequency of, 193–194
  historical perspective, 186–190, **186**, **188**,
      190
  non-coital, 197
  partners, number of, 193–194, 196–197
  sex surveys and, 175, 177
  sexual intercourse, age at first, **190**,
      191–199
  teenage pregnancy, 197–199
Premature ejaculation (PE), 88, 91
  ageing and, 240
  assessment, 371
  child sexual abuse (CSA) and, 497
  homosexual, 328–329, 376
  infertility and, 459
  in marriage, 319
  outcome studies, 357–358, 360
  Parkinson's disease (PD) and, 399
  rape and, 483
  serotonin re-uptake inhibitors (SSRIs)
      and, 305
  sexual interest, lack of and, 308, 323–324
  'squeeze technique', 323, 349, **350**
  'stop-start' technique, 323, 344
  treatment, 355, 363–364, 374
    in clinics, 314, **314**, 315–316
Pre-menstrual syndrome (PMS), 448, 449,
    450, 451
Preoccupation, sexual, 498
Pre-optic area (POA), 59, 126
Pre-puberty, hormone levels and, 28
President's Emergency Plan for AIDS Relief
    (PEPFAR) (US), 421–422, 425
Priapism, 363, 383
Primary affective disorder, 387
Primary syndrome, HIV/AIDS, 418
Primitive societies, 186
Problems, sexual, 303–339
  assessment, 306–307, 367–374
  barriers to sexual benefits, 338–339
  bisexual, 328–329
  causal mechanisms, 319
  child sexual abuse (CSA) and, 497
  classification, historical perspective,
      336–338
  clinics and, 313–316, **314**, **315**, 344
  community, prevalence in, 310–313,
      310, **312**

gender identity, 336
homosexual, 328–329
inhibition, role of, 305–307
laboratory investigations, 372–373
medicalization of, 304–305
multiple sclerosis (MS) and, 398
'problem clusters', brain systems and, 485
rape victims and, 490, 492
relationship context, 303–304
sexual behaviours, 329–335
sexual dysfunction, concept of, 306–307
sexual identity, 335–336
sexual interest, reduced, 307–310, 316–329
three windows approach, 306–307, 316–328, 338, 343, 346, 373–374
treatment see Treatment, sexual problems
vulnerability to, 319–327
Proceptive behaviours, in female, 132
Procidentia, 386
Procter & Gamble, 121
Profile of Female Sexual Function (PFSF), 115–116, 121, 245
Progesterone, 23, 439
pregnancy and, 41
role of, 30
Progestogen-only pill (POP), 449, 454
Progestogens, 22–23, 445–446, 450, 452
gender reassignment and, 292, 299
implants and, 452
long-acting injectable, 390
male contraception and, 453
management of sex offenders and, 502
Progression to AIDS, 418–419
Prolactin (PRL), 21, 384, 404
alcohol and, 406
breastfeeding and, 441
hyperprolactinaemia, 129, 328, 373, 384, 404
lactation and, 42
male/female effects, 87, 129–130
measurement, 372–373
oxytocin (OT) and, 130
refractory period and, 92–93, **92**
undernourishment and, 454
'Pro-life' movement, 457
Promiscuity, 320–321, 388
learning disabled (LD) and, 389
personality, incest and, 484
Promiscuous mating pattern, 477
Pro-opiomelanocortin (POMC), 130
Propanalol, 402
Prosecutions, 465
Prosocial activities, 158
Prostacyclin, 243
Prostaglandin E1, 363, 366
Prostate, **35**, 85
disease, 383
Prostatectomy, 87, 383
transurethral, 383
Prostatic pressure chamber, concept, 88
Prostatitis, 415
chronic (CP), 372, 383
Prostheses, 345
Prostitution, 189, 468
child, 467, 473–474
venereal disease (VD) and, 414
Protection hypothesis, brain oestrogens and, 51
Protective service agencies, 498
Protestantism, 217, 219
Provera, 124

Psychiatric classification systems, 336–337
Psychiatric treatment, child sexual abuse (CSA) victims and, 494
Psychiatry, 336, 387–390
Psychoanalysis, 256, 344
model of, 145
Psychoanalytic principles, 346
Psychogenic perspective
dysfunction, 304, 306
erections, 399
sexual development and, 479
stimulation, 399
Psychological Bulletin, 475, 495
Psychological factors
mechanisms, effects, 392
medical conditions and, 381
physical handicap and, 382
Psychological treatment
historical perspective, 345
/medical, integrated, 366–367
sex offenders and, 501, 503–505
Psychology, evolutionary, 9
Psychology Today, 407
Psychopathological theories of rape/sexual assault, 472
Psychosexual dysfunction, concept of, 337
Psychosomatic Circle of Sex, 17, 55–56, **56**, 99, 306, 307
Psychosurgery, 503
Psychotherapy, sex offenders and, 504
Psychotic illness, 484
Psychotropic medication, 403–405
sexual side-effects, 389
PT141 (bremelanotide), 130, 131, 362–363, 366
Puberty, 28–29
age of, 157, 474
attractiveness and, 485–486
early onset in girls, 32
hormone levels and, 28–29
see also Peri-pubertal entries
Public Broadcasting Service (US), 227
Public and Commercial Services Union (PCS), 467
Public Health Act 1917 (UK), 414
Punishment of Incest Act (1908), 467
Puritanism, 188–189, 217
Putamen, 57, 71, 73
Pyramidal abnormalities, 398

Q

Quadripartite model, child sexual abuse (CSA), 485
Quadriplegia, 399
'Queer theory', 261
Quetiapine, 405
Quinagolide, 364
Quinelorane, 362

R

Racial differences, 214–217
Radiotherapy, 387
Rape, 286, 464, 465, 466, 482–483
as act of sex or violence, 472–473
aggravated, 470, 490
causing sexual activity without consent, 466
child sexual abuse (CSA) victims and, 495
crisis centres, 491
exhibitionism/voyeurism and, 488

fantasies, 286
'no-crime' decisions, 465
rapists, 480–481
reporting, 465, 468, 470, 491
socio-cultural context, 471–473
statistics, 468–469
in United States (US), 470
victims, 489–492
Rape Myth Acceptance Scale, 224
Rapid eye movement (REM) sleep, 69–70, 110, 112, 391
Reactive inhibition, 346, 347
Reality, 6–7
Real-life test, gender reassignment, 297–298, 300
Reasoned Action, Theory of, 424
Reassignment surgery, sex see Gender reassignment
Receptive phase, 132
Rectal examination, 372
Rectal gonococcal infections, 415
Rectal gonorrhoea, 435
Rectal probing, pain threshold and, 95
Reductionism, 8
Reece, Carrol, 177
Referential system, emotional response, 100
Reflexive erections, 399
Refractory period, **56**, 84, 90–93, 152, 153
age-related, 91
gender differences and, 316
premature ejaculation (PE) and, 308
Regional cerebral blood flow (rCBF), 56, 71, 72, 104
Regressive behaviour, child sexual abuse (CSA) victims and, 493
Reitman, Helen, 257
Rejection, 351
fear of, 479
Relapse prevention techniques, 505
Relate, 316, 358
Relationships
ageing and, 243, 246, 249
barriers to rewarding, 338–339
breakup of, 424
close parent-child, 320
dyadic, 161, 264, 285, 336
importance of, 303–304
medical conditions and, 381
patient-therapist, 343, 347–348, 349, 353, 354, 503
pregnancy, impact on, 440
problems, 318, 348
risk management and, 435
role of sexuality in, 344
sexual problems in, 303–304, 367
see also Behaviours, sexual; Marriage/ Co-habitation
Relaxation
exercises, 354
progressive, 344
Releasing hormones, 21
Religion, 332
adolescence and, 158
contraception and, 443
heterosexuality and, 187–188, 195, 217–219
homosexuality and, 254, 258, 336
practices of, 474
see also Catholicism; Christian culture; Islamic culture; Jewish tradition; Protestantism
Re-offending, treatment and, 501, 505
Reparative therapy, 257, 258–259, 336, 377

Reporting, crime
  child sexual abuse (CSA), 493, 495
  rape, 465, 468, 470, 491
Reproductive infrastructure, 14
  components of, 14–15
  tract, steroid hormones and, 29–30
Resentment, 318, 319, 348, 352
Resistance, 333
  to abuse, 484
  to rape, 491
Respiratory excitement, 335
Response control models, 482
Response cycle, sexual, 309, 337
Responsibility
  for actions, 491
  adolescent, 158, 187, 192
  citizen, 255
  for contraception, 443, 445, 457
  cultural norms and, 474
  homosexuality and, 253, 258
Responsiveness, 160–161
  reduced, 307–310, 316–329
  see also Desire/interest, sexual; Genital
     response
Restrictive societies, 186
Retinopathy, 392
  diabetes mellitus (DM) and, 390–391
Retraction, child sexual abuse (CSA)
     accommodation syndrome,
     495–496
Retroviruses, 418
Reversion therapy, 256
Revolution, sexual, 175, 177, 185, 188, 197
Reward, 132, 144
  anticipation of, 90
  component, dopamine (DA) system, 89
  incentive and, 64–65
Ribonucleic acid (RNA), 126, 418
Riefenstein's syndrome, 49
Rigiscan devices, **96**, 362, 366, 373
Risk taking, sexual, 158
  adolescent, 479
  alcohol and, 406
  appraisal/management model, 429–434,
     430, 435
  autoerotic asphyxia (AEA) and, 334–335
  depression and, 110
  exhibitionism and, 487
  heterosexual women and, 432
  high-risk behaviour (HRSB), 329–330,
     332, 427, 428, 429, 434, 435
  child sexual abuse (CSA) and, 498–499,
     500
  HIV/AIDS and, 428, 431, 434–435
  homosexuality and, 272
  individual differences and, 429–435,
     430
  internet and, 227
  Kinsey Institute research, 183
  mood and, 111
  'out of control' see 'Out of control', sexual
     behaviour
  reduction, 196, 424
  sexual arousal and, 431
  sexually transmitted infections (STIs)
     and, 429–435
  theorizing on, 7–8
Rockefeller Foundation, 176–177
Role of Theory in Sex Research (Kinsey
     Institute workshop), 5, 7, 8, 13,
     159, 429
Roman Catholicism, 195, 208, 218–219, 267,
     282, 442–443, 454

Romantic love, 65, 220
  brain imaging and, 73–74
  homosexuality and, 255
  Kinsey ratings, **262**
  marriage and, 203–205
  sexual development and, 149–150,
     154–155
  stability of, 264–265, **265**
Royal College of Psychiatrists, 467
Royal Commission on Venereal Diseases
     (1871), 414
Rubberites, 285
'Rush' of addictive drugs, 89–90, 407

S

Sabbatsberg Sexual Self-Rating Scale,
     119, 125
Sadism, 286, 482
Sadomasochism, 164, 286–287, 487, 488
  determinants of, 286–287
  ritualized, 286
Sadomasochistic club, 284
Safe period, 454
Safe sex, 434
Safety
  interpersonal security, 316, 317, 348
  mechanisms, 334
Safety & Efficacy Task Force (WHO), 446
Salpingitis, 370
Salvarsan, 413
Same-sex attraction see Homosexuality;
     Lesbianism
San Francisco Sex Information Service, 262
Satcher, David, 8, 258, 445, 505
Satiation, 91–92
Satisfaction with life scale (SWLS), 205
Satisfaction, sexual, 228
Satyriasis, 330
Schachter, Stanley, 11
Schizophrenia, 307, 328, 388–389
  anti-psychotics and, 404–405
Schulte, Archbishop Paul, 176
Scopophilia (voyeurism), 470, 486–488
Scripting
  sexual see Sexual scripting theory; Sexual
     scripts
  social, 154, 156
Seasonal rhythm, 40
Secondary sexual characteristics, steroid
     hormones and, 29–30
Secrecy, child sexual abuse (CSA)
     accommodation syndrome,
     495–496
Security, interpersonal, 316, 317, 348
Sedatives, 403
Segregation, sexual, 266
Selective serotonin re-uptake inhibitors
     (SSRIs), 71, 87–88, 91–92
  anxiety/depression and, 305, 330
  ejaculation and, 305, 308, 323
  management of sex offenders and, 503
  'out of control' behaviour and, 376, 501,
     502–503
  side effects, sexual, 328, 330, 363, 403–404
Self-assertion, 316, 347, 348, 504
Self-awareness, 98
Self-blame
  child sexual abuse (CSA) victims and, 498
  rape victims and, 492
Self-control, 320–321, 330, 504
Self-deception, sex offenders and, 504
Self-discipline, 435

Self-esteem
  bolstering, 191, 192, 217, 319
  female, 459
  low, 317, 318, 348, 479, 493, 494
  male, 351
  rape victims and loss of, 490
  sex offenders and, 480, 498, 504
  sexual development and, 158, 167
  spinal cord injuries (SCI) and, 401
Self-harm
  child sexual abuse (CSA) victims and, 493
  juvenile female sex offenders and, 489
Self-image, 353
Self-labelling, 168
Self-protection, 316, 347, 348
Self-regulation, 332
Self-respect, 369
Self-stimulation techniques, 344
Semen
  emission, mechanisms underlying, 87–90
  'upsuck' of, 94
  see also Ejaculation; Orgasm
Semi-restrictive societies, 186
'Sensate focus', 347, **349**, 353, 354, 355
Sensation seekers, 431
Sensation Seeking Scales (SSS)
     (Zuckerman), 428, 431
Serotonergic (5HT) system, 63, 68–69, 71,
     90, 407
  5HT1A agonist, 404
  5HT2 antagonist, 403–404
Serotonin, 21, 68–69
  transporter gene markers, 332
  see also Selective serotonin re-uptake
     inhibitors (SSRIs)
Sertoli cells, 25, 241
Sertraline, 403, 503
Sex in Australia survey
  asexuality and, 282
  condom use and, 426
  homosexuality and, 269, 270, 274–275, 275
  masturbation and, 185
  sexually transmitted infections (STIs), 420
Sex education, 150, 192, 196, 467
  contraception and, 425, 426, 445
  learning disabled (LD) and, 390
  sex surveys and, 175
'Sex flush', 86
Sex hormone binding globulin (SHBG), 20,
     25, 29
  ageing and, 114, 241, 244, 392
  alcohol and, 406
  anti-convulsants and, 398, 405
  laboratory tests, 372
  obesity and, 392
  oestradiol and, 451
  sexual response and, 119, 120, 124
'Sex markets', 203
'Sex negativism', 176, 185, 255, 280, 505
'Sex positivism', 280, 282
Sex Problem Scale, 147
Sex therapy, 12, 325
  child sexual abuse (CSA) victims and, 501
  clearly defined tasks and, 347
  commitment to change, 352
  for couples, 346–353, 355–360, **356**, **357**,
     359
  emotion and, 352
  goals of treatment, 346–347
  for individual, 353–355
  outcome studies, 355–360, **356**, **357**
    controlled, 358–359
    uncontrolled, 355–358

patient-therapist relationship, 343, 347–348, 349, 353, 354
principles of, 345–346, 353–354
prognostic indicators, 359–360
psychotherapeutic component, 351–353
reality confrontation, 352
stages of treatment, 347–353, **349**, **350**
understanding and, 351–352
Sex Variant (Dickinson & Painter), 257
Sexual activity and attitudes measure, 498
Sexual Activity Log, 121
Sexual addictions: many conceptions, minimal data (Gold & Heffner), 330
Sexual Arousability Inventory (SAI), 229, 282
Sexual Arousal and Desire Inventory (SADI), 222
Sexual Arousal Inventory, 373
Sexual Behavior in the Human Female (Kinsey), 176
Sexual Behavior in the Human Male (Kinsey), 176
Sexual Conduct (Gagnon & Simon), 10
Sexual content-induced delay (SCID), 99–100, 102
Sexual Desire Inventory (SDI), 222, 282, 450
Sexual differentiation, anatomical, 24–25, **26**, **27**
anomalies of, 44–52
brain, 59–60, **60**
stages of, 24
see also Gender
Sexual Excitation/Sexual Inhibition Inventory for Women (SESII-W), 16–17, 67, 111, 201
homosexuality and, 264, 272
inhibition and, 326–327
personality and, 229, **231**
sexual risk taking and, 431, 432
Sexual Experience Scale, 113
Sexual function inventory (Derogatis), 394
Sexual Function Questionnaire, 387
Sexual Identity Conflict in Children and Adults (Green), 260
'Sexual impulsivity', 428
Sexual Inhibition/Sexual Excitation Scales (SIS/SES), 15–17
ageing and, 243, 244
condom use and (SIS1), 427
discontinuation, oral contraceptives and SES2, 447
erectile dysfunction (ED) and, 321–323, 329, 363
homosexuality and, 272, 282
mood and, 110–111, 330–331
personality and, 229, **230**
premature ejaculation (PE) and, 323–324, 329
psychometric assessment and, 373
safe sex and, 434
sex offenders and, 479–480
sex therapy and, 346
sexual risk taking and, 428, 431, 480
Sexual intercourse
age at first, 190, **190**, 195–196, 199, 214, 215
gender differences, 231
reduction in, 191–199, **193**, **194**, **195**, **196**, **197**
female superior position, **351**
illicit, 320
initiating, 208, 339, 347, 348, 351

post-partum, 439–440
sex therapy and, 350
Sexual Interest and Desire Inventory-Female (SIDI-F), 222
Sexual Offences Act
1956, 466
1976, 465
2003, 465, 466, 467–468
Sexual Offences Bill, 259
Sexual Opinion Survey (SOS), 99, 106, 228, 229, 264
Sexual Orientation Inventory, 373
Sexual response cycle, 309, 337
Sexual revolution, 175, 177, 185, 188, 197
Sexual scripting theory, 10–13, 182
Sexual scripts
adolescents and, 497
age-inappropriate, 499
child sexual abuse (CSA) and, 485
pre-pubertal school-aged child and, 497
Sexual strategy theory (SST), 8–10
Sexual variations, fetishism, sado-masochism and transvestism (Gosselin & Wilson), 281
Sexualization, 321
child sexual abuse (CSA) and, 479, 493, 496–497, 499–501
gender aspects of, 489
rape and, 482
traumatic, 499
Sexually dimorphic nucleus (SDN), 59–60
Sexually transmitted infections (STIs), 413–436
antibiotics and, 415, 416
antiviral drugs and, 417
bacterial infections, 414–415, 415–416
child sexual abuse (CSA) and, 497
clinics, 419–420
community, prevalence in, 419–420, **419**, **420**
concerns, 317
fungal infections, 414–415, 416–417
infertility and, 17, 66, 459
male condoms and, 454
medical practice and, 389
parasitic infections, 414, 416
sex surveys and, 175
sexual problems and, 328, 330, 381
sexual risk taking and, 429–435, **430**
venereal disease (VD), historical perspective, 413–414
viral infections, 414, 417–419
see also HIV/AIDS pandemic
Sherrington, Sir Charles Scott, 57
Short History of Marriage (Westermark), 476
Sickle cell disease, 383
Signals, sexual, 283
categories of, 283
visual, 200
Sildenafil, 78, 303, 393, 404
sexual interest, impaired and, 343, 360–361, 362, 364, 365
see also Viagra
Simon Population Trust, 456
Situationally contingent alternative strategies, 9
Skene's glands, 93
Skin colour, 201
Skin conductance (SC), 101, 105
Sleep
rapid eye movement (REM), 69–70, 110, 112, 384
non-rapid eye movement (REM), 242

Sleep erection *see* Nocturnal penile tumescence (NPT)
Sluice channels, 75
Smell, 96–97, 200, 320
impairment of, 384
Smoking, vascular impairment and, 392
Social class
contraception and, 443
impact of, 213–214
influence of, 189, 190, 195
lower, 175
middle, 175, 177, 184, 188, 189, 214, 317
sexual attraction and, 201, 204
sexual problems and, 317
working, 188–189, 213
Social Cognitive Theory, 424
Social construction theory, 6, 174, 260
Social factors
control, sex offenders and, 501
disruption, law and avoidance of, 464
history studies, 174, 187
learning, 144
phobia, 387
scripts, 154, 156
skills, 485, 504
Social network theory, 182
Social-labelling, 168
Society vs individual, 7–8
Socio-cultural factors
child sexual abuse (CSA) and, 473–474
contraception and, 442–443, 445
dimensions, 133
gender identity and, 289–291
homosexuality and, 261, 265
induced abortions and, 457
paedophilia and, 486
pregnancy and, 440
sexual offences and, 471–478
sexual problems and, 306
suppression, 255
see also Cultural factors; Taboos
Socio-economic factors, 215–216, 249
HIV/AIDS and, 422, 424
sterilization and, 455
Sociosexual Orientation Index, 264
Sodomy, 259
'Soft chancre', 413
Solicitation and pacing, 131, 132
Soliciting, 468
Solitary mating pattern, 477
Solitary scale, 222
Solitary tract, nucleus of, 59
Solly, Samuel, 413
South Africa, HIV/AIDS and, 422
Spasticity, 398, 400
Specificity vs novelty, attractiveness and, 485
Sperm, 25, 37, 91, 95, 384
spermatogenesis, 401, 453–454
see also Ejaculation
Spermicide, 454
Spielberger Trait Anxiety Inventory (STAI), 274, 321–322, 323, 327, 428, 431, 434
Spinal cord, 57
Spinal cord injuries (SCI), 74, 83, 88, 98, 328, 399–401
Spinal nucleus of bulbocavernosus, 59
Spirochaete, 413
Spitzer, Robert, 257
Spontaneity, 308, 309, 347, 368, 445, 454
'Squeeze' technique, 323, 349, **350**
SRY gene, 24, 25, 95

Standards, 332
  double, 189, 200, 212, 219, 337, 445, 482
Steinach, Eugen, 289
Stereotaxic hypothalamotomy, 503
Stereotyping, gender, 31–32, 271, 289, 290, 291
Sterilization, 442, 443, 454–457, **455**
  involuntary, 389
  spinal cord injuries (SCI) and, 401
Steroid hormones, 20, 22–24
  contra-indications, 299
  effects of, 29–30
  function of, 24
  gonadal, 111–114, **112**, **113**, 126–127
    receptors, 125
  intermediate stages, **23**
  pregnancy and, 50–51
  'steroid starvation', 247
  synthetic, 50
  see also Androgens; Oestrogens (E); Progestogens
Steroidal contraceptives, 427, 443, 445
  injectable forms of, 446
  medical practice and, 385
  sexual arousal and, 133
  sexual problems and, 328, 365
  spinal cord injuries (SCI) and, 401
  use in United Kingdom (UK), 443
  see also Oral contraceptives (OC)
Stigmatization
  child sexual abuse (CSA), 486, 496
  epilepsy, 397
  extramarital sex, 213
  gender dysphoria, 289
  HIV/AIDS, 424
  homosexuality, 168, 255–256, 259–260, 265, 271, 273, 275
  masturbation, 186, 219
  oral sex, 219
  peer group, 299
  rape victims, 472, 491
  sex surveys and, 178, 180
  sexual assault victims, 465
  venereal disease (VD), 414
Stimulation, sexual, 331
  brain imaging and, 71–73, 102–104, **103**
  clitoris, 122, 133
  see also Tactile stimulation; Vaginal stimulation (VS)
Stimuli, sexual
  genital response to, 96–98
  tactile, 98
  visual (VSS), 71, 72, 96, **96**, 102–104, **103**, 323, 362
  non-visual, 96–98
Stimulus control models, 482–483
'Stop-start' technique, 323, 344
'Storge' love, 204
Strangulation, 334, 335
Stratification, sexual, 266
Street children, 473
Streptococcus, 418
Stress, 110, 332
  conception and, 459
  disorders, acute, 494
Stria terminalis, bed nucleus of (BST), 59–60, 73, 89, 125–126, 404
Striatum, 57
Study of homosexual patterns (Henry), 256
Study of Women's Health Across the Nation (SWAN), 218, 250
Subliminal priming, 100
Subparafascial nucleus of thalamus, 404

Subparafascicular nucleus (SPFp), 89
Substance P, 83
Substance use disorders, 273, 330, 493
Substantia nigra, 57, 73
Subthalamic nuclei, 57
Suicide, 273–274, 334
  child sexual abuse (CSA) victims and, 493, 495
  juvenile female sex offenders and, 489
Superadded components, 133, 169, 186, 232, 249, 376
Surface electromyographic biofeedback, 385
Surgery, 345
  gynaecological, 385–386
  hysterectomy, 120–121, 300, 385–386
  intersex conditions and, 44
  ovariectomy, 117–118, 120–121
  prostate disease and, 383
  sex offenders and, 503
  vaginal repair, 386
  vascular, 384
  see also Gender reassignment
Survey Research Center (University of Michigan), 177
Surveys, sex, 174–183
  adolescents, 192–193, 194–195
  ageing and, 238–240, **239**, **240**, **241**, 243–244
  'branching', 180
  confidentiality/anonymity, 180, 182
  cross-cultural comparisons, 183
  data collection, 180–181
  design of, 179
  ethical implications, 181, 182
  interview methods, 180–181
    computer-assisted self (CASI), 180–181
      -audio (A-CASI), 180–181
    telephone, 180–181
      -audio-computer-assisted self (T-ACASI), 181, 227
  methodology of, 179–182
  participation biases, 180
  qualitative data, 183
  questionnaires, 180
  questions, 181–182
    'skip', 180
  random digit dialling (RDD), 180, 181
  samples, representative, 177, 180
  theoretical bases, 182–183
SWAN (Study of Women's Health Across the Nation), 218, 250
Sympathetic nervous system (SNS), 39, 58–59, 74, 75, 81
Synapses, excitatory/inhibitory, 61
Syphilis, 413, 414, 415–416, 422, 429
Syringe exchange programmes, PEPFAR and, 422

T

Taboos
  extramarital sex, 212
  incest and, 476–478
  masturbation, 184
  menstruation, 210
  pregnancy, sex during, 440
  premarital sex, 189, 190
  sexual development, 147, 149, 150–151, **152–153**
  sexually explicit behaviour, 497
  words, 354

Tactile stimulation, 98, 308, 309, 385, 398
  spinal cord injuries (SCI) and, 399
Tadalafil, 361, 404
Taoism, 219
Teenagers
  contraceptive use and, 182, 192, 198–199, 444–445
  indecent exposure and, 469
  males, sexual exploitation, 489
  pregnancy, 192, 197–199
    sex surveys and, 175, 177–178
    social class and, 214
  rape victims, 489
  sex offenders, 470
  see also Adolescence; Development, sexual
Temperamental syndrome, 167
Temporal lobe
  deactivation of, 89, 104
  epilepsy, 285, 397
Temporal lobectomy, 397
Terminology, sexual variations, 280–281
Testes, **35**, 37–38
  feminization of, 47
  size/consistency, 372
Testicular failure, 384
Testosterone (T), 23
  ageing and, 241–242, 243, 244–245, 246–247, 327
  alcohol and, 406
  anti-convulsants and, 405
  beta-endorphin and, 129
  brain localization of, 125–126
  breastfeeding and, **442**
  deficiency, 328, 384
  developmental aspects, 25–26, **27**, **28**, 29
  in female, 115–117, 118–119, 120–121, 124, 127–128, 133
  female-to-male transsexuals and, 296, 299
  homosexuality and, 256
  intersex conditions and, 45, 47, 49
  in male
    contraception, 453
    replacement, 111–114, **112**
    role, 114, 127
  measurement, 372–373
  mood and, 450–451
  opiates and, 407
  oral contraceptive-induced reduction, 451
  orgasm and, 94, 95
  outcome studies, 358
  passionate love and, 130
  post-natal levels, 25, 156
  production, 42
  progestogens and, 502
  replacement, 241, 364, 384, 502
  role of, 384
  sexual response and, 122
  therapy, 118, 364–365, 366
  see also Androgens
Textures, specific, 284
  leather, 284, 296
  rubber, 284, 285
Thalamus, 57, 130
  medial parvicellular subparafascicular nucleus, 404
Thatcher, Prime Minister Margaret, 179
Thematic apperception test (TAT) cards, 108
'Theorizing sexuality: evolution, culture and development' (conference), 5

Therapist-client relationship, 343, 347–348, 349, 353, 503
Thiazide diuretic, 402
'Third sex' concept, 260
'This is the night' syndrome, infertility and, 460
Thoracic cord, 399
Thoughts, sexual, **239**, 246, 312–313
  compulsive, 333
  frequency of, 221–222
  -induced orgasms, 89
  see also Desire/interest, sexual
Thousand marriages (Dickinson & Beam), 175, 257
Threats, sexual, 466
Three windows approach, 306–307, 316–328, 338, 343, 346, 373–374
Three-strand model, 145–146, **146**, 159–160, 168–169
  homosexuality and, 274–275
  sex offenders and, 478
  transgender identity and, 292
Thrush (Candida albicans), 326, 371, 372, 414, 416–417
Thymoxamine, **68**
Thyrotrophin-releasing hormone (TRH), 21
Tissot, Dr S.A.A.D., 184
Tomboys, 48, 294
'Tonic immobility reaction', 490
Toomey, State Representative, 179
Totem and Taboo (Freud), 477
Touching, sexual, 97–98
  armchair position, **349**
  with genital contact, 348–350
  for pleasure, 347, 348–350
  sensate focus, 347, **349**, 353, 354, 355
  teenage girls and, 470
  without consent, 466
Traditional Values Coalition, 179
Tranquillizers, 403
Transcendence, 332
Transference, 344
Transgender identity
  biological factors, 295–296
  gender reassignment, 290–291, 296–300
  incidence of, 291, **291**
  interactive explanation, 292–296
Transsexualism, 69, 162
  female-to-male, 265, 292, 294, 295, 296, 299
  historical perspective, 290
  homosexual, 290–291
  male-to-female, 292, 294–295, 299
  surgery, 300
  see also Gender reassignment
Transtheoretical Model of Behavior Change, 424
Transvestism, 104, 256, 289
  'double role' pattern, 293
  fetishistic, 290, 292–293, 295, 296, 297
  heterosexual fetishistic, 290
  see also Cross-gender behaviour
Tranylcypromine, 403
Trauma
  blunt, 383
  childhood, sexual, 111, 321, 335, 493, 497
  Freud, on sexual, 475
  hypogonadism and, 384
  legal process, 466
  perineal, 440
  rape, 472, 490, 491

sexual development and, 479
sexualization and, 499
see also Post-traumatic stress disorder (PTSD)
Traumagenic dynamics model, 145, 496
Trazadone, 70, 383, 403
Treatment, sexual problems, 343–377
  assessment for, 367–374
  case studies, 374–375
  current status, 367
  gender identity, 377
  historical perspective, 344–346
  'out of control' behaviour, 376
  pharmacological/hormonal, 360–366
  plans, 373–374
  psychological/medical, integrated, 366–367
  non-pharmacological, 366
  same-sex couples, 375–376
  sex therapy, 346–353, 353–355, 355–360, **356**, **367**
  sexual identity, 377
  sexual interest, impaired, 346–376
Treponema pallidum, 414
Trichomonas (Trichomoniasis), 371, 414, 415, 416
Tricyclic anti-depressants, 385, 403–404
Triple X (47-XXX) anomaly, 45
'Trough' reactions, child sexual abuse (CSA) and, 475
Trust
  breach of, 467
  capacity for, 145
  issues of, 348
  rape victims' loss of, 492
  in relationships, 316
Tubal ligation, 454, 456
Tuberculosis (TB), 418
Tubero-infundibular system, 62
Tunica albuginea, 74
  inflammation of connective tissue of, 382
Turner's syndrome (45-X0), 25, 45, **45**, 163–164
Twin Early Development Study (UK), 31
Twin Registers
  Australia, 157
  Finland, 157
  Netherlands, 31
  Vietnam era, 274

U

Uganda, 421
  HIV/AIDS programme, 423–424
Ulrichs, Karl, 260
Ultrasound, 80, 83, 370, 383, 384, 393
Unconscious processing, 99
Under-controlled behaviour, 435
'Unique invulnerability', 426
United Nations
  report on slavery (1993), 474
  UNAIDS, 421, 423, 424, 429
  UNICEF, on prostitution, 474
United Nations General Assembly, 421
Unmarried sex see Premarital sex
Unprotected anal intercourse (UAI), 426, 427, 428, 431, 432
'Upsuck' of semen, 94
Urbanization, 189–190
Urethra
  discharge from, 415
  female, 34, 83

infections of, 415
  male, 37
Urethritis, 415
Urine
  bacterial counts in, 415
  burning sensation, 415
  flow rates, 393
'Urnings' concept, 260
Uterus, 35, **35**
  bleeding, 385
  cancer of, 385
  orgasm and, 87
  prolapse of, 385
  retroversion, 328, 370–371

V

Vaccination, human papilloma virus (HPV), 417
Vacuum constriction devices (VCDs), 304, 345, 366, 393
Vagina
  ageing and, 247–248
  anatomy of, 34–35, **35**
  anterior wall erogenous complex, 83
  atrophy of, 246
  discharge from, 415
  'G' spot, 82–83, 87
  infection of, 324, 395
  nerve supply to, 326
  obstetric scarring, 371
  repairs, posterior wall, 345
  rings for, 446
  surgical repair, 386
  vault scarring, 371
  visual examination, 370
Vaginal blood flow (VBF), 79–82, 107, 130, 325, 333, 405
Vaginal dryness, 308
  ageing and, 240, 246, 247, 311, 325
  breastfeeding and, 441
  community, sexual problems and, 312
  diabetes mellitus (DM) and, 394, 395
  ischaemic heart disease (IHD) and, 395
  multiple sclerosis (MS) and, 398
Vaginal pulse amplitude (VPA)
  conditioned response and, 105
  diabetes mellitus (DM) and, 393, 394
  erotic stimuli and, 107–108, 119, 120, 132
  genital response and, 80–82, 97, 100
  melanocortins and, 130
  noradrenaline (NA) and, 70–71
  post-menopausal, 248–249
  sexual arousal and, 365
  spinal cord injuries (SCI) and, 400
Vaginal response, 79–83
  erotic sensitivity, 82–83
  orgasm and, 82, 86–87
  subjective arousal and, 80
  vaginal blood flow (VBF), 79–82, 107, 130, 325, 333, 405
Vaginal stimulation (VS), 82, 83, 133
  analgesic effect, 83, 325
  cervical and (VCS), 79, 89, 128
Vaginismus, 35, 309, 324–326, 344–345, 354
  cognitive behavioural technique (CBT) and, 359
  dilators and, 349
  infertility and, 459
  lesbianism and, 329
  outcome studies, 356–358, 360

Vaginismus *(Continued)*
  physical examination, 370
  treatment, 374
    in clinics, 315–316
Vaginitis, 416
Vaginosis, 415
Vagus (10th cranial) nerve, 58
Values *see* Attitudes, sexual; Moral values
van Ussel, Jos, 189
Vardenafil, 361
Variations, sexual, 280–287
  asexuality, 281–283
  fetishism, 283–286
  multivariant sexuality, 287
  sadomasochism, 286–287
  terminology, 280–281
Varicoceles, 372
Vas deferens, **35**, 85
Vas efferens, 85
Vascular disease, 243, 303, 307
  peripheral, 307, 328
Vascular impairment, 304, 328, 392, 395
  peripheral, 392
Vascular surgery
  corpora cavernosa and, 384
  for erectile problems, 345
Vasectomy, 449, 454, 456–457
Vasoactive intestinal polypeptide (VIP),
    63, 75, 78, 80
Vasopressin, 21
Velten Mood Induction Procedure, 107
Venereal disease (VD), 175
  historical perspective, 413–414
Venous drainage, 383
Ventral tegmental area (VTA), 73, 88, 129
Verapamil, **68**, 75, 382, 403
Vesiculitis, 372
Vestibulectomy, 385
Viagra, 76, 78, 303, 304, 338, 345, 360
  'for women', 305
  see also Sildenafil
Vibrators, 355, 366, 401
Victims
  child sexual abuse (CSA), 492–501
    helping, 500–501
  police and, 465
  rape, 489–492
  reporting crime, 465, 468, 470, 491, 493,
    495

Victorian Institute of Forensic Medicine,
    494
Victorian Psychiatric Case Register, 494
Vietnam Era Twin Registry, 274
Violence
  interpersonal, 471
  sexual, 286
  of war, 472
  see also Assault, sexual; Rape
Viral infections, 414, 417–419
Virginity, 265
  'census', 192
  importance of, 189
  'pledging', 158
Virginity ethic, 189, 191, 217, 445
Visual feedback, 98
Visual sexual stimuli (VSS), 71, 72, 96, **96**,
    102–104, **103**, 323, 362
Visual-evoked fields (VEF), 102
Vitality, 116
Vitamin E, 382
Vocabulary
  'bathroom', 150
  sexual, 147–148, 149
Voyeurism, 470, 486–488
'Vulnerability', 348
Vulva, 34
  cancer of, 386–387
  infection of, 324
  lesions of, 415
  nerve supply to, 326
  orgasm and, 87
Vulvar vestibulitis syndrome (VVS), 309,
    326, 359, 370, 374, 385
Vulvodynia, 324, 370, 385

W

Waist-to-hip ratio (WHR), 201
Wasserman blood test, 413
Wasserman test, 413
Weight
  body
    low, 202
      racial differences, 215
  body mass index (BMI), 201, 216
  gain, diabetes mellitus (DM) and, 390
  'ideal', 216
  loss, HIV and, 418

Weinberg, George, 268
Wellcome Foundation, 179
Wernicke, Carl, 57
Wernicke's encephalopathy, 406
Westphal, Carl, 253
Wet dreams, 371
Wish-fulfilling fantasy, Freud and, 475
Wolfenden Committee (1957), 255, 259,
    267, 464
Wolffian duct system, 25, 93–94, 95
World Health Organization (WHO)
  contraception and, 446, 448, 453, 454
  female circumcision and, 474
  HIV/AIDS and, 183, 423, 429
  menstruation and, 210

X

X chromosome, 163–164
45-XO anomaly (Turner's syndrome), 25,
    45, **45**, 163–164
47-XXX (Triple X) anomaly, 45
47-XXY anomaly (Klinefelter's syndrome),
    45–46, **46**
47-XYY anomaly, 46–47

Y

Y chromosome, 95
Yasmin, 449
Yeast infections, 385
Yohimbine, 70, 242, 361, 404
Yolles, Stanley, 178
YouGov survey, 267
Youth culture, 155, 195
Youth Risk Behavior Survey (YRBS), 155,
    194–195, **195**, **196**, 198, 215

Z

Zemore Depression Proneness Ratings
    (ZDPR), 274, 321–322
Zidovudine (AZT), 418
Zolpidem, 403
Zoophilia, 281
Zurich cohort study, 179, 387